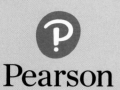

Pearson

New digital resources in concept-based nursing!

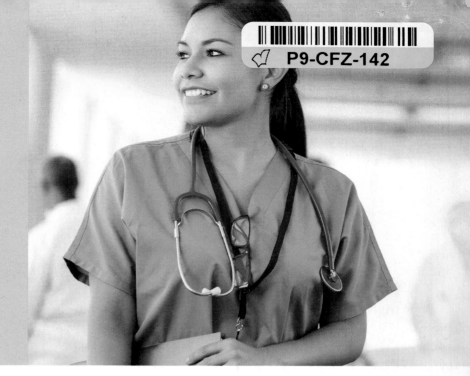

NEW! Skills Hub App

Helps students master essential nursing skills on their favorite mobile device

Offered in partnership with Skyscape, the Skills Hub app meets today's students where they are—on their smartphones and tablets—by providing procedural steps, skills videos, assessment, and progress tracking in one mobile application.

Learn more at **pearson.com/skills-hub-app**

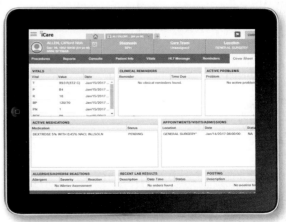

RealEHRPrep with iCare

Develop competency with documentation through an authentic EHR experience

Developed as a partnership between iCare and Pearson Education, RealEHRPrep with iCare is an authentic, evidence-based EHR learning system created by healthcare information technology and learning experts. Using RealEHRPrep with iCare, nursing students can improve their competency with documentation in preparation for clinical practice.

Learn more at **pearson.com/realehrprep**

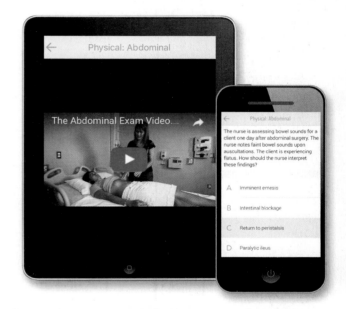

VOLUME 3

CLINICAL NURSING SKILLS

A Concept-Based Approach to Learning

Third Edition

Barbara Callahan, MEd, RN, NCC, CHSE
Lenoir Community College (Emerita)
La Grange, North Carolina

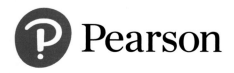

Vice President, Health Sciences and Teacher Education: Julie Levin Alexander
Director of Portfolio Management: Katrin Beacom
Executive Portfolio Manager: Lisa Rahn
Development Editor: Rachel Bedard
Portfolio Management Assistant: Taylor Scuglik
Vice President, Content Production and Digital Studio: Paul DeLuca
Managing Producer, Health Sciences: Melissa Bashe
Content Producer: Bianca Sepulveda
Diversity & Inclusion Specialists: Kendra R. Thomas, JD, and Chuin Phang
Operations Specialist: Maura Zaldivar-Garcia
Creative Director: Blair Brown
Creative Digital Lead: Mary Siener
Director of Digital Production, Digital Studio, Health Science: Amy Peltier
Digital Studio Producer, REVEL and eText 2.0: Jeff Henn
Digital Content Team Lead: Brian Prybella
Digital Content Project Lead: William Johnson
Vice President, Field Marketing: David Gesell
Executive Product Marketing Manager: Christopher Barry
Senior Field Marketing Manager: Brittany Hammond
Full-Service Project Management and Composition: iEnergizer Aptara®, Ltd.
Project Manager: Kelly Ricci
Inventory Manager: Vatche Demirdjian
Interior Design: Studio Montage
Cover Design: Studio Montage
Cover Art: Studio Montage
Printer/Binder: LSC Communications
Cover Printer: LSC Communications

Library of Congress Cataloging-in-Publication Data

Names: Callahan, Barbara, editor.
Title: Clinical nursing skills : a concept-based approach to learning /
   [edited by] Barbara Callahan, MEd, RN, NCC, CHSE, Lenoir Community
   College, Kinston, North Carolina.
Other titles: Clinical nursing skills (2017)
Description: Third edition. | Boston : Pearson, 2017. | Includes bibliographical references and index.
Identifiers: LCCN 2017044480 | ISBN 9780134616834 | ISBN 0134616839
Subjects: LCSH: Nursing.
Classification: LCC RT41 .C6715 2017 | DDC 610.73--dc23 LC record available at https://lccn.loc.gov/2017044480

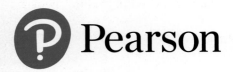

ISBN 13: 978-0-13-461683-4
ISBN 10:   0-13-461683-9

Preface

Nursing: A Concept-Based Approach to Learning is the number one choice for nursing schools employing a concept-based curriculum. The *only* true concept-based learning solution developed from the ground up, this three-volume learning suite equips you to deliver an effective concept-based program and to develop practice-ready nurses. Available as a digital or a print experience, this solution meets the needs of today's nursing student.

What Makes Pearson's Solution Different?

Nurses perform skills that apply knowledge, psychomotor dexterity, and critical thinking necessary for effective clinical practice. Pearson's *Nursing: A Concept-Based Approach to Learning*, Third Edition, is the *only* resource solution to dedicate a volume exclusively to nursing skills. Showcasing 277 skills with nearly 250 minor skills embedded in them, *Clinical Nursing Skills: A Concept-Based Approach to Learning*, the third volume in this suite, builds proficiency in the know-how and the rationales to execute psychomotor skills, delegate appropriately, provide patient teaching, and support individualized nursing care.

The previous edition of *Clinical Nursing Skills: A Concept-Based Approach to Learning* met the learning needs of tens of thousands of students and instructors in concept-based nursing programs. The Third Edition builds on that foundation and Pearson's commitment to excellence. We solicited and examined feedback on every skill and every feature that you—our customer—recommended in order to produce the best learning resource. This uniquely integrated solution provides students with a consistent design of content and assessment that specifically supports a concept-based curriculum.

Our goal for the Third Edition is to help students learn the essential knowledge they will need for patient care. The cover showcases a Möbius strip, which represents the relationships among the concepts and how they are all interconnected. By understanding important connections of concepts, students are able to relate topics to broader contexts.

Why Teach Concept-Based Learning?

University and college nursing programs across the United States and Canada evaluated how their programs can meet the needs of today's nursing students effectively. Nursing students felt overwhelmed by the amount of knowledge and skills they required to become proficient practitioners. As a result, many programs moved or are moving to the model of concept-based learning. A concept-based curriculum's streamlined approach helps nursing students to integrate concepts, apply information, and use clinical reasoning while minimizing content overload. Further, the model facilitates the transition from sage-on-the-stage teaching to engaging students in the learning process by doing meaningful, collaborative activities in lecture and the lab. Other benefits of conceptual learning in nursing programs –

- Concentrates on problems
- Fosters systematic observations
- Develops an understanding of relationships
- Focuses on nursing actions and interdisciplinary efforts
- Challenges students to think like a nurse

New to This Edition

- *Learning Outcomes* define measurable goals at the start of each chapter and align with end-of-chapter NCLEX-style questions and the test bank.
- *Concept of* … explains the chapter's theory that underpins the skill.
- *Review Questions* feature NCLEX-style questions that assess chapter-opening learning outcomes, answers, and rationales and serve not only as a self-review, but also as preparation for the licensing exam.
- *Enhanced eText*, available via *MyLab Nursing Concepts*, offers a rich and engaging learning experience with interactive activities and exercises. Note: Access requires an adoption of *MyLab Nursing Concepts*.
- *Instructor's Resource Manual* facilitates active learning in the classroom, lab, and clinical environment with class-tested interactive hands-on and cognitive exercises to help students apply concepts and exemplars.
- *Test Bank* offers test items written in NCLEX-like language.
- *Image Library* provides all the text's illustrations and photos to enhance your PowerPoint presentations and other materials.
- *New and Restructured Skills* 277 major skills with nearly 250 additional assessment, teaching, or care skills embedded in them. For example, *Skill 2.5 Hair: Caring for* includes the embedded skills of *Assessing and Treating Head Lice* and *Nits Infestation*.

More Changes for this Edition

- Integrates developmental ages across the lifespan throughout skills instead of having separate areas for different ages.
- Expands newborn, infant, and child procedural steps in the skills.
- Offers more photos and figures to improve learning through visual examples.

- Identifies common advanced skills students may have opportunities to observe or assist with following safety note perimeters – ex. "Paracentesis: Assisting" provides information about this procedure.
- Broadens teaching context to include the patient in the home environment after discharge.

New Skills

The following skills are new to the third edition:

- Colostomy: Irrigating, Skill 4.19
- Fall Prevention: Assessing and Managing, Skill 15.2
- Suicide: Caring for Suicidal Patient, Skill 15.4

Revised and Restructured Skills

The presentation of the following skills was re-envisioned for the third edition:

- Blood Transfusion: Administering, Skill 12.2
- Body Mass Index (BMI): Assessing, Skill 10.1
- Capillary Blood Specimen for Glucose: Measuring, Skill 8.4
- Cardiac Compressions, External: Performing, Skill 11.22
- Closed Wound Drains: Maintaining, Skill 16.3
- Ear Medication: Administering, Skill 2.17
- Feeding, Continuous, Nasointestinal/Jejunostomy with a Small-Bore Tube: Administering, Skill 10.6
- Implanted Vascular Access Devices: Managing, Skill 5.5
- Infusion Flow Rate Using Controller or IV Pump, Skill 5.7
- Intracranial Pressure: Monitoring and Caring for, Skill 7.2
- Nasogastric Tube: Inserting, Skill 10.11
- Newborn: Assessing, Skill 14.23
- Oxygen Delivery Systems: Using, Skill 11.8
- Range-of-Motion Exercises: Assisting, Skill 9.2
- Suctioning, Oropharyngeal and Nasopharyngeal: Newborn, Infant, Child, Adult, Skill 11.14
- Venipuncture: Initiating, Skill 5.15

Organization and Structure of *Clinical Nursing Skills*, Third Edition

Clinical Nursing Skills' chapters, listed alphabetically, support concepts in volumes 1 and 2. Within each chapter, associated skills appear in subgroups. Subgroups reflect the sequence of thinking, such as assessment skills appearing before intervention skills in the chapters. As an example, the path for finding the skill about using a nasal cannula for supplemental oxygen therapy is:

- Concept—Oxygenation, Chapter 11
- Subgroup—Supplemental Oxygen Therapy
- Skill—Oxygen Delivery Systems: Using, Skill 11.8
- VARIATIONS—Nasal Cannula/Simple Face Mask/ Partial Rebreather Mask, etc.

Skill Organization

- ***Delegation or Assignment*** offers guidelines when it is appropriate to delegate or assign skills to unlicensed assistive personnel (UAP).
- ***Equipment*** lists the apparatus required to perform the skill.
- ***Preparation*** includes safety, age, and cultural information for working with various patients.
- ***Procedure*** provides step-by-step best practice with rationales.
- ***Photos and illustrations*** depict critical steps visually.
- ***Documentation*** demonstrates what data to capture post-execution.
- ***Variation Skills*** present alternative methods for performing select skills.
- ***Embedded Skills*** (as appropriate) provide useful skills to enhance learning (such as USING A DOPPLER ULTRASOUND DEVICE in Skill 1.6, Pulse: Apical and Peripheral, Obtaining).

Chapter Organization

For the Third Edition, as shown in the Chapter at a Glance listed at the beginning of each chapter, each main section has a list of skills.

New! Each chapter contains **The Concept of …**, which explains the chapter's theoretical concept that underpins the skill, and a dedicated list of Learning Outcomes. The outcomes are reinforced by end-of-chapter review questions.

›› The Concept of Perfusion

Perfusion is the immersion of body cells in a fluid. Tissue perfusion refers to the movement of solutes such as oxygen, nutrients, and electrolytes in the blood through the vascular system to capillary networks. Tissue cells are bathed in solutes so they can readily cross cell membranes. Waste products of cellular metabolic activity pass into the interstitial fluid from the cells and are carried away from the cells. When tissue perfusion is diminished or absent, cells do not receive adequate oxygen, nutrients, or electrolytes. This may be manifested by a decrease in blood pressure, restlessness, confusion, cool extremities, pallor or cyanosis of distal extremities, faint peripheral pulses, slowed capillary refill, edema, or life-threatening conditions.

Learning Outcomes

12.1 Give examples of priority safety considerations when preparing and administering a unit of blood to a patient.

12.2 Support the benefits of applying sequential compression devices (SCDs) to promote circulation in the lower legs of an adult patient.

12.3 Summarize priority nursing actions if SCDs are being used on a patient, and the patient complains of numbness and tingling in one leg.

12.4 Explain proper placement of skin electrodes on the patient being monitored on telemetry to avoid artifacts on the monitor screen.

12.5 Differentiate the causes for different waves and intervals, the P wave, the PR interval, the QRS wave, the T wave, and the QT interval when interpreting an electrocardiogram (ECG) pattern.

12.6 Examine the arterial insertion site for signs and symptoms of bleeding, infection, or inflammation.

12.7 Explain why a transcutaneous pacemaker would be applied to a patient with a life-threatening dysrhythmia.

12.8 Explain what a pacemaker spike indicates in an ECG monitor pattern.

Skill Organization

Equipment provides a list of tools required to execute the skill.

Preparation includes safety, age, and cultural information for working with various clients.

Procedure provides step-by-step best practice with rationales.

Photos and illustrations depict crucial steps visually.

SKILL 12.7   Sequential Compression Devices: Applying

Sequential compression devices (SCDs) operate differently from pneumatic compression devices. SCDs use many inflatable compartments to compress the leg in a graduated sequential fashion. The compartment closest to the foot inflates first and the compartment closest to the thigh inflates last. The amount of pressure also differs in each compartment. The highest pressure is in the first compartment and the lowest in the last one. This creates a "milking" action to empty deeper veins of the lower leg to promote optimal blood flow.

Delegation or Assignment

The UAP often removes and reapplies SCDs when performing assigned or delegated hygiene care. The nurse should check that the UAP knows the correct application process for SCDs. Remind the UAP that the patient should not have SCDs removed for long periods of time because the purpose of the SCDs is to promote circulation. Note that state laws for UAPs vary, so this task might be assigned to the UAP or delegated.

Equipment

- Single-use tape measure (to prevent cross-infection)
- SCDs, including disposable sleeves, air pump, and tubing

Preparation

- Review healthcare provider's orders and the patient's nursing plan of care.
- Gather equipment and supplies.

Procedure

1. Introduce self and verify the patient's identity using two identifiers. Explain to the patient what you are going to do, why it is necessary, and the procedure for applying the sequential compression device. **Rationale:** *The patient's participation and comfort will be increased by understanding the reasons for applying the SCD.*
2. Perform hand hygiene and observe other appropriate infection control procedures.

Delegation or Assignment offers guidelines, when appropriate, to delegate or assign skills to unlicensed assistive personnel.

SKILL 12.7   Sequential Compression Devices: Applying *(continued)*

3. Provide for patient privacy and drape the patient appropriately. Assess legs for skin integrity and neurovascular status.
4. Prepare the patient. Position bed at correct height for procedure.
   - Place the patient in a dorsal recumbent or semi-Fowler position.
   - Measure the patient's legs as recommended by the manufacturer if a thigh-length sleeve is required. **Rationale:** *Foot and knee-length sleeves come in just one size; the thigh circumference determines the size needed for a thigh-length sleeve.*
5. Apply the sequential compression sleeves.
   - Place a sleeve under each leg with the opening at the knee ❶.
   - Wrap the sleeve securely around the leg, securing the Velcro tabs. Allow two fingers to fit between the leg and sleeve ❷. **Rationale:** *This amount of space ensures that the sleeve does not impair circulation when inflated. Ensure that there is no overlapping or increases in the SCD.* **Rationale:** *This prevents skin breakdown.*

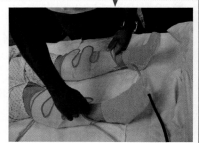

❷ Slip two fingers under wrap to ensure that it is not too tight.

Structures and Features

The Concepts are set up consistently throughout the program. This allows students to anticipate the learning they will experience. Special features recur in each chapter as well, which students can use for learning and review. The basic structure of each chapter is shown below with visuals and annotations describing the content.

Concepts Related to ...

Enhanced for the Third Edition, the Concepts Related to feature links to more concepts, relationships, and nursing implications.

Concepts Related to
Perfusion

CONCEPT	RELATIONSHIP TO PERFUSION	NURSING IMPLICATIONS
Cognition	Thought processing or mental status is affected if blood volume is decreased.	■ Monitor oxygen saturation, vital signs, and orientation status ■ Rule out physical reasons cognition may change
Comfort	Tissues not adequately oxygenated manifest pain.	■ Monitor pain and for signs of local and systemic hypoxia ■ Implement oxygen therapy as ordered ■ Monitor oxygen saturations and vital signs
Fluids and Electrolytes	Excess extracellular fluid volume causes lung congestion and impaired gas exchange.	■ Monitor fluid intake and output, vital signs, and oxygen saturation ■ Implement oxygen therapy as ordered ■ Administer medications as ordered
Intracranial Regulation	Blood flow volume to brain can change intracranial pressure (ICP).	■ Monitor vital signs, pupils, sensorium, and assess for motor or sensory neuro deficits
Tissue Integrity	Wound healing delayed without adequate perfusion to tissue.	■ Oxygen is needed for cell metabolism; hyperbaric oxygen therapy can be effective

Safety Note! and Icon ❶ ... Distinguishes skills that nursing students may observe or assist with only with faculty permission and while under direct supervision of faculty or another RN.

Safety Note! *During scheduled clinical time, nursing students may have a learning opportunity to observe or assist with this skill only with faculty permission and with direct supervision from faculty or another RN.*

Safety Considerations ... Identifies crucial safety information.

Safety Considerations

In addition to the usual blood components such as platelets and cryo-precipitate, modified blood products are becoming more popular. Washed, irradiated, or leukocyte-removed blood is being used for patients at risk because of multiple transfusions or a weakened immune system. Testing for cytomegalovirus and matching RBC or human leukocyte antigens is also done to ensure safe transfusions.

When infusing a blood product that has undergone leukocyte reduction, remember that it must be filtered again through a standard blood administration set in order to trap cellular debris that may have accumulated since the original filtration.

Patient Teaching ... Features teaching plans for patients and tips to assist patients in self-care.

Patient Teaching

Wearing Antiembolism Stockings at Home

■ Ensure the patient or caregiver knows how to apply antiembolism stockings.

■ Reinforce the importance and the rationales for no wrinkles and no rolling down of the stockings.

■ Reinforce the importance of removing the stockings daily and inspecting the skin on the legs.

■ Include instructions about:
 ● Laundering the stockings (air dry because putting them in a dryer can affect their elasticity.)
 ● Needing two pairs of stockings to allow one pair to be worn while the other is being laundered.
 ● Replacing the stockings when they lose their elasticity.

■ Reinforce knowledge about slipperiness of stockings if worn without slippers or shoes.
 ● If the patient is ambulatory, emphasize the need for footwear to prevent falling.

Lifespan Considerations ... Presents age-related content to alert learners to differences in caring for patients.

Lifespan Considerations
OLDER ADULTS

■ Because the elastic is quite strong in antiembolism stockings, older adults may need assistance putting on the stockings. Patients with arthritis may need to have another person put the stockings on for them.

■ Many older adults have circulation problems and wear antiembolism stockings. It is important to check for wrinkles in the stockings and to see if the stocking has rolled down or twisted. If so, correct it immediately. **Rationale:** *The stockings must be evenly distributed over the limb to promote—rather than hinder—circulation.*

■ Stockings should be removed at least once a day (check facility policy) so that a thorough assessment can be made of the legs and feet. **Rationale:** *Redness and skin breakdown on the heels can occur quickly and go undetected if not thoroughly assessed on a regular basis.*

■ Provide information about the importance of wearing the elastic stockings, how to wear them correctly, and how to take care of them.

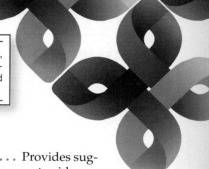

Caution! … Highlights key details for high-risk situations when performing the skill.

CAUTION! Dextrose solution (which causes lysis of RBCs), Ringer's solution, medications and other additives, and hyper-alimentation solutions are incompatible with blood or blood components.

EVIDENCE-BASED PRACTICE

Recommend Bed Rest for DVT?

Prolonged immobilization has been associated with DVT in critically ill patients. However, the value and safety of mobilizing patients with acute DVT has been a concern, largely because of the potential for venous thromboembolism (dislodging of the clot into the bloodstream) and life-threatening pulmonary embolism (PE).

A number of studies have shown that patients with acute DVT who use compression stockings and begin ambulating early after initiation of anticoagulant therapy experience several benefits from this approach. Benefits include reduced pain level, more rapid reduction in edema, increased strength maintenance, and improved flexibility. Early ambulation in these patients, with careful monitoring for any evidence of PE, resulted in no increase in incidence of PE. Conversely, bed rest and immobilization did not result in any reduction in incidence of PE. Therefore, the current recommendation of the American College of Chest Physicians is ambulation with compression as tolerated, after starting anticoagulation, in patients with acute DVT.

Source: Data from Christakou, A. (2015). *Effectiveness of early mobilization in hospitalized patients with deep venous thrombosis.* Retrieved from http://www.hospitalchronicles.gr/index.php/hchr/article/view/553.

Evidence-Based Practice … Provides suggestions for best practice from available, current evidence.

Critical Thinking Options for Unexpected Outcomes …
Demonstrates how evaluation can lead to further interventions for unexpected outcomes.

EXPECTED OUTCOME	UNEXPECTED OUTCOME	POSSIBLE INTERVENTIONS
General Assessment Height and weight are obtained and recorded.	Patient's weight varies more than expected from one day to the next.	■ Verify time of day weights were measured. ■ Verify if same scale was used for both weights. ■ Verify equipment's reliability. ■ Verify what clothing or linen was on the patient when weighed on both days. ■ Verify I&O record for sources of fluid loss or gain. ■ Verify MAR for medications that alter fluid balance (e.g., diuretics).
Vital Signs Temperature is within normal range.	Fever develops.	■ Verify possible sources of infection and take preventive measures. ■ Notify healthcare provider as needed. ■ Implement cooling methods if temperature is dangerously high, such as tepid sponge bath, cool oral fluids, ice packs, or antipyretic drugs as ordered. ■ Assess all vital signs.
Temperature is within normal range.	Temperature remains elevated because of bacterial-produced pyrogens.	■ Request order to obtain culture of possible sources of infection. ■ Give antipyretics and other drugs as ordered. ■ Decrease room temperature and remove excess covers. ■ Give tepid sponge bath.
	Temperature remains subnormal.	■ Assess for blood clots; extreme low temperature can cause vasoconstriction. ■ Implement measures to promote vasodilation (application of warmth). ■ If extremity is ischemic, monitor that heat source does not exceed body temperature.
Pulse is palpated without difficulty.	Apical, femoral, and carotid pulses are absent.	■ Assess all vital signs and status of the patient. ■ Immediately call for the rapid response team. ■ Initiate CPR immediately. ■ Use Doppler device to assess for presence of pulse.
	Peripheral pulse is absent.	■ Assess for other signs and symptoms of circulatory impairment.
Respiratory rate, rhythm, and depth are within normal limits.	Apnea (absence of breathing) occurs, may be intermittent.	■ Assess patient for pulse. ■ Begin rescue breathing at the rate of 12 per minute for an adult or 20 per minute for a child.
Labored, difficult, or noisy respirations are assessed.	Kussmaul respirations occur (deep and gasping breaths—more than 20 breaths/min).	■ Implement orders for diabetic ketoacidosis, renal failure, or septic shock.

New! Review Questions with answers and rationales feature NCLEX-style questions that relate to chapter-opening learning outcomes. They serve not only as a self-review, but also as preparation for the licensing exam. Answers and rationales for the review questions can be found in Appendix A or in the Pearson MyLab and eText.

REVIEW Questions

1. A client receiving a unit of packed red blood cells begins to vomit 15 minutes into the transfusion. What should the nurse do first?
   1. Call for help.
   2. Stop the transfusion.
   3. Provide an emesis basin.
   4. Increase infusing normal saline.

2. The nurse assigns the UAP to complete morning care for a client with a sequential compression device. What information should the nurse instruct the UAP to report to the nurse?
   1. Presence of pulses in the client's feet
   2. Condition of the skin under the devices
   3. Amount of time the devices were turned off
   4. Sensation and movement of the client's feet

3. A new graduate is using an automated external defibrillator (AED) for a client who was discovered without a pulse. For which reason should the charge nurse intervene?
   1. Resuming CPR after discharging the AED
   2. Loudly stating "Clear" before discharging the AED
   3. Stopping compressions for the AED to analyze the client's rhythm
   4. Placing electrode pads below the right clavicle and above the left nipple

4. The nurse evaluates the ability of the UAP to complete a 12-lead electrocardiogram for a client. Which lead placement should the nurse correct before the measurement is recorded?
   1. Green lead placed on the client's left leg
   2. White lead placed on the client's right wrist
   3. V2 placed at the fourth intercostal space, left sternal border
   4. V6 placed at the fifth intercostal space, left midclavicular line

5. A client is prescribed 3-lead telemetry to monitor atrial fibrillation. Which lead approach should the nurse use to obtain the best assessment of this client's atrial functioning?
   1. Lead I
   2. Lead II
   3. Lead III
   4. Lead aVL

6. The nurse notes the following when analyzing a client's cardiac rhythm strip: atrial rate 60; ventricular rate 42; QRS width 0.10 seconds. Which diagnostic test should the nurse anticipate to determine the best treatment for this client's rhythm?
   1. Digoxin level
   2. T3 and T4 levels
   3. Arterial blood gases
   4. Serum electrolyte levels

7. The nurse visits the home of a client with a newly inserted permanent pacemaker. Which observation indicates that the client would benefit from additional teaching about the device?
   1. Medical alert bracelet on the right wrist
   2. Telephone transmission device installed
   3. Pacemaker information card in the wallet
   4. Cell phone in shirt pocket over the pacemaker

8. A new graduate reports that a client's arterial blood pressure monitor reading is 20 mmHg higher than the measurement from the previous shift. What should the nurse assess *first* to determine the reason for the change in measurement?
   1. Calibration process
   2. Pressure bag setting
   3. Arterial site dressing
   4. Angle of the head of the bed

Resources

Instructor Resources

- **New! Instructor's Resource Manual** facilitates active learning in the classroom, lab, and clinical environment with class-tested interactive hands-on and cognitive exercises to help students apply concepts and exemplars.

- **New! Test Bank** offers test items written in NCLEX-like language.

- **New! Image Library** provides all the text's illustrations and photos to enhance your PowerPoint presentations and other materials.

- **Skills Checklists** deliver editable check-offs for each skill to assess students' competency, which can be used as is or can be tailored to meet local requirements.

Student Resources

- **New! Enhanced eText**, available via *MyLab Nursing Concepts*, offers a rich and engaging learning experience with interactive activities and exercises. Note: Access requires an adoption of *MyLab Nursing Concepts*.

- **RealEHRprep with iCare**, Developed as a partnership between iCare and Pearson Education, RealEHRPrep with iCare provides access to a real electronic health record system developed by healthcare information technology, and documentation activities created by education experts. Providing an environment that mirrors the point-of-care, students can document assessments, plan care, administer medications, communicate with other healthcare providers, and more.

  Access to RealEHRPrep with iCare may be packaged with Pearson materials or purchased as a standalone item.

- **Skills Hub,** The Skills Hub app meets students where they are - on their smartphones and tablets - by providing procedural steps, skills videos, assessment, and progress tracking in one mobile application. Access to Skills Hub may be packaged with Pearson materials or purchased as a standalone item.

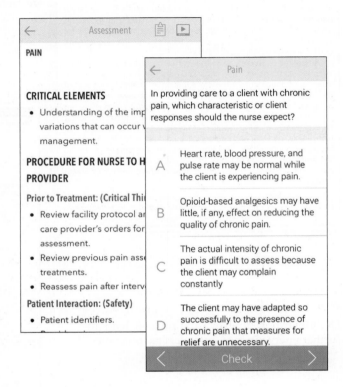

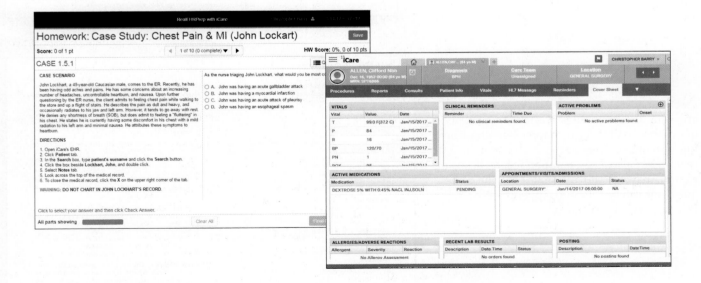

Acknowledgments

Foremost, my thanks to Pearson Education, Inc. for their continued support of concept-based nursing education and for the privilege of being one among so many involved in the production of this third edition of Volume 3 *Clinical Nursing Skills*. Much appreciation goes to Julie Alexander, Publisher, for her continued support and advocacy for concept-based learning; Lisa Rahn, Nursing Portfolio Manager/Editor, for her leadership, decision-making ability, and consistent encouragement; Rachel Bedard, Development Editor, for guidance through the development process and for being a great partner; Bianca Sepulveda, Content Producer in Nursing, for her organizational skills and many contributions to this edition and its eText version; Addy McCulloch and Laura Horowitz, Development Editors, for their availability to respond to questions and offer suggestions from a different perspective; and Mary Siener (and team) for the innovative cover, color scheme, and interior design of this edition. A special thanks goes to my husband for supporting me to do what I enjoy doing. Thank you, Pearson folks, for promoting a culture of professionalism and team effort during this fabulous adventure.

Barbara Callahan

Reviewers

Pearson thanks faculty who participated in pre-revision and manuscript reviews. We appreciate your thoughtful feedback, insights, and recommendations.

Stephanie Bailey, BA, RN, MHS
Nursing Instructor
British Columbia Institute of Technology
Burnaby, BC, Canada

Eleisa Bennett, RN, MSN
Instructor of Associate Degree Nursing
James Sprunt Community College
Kenansville, NC

Wendy I. Buchanan, RN, ADN, BS, BSN, MSN-E
Instructor of Nursing
Southwestern Community College
Sylva, NC

Marlena Bushway, PhD, MSNEd, RN, CNE
Professor of Nursing
New Mexico Junior College
Hobbs, NM

Kathleen Campbell, MSN, BSN
Instructor of Nursing
Hudson Valley Community College
Troy, NY

Darlene Clark, MS, RN
Professor of Nursing
The Pennsylvania State University
University Park, PA

Diane Cohen, MSN, RN
Professor of Nursing
MassBay Community College
Framingham, MA

Ann Marie Cote, MSN, RN, CEN
Professor of Nursing
Plymouth State University
Plymouth, NH

Ann Crawford, RN, PhD, CNS, CEN, CPEN
Professor, College of Nursing
University of Mary Hardin-Baylor
Belton, TX

Christy Dean, DNP, MSN, FNP-BC, CNE
Instructor of Nursing
University of Louisiana at Lafayette
Lafayette, LA

Michelle De Lima, DNP, APRN, CNOR, CNE
Associate Professor of Nursing
Delgado Community College
New Orleans, LA

James R. Fell, MSN, MBA, RN
Assistant Professor of Nursing
The Breen School of Nursing,
Ursuline University
Pepper Pike, OH

Charlene Beach Gagliardi, RN, MSN
Assistant Professor
Mount Saint Mary's University
Los Angeles, CA

Cathryn Jackson, MSN, RN
Instructor of Nursing and Associate Director of Undergraduate Programs
University of British Columbia
Vancouver, BC Canada

Carolyn Jones, BSN, MAEd, MSN
Professor of Nursing
Craven Community College
New Bern, NC

Christine Kleckner, MA, MAN, RN
Instructor of Nursing
Minneapolis Community and Technical College
Minneapolis, MN

Lynn Lowery, RN, ADN, BSN, MSN
Professor of Nursing
Delgado Community College
New Orleans, LA

Lauro Manolo, Jr., MSN
Professor of Nursing
Allan Hancock College
Santa Maria, CA

Christy McDonald Lenahan, DNP, MSN, FNP-BC, CNE
Assistant Professor of Nursing
University of Louisiana Lafayette
Lafayette, LA

Ellen Manieri, MN, MEd, RN, CMSRN
Professor of Nursing
Delgado Community College, Charity School of Nursing
New Orleans, LA

Janice Martin, MSN, BSN
Professor of Nursing
Southern Union State Community College
Opelika, AL

Amy Mersiovsky, DNP, RN, BC
Assistant Professor of Nursing
Scott and White College of Nursing,
University of Mary Hardin-Baylor
Belton, TX

Juleann H. Miller, PhD, RN, CNE
Professor of Nursing
St. Ambrose University
Davenport, IA

Linda Mollino, MSN, RN
Director of Career and Technical
Education (CTE) Programs
Oregon Coast Community College
Newport, OR

Michelle Natrop, MSN, BSN
Instructor of Nursing
Normandale Community College
Bloomington, MN

Karen Neighbors, RN
Professor of Nursing
Trinity Valley Community College
Athens, TX

Denise Owens, MS, BSN, CCRN
Instructor of Nursing
University of Maryland
Baltimore, MD

Allison Peters, AA, ADN, BSN, MSN, DNP
Professor of Nursing
University of Florida
Gainesville, FL

Katherine Poser, RN, BScN, MNEd
Professor of Nursing

St. Lawrence College School of
Baccalaureate Nursing
Kingston, ON

Margaret Prydun, PhD, RN, CNE
Professor of Nursing
University of Mary Hardin-Baylor
Belton, TX

Susan M. Randol, MSN, RN, CNE
Master Instructor of Nursing
University of Louisiana at Lafayette
Lafayette, LA

Marisue Rayno, EdD, RN
Professor of Nursing
Luzerene County CC
Nanticoke, PA

Lori-Ann D. Sarmiento, MSN, RN
Associate Professor of Nursing
Guilford Technical Community College
Jamestown, NC

Lisa S. Smith, DNP, MSN, RN
Instructor of Associate Degree Nursing
Sampson Community College
Clinton, NC

Tetsuya Umebayashi, DNP, RN
Director of Vocational Nursing Program
Tarrant County College—Trinity River East
Fort Worth, TX

Patricia Vasquez, MSN, RN
Professor of Nursing
Trinity Valley Community College
Athens, TX

Amanda Veesart, PhD, RN, CNE
Assistant Professor/Program Director
Texas Tech University
Lubbock, TX

Molly H. Wells, BSN, RN-BC, CEN
Instructor of Associate Degree Nursing
Beaufort County Community College
Washington, NC

Teri Wisdorf, RN
Professor of Nursing
Century College
White Bear Lake, MN

Lisa Zerby, MN, RN, CNOR
Adjunct Nursing Faculty
Shoreline Community College
Shoreline, WA and
Renton Technical College
Renton, WA

Megan Zerillo, MSN, RN
Professor of Nursing
University of Alabama
Birmingham, AL

Technical Reviewers

Pearson gratefully thanks those who checked the accuracy and currency of the nursing skills content during the production process. We appreciate you sharing your expertise and for your careful attention to detail.

Amanda Aird, RN, BScN
Instructor of Nursing
St. Lawrence College School of Bacca-
laureate Nursing
Kingston, ON

Stephanie Bailey, BA, RN, MHS
Nursing Instructor
British Columbia Institute of Technology
Burnaby, BC, Canada

Eleisa Bennett, RN, MSN
Instructor of Associate Degree Nursing

James Sprunt Community College
Kenansville, NC

Sherrilyn Coffman, PhD, RN, COI
Professor of Nursing
Nevada State College
Henderson, NV

Ann Crawford, RN, PhD, CNS, CEN,
CPEN
Professor, College of Nursing
University of Mary Hardin-Baylor
Belton, TX

Lynn Perkins, PhD, MSN, RN
Instructor of Nursing
Minneapolis Community and Technical
College
Minneapolis, MN

Katherine Poser, RN, BScN, MNEd
Professor of Nursing
St. Lawrence College School of Bacca-
laureate Nursing
Kingston, ON

SKILLS List by Key Word*

Items in black are major skills. Items in red are minor skills embedded within a major skill.

(continued on next page)

*Related Concepts can be found in *Nursing: A Concept-Based Approach to Learning*, Volumes 1 and 2, Third Edition.

(continued on next page)

(continued on next page)

Contents

❶ Nursing students may observe or assist with these skills only with faculty permission and while under direct supervision of faculty or another RN.

Chapter 3   Comfort   189

Chapter 4   Elimination   227

Chapter 5   Fluids and Electrolytes   291

Chapter 6   Infection 339

Chapter 7   Intracranial Regulation 361

Chapter 8   Metabolism 371

Chapter 9   Mobility 387

Chapter 10   Nutrition 435

● Nursing students may observe or assist with these skills only with faculty permission and while under direct supervision of faculty or another RN.

Chapter 1
Assessment

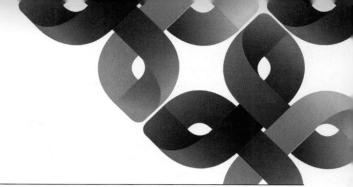

Chapter at a Glance

» The Concept of Assessment

Assessment provides nurses with information about the psychological, cognitive, and emotional well-being of patients that they can use to analyze the data critically, interpret it, and make clinical judgments to implement interventions for the best patient outcomes. Assessment includes many nursing skills and actions. It is the ability to observe and pay attention to significant signs that are seen, heard, smelled, and sensed by touch. Nurses use the techniques of palpation, auscultation, and percussion to perform physical assessment examinations. Nurses can measure and monitor temperatures, pulses, respirations, blood pressure readings, oxygen saturation, and pain. They can record and report data about the patient's history and current state of health, illness, home medications, cultural and spiritual beliefs, and acute and chronic conditions. Assessment tools can be scales and indexes (e.g., the Braden Scale to assess for risk of pressure injury, the Glasgow Coma Scale to assess consciousness, or a pain scale). Other tools such as the stethoscope, pulse oximeter, tape measure, thermometer, sphygmomanometer, and Doppler ultrasound (DUS) help nurses obtain assessment data.

Learning Outcomes

1.1 Summarize the role of observation when performing a general assessment.

1.2 Differentiate between normal and abnormal temperatures over the lifespan.

1.3 Support the reasoning of using a pulse oximeter for the patient with a respiratory problem.

1.4 Explain the examination procedures when doing a physical assessment using a head-to-toe framework.

1.5 Give examples of maneuvers used to test muscle strength throughout the body.

1.6 Explain lifespan considerations when performing a neurologic assessment on the older adult.

1.7 Differentiate between normal and abnormal breath sounds.

1.8 Demonstrate peripheral pulse assessment of an extremity.

The following feature links some, but not all, of the concepts related to assessment. They are presented in alphabetical order.

Concepts Related to
Assessment

CONCEPT	RELATIONSHIP TO ASSESSMENT	NURSING IMPLICATIONS
Caring Interventions	Individualize patient care to best meet needs of patient	■ Provide competent and compassionate nursing care to all patients ■ Build awareness of self-care
Clinical Decision Making	Utilize assessment data to make clinical judgments about patient and set priorities of care	■ Provide data to analyze, interpret, and implement nursing interventions to meet patient needs ■ Clarify priority order of care to provide a variety of patients
Health, Wellness, and Illness	Build self-awareness of health, wellness, and illness status	■ Provide support and encouragement to help patient change level of health, wellness, and illness
Safety	Support recognition of safety and quality care for patients and others	■ Provide data to ensure correction of unsafe conditions for patient and others in maintaining a safe environment ■ Include assessment techniques for patient and nurse safety
Skin Integrity	Observe any skin breakdown and monitor surgical wounds	■ Provide data to recognize skin integrity alterations ■ Monitor and evaluate healing progression resulting from nursing interventions

Health assessment, which is the collection and interpretation of data regarding the patient's previous and current health status, is one of the most important professional responsibilities of the registered nurse. Vigilance in performing relevant assessment techniques, determining the meaning of the findings, and taking appropriate action based on the evaluation of the data are central aspects of effective nursing care and cannot be delegated to those without the requisite skills and knowledge.

A holistic approach to assessment focuses on all aspects of the patient's mind and body to identify concerns that need to be addressed, including psychological, social, cultural, and spiritual health. Nurses gather subjective data from talking with the patient and or family and objective data from examining the patient. Experienced nurses may also use intuitive skills to notice significant cues about the patient.

Nurses can perform a comprehensive physical assessment of each individual body system. In practice, however, the generalist nurse performs a screening assessment of all systems (sometimes referred to as a head-to-toe assessment) when first encountering the patient and then more detailed focused assessments of particular systems as indicated by the patient's condition. Independent clinical judgment drives the selection of those components for which an assessment is indicated. **Box 1–1 》** presents the order generally followed in performing a *head-to-toe assessment*. Advance practice nurses such as nurse practitioners may perform much more in-depth assessments of specific systems.

The traditional vital signs are body temperature, pulse, respirations, and blood pressure. Some healthcare facilities refer to pain as a fifth vital sign. Remembering that pain is an individual experience for patients relative to their medical history and current health status, nurses individualize their interventions for each patient. In addition, the effectiveness of respirations and circulation is commonly measured noninvasively through pulse oximetry (see Skill 1.7) at the same time as other vital signs.

All these signs, when looked at both individually and collectively, enable nurses to monitor the functions of the body. Vital signs can reflect changes that otherwise might not be observed. Monitoring a patient's vital signs should not be an automatic or routine procedure; it should be a thoughtful scientific assessment. Vital signs should be evaluated with reference to the patient's present and prior health status and compared to accepted standards (**Box 1–2 》**). If findings appear inconsistent with those anticipated, they should immediately be rechecked. Some of the vital signs that are confirmed to vary from expected values may require nursing interventions, and a few represent medical emergencies.

Box 1–1
Head-to-Toe Framework

GENERAL SURVEY INCLUDING VITAL SIGNS

Areas below are assessed and include a determination of current complaints and inspection. Palpation, percussion, and auscultation are used if indicated.

- Head
  - Hair and face
  - Eyes and vision
  - Ears and hearing
  - Nose
  - Mouth and oropharynx
- Neck
  - Muscles
  - Lymph nodes
  - Trachea
  - Thyroid gland
  - Carotid arteries
  - Neck veins
- Upper extremities
  - Skin and nails
  - Muscle strength and tone
  - Joint range of motion
- Brachial and radial pulses
- Sensation
- Chest and back
  - Skin
  - Thorax shape and size
  - Lungs
  - Heart
  - Spinal column
  - Breasts and axillae
- Abdomen
  - Skin
  - Abdominal sounds
  - Femoral pulses
- External genitals
- Anus
- Lower extremities
  - Skin and toenails
  - Gait and balance; muscle strength and tone
  - Sensation
  - Joint range of motion
  - Popliteal, posterior tibial, and dorsalis pedis pulses

Box 1–2
Times to Assess Vital Signs

- On admission to a healthcare facility to obtain baseline data
- When a patient has a change in health status or reports symptoms such as chest pain or feeling hot or faint
- Before and after surgery or an invasive procedure
- Before and/or after the administration of a medication that could affect the respiratory or cardiovascular systems; for example, before giving a digitalis preparation
- Before and after any nursing intervention that could affect the vital signs (e.g., ambulating a patient who has been on bedrest)

>> General Assessment

Expected Outcomes

1. Assessment data of the patient's appearance reveal expected normal findings.
2. Height and weight are obtained and recorded.
3. Patient's weight shows expected losses, gains, or stabilization.

SKILL 1.1 Appearance and Mental Status: Assessing

This skill provides an overall initial impression or review of well-being by observing a patient for acute distress, general physical appearance, body structure, mobility, behavior, nonverbal communication, and body measurements. Measurements can be compared to standard expected measurements for age and gender across the lifespan.

Delegation or Assignment

The initial general survey assessment is completed by the nurse and not delegated or assigned to unlicensed assistive personnel (UAP). However, signs and symptoms of problems may be observed during usual care and may be recorded by individuals other than the nurse. Abnormal findings must be validated and interpreted by the nurse.

Unlicensed Assistive Personnel (UAP) are unlicensed healthcare workers trained to perform certain tasks delegated or assigned by nurses to help provide patient care as determined by facility policy. Nurses assess and evaluate the UAP's ability to complete a skill safely and accurately. The nurse remains responsible for the assessment, evaluation, and interpretation of abnormal findings and the determination

(continued on next page)

SKILL 1.1 Appearance and Mental Status: Assessing (*continued*)

of appropriate responses. There are many job titles for those considered a UAP, such as Patient Care Attendants, Home Health Aides, Certified Nursing Assistants, Medication Technicians, and Resident Assistants. Licensed Practical Nurses (LPN) and Licensed Vocational Nurses (LVN) are not UAPs. They are licensed nurses who work under a Registered Nurse (RN) and are regulated by state Boards of Nursing.

Equipment

■ No equipment is required.

Preparation

■ Observation of children's behavior can provide important data for the general survey, including physical development, neuromuscular function, and social and interactional skills.
■ Safety for newborns, infants, and children includes having an adult attending the child on an examination table or bed to avoid falls during the assessment.

■ It may be helpful to have parents hold older infants and very young children for part of the assessment.
■ Allow extra time for older patients to answer questions.
■ Adapt questioning techniques as appropriate for older patients with hearing or visual limitations.

Procedure

1. Prior to performing the procedure, introduce self and verify the patient's identity using two identifiers. Explain to the patient and parent (if appropriate) what you are going to do, why it is necessary, and how the patient can participate. Discuss how the results will be used in planning further care or treatments.
2. Perform hand hygiene and observe appropriate infection control procedures.
3. Provide for patient privacy.
4. Complete a general survey.

ASSESSMENT	NORMAL FINDINGS	DEVIATIONS FROM NORMAL
5. Observe body build, height, and weight in relation to the patient's age, lifestyle, and health.	Proportionate, varies with lifestyle	Excessively thin or obese
6. Observe patient's posture and gait, standing, sitting, and walking.	Relaxed, erect posture; coordinated movement	Tense, slouched, bent posture; uncoordinated movement; tremors, unbalanced gait
7. Observe patient's overall hygiene and grooming.	Clean, neat	Dirty, unkempt
8. Note body and breath odor in relation to activity level.	No body odor or minor body odor relative to work or exercise; no breath odor	Foul body odor; ammonia odor; acetone breath odor; foul breath
9. Observe for signs of distress in posture or facial expression.	No apparent distress	Bending over because of abdominal pain, wincing, frowning, or labored breathing
10. Note obvious signs of health or illness (e.g., in skin color or breathing).	Well developed, well nourished, intact skin, easy breathing	**Pallor** (paleness), weakness, lesions, cough
11. Assess the patient's attitude (frame of mind).	Cooperative, able to follow instructions	Negative, hostile, withdrawn, anxious
12. Note the patient's affect/mood; assess the appropriateness of the patient's responses.	Appropriate to situation	Inappropriate to situation, sudden mood changes, paranoia
13. Listen for speech quantity (amount and pace) and quality (loudness, clarity, inflection).	Understandable, moderate pace; clear tone and inflection	Rapid or slow pace; overly loud or soft
14. Listen for relevance and organization of thoughts.	Logical sequence, relevant answers, has sense of reality	Illogical sequence, flight of ideas, confusion, generalizations, vague
15. When procedure is completed, perform hand hygiene and leave patient safe and comfortable. Complete documentation using forms, checklists, or electronic dropdown lists supplemented by nurse's notes or additional comments as appropriate ❶.		

SKILL 1.1 Appearance and Mental Status: Assessing (continued)

ADMISSION DATA

Date 4-16-19 Time 3:15p.m. Primary Language English

Arrived Via: Wheelchair ☐ Stretcher ☐ Ambulatory ☑

From: ☐Admitting ☐ER ☑ Home ☐ Nursing Home ☐ Other

Admitting M.D. R. Katz   Time Notified 5 p.m.

ORIENTATION TO UNIT

	YES	NO		YES	NO
Arm Band Correct	☑	☐	Visiting Hours	☑	☐
Allergy Band	☑	☐	Smoking Policy	☑	☐
Telephone	☑	☐	TV, Lights, Bed Controls,		
Electrical Policy	☑	☐	Call Lights, Side Rails	☑	☐
Educational Mat'l	☑	☐	Nurses Station	☑	☐
(TV Brochure)	☑	☐			

Family M.D. R. Katz

Weight 125 lb. Height 5ft. 2in. BP:R — L 122/80

Temp. 103F Pulse 92, weak Resp 28, shallow

Source Providing Information ☑Patient ☐ Other

Unable to Obtain History ☐

Reason for Admission (Onset, Duration, Pt.'s Perception) "Chest cold" X2 weeks S.O.B on exertion. "Lung pain, fever," "Dr. says I have pneumonia."

ALLERGIES & REACTIONS

Drugs Penicillin

Food/Other None known

Signs & Symptoms rash, nausea

Blood Reaction ☐ Yes ☑No Dyes/Shellfish ☐ Yes ☑No

MEDICATIONS

Current Meds	Dose/Freq.	Last Dose
Synthroid	0.1 mg. daily	4-16, 8 a.m.

Disposition of Meds: ☑ Home ☐ Pharmacy ☐ Safe *At Bedside

MEDICAL HISTORY

☑ No Major Problems
☐ Cardiac
☐ Hyper/Hypotension
☐ Diabetes
☐ Cancer
☐ Respiratory
☐ Gastro
☐ Arthritis
☐ Stroke
☐ Seizures
☐ Glaucoma
☑ Other Childbirth-2003

Surgery/Procedures	Date
Appendectomy	1999
Partial thyroidectomy	2005

SPECIAL ASSISTIVE DEVICES

☐Wheelchair ☐Contacts ☐Venous ☐Dentures
☐Braces ☐Hearing Aid Access ☐Partial
☐Cane/Crutches ☐Prosthesis Device ☐Upper
☐Walker ☐Glasses ☐Epidural Catheter ☐Lower
☐Other None

VALUABLES

Patient informed Hospital not responsible for personal belongings.

Valuables Disposition: ☐ Patient ☐ Safe ☐ Given to

Patient/SO Signature None

PSYCHOSOCIAL HISTORY

Recent Stress None

Coping Mechanism Not assessed because of fatigue

Support System Husband, coworkers, friends

Calm: ☑Yes ☐No

Anxious: ☑Yes ☐No Facial muscles tense; trembling

Religion Catholic. Would want Last Rites

Tobacco Use: ☐Yes ☑No

Alcohol Use: ☐Yes ☑No

Drug Use: ☐Yes ☑No

NEUROLOGICAL

Oriented: ☑Person ☑Place ☑Time ☐Confused ☐Sedated
☐Alert ☐Restless ☑Lethargic ☐Comatose

Pupils: ☑Equal ☐Unequal ☑Reactive ☐Sluggish
☐Other 3mm.

Extremity Strength: ☑Equal ☐Unequal

Speech: ☑Clear ☐Slurred ☐Other

MUSCULO-SKELETAL

Normal ROM of Extremities ☑Yes ☐No

☑Weakness ☐Paralysis ☐Contractures ☐Joint Swelling ☑Pain
☐Other ↓ related to fatigue   when coughing

RESPIRATORY

Pattern: ☐Even ☐Uneven ☑Shallow ☑Dyspnea
☑Other diminished breath sounds (see NN)

Breathing Sounds: ☐Clear ☑Other inspiratory crackles

Secretions: ☐None ☑Other pink, thick sputum

Cough: ☐None ☑Productive ☐Nonproductive

CARDIOVASCULAR

Pulses: Apical Rate 92-W ☑Reg. ☐Irregular ☐Pacemaker
S = Strong W = Weak A = Absent D = Doppler

Radial R 92 L —   Pedal R — L —

Edema: ☑Absent ☐Present Site

Perfusion: ☐Warm ☐Dry ☑Diaphoretic ☐Cool (Hot)

GASTROINTESTINAL

Oral Mucosa ☐Normal ☑Other pale and dry

Bowel Sounds: ☑Normal ☐Other Abd. soft

Wt. Change: ☐☑N/V Stool Frequency/Character 1/day; soft

Last B/M 4-15-19 ☐Ostomy (type)

Equip. None

GENITOURINARY

Urine: Last Voided This morning

☐Normal ☐Anuria ☐Hematuria ☐Dysuria ☐Incontinent
☑Other ↓amount & frequency since ill
☐Catheter (type)   Other

LMP 4-1-19   ☐Vaginal/Penile Discharge

Equip. None

Other

SELF CARE

Need Assist with: ☐Ambulating ☐Elimination
☐Meals ☑Hygiene ☐Dressing
While fatigued

Amanda Aquilini [F age 37]
#4637651   DOB 11-02-82

⁂ NURSING ADMINISTRATION ASSESSMENT

❶ Nursing assessment form.

(continued on next page)

SKILL 1.1 Appearance and Mental Status: Assessing *(continued)*

NUTRITION

General Appearance: ☑ Well Nourished   ☐ Emaciated
☐ Other _____
Appetite: ☐ Good   ☐ Fair   ☑ Poor -x2 days
Diet _Liquid_   Meal Pattern _3/day_
☑ Feeds Self   ☐ Assist   ☐ Total Feed

SKIN ASSESSMENT

Color: ☐ Normal ☐ Flushed ☑ Pale ☐ Dusky ☐ Cyanotic
☐ Jaundiced ☑ Other _Cheeks flushed, hot_
General Description _Surgical scars:_
RLQ abdomen; anterior neck
_____
Note Cultures Obtained _____

PRESSURE SORE ™ AT RISK SCREENING CRITERIA

OVERALL SKIN CONDITION
Grade
	0	Turgor (elasticity adequate, skin warm and moist)
✓	1	Poor turgor, skin cold & dry
	2	Areas mottled, red or denuded
	3	Existing skin ulcer/lesions

BOWEL AND BLADDER CONTROL
Grade
✓	0	Always able to ask for bedpan
	1	Incontinence of urine
	2	Incontinence of feces
	3	Totally incontinent Confined to bed

REHABILITATIVE STATE
Grade
	0	Fully ambulatory
✓	1	Ambulated with assistance
	2	Chair to bed ambulation only
	3	Confined to bed
	4	Immobile in bed

NUTRITIONAL STATE
Grade
	0	Eats all
✓	1	Eats very little
	2	Refuses food often
	3	Tube feeding
	4	Intravenous feeding

MENTAL STATE
Grade
✓	0	Alert and clear
	1	Confused
	2	Disoriented/senile
	3	Stuporous
	4	Unconcious

CHRONIC DISEASE STATUS (i.e. COPD, ASCVD. Peripheral Vascular Disease, Diabetes, or Renal Disease, Cancer, Motor or Sensory Deficits, Elderly, Other)
Grade
✓	0	Absent
	1	One Present
	2	Two Present
	3	Three or more Present

TOTAL ___3___   Refer to Skin Care Protocol

FALLS SCREENING

If one or more of the following are checked institute fall precautions/plan of care
☐ History of Falls ☐ Unsteady Gait ☐ Confusion/Disorientation ☐ Dizziness
If two or more of the following are checked institute fall precautions/plan of care
☐ Age over 80   ☐ Utilizes cane, walker, w/c   ☐ Sleeplessness
☐ Impaired vision   ☐ Urgency/frequency in elimination
☐ Multiple Diagnoses   ☐ Impaired hearing   ☐ Medication/Sedative /Diuretic etc.
☐ Inability to understand or follow directions

NURSE SIGNATURE/TITLE	DATE	TIME
Mary Medina, RN	4-16-19	3:30pm
NURSE SIGNATURE/TITLE	DATE	TIME

EDUCATION/DISCHARGE PLANNING

1. What do you know about your present illness? "_Dr. says I have pneumonia._" "_I will have an I.V._"
2. What information do you want or need about your illness? "_How long do I have to stay here?_"
3. Would you like family/SO involved in your care? _Husband, Michael_
4. How long do you expect to be in the hospital? "_1-2 days_"
5. What concerns do you have about leaving the hospital? "_How long will I feel so tired all the time?_"

CHECK APPROPRIATE BOX
Will patient need post discharge assistance with ADLs/physical functioning? ☐ Yes ☑ No ☐ Unknown
Does patient have family capable of and willing to provide assistance post discharge?
☑ Yes ☐ No ☐ Unknown ☐ No family
Is assistance needed beyond that which family can provide?
☐ Yes ☑ No ☐ Unknown
Previous admission in the last six months?
☐ Yes ☑ No ☐ Unknown
Patient lives with _Husband and 1 child_
Planned discharge to _Home_
Comments: _Fatigue and anxiety may have interfered with learning. Re-teach anything covered at admission, later._

Social Services Notified   ☐ Yes ☑ No

NARRATIVE NOTES

S--c/o sharp chest pain when coughing and dyspnea on exertion. States unable to carry out regular daily exercise for past week. Coughing relieved "if I sit up and sit still." Nausea associated with coughing. Having occasional "chills." Occasionally becomes frightened, stating, "I can't breathe." Well groomed but "too tired to put on make-up." Assesses own supports as "good" (eg, relationship z husband). Is "worried" about daughter. States husband will be out of town until tomorrow. Left 13-year-old daughter with neighbor. Concerned too about her work (is attorney). "I'll never get caught up." Had water at noon—no food today.
O--Chest expansion < 3cm, no nasal flaring or use of accessory muscles. Breath sounds and insp. crackles in ℝ upper and lower chest. Capillary refill 5 seconds.

NURSING ADMINISTRATION ASSESSMENT

❶ Nursing assessment form *(continued)*

SKILL 1.1 Appearance and Mental Status: Assessing *(continued)*

Lifespan Considerations
INFANT

- Measure height of children under age 2 in the supine position with knees fully extended.
- Include measurement of head circumference until age 2 (standardized growth charts include head circumference up to age 3).

CHILD

- Anxiety in preschool-age children can be decreased by letting them handle and become familiar with examination equipment.
- School-age children may be very modest and shy about exposing parts of the body.
- Adolescents should be examined without parents present unless the adolescent requests their presence.
- Weigh children without shoes and with as little clothing as possible.

SKILL 1.2 Height: Newborn, Infant, Child, Adult, Measuring

A child's height measurement can be compared to a standard children's height and weight chart to evaluate growth and development with other children of the same age. Height measurement will change each year.

Delegation or Assignment

The nurse measures the height of newborns, infants, and small children (under the age of 2). Measuring height of the older child, adolescent, and adult may be delegated or assigned to the UAP. The nurse remains responsible for the assessment, interpretation of abnormal finds, and determination of appropriate actions. Note that state laws for UAPs vary, so this task might be assigned to the UAP rather than delegated.

Equipment

- Stadiometer or platform scale with stature-measuring device
- Measuring board or other length-measuring device for newborn, infant, and small child

Preparation

- Have the child remove shoes and hat.
- Have the parent remove hat or shoes the newborn or infant is wearing.
- Because older adults with osteoporosis can lose several inches in height, be sure to document height and ask if they are aware of becoming shorter.
- Keep children safe when using the stadiometer or platform scale by helping them stand with stability when measuring them.

Procedure

1. Introduce self and verify the patient's identity using two identifiers. Explain to the patient and parent what you are going to do, why it is necessary, and how the patient can participate. Discuss how the results will be used in planning further care or treatments with parent.
2. Perform hand hygiene and observe appropriate infection control procedures.
3. Provide for patient privacy.

NEWBORN, INFANT, OR SMALL CHILD

4. When using a measuring board for a newborn, infant, or small child (under age of 2), place the head against the top of the board.

5. After positioning the head, gently push down on the knees until the legs are straight ❶. **Rationale:** *Because of their normally flexed posture, the bodies of infants and small children must be extended to obtain an accurate measurement.*

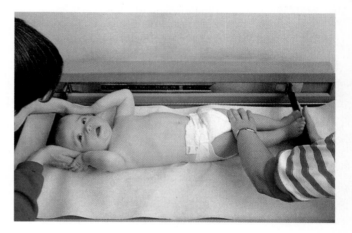

❶ Measuring an infant's length.

6. Position the heels of the feet on the footboard, and record the length to the nearest 0.6 cm or ¼ in.
7. Repeat the measurement for accuracy. If a difference between the two readings is found, take the average reading for documentation.
   Note: If such a measuring device is not available, place the newborn or infant on a paper sheet, stabilizing in the same manner as when using the board. Carefully holding the pen that touches the child's head and feet at a right angle to the surface, make one mark at the vertex of the head and another at the heel. Then measure the distance between the two marks. Record the length in centimeters or inches.
8. Plot the measurement for the child's age on the standardized growth curve and proceed to step 9 below.

OLDER CHILD OR ADULT

4. Have the patient stand straight with their back to the wall. The head should be held erect and in the midline position.

(continued on next page)

SKILL 1.2 Height: Newborn, Infant, Child, Adult, Measuring *(continued)*

5. The shoulders, buttocks, and heels should touch the wall. ❷ The outer canthus of the eyes should be on the same horizontal plane as the external auditory canals. **Rationale:** *Positioning the head properly helps ensure consistency in placement of the headpiece on the crown of the head.*
6. Move the headpiece down to touch the crown.
7. Make the height reading to the nearest 0.6 cm or ¼ in.
8. For a child, plot the measurement for the child's age on the standardized growth curve.
   Note: In the older child and adolescent, as well as in adults, height is often measured using a platform scale with an attached stature-measuring device. Have the child stand erect, facing forward. Move the stature-measuring device to the top of the head. Have the child step off the scale, and read the height in centimeters or inches.
9. When the procedure is complete, perform hand hygiene and leave patient safe and comfortable.
10. Complete documentation using forms, checklists, or electronic dropdown lists supplemented by nurse's notes or additional comments as appropriate.

SAMPLE DOCUMENTATION

[date] 0900 Height measurement 43 inches on platform scale; tolerated well with mother holding his hand. *R. Cummings*

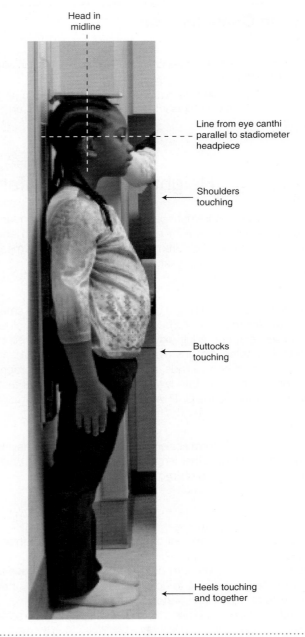

❷ Measuring a child's height. Position the head in an erect and midline position while the shoulders, buttocks, and heels touch the wall. Move the headpiece down to touch the crown.

SKILL 1.3 Newborn's or Infant's Head, Chest, and Abdomen: Measuring

The head circumference usually is greater than the chest circumference of a newborn and infant during the first year. The abdomen is measured to detect abdominal distention. These measurements reflect growth levels and development and can also suggest any potential alterations, such as hydrocephalus.

Delegation or Assignment

This skill is not delegated or assigned to the UAP. However, many aspects are observed during usual care and may be recorded by individuals other than the nurse. Abnormal findings must be validated and interpreted by the nurse.

SKILL 1.3 Newborn's or Infant's Head, Chest, and Abdomen: Measuring (*continued*)

Equipment

- Disposable, nonstretching measuring tape with centimeter and millimeter markings

Preparation

- For head measurement, remove any hat, braids, or barrettes the newborn or infant is wearing.
- For chest measurement, remove all clothing from the child's chest.
- For abdominal measurement, remove all clothing from the abdomen.
- Include measurement of head circumference for small child until age 2.
- Standardized growth charts include head circumference up to age 3.
- Newborn, infant, or small child should be stabilized by adult during measuring for safety.

Procedure

1. Introduce self to parent and verify the patient's identity using two identifiers. Explain to the parent what you are going to do, why it is necessary, and how the patient can participate. Discuss how the results will be used in planning further care or treatments.
2. Perform hand hygiene and observe appropriate infection control procedures.
3. Provide for patient privacy.

HEAD CIRCUMFERENCE

4. Wrap the tape around the head at the supraorbital prominence above the eyebrows, above the ears, and around the occipital prominence ❶. Be sure to prevent the tape from slipping or causing a paper cut. **Rationale:** *This is usually the point of largest circumference of the head.*

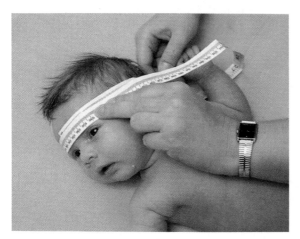

Source: George Dodson/Pearson Education, Inc.

❶ Measuring head circumference.

5. Record the circumference to the nearest 0.3 cm or ⅛ in. Repeat the measurement to confirm the reading.
6. Plot the measurement for the child's exact age in months on the standardized growth curve.

CHEST CIRCUMFERENCE

7. Wrap the tape measure around the chest, placed just under the axilla and at the nipple line ❷.

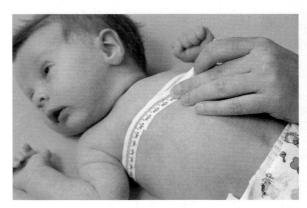

Source: George Dodson/Pearson Education, Inc.

❷ Measuring chest circumference.

8. Record the circumference measurement to the nearest 0.3 cm or ⅛ in.
9. Compare the chest circumference to the head circumference measurement.

ABDOMEN CIRCUMFERENCE

10. Wrap the tape around the abdomen at the level of the umbilicus, taking care to prevent a paper cut.
11. If the measurement is taken at another location on the abdomen, place ink marks at the location of the measurement. **Rationale:** *This action will enable you or another nurse to take a future measurement at the same location.*
12. Record the measurement to the nearest 0.6 cm or ¼ in. Compare the reading to those taken previously to determine a change in size.
13. When the procedure is complete, perform hand hygiene and leave patient safe and comfortable.
14. Complete documentation using forms, checklists, or electronic dropdown lists supplemented by nurse's notes or additional comments as appropriate.

SAMPLE DOCUMENTATION

[date] 0900 Circumference measurements: head 45.7 cm (18¼ in.), chest 45 cm (18 in.), abd 44.4 cm (17½ in.); tolerated well with mother holding his hands. *R. Cummings*

SKILL 1.4 Weight: Newborn, Infant, Child, Adult, Measuring

A child's weight measurement can be compared to a standard children's height and weight chart to evaluate growth and development with other children of the same age. Weight measurements will change each year.

Delegation or Assignment

The nurse measures the weight of newborns or infants. Weight measurement of child, adolescent, and adult may be delegated or assigned to the UAP. The nurse remains responsible for the assessment, interpretation of abnormal finds, and determination of appropriate actions. Note that state laws for UAPs vary, so this task might be assigned to the UAP rather than delegated.

Equipment

- Infant scale for newborns or infants
- Paper
- Standing scale for older children and adults

Preparation

- Check the balance of the scale before using it.
- Have the parent or assistant remove all of the newborn's or infant's clothing and diaper. Weigh toddlers in their underclothes. Weigh older children and adults in their street clothes with heavy clothing and shoes removed. Newborns or infants with acute diarrheal disease or a chronic health problem may need to be weighed nude for accuracy. **Rationale:** *It is important to try to minimize the amount of clothing worn by children when weighing them to improve comparisons with previous weights taken.*
- Clean the infant scale tray between uses. Place a paper cover over the scale tray.
- When asking an adolescent or adult about weight loss, be specific about amount and time frame, for example, "Have you lost more than five pounds in the last two months?"

Procedure

1. Introduce self to patient (and parent) and verify the patient's identity using two identifiers. Explain to the patient (and parent) what you are going to do, why it is necessary, and how the patient can participate. Discuss how the results will be used in planning further care or treatments.
2. Perform hand hygiene and observe appropriate infection control procedures.
3. Provide for patient privacy.

NEWBORN OR INFANT

4. Place the newborn or infant on the scale and keep a hand close ❶. **Rationale:** *Newborns or infants may move quickly, and it is essential to protect them from falling.*

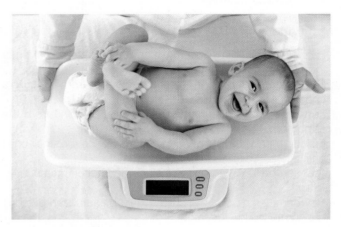

Source: Didesign021/Shutterstock

❶ A platform scale is used to weigh an infant.

5. Distract the infant, and take the reading when the infant stops moving. **Rationale:** *It takes a few seconds of inactivity for the scale to settle on the infant's actual weight.* Record the weight to the nearest 10 g or ½ oz.
6. Plot the measurement for the child's age in months on the standardized growth curve and proceed to step 7.

OLDER CHILD OR ADULT

4. Have the older child or adult stand still on the scale.
5. View the digital reading or move the weights until the scale is balanced.
6. Record the weight to the nearest 0.1 kg or ¼ lb.
7. When procedure is complete, perform hand hygiene. Leave patient safe and comfortable.
8. Complete documentation using forms, checklists, or electronic dropdown lists supplemented by nurse's notes or additional comments as appropriate.

SAMPLE DOCUMENTATION

[date] 0800 Weight per bed scale 147 kg (324 lb); tolerated without complaint. *R. Cummings*

>> Vital Signs

Expected Outcomes

1. Temperature is within normal range.
2. Appropriate method of temperature taking is determined for each patient.
3. Pulse is palpated without difficulty.
4. Pulse rate is within normal range and rhythm is regular.
5. Respiratory rate, rhythm, and depth are within normal limits.

6. Labored, difficult, or noisy respirations are assessed.
7. Accurate blood pressure readings are taken by using the correct cuff size and procedure.

8. The presence of factors that can alter blood pressure readings is identified.

Provide initial and serial objective measurements of body function to monitor patient status. The normal ranges for vital signs will vary with age, weight, gender, and overall health.

SKILL 1.5 Blood Pressure: Newborn, Infant, Child, Adult, Obtaining

Delegation or Assignment

Blood pressure measurement may be delegated or assigned to the UAP. The interpretation of abnormal blood pressure readings and determination of appropriate responses are done by the nurse. Note that state laws for UAPs vary, so this task might be assigned to the UAP rather than delegated.

Equipment

- Stethoscope
- Doppler ultrasound (DUS) as needed
- Blood pressure cuff of appropriate size

The blood pressure cuff consists of a rubber bag called a bladder that can be inflated with air ❶. It is covered with cloth and has two tubes attached to it. One tube connects to a rubber bulb that inflates the bladder. A small valve on the side of this bulb traps and releases the air in the bladder. The other tube is attached to a sphygmomanometer.

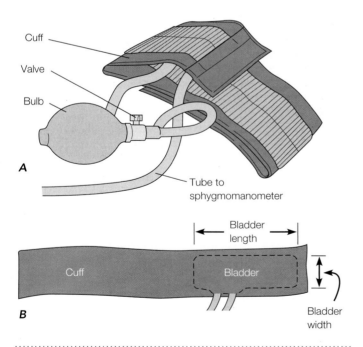

❶ **A,** Blood pressure cuff and bulb; **B,** The bladder inside the cuff.

Blood pressure cuffs come in various sizes (newborn, infant, child, small adult, adult, large adult, thigh). The bladder must be the correct width and length for the patient's arm. The width should be 40% of the circumference, or 20% wider than the diameter of the midpoint, of the arm on which it is used. Arm circumference, not the age of the patient, should always

be used to determine bladder size. Lay the cuff lengthwise at the midpoint of the upper arm, and hold the outermost side of the bladder edge laterally on the arm. With the other hand, wrap the width of the cuff around the arm, and ensure that the width is 40% of the arm circumference ❷.

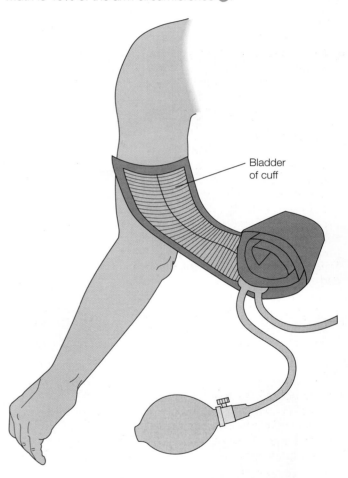

❷ Determining that the bladder of a blood pressure cuff is 40% of the arm circumference or 20% wider than the diameter of the midpoint of the limb.

The length of the bladder also affects the accuracy of measurement. The bladder should be sufficiently long to cover at least two thirds of the arm's circumference.

Blood pressure cuffs are made of nondistensible material so that an even pressure is exerted around the arm. Most cuffs are held in place by hooks, snaps, or Velcro. Others have a cloth bandage that is long enough to encircle the limb several

(continued on next page)

SKILL 1.5 Blood Pressure: Newborn, Infant, Child, Adult, Obtaining (*continued*)

times; this type is closed by tucking the end of the bandage into one of the bandage folds.

- Sphygmomanometer

The sphygmomanometer indicates the pressure of the air within the bladder. The aneroid sphygmomanometer is a calibrated dial with a needle that points to the calibrations ❸. Many agencies use digital (electronic) sphygmomanometers ❹, which eliminate the need to listen for the sounds of the patient's systolic and diastolic blood pressures through a stethoscope. Electronic blood pressure devices should be calibrated periodically to check accuracy. All healthcare facilities should have manual blood pressure equipment available as backup.

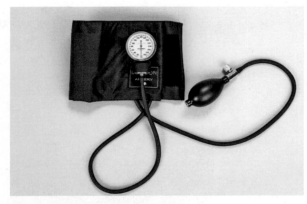

Source: Rick Brady/Pearson Education, Inc.

❸ Blood pressure equipment: an aneroid sphygmomanometer and cuff.

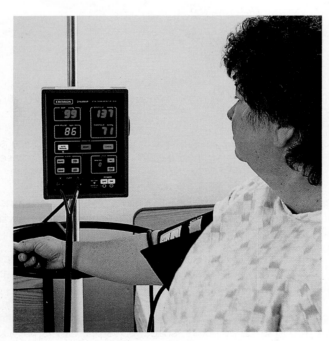

Source: Ronald May/Pearson Education, Inc.

❹ Electronic blood pressure monitors register blood pressures.

Preparation

- Ensure that the equipment is intact and functioning properly. Check for leaks in the tubing of the sphygmomanometer and report any equipment that is in need of repair.
- Explain to the patient and family what the equipment actually does and the information it provides.
- Determine if the adult patient is taking antihypertensive medications and, if so, when the last dose was taken.
- Make sure that the adult patient has not smoked or ingested caffeine within 30 minutes prior to measurement. **Rationale:** *Smoking constricts blood vessels, and caffeine increases the pulse rate. Both of these cause a temporary increase in blood pressure.*
- When using a site other than the upper arm, include the site of the blood pressure reading in the documentation to give the results more meaning. The ideal is to use the same site for trending blood pressure results.
- For accurate identification of systolic and diastolic sounds, remember Korotkoff sounds (blood pressure sounds): Phase 1 is the systolic pressure; phases 2 and 3 reflect blood flow in arteries; phase 4 reflects muffled blood flow; and phase 5 is the diastolic pressure (some professionals record diastolic during phases 4 and 5).

NEWBORN, INFANT, OR CHILD

Preparation

- To select the proper cuff size for a newborn, measure the newborn's arm (leg) circumference with a measuring tape around the midpoint of the arm (leg) used. If the blood pressure cuff has marks to determine fit, use these lines to ensure that the cuff is not too small. The cuff width should not extend to or beyond any joint on the arm (leg) used. Make sure the artery mark on the cuff is placed over the brachial artery.
- To select the proper cuff size for a child, compare the cuff to the size of the child's upper arm or thigh. The bladder of the cuff should encircle 80–100% of the extremity used.
- Use a pediatric stethoscope with a small diaphragm for the newborn or infant.
- With the child, explain each step of the process and what it will feel like. Demonstrate on a doll.
- Remember to include the site of the blood pressure reading to give the results more meaning when using a site other than the upper arm.

Equipment

- Various sizes blood pressure cuffs ❺
- Electronic blood pressure monitor
- Sphygmomanometer and stethoscope
- Blood pressure values by age, sex, and height percentiles

Oscillometry

Procedure

Electronic equipment is often used to obtain the systolic blood pressure for newborns, infants, and young children. With this

SKILL 1.5 Blood Pressure: Newborn, Infant, Child, Adult, Obtaining (*continued*)

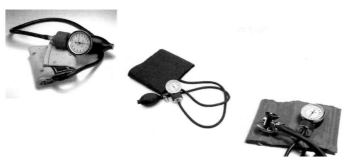

Source: Daniel Templeton/Alamy Stock Photo; Karen roach/Shutterstock; Henrik Dolle/Shutterstock

⑤ Blood pressure cuffs are available in various types and sizes for pediatric patients.

technique, a transducer uses pressure oscillations received and transmitted by the blood pressure cuff to identify the mean pressure and estimate the systolic and diastolic blood pressure. **⑥**

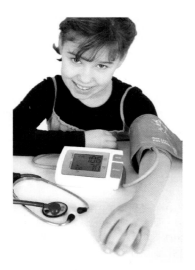

Source: St-fotograf/Fotolia

⑥ Measuring blood pressure using oscillometric technique.

1. Wrap the cuff around the right arm or upper leg directly against the skin with the center of the bladder over the artery of the extremity. The lower edge of the cuff should be 2–3 cm (about 1 in.) above the antecubital or popliteal fossa. **Rationale:** *The right arm is preferred, as this is the extremity used for standardizing the blood pressure tables. The upper leg is not a preferred site to obtain the blood pressure. It is used to measure the blood pressure and contrast with the arm blood pressure to detect coarctation of the aorta, a congenital heart defect.*
2. Place the arm with the antecubital fossa at heart level with muscles relaxed. Stabilize the arm, because movement interferes with the reading.

3. Ensure that the tubing is free of kinks, and activate the equipment according to the manufacturer's recommendations.
4. Pressure is recorded as the number over "D."
5. Document the blood pressure reading and compare values for age, sex, and height percentile.

Manual Sphygmomanometer

Procedure

1. Wrap the cuff snugly around the desired extremity directly against the skin with the bladder centered over the extremity's artery.
2. Hold the arm with the antecubital fossa at heart level **⑦**. If taking the blood pressure in the thigh, the child should be lying flat.

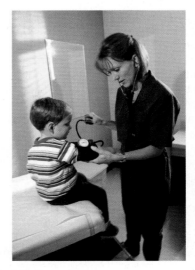

Source: Thinkstock/Getty Images

⑦ Measuring blood pressure with a manual cuff. Note the arm is at the same level as the heart.

3. Palpate for the pulse and inflate the cuff until the pulse is occluded and no longer felt. Note the reading. Release the cuff pressure. This is the palpated systolic blood pressure, and it can be recorded as blood pressure over "P."
4. Wait a minute and place the stethoscope over the pulse area. To improve the quality of sounds heard, avoid using too much pressure against the pulse area.
5. Close the air escape valve. Pump the cuff with the bulb until the gauge rises 30 mmHg above the level of the palpated systolic blood pressure. Slowly release the air through the valve at 2–3 mm/sec while watching the falling gauge. **Rationale:** *The palpated reading helps improve accuracy in the recognition of the first Korotkoff sound.*
6. Continue slowly releasing the air. The fifth Korotkoff sound (the disappearance of all sound) is the diastolic pressure. It may be

(*continued on next page*)

SKILL 1.5 Blood Pressure: Newborn, Infant, Child, Adult, Obtaining (*continued*)

0 in children under age 12 years. For these children the fourth Korotkoff sound is considered the diastolic pressure.

7. Document the blood pressure reading and compare to values for age, sex, and height percentile.

ADOLESCENT OR ADULT

Procedure

1. Prior to performing the procedure, introduce self and verify the patient's identity using two identifiers. Explain to the patient what you are going to do, why it is necessary, and how the patient can participate. Discuss how the results will be used in planning further care or treatments.
2. Perform hand hygiene and observe other appropriate infection control procedures.
3. Provide for patient privacy.
4. Position the patient appropriately.
   - The adult patient should be sitting with back straight and feet flat on the floor, not crossed. **Rationale:** *Sitting with legs crossed at the knee results in elevated systolic and diastolic blood pressures.*
   - The patient's arm to which the cuff will be applied should be supported on a flat surface, like the bedside table, with the upper arm at heart level (American Heart Association, 2014).
   - Expose the upper arm.
5. Wrap the deflated cuff evenly around the upper arm. Locate the brachial artery. Apply the center of the bladder directly over the artery. **Rationale:** *The bladder inside the cuff must be directly over the artery to be compressed if the reading is to be accurate.*
   - For an adult, place the lower border of the cuff approximately 2.5 cm (1 in.) above the antecubital space.
6. If this is the patient's initial examination, perform a preliminary palpatory determination of systolic pressure. **Rationale:** *The initial estimate tells the nurse the maximal pressure to which the sphygmomanometer needs to be elevated in subsequent determinations. It also prevents underestimation of the systolic pressure or overestimation of the diastolic pressure should an auscultatory gap occur.*
   - Palpate the brachial artery with the fingertips.
   - Close the valve on the bulb.
   - Pump up the cuff until you no longer feel the brachial pulse. At that pressure, the blood cannot flow through the artery. Note the pressure on the sphygmomanometer at which the pulse is no longer felt. **Rationale:** *This gives an estimate of the systolic pressure.*
   - Release the pressure completely in the cuff, and wait 1–2 min before making further measurements. **Rationale:** *A waiting period gives the blood trapped in the veins time to be released. Otherwise, falsely high systolic readings will occur.*
7. Position the stethoscope appropriately.
   - Cleanse the earpieces with antiseptic wipe.
   - Insert the ear attachments of the stethoscope in your ears so that they tilt slightly forward. **Rationale:** *Sounds are heard more clearly when the ear attachments follow the direction of the ear canal.*
   - Ensure that the stethoscope hangs freely from the ears to the diaphragm. **Rationale:** *If the stethoscope tubing rubs against an object, the noise can block the sounds of the blood within the artery.*
   - Place the bell side of the amplifier of the stethoscope over the brachial pulse site. **Rationale:** *Because the blood pressure is a low-frequency sound, it is best heard with the bell-shaped diaphragm.*
   - Place the stethoscope directly on the skin, not on clothing over the site. **Rationale:** *This is to avoid noise made from rubbing the amplifier against cloth.*
   - Hold the diaphragm with the thumb and index finger.
8. Auscultate the patient's blood pressure.
   - Pump up the cuff until the sphygmomanometer reads 30 mmHg above the point where the brachial pulse disappeared.
   - Release the valve on the cuff carefully so that the pressure decreases at the rate of 2–3 mmHg per second. **Rationale:** *If the rate is faster or slower, an error in measurement may occur.*
   - As the pressure falls, identify the manometer reading at Korotkoff phases 1, 4, and 5. **Rationale:** *There is no clinical significance to phases 2 and 3.*

CAUTION! The American Heart Association recommends routine use of the *bell* of the stethoscope for blood pressure (Korotkoff sounds) auscultation.

   - Deflate the cuff rapidly and completely. Document the results.
   - Wait 1–2 min before making further determinations. **Rationale:** *This permits blood trapped in the veins to be released.*
   - Repeat the above steps to confirm the accuracy of the reading—especially if it falls outside the normal range (although this may not be a routine procedure for hospitalized or well patients). If the difference between the two readings is greater than 5 mmHg, additional measurements may be taken and the results averaged. Selected sources of error are listed in **Table 1–1 》**.
9. If this is the patient's initial examination, repeat the procedure on the patient's other arm. There should be a difference of no more than 10 mmHg between the arms. The arm found to have the higher pressure should be used for subsequent examinations. Approximate values by age are shown in **Table 1–2 》**.

OBTAINING BLOOD PRESSURE BY THE PALPATION METHOD

■ If it is not possible to use a stethoscope to obtain the blood pressure or if Korotkoff sounds cannot be heard, palpate the

SKILL 1.5 Blood Pressure: Newborn, Infant, Child, Adult, Obtaining (*continued*)

TABLE 1–1 Selected Sources of Error in Blood Pressure Assessment

Error	Effect
Bladder cuff too narrow	Erroneously high
Bladder cuff too wide	Erroneously low
Arm unsupported	Erroneously high
Insufficient rest before the assessment	Erroneously high
Repeating assessment too quickly	Erroneously high systolic or low diastolic readings
Cuff wrapped too loosely or unevenly	Erroneously high
Deflating cuff too quickly	Erroneously low systolic and high diastolic readings
Deflating cuff too slowly	Erroneously high diastolic reading
Failure to use the same arm consistently	Inconsistent measurements
Arm above level of the heart	Erroneously low
Arm below heart level	Erroneously high
Assessing immediately after a meal or while patient smokes or has pain	Erroneously high
Failure to identify auscultatory gap	Erroneously low systolic pressure and erroneously low diastolic pressure

radial or brachial pulse site as the cuff pressure is released. The manometer reading at the point where the pulse reappears is an estimate of the systolic blood pressure.

TAKING A THIGH BLOOD PRESSURE

- Help the patient to assume a prone or supine position. If the patient cannot assume a prone position, measure the blood pressure while the patient is in a supine position with the knee slightly flexed. Slight flexing of the knee will facilitate placing the stethoscope on the popliteal space.
- Expose the thigh, taking care not to expose the patient unduly.
- Locate the popliteal artery.

TABLE 1–2 Approximate Blood Pressure by Age

Age Range	Systolic Range	Diastolic Range
Newborn	60–70	30–45
0–6 months	70–90	45–65
6–12 months	80–100	50–70
1–3 years	80–110	50–75
3–6 years	90–110	55–70
6–12 years	95–116	60–70
12 years and older	100–119	65–79
Adult	110–119	70–79

- Wrap the cuff evenly around the mid-thigh with the compression bladder over the posterior aspect of the thigh and the bottom edge above the knee. **Rationale:** *The bladder must be directly over the posterior popliteal artery if the reading is to be accurate.*
- If this is the patient's initial examination, perform a preliminary palpatory determination of systolic pressure while palpating the popliteal artery.
- In adults, the systolic pressure in the popliteal artery is often 20–30 mmHg higher than that in the brachial artery; the diastolic pressure is usually the same.

USING ELECTRONIC BLOOD PRESSURE MONITORING DEVICE

- Place the blood pressure cuff on the extremity according to the manufacturer's guidelines.
- Turn on the blood pressure switch.
- If appropriate, set the device for the desired number of minutes between blood pressure determinations.
- Instruct patient to keep the elbow extended when the cuff inflates.
- When the device has determined the blood pressure reading, note the digital results.
- Electronic/automatic blood pressure cuffs can be left in place for many hours. Remove the cuff and check skin condition periodically or follow facility policy.

10. Remove the cuff from the patient's arm.
11. Wipe the cuff with an approved disinfectant. **Rationale:** *Cuffs can become significantly contaminated.* Many institutions use disposable blood pressure cuffs. The patient uses a disposable cuff for the length of stay and then it is discarded. **Rationale:** *This decreases the risk of spreading infection by sharing cuffs.*
12. When the procedure is complete, perform hand hygiene. Leave patient safe and comfortable.
13. Complete documentation using forms, checklists, or electronic dropdown lists supplemented by nurse's notes or additional comments as appropriate. Record two pressures in the form "130/80," where "130" is the systolic (phase 1) and "80" is the diastolic (phase 5) pressure. Record three pressures in the form "130/90/0," where "130" is the systolic, "90" is the first diastolic (phase 4), and sounds are audible even after the cuff is completely deflated. Use the abbreviations RA or RL for right arm or right leg, respectively, and LA or LL for left arm or left leg, respectively. Record a difference of greater than 10 mmHg between the two arms or legs.

SAMPLE DOCUMENTATION

[date] 0730 Sitting in chair BP 126/82 RA; tolerated without complaint. *K. Burger*

SKILL 1.5 Blood Pressure: Newborn, Infant, Child, Adult, Obtaining (*continued*)

Lifespan Considerations

NEWBORN OR INFANT

- The lower edge of the blood pressure cuff can be closer to the antecubital space of a newborn or infant.
- Use the palpation method if auscultation with a stethoscope or DUS is unsuccessful.
- Arm and thigh pressures are equivalent in children under 1 year of age.
- Blood pressure ranges depend on gestational age and health of newborn at time of delivery.

CHILD

- Blood pressure should be measured in all children over 3 years of age and in children less than 3 years of age with certain medical conditions (e.g., congenital heart disease, renal malformation, or medications that affect blood pressure).
- Use the palpation technique for children under 3 years old.
- Cuff bladder width should be 40% and length should be 80–100% of the arm circumference. **Rationale:** *If the bladder is too small,*

the blood pressure reading will be falsely high; if it is too large, the pressure will be falsely low.

- Take the blood pressure prior to other uncomfortable procedures so that the blood pressure is not artificially elevated by the discomfort.
- In children, the diastolic pressure is considered to be the onset of phase 4, where the sounds become muffled.
- In children, the thigh pressure is about 10 mmHg higher than the arm.

OLDER ADULT

- Skin may be very fragile. Do not allow cuff pressure to remain high any longer than necessary.
- Medications that cause vasodilation (antihypertensive medications) along with the loss of baroreceptor efficiency in older adults place them at increased risk for having orthostatic hypotension (significant fall in blood pressure when changing from supine to sitting or standing). Measuring blood pressure while the patient is in the lying, sitting, and standing positions—and noting any changes—can determine this.
- If the patient has arm contractures, assess the blood pressure by palpation, with the arm in a relaxed position. If this is not possible, take a thigh blood pressure.

SKILL 1.6 Pulse, Apical and Peripheral: Obtaining

Delegation or Assignment

Measurement of the patient's radial or brachial pulse can be delegated or assigned to the UAP. Reports of abnormal pulse rates or rhythms require reassessment by the nurse, who also determines appropriate action if the abnormality is confirmed. UAPs are generally not delegated these assessment techniques due to the skill required in locating and interpreting peripheral pulses other than the radial or brachial artery and in using Doppler ultrasound (DUS) devices. Due to the degree of skill and knowledge required, UAPs are generally not responsible for assessing apical pulses. Note that state laws for UAPs vary, so this task might be assigned to the UAP rather than delegated.

Equipment

- Watch with a second hand or indicator
- Stethoscope
- Antiseptic wipes
- If using a DUS, the transducer probe, the stethoscope headset, transmission gel, and tissues/wipes

Preparation

- If using the DUS, check that the equipment is functioning normally.
- Verify the adult patient has not smoked or ingested caffeine within 30 minutes prior to measurement. **Rationale:** *Smoking constricts blood vessels, and caffeine increases the pulse rate.*
- Include the site of the pulse reading in documentation to give the results more meaning when using a site other than the radial artery.
- To ensure accuracy of pulse rate, the apical pulse site is preferred when the patient's pulse is irregular.

APICAL PULSE

Procedure

1. Prior to performing the procedure, introduce self and verify the patient's identity using two identifiers. Explain to the patient what you are going to do, why it is necessary, and how the patient can participate. Discuss how the results will be used in planning further care or treatments.
2. Perform hand hygiene and observe other appropriate infection control procedures.
3. Provide for patient privacy.
4. Position the patient appropriately in a comfortable supine position or in a sitting position. Expose the area of the chest over the apex of the heart.
5. Locate the apical impulse ❶. This is the point over the apex of the heart where the apical pulse can be most clearly heard.
   - Palpate the angle of Louis (the angle between the manubrium, the top of the sternum, and the body of the sternum). It is palpated just below the suprasternal notch and is felt as a prominence.
   - Slide your index finger just to the left of the sternum and palpate the second intercostal space ❷. The left intercostal space is the pulmonic area.
   - Place your middle or next finger in the third intercostal space ❸, and continue palpating downward until you locate the fifth intercostal space.
   - Move your index finger laterally along the fifth intercostal space toward the midclavicular line (MCL) for the right ventricular area. Then move fingertips laterally 5–7.6 cm (2–3 in.) to the left midclavicular line for the apical impulse or point of maximal impulse (PMI) ❹.

SKILL 1.6 Pulse, Apical and Peripheral: Obtaining *(continued)*

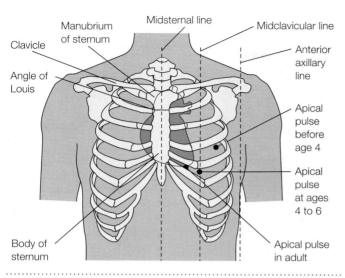

Clavicle · Manubrium of sternum · Midsternal line · Midclavicular line · Angle of Louis · Anterior axillary line · Apical pulse before age 4 · Apical pulse at ages 4 to 6 · Body of sternum · Apical pulse in adult

❶ Location of apical pulse for a child under 4 years, a child 4 to 6 years, and an adult.

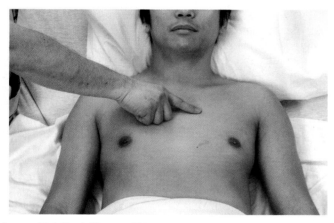

Source: Rick Brady/Pearson Education, Inc.

❷ Palpating the second intercostal space.

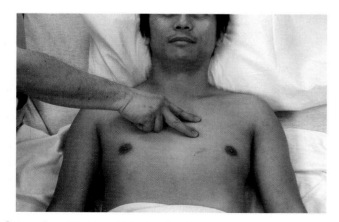

Source: Rick Brady/Pearson Education, Inc.

❸ Third intercostal space.

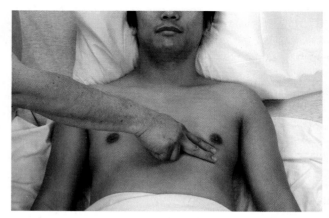

Source: Rick Brady/Pearson Education, Inc.

❹ Fifth intercostal space midclavicular line.

6. Auscultate and count heartbeats (**Table 1–3 》**).
   - Use antiseptic wipes to clean the earpieces and diaphragm of the stethoscope if their cleanliness is in doubt. **Rationale:** *The diaphragm needs to be cleaned and disinfected if soiled with body substances.*
   - Warm the diaphragm of the stethoscope by holding it in the palm of the hand for a moment. **Rationale:** *The metal of the diaphragm is usually cold and can startle the patient when placed immediately on the chest.*
   - Insert the earpieces of the stethoscope into your ears in the direction of the ear canals, or slightly forward. **Rationale:** *This position facilitates hearing.*
   - Tap your finger lightly on the diaphragm. **Rationale:** *This is to be sure it is the active side of the stethoscope head.* If necessary, rotate the head to select the diaphragm side ❺.

TABLE 1–3 Approximate Heart Rate by Age

Age Range	Heart Rate Range (Beats/Minute)
Newborn	100–170
6–12 months	80–130
1–3 years	70–120
3–6 years	65–110
6–10 years	70–110
10–16 years	60–100
17 years and older	60–100
Adult	55–85
Older adult	60–80

(continued on next page)

SKILL 1.6 Pulse, Apical and Peripheral: Obtaining (*continued*)

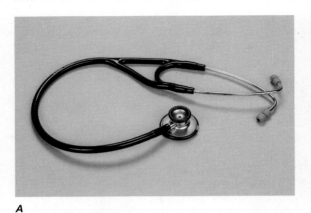

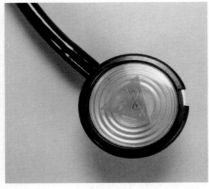

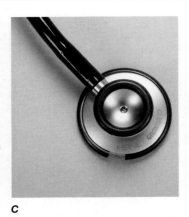

A   *B*   *C*

*Sources: **A**, **B**,* and ***C**,* Rick Brady/Pearson Education, Inc.

⑤ *A*, Stethoscope with both a bell and diaphragm; ***B*,** close-up of a diaphragm; ***C*,** close-up of a bell.

- Place the diaphragm of the stethoscope over the apical impulse and listen for the normal S_1 and S_2 heart sounds, which are heard as "lub-dub" **⑥ Rationale:** *The heartbeat is normally loudest over the apex of the heart.* Each lub-dub is counted as one heartbeat. **Rationale:** *The two heart sounds are produced by closure of the heart valves. The S_1 heart sound (lub) occurs when the atrioventricular valves close after the ventricles have been sufficiently filled. The S_2 heart sound (dub) occurs when the semilunar valves close after the ventricles empty.*

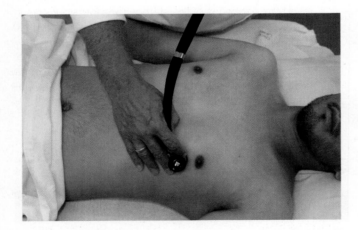

⑥ Taking an apical pulse using the diaphragm of the stethoscope. Note how the diaphragm is held against the chest.

- If you have difficulty hearing the apical pulse, ask the supine patient to roll onto the left side or the sitting patient to lean slightly forward. **Rationale:** *This positioning moves the apex of the heart closer to the chest wall.*
- If the rhythm is regular, count the heartbeats for 30 seconds and multiply by 2. If the rhythm is irregular or for giving certain medications such as digoxin, count the

beats for 60 seconds. **Rationale:** *A 60-second count provides a more accurate assessment of an irregular pulse than a 30-second count.*

7. Assess the rhythm and the strength of the heartbeat.
   - Assess the rhythm of the heartbeat by noting the pattern of intervals between the beats. A normal pulse has equal time periods between beats.
   - Assess the strength (volume) of the heartbeat. Normally, the heartbeats are equal in strength and can be described as strong or weak.
8. When the procedure is complete, perform hand hygiene. Leave the patient safe and comfortable. Complete documentation using forms, checklists, or electronic dropdown lists supplemented by nurse's notes or additional comments as appropriate. Also record pertinent related data such as variation in pulse rate compared to normal for the patient and abnormal skin color and skin temperature.

SAMPLE DOCUMENTATION

[date] 1000 Radial pulse 116 and & irregular; had been 82 & regular at 0600; T, R, & BP within patient's usual range; C/o slight dizziness; Skin warm & dry; Apical pulse 120, irregular, with slight pause after every 3rd beat; Dr. Jones notified & ECG ordered. *G. Chapman*

PERIPHERAL PULSES

Procedure

1. Prior to performing the procedure, introduce self and verify the patient's identity using two identifiers. Explain to the patient what you are going to do, why it is necessary, and how the patient can participate. Discuss how the results will be used in planning further care or treatments.
2. Perform hand hygiene and observe other appropriate infection control procedures.
3. Provide for patient privacy.

SKILL 1.6 Pulse, Apical and Peripheral: Obtaining (*continued*)

4. Select the pulse point. Normally, the radial pulse is taken, unless it cannot be exposed or circulation to another body area is to be assessed.

5. Assist the patient to a resting position. When the radial pulse is assessed, with the palm facing inward, the patient's arm can rest alongside the body, or the forearm can rest at a 90-degree angle across the chest. For the patient who can sit, the forearm can rest across the thigh, with the palm of the hand facing downward or inward.

6. Palpate and count the pulse. Place two or three middle fingertips lightly and squarely over the pulse point ➐. *Rationale: Use of the thumb is contraindicated because the nurse's thumb has a pulse that could be mistaken for the patient's pulse.*
   - Count for 15 seconds and multiply by 4, or follow facility policy. Record the pulse in beats per minute on your worksheet. Count for a full minute if taking a patient's pulse for the first time, when obtaining baseline data, or if the pulse is irregular. If an irregular pulse is found, also take the apical pulse.

7. Assess the pulse rhythm and volume.
   - Assess the pulse rhythm by noting the pattern of the intervals between the beats. A normal pulse has equal time periods between beats. If this is an initial assessment, assess for 1 minute.
   - Assess the pulse volume, also called *amplitude* or *degree of expansion*. A normal pulse can be felt with moderate pressure, and the pressure is equal with each beat. A forceful pulse volume is full; an easily obliterated pulse is weak. Record the rhythm and volume on your worksheet.

8. Document the pulse rate, rhythm, and volume and your actions in the patient record. Also record in the nurse's notes pertinent related data such as variation in pulse rate compared to normal for the patient, as well as abnormal skin color and skin temperature.

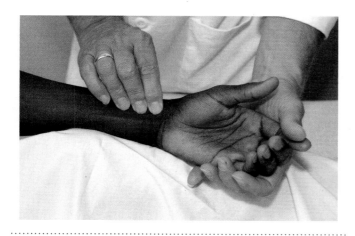

➐ *A,* radial

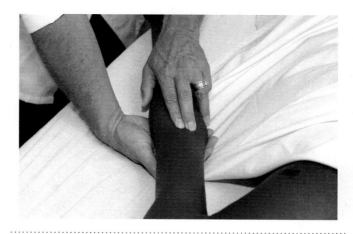

➐ *B,* brachial

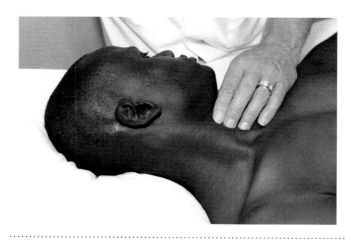

➐ *C,* carotid

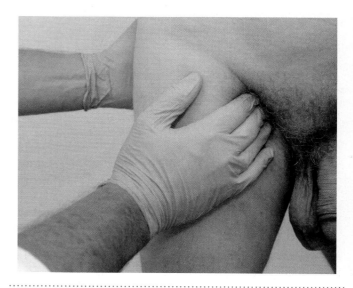

➐ *D,* femoral

(*continued on next page*)

SKILL 1.6 Pulse, Apical and Peripheral: Obtaining (*continued*)

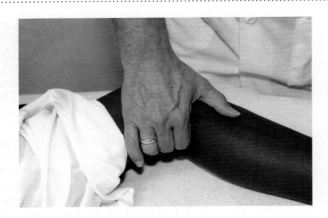

7 **E,** popliteal

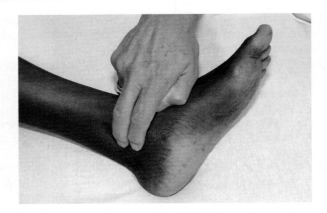

7 **F,** posterior tibial

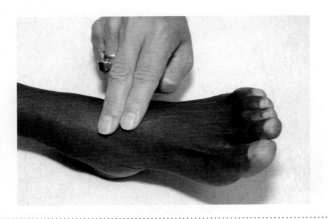

7 **G,** pedal (dorsalis pedis)

USING A DOPPLER ULTRASOUND DEVICE

- If used, plug the stethoscope headset into one of the two output jacks located next to the volume control **8**.
- Apply transmission gel either to the probe at the narrow end of the plastic case housing the transducer, or to the patient's skin. **Rationale:** *Ultrasound beams do not travel well through air. The gel makes an airtight seal, which then promotes optimal ultrasound wave transmission.*
- Press the "on" button.
- Hold the probe against the skin over the pulse site. Use a light pressure, and keep the probe in contact with the skin **9**. **Rationale:** *Too much pressure can stop the blood flow and obliterate the signal.*
- Adjust the volume if necessary. Distinguish artery sounds from vein sounds. The artery sound (signal) is distinctively pulsating and has a pumping quality. The venous sound is intermittent and varies with respirations. Both artery and vein sounds are heard simultaneously through the DUS because major arteries and veins are situated close together throughout the body. If arterial sounds cannot be easily heard, reposition the probe.
- After assessing the pulse, remove all gel from the probe to prevent damage to the surface. Clean the transducer with

water-based solution. **Rationale:** *Alcohol or other disinfectants may damage the face of the transducer. Remove all gel from the patient.*
- When the procedure is complete, perform hand hygiene. Leave patient safe and comfortable.
- Complete documentation using forms, checklists, or electronic dropdown lists supplemented by nurse's notes or additional comments as appropriate.

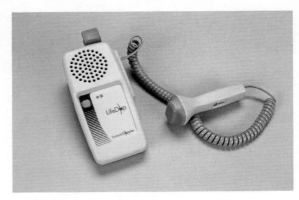

Source: Rick Brady/Pearson Education, Inc.

8 A Doppler ultrasound (DUS) stethoscope.

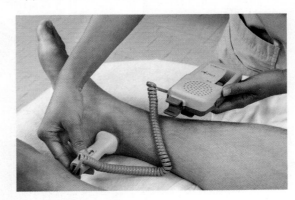

Source: Rick Brady/Pearson Education, Inc.

9 Using a DUS to assess the posterior tibial pulse.

SKILL 1.7 Pulse Oximeter: Using

This skill provides a noninvasive method of measuring oxygenation, or oxygen saturation, in the blood and provides a pulse reading. It is especially helpful for the patient with a respiratory illness or disease.

Delegation or Assignment

Application of the pulse oximeter sensor and recording of the oxygen saturation (SpO_2) value may be delegated or assigned to the UAP. The interpretation of the SpO_2 value and determination of appropriate responses are done by the nurse. Note that state laws for UAPs vary, so this task might be assigned to the UAP rather than delegated.

Equipment

- Nail polish remover as needed
- Alcohol wipe
- Sheet or towel
- Pulse oximeter

Pulse oximeters with various types of sensors are available from several manufacturers. The *oximeter unit* consists of an inlet connection for the sensor cable, a faceplate that indicates (a) the oxygen saturation measurement (expressed as a percentage) and (b) the pulse rate. Cordless units are also available. A preset alarm system signals high and low SpO_2 measurements and a high and low pulse rate. The high and low SpO_2 levels are generally preset at 100% and 85%, respectively, for adults. The high and low pulse rate alarms are usually preset at 140 bpm and 50 bpm for adults. These alarm limits can, however, be changed according to the manufacturer's directions.

Preparation

- Check that the oximeter equipment is functioning normally.
- Always remember to include percentage of oxygen patient is receiving when documenting a SpO_2. If patient is not on supplemental oxygen therapy, document reading is on *room air*.
- If an appropriate-size finger or toe sensor is not available, consider using an earlobe or forehead sensor for a newborn or infant.
- The high and low SpO_2 alarm levels are generally preset at 95% and 80% for neonates.
- The high and low pulse rate alarms are usually preset at 200 and 100 for neonates.
- The oximeter may need to be taped, wrapped with an elastic bandage, or covered by a stocking to keep it in place on a newborn or infant.
- Instruct the child that the sensor does not hurt. Disconnect the probe whenever possible to allow for movement.

Procedure

1. Prior to performing the procedure, introduce self and verify the patient's identity using two identifiers. Explain to the patient what you are going to do, why it is necessary, and how the patient can participate. Discuss how the results will be used in planning further care or treatments.
2. Perform hand hygiene and observe other appropriate infection control procedures.
3. Provide for patient privacy.
4. Choose a sensor appropriate for the patient's weight, size, and desired location ❶. Because weight limits of sensors overlap, a pediatric sensor could be used for a small adult.
   - If the patient is allergic to adhesive, use a clip or sensor without adhesive. If using an extremity, assess the proximal pulse and capillary refill at the point closest to the site.
   - If the patient has low tissue perfusion due to peripheral vascular disease or therapy using vasoconstrictive medications, use a nasal sensor or a reflectance sensor on the forehead. Avoid using lower extremities that have compromised circulation and extremities that are used for infusions or other invasive monitoring.

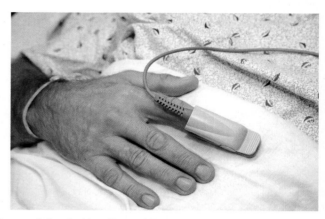

Source: Celina Burkhart/Pearson Education, Inc.

❶ Fingertip oximeter sensor provides continuous oximeter unit display of hemoglobin oxygen saturation (SpO_2) and pulse rate.

5. Prepare the site.
   - Clean the site with an alcohol wipe before applying the sensor.
   - It may be necessary to remove a patient's dark nail polish. **Rationale:** *It can interfere with accurate measurements.*
   - Alternatively, position the sensor on the side of the finger rather than perpendicular to the nail bed.
6. Apply the sensor, and connect it to the pulse oximeter.
   - Make sure the LED and photodetector are accurately aligned, that is, opposite each other on either side of the finger, toe, nose, or earlobe. Many sensors have markings to facilitate correct alignment of the LEDs and photodetector.
   - Attach the sensor cable to the connection outlet on the oximeter. Turn on the machine according to the manufacturer's directions. Appropriate connection will be confirmed by an audible beep indicating each arterial pulsation. Some devices have a wheel that can be turned clockwise to increase the pulse volume and counterclockwise to decrease it.
   - Ensure that the bar of light or waveform on the face of the oximeter fluctuates with each pulsation.

(continued on next page)

SKILL 1.7 Pulse Oximeter: Using (continued)

7. Set and turn on the alarm when using continuous monitoring.
   - Check the preset alarm limits for high and low oxygen saturation and high and low pulse rates. Change these alarm limits according to the manufacturer's directions as indicated. Ensure that the audio and visual alarms are on before you leave the patient. A tone will be heard and a number will blink on the faceplate.
8. Ensure patient safety.
   - Inspect and/or move or change the location of an adhesive toe or finger sensor every 4 hours and a spring-tension sensor every 2 hours.
   - Inspect the sensor site tissues for irritation from adhesive sensors.
9. Ensure the accuracy of measurement.
   - Minimize motion artifacts by using an adhesive sensor, or immobilize the patient's monitoring site. **Rationale:** *Movement of the patient's finger or toe may be misinterpreted by the oximeter as arterial pulsations.*

   - If indicated, cover the sensor with a sheet or towel to block large amounts of light from external sources (e.g., sunlight, procedure lamps, bilirubin lights in the nursery). **Rationale:** *Bright room light may be sensed by the photodetector and alter the SpO_2 value.*
   - Compare the pulse rate indicated by the oximeter to the radial pulse periodically. **Rationale:** *A large discrepancy between the two values may indicate oximeter malfunction.*
10. When the procedure is complete, perform hand hygiene. Leave the patient safe and comfortable.
11. Complete documentation using forms, checklists, or electronic dropdown lists supplemented by nurses notes or additional comments as appropriate.

> **SAMPLE DOCUMENTATION**
>
> Date 0800 SpO_2 97% on room air; no complaints of SOB. *K. Dater*

SKILL 1.8 Respirations: Newborn, Infant, Child, Adult, Obtaining

Delegation or Assignment

Counting and observing respirations may be delegated or assigned to the UAP. The follow-up assessment, interpretation of abnormal respirations, and determination of appropriate responses are done by the nurse. Note that state laws for UAPs vary, so this task might be assigned to the UAP rather than delegated.

Equipment

- Watch with a second hand or indicator

Preparation

- For a routine assessment of respirations, determine the patient's activity schedule and choose a suitable time to monitor the respirations. A patient who has been exercising will need to rest for a few minutes to permit the accelerated respiratory rate to return to normal.
- A newborn, infant, or child who is crying will have an abnormal respiratory rate and rhythm and needs to be quieted before respirations can be accurately assessed.
- Have an adult hold a child gently to reduce movement while counting respirations.
- Because young children are diaphragmatic breathers, observe the rise and fall of the abdomen. If necessary, place your hand gently on the abdomen to feel the rapid rise and fall during respirations.
  - Abdominal movement in a child will be irregular.
  - Count breaths for 1 full minute, or count for 30 seconds and multiply by 2. Approximate respiratory rates by age are shown in **Table 1–4 ⟩⟩**.

Procedure

1. Prior to performing the procedure, introduce self and verify the patient's identity using two identifiers. Explain to the patient and parent what you are going to do, why it is necessary, and

TABLE 1–4 Approximate Respiratory Rate by Age

Age Range	Respiratory Range (Respirations/Minute)
Newborn	30–60
0–1 year	20–40
1–3 years	20–30
3–6 years	20–30
6–10 years	15–30
10–15 years	15–20
15 years and older	12–20

how the patient can participate. Discuss how the results will be used in planning further care or treatments.
2. Perform hand hygiene and observe other appropriate infection control procedures.
3. Provide for patient privacy.

NEWBORN, INFANT, OR CHILD

4. Observe or palpate and count the respiratory rate.
   - Observe the abdomen, rather than the chest, rise and fall in a newborn, infant, or child under the age of 3. **Rationale:** *Because a newborn's, infant's, and young child's respirations are diaphragmatic, the abdomen moves more than the chest with breathing.*
   - Abdominal movement in a newborn, infant, or child will be irregular.
   - The child's awareness that the nurse is counting the respiratory rate could cause the child to purposefully alter the respiratory pattern. If you anticipate this, place a hand against the child's abdomen to feel the abdominal

SKILL 1.8 Respirations: Newborn, Infant, Child, Adult, Obtaining (continued)

movements with breathing, or place the child's arm across the abdomen and observe the abdominal movements while supposedly taking the radial pulse.

- Count breaths for 1 full minute, or count for 30 seconds and multiply by 2, then proceed to step 5 below.

ADULT

4. The procedure for measuring an adult's respiratory rate is essentially the same as for a newborn, infant, or child. However, keep in mind these points:
   - Observe the chest, rather than the abdomen, rise and fall.
   - Count breaths for 1 full minute, or count for 30 seconds and multiply by 2.
   - The patient's awareness that the nurse is counting the respiratory rate could cause the patient to purposefully alter the respiratory pattern. If you anticipate this, place a hand against the patient's chest to feel the chest movements with breathing, or place the patient's arm across the chest and observe the chest movements while supposedly taking the radial pulse.

- Count the respiratory rate for 30 seconds if the respirations are regular. Count for 60 seconds if they are irregular. An inhalation and an exhalation count as one respiration.
5. Observe the depth, rhythm, and character of respirations.
   - Observe the respirations for depth by watching the movement of the chest. **Rationale:** *During deep respirations, a large volume of air is exchanged; during shallow respirations, a small volume is exchanged.*
   - Observe the respirations for regular or irregular rhythm. **Rationale:** *Normally, respirations are evenly spaced.*
   - Observe the character of respirations: the sound they produce and the effort they require. **Rationale:** *Normally, respirations are silent and effortless.* **Table 1–5 》》** describes altered breathing patterns and sounds.
6. When the procedure is complete, perform hand hygiene. Leave the patient safe and comfortable. Complete the documentation using forms, checklists, or electronic dropdown lists supplemented by nurse's notes or additional comments as appropriate. Document the respiratory rate, depth, rhythm, and character on the appropriate record.

TABLE 1–5 Altered Breathing Patterns and Sounds

Breathing Patterns	Breath Sounds
Rate	**Audible without Amplification**
■ Tachypnea—quick, shallow breaths	■ Stridor—a shrill, harsh sound heard during inspiration with laryngeal obstruction
■ Bradypnea—abnormally slow breathing	■ Stertor—snoring or sonorous respiration, usually due to a partial obstruction of the upper airway
■ Apnea—cessation of breathing	
Volume	■ Wheeze—continuous, high-pitched musical squeak or whistling sound occurring on expiration and sometimes on inspiration when air moves through a narrowed or partially obstructed airway
■ Hyperventilation—overexpansion of the lungs characterized by rapid and deep breaths	
■ Hypoventilation—under-expansion of the lungs, characterized by shallow respirations	■ Bubbling—gurgling sounds heard as air passes through moist secretions in the respiratory tract
Rhythm	**Chest Movements**
■ Cheyne-Stokes breathing—rhythmic waxing and waning of respirations, from very deep to very shallow breathing and temporary apnea	■ Intercostal retraction—indrawing between the ribs
	■ Substernal retraction—indrawing beneath the breastbone
Ease or Effort	■ Suprasternal retraction—indrawing above the clavicles
■ Dyspnea—difficult and labored breathing during which the individual has a persistent, unsatisfied need for air and feels distressed	**Secretions and Coughing**
	■ Hemoptysis—the presence of blood in the sputum
■ Orthopnea—ability to breathe only in upright sitting or standing positions	■ Productive cough—a cough accompanied by expectorated secretions
	■ Nonproductive cough—a dry, harsh cough without secretions

CAUTION! Monitor the respiratory rate following the administration of medications that are respiratory depressants, such as morphine.

SAMPLE DOCUMENTATION

[date] 1320 Respirations irregular, varying from 18–34/min in past hour (see vital signs sheet); shallower resp. during tachypnea; slight wheezing noted; respiratory therapist called to provide treatment. *D. Katano*

Lifespan Considerations
NEWBORNS AND INFANTS

- Newborns and infants use their diaphragms for inhalation and exhalation. If necessary, place your hand gently on the newborn's or infant's abdomen to feel the rapid rise and fall during respirations.
- Most newborns are complete nose breathers, and nasal obstruction can be life threatening.
- Some newborns display "periodic breathing" in which they pause for a few seconds between respirations. This condition can be normal, but parents should be alert to prolonged or frequent pauses (apnea) that require medical attention.
- Compared to adults, newborns and infants have fewer alveoli and their airways have a smaller diameter. As a result, the respiratory

SKILL 1.8 Respirations: Newborn, Infant, Child, Adult, Obtaining (*continued*)

rate and effort of breathing will increase in newborns and infants with respiratory infections.

CHILDREN

- Count respirations prior to other uncomfortable procedures so that the respiratory rate is not artificially elevated by the discomfort.

OLDER ADULTS

- Ask the patient to remain quiet, or count respirations after taking the pulse.
- Older adults may experience anatomical and physiological changes that cause the respiratory system to be less efficient. Any changes in rate or type of breathing should be reported immediately.

SKILL 1.9 Temperature: Newborn, Infant, Child, Adult, Obtaining

Delegation or Assignment

Routine measurement of the patient's temperature can be delegated or assigned to the UAP. The nurse must explain the appropriate type of thermometer and site to be used and ensure that the person knows when to report an abnormal temperature and how to record the finding. The interpretation of an abnormal temperature and determination of appropriate responses are done by the nurse. Note that state laws for UAPs vary, so this task might be assigned to the UAP rather than delegated.

Equipment

- Digital or electronic thermometer or scanner thermometer ① ②
- Disposable thermometer probe sheath or cover
- Water-soluble lubricant for a rectal temperature
- Clean gloves for a rectal temperature
- Towel for axillary temperature
- Tissues/wipes

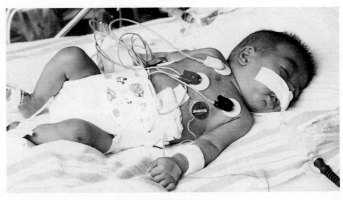

Source: Rick Brady/Pearson Education, Inc.

② The new scanner method is often used for children who are unconscious, have seizures, or have a structural abnormality.

Preparation

- Check that all equipment is functioning normally.
- Consider whether environmental conditions such as lack of heat or air conditioning are affecting the patient's temperature or temperature measurement.
- Ensure that only water-soluble lubricant is used for a rectal thermometer.
- Temperature varies with the time of day: It is highest between 5–7 p.m. and lowest between 2–6 a.m. This variation is termed *circadian thermal rhythm*. A consistent method of body temperature measurement should be used so that readings are comparable.
- The temperature of an unconscious patient is never taken by mouth. The rectal, tympanic, or scanner method is preferred.
- Temperature measurements vary with the location they are obtained. Common approximate correlation of temperature results is: average normal oral temperature is 37°C (98.6°F); a rectal temperature and a tympanic (ear) temperature are both approximately 0.5°C (1°F) higher than an oral temperature; an axillary (armpit) temperature and a temporal (forehead) scanned temperature are both approximately 0.5°C (1°F) lower than an oral temperature.
- Identify appropriate thermometer and route for each patient (**Box 1–3** ⟫). Recognize possible disadvantages of different sites (**Table 1–6** ⟫)

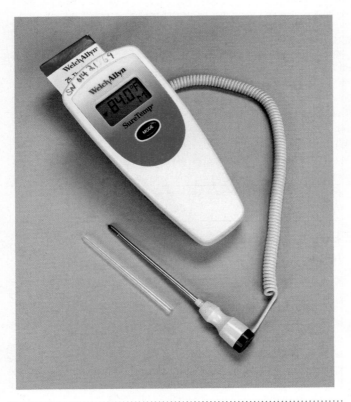

① An electronic thermometer. Note the probe and probe cover.

SKILL 1.9 Temperature: Newborn, Infant, Child, Adult, Obtaining (*continued*)

Box 1–3
Thermometer Placement

ORAL

- Place the bulb on either side of the frenulum Ⓐ.

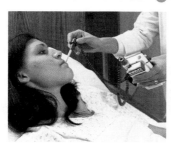

Ⓐ Oral thermometer placement.

RECTAL

- Apply clean gloves.
- Instruct the patient to take a slow, deep breath during insertion Ⓑ.
- Never force the thermometer if resistance is felt.
- Insert 3.8 cm (1.5 in.) in adults.

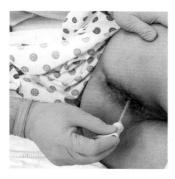

Source: Rick Brady/Pearson Education, Inc.

Ⓑ Inserting a rectal thermometer.

AXILLARY

- Pat the axilla dry if very moist.
- Place the bulb in the center of the axilla Ⓒ.

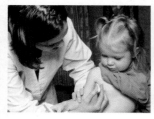
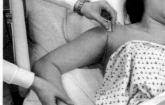

Sources: George Dodson/Pearson Education, Inc.; Rick Brady/Pearson Education, Inc.

Ⓒ Placing the bulb of the thermometer in the center of the axilla.

TYMPANIC MEMBRANE

- Pull the pinna slightly down and back for children younger than 3 years, and slightly upward and backward for a patient 3 years and older Ⓓ.
- Point the probe slightly anteriorly, toward the eardrum.
- Insert the probe slowly using a circular motion until snug.

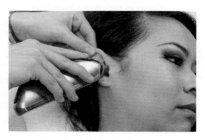

Source: Rick Brady/Pearson Education, Inc.

Ⓓ On patients 3 years or older, pull the pinna of the ear up and back while inserting the tympanic thermometer.

TEMPORAL ARTERY

- Brush hair aside if covering the temporal artery area.
- With the probe flush on the center of the forehead, depress the red button; keep depressed.
- Slowly slide the probe midline across the forehead to the hairline, not down the side of the face.
- Lift the probe from the forehead and touch on the neck just behind the earlobe. Release the button Ⓔ.

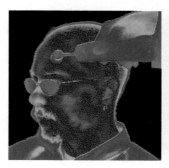
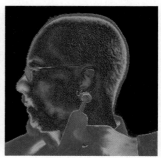

Source: Courtesy of Exergen Corporation

Ⓔ Positioning a temporal artery thermometer.

NONCONTACT INFRARED THERMOMETER

- Measures infrared energy coming off the body without any contact with skin.
- Forehead skin needs to be dry with hair pushed aside (can also use neck or other body surfaces, depending on manufacturer).
- Thermometer held 5–15 cm (2–6 in.) away from body surface.
- Aim lens then press and hold scanner button for reading.

(*continued on next page*)

SKILL 1.9 Temperature: Newborn, Infant, Child, Adult, Obtaining *(continued)*

TABLE 1–6 Potential Disadvantages of Sites for Body Temperature Measurement

Site	Disadvantages
Oral	Inaccurate if patient has just ingested hot or cold food or fluid or smoked.
	Could injure the mouth following oral surgery.
Rectal	Inconvenient and more unpleasant for patients; difficult for patient who cannot turn to the side.
	Could injure the rectum following rectal surgery.
	Presence of stool may interfere with thermometer placement and accuracy of reading.
Axillary	The thermometer must be left in place 3–5 min to obtain an accurate measurement.
Tympanic membrane	Can be uncomfortable and involves risk of injuring the membrane if the probe is inserted too far.
	Right and left measurements can differ.
	Presence of cerumen can affect the reading.
Temporal scanner	Requires electronic equipment that may be expensive or unavailable; variation in technique needed if the patient has perspiration on the forehead.
Skin scanner	Requires dry, nonhairy skin area like the forehead in a constant environmental temperature with low humidity.

Procedure

1. Determine appropriate thermometer and route for the patient. **Rationale:** *Oral route is appropriate for a child over 3 years of age and an electronic, nonbreakable thermometer is preferred.*
2. Perform hand hygiene and identify patient with two forms of identifiers.
3. Explain the procedure at patient's level of understanding and to parent.
4. Remove probe from cover or attach probe tip to electronic thermometer.

ORAL ROUTE

a. Use only for child who is age 3 or older.
b. Place probe under patient's tongue, one side or the other of the frenulum.
c. Have patient close mouth and either hold thermometer in place or monitor while taking temperature.
d. Leave digital thermometer in place 45–90 seconds or remove electronic thermometer when audible signal occurs. Proceed to step 5.

RECTAL ROUTE

a. Place patient in prone or side-lying position.
b. Lubricate probe.
c. Insert thermometer 0.6–1.3 cm (¼–½ in.) into rectum for newborn or infant or 1.3–2.5 cm (½–1 in.) for child, and hold in place.
d. Turn on scanner and follow directions.
e. Remove probe when tone or beep is heard.

f. Only use patient's own dedicated electronic thermometer (including rectal and oral) if diagnosis includes *Clostridium difficile*–associated diarrhea because of the potential for spreading the bacteria and increasing the risk of transmitting a healthcare-associated infection (HAI) to others. Proceed to step 5.

AXILLARY ROUTE

a. Assist patient to a comfortable position and expose axilla.
b. Dry axilla if necessary. **Rationale:** *A moist axillary area can produce a false low reading.*
c. Place thermometer in center of axilla. Lower patient's arm down and across the chest. **Rationale:** *This position ensures that the thermometer remains in contact with large vessels of the axilla.*
d. Leave in place 1–2 min or until tone is heard. **Rationale:** *Axillary temperature readings take longer to register than oral or rectal.*

5. Read and record temperature, indicating method.
6. Discard probe cover into trash by pushing ejection button, or return digital thermometer to its case.

TYMPANIC TEMPERATURE

Note: A tympanic thermometer measures the infrared energy that naturally radiates from the tympanic membrane and surrounding tissues.

- Perform hand hygiene and identify the patient with two identifiers.
- Attach disposable cover centering probe on film and press firmly until backing frame of probe cover engages base of probe. **Rationale:** *Cover protects patient from transmission of microorganisms.*
- Turn the patient's head to one side and stabilize the patient's head.
- Pull pinna upward and backward for an adult ❸ and child 3 years of age and older, and down and back for a child less than 3 years old. **Rationale:** *This procedure provides better access to the ear canal and tympanic membrane.*

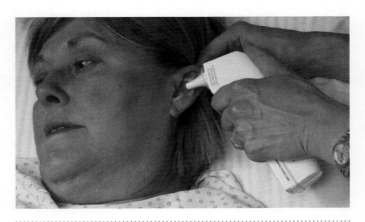

❸ Position adult patient so ear canal is easily seen and pull pinna back and up.

SKILL 1.9 Temperature: Newborn, Infant, Child, Adult, Obtaining *(continued)*

■ Center probe or enter at right side (follow manufacturer's guidelines) and gently advance into ear canal to make a firm seal, directing probe toward tympanic membrane. **Rationale:** *Pressure close to the tympanic membrane seals ear canal and allows for accurate reading.*

CAUTION!

Correct Technique for Taking a Tympanic Temperature

The ear tug (pulling the pinna upward and backward for an adult and down and backward for a child) is essential for an accurate reading. Eliminating this step will not allow the thermometer to be aimed directly at the tympanic membrane.

Do not use an ear thermometer in an infected or draining ear or if an adjacent lesion or incision exists.

■ Press and hold temperature switch until green light flashes and temperature reading displays (approximately 3 seconds). **Rationale:** *Method records core body temperature.*
■ Remove thermometer. Discard probe cover.
■ Return thermometer to home base or storage unit for recharge.
■ Keep lens clean using lint-free wipe or alcohol swab, then wipe dry. Do not use povidone-iodine (Betadine).
■ Perform hand hygiene.
■ May be used for patients over 3 months of age.

INFRARED SCANNER THERMOMETER

■ Check orders for scanner device (may be used with children to check temperature without waking) ❹.
■ Press power button to turn device on. Check to see thermometer is in person mode (see symbol in window).
■ Press and hold scan button; "00" will be displayed.
■ Aim infrared lens at patient's forehead, holding thermometer 5–7.6 cm (2–3 in.) away.
■ Release scan button and note reading that is displayed.
■ Clean device with antiseptic wipe.

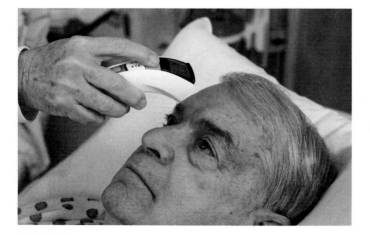

❹ Follow manufacturer's directions for scanner device.

EVIDENCE-BASED PRACTICE

Noncontact Infrared Thermometers (NCITs)

Problem

Emerging infectious diseases continue to present worldwide challenges to contain outbreaks and prevent the transmission of disease from infected travelers going from country to country. Health officials use current evidence and technology to implement improved methods to do this and protect people around the world. One device that has gained much attention and popularity is the noncontact infrared thermometer. This thermometer offers a noncontact method of accurate, low-cost, easily implemented screening for large numbers of people who are entering and leaving countries. Public health officials and airport authorities are now using them as part of port-of-entry screening. Screening can occur before travelers leave countries with active disease outbreaks or before they are allowed to enter other countries at the port of entry.

Some Asian airports used thermometers as part of their screening of passengers for symptoms of severe acute respiratory syndrome, or SARS, in 2003. In 2009, airports were checking temperatures of individuals flying for early symptoms of H1N1 flu. Ebola outbreaks in Africa in 2014 also prompted airports to check for elevated temperatures for those traveling out of outbreak areas in Africa to other countries.

Evidence

The FDA does not directly test products, but they do analyze evidence from clinical testing. The testing is done by company manufacturers in laboratories using animals and humans. The FDA determined that the noncontact infrared thermometer is as safe and effective as other thermometer products used for oral, axillary, tympanic, and forehead measurements currently on the market. The European Union also approved with CE-Marking that the product complies with European safety standards. While it is not a sole primary screening or diagnostic tool, it has much value in the initial screening of an elevated body temperature indicative of a fever condition. These devices are cleared by the FDA and CE-Marking for adjunctive use in measuring temperature in addition to other clinical diagnostic data.

The risk of cross-infection is low because the noncontact thermometers do not touch any body surfaces. The thermometer works by measuring the infrared energy coming off the body. Best temperature readings result when forehead skin is dry and non-hairy in a draft-free, constant temperature environment. Some of these electronic thermometers are calibrated to convert the temperature taken from the forehead into an oral equivalent.

Implications

Initial screening using noncontact thermometers for early detection of a fever condition, a symptom of individuals who might be sick, can help identify individuals with early stage infectious disease that need to be separated from general populations to avoid disease transmission to uninfected people. The Centers for Disease Control and Prevention (CDC) guidance for public screening of fever includes the need for medical follow-up for an individual having a body temperature elevation higher than 38°C F (100.4°), and who may have been exposed to an outbreak disease, such as Ebola. Additional screening may include general observations, health questionnaires, interviews, and serial temperature readings.

Health organizations, such as the World Health Organization, encourage countries to use the technology of noncontact temperature measurement electronic devices for screening of some travelers

(continued on next page)

SKILL 1.9 Temperature: Newborn, Infant, Child, Adult, Obtaining (continued)

to prevent infectious disease transmission. Detecting earliest symptoms, such as an elevated body temperature, before individuals even realize they are sick and following up with additional clinical diagnostic procedures can help prevent international spreading of infectious diseases. Some larger airports in the United States are now using non-contact thermometers for public screening.

Source: Data from Centers for Disease Control (CDC). (2014). *Non-Contact Temperature Measurement Devices: Considerations for Use in Port of Entry Screening Activities.* Retrieved from http://wwwnc.cdc.gov/travel/files/ebola-non-contact-temperature-measurement-guidance.pdf?action=NotFound&controller=Utility NPR, Shots Health News from NPR. (2014).

HEAT-SENSITIVE WEARABLE THERMOMETER

■ Check orders for continuous-reading thermometer and identify the patient with two forms of identification.
■ Dry forehead or axilla area, if necessary.
■ Place strip on forehead or deep in patient's axilla—may stay in place for 2 days ❺ ❻.
■ Read correct temperature by checking color changes or dots that turn from green to black.
■ Record temperature on appropriate form or record.

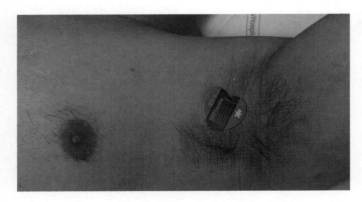

❺ Place a continuous-reading wearable thermometer deep in the patient's axilla.

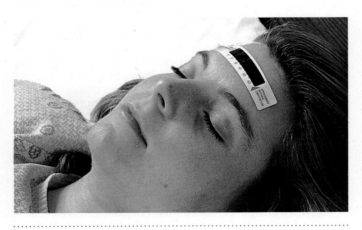

❻ Liquid crystal thermometer is placed against lower forehead for 15 seconds. The temperature is read by noting color changes on the device.

Documentation for Temperature

■ Site designated: "O" (oral), "R" or Ⓡ (rectal), "A" (axillary), "T" (tympanic), or "S" (scanner) ❼
■ Temperature recorded on temp sheet and graph
■ Nursing interventions used for alterations in temperature
■ Condition of skin related to alterations from normothermia (e.g., diaphoresis)
■ Signs and symptoms associated with alterations in temperature (e.g., shivering, dehydration)

CAUTION! Be sure to record the temperature from an electronic thermometer before replacing the probe into the charging unit. With many models, replacing the probe erases the temperature from the display.

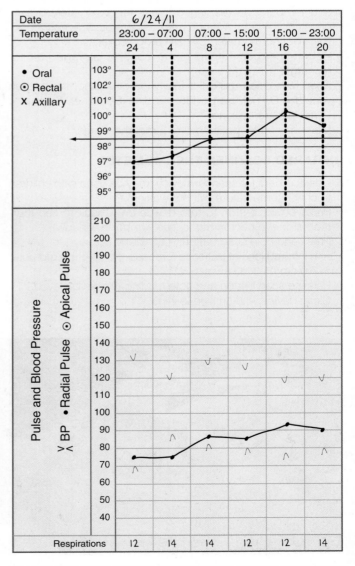

❼ Vital signs graphic record.

SKILL 1.9 Temperature: Newborn, Infant, Child, Adult, Obtaining (*continued*)

7. Wash the thermometer if necessary and return it to the storage or recharging location.
8. When the procedure is complete, perform hand hygiene. Leave patient safe and comfortable.
9. Complete documentation using forms, checklists, or electronic dropdown lists supplemented by nurse's notes or additional comments as appropriate.

SAMPLE DOCUMENTATION

[date] 0800 Temperature 37.5°C (99.2°F) (O) tolerated without concern. *C. Putney*

Patient Teaching

- Teach the patient accurate use and reading of the type of thermometer to be used. Examine the thermometer used by the patient in the home for safety and proper functioning. Facilitate the replacement of mercury thermometers with nonmercury ones.
- Observe the patient/caregiver taking and reading a temperature. Reinforce the importance of reporting the site and type of thermometer used and the value of using the same thermometer consistently.
- Discuss means of keeping the thermometer clean, such as warm water and soap, and avoiding cross-contamination.
- Instruct the patient or family member to notify the healthcare provider if the temperature is higher than a specified level, for example, 38.5°C (101.3°F).
- Check that the patient knows how to record the temperature. Provide a recording chart/table if indicated.
- Discuss environmental control modifications that should be taken during illness or extreme climate conditions (e.g., heating, air conditioning, appropriate clothing, and bedding).
- Pacifier thermometers for children under 2 years old have instructions that must be followed carefully because many require adding about 0.25°C (0.5°F) in order to estimate rectal temperature.

Lifestyle Considerations

NEWBORNS AND INFANTS

- The body temperature of newborns is extremely labile (changeable), and newborns must be kept warm and dry to prevent hypothermia.
- Using the axillary site, you need to hold the newborn's or infant's arm against the chest to keep the thermometer in place.

- The axillary route may not be as accurate as other routes for detecting fevers in children.
- The tympanic route is fast and convenient. Place the newborn or infant supine and stabilize the head. Pull the pinna straight back and slightly downward. Remember that the pinna is pulled upward for children over 3 years of age and adults but downward for children younger than 3. Direct the probe tip anteriorly and insert far enough to seal the canal. The tip will not touch the tympanic membrane.
- Avoid the tympanic route in a child with active ear infections or tympanic membrane drainage tubes.
- The tympanic membrane route may be more accurate in determining temperature in febrile newborns or infants.
- When using a temporal artery thermometer, touching only the forehead or behind the ear is needed.
- The rectal route is least desirable in newborns or infants.

CHILDREN

- Tympanic or temporal artery sites are preferred.
- For the tympanic route, have an adult hold the child in his or her lap with the child's head held gently against the adult for support. Pull the pinna straight back and upward for children over age 3.
- Avoid the tympanic route in a child with active ear infections or tympanic membrane drainage tubes.
- The oral route may be used for children over age 3, but nonbreakable, electronic thermometers are recommended.
- For a rectal temperature, place the child prone across your lap or in a side-lying position with the knees flexed. Insert the thermometer 2.5 cm (1 in.) into the rectum.

OLDER ADULTS

- Temperatures tend to be lower than those of middle-aged adults.
- Temperatures are strongly influenced by both environmental and internal temperature changes. Their thermoregulation control processes are not as efficient as when they were younger, and they are at higher risk for both hypothermia and hyperthermia.
- Significant buildup of ear cerumen can develop and interfere with tympanic thermometer readings.
- Older adults are more likely to have hemorrhoids. Inspect the anus before taking a rectal temperature.
- Temperatures may not be a valid indication of the seriousness of the pathology of a disease. Older adults may have pneumonia or a urinary tract infection and have only a slight temperature elevation. Other symptoms, such as confusion and restlessness, may be displayed and need follow-up to determine if there is an underlying process.

» Physical Assessment

Expected Outcomes

1. Assessment data include nursing history and behavioral and physical data.
2. Physical assessment data are collected through inspection, palpation, percussion, and auscultation.
3. A *head-to-toe physical assessment* is done when assessing all body systems to identify and prioritize patient needs (see framework for this type of assessment in Box 1–1 given earlier in the chapter's introduction).

4. A *focused physical assessment* is done detailing data of a specific system or area of the body relative to the patient's current concern to evaluate effectiveness of nursing interventions.
5. Normal and abnormal assessment data are documented.
6. Assessment data documentation is available to other disciplines taking care of the patient.
7. Lifespan considerations are made for the newborn, infant, child, and older adult.

SKILL 1.10 Abdomen: Assessing

This skill is performed using inspection, auscultation, percussion, and palpation to evaluate the functions of ingestion, digestion, and elimination. Preexisting concerns can be exacerbated or new conditions develop when illness occurs in other body systems.

Delegation or Assignment

Assessment of the abdomen is not delegated or assigned to the UAP. However, signs and symptoms of problems may be observed during usual care and may be recorded by individuals other than the nurse. Abnormal findings must be validated and interpreted by the nurse.

Equipment

- Examining light
- Tape measure (metal or nonstretchable cloth)
- Water-soluble skin-marking pencil
- Stethoscope
- Extra pillows to position patient

Preparation

- Gather needed equipment and supplies.
- Peristaltic waves may be more visible in children than in adults.
- Children may not be able to pinpoint areas of tenderness; by observing facial expressions the examiner can determine areas of maximum tenderness.
- If the child is ticklish, guarding, or fearful, use a task that requires concentration (such as squeezing the hands together) to distract the child, or have the child place his or her hands on yours as you palpate the abdomen, "helping" you to do the exam.
- The pain threshold in older adults is often higher than that of younger adults; major abdominal problems such as appendicitis or other acute emergencies may therefore go undetected.

- Gastrointestinal pain in adults needs to be differentiated from cardiac pain. Factors aggravating gastrointestinal pain are usually related to either ingestion or lack of food intake; gastrointestinal pain is usually relieved by antacids, food, or assuming an upright position.
- When assessing for constipation, the nurse must consider the adult patient's diet, activity, medications, and characteristics and ease of passage of feces, as well as the frequency of bowel movements.

Procedure

1. Prior to performing the procedure, introduce self and verify the patient's identity using two identifiers. Explain to the patient what you are going to do, why it is necessary, and how the patient can participate. Discuss how the results will be used in planning further care or treatments.
2. Perform hand hygiene and observe other appropriate infection control procedures.
3. Provide for patient privacy.
4. Inquire if the patient has any history of the following: incidence of abdominal pain; its location, onset, sequence, and chronology; its quality (description); its frequency; associated symptoms (e.g., nausea, vomiting, diarrhea); bowel habits; incidence of constipation or diarrhea (have patient describe what patient means by these terms); change in appetite, food intolerances, and foods ingested in past 24 hours; specific signs and symptoms (e.g., heartburn, flatulence and/or belching, difficulty swallowing, hematemesis [vomiting blood], blood or mucus in stools, and aggravating and alleviating factors); previous problems and treatment (e.g., stomach ulcer, gallbladder surgery, history of jaundice).
5. Assist the patient to a supine position, with the arms placed comfortably at the sides. Place small pillows beneath the knees and the head to reduce tension in the abdominal muscles. Expose the patient's abdomen only from the chest to the pubic area to avoid chilling and shivering, which can tense the abdominal muscles.

ASSESSMENT	NORMAL FINDINGS	DEVIATIONS FROM NORMAL
Inspection of the Abdomen		
6. Inspect the abdomen for skin integrity (refer to the discussion of skin assessment in Chapter 18, Tissue Integrity).	Unblemished skin Uniform color Silver-white striae (stretch marks) or surgical scars	Presence of rash or other lesions Tense, glistening skin (may indicate ascites, edema) Purple striae (associated with Cushing disease or rapid weight gain and loss)

SKILL 1.10 Abdomen: Assessing *(continued)*

ASSESSMENT	NORMAL FINDINGS	DEVIATIONS FROM NORMAL
7. Inspect the abdomen for contour and symmetry: ▪ Observe the abdominal contour (profile line from the rib margin to the pubic bone) while standing at the patient's side when the patient is supine. ▪ Ask the patient to take a deep breath and to hold it. **Rationale:** *This makes an enlarged liver or spleen more obvious.* ▪ Assess the symmetry of contour while standing at the foot of the bed. ▪ If distention is present, measure the abdominal girth by placing a tape around the abdomen at the level of the umbilicus ❶. If girth will be measured repeatedly, use an indelible skin marker to outline the upper and lower margins of the tape placement for consistency of future measurements.	Flat, rounded (convex), or scaphoid (concave) No evidence of enlargement of liver or spleen Symmetric contour	Distended Evidence of enlargement of liver or spleen Asymmetric contour (e.g., localized protrusions around umbilicus, inguinal ligaments, or scars from possible hernia or tumor) 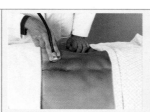 *Source:* Rick Brady/Pearson Education, Inc. ❶ Measuring abdominal girth.
8. Observe abdominal movements associated with respiration, peristalsis, or aortic pulsations.	Symmetric movements caused by respiration Visible peristalsis in very lean people Aortic pulsations in thin people at the epigastric area	Limited movement due to pain or disease process Visible peristalsis in nonlean patients (possible bowel obstruction) Marked aortic pulsations
9. Observe the vascular pattern.	No visible vascular pattern	Visible venous pattern (dilated veins) that is associated with liver disease, ascites, and venacaval obstruction

Auscultation of the Abdomen

10. Auscultate the abdomen for bowel sounds, vascular sounds, and peritoneal friction rubs ❷. Warm the hands and the stethoscope diaphragm and bell. **Rationale:** *Cold hands and a cold stethoscope may cause the patient to contract the abdominal muscles, and these contractions may be heard during auscultation.*		*Source:* Richard Tauber/Pearson Education, Inc. ❷ Auscultating the abdomen for bowel sounds.

For Bowel Sounds

▪ Use the diaphragm. **Rationale:** *Intestinal sounds are relatively high pitched and best transmitted by the diaphragm. Light pressure with the stethoscope is adequate.* ▪ Ask when the patient last ate. **Rationale:** *Bowel sounds may increase shortly after or long after eating.* They are loudest when a meal is long overdue. Four to 7 hours after a meal, bowel sounds may be heard continuously over the ileocecal valve area while the digestive contents from the small intestine empty through the valve into the large intestine. ▪ Place diaphragm of the stethoscope in each of the four quadrants of the abdomen over the auscultatory sites shown in ❸. ▪ Listen for active bowel sounds—irregular gurgling noises occurring about every 5–20 sec. The duration of a single sound may range from less than a second to more than several seconds.	Audible bowel sounds	Hypoactive, i.e., extremely soft and infrequent (e.g., one per minute) Hypoactive sounds indicate decreased motility and are usually associated with manipulation of the bowel during surgery, inflammation, paralytic ileus, or late bowel obstruction. Hyperactive/increased, i.e., high-pitched, loud, rushing sounds that occur frequently in the intestines made by fluid and gas movement (e.g., every 3 seconds); also known as borborygmi Hyperactive sounds indicate increased intestinal motility and are usually associated with diarrhea, an early bowel obstruction, or the use of laxatives. True absence of sounds (none heard in 3–5 min) indicates a cessation of intestinal motility.

(continued on next page)

SKILL 1.10 Abdomen: Assessing (continued)

ASSESSMENT	NORMAL FINDINGS	DEVIATIONS FROM NORMAL
Source: Ollyy/Shutterstock ❸ Sites for auscultating the abdomen.		

For Vascular Sounds

■ Use the bell of the stethoscope over the aorta, renal arteries, iliac arteries, and femoral arteries. ■ Listen for bruits.	Absence of arterial bruits	Loud bruit over aortic area (possible aneurysm) Bruit over renal or iliac arteries

Peritoneal Friction Rubs

■ Peritoneal friction rubs are rough, grating sounds like two pieces of leather rubbing together. Friction rubs may be caused by inflammation, infection, or abnormal growths. ■ To auscultate the splenic site, place the stethoscope over the left lower rib cage in the anterior axillary line, and ask the patient to take a deep breath. A deep breath may accentuate the sound of a friction rub area. ■ To auscultate the liver site, place the stethoscope over the lower right rib cage.	Absence of friction rub	Friction rub

Percussion of the Abdomen

11. Percuss several areas in each of the four quadrants to determine the presence of tympany (gas in stomach and intestines) and dullness (decrease, absence, or flatness of sound over solid masses or fluid). Use a systematic pattern: Begin in the lower right quadrant, proceed to the upper right quadrant, then the upper left quadrant, and last the lower left quadrant ❹.	Tympany over the stomach and gas-filled bowels; dullness, especially over the liver and spleen, or a full bladder Source: Ollyy/Shutterstock ❹ Systematic percussion sites for all four abdominal quadrants.	Large dull areas (associated with presence of fluid or a tumor)

SKILL 1.10 Abdomen: Assessing (*continued*)

ASSESSMENT	NORMAL FINDINGS	DEVIATIONS FROM NORMAL
Palpation of the Abdomen		
12. Perform light palpation first to detect areas of tenderness and/or muscle guarding. Systematically explore all four quadrants. Ensure that the patient's position is appropriate for relaxation of the abdominal muscles, and warm the hands. **Rationale:** *Cold hands can elicit muscle tension and thus impede palpatory evaluation.*	No tenderness; relaxed abdomen with smooth, consistent tension	Tenderness and hypersensitivity Superficial masses Localized areas of increased tension
Light Palpation		
▪ Hold the palm of your hand slightly above the patient's abdomen, with your fingers parallel to the abdomen. ▪ Depress the abdominal wall lightly, about 1 cm or to the depth of the subcutaneous tissue, with the pads of your fingers ⑤. ▪ Move the finger pads in a slight circular motion. ▪ Note areas of tenderness or superficial pain, masses, and muscle guarding. To determine areas of tenderness, ask the patient to tell you about them and watch for changes in the patient's facial expressions. ▪ If the patient is excessively ticklish, begin by pressing your hand on top of the patient's hand while pressing lightly. Then slide your hand off the patient's and onto the abdomen to continue the examination.	No bulges felt No masses felt *Source:* Richard Tauber/Pearson Education, Inc. ⑤ Light palpation of the abdomen.	Rigid, tender muscles or pain may be due to presence of muscle spasm, inflammation, or infection (peritonitis). Pain or tenderness with quick release of pressure indicates rebound tenderness suggesting peritoneal inflammation. If hernia is suspected, have patient raise head and shoulders and observe for abdominal bulge.
Palpation of the Bladder		
13. Palpate the area above the pubic symphysis if the patient's history indicates possible urinary retention ⑥.	Not palpable	Distended and palpable as smooth, round, tense mass (indicates urinary retention)
14. When the procedure is complete, perform hand hygiene. Leave patient safe and comfortable. Complete documentation using forms, checklists, or electronic dropdown lists supplemented by nurse's notes or additional comments as appropriate.	*Source:* Richard Tauber/Pearson Education, Inc. ⑥ Palpating the bladder.	

SAMPLE DOCUMENTATION

[date] 0945 c/o "gassy" pain lower right quadrant; no bowel movement × 48 hr; ate 75% regular diet yesterday; abdomen flat; active bowel sounds all 4 quadrants; tympany above umbilicus, dull below; no masses felt on palpation; 30 mL Milk of Magnesia given po per order. *N. Schmidt*

(*continued on next page*)

SKILL 1.10 Abdomen: Assessing (*continued*)

Patient Teaching

Tips to Help Prevent Constipation

- Eat breakfast every morning.
- Assume a squatting position when sitting on the toilet by placing a stool under your feet, lean forward, and place elbows on thighs.
- Increase water intake if not contraindicated.
- Increase dietary fiber.
- Become more active physically.
- Avoid using stimulant laxatives.

Lifespan Considerations

NEWBORNS AND INFANTS

- Internal organs of newborns and infants are proportionally larger than those of older children and adults, so their abdomens are rounded and tend to protrude.
- Umbilical hernias may be present at birth.

CHILDREN

- Toddlers have a characteristic "pot belly" appearance, which can persist until age 3–4 years.
- Late preschool and school-age children are leaner than toddlers and have a flat abdomen.

OLDER ADULTS

- The rounded abdomens of some older adults may be due to an increase in adipose tissue and a decrease in muscle tone.
- The abdominal wall is slacker and thinner, making palpation easier and more accurate than in younger patients. Muscle wasting and loss of fibroconnective tissue occur.
- Stool passes through the intestines at a slower rate in older adults, and the perception of stimuli that produce the urge to defecate often diminishes.
- Fecal incontinence may occur in older adults who are confused or neurologically impaired.
- The incidence of colon cancer is higher among older adults than younger adults. Symptoms include a change in bowel function, rectal bleeding, and weight loss. Changes in bowel function, however, are associated with many factors, such as diet, exercise, and medications.
- Decreased absorption of oral medications often occurs with aging.
- In the liver, impaired metabolism of some drugs may occur with aging.

SKILL 1.11 Anus: Assessing

Nurses will usually only include this assessment in the initial complete examination when the patient has a medical or surgical problem of the perianal area or anus.

Delegation or Assignment

Assessment of the anus is not delegated or assigned to the UAP. However, the condition of the anal area may be observed during usual care and may be recorded by individuals other than the nurse. Abnormal findings must be validated and interpreted by the nurse.

Equipment

- Clean gloves

Preparation

- Lightly touching the anus of a newborn or infant should result in a brief anal contraction ("wink" reflex).
- Erythema and scratch marks around the anus may indicate a pinworm parasite. Children with this condition may be disturbed by itching during sleep.

Procedure

1. Prior to performing the procedure, introduce self and verify the patient's identity using two identifiers. Explain to the patient what you are going to do, why it is necessary, and how the patient can participate. Discuss how the results will be used in planning further care or treatments.
2. Perform hand hygiene, apply gloves, and observe other appropriate infection control procedures for all rectal examinations.
3. Provide for patient privacy. Drape the patient appropriately to prevent undue exposure of body parts.
4. Inquire if the patient has any history of the following: bright blood in stools, tarry black stools, diarrhea, constipation, abdominal pain, excessive gas, hemorrhoids, or rectal pain; family history of colorectal cancer; when last stool specimen for occult blood was performed and the results; and for males, if not obtained during the genitourinary examination, signs or symptoms of prostate enlargement (e.g., slow urinary stream, hesitancy, frequency, dribbling, and nocturia).
5. Position the patient in a left lateral or Sims position with the upper leg acutely flexed. A dorsal recumbent position with hips externally rotated and knees flexed may also be used. For males, a standing position while the patient bends over the examining table may also be used.

SKILL 1.11 Anus: Assessing (*continued*)

ASSESSMENT	NORMAL FINDINGS	DEVIATIONS FROM NORMAL
6. Inspect the anus and surrounding tissue for color, integrity, and skin lesions. Then, ask the patient to bear down as though defecating. Bearing down creates slight pressure on the skin that may accentuate rectal fissures, rectal prolapse, polyps, or internal hemorrhoids. Describe the location of all abnormal findings in terms of a clock, with the 12 o'clock position toward the pubic symphysis.	Intact perianal skin; usually slightly more pigmented than the skin of the buttocks Anal skin is normally more pigmented, coarser, and moister than perianal skin and is usually hairless.	Presence of fissures (cracks), ulcers, excoriations, inflammations, abscesses, protruding hemorrhoids (dilated veins seen as reddened protrusions of the skin), lumps or tumors, fistula openings, or rectal prolapse (varying degrees of protrusion of the rectal mucous membrane through the anus)
7. Remove and discard gloves. Perform hand hygiene. Leave the patient safe and comfortable.		
8. Complete documentation using forms, checklists, or electronic dropdown lists supplemented by nurse's notes or additional comments as appropriate.		

SAMPLE DOCUMENTATION

[date] 1430 Intact perianal skin; no external hemorrhoids noted; able to bear down without discomfort; no bleeding or stool noted. *T. Rales*

Lifespan Considerations
OLDER ADULTS

- Chronic constipation and straining at stool may cause an increase in the frequency of hemorrhoids and rectal prolapse.

SKILL 1.12 Breasts and Axillae: Assessing

Nurses will usually only include this assessment in the initial complete examination when the patient has a medical or surgical problem of the breasts or axillae.

Delegation or Assignment

Assessment of the breasts and axillae is not delegated or assigned to the UAP. However, individuals other than the nurse may record aspects observed during usual care. Abnormal findings must be validated and interpreted by the nurse.

Equipment

- Centimeter ruler

Preparation

- Newborns, both boys and girls, up to 2 weeks of age may have breast enlargement and white discharge from the nipples ("witch's milk").
- Boys may develop breast buds and have slight enlargement of the areola in early adolescence. Further enlargement of breast tissue (gynecomastia) can occur. This growth is transient, usually lasting about 2 years, resolving completely by late puberty.
- In older adults, the presence of breast lesions may be detected more readily because of the decrease in connective tissue.

Procedure

1. Prior to performing the procedure, introduce self and verify the patient's identity using two identifiers. Explain to the patient what you are going to do, why it is necessary, and how the patient can participate. Inquire whether the patient has ever had a clinical breast exam. Discuss how the results will be used in planning further care or treatments.
2. Perform hand hygiene and observe other appropriate infection control procedures.
3. Provide for patient privacy.
4. Inquire if the patient has any history of the following: breast masses and what was done about them; pain or tenderness in the breasts in relation to the woman's menstrual cycle; discharge from the nipple; medication history (some medications—e.g., oral contraceptives, steroids, digitalis, and diuretics—may cause nipple discharge; estrogen replacement therapy may be associated with the development of cysts or cancer); risk factors that may be associated with development of breast cancer (e.g., mother, sister, aunt with breast cancer; alcohol consumption, high-fat diet, obesity, use of oral contraceptives, menarche before age 12, menopause after age 55, age 30 or older at first pregnancy). Inquire if the patient performs breast self-examination, the technique used, and when performed in relation to the menstrual cycle.

(*continued on next page*)

SKILL 1.12 Breasts and Axillae: Assessing (continued)

ASSESSMENT	NORMAL FINDINGS	DEVIATIONS FROM NORMAL
5. Inspect the breasts for size, symmetry, and contour or shape while the patient is in a sitting position.	*Females:* rounded shape; slightly unequal in size; generally symmetric *Males:* breasts even with the chest wall; if obese, may be similar in shape to female breasts	Recent change in breast size; swellings; marked asymmetry
6. Inspect the skin of the breast for localized discolorations or hyperpigmentation, retraction or dimpling, localized hypervascular areas, swelling, or edema ①.	Skin uniform in color (same in appearance as skin of abdomen or back) Skin smooth and intact Diffuse symmetric horizontal or vertical vascular pattern in light-skinned people Striae (stretch marks); moles and nevi	Localized discolorations or hyperpigmentation Retraction or dimpling (result of scar tissue or an invasive tumor) Unilateral, localized hypervascular areas (associated with increased blood flow) Swelling or edema appearing as pig skin or orange peel due to exaggeration of the pores

Retraction

Lesion

① A lesion causing retraction of the skin.

7. Emphasize any retraction by having the patient: ▪ Raise the arms above the head. ▪ Push the hands together, with elbows flexed ②. ▪ Press the hands down on the hips ③.	Skin and tissue follow patient motion.	Retraction or dimpling, and skin or underlying tissue does not move freely

Source: Pat Watson/Pearson Education, Inc.

② Pushing the hands together to accentuate retraction of breast tissue.

Source: Southern Illinois University/Science Source

③ Pressing the hands down on the hips to accentuate retraction of the breast tissue.

8. Inspect the areola area for size, shape, symmetry, color, surface characteristics, and any masses or lesions.	Round or oval and bilaterally the same Color varies widely, from light pink to dark brown Irregular placement of sebaceous glands on the surface of the areola (Montgomery tubercles)	Any asymmetry, mass, or lesion

SKILL 1.12 Breasts and Axillae: Assessing (*continued*)

ASSESSMENT	NORMAL FINDINGS	DEVIATIONS FROM NORMAL
9. Inspect the nipples for size, shape, position, color, discharge, and lesions.	Round, everted, and equal in size; similar in color; soft and smooth; both nipples point in same direction (out in young women and men, downward in older women) No discharge, except from pregnant or breastfeeding females Inversion of one or both nipples that is present from puberty	Asymmetrical size and color Presence of discharge, crusts, or cracks Recent inversion of one or both nipples
10. Palpate the axillary, subclavicular, and supraclavicular lymph nodes ④ while the patient sits with the arms abducted and supported on the nurse's forearm. For palpation of clavicular lymph nodes, use the flat surfaces of all fingertips to palpate the four areas of the axilla: ▪ The edge of the greater pectoral muscle along the anterior axillary line ▪ The thoracic wall in the midaxillary area ▪ The upper part of the humerus ▪ The anterior edge of the latissimus dorsi muscle along the posterior axillary line.	No tenderness, masses, or nodules **A** **B** *Source:* **B,** Pat Watson/Pearson Education, Inc. ④ Location and palpation of the lymph nodes that drain the lateral breast: **A,** lymph nodes; **B,** palpating the axilla.	Tenderness, masses, or nodules

11. Palpate the breast for masses, tenderness, and any discharge from the nipples. Palpation of the breast is generally performed while the patient is supine. **Rationale:** *In the supine position, the breasts flatten evenly against the chest wall, facilitating palpation.* For patients who have a past history of breast masses, who are at high risk for breast cancer, or who have pendulous breasts, examination in both a supine and a sitting position is recommended.
 ▪ If the patient reports a breast lump, start with the "normal" breast to obtain baseline data that will serve as a comparison to the involved breast.
 ▪ To enhance flattening of the breast, instruct the patient to abduct the arm and place her hand behind her head. Then place a small pillow or rolled towel under the patient's shoulder.
 ▪ For palpation, use the palmar surface of the middle three fingertips (held together) and make a gentle rotary motion on the breast.
 ▪ Choose one of three patterns for palpation:
  a. Hands-of-the-clock or spokes-on-a-wheel ⑤
  b. Concentric circles ⑥
  c. Vertical strips pattern ⑦
 ▪ Start at one point for palpation, and move systematically to the end point to ensure that all breast surfaces are assessed.
 ▪ Pay particular attention to the upper, outer quadrant area and the tail of Spence.
	No tenderness, masses, nodules, or nipple discharge	Tenderness, masses, nodules, or nipple discharge
		If you detect a mass, record the following data:
		 ▪ *Location:* the exact location relative to the quadrants and axillary tail or a clock face, plus the distance from the nipple in centimeters
		 ▪ *Size:* the length, width, and thickness of the mass in centimeters. If you are able to determine the discrete edges, record this fact.
		 ▪ *Shape:* whether the mass is round, oval, lobulated, indistinct, or irregular
		 ▪ *Consistency:* whether the mass is hard or soft
		 ▪ *Mobility:* whether the mass is movable or fixed
		 ▪ *Skin over the lump:* whether it is reddened, dimpled, or retracted
		 ▪ *Nipple:* whether it is displaced or retracted
		 ▪ *Tenderness:* whether palpation is painful

(*continued on next page*)

SKILL 1.12 Breasts and Axillae: Assessing *(continued)*

ASSESSMENT	NORMAL FINDINGS	DEVIATIONS FROM NORMAL

⑤ Hands-of-the-clock or spokes-on-a-wheel pattern of breast palpation.

⑥ Concentric circles pattern of breast palpation.

⑦ Vertical strips pattern for breast palpations.

ASSESSMENT	NORMAL FINDINGS	DEVIATIONS FROM NORMAL
12. Palpate the areola and the nipples for masses. Compress each nipple to determine the presence of any discharge. If discharge is present, milk the breast along its radius to identify the discharge-producing lobe. Assess any discharge for amount, color, consistency, and odor. Note also any tenderness on palpation.	No tenderness, masses, nodules, or nipple discharge	Tenderness, masses, nodules, or nipple discharge
13. Teach the patient the technique of breast self-examination (BSE).		
14. When the procedure is complete, perform hand hygiene. Leave patient safe and comfortable. Complete documentation using forms, checklists, or electronic dropdown lists supplemented by nurse's notes or additional comments as appropriate.		

SAMPLE DOCUMENTATION

[date] 1500 Breast exam demonstrates equal size and shape; 2 cm smooth, slightly raised mole noted on left breast upper outer area; areola areas oval and same bilaterally, both nipples everted and equal in size, smooth and soft without discharge. No tenderness or masses noted in axillary lymph nodes or throughout breast tissue bilaterally. *H. Hayes*

Patient Teaching

Doing a Breast Self-Examination (BSE)

Instruct the patient to perform the following steps.

Inspection before a Mirror

Look for any change in size or shape; lumps or thickenings; any rashes or other skin irritations; dimpled or puckered skin; any discharge or change in the nipples (e.g., position or asymmetry). Inspect the breasts in all of the following positions:

- Stand and face the mirror with your arm relaxed at your sides or hands resting on the hips; then turn to the right and then the left for a side view (look for any flattening in the side view).

- Bend forward from the waist with arms raised over the head.
- Stand straight with the arms raised over the head and move the arms slowly up and down at the sides. (Look for free movement of the breasts over the chest wall.)
- Press your hands firmly together at chin level while the elbows are raised to shoulder level.

Palpation: Lying Position

- Place a pillow under your right shoulder and place your right hand behind your head. This position distributes breast tissue more evenly on the chest.

SKILL 1.12 Breasts and Axillae: Assessing (*continued*)

- Use the finger pads (tips) of the three middle fingers (held together) on your left hand to feel for lumps in the right breast.
- Press the breast tissue against the chest wall firmly enough to know how your breast feels. A ridge of firm tissue in the lower curve of each breast is normal.
- Use small circular motions along one arrow in your chosen pattern. Then move your fingers about 2 cm and feel along the next arrow. Repeat this action as many times as necessary until the entire breast is covered.
- Bring your arm down to your side and feel under your armpit, where breast tissue is also located.

- Repeat the exam on your left breast, using the finger pads of your right hand.

Palpation: Standing or Sitting

- Repeat the examination of both breasts while upright with one arm behind your head. This position makes it easier to check the area where a large percentage of breast cancers are found, the upper outer part of the breast and toward the armpit.
- Optional: Do the upright BSE in the shower. Soapy hands glide more easily over wet skin. Report any changes to your healthcare provider promptly.

Lifespan Considerations

NEWBORNS AND INFANTS

- Supernumerary ("extra") nipples infrequently are present along the mammary chain; these may be associated with renal anomalies.

CHILDREN

- Female breast development begins between 9 and 13 years of age and occurs in five stages (Tanner stages). One breast may develop more rapidly than the other, but at the end of development, they are more or less the same size.

  Stage 1: Prepubertal with no noticeable change

  Stage 2: Breast bud with elevation of nipple and enlargement of the areola

  Stage 3: Enlargement of the breast and areola with no separation of contour

  Stage 4: Projection of the areola and nipple

  Stage 5: Recession of the areola by about age 14 or 15, leaving only the nipple projecting.

- Boys may develop breast buds and have slight enlargement of the areola in early adolescence. Further enlargement of breast tissue (gynecomastia) can occur. This growth is transient, usually lasting about 2 years, resolving completely by late puberty.

PREGNANT FEMALES

- Breast, areola, and nipple size increase.
- The areolae and nipples darken; nipples may become more erect; areolae contain small, scattered, elevated Montgomery glands.
- Superficial veins become more prominent, and jagged linear stretch marks may develop.
- A thick yellow fluid (colostrum) may be expressed from the nipples after the first trimester.

OLDER ADULTS

- In the postmenopausal female, breasts change in shape and often appear pendulous or flaccid; they lack the firmness they had in younger years.
- General breast size remains the same. Although glandular tissue atrophies, the amount of fat in breasts (predominantly in the lower quadrants) increases in most women.

SKILL 1.13 Ears: Hearing Acuity, Assessing

Nursing assessment of the ears can be done with examination and hearing assessed by using gross hearing acuity tests, some of which require a tuning fork. Additional assessment, usually by an advanced practice nurse, can be done using an otoscope. Each state has specific laws mandating when children attending school should be screened for hearing acuity, and the hertz and decibel levels to be included.

Delegation or Assignment

Assessment of the ears and hearing is not delegated or assigned to the UAP. However, many aspects of ear function are observed during usual care and may be recorded by individuals other than the nurse. Abnormal findings must be validated and interpreted by the nurse.

Equipment

- Penlight
- Tuning fork
- Otoscope with several sizes of ear specula (option)

Preparation

- To assess gross hearing, ring a bell from behind the newborn or infant or have the parent call the child's name to check for a response. Newborns will quiet to the sound and may open their eyes wider. By 3–4 months of age, the child will turn head and eyes toward the sound.
- All newborns should have their hearing assessed using auditory brain response testing prior to discharge from the hospital.

(*continued on next page*)

SKILL 1.13 Ears: Hearing Acuity, Assessing (*continued*)

- If necessary, ask the adult present with a newborn, infant, or child to assist in holding the child still during the examination.
- With pure tone audiometry, if the young child does not seem to understand what to do once screening begins, remove the headphones and practice more. Have blocks ready and instruct the child to place a block in a basket when hearing the sound. Turn up the decibel level slightly and practice until the child understands. Then turn the decibel level back to the appropriate screening level.
- Sensorineural hearing loss occurs in older adults. Generalized hearing loss (presbycusis) occurs in all frequencies, although the first symptom is the loss of high-frequency sounds: the *f*, *s*, *sh*, and *ph* sounds. For such individuals, conversation can be distorted and result in what appears to be inappropriate or confused behavior.
- Ensure that the examination is conducted in a quiet place. In particular, older adults may have difficulty accurately reporting results of hearing tests if there is excessive outside noise.

Procedure

1. Prior to performing the procedure, introduce self and verify the patient's identity using two identifiers. Explain to the patient what you are going to do, why it is necessary, and how the patient can participate. Discuss how the results will be used in planning further care or treatments.
2. Perform hand hygiene and observe other appropriate infection control procedures.
3. Provide for patient privacy.
4. Inquire if the patient has any history of the following: family history of hearing problems or loss; presence of ear problems or pain; medication history, especially if there are complaints of ringing in ears (tinnitus); hearing difficulty (its onset, factors contributing to it, and how it interferes with activities of daily living); use of a corrective hearing device (when and from whom it was obtained).
5. Position the patient comfortably, seated if possible.

ASSESSMENT	NORMAL FINDINGS	DEVIATIONS FROM NORMAL
Auricles		
6. Inspect the auricles for color, symmetry of size, and position. To inspect position, note the level at which the superior aspect of the auricle attaches to the head in relation to the eye.	Color same as facial skin Symmetrical Auricle aligned with outer canthus of eye, about 10 degrees from vertical ❶	Bluish color of earlobes (e.g., cyanosis); pallor (e.g., frostbite); excessive redness (inflammation or fever) Asymmetry Low-set ears (associated with a congenital abnormality, such as Down syndrome)

Normal alignment

Low-set ears and deviation in alignment

❶ Alignment of ears.

7. Palpate the auricles for texture, elasticity, and areas of tenderness.
  ▪ Gently pull the auricle upward, downward, and backward.
  ▪ Fold the pinna forward (it should recoil).
  ▪ Push in on the tragus.
  ▪ Apply pressure to the mastoid process.
	Mobile, firm, and not tender; pinna recoils after it is folded.	Lesions (e.g., cysts); flaky, scaly skin (e.g., seborrhea); tenderness when moved or pressed (may indicate inflammation or infection of external ear)

Gross Hearing Acuity Tests		
8. Assess patient's response to normal voice tones. If patient has difficulty hearing the normal voice, proceed with the following tests.	Normal voice tones audible	Normal voice tones not audible (e.g., requests nurse to repeat words or statements, leans toward the speaker, turns the head, cups the ears, or speaks in loud tone of voice)

SKILL 1.13 Ears: Hearing Acuity, Assessing *(continued)*

ASSESSMENT	NORMAL FINDINGS	DEVIATIONS FROM NORMAL
9A. *Watch tick test.* Perform the watch tick test. The ticking of a watch has a higher pitch than the human voice. ▪ Have the patient occlude one ear. Out of the patient's sight, place a ticking watch 2.5–5 cm (1–2 in.) from the unoccluded ear. ▪ Ask what the patient can hear. ▪ Repeat with the other ear.	Able to hear ticking in both ears	Unable to hear ticking in one or both ears
9B. *Tuning fork tests.* Perform Weber's test to assess bone conduction by examining the lateralization (sideward transmission) of sounds. ▪ Hold the tuning fork at its base. Activate it by tapping the fork gently against the back of your hand near the knuckles or by stroking the fork between your thumb and index fingers. It should be made to ring softly. ▪ Place the base of the vibrating fork on top of the patient's head ❷ and ask where the patient hears the noise. ▪ For Rinne test, hold the handle of the activated tuning fork on the mastoid process of one ear ❸ until the patient states that the sound can no longer be heard. ▪ Immediately hold the still-vibrating fork prongs in front of the patient's ear canal. Push aside the patient's hair if necessary. Ask whether the patient now hears the sound. Sound conducted by air is heard more readily than sound conducted by bone. The tuning fork vibrations conducted by air are normally heard longer.	Sound is heard in both ears or is localized at the center of the head (Weber negative). Air-conducted (AC) hearing is greater than bone-conducted (BC) hearing, that is, AC > BC (positive Rinne). *Source:* Pat Watson/Pearson Education, Inc. ❷ Placing the base of the tuning fork on the patient's skull (Weber's test).	Sound is heard better in impaired ear, indicating a bone-conductive hearing loss; or sound is heard better in ear without a problem, indicating a sensorineural disturbance (Weber positive). Bone conduction time is equal to or longer than the air conduction time, that is, BC > AC or BC = AC (negative Rinne; indicates a conductive hearing loss). *A* *B* *Sources: A,* and *B,* Pat Watson/Pearson Education, Inc. ❸ Rinne test tuning fork placement: *A,* Base of the tuning fork on the mastoid process; *B,* tuning fork prongs placed in front of the patient's ear.
10. When the procedure is complete, perform hand hygiene. Leave patient safe and comfortable. Complete documentation using forms, checklists, or electronic dropdown lists supplemented by nurse's notes or additional comments as appropriate.		

EXAMINATION USING AN OTOSCOPE: POSITIONING A CHILD

▪ Exam is not usually done by a generalist nurse.

▪ If the parent is present, discuss the parent's role (e.g., holding the child or providing distraction or comfort during the procedure).

▪ Make sure the person positioning and holding the child (parent or other assistant) clearly understands what body parts must be held still and how to do this safely.

For Supine Position

1. Place the child in a supine position on a bed or stretcher. Have the parent, a nurse, or an assistant lean over the child to position and hold the child's arms and body. The assistant may also assist with stabilizing the child's head.

2. Hold the otoscope in the hand closest to the child's face. When the child is cooperative, rest the back of your hand against the child's head. **Rationale:** *This action provides*

(continued on next page)

SKILL 1.13 Ears: Hearing Acuity, Assessing *(continued)*

additional stabilization of the child's head to prevent pain and injury when the otoscope earpiece is inserted into the auditory canal.

3. Use your other hand to pull the pinna toward the back of the head and either up or down.

For Sitting Position

1. Have the child sit on the parent's or assistant's lap with his or her legs held firmly between the assistant's legs.

The child's arms can be wrapped around the parent's or assistant's waist.

2. Have the parent or assistant hold the child's head firmly against the chest with one arm while the other arm holds the arms and upper chest. **Rationale:** *This position provides comfort to the child while securing the head.*

External Ear Canal and Tympanic Membrane

ASSESSMENT	NORMAL FINDINGS	DEVIATIONS FROM NORMAL
1. Inspect the external ear canal for cerumen, skin lesions, pus, and blood.	Distal third contains hair follicles and glands. Dry cerumen, grayish-tan color; or sticky, wet cerumen in various shades of brown	Redness and discharge Scaling Excessive cerumen obstructing canal
2. Visualize the tympanic membrane using an otoscope. 　■ Attach a speculum to the otoscope. Use the largest diameter that will fit the ear canal without causing discomfort. **Rationale:** *This achieves maximum vision of the entire ear canal and tympanic membrane.* 　■ Tip the patient's head away from you, and straighten the ear canal. For an adult, straighten the ear canal by pulling the pinna up and back. **Rationale:** *Straightening the ear canal facilitates vision of the ear canal and the tympanic membrane.* 　■ Hold the otoscope either (a) right side up, with your fingers between the otoscope handle and the patient's head, or (b) upside down, with your fingers and the ulnar surface of your hand against the patient's head ④. **Rationale:** *These positions stabilize the head and protect the eardrum and canal from injury if a quick head movement occurs.* 　■ Gently insert the tip of the otoscope into the ear canal, avoiding pressure by the speculum against either side of the ear canal. **Rationale:** *The inner two thirds of the ear canal is bony; if the speculum is pressed against either side, the patient will experience discomfort.*	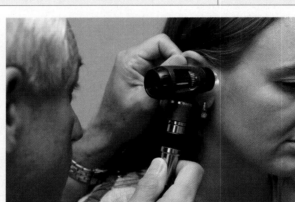 *Source:* Pat Watson/Pearson Education, Inc. ④ Inserting an otoscope.	
3. Inspect the tympanic membrane for color and gloss. Check for bulging of the tympanic membrane.	Pearly gray color, semitransparent ⑤ 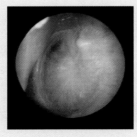 *Source:* CNRI/Science Source ⑤ Normal tympanic membrane.	Pink to red, some opacity Yellow-amber White Blue or deep red Dull surface Bulging of the tympanic membrane may indicate infection or fluid behind it.

SKILL 1.13 Ears: Hearing Acuity, Assessing *(continued)*

External Ear Canal and Tympanic Membrane

ASSESSMENT	NORMAL FINDINGS	DEVIATIONS FROM NORMAL
4. When the procedure is complete, perform hand hygiene. Leave patient safe and comfortable. Complete documentation using forms, checklists, or electronic dropdown lists supplemented by nurse's notes or additional comments as appropriate.		

HEARING ACUITY SCREENING: CHILD

Performance of a hearing acuity screening is important to ensure that the child is able to hear so that speech and language development can occur. Newborn and infant hearing screening is performed using evoked otoacoustic emission and auditory brainstem response. Several procedures may be used to screen hearing acuity in children. Various conditions during childhood, such as frequent ear infections, could result in a hearing loss.

Pure Tone Audiometry

The sounds of the audiometer are delivered at hertz (Hz) levels, or the frequency of sound in cycles per second. Lower numbers indicate lower sounds, such as speech tones. Higher numbers indicate higher sounds, such as those heard in music. The decibels (loudness of the sounds) can also be controlled by the audiometer.

Equipment

- Calibrated audiometer
- Scoring sheet
- Alcohol swabs

Preparation

- When screening a large group of children, such as in a school, the machine may be taken to the classroom for demonstration and practice.
- Check the transmission of sound to be sure both earphones work properly.
- Explain the procedure in terms the child can understand. Show the earphones. Turn the sound loud enough for the child to hear and practice raising a hand or putting a block in a basket in response to the sound, which will improve test accuracy.
- If a soundproof room is not available, the audiometer should be set up in a quiet environment. **Rationale:** *It is important to reduce exposure to other sources of sound that could interfere with the child's response to the audiometer's sounds.*
- Clean the earphones with alcohol swabs between children. **Rationale:** *This practice removes most microorganisms for infection control between children.*

Procedure

1. Position the child so that his or her back is toward the machine and faced away from the tester. **Rationale:** *This*

position ensures that the child cannot see the examiner press the lever to present the sound and cannot receive visual cues from the examiner's face when the sound is presented.

2. Place the headset on the child's head and adjust for a proper fit. Note the right and left indicators on the earphones.

3. Follow directions for using the audiometer. Deliver sounds and watch for the child to raise a hand or put a block in a basket when heard. The sound cue is given to the child using a random order when testing the ears. **Rationale:** *A random order ensures that the child cannot anticipate the sound and potentially cause an inaccurate interpretation of the screening test.*

4. Test each ear at the following pitches: 500, 1000, 2000, and 4000 Hz at increasing levels of loudness (decibels).

5. If the child does not pass the screening with both ears, retest the child in 2 weeks. If the child still does not pass, refer for further evaluation. **Rationale:** *The child with an upper respiratory infection may not hear well and needs time for the infection to improve.* Continued failure of the screening may indicate a hearing problem.

6. Document the results of the hearing test.

SAMPLE DOCUMENTATION

[date] 1345 Ear auricles symmetrical and aligned; moves firm, denies tenderness; acuity demonstrates response to questions with voice and whisper bilaterally; outer external ear canal clear of drainage and cerumen; tolerated without complaint. *B. Terry*

Lifespan Considerations
CHILDREN

- To inspect the external canal and tympanic membrane in children less than 3 years old, pull the pinna down and back. Insert the otoscopic speculum only 0.6–1.25 cm (¼–½ in.).
- Perform routine hearing checks and follow up on abnormal results. In addition to congenital or infection-related causes of hearing loss, noise-induced hearing loss is becoming more common in

(continued on next page)

SKILL 1.13 Ears: Hearing Acuity, Assessing (*continued*)

adolescents and young adults as a result of exposure to loud music and prolonged use of headsets at loud volumes. Teach that music loud enough to prevent hearing a normal conversation can damage hearing.

- With pure tone audiometry, if the young child does not seem to understand what to do once screening begins, remove the headphones and practice more. Have blocks ready and instruct the child to place a block in a basket when hearing the sound. Turn up the decibel level slightly and practice until the child understands. Then turn the decibel level back to the appropriate screening level.

OLDER ADULTS

- The skin of the ear may appear dry and be less resilient because of the loss of connective tissue.
- Increased coarse and wire-like hair growth occurs along the helix, antihelix, and tragus.
- The pinna increases in both width and length, and the earlobe elongates.
- Earwax is drier.
- The tympanic membrane is more translucent and less flexible. The intensity of the light reflex may diminish slightly.

SKILL 1.14 Eyes: Visual Acuity, Assessing

Vision acuity screening should begin at about 3 years of age, when the child can cooperate with the procedure. Several procedures may be used to screen visual acuity in children.

Most states have laws regulating the ages or grades at which children must have vision screening performed, and what passing standards are accepted.

Delegation or Assignment

Due to the substantial knowledge and skill required, assessment of the eyes and vision is not delegated or assigned to the UAP. However, many aspects of eye function are observed during usual care and may be recorded by individuals other than the nurse. Abnormal findings must be validated and interpreted by the nurse.

Equipment

- Millimeter ruler
- Penlight
- Snellen, E, or picture chart
- Opaque card

Preparation

- Lay out about 6 m (20 ft) for distance vision testing.
- Infants 4 weeks of age should gaze at and follow objects.

- Preschool children's acuity can be checked with picture cards or the E chart. Acuity should approach 20/20 by 6 years of age.
- Always perform the acuity test with glasses on if a child has a prescription to wear lenses.
- In the older adult, visual acuity decreases as the lens of the eye ages and becomes more opaque and loses elasticity.

Procedure

1. Prior to performing the procedure, introduce self and verify the patient's identity using two identifiers. Explain to the patient what you are going to do, why it is necessary, and how the patient can participate. Discuss how the results will be used in planning further care or treatments.
2. Perform hand hygiene and observe other appropriate infection control procedures.
3. Provide for patient privacy.
4. Inquire if the patient has any history of the following: family history of diabetes, hypertension, blood dyscrasia, or eye disease, injury, or surgery; patient's last visit to an ophthalmologist; current use of eye medications; use of contact lenses or eyeglasses; hygienic practices for corrective lenses; current symptoms of eye problems (e.g., changes in visual acuity, blurring of vision, tearing, spots, photophobia, itching, or pain).

ASSESSMENT	NORMAL FINDINGS	DEVIATIONS FROM NORMAL
External Eye Structures		
5. Inspect the eyebrows for hair distribution, alignment, skin quality, and movement (ask patient to raise and lower the eyebrows).	Hair evenly distributed; skin intact Eyebrows symmetrically aligned; equal movement	Loss of hair; scaling and flakiness of skin Unequal alignment and movement of eyebrows
6. Inspect the eyelashes for evenness of distribution and direction of curl.	Equally distributed; curled slightly outward	Turned inward

SKILL 1.14 Eyes: Visual Acuity, Assessing (*continued*)

ASSESSMENT	NORMAL FINDINGS	DEVIATIONS FROM NORMAL
7. Inspect the eyelids for surface characteristics (e.g., skin quality and texture), position in relation to the cornea, ability to blink, and frequency of blinking. Inspect the lower eyelids while the patient's eyes are closed.	Skin intact; no discharge; no discoloration Lids close symmetrically Approximately 15–20 involuntary blinks per minute; bilateral blinking When lids open, no visible sclera above corneas, and upper and lower borders of cornea are slightly covered.	Redness, swelling, flaking, crusting, plaques, discharge, nodules, lesions Lids close asymmetrically, incompletely, or painfully Rapid, monocular, absent, or infrequent blinking Ptosis, ectropion, or entropion; rim of sclera visible between lid and iris
8. Inspect the bulbar conjunctiva (lying over the sclera) for color, texture, and the presence of lesions.	Transparent; capillaries sometimes evident; sclera appears white (darker or yellowish and with small brown macules in dark-skinned patients)	Jaundiced sclera (e.g., in liver disease); excessively pale sclera (e.g., in anemia); reddened sclera (e.g., marijuana use, rheumatoid disease); lesions or nodules (may indicate damage by mechanical, chemical, allergenic, or bacterial agents)
9. Inspect the cornea for clarity and texture. Ask the patient to look straight ahead. Hold a penlight at an oblique angle to the eye, and move the light slowly across the corneal surface.	Transparent, shiny, and smooth; details of the iris are visible. In older people, a thin, grayish white ring around the margin, called arcus senilis, may be evident.	Opaque; surface not smooth (may be the result of trauma or abrasion) Arcus senilis in patients under age 40
10. Inspect the pupils for color, shape, and symmetry of size. Pupil charts are available in some agencies. See ① for variations in pupil diameters. · • • ● ● ● ⬤ ⬤ ⬤ ⬤ 1 2 3 4 5 6 7 8 9 10 ① Variations in pupil diameters in millimeters.	Black in color; equal in size; normally 3–7 mm in diameter; round, smooth border, iris flat and round	Cloudiness, mydriasis, miosis, anisocoria; bulging of iris toward cornea; pupils less than 3 or greater than 7 mm in normal light conditions; unequal pupil size
11. Assess each pupil's direct and consensual reaction to light to determine the function of the third (oculomotor) cranial nerve. ■ Partially darken the room. ■ Ask the patient to look straight ahead. ■ Using a penlight and approaching from the side, shine a light on the pupil. ■ Observe the response of the illuminated pupil. It should constrict (direct response). ■ Shine the light on the pupil again, and observe the response of the other pupil. It should also constrict (consensual response).	Illuminated pupil constricts (direct response) Nonilluminated pupil constricts (consensual response)	Neither pupil constricts Unequal responses Absent responses
12. Assess each pupil's reaction to accommodation. ■ Hold an object (a penlight or pencil) about 10 cm (4 in.) from the bridge of the patient's nose. ■ Ask the patient to look first at the top of the object and then at a distant object (e.g., the far wall) behind the penlight. Alternate the gaze from the near to the far object. ■ Observe the pupil response. The pupils should constrict when looking at the near object and dilate when looking at the far object. ■ Next, move the penlight or pencil toward the patient's nose. The pupils should converge. To record normal assessment of the pupils, use the abbreviation **PERRLA** (pupils equally round and react to light and accommodation).	Pupils constrict when looking at near object; pupils dilate when looking at far object; pupils converge when near object is moved toward nose.	One or both pupils fail to constrict, dilate, or converge.

(*continued on next page*)

SKILL 1.14 Eyes: Visual Acuity, Assessing *(continued)*

ASSESSMENT	NORMAL FINDINGS	DEVIATIONS FROM NORMAL
Visual Fields		

13. Assess peripheral visual fields to determine function of the retina and neuronal visual pathways to the brain and second (optic) cranial nerve.
▪ Have the patient sit directly facing you at a distance of 60–90 cm (2–3 ft).
▪ Ask the patient to cover the right eye with a card and look directly at your nose.
▪ Cover or close your eye directly opposite the patient's covered eye (i.e., your left eye), and look directly at the patient's nose.
▪ Hold an object (e.g., a penlight or pencil) in your fingers, extend your arm, and move the object into the visual field from various points in the periphery. The object should be at an equal distance from the patient and yourself. Ask the patient to tell you when the moving object is first spotted.
  a. To test the temporal field of the left eye, extend and move your right arm in from the patient's right periphery.
  b. To test the upward field of the left eye, extend and move the right arm down from the upward periphery.
  c. To test the downward field of the left eye, extend and move the right arm up from the lower periphery.
  d. To test the nasal field of the left eye, extend and move your left arm in from the periphery ②.
▪ Repeat the above steps for the right eye, reversing the process.
	When looking straight ahead, patient can see objects in the periphery.
	Temporally, peripheral objects can be seen at right angles (90 degrees) to the central point of vision.
	The upward field of vision is normally 50 degrees because the orbital ridge is in the way.
	The downward field of vision is normally 70 degrees because the cheekbone is in the way.
	The nasal field of vision is normally 50 degrees away from the central point of vision because the nose is in the way.
	
	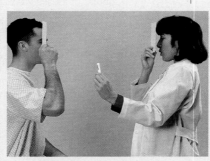
	Source: Richard Tauber/Pearson Education, Inc.
	
	② Assessing the patient's left peripheral vision field.
		Visual field smaller than normal (possible glaucoma); one half vision in one or both eyes (possible nerve damage)

Extraocular Muscle Tests		
14. Assess six ocular movements to determine eye alignment and coordination ③. These can be performed on patients over 6 months of age. ▪ Stand directly in front of the patient and hold the penlight at a comfortable distance, such as 30 cm (1 ft) in front of the patient's eyes. ▪ Ask the patient to hold the head in a fixed position facing you and to follow the movements of the penlight with the eyes only. ▪ Move the penlight in a slow, orderly manner through the six cardinal fields of gaze; that is, from the center of the eye along the lines of the arrows in and back to the center. ▪ Stop the movement of the penlight periodically so that nystagmus can be detected.	Both eyes coordinated, move in unison, with parallel alignment 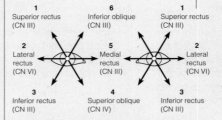 *Source:* (Right), Pat Watson/Pearson Education, Inc. ③ The six muscles that govern eye movement.	Eye movements not coordinated or parallel; one or both eyes fail to follow a penlight in specific directions (e.g., **strabismus** [cross-eye]). **Nystagmus** (rapid involuntary rhythmic eye movement) other than at end point may indicate neurological impairment.
15. Assess for location of light reflex by shining penlight on pupil in corneal surface (Hirschberg test).	Light falls symmetrically on both pupils (e.g., at "6 o'clock" on both pupils).	Light falls off center on one eye (indicates misalignment).
16. Have patient fixate on a near or far object. Cover one eye and observe for movement in the uncovered eye (cover test).	Uncovered eye does not move.	If misalignment is present, when dominant eye is covered, the uncovered eye will move to focus on object

SKILL 1.14 Eyes: Visual Acuity, Assessing (continued)

ASSESSMENT	NORMAL FINDINGS	DEVIATIONS FROM NORMAL
Visual Acuity		
17. Assess near vision by providing adequate lighting and asking the patient to read from a magazine or newspaper held at a distance of 36 cm (14 in.). If the patient normally wears corrective lenses, the glasses or lenses should be worn during the test.	Able to read newsprint	Difficulty reading newsprint unless due to aging process
18. Assess distance vision by asking the patient to wear corrective lenses, unless they are used for reading only, that is, for distances of only 30–36 cm (12–14 in.). ▪ Ask the patient to stand or sit about 6 m (20 ft) from a Snellen or character chart ❹, cover the eye not being tested, and identify the letters or characters on the chart. ▪ Take three readings: right eye, left eye, both eyes. ▪ Record the readings of each eye and both eyes (i.e., the smallest line from which the person is able to read one half or more of the letters). At the end of each line of the chart are standardized numbers (fractions). The top line is 20/200. The numerator (top number) is always 20, the distance the person stands from the chart. The denominator (bottom number) is the distance from which the normal eye can read the chart. Therefore, an individual who has 20/40 vision can see at 20 ft from the chart what a normal-sighted person can see at 40 ft from the chart. Visual acuity is recorded as "s̄–c" (without correction), or "c̄–c" (with correction). You can also indicate how many letters were misread in the line, for example, "visual acuity 20/40-2 c̄–c" indicates that two letters were misread in the 20/40 line by a patient wearing corrective lenses.	20/20 vision on Snellen-type chart *Source:* Richard Tauber/Pearson Education, Inc. ❹ Testing distance vision.	Denominator of 40 or more on Snellen-type chart with corrective lenses
19. If the patient is unable to see even the top line (20/200) of the Snellen-type chart, perform one or more of the following functional vision tests.	Able to read top line (20/200) of the Snellen-type chart	Functional vision only (e.g., light perception, hand movements, counting fingers at 30 cm [1 ft])
Light Perception		
20. Shine a penlight into the patient's eye from a lateral position, and then turn the light off. Ask the patient to tell you when the light is on or off.	Able to tell when the light is on or off	Difficulty in knowing when the light is on or off
Hand Movements		
21. Hold your hand 30 cm (1 ft) from the patient's face and move it slowly back and forth, stopping it periodically. Ask the patient to tell you when your hand stops moving.	Able to tell when the hand stops moving	Difficulty in knowing when the hand stops moving
Counting Fingers		
22. Hold up some of your fingers 30 cm (1 ft) from the patient's face, and ask the patient to count your fingers.	Able to count the number of fingers	Difficulty in counting the number of fingers
23. When the procedure is complete, perform hand hygiene. Leave patient safe and comfortable. Complete documentation using forms, checklists, or electronic dropdown lists supplemented by nurse's notes or additional comments as appropriate.		

(continued on next page)

SKILL 1.14 Eyes: Visual Acuity, Assessing (*continued*)

SNELLEN LETTER CHART

The Snellen letter (alphabet) chart is the most commonly used assessment tool for visual acuity. It consists of lines of letters in decreasing size ❺.

- As described, most charts are designed for reading from a distance of about 6 m (20 ft). When the child reads the line designated "20 ft" while standing 20 ft away, vision is 20/20. If, however, the child can only read the line labeled "40 ft" while standing 20 ft away, vision is 20/40.
- Charts are also available that can be used at a distance of about 3 m (10 ft). A child who stands 10 ft from this chart and reads the 10-ft line (10/10) has vision equivalent to that of 20/20 when using the 20-ft chart.

HOTV, SNELLEN E, OR PICTURE CHART

For toddlers and children who have not yet mastered the alphabet, the HOTV, Snellen E, or picture chart may be used, positioned either about 3 or 6 m (10 or 20 ft) away, matching the guidelines on the chart.

- The HOTV test uses a chart with the letters H, O, T, and V used in random order on lines in decreasing size. The child either names the letters or points to them on a card held close by. The procedure followed is the same as with the Snellen test, but because children can point to the letters on the chart in front of them, they do not need to know the alphabet. The HOTV test can also be used, after a practice session, with children who do not speak English.
- In the Snellen E chart, the capital letter E is shown facing in different directions. The child is asked to point in the direction of the "legs" of the E. Another option is to give the child a paper with an E on it and have the child turn it in the direction the E is pointing on the chart.
- The Lea Symbols are commonly identified simple pictures (e.g., heart, square, circle, house). The child is asked to identify the pictures or point to the picture on a card held close by.

Preparation

- The procedure is explained to the child and parent. With a young child, make a game of identifying the letter, direction of the E, or the picture. Practice with the child before starting, providing positive feedback for correct responses. **Rationale:** *This ensures that the child understands the directions for the test so as to improve the chances of an accurate screening test result.*
- Place the chart at the child's eye level and ensure that it is well lit.

Equipment

- Screening chart
- Card or other item to cover one eye
- Card with HOTV letters, E, or Lea Symbols

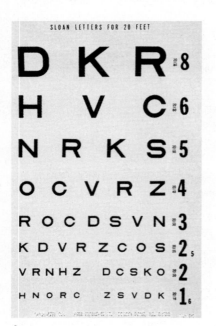

HOTV CHART FOR 10 FEET

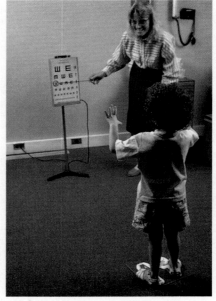

A   *B*   *C*

*Sources: **A,** and **B,** Courtesy of the National Society to Prevent Blindness.*

❺ Visual acuity charts. **A,** Snellen letter chart; **B,** HOTV chart; **C,** Snellen E chart. (A and B courtesy of the National Society to Prevent Blindness)

SKILL 1.14 Eyes: Visual Acuity, Assessing (*continued*)

Procedure

1. Place the heels of the child at the correct distance from the chart about 6 m (20 ft) or about 3 m (10 ft if using that chart).
2. Assess each eye separately and then both together. If the child wears glasses, check the vision both with and without glasses. If the child is wearing contacts, leave them in and note that the results were taken with contacts in place. **Rationale:** *It is important to detect significant differences in visual acuity of the eyes of children under 5 years of age.* When one eye has poorer vision than the other, the brain may decide to stop using the eye with poor vision, leading to further vision deterioration. Corrective lenses are required to enable the child to use both eyes and to preserve vision.
3. While one eye is being tested, use the child's hand, a patch, or a piece of cardboard to cover the other eye. Tell the child to keep the covered eye open during the testing. Use a different eye cover for each child to minimize the spread of infection among children.
4. Observe for squinting, moving the head forward (to be closer to the chart), excessive blinking, or tearing during the examination. **Rationale:** *These may be signs that the child has a vision problem.*
5. Document the last line the child can read correctly (i.e., the smallest line on which the child reads at least three of five symbols).
6. Emphasis should be directed to screening high-risk newborns, infants, and children with a family history of eye disorders such as cataracts and strabismus, eye surgery, and use of glasses during childhood. When necessary, screeners should readily refer such children to an ophthalmologist for a comprehensive eye evaluation.

Lifespan Considerations
NEWBORNS AND INFANTS

- Ability to focus with both eyes should be present by 6 months of age.
- Newborns and infants do not have tears until about 3 months of age.
- Visual acuity is about 20/300 at 4 months and progressively improves.

CHILDREN

- Epicanthal folds, common in many people of Asian heritage, may cover the medial canthus and cause eyes to appear misaligned. Epicanthal folds may also be seen in young children of any heritage before the bridge of the nose begins to elevate.
- Children should be tested for color vision deficit. Eight percent of males and 0.5% of women with Northern European ancestry have red-green color blindness (NEI, 2015). The Ishihara or Hardy-Rand-Rittler test can be used.

OLDER ADULTS

- The ability of the iris to accommodate to darkness and dim light diminishes.
- Peripheral vision diminishes.
- The adaptation to light (glare) and dark decreases.
- Accommodation to far objects often improves, but accommodation to near objects decreases.
- Color vision declines; older people are less able to perceive purple colors and to discriminate pastel colors.
- Many older adults wear corrective lenses; they are most likely to have hyperopia. Visual changes are due to loss of elasticity (presbyopia) and diminishing transparency of the lens.
- Pupil reaction to light and accommodation is normally symmetrically equal but may be less brisk.

SKILL 1.15 Genitals and Inguinal Area: Assessing

Nurses will usually only include this assessment in the initial complete examination when the patient has a medical or surgical problem of the genitals or inguinal area.

Delegation or Assignment

Due to the substantial knowledge and skill required, assessment of the genitals and inguinal area of the female or male is not delegated or assigned to the UAP. However, individuals other than the nurse may record any aspect of the genital system that is observed during usual care. Abnormal findings must be validated and interpreted by the nurse.

Equipment

- Clean gloves
- Drape
- Supplemental lighting, as needed

FEMALE

Preparation

- Newborns and infants can be held in a supine position on the parent's lap with the knees supported in a flexed position and separated. Assess the newborn or infant female's mons pubis and newborn or infant male and female inguinal area for swelling or tenderness that may indicate the presence of an inguinal hernia.
- Ensure that you have the parent or guardian's approval to perform the examination and then tell the child what you are going to do. Preschool children are taught not to allow others to touch their "private parts."
- In older women, ovulation and estrogen production cease so vaginal bleeding unrelated to estrogen therapy is abnormal.

(*continued on next page*)

SKILL 1.15 Genitals and Inguinal Area: Assessing (continued)

Procedure

1. Prior to performing the procedure, introduce self and verify the patient's identity using two identifiers. Explain to the patient what you are going to do, why it is necessary, and how she can participate. Discuss how the results will be used in planning further care or treatments.
2. Perform hand hygiene, apply gloves, and observe other appropriate infection control procedures.
3. Provide for patient privacy. Request the presence of another woman if desired, required by facility policy, or requested by the patient.

4. Inquire regarding the following: age of onset of menstruation, date of last menstrual period (LMP), regularity of cycle, duration, amount of daily flow, and whether menstruation is painful; incidence of pain during intercourse; vaginal discharge; number of pregnancies, number of live births, labor or delivery complications; urgency and frequency of urination at night; blood in urine, painful urination, incontinence; history of sexually transmitted infection, past and present.
5. Cover the pelvic area with a sheet or drape at all times when not actually being examined. Position the patient supine.

ASSESSMENT	NORMAL FINDINGS	DEVIATIONS FROM NORMAL
6. Inspect the distribution, amount, and characteristics of pubic hair.	There are wide variations: generally kinky in the menstruating adult, thinner and straighter after menopause. Distributed in the shape of an inverse triangle	Scant pubic hair (may indicate hormonal problem) Hair growth should not extend over the abdomen.
7. Inspect the skin of the pubic area for parasites, inflammation, swelling, and lesions. To assess pubic skin adequately, separate the labia majora and labia minora.	Pubic skin intact, no lesions Skin of vulva area slightly darker than the rest of the body Minimal odor Labia round, full, and relatively symmetric in adult females	Lice, lesions, scars, fissures, swelling, erythema, excoriations, varicosities, or leukoplakia Malodorous discharge; thin, friable labia; protruding uterus
8. Palpate the inguinal lymph nodes ❶. Use the pads of the fingers in a rotary motion, noting any enlargement or tenderness. ❶ Lymph nodes of the groin area.	No enlargement or tenderness	Enlargement and tenderness
9. Remove and discard gloves. Perform hand hygiene.		
10. When the procedure is complete, leave patient safe and comfortable. Complete documentation using forms, checklists, or electronic dropdown lists supplemented by nurse's notes or additional comments as appropriate.		

Superior or horizontal group

Inferior or vertical group

SKILL 1.15 Genitals and Inguinal Area: Assessing (continued)

Lifespan Considerations

NEWBORNS AND INFANTS

- In newborns, because of maternal estrogen, the labia and clitoris may be edematous and enlarged, and there may be a small amount of white or bloody vaginal discharge.

CHILDREN

- Girls should be assessed for Tanner staging of pubertal development. (**Table 1–7 》**).
- Girls should be referred to a healthcare provider for a Papanicolaou (Pap) test if sexually active, or by age 18 years.
- The clitoris is a common site for syphilitic chancres in younger females.

OLDER ADULTS

- Labia are atrophied and flatter in older females.
- The clitoris is a potential site for cancerous lesions in older females.
- The vulva atrophies as a result of a reduction in vascularity, elasticity, adipose tissue, and estrogen levels. Because the vulva is more fragile, it is more easily irritated.
- The vaginal environment becomes drier and more alkaline, resulting in an alteration of the type of flora present and a predisposition to vaginitis. Dyspareunia (difficult or painful intercourse) is also a common occurrence.
- The cervix and uterus decrease in size.
- The fallopian tubes and ovaries atrophy.
- Ovulation and estrogen production cease.

MALE

Preparation

- Assess newborn for placement of the urethral meatus.
- Assess newborn's or infant's inguinal area for swelling or tenderness that may indicate presence of an inguinal hernia.
- Ensure that you have the parent or guardian's approval to perform the examination and then tell the child what you are going to do. Preschool children are taught not to allow others to touch their "private parts."
- In young boys, the cremasteric reflex can cause the testes to ascend into the inguinal canal. If possible, have the boy sit cross-legged; this stretches the muscle and decreases the reflex.

Procedure

1. Prior to performing the procedure, introduce self and verify the patient's identity using two identifiers. Explain to the patient what you are going to do, why it is necessary, and how he can participate. Discuss how the results will be used in planning further care or treatments.

TABLE 1–7 Tanner's Five Stages of Pubic Hair Development in Females

Stage 1	Preadolescence. No pubic hair except for fine body hair.	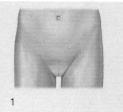 1
Stage 2	Usually occurs at ages 11 and 12. Sparse, long, slightly pigmented curly hair develops along the labia.	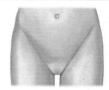 2
Stage 3	Usually occurs at ages 12 and 13. Hair becomes darker in color and curlier and develops over the pubic symphysis.	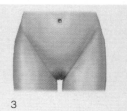 3
Stage 4	Usually occurs between ages 13 and 14. Hair assumes the texture and curl of the adult but is not as thick and does not appear on the thighs.	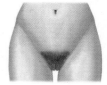 4
Stage 5	Sexual maturity. Hair assumes adult appearance and appears on the inner aspect of the upper thighs.	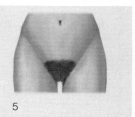 5

2. Perform hand hygiene, apply gloves, and observe other appropriate infection control procedures.
3. Provide for patient privacy. Request the presence of another person if desired, required by facility policy, or requested by the patient.
4. Inquire about the following: usual voiding patterns and changes, bladder control; history of urinary incontinence, frequency, urgency, abdominal pain; symptoms of sexually transmitted infection; swellings that could indicate presence of hernia; family history of nephritis, malignancy of the prostate, or malignancy of the kidney.
5. Cover the pelvic area with a sheet or drape at all times when not actually being examined.

(continued on next page)

SKILL 1.15 Genitals and Inguinal Area: Assessing (continued)

ASSESSMENT	NORMAL FINDINGS	DEVIATIONS FROM NORMAL
Pubic Hair		
6. Inspect the distribution, amount, and characteristics of pubic hair.	Triangular distribution, often spreading up the abdomen	Scant amount or absence of hair
Penis		
7. Inspect the penile shaft and glans penis for lesions, nodules, swellings, and inflammation.	Penile skin intact Appears slightly wrinkled and varies in color as widely as other body skin Foreskin easily retractable from the glans penis is not circumcised Small amount of thick white smegma between the glans and foreskin	Presence of lesions, nodules, swellings, or inflammation
8. Inspect the urethral meatus for swelling, inflammation, and discharge. ▪ Compress or ask the patient to compress the glans slightly to open the urethral meatus to inspect it for discharge.	Pink and slit-like appearance Positioned at the tip of the penis	Inflammation; discharge Variation in meatal locations (e.g., hypospadias, on the underside of the penile shaft, and epispadias, on the upper side of the penile shaft)
Scrotum		

9. Inspect the scrotum for appearance, general size, and symmetry.
  ▪ To facilitate inspection of the scrotum during a physical examination, ask the patient to hold the penis out of the way.
  ▪ Inspect all skin surfaces by spreading the rugated surface skin and lifting the scrotum as needed to observe posterior surfaces.
	Scrotal skin is darker in color than that of the rest of the body and is loose.
	Size varies with temperature changes (the dartos muscles contract when the area is cold and relax when the area is warm).
	Scrotum appears asymmetric (left testis is usually lower than right testis).
		Discolorations; any tightening of skin (may indicate edema or mass)
		Marked asymmetry in size

Inguinal Area		

10. Inspect both inguinal areas for bulges while the patient is standing, if possible.
  ▪ First, have the patient remain at rest.
  ▪ Next, have the patient hold his breath and strain or bear down as though having a bowel movement. Bearing down may make the hernia more visible.
	No swelling or bulges	Swelling or bulge (possible inguinal or femoral hernia)

11. Teach the patient the technique of testicular self-examination. (See Patient Teaching below.)		
12. Remove and discard gloves. Perform hand hygiene.		
13. Document findings in the patient record using forms or checklists supplemented by narrative notes when appropriate.		

SAMPLE DOCUMENTATION

[date] 1630 Circumcised with no inflammation or lesions noted on penis or drainage from meatus; scrotum is asymmetric with left testis slightly lower than right; no swelling noted at inguinal areas; no tenderness expressed; tolerated without complaint. P. Daniels

SKILL 1.15 Genitals and Inguinal Area: Assessing (continued)

Patient Teaching

Testicular Self-Exam

Instruct the patient to perform the following steps monthly.

- Inspection in front of a mirror. Look for any swelling on the skin of the scrotum.
- The best time to do the self-exam is after a shower or bath, when the scrotum is relaxed.
- Move the penis out of the way, and place your index and middle fingers of both hands under one testicle and both thumbs on top. Gently roll the testicle between the fingers feeling for any smooth rounded bumps, irregularities of the skin, and texture of the testicle.
- It is normal for one testicle to be slightly larger than the other or one testicle to hang slightly lower than the other. There is a soft tubelike structure called the epididymis normally found at the back of the testicle.
- You want to look and feel for any hard lumps, change in size, shape, or consistency of both testicles.
- If you notice any changes, irregularities, or hard lumps see a doctor right away. If you have any concerns, ask your doctor about them.

As you check your testicles more, you will learn what is normal for you and be able to tell when something changes.

Lifespan Considerations

NEWBORNS AND INFANTS

- Assess for placement of the urethral meatus.
- Assess the inguinal area for swelling or tenderness that may indicate presence of an inguinal hernia.

CHILDREN

- **Table 1–8 »** shows the five Tanner stages of development of pubic hair, penis, testes, and scrotum.

OLDER ADULTS

- The penis decreases in size with age; the size and firmness of the testes decrease.
- Testosterone is produced in smaller amounts.

TABLE 1–8 Tanner's Stages of Male Pubic Hair and External Genital Development

Stage	Pubic Hair	Penis	Testes/Scrotum
1	None, except for body hair like that on the abdomen	Size is relative to body size, as in childhood.	Size is relative to body size, as in childhood.
2	Scant, long, slightly pigmented at base of penis	Slight enlargement occurs	Becomes reddened in color and enlarged
3	Darker, begins to curl and becomes coarser; extends over pubic symphysis	Elongation occurs	Continuing enlargement
4	Continues to darken and thicken; extends on the sides, above and below	Increase in both breadth and length; glans develops	Continuing enlargement; color darkens
5	Adult distribution that extends to inner thighs, umbilicus, and anus	Adult appearance	Adult appearance

- More time and direct physical stimulation are required for an older man to achieve an erection, but he can maintain the erection for a longer period before ejaculation than he could at a younger age.
- Seminal fluid is reduced in amount and viscosity.
- Urinary frequency, nocturia, dribbling, and problems with beginning and ending the stream are usually the result of prostatic enlargement.

SKILL 1.16 Hair: Assessing

Delegation or Assignment

Assessment of the hair is not delegated or assigned to the UAP. However, many aspects are observed during usual care and may be recorded by individuals other than the nurse. Abnormal findings must be validated and interpreted by the nurse.

Equipment

- Clean gloves
- Pen light

Preparation

- Have patient remove any clips or hat.
- Remove or ask parent to remove any clasps or hat from newborn's or infant's head.
- Have extra lighting available as needed.

Procedure

1. Prior to performing the procedure, introduce self and verify the patient's identity using two identifiers. Explain to the

(continued on next page)

SKILL 1.16 Hair: Assessing (*continued*)

patient what you are going to do, why it is necessary, and how the patient can participate. Discuss how the results will be used in planning further care or treatments.

2. Perform hand hygiene, apply gloves, and observe other appropriate infection control procedures.

3. Provide for patient privacy.

4. Inquire if the patient has any history of the following: recent use of hair dyes, rinses, or curling or straightening preparations; chemotherapy; and the presence of acute or chronic conditions.

ASSESSMENT	NORMAL FINDINGS	DEVIATIONS FROM NORMAL
5. Inspect the evenness of growth over the scalp.	Evenly distributed hair	Patches of hair loss (i.e., alopecia)
6. Inspect hair thickness or thinness.	Thick hair	Very thin hair
7. Inspect hair texture and oiliness.	Silky, resilient hair	Brittle hair, excessively oily or dry hair
8. Note presence of infections or infestations by parting the hair in several areas, checking behind the ears and along the hairline at the neck.	No infection or infestation	Flaking, sores, lice, nits (louse eggs), and ringworm
9. Inspect amount of body hair.	Variable	Hirsutism (abnormal hairiness) Absent or sparse leg hair
10. Provide education regarding hygiene of the hair and scalp, appropriate combs and brushes, and safety in using electric hair-styling appliances such as hair dryers.		
11. Remove and discard gloves. Perform hand hygiene.		
12. Leave patient safe and comfortable. Complete documentation using forms, checklists, or electronic dropdown lists supplemented by nurse's notes or additional comments as appropriate.		

SAMPLE DOCUMENTATION

[date] 0730 Hair groomed; no scalp irritations noted; no tenderness expressed; tolerated without concern. *R. Finley*

Lifespan Considerations

NEWBORNS AND INFANTS

- Newborns and infants exhibit a wide variation of normal hair distribution that can range from very little or none to a great deal of body and scalp hair.

CHILDREN

- As puberty approaches, axillary and pubic hair will appear.

OLDER ADULTS

- Older adults may experience a loss of scalp, pubic, and axillary hair.
- Hairs of the eyebrows, ears, and nostrils become bristle-like and coarse.

SKILL 1.17 Heart and Central Vessels: Assessing

Delegation or Assignment

Assessment of the heart and central vessels is not delegated or assigned to the UAP. However, many aspects of cardiac function are observed during usual care and may be recorded by individuals other than the nurse. Abnormal findings must be validated and interpreted by the nurse.

Equipment

- Stethoscope
- Centimeter ruler

Preparation

- Murmurs may be heard in newborns as the structures of fetal circulation close, especially the ductus arteriosus.
- The PMI is higher and more medial in children under 8 years old.
- A S_4 heart sound is commonly heard in older adults, indicating a change in the left ventricle.

Procedure

1. Prior to performing the procedure, introduce self and verify the patient's identity using two identifiers. Explain to the

SKILL 1.17 Heart and Central Vessels: Assessing (*continued*)

patient what you are going to do, why it is necessary, and how the patient can participate. Discuss how the results will be used in planning further care or treatments.

2. Perform hand hygiene and observe other appropriate infection control procedures.

3. Provide for patient privacy.

4. Inquire if the patient has any history of the following: family history of incidence of heart disease, high cholesterol levels, high blood pressure, stroke, obesity, congenital heart disease, arterial disease, hypertension, and rheumatic fever and age at which event occurred; patient's past history of rheumatic fever, heart murmur, heart attack, varicosities, or heart failure; present symptoms indicative of heart disease (e.g., fatigue, dyspnea, orthopnea, edema, cough, chest pain, palpitations, syncope, hypertension, wheezing, hemoptysis); presence of diseases that affect heart (e.g., obesity, diabetes, lung disease, endocrine disorders); lifestyle habits that are risk factors for cardiac disease (e.g., smoking, alcohol intake, eating and exercise patterns, areas and degree of stress perceived).

ASSESSMENT	NORMAL FINDINGS	DEVIATIONS FROM NORMAL
5. Simultaneously inspect and palpate the precordium for the presence of abnormal pulsations, lifts, or heaves. Locate the valve areas of the heart: ▪ Locate the angle of Louis. It is felt as a prominence on the sternum. ▪ Move your fingertips down each side of the angle until you can feel the second intercostal spaces. The patient's right second intercostal space is the aortic area, and the left second intercostal space is the pulmonic area ❶. ▪ From the pulmonic area, move your fingertips down three left intercostal spaces along the side of the sternum. The left fifth intercostal space close to the sternum is the tricuspid or right ventricular area. ▪ From the tricuspid area, move your fingertips laterally 5–7.6 cm (2–3 in.) to the left midclavicular line (MCL) ❷. This is the apical or mitral area, or point of maximal impulse (PMI). If you have difficulty locating the PMI, have the patient roll onto the left side to move the apex closer to the chest wall. ▪ Inspect and palpate the aortic and pulmonic areas, observing them at an angle and to the side, to note the presence or absence of pulsations. ▪ Observing these areas at an angle increases the likelihood of seeing pulsations. ▪ Inspect and palpate the tricuspid area for pulsations and heaves or lifts. ▪ Inspect and palpate the apical area for pulsation, noting its specific location (it may be displaced laterally or lower) and diameter. If displaced laterally, record the distance between the apex and the MCL in centimeters. ▪ Inspect and palpate the epigastric area at the base of the sternum for abdominal aortic pulsations.	No pulsations No lift or heave Pulsations visible in 50% of adults and palpable in most PMI in fifth left intercostal space (LICS) at or medial to MCL Diameter of 0.8–1.3 cm (⅓ – ½ in.). No lift or heave Aortic pulsations	Pulsations Diffuse lift or heave, indicating enlarged or overactive right ventricle PMI displaced laterally or lower (indicates enlarged heart) Diameter over 1.3 cm (½ in.); indicates enlarged heart or aneurysm Diffuse lift or heave lateral to apex; indicates enlargement or overactivity of left ventricle Bounding abdominal pulsations (e.g., aortic aneurysm)

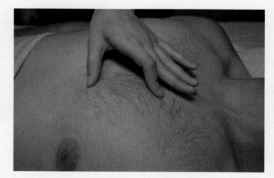

Source: Ronald May/Pearson Education, Inc.

❶ The second intercostal space.

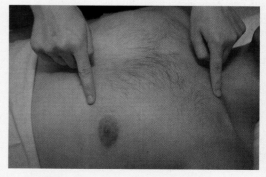

Source: Ronald May/Pearson Education, Inc.

❷ Midclavicular line, fifth intercostal space.

(*continued on next page*)

SKILL 1.17 Heart and Central Vessels: Assessing *(continued)*

ASSESSMENT	NORMAL FINDINGS	DEVIATIONS FROM NORMAL
6. Auscultate the heart in all four anatomical sites: aortic, pulmonic, tricuspid, and apical (mitral) ❸. Auscultation need not be limited to these areas; the nurse may need to move the stethoscope to find the most audible sounds for each patient. ■ Eliminate all sources of room noise. **Rationale:** *Heart sounds are of low intensity, and other noise hinders the nurse's ability to hear them.* ■ Keep the patient in a supine position with head elevated 30–45 degrees. ■ Use both the diaphragm and the bell to listen to all areas. ■ In every area of auscultation, distinguish both S_1 and S_2 sounds. ■ When auscultating, concentrate on one particular sound at a time in each area: the first heart sound, followed by systole, then the second heart sound, then diastole. Systole and diastole are normally silent intervals. ■ Later, reexamine the heart while the patient is in the upright sitting position. **Rationale:** *Certain sounds are more audible in certain positions.*	S_1: Usually heard at all sites Usually louder at apical area S_2: Usually heard at all sites; well heard at Erb's point (third intercostal space on left sternal border); S_2 usually louder at base of heart *Systole:* silent interval; slightly shorter duration than diastole at normal heart rate (60–90 beats/min) *Diastole:* silent interval; slightly longer duration than systole at normal heart rates S_3 in children and young adults S_4 in many older adults	Increased or decreased intensity Varying intensity with different beats Increased intensity at aortic area Increased intensity at pulmonic area Sharp-sounding ejection clicks S_3 in older adults S_4 may be a sign of hypertension.

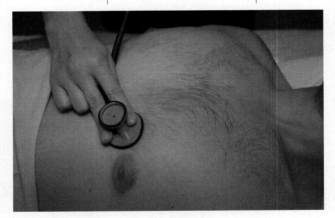

Source: Ronald May/Pearson Education, Inc.

❸ Apical pulse is best found in fifth intercostal space, left of sternum at midclavicular line or mitral area.

Carotid Arteries

7. Palpate the carotid artery, using extreme caution. ■ Palpate only one carotid artery at a time. **Rationale:** *This ensures adequate blood flow through the other artery to the brain.* ■ Avoid exerting too much pressure and massaging the area. **Rationale:** *Pressure can occlude the artery, and carotid sinus massage can precipitate bradycardia. The carotid sinus is a small dilation at the beginning of the internal carotid artery just above the bifurcation of the common carotid artery, in the upper third of the neck.* ■ Ask the patient to turn the head slightly toward the side being examined. This makes the carotid artery more accessible.	Symmetric pulse volumes Full pulsations, thrusting quality Quality remains same when patient breathes, turns head, and changes from sitting to supine position Elastic arterial wall	Asymmetric volumes (possible stenosis or thrombosis) Decreased pulsations (may indicate impaired left cardiac output) Increased pulsations Thickening, hard, rigid, beaded, inelastic walls (indicates arteriosclerosis)

SKILL 1.17 Heart and Central Vessels: Assessing (*continued*)

ASSESSMENT	NORMAL FINDINGS	DEVIATIONS FROM NORMAL
8. Auscultate the carotid artery. • Turn the patient's head slightly away from the side being examined. **Rationale:** *This facilitates the placement of the stethoscope.* • Auscultate the carotid artery on one side and then the other using the bell side of the stethoscope. • Listen for the presence of a bruit (an abnormal sound heard with a stethoscope indicating turbulent blood flow and carotid artery disease). If you hear a bruit, gently palpate the artery to determine the presence of a thrill (a vibration felt indicating turbulent blood flow and carotid artery disease).	No sound heard on auscultation	Presence of bruit in one or both arteries (suggests occlusive artery disease)

Jugular Veins

ASSESSMENT	NORMAL FINDINGS	DEVIATIONS FROM NORMAL
9. Inspect the jugular veins for distention while the patient is placed in a semi-Fowler's position (15–45 degree angle), with the head supported on a small pillow.	Veins not visible (indicating right side of heart is functioning normally)	Veins visibly distended (indicating advanced cardiopulmonary disease)
10. If jugular distention is present, assess the jugular venous pressure (JVP). • Locate the highest visible point of distention of the internal jugular vein. Although either the internal or the external jugular vein can be used, the internal jugular vein is more reliable. **Rationale:** *The external jugular vein is more easily affected by obstruction or kinking at the base of the neck.* • Measure the vertical height of this point in centimeters from the sternal angle, the point at which the clavicles meet ④. • Repeat the preceding steps on the other side.		Bilateral measurements above 3–4 cm (1¼–1½ in.) are considered elevated (may indicate right-sided heart failure). Unilateral distention (may be caused by local obstruction)

Level of the highest visible point of distention

The vertical distance between the sternal angle and the highest level of jugular distention

Level of the sternal angle (angle of Louis)

External jugular vein

Internal jugular vein

15° – 45°

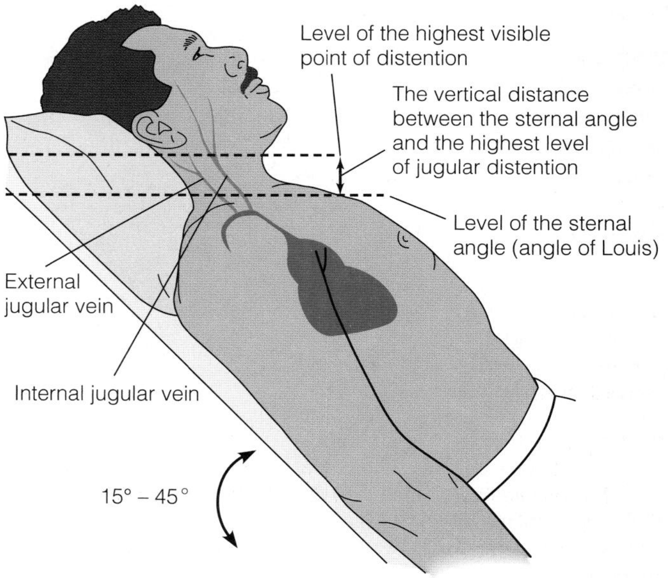

④ Assessing the highest point of distention of the jugular vein.

| 11. When the procedure is complete, perform hand hygiene. Leave patient safe and comfortable.
  Complete documentation using forms, checklists, or electronic dropdown lists supplemented by nurse's notes or additional comments as appropriate. | | |

(*continued on next page*)

SKILL 1.17 Heart and Central Vessels: Assessing (*continued*)

Lifespan Considerations

NEWBORNS AND INFANTS

- Physiological splitting of the second heart sound (S_2) may be heard when the newborn or infant takes a deep breath and the aortic valve closes a split second before the pulmonic valve. If splitting of S_2 is heard during normal respirations, it is abnormal and may indicate an atrial–septal defect, pulmonary stenosis, or another heart problem.

- Newborns or infants may normally have sinus arrhythmia that is related to respiration. The heart rate slows during expiration and increases when the child breathes in.

CHILDREN

- Heart sounds may be louder because of the thinner chest wall.
- A third heart sound (S_3), caused as the ventricles fill, is best heard at the apex and is present in about one third of all children.

OLDER ADULTS

- If no disease is present, heart size remains the same size throughout life.
- Cardiac output and strength of contraction decrease, thus lessening the older person's activity tolerance.
- The heart rate returns to its resting rate more slowly after exertion than it did when the individual was younger.
- Extra systoles commonly occur. Ten or more extra systoles per minute are considered abnormal.
- Sudden emotional and physical stress may result in cardiac arrhythmias and heart failure.

SKILL 1.18 Mouth and Oropharynx: Assessing

Delegation or Assignment

Assessment of the mouth and oropharynx is not delegated or assigned to the UAP. However, many aspects of mouth function are observed during usual care and may be recorded by individuals other than the nurse. Abnormal findings must be validated and interpreted by the nurse.

Equipment

- Clean gloves
- Tongue depressor
- 2 × 2 gauze pads
- Penlight

Preparation

- Newborns may have a pearly white nodule on their gums, which resolves without treatment.
- White spots on the child's teeth may indicate excessive fluoride ingestion.

- Tiny purple or bluish-black swollen areas (varicosities) under the tongue, known as caviar spots, are not uncommon in the older adult.
- The gag reflex may be slightly sluggish in the older adult.

Procedure

1. Prior to performing the procedure, introduce self and verify the patient's identity using two identifiers. Explain to the patient what you are going to do, why it is necessary, and how the patient can participate. Discuss how the results will be used in planning further care or treatments.
2. Perform hand hygiene and observe other appropriate infection control procedures.
3. Provide for patient privacy.
4. Inquire if the patient has any history of the following: routine pattern of dental care, last visit to dentist; length of time ulcers or other lesions have been present; denture discomfort; medications patient is receiving.
5. Position the patient comfortably, seated if possible.

ASSESSMENT	NORMAL FINDINGS	DEVIATIONS FROM NORMAL
Lips and Buccal Mucosa		
6. Inspect the outer lips for symmetry of contour, color, and texture. Ask the patient to purse the lips as if to whistle.	Uniform pink color (darker, e.g., bluish hue, in Mediterranean groups and dark-skinned patients) Soft, moist, smooth texture Symmetry of contour Ability to purse lips	Pallor; cyanosis Blisters; generalized or localized swelling; fissures, crusts, or scales (may result from excessive moisture, nutritional deficiency, or fluid deficit) Inability to purse lips (may indicate facial nerve damage)

SKILL 1.18 Mouth and Oropharynx: Assessing (*continued*)

ASSESSMENT	NORMAL FINDINGS	DEVIATIONS FROM NORMAL

7. Inspect the inner lips and buccal mucosa for color, moisture, texture, and the presence of lesions.
  ▪ Apply clean gloves.
  ▪ Ask the patient to relax the mouth, and, for better visualization, pull the lip outward and away from the teeth.
  ▪ Grasp the lip on each side between the thumb and index finger ❶.
	Uniform pink color (freckled brown pigmentation in dark-skinned patients)
	Moist, smooth, soft, glistening, and elastic texture (drier oral mucosa in older adults due to decreased salivation)
	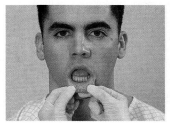
	Source: Richard Tauber/Pearson Education, Inc.
	❶ Inspecting the mucosa of the lower lip.
		Pallor; leukoplakia (white patches), red, bleeding
		Excessive dryness
		Mucosal cysts; irritations from dentures; abrasions, ulcerations; nodules

Teeth and Gums

8. Inspect the teeth and gums while examining the inner lips and buccal mucosa.
  ▪ Ask the patient to open the mouth. Using a tongue depressor, retract the cheek ❷. View the surface buccal mucosa from top to bottom and back to front. A flashlight or penlight will help illuminate the surface.
    Repeat the procedure for the other side.
  ▪ Examine the back teeth. For proper vision of the molars, use the index fingers of both hands to retract the cheek ❸. Ask the patient to relax the lips and first close, then open, the jaw. **Rationale:** *Closing the jaw assists in observation of tooth alignment and loss of teeth; opening the jaw assists in observation of dental fillings and caries.* Observe the number of teeth, tooth color, the state of fillings, dental caries, and tartar along the base of the teeth. Note the presence and fit of partial or complete dentures. To remove dentures to inspect the gums (a) have patient rinse mouth with warm water, (b) remove top dentures by pressing your thumb against the inside of the front teeth and then push up and outward toward the nose, (c) remove lower dentures by slowly pulling them with a rocking up and down motion.
  ▪ Inspect the gums around the molars. Observe for bleeding, color, retraction (pulling away from the teeth), edema, and lesions.
	Thirty-two adult teeth
	Smooth, white, shiny tooth enamel
	Pink gums (bluish or brown patches in dark-skinned patients)
	Moist, firm texture to gums
	No retraction of gums (pulling away from the teeth)
	
	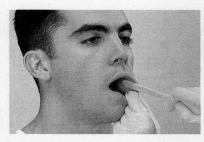
	Source: Richard Tauber/Pearson Education, Inc.
	❷ Inspecting the buccal mucosa using a tongue depressor.
		Missing teeth; ill-fitting dentures
		Brown or black discoloration of the enamel (may indicate staining or the presence of caries)
		Excessively red gums
		Spongy texture; bleeding; tenderness (may indicate periodontal disease)
		Receding, atrophied gums; swelling that partially covers the teeth
		
		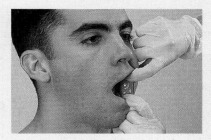
		Source: Richard Tauber/Pearson Education, Inc.
		❸ Inspecting the back teeth.

9. Inspect the dentures. Remove or have patient remove complete or partial dentures. Inspect their condition, noting in particular broken or worn areas.	Smooth, intact dentures	Ill-fitting dentures; irritated and excoriated area under dentures

(*continued on next page*)

SKILL 1.18 Mouth and Oropharynx: Assessing (*continued*)

ASSESSMENT	NORMAL FINDINGS	DEVIATIONS FROM NORMAL
Tongue/Floor of the Mouth		
10. Inspect the surface of the tongue for position, color, and texture. Ask the patient to protrude the tongue.	Central position Pink color (some brown pigmentation on tongue borders in dark-skinned patients); moist; slightly rough; thin whitish coating Smooth, lateral margins; no lesions Raised papillae (taste buds)	Deviated from center (may indicate damage to hypoglossal [twelfth cranial] nerve); excessive trembling Smooth red tongue (may indicate iron, vitamin B_{12}, or vitamin B_3 deficiency) Dry, furry tongue (associated with fluid deficit), white coating (may be oral yeast infection) Nodes, ulcerations, discolorations (white or red areas); areas of tenderness
11. Inspect tongue movement. Ask the patient to roll the tongue upward and move it from side to side.	Moves freely; no tenderness	Restricted mobility
12. Inspect the base of the tongue, the mouth floor, and the frenulum. Ask the patient to place the tip of the tongue against the roof of the mouth.	Smooth tongue base with prominent veins	Swelling, ulceration
Palates and Uvula		
13. Inspect the hard and soft palate for color, shape, texture, and the presence of bony prominences. Ask the patient to open the mouth wide and tilt the head backward. Then, depress tongue with a tongue depressor as necessary, and use a penlight for appropriate visualization.	Light pink, smooth, soft palate Lighter pink, hard palate, more irregular texture	Discoloration (e.g., jaundice or pallor) Palates the same color Irritations Exostoses (bony growths) growing from the hard palate
14. Inspect the uvula for position and mobility while examining the palates. To observe the uvula, ask the patient to say "ah" so that the soft palate rises.	Positioned in midline of soft palate	Deviation to one side from tumor or trauma; immobility (may indicate damage to trigeminal [fifth cranial] nerve or vagus [tenth cranial] nerve)
Oropharynx and Tonsils		
15. Inspect the oropharynx for color and texture. Inspect one side at a time to avoid eliciting the gag reflex. To expose one side of the oropharynx, press a tongue depressor against the tongue on the same side about halfway back while the patient tilts the head back and opens the mouth wide. Use a penlight for illumination, if needed.	Pink and smooth posterior wall	Reddened or edematous; presence of lesions, plaques, or drainage
16. Inspect the tonsils (behind the fauces [throat]) for color, discharge, and size.	Pink and smooth No discharge Of normal size or not visible *Grade 1 (normal):* The tonsils are behind the tonsillar pillars (the soft structures supporting the soft palate).	Inflamed Presence of discharge Swollen *Grade 2:* The tonsils are between the pillars and the uvula. *Grade 3:* The tonsils touch the uvula. *Grade 4:* One or both tonsils extend to the midline of the oropharynx.
17. Remove and discard gloves. Perform hand hygiene.		
18. Leave patient safe and comfortable. Complete documentation using forms, checklists, or electronic dropdown lists supplemented by nurse's notes or additional comments as appropriate.		

SKILL 1.18 Mouth and Oropharynx: Assessing *(continued)*

[date]0725 Inspection of mouth shows missing incisor tooth right side; no lesions or irritation noted, gums pink, full movement tongue and lips; tolerated well without incident; dad talking with child. *O. Hughes*

Patient Teaching

- Although patients may be sensitive to discussion of their personal hygiene practices, use the assessment as an opportunity to provide teaching about appropriate oral and dental care for the entire family. Refer patients to a dentist if indicated.

Lifespan Considerations

NEWBORNS AND INFANTS

- Inspect the palate and uvula for a cleft. A bifid (forked) uvula may indicate an undetected cleft palate (i.e., a cleft in the cartilage that is covered by skin).
- The first teeth erupt at about 6–7 months of age. Assess for dental hygiene; parents should cleanse the infant's teeth daily with a soft cloth or soft toothbrush.
- Fluoride supplements should be given by 6 months if the child's drinking water contains less than 0.3 part per million (ppm) fluoride.
- Children should see a dentist by 1 year of age.

CHILDREN

- Tooth development should be appropriate for age.
- Drooling is common up to 2 years of age.
- The tonsils are normally larger in children than in adults and commonly extend beyond the palatine arch until the age of 11 or 12 years.

OLDER ADULTS

- The oral mucosa may be drier than that of younger individuals because of decreased salivary gland activity. Decreased salivation occurs in older adults taking prescribed medications such as antidepressants, antihistamines, decongestants, diuretics, antihypertensives, tranquilizers, antispasmodics, and antineoplastics. Extreme dryness is associated with dehydration.
- Some receding of the gums occurs, giving an appearance of increased tooth size.
- Taste sensations diminish. Sweet and salty tastes are lost first. Older adults may add more salt and sugar to food than they did when they were younger. Diminished taste sensation is due to atrophy of the taste buds and a decreased sense of smell. It indicates diminished function of the seventh and ninth cranial nerves.
- The teeth may show signs of staining, erosion, chipping, and abrasions due to loss of dentin.
- Tooth loss occurs as a result of dental disease but is preventable with good dental hygiene.
- Older adults who are homebound or are in long-term care facilities often have teeth or dentures in need of repair, due to the difficulty of obtaining dental care in these situations. Do a thorough assessment of missing teeth and those in need of repair, whether they are natural teeth or dentures.

SKILL 1.19 Musculoskeletal System: Assessing

This skill allows the evaluation of the function and strength of individual muscles and muscle groups based on the patient's ability to perform range of movements in relation to the forces of gravity and manual resistance.

Delegation or Assignment

Assessment of the musculoskeletal system is not delegated or assigned to the UAP. However, many aspects of its functioning are observed during usual care and may be recorded by individuals other than the nurse. Abnormal findings must be validated and interpreted by the nurse.

Equipment

- *Goniometer* (a joint angle-measuring device)
- Tape measure

Preparation

- When the arms and legs of newborns are pulled to extension and released, newborns naturally return to the flexed fetal position.
- Infants should be able to sit without support by 8 months of age, crawl by 7–10 months, and walk by 12–15 months.
- Observe the child in normal activities to determine motor function.
- In most older adults, osteoarthritic changes in the joints can be observed.
- Note any surgical scars from joint replacement surgeries in the older adult.

Procedure

1. Prior to performing the procedure, introduce self and verify the patient's identity using two identifiers. Explain to the

(continued on next page)

SKILL 1.19 Musculoskeletal System: Assessing (continued)

patient what you are going to do, why it is necessary, and how the patient can participate. Discuss how the results will be used in planning further care or treatments.

2. Perform hand hygiene and observe other appropriate infection control procedures.

3. Provide for patient privacy.

4. Inquire if the patient has any history of the following: presence of muscle or joint pain: onset, location, character, associated phenomena (e.g., redness and swelling of joints), and aggravating and alleviating factors; limitations to movement or inability to perform activities of daily living; previous sports injuries; loss of function without pain.

ASSESSMENT	NORMAL FINDINGS	DEVIATIONS FROM NORMAL
Muscles		
5. Inspect the muscles for size. Compare the muscles on one side of the body (e.g., of the arm, thigh, and calf) to the same muscle on the other side. For any discrepancies, measure the muscles with a tape.	Equal size on both sides of body	Atrophy (a decrease in size) or hypertrophy (an increase in size) Asymmetry
6. Inspect the muscles and tendons for contractures (shortening).	No contractures	Malposition of body part, (e.g., foot drop, in which the foot is flexed downward)
7. Inspect the muscles for tremors, for example, by having the patient hold the arms out in front of the body.	No tremors	Presence of tremor
8. Test muscle strength. Compare the right side with the left side. *Sternocleidomastoid:* Patient turns the head to one side against the resistance of your hand. Repeat with the other side. *Trapezius:* Patient shrugs the shoulders against the resistance of your hands. *Deltoid:* Patient holds arm up and resists while you try to push it down. *Biceps:* Patient fully extends each arm and tries to flex it while you attempt to hold arm in extension. *Triceps:* Patient flexes each arm and then tries to extend it against your attempt to keep arm in flexion. *Wrist and finger muscles:* Patient spreads the fingers and resists as you attempt to push the fingers together. *Grip strength:* Patient grasps your index and middle fingers while you try to pull the fingers out. *Hip muscles:* Patient is supine, both legs extended; patient raises one leg at a time while you attempt to hold it down. *Hip abduction:* Patient is supine, both legs extended. Place your hands on the lateral surface of each knee; patient spreads the legs apart against your resistance. *Hip adduction:* Patient is in same position as for hip abduction. Place your hands between the knees; patient brings the legs together against your resistance. *Hamstrings:* Patient is supine, both knees bent. Patient resists while you attempt to straighten the legs. *Quadriceps:* Patient is supine, knee partially extended; patient resists while you attempt to flex the knee. *Muscles of the ankles and feet:* Patient resists while you attempt to dorsiflex the foot and again resists while you attempt to flex the foot.	Equal strength on each body side	Muscle grading 25% or less of normal strength **Grading Muscle Strength Scale** **0:** 0% of normal strength; complete paralysis **1:** 10% of normal strength; no movement, contraction of muscle is palpable or visible **2:** 25% of normal strength; full muscle movement against gravity, with support **3:** 50% of normal strength; normal movement against gravity **4:** 75% of normal strength; normal full movement against gravity and against minimal resistance **5:** 100% of normal strength; normal full movement against gravity and against full resistance

SKILL 1.19 Musculoskeletal System: Assessing (*continued*)

ASSESSMENT	NORMAL FINDINGS	DEVIATIONS FROM NORMAL
Bones		
9. Inspect the skeleton for structure.	No deformities	Bones misaligned
10. Palpate the bones to locate any areas of edema or tenderness.	No tenderness or swelling	Presence of tenderness or swelling (may indicate fracture, necplasms, or osteoporosis)
Joints		
11. Inspect the joint for swelling. Palpate each joint for tenderness, smoothness of movement, swelling, crepitation, and presence of nodules.	No swelling No tenderness, swelling, crepitation or nodules Joints move smoothly.	One or more swollen joints Presence of tenderness, swelling, crepitation, or nodules
12. Assess joint range of motion. Ask the patient to move selected body parts. The amount of joint movement can be measured by a goniometer (a device that measures in degrees the angle of the joint). ❶	Varies to some degree in accordance with person's genetic makeup and degree of physical activity. *Source:* Pat Watson/ Pearson Education, Inc. ❶ A goniometer used to measure joint angle.	Limited range of motion in one or more joints
13. When the procedure is complete, perform hand hygiene. Leave patient safe and comfortable. Complete documentation using forms, checklists, or electronic dropdown lists supplemented by nurse's notes or additional comments as appropriate.		

SAMPLE DOCUMENTATION

[date] 1030 Able to move full range of motion (FROM) all extremities; denies tenderness of joints; grips and strength equal both sides; no deformities noted; tolerated without complaint. *L. Moores*

Lifespan Considerations

NEWBORNS AND INFANTS

- Palpate the clavicles of newborns. A mass and crepitus may indicate a fracture experienced during vaginal delivery. The newborn may also have limited movement of the arm and shoulder on the affected side.

- Check muscle strength by holding the newborn or infant lightly under the arms with feet placed lightly on a table. Newborns or infants should not fall through the hands and should be able to bear body weight on their legs if normal muscle strength is present.

- Check newborns or infants for developmental dysplasia of the hip (congenital dislocation) by examining for asymmetric gluteal folds, asymmetric abduction of the legs (Ortolani and Barlow tests), or apparent shortening of the femur.

- Observe for symmetry of muscle mass, strength, and function.

CHILDREN

- Pronation and "toeing in" of the feet are common in children between 12–30 months of age.

(continued on next page)

SKILL 1.19 Musculoskeletal System: Assessing (*continued*)

- Genu varum (bowleg) is normal in children for about 1 year after beginning to walk.
- Genu valgus (knock-knee) is normal in preschool and early school-age children.
- Lordosis (swayback) is common in children before age 5.
- During the rapid growth spurts of adolescence, spinal curvature and rotation (scoliosis) may appear. Children should be assessed for scoliosis by age 12 and annually until their growth slows. Curvature greater than 10% should be referred for further medical evaluation.
- Muscle mass increases in adolescence, especially as children engage in strenuous physical activity, and requires increased nutritional intake.
- Children are at risk for injury related to physical activity and should be assessed for nutritional status, physical conditioning, and safety precautions in order to prevent injury.

- Adolescent girls who participate in strenuous athletic activities are at risk for delayed menses, osteoporosis, and eating disorders; assessment should include a history of these factors.

OLDER ADULTS

- Muscle mass decreases progressively with age, but there are wide variations among individuals.
- The decrease in speed, strength, resistance to fatigue, reaction time, and coordination in the older person is due to a decrease in nerve conduction and muscle tone.
- The bones become more fragile and osteoporosis may occur, with a loss of total bone mass. As a result, older adults are predisposed to fractures and compressed vertebrae.

SKILL 1.20 Nails: Assessing

Delegation or Assignment

Due to the substantial knowledge required, assessment of the nails is not delegated or assigned to the UAP. However, many nail characteristics are observed during usual care and may be recorded by individuals other than the nurse. Abnormal findings must be validated and interpreted by the nurse.

Equipment

No equipment is needed for this skill.

Preparation

- Bent, bruised, or ingrown toenails may indicate that shoes are too tight.
- Toenail fungus is more common and difficult to eliminate (although not dangerous to health) in the older adult.

Procedure

1. Prior to performing the procedure, introduce self and verify the patient's identity using two identifiers. Explain to the patient what you are going to do, why it is necessary, and how the patient can participate. Discuss how the results will be used in planning further care or treatments. In most situations, patients with artificial nails or polish on fingernails or toenails are not required to remove these for assessment. If the assessment cannot be conducted due to the presence of polish or artificial nails, document this in the record.
2. Perform hand hygiene and observe other appropriate infection control procedures.
3. Provide for patient privacy.
4. Inquire if the patient has any history of the following: presence of diabetes mellitus, peripheral circulatory disease, previous injury, or severe illness.

ASSESSMENT	NORMAL FINDINGS	DEVIATIONS FROM NORMAL
5. Inspect fingernail plate shape to determine its curvature and angle.	Convex curvature; angle of nail plate about 160 degrees ❶ (see A)	Spoon nail (see 1B); clubbing (180 degrees or greater) (see 1C and D)

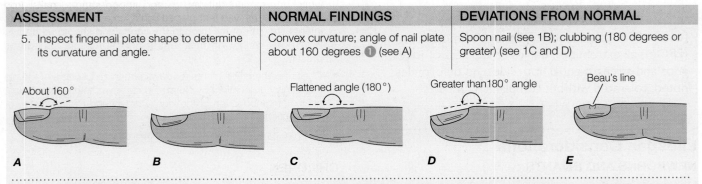

❶ **A,** A normal nail, showing the convex shape and the nail plate angle of about 160 degrees; **B,** a spoon-shaped nail, which may be seen in patients with iron deficiency anemia; **C,** early clubbing; **D,** late clubbing (may be caused by long-term lack of oxygen); **E,** Beau's line on nail (may result from severe injury or illness).

SKILL 1.20 Nails: Assessing *(continued)*

ASSESSMENT	NORMAL FINDINGS	DEVIATIONS FROM NORMAL
6. Inspect fingernail and toenail texture.	Smooth texture	Excessive thickness or thinness or presence of grooves or furrows; Beau's lines (see 1E); discolored or detached nail (often due to fungus or injury)
7. Inspect fingernail and toenail bed color.	Highly vascular and pink in light-skinned patients; dark-skinned patients may have brown or black pigmentation in longitudinal streaks.	Bluish or purplish tint (may reflect cyanosis); pallor (may reflect poor arterial circulation)
8. Inspect tissues surrounding nails. If indicated, teach the patient or family member about proper nail care including how to trim and shape the nails to avoid paronychia.	Intact epidermis	Hangnails; paronychia (inflammation)
9. Perform blanch test of capillary refill. Press two or more nails between your thumb and index finger; look for blanching and return of pink color to nail bed. Count in seconds the time for the color to return completely.	Prompt return of pink or usual color (generally less than 2 seconds)	Delayed return of pink or usual color (may indicate circulatory impairment)
10. If eyesight, fine motor control, or cognition prevents the patient from safely trimming the nails, refer the patient to a podiatrist or manicurist.		
11. When the procedure is complete, perform hand hygiene. Leave patient safe and comfortable. Complete documentation using forms, checklists, or electronic dropdown lists supplemented by nurse's notes or additional comments as appropriate.		

SAMPLE DOCUMENTATION

[date] 1335 Finger nails smooth, pale pink; capillary refill brisk; toe nails smooth; right great toe has tissue redness with some tenderness right side. States has been like that for about 2 weeks. Nail hygiene adequate; tolerated without incident. *B. Collins*

Lifespan Considerations
NEWBORNS AND INFANTS

- Newborns' nails grow very quickly, are extremely thin, and tear easily.

CHILDREN

- Nail biting should be discussed with an adult family member because it may be a symptom of stress.

OLDER ADULTS

- The nails grow more slowly and thicken.
- Longitudinal bands commonly develop, and the nails tend to split.
- Bands across the nails may indicate protein deficiency; white spots, zinc deficiency; and spoon-shaped nails, iron deficiency.

SKILL 1.21 Neck: Assessing

Delegation or Assignment

Assessment of the neck is not delegated or assigned to the UAP. However, many aspects of the neck are observed during usual care and may be recorded by individuals other than the nurse. Abnormal findings must be validated and interpreted by the nurse.

Equipment

No equipment is required for this skill to be completed.

Preparation

- Have worksheet and pen available to make notes on movement restrictions, location of nodes palpated, and trachea location.
- Face the older adult when speaking in order to improve communication.

(continued on next page)

SKILL 1.21 Neck: Assessing (continued)

Procedure

1. Prior to performing the procedure, introduce self and verify the patient's identity using two identifiers. Explain to the patient what you are going to do, why it is necessary, and how the patient can participate. Discuss how the results will be used in planning further care or treatments.

2. Perform hand hygiene and observe other appropriate infection control procedures.
3. Provide for patient privacy.
4. Inquire if the patient has any history of the following: problems with neck lumps; neck pain or stiffness; when and how any lumps occurred; previous diagnoses of thyroid problems; and other treatments provided (e.g., surgery, radiation).

ASSESSMENT	NORMAL FINDINGS	DEVIATIONS FROM NORMAL
Neck Muscles		
5. Inspect the neck muscles (sternocleidomastoid and trapezius) for abnormal swellings or masses. Ask the patient to hold the head erect.	Muscles equal in size; head centered	Unilateral neck swelling; head tilted to one side (indicates presence of masses, injury, muscle weakness, shortening of sternocleidomastoid muscle, scars)
6. Observe head movement. Ask patient to: ■ Move the chin to the chest. **Rationale:** *This determines function of the sternocleidomastoid muscle.* ■ Move the head back so that the chin points upward. **Rationale:** *This determines function of the trapezius muscle.* ■ Move the head so that the ear is moved toward the shoulder on each side. **Rationale:** *This determines function of the sternocleidomastoid muscle.* ■ Turn the head to the right and to the left. **Rationale:** *This determines function of the sternocleidomastoid muscle.*	Coordinated, smooth movements with no discomfort Head flexes 45 degrees Head hyperextends 60 degrees Head laterally flexes 40 degrees Head laterally rotates 70 degrees	Muscle tremor, spasm, or stiffness Limited range of motion; painful movements; involuntary movements (e.g., up-and-down nodding movements associated with Parkinson's disease) Head hyperextends less than 60 degrees Head laterally flexes less than 40 degrees Head laterally rotates less than 70 degrees
7. Assess muscle strength. ■ Ask the patient to turn the head to one side against the resistance of your hand. Repeat with the other side. **Rationale:** *This determines the strength of the sternocleidomastoid muscle.* ■ Ask the patient to shrug the shoulders against the resistance of your hands. **Rationale:** *This determines the strength of the trapezius muscles.*	Equal strength Equal strength	Unequal strength Unequal strength
Lymph Nodes		
8. Palpate the entire neck for enlarged lymph nodes. ■ Face the patient, and bend the patient's head forward slightly or toward the side being examined. **Rationale:** *This relaxes the soft tissue and muscles.* ■ Palpate the nodes using the pads of the fingers. Move the fingertips in a gentle rotating motion. ■ When examining the submental and submandibular nodes, place the fingertips under the mandible on the side nearest the palpating hand, and pull the skin and subcutaneous tissue laterally over the mandibular surface so that the tissue rolls over the nodes.	Not palpable	Enlarged, palpable, possibly tender (associated with infection and tumors)

SKILL 1.21 Neck: Assessing (continued)

ASSESSMENT	NORMAL FINDINGS	DEVIATIONS FROM NORMAL
▪ When palpating the supraclavicular nodes, have the patient bend the head forward to relax the tissues of the anterior neck and to relax the shoulders so that the clavicles drop. Use your hand nearest the side to be examined when facing the patient (i.e., your left hand for the patient's right nodes). Use your free hand to flex the patient's head forward if necessary. Hook your index and third fingers over the clavicle lateral to the sternocleidomastoid muscle ❶. ▪ When palpating the anterior cervical nodes and posterior cervical nodes, move your fingertips slowly in a forward circular motion against the sternocleidomastoid and trapezius muscles, respectively. ▪ To palpate the deep cervical nodes, bend or hook your fingers around the sternocleidomastoid muscle.	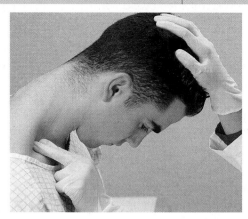 *Source:* Richard Tauber/Pearson Education, Inc. ❶ Palpating the supraclavicular lymph nodes.	

Trachea

9. Palpate the trachea for lateral deviation. Place your fingertip or thumb on the trachea in the suprasternal notch and then move your finger laterally to the left and the right in spaces bordered by the clavicle, the anterior aspect of the sternocleidomastoid muscle, and the trachea.	Central placement in midline of neck; spaces are equal on both sides	Deviation to one side, indicating possible neck tumor; thyroid enlargement; enlarged lymph nodes
10. When the procedure is complete, perform hand hygiene. Leave patient safe and comfortable. Complete documentation using forms, checklists, or electronic dropdown lists supplemented by nurse's notes or additional comments as appropriate.		

Lifespan Considerations
NEWBORNS, INFANTS, AND CHILDREN

▪ Examine the neck while the newborn, infant, or child is lying supine. Lift the head and turn it from side to side to determine neck mobility.

▪ A newborn's or infant's neck is normally short, lengthening by about age 3 years. This makes palpation of the trachea difficult.

SKILL 1.22 Neurologic Status: Assessing

This skills is performed to evaluate neurologic status and changes in mental status for early recognition of potential neurologic deterioration. Physical assessment is done to identify clinical changes in the neurologic functioning of the body that may be manifestations of neurologic injury or disease.

Delegation or Assignment

Due to the substantial knowledge and skill required, assessment of the neurologic system is not delegated or assigned to

(continued on next page)

SKILL 1.22 Neurologic Status: Assessing (*continued*)

the UAP. However, many aspects of neurologic behavior are observed during usual care and may be recorded by individuals other than the nurse. Abnormal findings must be validated and interpreted by the nurse.

Equipment (Depending on Components of Examination)

- Percussion hammer
- Wisps of cotton to assess light-touch sensation
- Sterile safety pin for tactile discrimination

Preparation

- All questions and tests used must be individualized to the patient's age, language, education level, and culture to have accurate assessment and patient responses.
- A full neurologic assessment can be lengthy. Conduct in several sessions if indicated, and cease the tests if the patient is noticeably fatigued.
- Present the procedures as games to a child whenever possible.
- Note the child's ability to understand and follow directions.
- Many older adults have some impairment of hearing, vision, smell, temperature and pain sensation, memory, and mental endurance.

Procedure

1. Prior to performing the procedure, introduce self and verify the patient's identity using two identifiers. Explain to the patient what you are going to do, why it is necessary, and how the patient can participate. Discuss how the results will be used in planning further care or treatments.
2. Perform hand hygiene and observe other appropriate infection control procedures.
3. Provide for patient privacy.
4. Inquire if the patient has any history of the following: presence of pain in the head, back, or extremities, as well as onset and aggravating and alleviating factors; disorientation to time, place, or person; speech disorder; history of loss of consciousness, fainting, convulsions, trauma, tingling or numbness, tremors or tics, limping, paralysis, uncontrolled muscle movements, loss of memory, mood swings, or problems with smell, vision, taste, touch, or hearing.

LANGUAGE

5. If the patient displays difficulty speaking:
   - Point to common objects and ask the patient to name them.
   - Ask the patient to read some words and to match the printed and written words with pictures.
   - Ask the patient to respond to simple verbal and written commands, for example, "point to your toes" or "raise your left arm."

ORIENTATION

6. Determine the patient's orientation to *time, place,* and *person* by tactful questioning. Ask the patient the time of day, date, day of the week, city and state of residence, duration of illness, and names of family members. Ask the patient the reason for seeing a healthcare provider. Orientation is lost gradually, and early disorientation may be very subtle. "Why" questions may elicit a more accurate clinical picture of the patient's orientation status than questions directed to time, place, and person. To evaluate the response, you must know the correct answer.

More direct questioning may be necessary for some people, for example, "Where are you now?" "What day is it today?" Most people readily accept these questions if initially the nurse asks, "Do you get confused at times?" If the patient cannot answer these questions regarding place and time accurately, also include assessment of the *self* by asking the patient to state his or her full name.

MEMORY

7. Listen for lapses in memory. Ask the patient about difficulty with memory. If problems are apparent, three categories of memory are tested: immediate recall, recent memory, and remote memory.

To assess immediate recall:

- Ask the patient to repeat a series of three digits (e.g., 7–4–3), spoken slowly.
- Gradually increase the number of digits (e.g., 7–4–3–5, 7–4–3–5–6, and 7–4–3–5–6–7), until the patient fails to repeat the series correctly.
- Start again with a series of three digits, but this time ask the patient to repeat them backward. The average person can repeat a series of five to eight digits in sequence and four to six digits in reverse order.

To assess recent memory:

- Ask the patient to recall the recent events of the day, such as how the patient got to the clinic. This information must be validated, however.
- Ask the patient to recall information given early in the interview (e.g., the name of a physician).
- Provide the patient with three facts to recall (e.g., a color, an object, and an address), and ask the patient to repeat all three. Later in the interview, ask the patient to recall all three items.

To assess remote memory, ask the patient to describe a previous illness or surgery (e.g., 5 years ago) or a birthday or anniversary. Generally remote memory will be intact until late in neurological pathology. It is least useful to assess for acute neurological problems.

ATTENTION SPAN AND CALCULATION

8. Test the ability to concentrate or maintain *attention span* by asking the patient to recite the alphabet or to count backward from 100. Test the ability to calculate by asking the patient to subtract 7 or 3 progressively from 100, that is, 100, 93, 86, 79, or 100, 97, 94, 91 (referred to as *serial sevens* or *serial threes*). Normally, an adult can complete the serial sevens test in about 90 seconds with three or fewer errors. Because educational level, language, or

SKILL 1.22 Neurologic Status: Assessing (continued)

cultural differences affect calculating ability, this test may be inappropriate for some people.

LEVEL OF CONSCIOUSNESS

9. Apply the Glasgow Coma Scale: eye response, motor response, and verbal response. An assessment totaling 15 points indicates the patient is alert and completely oriented. A comatose patient scores 8 or less.

CRANIAL NERVES

10. For the specific functions and assessment methods of each cranial nerve, see **Table 1–9** 》. Test each nerve not already evaluated in another component of the health assessment. A quick way to test cranial nerve I is shown in ①.

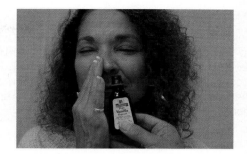

Source: Pat Watson/Pearson Education, Inc.

① Cranial nerves are tested for normal or abnormal response. For example, cranial nerve I (smell) can be tested by having the patient close his or her eyes and identify different mild, familiar scents.

TABLE 1–9 Cranial Nerve Functions and Assessment Methods

Cranial Nerve	Name	Type	Function	Assessment Method
I	Olfactory	Sensory	Smell	Ask patient to close eyes and identify different mild aromas such as coffee, vanilla, peanut butter, orange/lemon, chocolate.
II	Optic	Sensory	Vision and visual fields	Ask patient to read Snellen-type chart; check visual fields by confrontation; and conduct an ophthalmoscopic examination (also see Skill 1.14).
III	Oculomotor	Motor	Extraocular eye movement (EOM); movement of sphincter of pupil; movement of ciliary muscles of lens	Assess six ocular movements and pupil reaction (also see Skill 1.14).
IV	Trochlear	Motor	EOM; specifically, moves eyeball downward	Assess six ocular movements (also see Skill 1.14).
V	Trigeminal ophthalmic branch	Sensory	Sensation of cornea, skin of face, and nasal mucosa	While patient looks upward, lightly touch the lateral sclera of the eye with sterile gauze to elicit blink reflex. To test light sensation, have patient close eyes, wipe a wisp of cotton over patient's forehead and paranasal sinuses.
	Maxillary branch	Sensory	Sensation of skin of face and anterior oral cavity (tongue and teeth)	Assess skin sensation as for ophthalmic branch above.
	Mandibular branch	Motor and sensory	Muscles of mastication; sensation of skin of face	Ask patient to clench teeth.
VI	Abducens	Motor	EOM; moves eyeball laterally	Assess directions of gaze.
VII	Facial	Motor and sensory	Facial expression; taste (anterior two thirds of tongue)	Ask patient to smile, raise the eyebrows, frown, puff out cheeks, close eyes tightly. Ask patient to identify various tastes placed on the tip and sides of tongue: sugar (sweet), salt, lemon juice (sour), and quinine (bitter); identify areas of taste.
VIII	Cochlear branch Sensory hearing Assess patient's ability to hear spoken word and vibrations of tuning fork.	Sensory	Hearing: air-conduction and bone-conduction	Gross hearing acuity tests Normal tone, whisper tone Weber's test, and Rinne test with tuning fork (also see Skill 1.13)
	Vestibular branch	Sensory	Equilibrium	Romberg test (see page 70)
	Cochlear branch	Sensory	Hearing	Assess patient's ability to hear spoken word and vibrations of tuning fork.
IX	Glossopharyngeal	Motor and sensory	Swallowing ability, tongue movement, taste (posterior tongue)	Apply tastes on posterior tongue for identification. Ask patient to move tongue from side to side and up and down.
X	Vagus	Motor and sensory	Sensation of pharynx and larynx; swallowing; vocal cord movement	Assessed with cranial nerve IX; assess patient's speech for hoarseness.
XI	Accessory	Motor	Head movement; shrugging of shoulders	Ask patient to shrug shoulders against resistance from your hands and turn head to side against resistance from your hand (repeat for other side). (Also see Skills 1.19 and 1.21.)
XII	Hypoglossal	Motor	Protrusion of tongue; moves tongue up and down and side to side	Ask patient to protrude tongue at midline, then move it side to side. (Also see Skill 1.18.)

(continued on next page)

SKILL 1.22 Neurologic Status: Assessing (continued)

REFLEXES

11. Generalist nurses do not commonly assess each of the deep tendon reflexes except for the plantar (Babinski) reflex, indicative of possible spinal cord injury. Reflexes are reported using the scale below, comparing one side of the body with the other to evaluate the symmetry of response.

     0 No reflex response
     +1 Minimal activity (hypoactive)
     +2 Normal response
     +3 More active than normal
     +4 Maximal activity (hyperactive)

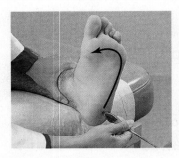

Source: Richard Tauber/Pearson Education, Inc.

❷ Testing plantar (Babinski) reflexes.

BABINSKI REFLEX

- Use a moderately sharp object, such as the handle of the percussion hammer, a key, or an applicator stick.
- Stroke the lateral border of the sole of the patient's foot, starting at the heel, continuing to the ball of the foot, and then proceeding across the ball of the foot toward the big toe ❷.
- Observe the response. Normally, in the child more than 2 years old and the adult, all five toes bend downward; this reaction is called a negative Babinski. In an abnormal

(positive) Babinski response, the toes spread outward and the big toe moves upward and backward, indicative of an upper motor neuron dysfunction in the child more than 2 years old and the adult.

In the newborn, infant, and child less than 2 years old, the opposite is true. It is normal for a newborn, infant, or child less than 2 years old to have a positive Babinski response, meaning the toes spread outward and the big toe moves upward and backward. It would be abnormal for the toes to bend downward.

MOTOR FUNCTION

ASSESSMENT	NORMAL FINDINGS	DEVIATIONS FROM NORMAL
12. *Gross Motor and Balance Tests:* Generally, the Romberg test and one other gross motor function and balance tests are used.		

Walking Gait

Ask the patient to walk across the room and back, and assess the patient's gait.	Has upright posture and steady gait with opposing arm swing; walks unaided, maintaining balance	Has poor posture and unsteady, irregular, staggering gait with wide stance; bends legs only from hips; has rigid or no arm movements

Romberg Test

Ask the patient to stand with feet together and arms resting at the sides, first with eyes open, then closed. Stand close during this test. **Rationale:** *This prevents the patient from falling.*	*Negative Romberg:* may sway slightly but is able to maintain upright posture and foot stance	*Positive Romberg:* cannot maintain foot stance; moves the feet apart to maintain stance If patient cannot maintain balance with the eyes shut, patient may have sensory ataxia (lack of coordination of the voluntary muscles). If balance cannot be maintained whether the eyes are open or shut, patient may have cerebellar ataxia.

Standing on One Foot with Eyes Closed

Ask the patient to close the eyes and stand on one foot. Repeat on the other foot. Stand close to the patient during this test.	Maintains stance for at least 5 seconds	Cannot maintain stance for 5 seconds

SKILL 1.22 Neurologic Status: Assessing *(continued)*

ASSESSMENT	NORMAL FINDINGS	DEVIATIONS FROM NORMAL
Heel–Toe Walking		
Ask the patient to walk a straight line, placing the heel of one foot directly in front of the toes of the other foot ❸. *Source:* Pat Watson/Pearson Education, Inc. ❸ Heel-toe walking test.	Maintains heel–toe walking along a straight line	Assumes a wider foot gait to stay upright
Toe or Heel Walking		
Ask the patient to walk several steps on the toes and then on the heels.	Able to walk several steps on toes or heels	Cannot maintain balance on toes and heels
13. *Fine Motor Tests for the Upper Extremities:*		
Finger-to-Nose Test		
Ask the patient to abduct and extend the arms at shoulder height and then rapidly touch the nose alternately with one index finger and then the other. The patient repeats the test with the eyes closed if the test is performed easily ❹. *Source:* Richard Tauber/Pearson Education, Inc. ❹ Finger-to-nose test.	Repeatedly and rhythmically touches the nose	Misses the nose or gives slow response
Alternating Supination and Pronation of Hands on Knees		
Ask the patient to pat both knees with the palms of both hands and then with the backs of the hands alternately at an ever-increasing rate ❺.	Can alternately supinate and pronate hands at rapid pace	Performs with slow, clumsy movements and irregular timing; has difficulty alternating from supination to pronation

(continued on next page)

SKILL 1.22 Neurologic Status: Assessing *(continued)*

ASSESSMENT	NORMAL FINDINGS	DEVIATIONS FROM NORMAL

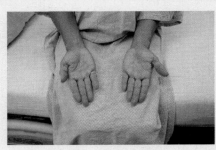 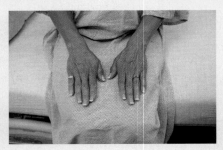

Sources: (Left and Right) Pat Watson/Pearson Education, Inc.

⑤ Alternating supination and pronation of hands on knees test.

Finger to Nose and to the Nurse's Finger

Ask the patient to touch the nose and then your index finger, held at a distance of about 45 cm (18 in.), at a rapid and increasing rate ⑥.	Performs with coordination and rapidity	Misses the finger and moves slowly

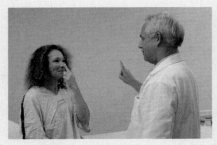 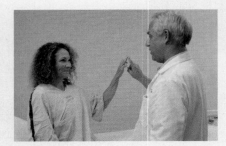

Sources: (Left and Right) Pat Watson/Pearson Education, Inc.

⑥ Finger-to-nose and to the nurse's finger test.

Fingers to Fingers

Ask the patient to spread the arms broadly at shoulder height and then bring the fingers together at the midline, first with the eyes open and then closed, first slowly and then rapidly.	Performs with accuracy and rapidity	Moves slowly and is unable to touch fingers consistently

Fingers to Thumb (Same Hand)

Ask the patient to touch each finger of one hand to the thumb of the same hand as rapidly as possible ⑦.	Rapidly touches each finger to thumb with each hand	Cannot coordinate this fine discrete movement with either one or both hands

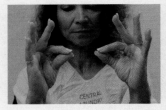 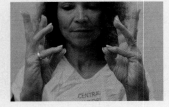

Sources: (Left and Right) Pat Watson/Pearson Education, Inc.

⑦ Fingers-to-thumb (same hand) test.

14. *Fine Motor Tests for the Lower Extremities:* Ask the patient to perform this test.		

SKILL 1.22 Neurologic Status: Assessing *(continued)*

ASSESSMENT	NORMAL FINDINGS	DEVIATIONS FROM NORMAL
Heel Down Opposite Shin		
Ask the patient to place the heel of one foot just below the opposite knee and run the heel down the shin to the foot. Repeat with the other foot. The patient may also use a sitting position for this test ⑧.	Demonstrates bilateral equal coordination *Source:* Pat Watson/Pearson Education, Inc. ⑧ Heel down opposite shin.	Has tremors or is awkward; heel moves off shin
15. *Light-Touch Sensation:* Compare the light-touch sensation of symmetric areas of the body. **Rationale:** *Sensitivity to touch varies among different skin areas.* ▪ Ask the patient to close the eyes and to respond by saying "yes" or "now" whenever the patient feels the cotton wisp touching the skin. ▪ With a wisp of cotton, lightly touch one specific spot and then the same spot on the other side of the body ⑨. ▪ Test areas on the forehead, cheek, hand, lower arm, abdomen, foot, and lower leg. Check a distal area of the limb first (i.e., the hand before the arm and the foot before the leg). **Rationale:** *The sensory nerve may be assumed to be intact if sensation is felt at its most distal part.* ▪ If areas of sensory dysfunction are found, determine the boundaries of sensation by testing responses about every 2.5 cm (1 in.) in the area. Make a sketch of the sensory loss area for recording purposes.	Light tickling or touch sensation *Source:* Pat Watson/Pearson Education, Inc. ⑨ Assessing light-touch sensation.	Loss of sensation (**anesthesia**); more than normal sensation (**hyperesthesia**); less than normal sensation (**hypoesthesia**); or an abnormal sensation such as burning, pain, or an electric shock (**paresthesia**)
16. *Pain Sensation* Assess pain sensation as follows: ▪ Ask the patient to close the eyes and to say "sharp," "dull," or "don't know" when the sharp or dull end of a safety pin is felt. ▪ Alternately, use the sharp and dull end to lightly prick designated anatomical areas at random (e.g., hand, forearm, foot, lower leg, abdomen). The face is not tested in this manner. ▪ Allow at least 2 seconds between each test to prevent summation effects of stimuli (i.e., several successive stimuli perceived as one stimulus).	Able to discriminate "sharp" and "dull" sensations	Areas of reduced, heightened, or absent sensation (map them out for recording purposes)

(continued on next page)

SKILL 1.22 Neurologic Status: Assessing (continued)

ASSESSMENT	NORMAL FINDINGS	DEVIATIONS FROM NORMAL
17. *Position or Kinesthetic Sensation:* Commonly, the middle fingers and the large toes are tested for the kinesthetic sensation (sense of position). ■ To test the fingers, support the patient's arm and hand with one hand. To test the toes, place the patient's heels on the examining table. ■ Ask the patient to close the eyes. ■ Grasp a middle finger or a big toe firmly between your thumb and index finger, and exert the same pressure on both sides of the finger or toe while moving it. ■ Move the finger or toe until it is up, down, or straight out, and ask the patient to identify the position ⑩. ■ Use a series of brisk up-and-down movements before bringing the finger or toe suddenly to rest in one of the three positions.	Can readily determine the position of fingers and toes *Source:* Pat Watson/Pearson Education, Inc. ⑩ Position or kinesthetic sensation.	Unable to determine the position of one or more fingers or toes
18. When the procedure is complete, perform hand hygiene. Leave patient safe and comfortable. Complete documentation using forms, checklists, or electronic dropdown lists supplemented by nurse's notes or additional comments as appropriate. Describe any abnormal findings in objective terms, for example, "When asked to count backward by threes, patient made seven errors and completed the task in 4 minutes."		

Lifespan Considerations

NEWBORNS AND INFANTS

■ Reflexes commonly tested in newborns include the following:
- Rooting: Stroke the side of the face near mouth; newborn or infant opens mouth and turns to the side that is stroked.
- Sucking: Place nipple or finger 3–4 cm (about 1–1½ in.) into mouth; newborn or infant sucks vigorously.
- Tonic neck: Place newborn or infant supine, turn head to one side; arm on side to which head is turned extends; on opposite side, arm curls up (fencer's pose).
- Palmar grasp: Place finger in newborn's or infant's palm and press; newborn or infant curls fingers around.
- Stepping: Hold infant as if weight bearing on surface; infant steps along, one foot at a time.
- Moro: Present loud noise or unexpected movement; newborn or infant spreads arms and legs, extends fingers, then flexes and brings hands together; may cry.

■ Most of these reflexes disappear between 4–6 months of age.

CHILDREN

■ Positive Babinski reflex is abnormal after the child ambulates or at age 2.

■ For children under age 5, the Denver Developmental Screening Test II provides a comprehensive neurological evaluation—particularly for motor function.

■ Assess immediate recall or recent memory by using names of cartoon characters.

■ Assess for signs of hyperactivity or abnormally short attention span.

■ Children should be able to walk backward by age 2, balance on one foot for 5 seconds by age 4, heel–toe walk by age 5, and heel–toe walk backward by age 6.

■ The Romberg test is appropriate over age 3.

OLDER ADULTS

■ A decline in mental status is not a normal result of aging. Changes are more the result of physical or psychological disorders (e.g., fever, fluid and electrolyte imbalances, medications). Chronic subtle insidious mental health changes are usually caused by dementia and are usually irreversible.

■ Short-term memory is often less efficient. Long-term memory is usually unaltered.

SKILL 1.22 Neurologic Status: Assessing (*continued*)

- Because old age is often associated with loss of support individuals, depression is a common disorder. Mood changes, weight loss, anorexia, constipation, and early morning awakening may be symptoms of depression.
- The stress of being in unfamiliar situations can cause confusion in older adults.
- Impulse transmission and reaction to stimuli are slower.

- Coordination changes, including a reduced speed of fine finger movements.
- When testing sensory function, the nurse needs to give older adults time to respond. Normally, older adults have unaltered perception of light touch and superficial pain, decreased perception of deep pain, and decreased perception of temperature stimuli.

SKILL 1.23 Nose and Sinuses: Assessing

Nursing assessment of the nose and sinuses can be done with examination and palpation. Additional assessment, usually by an advanced practice nurse, can be done using a nasal speculum.

Delegation or Assignment

Assessment of the nose and sinuses is not delegated or assigned to the UAP. However, many aspects of nasal function are observed during usual care and may be recorded by individuals other than the nurse. Abnormal findings must be validated and interpreted by the nurse.

Equipment

- Flashlight/penlight
- Nasal speculum (option)

Preparation

- Don clean gloves when there is discharge from the nares.

- To examine the septum, turbinates, and vestibule of the newborn, infant, or child, push the tip of the nose upward with the thumb and shine a light into the nares.

Procedure

1. Prior to performing the procedure, introduce self and verify the patient's identity using two identifiers. Explain to the patient what you are going to do, why it is necessary, and how the patient can participate. Discuss how the results will be used in planning further care or treatments.
2. Perform hand hygiene and observe other appropriate infection control procedures.
3. Provide for patient privacy.
4. Inquire if the patient has any history of the following: allergies, difficulty breathing through the nose, sinus infections, injuries to nose or face, nosebleeds; medications taken; changes in sense of smell.
5. Position the patient comfortably, seated if possible.

ASSESSMENT	NORMAL FINDINGS	DEVIATIONS FROM NORMAL
Nose		
6. Inspect the external nose for any deviations in shape, size, or color and flaring or discharge from the nares.	Symmetric and straight No discharge or flaring Uniform color	Asymmetric Discharge from nares Localized areas of redness or presence of skin lesions
7. Lightly palpate the external nose to determine any areas of tenderness, masses, and displacements of bone and cartilage.	Not tender; no lesions	Tenderness on palpation; presence of lesions
8. Determine patency of both nasal cavities. Ask the patient to close the mouth, exert pressure on one naris, and breathe through the opposite naris. Repeat the procedure to assess patency of the opposite naris.	Air moves freely as the patient breathes through the nares.	Air movement is restricted in one or both nares.

(*continued on next page*)

SKILL 1.23 Nose and Sinuses: Assessing *(continued)*

ASSESSMENT	NORMAL FINDINGS	DEVIATIONS FROM NORMAL

9. Inspect the nasal cavities using a flashlight.
  ■ Inspect each of the nasal cavities.
  ■ Tip the patient's head back for better visualization ❶.
  ■ Inspect the floor of the nose (vestibule), the anterior portion of the septum, the middle meatus, and the middle turbinates. The posterior turbinate is rarely visualized because of its position ❷.
  (A generalist nurse usually does not use a nasal speculum for inspection. If one is used, it is stabilized with the index finger against the side of the nose and the other hand used to position the head and then to hold the light. The speculum is opened as much as possible for inspection.)
  ■ Inspect the lining of the nares and the integrity and the position of the nasal septum.
	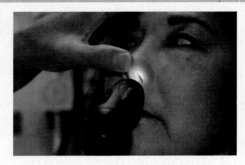
	Source: Pat Watson/Pearson Education, Inc.
	
	❶ Using a light to inspect the nasal passages.
	
	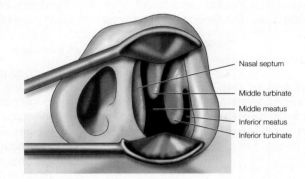
	Nasal septum
	Middle turbinate
	Middle meatus
	Inferior meatus
	Inferior turbinate
	
	❷ The inferior and middle turbinates of the nasal passage.	

10. Observe for the presence of redness, swelling, growths, and discharge.	Mucosa pink Clear, watery discharge No lesions	Mucosa red, edematous Abnormal discharge (e.g., pus) Presence of lesions (e.g., polyps)
11. Inspect the nasal septum between the nasal chambers.	Nasal septum intact and in midline	Septum deviated to the right or to the left or septum eroded
Facial Sinuses		
12. Palpate the maxillary and frontal sinuses for tenderness.	Not tender	Tenderness in one or more sinuses
13. When the procedure is complete, perform hand hygiene. Leave patient safe and comfortable. Complete documentation using forms, checklists, or electronic dropdown lists supplemented by nurse's notes or additional comments as appropriate.		

SAMPLE DOCUMENTATION

[date] 1320 Nose is straight and midline in face; no flaring of nostrils noted; no discharge or tenderness of nasal passageway; no lesions noted; pink mucosa; no tenderness or swelling over sinuses; tolerated without concern; dad held patient's hand. *G. Dawson*

Lifespan Considerations

NEWBORNS AND INFANTS

■ Ethmoid and maxillary sinuses are present at birth; frontal sinuses begin to develop by 1–2 years of age; and sphenoid sinuses develop later in childhood. Infants and young children have fewer sinus problems than older children and adolescents.

SKILL 1.23 Nose and Sinuses: Assessing (*continued*)

CHILDREN

- Ethmoid sinuses continue to develop until age 12. Sinus problems in children under this age are rare.
- Cough and runny nose are the most common signs of sinusitis in preadolescent children.
- Adolescents may have headaches, facial tenderness, and swelling, similar to the signs seen in adults.

OLDER ADULTS

- The sense of smell markedly diminishes because of a decrease in the number of olfactory nerve fibers and atrophy of the remaining fibers. Older adults are less able to identify and discriminate odors.
- Nosebleeds may result from hypertensive disease or other arterial vessel changes.

SKILL 1.24 Peripheral Vascular System: Assessing

Delegation or Assignment

Due to the substantial knowledge and skill required, assessment of the peripheral vascular system is not delegated or assigned to the UAP. However, many aspects of the vascular system are observed during usual care and may be recorded by individuals other than the nurse. Abnormal findings must be validated and interpreted by the nurse.

Equipment

No equipment is needed for this skill.

Preparation

- Have access to all peripheral pulse points before the procedure begins but keep drape in place until ready to evaluate them.

- Let the patient know when you are going to touch his or her pulse points, avoiding excessive touching which may be offensive in some cultures.

Procedure

1. Prior to performing the procedure, introduce self and verify the patient's identity using two identifiers. Explain to the patient what you are going to do, why it is necessary, and how the patient can participate. Discuss how the results will be used in planning further care or treatments.
2. Perform hand hygiene and observe other appropriate infection control procedures.
3. Provide for patient privacy.
4. Inquire if the patient has any history of the following: past history of heart disorders, varicosities, arterial disease, and hypertension; lifestyle habits such as exercise patterns, activity patterns and tolerance, smoking, and use of alcohol.

ASSESSMENT	NORMAL FINDINGS	DEVIATIONS FROM NORMAL
Peripheral Pulses		
5. Simultaneously and systematically palpate the peripheral pulses on both sides of the patient's body individually (except the carotid pulse), to determine the symmetry of pulse volume. If you have difficulty palpating some of the peripheral pulses, use a Doppler ultrasound (DUS) probe.	Symmetric pulse volumes Full pulsations	Asymmetric volumes (indicate impaired circulation) Absence of pulsation (indicates arterial spasm or occlusion) Decreased, weak, thready pulsations (indicate impaired cardiac output) Increased pulse volume (may indicate hypertension, high cardiac output, or circulatory overload)
Peripheral Veins		
6. Inspect the peripheral veins in the arms and legs for the presence and/or appearance of superficial veins when limbs are dependent and when limbs are elevated.	In dependent position, there is presence of distention and nodular bulges at calves. When limbs are elevated, veins collapse (veins may appear tortuous or distended in older people).	Distended veins in the thigh and/or lower leg or on posterolateral part of calf from knee to ankle

(*continued on next page*)

SKILL 1.24 Peripheral Vascular System: Assessing (*continued*)

ASSESSMENT	NORMAL FINDINGS	DEVIATIONS FROM NORMAL

7. Assess the peripheral leg veins for signs of phlebitis.
  ▪ Inspect the calves for redness and swelling over vein sites.
  ▪ Palpate the calves for firmness or tension of the muscles, the presence of edema over the dorsum of the foot, and areas of localized warmth. **Rationale:** *Palpation augments inspection findings, particularly for greater pigmented people in whom redness may not be visible.*
  ▪ Push the calves from side to side to test for tenderness.
  ▪ Firmly dorsiflex the patient's foot while supporting the entire leg in extension (Homans test), or have the person stand or walk.
	Limbs not tender
	Symmetric in size
		Tenderness on palpation
		Pain in calf muscles with forceful dorsiflexion of the foot (positive Homans test)
		Warmth and redness over vein
		Swelling of one calf or leg
		No one sign or symptom consistently confirms or excludes presence of phlebitis or a deep venous thrombosis. Pain, tenderness, and swelling are the most predictive.

Peripheral Perfusion

ASSESSMENT	NORMAL FINDINGS	DEVIATIONS FROM NORMAL
8. Inspect the skin of the hands and feet for color, temperature, edema, and skin changes.	Skin color pink Skin temperature not excessively warm or cold No edema Skin texture resilient and moist	Cyanotic (venous insufficiency) Pallor that increases with limb elevation Dependent rubor, a dusky red color when limb is lowered (arterial insufficiency) Brown pigmentation around ankles (arterial or chronic venous insufficiency) Cool skin (arterial insufficiency) Marked edema (venous insufficiency) Mild edema (arterial insufficiency) Skin thin and shiny or thick, waxy, shiny, and fragile, with reduced hair and/or ulceration (venous or arterial insufficiency)
9. Assess the adequacy of arterial flow if arterial insufficiency is suspected.		

Capillary Refill Test

ASSESSMENT	NORMAL FINDINGS	DEVIATIONS FROM NORMAL
▪ Squeeze the patient's fingernail and toenail between your fingers sufficiently to cause blanching (about 5 seconds). ▪ Release the pressure, and observe how quickly normal color returns. Color normally returns immediately (less than 2 seconds).	Immediate return of color	Delayed return of color (arterial insufficiency)

Other Assessments

ASSESSMENT	NORMAL FINDINGS	DEVIATIONS FROM NORMAL
▪ Inspect the fingernails for changes indicative of circulatory impairment. (Also see Skill 1.20 on assessment of nails.)		
10. When the procedure is complete, perform hand hygiene. Leave patient safe and comfortable. Complete documentation using forms, checklists, or electronic dropdown lists supplemented by nurse's notes or additional comments as appropriate.		

SKILL 1.24 Peripheral Vascular System: Assessing (*continued*)

Patient Teaching

- Use the assessment as an opportunity to provide teaching regarding appropriate care of the extremities in those at high risk for or with actual vascular impairment. Educate patients and families about skin and nail care, exercise, and positioning to promote circulation.

Lifespan Considerations

NEWBORNS AND INFANTS

- Screen for coarctation of the aorta by palpating the peripheral pulses and comparing the strength of the femoral pulses with the radial pulses and apical pulse. If coarctation is present, femoral pulses will be diminished and radial pulses will be stronger.

CHILDREN

- Changes in the peripheral vasculature, such as bruising, petechiae, and purpura, can indicate serious systemic diseases in children (e.g., leukemia, meningococcemia).

OLDER ADULTS

- The overall effectiveness of blood vessels decreases as smooth muscle cells are replaced by connective tissue. The lower extremities are more likely to show signs of arterial and venous impairment because of the more distal and dependent position.
- Peripheral vascular assessment should always include upper and lower extremities' temperature, color, pulses, edema, skin integrity, and sensation. Any differences in symmetry of these findings should be noted.
- Blood vessels lengthen and become more twisted and prominent. Varicosities occur more frequently.
- The most distal pulses of the lower extremities are more difficult to palpate because of decreased arterial perfusion.
- Systolic and diastolic blood pressures increase, but the increase in the systolic pressure is greater. As a result, the pulse pressure widens. Any patient with a blood pressure reading above 140/90 should be referred for follow-up assessments.
- Peripheral edema is frequently observed and is most commonly the result of chronic venous insufficiency or low protein levels in the blood (hypoproteinemia).

SKILL 1.25 Skin: Assessing

Inspection and palpation of the skin is performed to identify cutaneous problems as well as systemic diseases.

Delegation or Assignment

Due to the substantial knowledge and skill required, assessment of the skin is not delegated or assigned to the UAP. However, the skin is observed during usual care and the UAP should record their findings. Abnormal findings must be validated and interpreted by the nurse.

Equipment

- Millimeter ruler
- Clean gloves
- Magnifying glass

Preparation

- If a rash is present on newborn, infant, or child, inquire in detail about immunization history.
- Assess skin turgor by pinching the skin on the abdomen of a child.

- Due to the normal loss of peripheral skin turgor in older adults, assess for hydration by checking skin turgor over the sternum or clavicle.

Procedure

1. Prior to performing the procedure, introduce self and verify the patient's identity using two identifiers. Explain to the patient what you are going to do, why it is necessary, and how the patient can participate. Discuss how the results will be used in planning further care or treatments.
2. Perform hand hygiene and observe other appropriate infection control procedures.
3. Provide for patient privacy.
4. Inquire if the patient has any history of the following: pain or itching; presence and spread of lesions, bruises, abrasions, pigmented spots; previous experience with skin problems; associated clinical signs; family history; presence of problems in other family members; related systemic conditions; use of medications, lotions, home remedies; excessively dry or moist feel to the skin; tendency to bruise easily; association of the problem with season of year, stress, occupation, medications, recent travel, housing, and so on; recent contact with allergens (e.g., metal paint).

(*continued on next page*)

SKILL 1.25 Skin: Assessing (continued)

ASSESSMENT	NORMAL FINDINGS	DEVIATIONS FROM NORMAL
5. Inspect skin color (best assessed under natural light and on areas not exposed to the sun).	Varies from light to deep brown or black; from light pink to ruddy pink; from yellow overtones to olive	Pallor, cyanosis, jaundice, erythema
6. Inspect uniformity of skin color.	Generally uniform except in areas exposed to the sun; areas of lighter pigmentation (palms, lips, nail beds) in dark-skinned people	Areas of either hyperpigmentation or hypopigmentation
7. Assess edema, if present (i.e., location, color, temperature, shape, and the degree to which the skin remains indented or pitted when pressed by a finger) ❶. Measuring the circumference of the extremity with a millimeter tape may be useful for future comparison.	No edema	See the scale for describing edema.
8. Inspect, palpate, and describe skin lesions ❷. Don gloves if lesions are open or draining. Palpate lesions to determine shape and texture (**Table 1–10 》**). Describe lesions according to location, distribution, color, configuration, size, shape (**Table 1–11 》**; see **Box 1–4 》**). Use the millimeter ruler to measure lesions. If gloves were applied, remove and discard gloves. Perform hand hygiene.	Freckles, pigmented birthmarks that have not changed since childhood, and some long-standing vascular birthmarks such as strawberry or port-wine hemangiomas, some flat and raised nevi (moles); no abrasions or other lesions	Various interruptions in skin integrity; irregular, multicolored, or raised nevi, some pigmented birthmarks such as melanocytic nevi, and some vascular birthmarks such as cavernous hemangiomas. Even these deviations from normal may not be dangerous or require treatment. Assessment by an advanced-level practitioner is required.

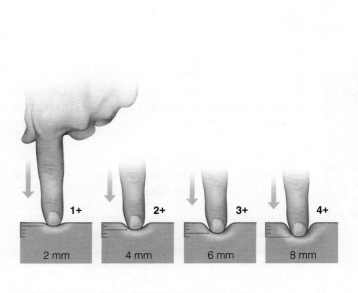

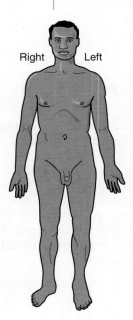

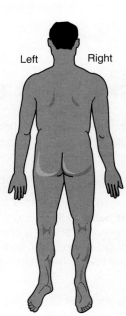

❶ Scale for grading edema.

❷ Diagram for charting skin lesions.

ASSESSMENT	NORMAL FINDINGS	DEVIATIONS FROM NORMAL
9. Observe and palpate skin moisture.	Moisture in skinfolds and the axillae (varies with environmental temperature and humidity, body temperature, and activity)	Excessive moisture (e.g., in hyperthermia); excessive dryness (e.g., in dehydration)
10. Palpate skin temperature. Compare the two feet and the two hands, using the backs of your fingers.	Uniform; within normal range	Generalized hyperthermia (e.g., in fever); generalized hypothermia (e.g., in shock); localized hyperthermia (e.g., in infection); localized hypothermia (e.g., in arteriosclerosis)

SKILL 1.25 Skin: Assessing (continued)

TABLE 1–10 Primary Skin Lesions

Macule, Patch

Source: Michael P. Gadomski / Science Source

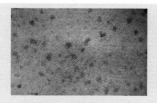

A. Multiple café-au-lait macules

Flat, unelevated change in color. Macules are 1 mm to 1 cm (0.04 to 0.4 in.) in size and circumscribed. Examples: freckles, measles, petechiae, flat moles.

Patches are larger than 1 cm (0.4 in.) and may have an irregular shape. Examples: port-wine birthmark, vitiligo (white patches), rubella.

Papule

Source: Hercules Robinson/Alamy Stock Photo

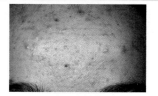

B. Papular drug eruption

Circumscribed, solid elevation of skin. Papules are less than 1 cm (0.4 in.). Examples: warts, acne, pimples, elevated moles.

Plaque

Source: Olavs Silis/Alamy Stock Photo

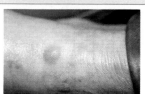

C. Psoriasis vulgaris

Plaques are larger than 1 cm (0.4 in.). Examples: psoriasis, rubeola.

Nodule, Tumor

Source: DermPics / Science Source

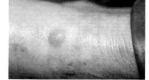

D. Peripheral neurofibromas

Elevated, solid, hard mass that extends deeper into the dermis than a papule.

Nodules have a circumscribed border and are 0.5 to 2 cm (0.2 to 0.8 in.). Examples: squamous cell carcinoma, fibroma. Tumors are larger than 2 cm (0.8 in.) and may have an irregular border. Examples: malignant melanoma, hemangioma.

Pustule

Source: Dr. Harout Tanielian / Science Source

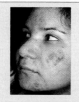

E. Chronic pustular psoriasis

Vesicle or bulla filled with pus. Examples: acne vulgaris, impetigo.

Vesicle, Bulla

Source: Scott Camazine / Science Source

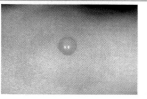

F. Bullous pemphigoid

A circumscribed, round or oval, thin translucent mass filled with serous fluid or blood.

Vesicles are less than 0.5 cm (0.2 in.).

Examples: herpes simplex, early chickenpox, small burn blister.

Bullae are larger than 0.5 cm (0.2 in.).

Examples: large blister, seconddegree burn, herpes simplex.

Cyst

Source: Mediscan/Alamy Stock Photo

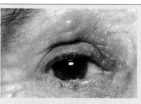

G. Digital mucous cyst

A 1-cm (0.4 in.) or larger, elevated, encapsulated, fluid-filled or semi-solid mass arising from the subcutaneous tissue or dermis. Examples: sebaceousand epidermoid cysts, chalazion of the eyelid.

Wheal

Source: Ted Kinsman / Science Source

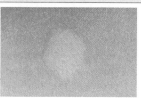

H. Allergic wheals, urticaria

A reddened, localized collection of edema fluid; irregular in shape. Size varies. Examples: hives, mosquito bites.

(continued on next page)

SKILL 1.25 Skin: Assessing (continued)

ASSESSMENT	NORMAL FINDINGS	DEVIATIONS FROM NORMAL
11. Note skin turgor (fullness or elasticity) by lifting and pinching the skin on an extremity.	When pinched, skin springs back to previous state; may be slower in older adults.	Skin stays pinched or tented or moves back slowly (e.g., in dehydration). Count in seconds how long the skin remains tented.
12. When the procedure is completed, perform hand hygiene. Leave patient safe and comfortable. Complete documentation using forms, checklists, or electronic dropdown lists supplemented by nurse's notes or additional comments as appropriate. If possible and the patient agrees, take a digital or instant photograph of significant skin lesions for the patient record. Include a measuring guide (ruler or tape) in the picture to indicate lesion size. If not possible, draw location of skin lesions on body surface diagrams.		

SAMPLE DOCUMENTATION

[date] 1000 Skin tone deep brown and even throughout; warm and dry to touch; turgor non-tenting; no signs of breakdown or edema noted; dark pigmented birthmark on left posterior shoulder; scattered small moles noted on both arms; no areas of tenderness tolerated without complaint. *R. Graves*

Box 1–4
Describing Skin Lesions

- **Type or structure.** Skin lesions are classified as primary (those that appear initially in response to some change in the external or internal environment of the skin) and secondary (those that do not appear initially but result from modifications such as chronicity, trauma, or infection of the primary lesion). For example, a vesicle (primary lesion) may rupture and cause an erosion (secondary lesion).
- **Size, shape, and texture.** Note size in millimeters and whether the lesion is circumscribed or irregular; round or oval shaped; flat, elevated, or depressed; solid, soft, or hard; rough or thickened; fluid filled or has flakes.
- **Color.** There may be no discoloration, one color (e.g., red, brown, or black), or several colors, as with ecchymosis (a bruise), in which an initial dark red or blue color fades to a yellow color. When color changes are limited to the edges of a lesion, they are described as circumscribed; when spread over a large area, they are described as diffuse.
- **Distribution.** Distribution is described according to the location of the lesions on the body and symmetry or asymmetry of findings in comparable body areas.
- **Configuration.** Configuration refers to the arrangement of lesions in relation to each other. Configurations of lesions may be annular (arranged in a circle), clustered together or grouped, linear (arranged in a line), arc or bow shaped, or merged together or indiscrete. They may follow the course of cutaneous nerves, or be meshed in the form of a network.

Lifespan Considerations
NEWBORNS AND INFANTS

- *Physiological* jaundice may appear in newborns 2–3 days after birth and usually lasts about 1 week. Pathological jaundice, or that which indicates a disease, appears within 24 hours of birth and may last more than 8 days.
- Newborns may have milia (whiteheads), tiny white nodules over the nose and face, and vernix caseosa (white, cheesy, greasy material on the skin).
- Premature newborns and infants may have lanugo, a fine downy hair covering their shoulders and back.
- In dark-skinned newborns or infants, areas of hyperpigmentation may be found, especially on the back, in the sacral area.
- Diaper dermatitis (a rash in the groin area) may be seen in newborns or infants.

CHILDREN

- Children normally have minor skin lesions (e.g., bruising or abrasions) on arms and legs due to their high activity level. Lesions on other parts of the body may be signs of disease or abuse, and a thorough history should be taken.
- Secondary skin lesions may occur frequently as children scratch or expose a primary lesion to microbes.
- With puberty, oil glands become more productive, and children may develop acne. Most individuals of age 12–24 have some acne.
- In dark-skinned children, areas of hyperpigmentation may be found on the back, especially in the sacral area.

SKILL 1.25 Skin: Assessing (continued)

TABLE 1–11 Secondary Skin Lesions

Atrophy

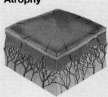

A translucent, dry, paper-like, sometimes wrinkled skin surface resulting from thinning or wasting of the skin due to loss of collagen and elastin.

Examples: Striae, aged skin

Ulcer

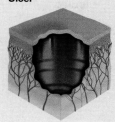

Deep, irregularly shaped area of skin loss extending into the dermis or subcutaneous tissue. May bleed. May leave scar.

Examples: Pressure ulcers, stasis ulcers, chancres

Erosion

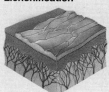

Wearing away of the superficial epidermis causing a moist, shallow depression. Because erosions do not extend into the dermis, they heal without scarring.

Examples: Scratch marks, ruptured vesicles

Fissure

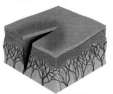

Linear crack with sharp edges, extending into the dermis.

Examples: Cracks at the corners of the mouth or in the hands, athlete's foot

Lichenification

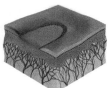

Rough, thickened, hardened area of epidermis resulting from chronic irritation such as scratching or rubbing.

Examples: Chronic dermatitis

Scar

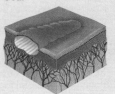

Flat, irregular area of connective tissue left after a lesion or wound has healed. New scars may be red or purple; older scars may be silvery or white.

Examples: Healed surgical wound or injury, healed acne

Scales

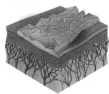

Shedding flakes of greasy, keratinized skin tissue. Color may be white, gray, or silver. Texture may vary from fine to thick.

Examples: Dry skin, dandruff, psoriasis, and eczema

Keloid

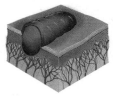

Elevated, irregular, darkened area of excess scar tissue caused by excessive collagen formation during healing. Extends beyond the site of the original injury. Higher incidence in people of African descent.

Examples: Keloid from ear piercing or surgery

Crust

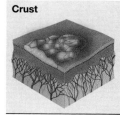

Dry blood, serum, or pus left on the skin surface when vesicles or pustules burst. Can be red-brown, orange, or yellow. Large crusts that adhere to the skin surface are called scabs.

Examples: Eczema, impetigo, herpes, or scabs following abrasion

Excoriation

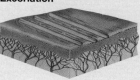

Linear erosion.

Examples: Scratches, some chemical burns

OLDER ADULTS

- The skin loses its elasticity and develops wrinkles. Wrinkles first appear on the skin of the face and neck, which are abundant in collagen and elastic fibers.
- The skin becomes dry and flaky because sebaceous and sweat glands are less active. Dry skin is more prominent over the extremities.
- The skin takes longer to return to its natural shape after being pinched between the thumb and finger. This is called tenting.
- Flat tan to brown-colored macules, referred to as senile lentigines or melanotic freckles, are normally apparent on the back of the hand and other skin areas that are exposed to the sun.

- Cutaneous tags (acrochordons) are most commonly seen in the neck and axillary regions. These skin lesions vary in size and are soft, often flesh colored, and pedicled.
- Visible, bright red, fine dilated blood vessels commonly occur as a result of the thinning of the dermis and the loss of support for the blood vessel walls.
- Pink to slightly red lesions with indistinct borders (actinic keratoses) may appear at about age 50, often on the face, ears, backs of the hands, and arms. They may become malignant if untreated.

SKILL 1.26 Skull and Face: Assessing

Delegation or Assignment

Due to the substantial knowledge and skill required, assessment of the skull and face is not delegated or assigned to the UAP. However, many aspects of the skull and face are observed during usual care and may be recorded by individuals other than the nurse. Abnormal findings must be validated and interpreted by the nurse.

Equipment

No equipment is required for this skill.

Preparation

- Move hair away from face for better observation.
- Be aware of eye contact, some cultures avoid it as a sign of respect for the other individual.

Procedure

1. Prior to performing the procedure, introduce self and verify the patient's identity using two identifiers. Explain to the patient what you are going to do, why it is necessary, and how the patient can participate. Discuss how the results will be used in planning further care or treatments.
2. Perform hand hygiene and observe other appropriate infection control procedures.
3. Provide for patient privacy.
4. Inquire if the patient has any history of the following: past problems with lumps or bumps, itching, scaling, or dandruff; history of loss of consciousness, dizziness, seizures, headache, facial pain, or injury; when and how any lumps occurred; length of time any other problem existed; any known cause of problem; associated symptoms, treatment, and recurrences.

ASSESSMENT	NORMAL FINDINGS	DEVIATIONS FROM NORMAL
5. Inspect the skull for size, shape, and symmetry.	Rounded (normocephalic and symmetric, with frontal, parietal, and occipital prominences); smooth skull contour	Lack of symmetry; increased skull size with more prominent nose and forehead; longer mandible (may indicate excessive growth hormone or increased bone thickness)
6. Inspect the facial features (e.g., symmetry of structures and of the distribution of hair).	Symmetric or slightly asymmetric facial features, palpebral fissures equal in size, symmetric nasolabial folds	Increased facial hair, low hair line, thinning of eyebrows, asymmetric features, exophthalmos, myxedema facies, moon face
7. Inspect the eyes for edema and hollowness.	No edema	Periorbital edema; sunken eyes
8. Note symmetry of facial movements. Ask the patient to elevate the eyebrows, frown, or lower the eyebrows, close the eyes tightly, puff the cheeks, and smile and show the teeth.	Symmetric facial movements	Asymmetric facial movements (e.g., eye on affected side cannot close completely); drooping of lower eyelid and mouth; involuntary facial movements (i.e., tics or tremors)
9. When the procedure is complete, perform hand hygiene. Leave patient safe and comfortable. Complete documentation using forms, checklists, or electronic dropdown lists supplemented by nurse's notes or additional comments as appropriate.		

SAMPLE DOCUMENTATION

[date] 1720 Rounded smooth skull contour; symmetric facial features; no edema or tenderness to touch; facial movements equal bilaterally; tolerated without crying with mom holding child. *T. Graham*

Lifespan Considerations
NEWBORNS AND INFANTS

- Newborns delivered vaginally can have elongated, molded heads, which take on more rounded shapes after a week or two. Newborns born by cesarean section tend to have smooth, rounded heads.

- The posterior fontanel (soft spot) is about 1 cm in size and usually closes by 8 weeks. The anterior fontanel is larger, about 2–3 cm in size. It closes by 18 months.

- Newborns can lift their heads slightly and turn them from side to side. Voluntary head control is well established by 4–6 months.

SKILL 1.27 Thorax and Lungs: Assessing

Clinical examination involves inspection, palpation, percussion, and auscultation of the chest to evaluate the performance of respiratory and ventilatory functioning and determine the state of underlying tissues. Further investigation of potential pulmonary disease may also be done.

Delegation or Assignment

Assessment of the thorax and lungs is not delegated or assigned to the UAP. However, many aspects of breathing are observed during usual care and may be recorded by individuals other than the nurse. Abnormal findings must be validated and interpreted by the nurse.

Equipment

- Stethoscope
- Skin marker/pencil
- Centimeter ruler

Preparation

- To assess tactile fremitus, place your hand over the crying newborn's or infant's thorax.

- Children tend to breathe more abdominally than thoracically up to age 6 years, so your hand on abdomen may help measure respirations.
- In older adults, breathing rate and rhythm are unchanged at rest; the rate normally increases with exercise but may take longer to return to the pre-exercise rate.

Procedure

1. Prior to performing the procedure, introduce self and verify the patient's identity using two identifiers. Explain to the patient what you are going to do, why it is necessary, and how the patient can participate. Discuss how the results will be used in planning further care or treatments.
2. Perform hand hygiene and observe other appropriate infection control procedures.
3. Provide for patient privacy. In women, drape the anterior thorax when it is not being examined.
4. Inquire if the patient has any history of the following: family history of illness, including cancer, allergies, tuberculosis; lifestyle habits such as smoking and occupational hazards (e.g., inhaling fumes); medications being taken; current problems (e.g., swellings, coughs, wheezing, pain).

ASSESSMENT	NORMAL FINDINGS	DEVIATIONS FROM NORMAL
Posterior Thorax		
5. Inspect the shape and symmetry of the thorax from posterior and lateral views. Compare the anteroposterior diameter to the transverse diameter.	Anteroposterior to transverse diameter in ratio of 1:2 Thorax symmetric	Barrel chest; increased anteroposterior to transverse diameter Thorax asymmetric
6. Inspect the spinal alignment for deformities. Have the patient stand. From a lateral position, observe the three normal curvatures: cervical, thoracic, and lumbar. ■ To assess for lateral deviation of the spine (scoliosis), observe the standing patient from the rear. Have the patient bend forward at the waist and observe from behind.	Spine vertically aligned Spinal column is straight; right and left shoulders and hips are at same height.	Exaggerated spinal curvatures (kyphosis, lordosis) Spinal column deviates to one side, often accentuated when bending over. Shoulders or hips not even (level)
7. Palpate the posterior thorax. ■ For patients who have no respiratory complaints, rapidly assess the temperature and integrity of all thorax skin. ■ For patients who do have respiratory complaints, palpate all areas for bulges, tenderness, or abnormal movements. Avoid deep palpation for painful areas, especially if a fractured rib is suspected. In such a case, deep palpation could lead to displacement of the bone fragment against the lungs.	Skin intact; uniform temperature Thorax intact; no tenderness; no masses	Skin lesions; areas of hyperthermia Lumps, bulges; depressions; areas of tenderness; movable structures (e.g., rib)

(continued on next page)

SKILL 1.27 Thorax and Lungs: Assessing *(continued)*

ASSESSMENT	NORMAL FINDINGS	DEVIATIONS FROM NORMAL
8. Palpate the posterior thorax for respiratory excursion (thoracic expansion). Place the palms of both your hands over the lower thorax with your thumbs adjacent to the spine and your fingers stretched laterally ❶. Ask the patient to take a deep breath while you observe the movement of your hands and any lag in movement.	Full and symmetric thorax expansion (When the patient takes a deep breath, your thumbs should move apart an equal distance and at the same time; normally the thumbs separate 3–5 cm [1.5–2 in.] during deep inspiration.)	Asymmetric and/or decreased thorax expansion 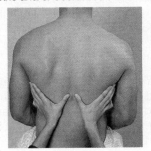 *Source:* Richard Tauber/Pearson Education, Inc. ❶ Position of the nurse's hands when assessing posterior respiratory excursion on the posterior thorax.
9. Palpate the posterior thorax for vocal (tactile) **fremitus**, the faintly perceptible vibration felt through the chest wall when the patient speaks. ▪ Place the palmar surfaces of your fingertips or the ulnar aspect of your hand or closed fist on the posterior thorax, starting near the apex of the lungs ❷, position A. ▪ Ask the patient to repeat such words as "blue moon" or "one, two, three." ▪ Repeat the two steps, moving your hands sequentially to the base of the lungs, through positions B–E in ❷. ▪ Compare the fremitus on both lungs and between the apex and the base of each lung, using either one hand and moving it from one side of the patient to the corresponding area on the other side *or* using two hands that are placed simultaneously on the corresponding areas of each side of the thorax.	Bilateral symmetry of vocal fremitus Fremitus is heard most clearly at the apex of the lungs. Low-pitched voices of males are more readily palpated than higher-pitched voices of females.	Decreased or absent fremitus (associated with pneumothorax) Increased fremitus (associated with consolidated lung tissue, as in pneumonia) 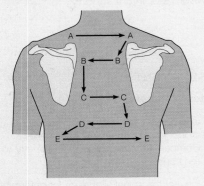 ❷ Areas and sequence for palpating tactile fremitus on the posterior chest.
10. Percuss the thorax. Percussion of the thorax is performed to determine whether underlying lung tissue is filled with air, liquid, or solid material and to determine the positions and boundaries of certain organs. Because percussion penetrates to a depth of 5–7.6 cm (2–3 in.), it detects superficial rather than deep lesions ❸. ▪ Ask the patient to bend the head and fold the arms forward across the chest. **Rationale:** *This separates the scapula and exposes more lung tissue to percussion.* ▪ Percuss in the intercostal spaces at about 5-cm (2-in.) intervals in a systematic sequence ❹. ▪ Compare one side of the lung with the other. ▪ Percuss the lateral thorax every few inches, starting at the axilla and working down to the eighth rib.	Percussion notes resonate, except over scapula. Lowest point of resonance is at the diaphragm (i.e., at the level of the eighth to tenth rib posteriorly). *Note:* Percussion on a rib normally elicits dullness. 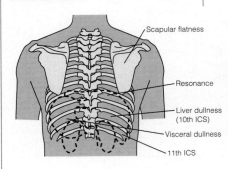 ❸ Normal percussion sounds on the posterior chest.	Asymmetry in percussion Areas of dullness or flatness over lung tissue (associated with fluid, consolidation of lung tissue, or a mass) 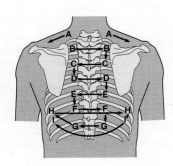 ❹ Sequence for posterior chest percussion.

SKILL 1.27 Thorax and Lungs: Assessing (continued)

ASSESSMENT	NORMAL FINDINGS	DEVIATIONS FROM NORMAL
11. Auscultate the thorax using the diaphragm of the stethoscope. **Rationale:** *The diaphragm of the stethoscope is best for transmitting the high-pitched breath sounds.* ■ Use the systematic zigzag procedure used in percussion. ■ Ask the patient to take slow, deep breaths through the mouth. Listen at each point to the breath sounds during a complete inspiration and expiration. ■ Compare findings at each point with the corresponding point on the opposite side of the thorax.	Vesicular and bronchovesicular breath sounds	Adventitious breath sounds (e.g., crackles, gurgles, friction rub, wheeze) on inspiration and/or expiration Absence of breath sounds
12. Inspect breathing patterns (e.g., respiratory rate and rhythm).	Quiet, rhythmic, and effortless respirations	See Table 1–5 for altered breathing patterns and sounds.
13. Inspect the costal angle (angle formed by the intersection of the costal margins) and the angle at which the ribs enter the spine.	Costal angle is less than 90 degrees, and the ribs insert into the spine at an approximate 45-degree angle.	Costal angle is widened (associated with chronic obstructive pulmonary disease [COPD]).
14. Palpate the anterior thorax (also see posterior thorax palpation).		
15. Palpate the anterior thorax for respiratory excursion. ■ Place the palms of both hands on the lower thorax, with your fingers laterally along the lower rib cage and your thumbs along the costal margins ⑤. ■ Ask the patient to take a deep breath while you observe the movement of your hands.	Full symmetric excursion; thumbs normally separate 3–5 cm (1.5–2 in.) *Source:* Richard Tauber/Pearson Education, Inc. ⑤ **Position of the nurse's hands when assessing respiratory excursion on the anterior thorax.**	Asymmetric and/or decreased respiratory excursion
16. Palpate anterior tactile fremitus in the same manner as for the posterior thorax and using the sequence shown in ⑥. If the breasts are large and cannot be retracted adequately for palpation, this part of the examination is usually omitted.	Same as posterior vocal fremitus; fremitus is normally decreased over heart and breast tissue.	Same as posterior fremitus ⑥ **Areas and sequence for palpating tactile fremitus on the anterior thorax.**

(continued on next page)

SKILL 1.27 Thorax and Lungs: Assessing (continued)

ASSESSMENT	NORMAL FINDINGS	DEVIATIONS FROM NORMAL
17. Percuss the anterior thorax systematically. ■ Begin above the clavicles in the supraclavicular space, and proceed downward to the diaphragm ❼. ■ Compare one side of the lung to the other. ■ Displace female breast to facilitate percussion of the lungs.	Percussion notes resonate down to the sixth rib at the level of the diaphragm but are flat over areas of heavy muscle and bone, dull on areas over the heart and the liver, and tympanic over the underlying stomach ❽.	Asymmetry in percussion notes Areas of dullness or flatness over lung tissue

❼ Sequence for anterior thorax percussion.

Flatness over heavy muscles and bones
Resonance
Cardiac dullness
5th ICS
Liver dullness
Costal margin
Stomach tympany (6th ICS)

❽ Normal percussion sounds on the anterior thorax.

ASSESSMENT	NORMAL FINDINGS	DEVIATIONS FROM NORMAL
18. Auscultate the trachea.	Bronchial and tubular breath sounds (see normal breath sounds in **Table 1–12 ≫**)	Adventitious breath sounds (see adventitious breath sounds in **Table 1–13 ≫**)
19. Auscultate the anterior thorax. Use the sequence used in percussion, beginning over the bronchi between the sternum and the clavicles.	Bronchovesicular and vesicular breath sounds	Adventitious breath sounds
20. When the procedure is complete, perform hand hygiene. Leave patient safe and comfortable. Complete documentation using forms, checklists, or electronic dropdown lists supplemented by nurse's notes or additional comments as appropriate.		

TABLE 1–12 Normal Breath Sounds

Type	Description	Location	Characteristics
Vesicular	Soft-intensity, low-pitched, "gentle sighing" sounds created by air moving through smaller airways (bronchioles and alveoli)	Over peripheral lung; best heard at base of lungs	Best heard on inspiration, which is about 2.5 times longer than the expiratory phase (5:2 ratio)
Bronchovesicular	Moderate-intensity and moderate-pitched "blowing" sounds created by air moving through larger airways (bronchi)	Between the scapulae and lateral to the sternum at the first and second intercostal spaces	Equal inspiratory and expiratory phases (1:1 ratio)
Bronchial (tubular)	High-pitched, loud, "harsh" sounds created by air moving through the trachea	Anteriorly over the trachea; not normally heard over lung tissue	Louder than vesicular sounds; have a short inspiratory phase and long expiratory phase (1:2 ratio)

SKILL 1.27 Thorax and Lungs: Assessing (*continued*)

TABLE 1–13 Adventitious Breath Sounds

Name	Description	Cause	Location
Crackles (rales)	Fine, short, interrupted crackling sounds; alveolar rales are high pitched. Sound can be simulated by rolling a lock of hair near the ear. Best heard on inspiration but can be heard on both inspiration and expiration. May not be cleared by coughing	Air passing through fluid or collapsed smaller air passages or alveoli	Most commonly heard in the bases of the lower lung lobes
Gurgles (rhonchi)	Continuous, low-pitched, coarse, gurgling, harsh, louder sounds with a moaning or snoring quality Best heard on expiration, but can be heard on both inspiration and expiration.	Air passing through narrowed air passages as a result of secretions, swelling, tumors	Loud sounds can be heard over most lung areas but dominate over the trachea and bronchi. May be altered by coughing
Friction rub	Superficial grating or creaking sounds heard during inspiration and expiration Not relieved by coughing.	Rubbing together of inflamed pleural surfaces	Heard most often in areas of greatest thoracic expansion (e.g., lower anterior and lateral thorax)
Wheezes	Continuous, high-pitched, squeaky musical sounds Best heard on expiration Not usually altered by coughing	Air passing through a constricted bronchus as a result of secretions, swelling, tumors	Heard over all lung fields

SAMPLE DOCUMENTATION

[date] 0830 Bilateral upper lobes clear to auscultation; fine crackles both lower lobes. Temp. 99.2°F (37.3°C) (O); pulse 78 bpm; respiration 20/min; BP 134/82; O₂ Sat. 95% on room air. Rarely moves in bed. Assisted to a chair. Reviewed deep breathing exercises. Effective return demonstration. *N. Schmidt*

Lifespan Considerations

NEWBORNS AND INFANTS

- The thorax is rounded; that is, the diameter from the front to the back (anteroposterior) is equal to the transverse diameter. It is also cylindrical, having a nearly equal diameter at the top and the base. This makes it harder for newborns or infants to expand their thoracic space **9**.

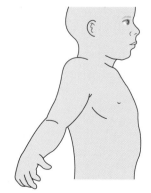
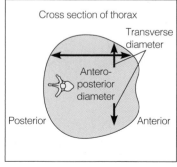

Clinical appearance

Cross section of thorax

Transverse diameter

Antero-posterior diameter

Posterior   Anterior

9 Configurations of the child's thorax showing anteroposterior diameter and transverse diameter.

- Newborns or infants tend to breathe using their diaphragm; assess rate and rhythm by watching the abdomen, rather than the thorax, rise and fall.
- The right bronchial branch is short and angles downward as it leaves the trachea, making it easy for small objects to be inhaled. Sudden onset of cough or other signs of respiratory distress may indicate that the newborn or infant has inhaled a foreign object.

CHILDREN

- By about 6 years of age, the anteroposterior diameter has decreased in proportion to the transverse diameter, with a 1:2 ratio present.
- During the rapid growth spurts of adolescence, spinal curvature and rotation (scoliosis) may appear. Children should be assessed for scoliosis by age 12 and annually until their growth slows. Curvature greater than 10% should be referred for further medical evaluation.

OLDER ADULTS

- The thoracic curvature may be accentuated (kyphosis) because of osteoporosis and changes in cartilage, resulting in collapse of the vertebrae. This can also compromise and decrease normal respiratory effort **10**.
- Kyphosis and osteoporosis alter the size of the chest cavity as the ribs move downward and forward.
- The anteroposterior diameter of the thorax widens, giving the person a barrel-chested appearance. This is due to loss of skeletal muscle strength in the thorax and diaphragm and constant lung inflation from excessive expiratory pressure on the alveoli.
- Inspiratory muscles become less powerful, and the inspiratory reserve volume decreases. A decrease in depth of respiration is therefore apparent.
- Expiration may require the use of accessory muscles. The expiratory reserve volume significantly increases because of the

(*continued on next page*)

SKILL 1.27 Thorax and Lungs: Assessing (continued)

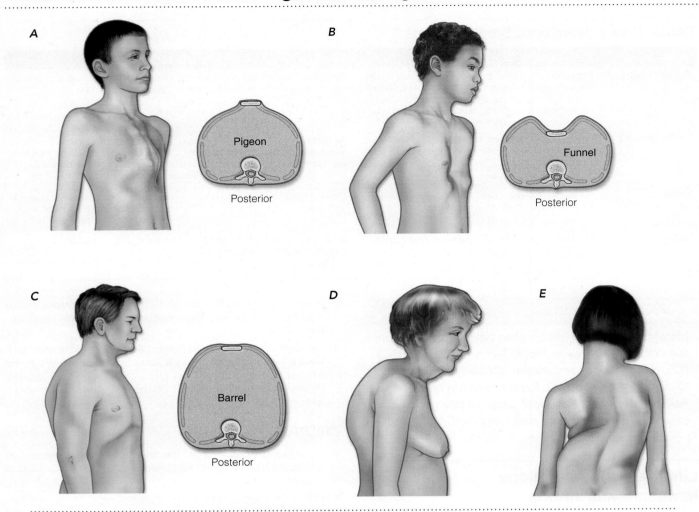

⑩ Chest deformities: **A,** pigeon chest; **B,** funnel chest; **C,** barrel chest; **D,** kyphosis; **E,** scoliosis.

increased amount of air remaining in the lungs at the end of a normal breath.

■ Small airways lose their cartilaginous support and elastic recoil; as a result, they tend to close, particularly in basal or dependent portions of the lung.

■ Elastic tissue of the alveoli loses its ability to stretch and changes to fibrous tissue. Exertional capacity decreases.

■ Cilia in the airways decrease in number and are less effective in removing mucus; older patients are therefore at greater risk for pulmonary infections.

›› Physical Assessment for the Newborn

For physical assessment of the newborn, see Chapter 14 on Reproduction.

›› Critical Thinking Options for Unexpected Outcomes

Not all unexpected outcomes require nursing intervention; however, many times they do. When the patient demonstrates a change in signs or symptoms indicating an emerging problem, the nurse should immediately assess and troubleshoot what is happening. The assess-ment data must be processed quickly to formulate a hypothesis so the nurse can make a clinical judgment. The nurse then decides how best to resolve the problem and improve the patient's situation for a better outcome.

EXPECTED OUTCOME	UNEXPECTED OUTCOME	POSSIBLE INTERVENTIONS
General Assessment Height and weight are obtained and recorded.	Patient's weight varies more than expected from one day to the next.	■ Verify time of day weights were measured. ■ Verify if same scale was used for both weights. ■ Verify equipment's reliability. ■ Verify what clothing or linen was on the patient when weighed on both days. ■ Verify I&O record for sources of fluid loss or gain. ■ Verify MAR for medications that alter fluid balance (e.g., diuretics).
Vital Signs Temperature is within normal range.	Fever develops.	■ Verify possible sources of infection and take preventive measures. ■ Notify healthcare provider as needed. ■ Implement cooling methods if temperature is dangerously high, such as tepid sponge bath, cool oral fluids, ice packs, or antipyretic drugs as ordered. ■ Assess all vital signs.
Temperature is within normal range.	Temperature remains elevated because of bacterial-produced pyrogens.	■ Request order to obtain culture of possible sources of infection. ■ Give antipyretics and other drugs as ordered. ■ Decrease room temperature and remove excess covers. ■ Give tepid sponge bath.
	Temperature remains subnormal.	■ Assess for blood clots; extreme low temperature can cause vasoconstriction. ■ Implement measures to promote vasodilation (application of warmth). ■ If extremity is ischemic, monitor that heat source does not exceed body temperature.
Pulse is palpated without difficulty.	Apical, femoral, and carotid pulses are absent.	■ Assess all vital signs and status of the patient. ■ Immediately call for the rapid response team. ■ Initiate CPR immediately. ■ Use Doppler device to assess for presence of pulse.
	Peripheral pulse is absent.	■ Assess for other signs and symptoms of circulatory impairment.
Respiratory rate, rhythm, and depth are within normal limits.	Apnea (absence of breathing) occurs, may be intermittent.	■ Assess patient for pulse. ■ Begin rescue breathing at the rate of 12 per minute for an adult or 20 per minute for a child.
Labored, difficult, or noisy respirations are assessed.	Kussmaul respirations occur (deep and gasping breaths—more than 20 breaths/min).	■ Implement orders for diabetic ketoacidosis, renal failure, or septic shock.
The presence of factors that can alter blood pressure readings is identified.	Blood pressure reading is abnormally high without apparent physiological cause.	■ Verify that proper BP cuff size was used. ■ Verify BP cuff was snug. ■ Ask if patient has pain, was anxious, had just consumed caffeine, or had just exercised. ■ Verify blood pressure on both arms. The normal difference from arm to arm is usually about 5 mmHg. ■ Ask patient to sit and rest for 15 minutes and then retake blood pressure reading.
Accurate readings are taken by using the correct BP cuff size and procedure.	Blood pressure cannot be measured on upper extremity due to casts, dialysis shunt, or surgical procedure.	■ Use thigh of lower extremity to obtain blood pressures. ■ Be sure to document site where blood pressure reading was obtained.
	Hypotension (systolic pressure less than 90 mmHg) develops.	■ Take all vital signs more frequently until condition has stabilized. ■ Place patient in supine position with lower extremities elevated 45 degrees. ■ Assess cause of hypotension, and notify healthcare provider. ■ Increase or administer fluids as ordered by healthcare provider. ■ Observe postoperative patients for signs of bleeding. ■ Administer oxygen.

REVIEW Questions

1. A 1-month-old baby is having a wellness examination. Which approach indicates that the nurse correctly measured this client's abdomen?
   1. Wrapped the measuring tape above the bladder
   2. Recorded the measurement to the nearest ¼ inch
   3. Recorded the measurement to the nearest ⅛ inch
   4. Wrapped the measuring tape below the nipple line

2. The mother of a new pediatric client asks why her preschool age child's blood pressure equipment was pumped up twice. Which would be the best response for the nurse to make to the mother?
   1. "I wanted to validate the reading."
   2. "All blood pressure measurements should be done twice."
   3. "The child moved and I was not able to measure the first reading accurately."
   4. "The first measurement was to help determine how high to pump the blood pressure cuff."

3. A neonate receiving phototherapy is prescribed pulse oximetry measurements every 2 hours. Which nursing action ensures that the measurement will be accurate?
   1. Covers the sensor with a blanket
   2. Applies the sensor to the right great toe
   3. Changes the location of the sensor every hour
   4. Ensures the high and low settings are at 100% and 85%

4. A client who consumed breakfast at 0800 hours has loud and frequent bowel sounds at 1330 hours. Which of the following options is most likely?
   1. Normal expected bowel sounds
   2. Development of a paralytic ileus
   3. Evidence of a late bowel obstruction
   4. Evidence of an early bowel obstruction

5. The nurse notes that a preschool child is able to read the 10th line on the HOTV eye chart with the right eye and the 5th line with the left eye. Which of the following should the nurse expect to be prescribed for this client?
   1. CT scan of the head
   2. Corrective eyeglasses
   3. Medication to dilate the pupil
   4. Medication to constrict the pupil

6. The nurse suspects that a client in the intensive care unit is experiencing a reaction to carotid sinus massage. Which finding did the nurse observe to make this clinical determination?
   1. Client complained of having palpitations
   2. Continuous cardiac monitor alarmed "low pulse"
   3. Radial pulse rate 10 bpm less than apical heart rate
   4. Point of maximum impulse displaced 2 cm laterally

7. A client is able to shrug the shoulders at the level of normal movement against gravity. Which notation should the nurse make to document this finding?
   1. Grip strength grade 5
   2. Deltoid muscles grade 2
   3. Trapezius muscles grade 3
   4. Sternocleidomastoid muscles grade 4

8. The nurse is assessing a client's neck with the chin bent down over the chest. Which approach should be used to palpate the client's supraclavicular nodes?
   1. With client's head forward, bend the fingers around the sternocleidomastoid muscle.
   2. With client's head bent back, place the fingertips under the mandible and pull the skin and subcutaneous tissue laterally.
   3. With client's head forward, hook the index and third fingers over the clavicle lateral to the sternocleidomastoid muscle.
   4. With client's head tilted back, move the fingertips in a forward circular motion against the sternocleidomastoid and trapezius muscles.

9. A client is unable to feel the nurse lightly touching the lower legs. How should the nurse document this finding?
   1. Hypoesthesia both legs
   2. Paresthesia present in legs
   3. Hyperesthesia bilateral legs
   4. Anesthesia bilateral lower legs

10. The nurse suspects that an older client has chronic venous insufficiency. What did the nurse assess to make this clinical determination?
    1. Dusky-red lower legs and cool skin
    2. Mild ankle edema and thin, shiny skin of the lower legs
    3. Pallor with limb elevation and lower leg muscle atrophy
    4. Brown hyperpigmentation of the lower legs and edema of the ankles

11. The nurse auscultates a client's breath sounds. Which sounds should the nurse report to the healthcare provider?
    1. High-pitched loud sounds heard over the trachea
    2. Soft, low-pitched sounds heard at the lung bases
    3. Low-pitched, continuous snoring heard over the trachea
    4. Moderate-pitched blowing sounds heard between the scapulae

12. The nurse is reviewing tasks that need to be completed over the next shift. Which peripheral pulse assessment should the nurse delegate to the unlicensed assistive personnel (UAP) to complete?
    1. Apical
    2. Brachial
    3. Femoral
    4. Popliteal

Note: For answers and rationales for the review questions, go to Appendix A or your Pearson MyLab Nursing and eText.

Chapter 2
Caring Interventions

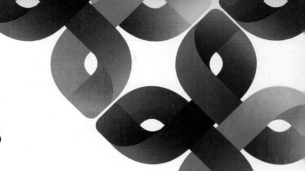

Chapter at a Glance

❶ Nursing students may observe or assist with the following skills only with faculty permission and while under direct supervision of faculty or another RN.

❯❯ The Concept of Caring Interventions

Caring interventions are evidence-based actions and behaviors implemented to assist patients and their families in meeting their needs. These interventions include independent and dependent actions the nurse does directly or indirectly for best patient outcomes. Caring interventions are done with a supportive, nurturing, patient-centered approach that respects cultural differences and patient choices as appropriate for the clinical setting. There is a responsibility of trust by the patient that the nurse is knowledgeable and will perform quality and safe interventions competently. A nursing plan of care is developed to assist patients in achieving goals to maintain or improve health conditions and prevent complications with caring interventions.

Learning Outcomes

2.1 Differentiate advantages and disadvantages between changing an occupied bed and an unoccupied bed.

2.2 Give examples of safety considerations when providing oral care to a patient who is unconscious or debilitated.

2.3 Summarize the steps in bathing an adult patient.

2.4 Explain how rights of medication administration can prevent medication errors.

2.5 Give examples of five common "Do's and Don'ts" of safety during the preparation of oral medications.

2.6 Show how to find the appropriate sites for safe administration of intramuscular injections.

2.7 Demonstrate how to safely remove medication from a vial container using a syringe.

2.8 Explain four methods of administering intravenous medications to a patient.

The following feature links some, but not all, of the concepts related to assessment. They are presented in alphabetical order.

Concepts Related to
Caring Interventions

CONCEPT	RELATIONSHIP TO CARING INTERVENTIONS	NURSING IMPLICATIONS
Culture and Diversity	May avoid asking for help when needed or not understand Western medication therapy	■ Build rapport with respect to cultural differences ■ Assist with personal care as needed ■ Explain medication therapy utilizing resources as needed
Infection	Maintain a clean environment and support personal hygiene to promote health and well-being.	■ Use standard precautions and other precautions to prevent transmission of pathogens ■ Follow appropriate techniques of medication administration
Professional Behaviors	Provide equal level of care to all patients.	■ Provide sustained quality of care for all patients ■ Build cultural awareness and sensitivity
Safety	Promotion of a safe environment and safety of interventions provided	■ Follow rights of medication administration ■ Maintain safe practice when providing care
Teaching and Learning	Promote health teaching and care in preparation of continuing care at home.	■ Provide teaching materials in patient's primary language, demonstration and return of procedures, and answer questions in preparation of discharge ■ Use an interpreter as needed

Because people are usually confined to bed when ill, sometimes for a long period, the bed becomes an important element in the patient's life. A place that is clean, safe, and comfortable contributes to the patient's ability to rest and sleep and to a sense of well-being. From a holistic perspective, bedmaking can be viewed as the preparation of a healing space. Basic furniture in a healthcare facility includes the bed, bedside cabinet, overbed table, one or more chairs, and a storage space for clothing. Most bed units also have a call light, light fixtures, electric outlets, and hygienic equipment in a bedside cabinet. Four types of equipment often installed in an acute care facility are a suction outlet for several types of suction, an air outlet that can humidify air, an oxygen outlet for supplemental oxygen systems, and a sphygmomanometer to measure the patient's blood pressure. Some long-term care agencies also permit patients to have personal furniture, such as a television, a chair, and lamps, at the bedside. In the home a patient often has personal and medical equipment near the bed.

Personal hygiene is the self-care by which people attend to such functions as bathing, toileting, general body hygiene, and grooming. Hygiene is a highly personal matter determined by various factors, including individual and cultural values and practices. It involves care of the skin, hair, nails, teeth, oral and nasal cavities, eyes, ears, and perineal-genital areas.

There are many factors to consider when planning personal hygiene interventions for patients. Nurses will discuss patient habits and preferences for personal care, hygiene, and grooming with patients or family to determine how much assistance the patient may need while in the healthcare facility. Patients may be able to independently provide all of their own care and need very little assistance. Other patients may require partial care to assist them with hygienic care, and some patients require complete care and are totally dependent on others to provide their personal care, hygiene, and grooming. In addition, cultural beliefs and practices can influence hygienic care. **Table 2–1 »** lists factors that influence hygienic practices.

There are common times during the day that patients may need assistance in meeting their toileting and hygienic needs: (a) Upon waking up in the morning before breakfast, many patients have toileting needs such as assistance to go

TABLE 2–1 Factors That Influence Individual Hygienic Practices

Factor	Variables
Culture	Cultures define cleanliness in different ways. Cultures and subcultures can have varying attitudes around hygiene and cleanliness. For example, some cultures value body cleanliness and the absence of body odor. Some value the use of perfume, deodorants, and after-shave lotions as a major part of their hygienic care. In other cultures, natural body odor is thought to have sex appeal.
Religion	Ceremonial washings are practiced by some religions. Some religions do not allow members of the opposite sex to see them from the waist to the knees.
Environment	Finances may affect the availability of facilities for bathing. For example, homeless people may not have warm water available; soap, shampoo, shaving lotion, and deodorants may be too expensive for people who have limited resources. Some underdeveloped countries have limited access to fresh water and, therefore, may not wash clothes as frequently.
Developmental level	Children learn hygiene in the home.
	Practices vary according to the individual's age; for example, preschoolers can carry out most tasks independently with encouragement.
Health and energy	Ill people may not have the motivation or energy to attend to hygiene. Some patients who have neuromuscular impairments may be unable to perform hygienic care.
Personal preferences	Some people prefer a shower to a tub bath. People have different preferences regarding the time of bathing (e.g., morning versus evening). Women in some cultures have a strong sense of modesty and do not want healthcare workers to see them unclothed.

to the bathroom, to get up to a commode chair, or help with a urinal or bedpan. They may want to wash their face and hands and do oral care for refreshment before eating breakfast. (b) Some patients may want to have their baths completed and beds made before breakfast, while others will want to wait until after breakfast. Bathing can be done in a shower, tub, chair, or bed and generally includes grooming activities. (c) At the end of the day, in preparation for sleep, patients may have toileting needs, may want to wash their face and hands, and do oral care before going to sleep. A back massage may be done to help patients relax. Some patients prefer bathing in the evening; as appropriate, the nurse needs to accommodate the patient's routine schedule for personal hygiene. (d) The last common need for personal hygiene care is as-needed (PRN) care. These are unscheduled times when patients require hygienic help, such as after urinating or defecating, after vomiting, and whenever they become soiled, for example, from wound drainage or from perspiration. They may need bathing and changing of clothing and linen.

» Bed Care and Activities of Daily Living (ADLs)

Expected Outcomes

1. Bed remains clean, dry, and free of wrinkles.
2. Transmission of pathogenic microorganisms is prevented with standard precautions.
3. Bathing and hygiene care are completed without incidence.
4. Patient's skin, hair, nails, and mouth are clean, odor free, and without irritation.
5. Patient is comfortable with safety measures implemented.
6. Eyes and surrounding area are clean and free from crustation.

SKILL 2.1 Bathing: Newborn, Infant, Child, Adult

There are a variety of differences in the habits and products used for hygiene and grooming. Having a clean and neat appearance is important to individuals in maintaining their dignity and self-esteem. Cleanliness and hygiene for all ages of patients combined with a clean, safe environment that healthcare facilities strive to maintain can help to lower rates of infection. Providing assistance to patients includes taking the individual's choices into consideration, such as their preference of clothing and hairstyle. When providing hygienic care for patients, the nurse needs to assess the patient's usual pattern of bathing, hygienic products usually used, and cultural rituals and beliefs.

Delegation or Assignment

The nurse often delegates or assigns the skill of bathing to the unlicensed assistive personnel (UAP). However, the nurse remains responsible for assessment and patient care. The nurse needs to do the following:

- Inform the UAP of the type of bath appropriate for the patient and precautions, if any, specific to the needs of the patient.
- Remind the UAP to notify the nurse of any concerns or changes (e.g., redness, skin breakdown, rash) so the nurse can assess, intervene if needed, and document.
- Instruct the UAP to encourage the patient to perform as much self-care as appropriate in order to promote independence and self-esteem.
- Obtain a complete report about the bathing experience from the UAP.

(continued on next page)

SKILL 2.1 Bathing: Newborn, Infant, Child, Adult (continued)

Equipment

- Basin or sink with warm water between 43°C–46°C (110°–115°F) and water temperature 37.8°C (100°F) (for newborn or infant only)
- Soap and soap dish (mild soap for newborn or infant)
- Suction bulb (for newborn or infant only)
- Cotton balls (for newborn or infant only)
- Linens: bath blanket, two bath towels, washcloth, clean gown or clothes as needed, additional bed linen and towels, if required
- Clean gloves, if appropriate (e.g., presence of body fluids or open lesions)
- Commercial cleansing pack (for disposable bath only)
- Personal hygiene articles (e.g., deodorant, powder, lotions)
- Shaving equipment (for adult only)
- Table for bathing equipment
- Laundry bag

Preparation

- Provide a comfortable room environment (i.e., comfortable temperature, lighting).
- Collect necessary equipment, and place articles within reach.
- Position the bed at a comfortable working height.
- Before bathing a patient, determine (a) the purpose and type of bath the patient needs; (b) self-care ability of the patient; (c) any movement or positioning precautions specific to the patient; (d) other care the patient may be receiving, such as physical therapy or x-rays, in order to coordinate all aspects of healthcare and prevent unnecessary fatigue; (e) the patient's comfort level with being bathed by someone else; and (f) necessary bath equipment and linens.
- Caution is needed when bathing patients who are receiving intravenous (IV) therapy. Easy-to-remove gowns that have Velcro or snap fasteners along the sleeves may be used. If a special gown is not available, the nurse needs to pay special attention when changing the patient's gown after the bath (or whenever the gown becomes soiled). In addition, special attention is needed to reassess the IV site for security of IV connections and appropriate taping around the IV site.
- The nurse should use standard precautions when bathing a patient, particularly when performing perineal care or there is a risk of exposure to other body secretions. It is not always necessary, however, to wear gloves while bathing other areas of the body. The nurse should use clinical judgment to make this decision.

NEWBORN OR INFANT

Procedure

1. Prior to performing the procedure, introduce self to the patient and parent and verify the patient's identity using two identifiers or follow facility protocol. Explain to the parent what you are going to do, why it is necessary, and how the parent can participate. Discuss with the parent preferences for bathing and explain any unfamiliar procedures to them.

2. Perform hand hygiene and observe other appropriate infection control procedures (e.g., clean gloves).
3. Provide for patient privacy by drawing the curtains around the bed or closing the door to the room. Some agencies provide signs indicating the need for privacy. **Rationale:** *Hygiene is a personal matter.*
4. Test water temperature with your wrist or elbow.
5. Lift newborn or infant using football hold.
6. Remove all clothing except shirt and diaper.
7. Cover newborn or infant with towel or blanket. Never let go of the newborn or infant during the bath. **Rationale:** *This is a safety intervention to prevent falls or other injury.*
8. Clean newborn's or infant's eyes, using a cotton ball moistened with water or moist washcloth. Wipe from inner to outer canthus, using a new moistened cotton ball or moist washcloth section for each eye. **Rationale:** *This procedure prevents water and particles from entering the lacrimal duct.*

CAUTION! Discharge from the eyes may be present for 2–3 days due to prophylactic eyedrops administered at birth.

---

9. Make a mitt with the washcloth.
10. Wash newborn's or infant's face with water.
11. Suction nose, if necessary, by compressing suction bulb prior to placing it in nostril. **Rationale:** *This prevents aspiration of moisture. Gently release bulb after it is placed in nostril.*
12. Wash newborn's or infant's ears and neck, paying attention to folds; dry all areas thoroughly. Use mild soap and rinse.
13. Remove shirt or gown.
14. Remove diaper by picking up newborn's or infant's ankles in your hand.
15. Pick up newborn or infant and place feet first into basin or tub. Immerse newborn or infant in tub of water only after umbilical cord has healed. Pick up newborn or infant by placing your hand and arm around newborn or infant, cradling the newborn's or infant's head and neck in your elbow. Grasp the newborn's or infant's thigh with your hand. **Rationale:** *The umbilical cord is kept dry to prevent infection.*
16. Wash and rinse the newborn's or infant's body, especially the skinfolds ❶. Baby may be bathed on a firm surface for safety.
    Note: Some facilities use disposable cleansing systems to bathe newborns and infants.

    There are infant-size washcloths for newborns or infants up to 11.3 kg (25 lb). The bathing procedure is the same for newborns, infants, and adults.

17. Washing newborn's or infant's genitalia (if done outside bath):
    - For a female newborn or infant: Separate labia and with a cotton ball moistened with soap and water, cleanse downward once on each side. Use a new piece of cotton on each side.
    - For an uncircumcised male newborn or infant: Do not force foreskin back. Gently cleanse the exposed surface with a cotton ball moistened with soap and water.
    - For a circumcised male newborn or infant: Gently cleanse with plain water.

SKILL 2.1 Bathing: Newborn, Infant, Child, Adult (continued)

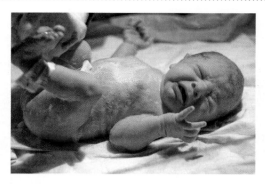

Source: Vivid Pixels/Shutterstock

❶ Bathing a newborn or infant

18. Wrap the newborn or infant in a towel and use a football hold when washing a newborn's or infant's head. Soap your own hands and wash newborn's or infant's hair and scalp paying attention to the nape of the neck and using a circular motion. Rinse hair and scalp thoroughly. **Rationale:** *Football hold is the most secure for active newborns or infants.*

19. Place newborn or infant on a clean, dry towel with head facing the top corner and wrap newborn or infant.

20. Use the corner of the towel to dry newborn's or infant's head with gentle, yet firm, circular movements.

21. Replace newborn's or infant's diaper and redress in a new gown or shirt.

22. Provide comfort by holding the newborn or infant for a time following the bath procedure.

23. Perform hand hygiene. Leave the patient safe and comfortable.

24. Documentation is completed using forms, checklists, or electronic dropdown lists supplemented by nurse's notes or additional comments as appropriate.

CHILD OR ADULT

Procedure

1. Prior to performing the procedure, introduce self and verify the patient's identity using two identifiers or follow facility protocol. Explain to the patient what you are going to do, why it is necessary, and how the patient can participate. Discuss with the patient preferences for bathing and explain any unfamiliar procedures to the patient.

2. Perform hand hygiene and observe other appropriate infection control procedures (e.g., clean gloves).

3. Provide for patient privacy by drawing the curtains around the bed or closing the door to the room. Some agencies provide signs indicating the need for privacy. **Rationale:** *Hygiene is a personal matter.*

4. Prepare the patient and the environment.
   - Invite a family member or significant other to participate if desired or requested by the patient.
   - Close the door to ensure the room is a comfortable temperature. **Rationale:** *Air currents increase loss of heat from the body by convection.*
   - Offer the patient a bedpan or urinal or ask whether the patient wishes to use the toilet or commode.

Rationale: *Warm water and activity can stimulate the need to void. The patient will be more comfortable after voiding, and voiding before cleaning the perineum is advisable.*
   - Encourage the patient to perform as much personal self-care as possible. **Rationale:** *This promotes independence, exercise, and self-esteem.*
   - During the bath, assess each area of the skin carefully.

For a Bed Bath

5. Prepare the bed and position the patient appropriately.
   - Lower the side rail on the side close to you. Keep the other side rail *up.* Assist the patient to move near you. **Rationale:** *This avoids undue reaching and straining and promotes good body mechanics, and allows the nurse to wash both sides of the patient's body without moving around the bed. It also ensures patient safety.*
   - Place a bath blanket over the top sheet. Remove the top sheet from under the bath blanket by starting at the patient's shoulders and moving linen down toward the patient's feet ❷. Ask the patient to grasp and hold the top of the bath blanket while pulling linen to the foot of the bed. **Rationale:** *The bath blanket provides comfort, warmth, and privacy.*

   Note: If the bed linen is to be reused, place it over the bedside chair. If it is to be changed, place it in the linen hamper, not on the floor. **Rationale:** *Placing used linens in the linen hamper rather than on the floor prevents the spread of microorganisms.*

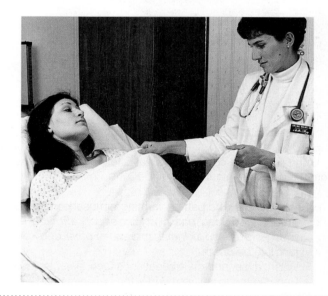

❷ Remove top sheet from under the bath blanket.

   - Remove the patient's gown while keeping the patient covered with the bath blanket. Place gown in linen hamper.

6. Make a bath mitt with the washcloth ❸. **Rationale:** *A bath mitt retains water and heat better than a cloth loosely held and prevents the ends of the washcloth from dragging across the skin.*

(continued on next page)

SKILL 2.1 Bathing: Newborn, Infant, Child, Adult (*continued*)

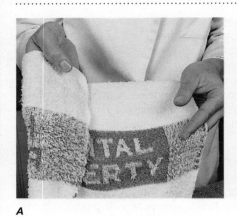

A

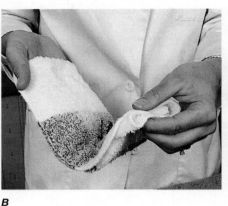

B

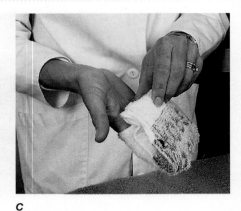

C

③ Making a bath mitt, rectangular method: *A,* Wrap one edge of cloth around palm and fingers; *B,* wrap cloth around hand and anchor with thumb; *C,* tuck far edge of cloth under edge in palm of hand.

7. Wash the face. **Rationale:** *Begin the bath at the cleanest area and work downward toward the feet.*
   - Place a towel under the patient's head.
   - Wash the patient's eyes with water only and dry them well. Wipe from the inner to the outer canthus ④. **Rationale:** *This prevents secretions from entering the nasolacrimal ducts.* Use a separate corner of the washcloth for each eye. **Rationale:** *Using separate corners prevents transmitting microorganisms from one eye to the other.*

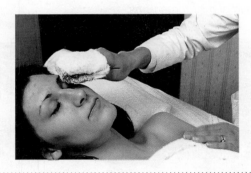

④ Using a separate corner of the washcloth for each eye, wipe from the inner to the outer canthus.

   - Ask whether the patient wants soap used on the face. **Rationale:** *Soap has a drying effect, and the face, which is exposed to the air more than other body parts, tends to be drier.*
   - Wash, rinse, and dry the patient's face, ears, and neck.
   - Remove the towel from under the patient's head.
8. Wash the arms and hands. (Omit the arms for a partial bath.)
   - Place a towel lengthwise under the arm away from you. **Rationale:** *It protects the bed from becoming wet.*
   - Wash, rinse, and dry the arm by elevating the patient's arm and supporting the patient's wrist and elbow. Use long, firm strokes from wrist to shoulder, including the axillary area ⑤. **Rationale:** *Firm strokes from distal to proximal areas promote circulation by increasing venous blood return.*

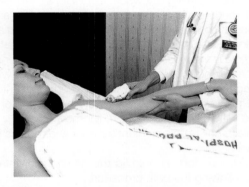

⑤ Washing the far arm using long, firm strokes from wrist to shoulder area.

   - Apply deodorant if desired. Special caution is needed for patients with respiratory alterations. **Rationale:** *Powder is not recommended due to potential adverse respiratory effects.*
   - *Optional:* Place a towel on the bed and put a washbasin on it. Place the patient's hands in the basin ⑥. **Rationale:** *Many patients enjoy immersing their hands in the basin and washing them themselves. Soaking loosens dirt under*

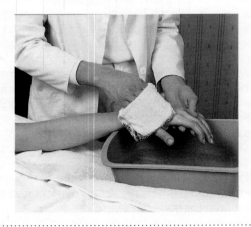

⑥ Wash hands by soaking them in a basin.

SKILL 2.1 Bathing: Newborn, Infant, Child, Adult (continued)

the nails. Assist the patient as needed to wash, rinse, and dry the hands, paying particular attention to the spaces between the fingers.

- Repeat for hand and arm nearest you. Exercise caution if an intravenous infusion is present, and check its flow after moving the arm. Avoid submersing the IV site.

9. Wash the chest and abdomen. (Omit the chest and abdomen for a partial bath. However, the areas under a woman's breast may require bathing if this area is irritated or if the patient has significant perspiration under the breasts.)
   - Place the bath towel lengthwise over the chest. Fold the bath blanket down to the patient's pubic area. **Rationale:** *This keeps the patient warm while preventing unnecessary exposure of the chest* ⑦.

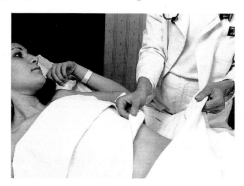

⑦ Place the bath towel across the patient's chest.

- Lift the bath towel off the chest, and bathe the chest and abdomen with your mitted hand using long, firm strokes. Give special attention to the skin under the breasts and any other skinfolds, particularly if the patient is overweight. Rinse and dry well.
- Replace the bath blanket when the areas have been dried.

10. Wash the legs and feet. (Omit legs and feet for a partial bath.)
    - Expose the leg farthest from you by folding the bath blanket toward the other leg, being careful to keep the perineum covered. **Rationale:** *Covering the perineum promotes privacy and maintains the patient's dignity.*
    - Lift leg and place the bath towel lengthwise under the leg. Wash, rinse, and dry the leg using long, smooth, firm strokes from the ankle to the knee to the thigh ⑧.

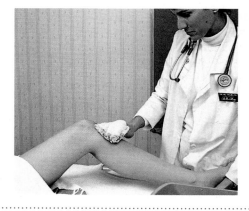

⑧ Washing the patient's leg.

Rationale: *Washing from the distal to proximal areas promotes circulation by stimulating venous blood flow.*
- Reverse the coverings and repeat for the other leg.
- Wash the feet by placing them in a basin of water ⑨.

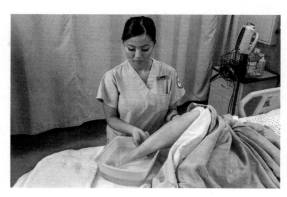

⑨ Soaking a foot in a basin.

- Dry each foot. Pay particular attention to the spaces between the toes. If preferred, wash one foot after that leg before washing the other leg.
- Obtain fresh, warm bathwater now or when necessary. **Rationale:** *Water may become dirty or cold.* Because surface skin cells are removed with washing, the bathwater from dark-skinned patients may be dark; however, this does not mean the patient is dirty. Lower the bed and raise the side rails when refilling basin. **Rationale:** *This ensures the safety of the patient.*

11. Wash the back and then the perineum ⑩.
    - Assist the patient into a prone or side-lying position facing away from you. Place the bath towel lengthwise alongside the back and buttocks while keeping the patient covered with the bath blanket as much as possible. **Rationale:** *This provides warmth and prevents undue exposure.*

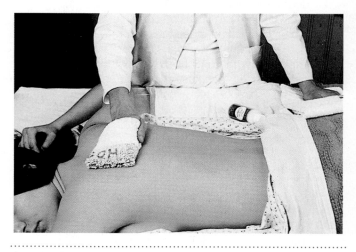

⑩ Washing the back.

(continued on next page)

SKILL 2.1 Bathing: Newborn, Infant, Child, Adult (continued)

- Wash and dry the patient's back, moving from the shoulders to the buttocks, and upper thighs, paying attention to the gluteal folds. **Rationale:** *Wash from the area of least contamination (the back) to that of greatest (gluteal folds).*
- Remove and discard gloves if used.
- Assist the patient to the supine position and determine whether the patient can wash the perineal area independently. If the patient cannot do so, drape the patient and wash the area (see Skill 2.8).
12. Assist the patient with grooming aids such as lotion or deodorant.
- Use any powder very sparingly. Release as little as possible into the atmosphere. **Rationale:** *This will avoid irritation of the respiratory tract by powder inhalation. Excessive powder can cause caking, which leads to skin irritation.*
- Help the patient put on a clean gown or pajamas.
- Assist the patient to care for hair, mouth, and nails. Some people prefer or need mouth care prior to their bath.
- Proceed to step13.

For a Tub Bath or Shower

5. Prepare the patient and the tub.
- Fill the tub about one third to one half full of water at 43°C–46°C (110°F–115°F). **Rationale:** *Sufficient water is needed to cover the perineal area.*
- Cover all intravenous catheters or wound dressings with plastic coverings, and instruct the patient to prevent wetting these areas if possible.
- Put a rubber bath mat or towel on the floor of the tub if safety strips are not on the tub floor. **Rationale:** *These prevent slippage of the patient during the bath or shower.*
6. Assist the patient into the shower or tub.
- Assist the patient taking a standing shower with the initial adjustment of the water temperature and water flow pressure, as needed. Some patients need a chair to sit on in the shower because of weakness. Hot water can cause older adults to feel faint due to vasodilation and decreased blood pressure from positional changes.
- If the patient requires considerable assistance with a tub bath, a hydraulic bathtub chair may be required (see Hydraulic Bathtub Chair section later in this skill).
- Explain how the patient can signal for help, leave the patient for 2–5 minutes, and place an "Occupied" sign on the door. For safety reasons, do not leave a patient with decreased cognition or patients who may be at risk (e.g., history of seizures, syncope).
7. Assist the patient with washing and getting out of the tub.
- Wash the patient's back, lower legs, and feet, if necessary.
- Assist the patient out of the tub. If the patient is unsteady, place a bath towel over the patient's shoulders and drain the tub of water before the patient attempts to get out of it. **Rationale:** *Draining the water first lessens the likelihood of a fall. The towel prevents chilling.*

8. Dry the patient, and assist with follow-up care.
- Assist the patient back to bed.
- Clean the tub or shower in accordance with facility practice, discard the used linen in the laundry hamper, and place the "Unoccupied" sign on the door.
9. Perform hand hygiene. Leave the patient safe and comfortable. Proceed to step 13.
13. Document the following:
- Type of bath given (i.e., complete, partial, or self-help). This is usually recorded on a flow sheet
- Skin assessment, such as excoriation, erythema, exudates, rashes, drainage, or skin breakdown
- Nursing interventions related to skin integrity
- Ability of the patient to assist or cooperate with bathing
- Patient response to bathing, and document the need for reassessment of vital signs if appropriate
- Educational needs regarding hygiene
- Information or teaching shared with the patient or the family.

SAMPLE DOCUMENTATION

[date] 0735 Assisted bath given, able to complete upper body bathing, no redden skins areas noted, small amount of fatigue voiced by patient, after short rest, stated she felt much better, denies any tenderness of joints, smiling, states "I'm ready for the day now." *T. Ross*

CHANGING GOWN FOR PATIENT WITH AN IV

Procedure

1. Check patient care plan for infusion drip rate, type of solution, and any special considerations.
2. Perform hand hygiene.
3. Identify patient using two descriptors.
4. Take equipment to patient's room and explain procedure to patient.
5. Untie back of gown, and remove gown from unaffected arm.
6. Support arm with IV and slip gown down arm to IV tubing.
7. Place clean gown over patient's chest and abdomen.
8. Use tubing clamp to slow infusion to "keep-open" rate and remove tubing from infusion pump if in use.
9. Remove IV bag from hook and slip sleeve over bag, keeping bag above patient's arm. **Rationale:** *This prevents backflow of blood into tubing. Do not jar or pull tubing. IV tubing may become dislodged and infiltrate into surrounding tissue.*
10. Place your hand up through distal end of clean gown sleeve and grasp IV bag. Pull bag and tubing out through clean gown sleeve.
11. Rehang bag on hook, and check to see that infusion is running according to ordered drip rate.

SKILL 2.1 Bathing: Newborn, Infant, Child, Adult (*continued*)

12. Replace tubing into infusion pump, unclamp, and reestablish prescribed infusion flow rate.
13. Guide sleeve of gown up patient's arm to shoulder.
14. Assist patient to put other arm through remaining sleeve.
15. Tie gown at the back.
16. Check IV infusion rate and IV tubing to determine that solution is flowing unimpeded into patient's vein. **Rationale:** *Kinks in tubing impede solution flow.*
17. Return bed to comfortable position for patient.
18. Remove dirty linen from room.
19. Perform hand hygiene.
    Note: Most facilities provide "IV gowns" that snap from the shoulder down the sleeve of the gown for ease in removal without disturbing the IV.

USING A HYDRAULIC BATHTUB CHAIR

A hydraulic lift, often used in long-term care or rehabilitation settings, can facilitate the transfer of a patient who is unable to ambulate to a tub. The lift also helps eliminate strain on the nurse's back.

1. Bring the patient to the tub room in a wheelchair or shower chair.
2. Fill the tub and check the water temperature with a bath thermometer. **Rationale:** *This avoids thermal injury to the patient.*
3. Lower the hydraulic chair lift to its lowest point, outside the tub.
4. Transfer the patient to the chair lift and secure the seat belt ⓫.
5. Raise the chair lift above the tub.
6. Support the patient's legs as the chair is moved over the tub. **Rationale:** *This avoids injury to the legs.*
7. Position the patient's legs down into the water and slowly lower the chair lift into the tub.
8. Assist in bathing the patient, if appropriate.
9. Reverse the procedure when taking the patient out of the tub.
10. Dry the patient and transport him or her to the room.

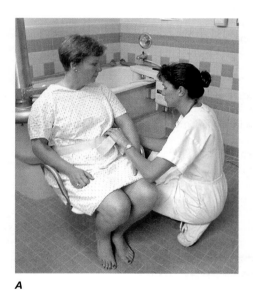

A

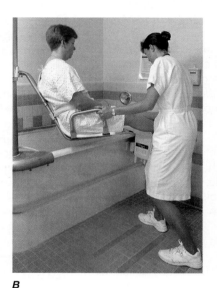

B

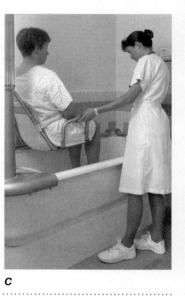

C

⓫ *A,* Attach seat belt before swinging chair over the tub. *B,* Support the patient in the chair as the chair is swung over tub. *C,* Lower chair into tub filled with water.

Safety Considerations

BATHING PATIENTS WITH DEMENTIA

1. Focus on the patient rather than the task.
   - Evaluate to determine if the patient needs pain control before the bath.
   - Time the bath to fit the patient's history, preferences, and mood.
   - Cover the patient! Keep the patient covered as much as possible to keep him or her warm.
   - Move slowly and let the patient know when you are going to move or touch him or her.
   - Use a gentle touch. Use soft cloths. Pat dry rather than rubbing.
   - Consider adapting your methods (e.g., distracting the patient with singing while bathing), the environment (e.g., correct size of shower chair, reducing noise, playing music), and the procedure (e.g., consistently assigning same caregiver, inviting family to help).
   - Encourage flexibility in scheduling of the bath based on patient's preference.
2. Use persuasion, not coercion.
   - Give choices and respond to individual requests.
   - Help the patient feel in control.
   - Use a supportive, calm approach and praise the patient often.
3. Be prepared.
   - Gather everything that you will need for the bath (e.g., towels, washcloths, clothes) before approaching the patient.

(continued on next page)

SKILL 2.1 Bathing: Newborn, Infant, Child, Adult (continued)

4. Stop when a patient becomes distressed. It is not normal to have cries, screams, or protests from the patient.
   * Stop what you are doing and assess for causes of the distress.
   * Adjust your approach.
   * Shorten or stop the bath.
   * Try to end on a positive note.
   * Return later to wash critical areas if necessary.
5. Ask for help.
   * Talk with others, including the family, about different ways to help make the bath more comfortable for the patient.

USING A DISPOSABLE BATH PACK

1. Obtain package with cleansing cloths. Cloths are pre-moistened with an aloe and vitamin E formula. **Rationale:** *The cleansing cloths are less drying as they maintain the skin at a pH of 4.7–4.9.*
2. Heat package in microwave for no more than 45 seconds. Check temperature before applying to skin. **Rationale:** *Increased time could lead to excessive heat and burning of the skin. The commercial system can be used at room temperature.*
3. Explain procedure to patient. **Rationale:** *This procedure may be new to the patient and an explanation is needed to ensure patient understands the difference between a bed bath and a bath using a cleansing system. The patient may not think he has had a complete bath but only a "sponge bath."*
4. Perform hand hygiene.
5. Don gloves if there is a risk of contact with body secretions.
6. Replace top linen and gown with bath blanket or top sheet if bath blanket is not available.
7. Open package and remove one cloth at a time.
8. Remove bath blanket at each site when cleansing with cloth.
9. Replace bath blanket when cloth is removed. **Rationale:** *This prevents patient chilling.*
10. Use a new cloth for each section of the body as follows:
    * Face, neck, and chest
    * Right arm and axilla
    * Left arm and axilla
    * Perineum
    * Right leg
    * Left leg
    * Back
    * Buttocks
11. Discard cloth after cleansing each area. Do not flush down toilet. Rinsing is not required with this system. Replace bath blanket or sheet over each part of the body after it has been cleaned. **Rationale:** *This prevents the patient from becoming chilled.*
12. Place clean gown on patient.
13. Place patient in comfortable position.
14. Discard cloths in appropriate receptacle.
15. Perform hand hygiene. Leave patient safe and comfortable.
16. Complete documentation using forms, checklists, or electronic dropdown lists supplemented by nurse's notes or additional comments as appropriate.

Patient Teaching

Dry Skin
* When bathing, use a cleansing cream to clean the skin rather than soap or detergent, which cause drying and, in some cases, allergic reactions.
* Bathe less frequently using a soap product.
* Increase fluid intake unless contraindicated.
* Eat a diet that includes all nutrients and proteins.
* Daily use of moisturizing or emollient creams that contain lanolin, petroleum jelly, or cocoa butter is recommended to retain skin moisture.

Skin Rashes
* Keep the area clean by washing it with a mild soap. Rinse the skin well, and pat it dry.
* To relieve itching, try a tepid bath or soak. Some over-the-counter preparations, such as calamine (Caladryl) lotion, may help but should be used with full knowledge of the product.
* Avoid scratching the rash to prevent inflammation, infection, and further skin lesions.
* Choose clothing that is loose-fitting and not binding on the rash area.

Acne
* Wash the face frequently with soap or detergent and warm water to remove oil and dirt.
* Avoid using oil-based creams, which aggravate the condition.
* Avoid using heavy cosmetic products that block the ducts of the sebaceous glands and the hair follicles.
* Don't squeeze or pick at the lesions because this increases the potential for infection and scarring.
* If there is no relief when using over-the-counter products, follow-up with a healthcare provider for further treatment.

Lifespan Considerations

FACTORS THAT CAN INCREASE RISK OF SKIN BREAKDOWN AND DELAY WOUND HEALING
* Inadequate nutritional intake
* Compromised immune system
* Compromised circulatory and respiratory systems
* Poor hydration
* Decreased mobility and activity
* Bowel and/or bladder incontinence

SKIN CHANGES WITH AGE
* There is delayed cellular migration and proliferation.
* Skin is less effective as a barrier and slow to heal.
* There is increased vulnerability to trauma.
* There is less ability to retain water.
* The skin of older adults may be dry (xeroderma) due to decreased endocrine secretion and loss of elastin. This can cause pruritus, which could lead to skin ulceration.

SKILL 2.1 Bathing: Newborn, Infant, Child, Adult (*continued*)

- Increased skin susceptibility to shearing stress leads to blister formation and skin tears.
- There is increased vascular fragility.

NEED FOR ASSESSMENT OF THE SKIN OF OLDER ADULTS

- Decreased temperature, degree of moisture, dryness resulting from decreased dermal vascularity
- Skin not intact, open lesions, tears, pressure ulcers as a result of increased skin fragility
- Decreased turgor, dehydration as a result of decreased oil and sweat glands
- Pigmentation alterations, potential cancer
- Pruritus—dry skin most common cause because of decreased oil and sweat glands
- Bruises, scars from increased skin fragility

BATHING ADAPTATIONS TO MINIMIZE DRYNESS

- Have patient take complete bath only twice a week.
- Use super-fatted or mild soap or lotions to aid in moisturizing.
- Use tepid, not hot, water.
- Apply emollient (lanolin) to skin after bathing.

NEWBORNS AND INFANTS

- Sponge baths are suggested for the newborn because daily tub baths are not considered necessary. After the bath, the newborn or infant should be immediately dried and wrapped. Parents need to be advised that the newborn's or infant's ability to regulate body temperature has not yet fully developed and newborns' bodies lose heat readily.

CHILDREN

- Encourage a child's participation as appropriate for developmental level.
- Closely supervise children in the bathtub. Do not leave them unattended.

ADOLESCENTS

- Assist adolescents as needed to choose deodorants and antiperspirants. Secretions from newly active sweat glands react with bacteria on the skin, causing a pungent odor.

OLDER ADULTS

- Changes of aging can decrease the protective function of the skin in older adults. These changes include fragile skin, less oil and moisture, and a decrease in elasticity.
- To minimize skin dryness in older adults, avoid excessive use of soap.
- The ideal time to moisturize the skin is immediately after bathing.
- Avoid powder because it causes moisture loss and is a hazardous inhalant. Cornstarch should also be avoided because in the presence of moisture it breaks down into glucose and can facilitate the growth of organisms.
- Protect older adults and children from injury related to hot water burns.

SKILL 2.2 Bedmaking: Occupied, Unoccupied

Bedmaking time can be an opportunity to assess and meet the patient's needs. A wrinkle-free safe and clean comfortable bed will ensure rest and sleep and will help prevent several complications in bedridden patients, such as foot drop and pressure injury.

Delegation or Assignment

Bedmaking is usually delegated or assigned to the UAP. Inform the UAP to what extent the patient can assist or if another person will be needed to assist the UAP. Instruct the UAP about the handling of any dressings and/or tubes of the patient and also the need for special equipment (e.g., footboard, heel protectors), if appropriate. When making an unoccupied bed, ask the UAP to inform you immediately if any tubes or dressings become dislodged or removed when the patient gets out of bed. Stress the importance of the call light being readily available while the patient is out of bed. Note that state laws for UAPs vary, so this task might be assigned to the UAP rather than delegated.

Equipment

- Clean gloves, as needed
- Two flat sheets or one fitted and one flat sheet
- Cloth drawsheet (optional)
- One blanket
- One bedspread
- Incontinent pads (optional)
- Pillowcase(s) for the head pillow(s)
- Laundry bag or portable linen hamper (follow facility guidelines)

Preparation

- Determine what linens the patient may already have in the room. **Rationale:** *This avoids stockpiling of unnecessary extra linens.*
- Linen for one patient is never (even momentarily) placed on another patient's bed or on the floor.
- Do not shake soiled linen in the air because shaking can disseminate secretions and excretions and the microorganisms they contain.
- Assess and discuss with the caregiver the following: need for linens (e.g., incontinence, drainage), available linen supply, and laundry accommodations.
- Determine the need for a second person to help patient move from side to side while changing the linen. Move the patient gently and smoothly. Rough handling can cause the patient discomfort and abrade the skin.

(*continued on next page*)

SKILL 2.2 Bedmaking: Occupied, Unoccupied (*continued*)

OCCUPIED BED

Procedure

1. Prior to performing the procedure introduce self and verify the patient's identity using two identifiers. Explain to the patient what you are going to do, why it is necessary, and how the patient can participate.
2. Perform hand hygiene and observe other appropriate infection control procedures. Put on disposable clean gloves if linen is soiled with body fluids.
3. Provide for patient privacy.
4. Remove the top bedding.
   - Remove any equipment attached to the bed linen, such as a signal light.
   - Loosen all top linen at the foot of the bed, and remove the spread and the blanket.
   - Leave the top sheet over the patient (the top sheet can remain over the patient if it is being changed and if it will provide sufficient warmth), or replace it with a bath blanket as follows:
     a. Spread the bath blanket over the top sheet.
     b. Ask the patient to hold the top edge of the blanket.
     c. Reaching under the blanket from the side, grasp the top edge of the sheet and draw it down to the foot of the bed, leaving the blanket in place ❶.
     d. Remove the sheet from the bed and place it in the soiled hamper.
5. Change the bottom sheet and drawsheet.
   - Raise the side rail that the patient will turn toward. **Rationale:** *This protects patients from falling and allows them to support themselves in the side-lying position.* If there is no side rail, have another nurse support the patient at the edge of the bed.
   - Assist the patient to turn on the side away from the nurse and toward the raised side rail.
   - Loosen the bottom linens on the side of the bed near the nurse.

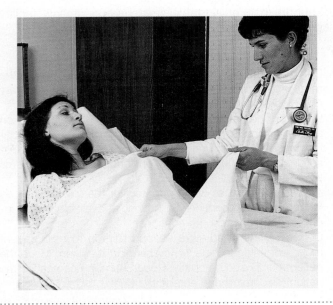

❶ Remove top linen and replace with a bath blanket.

- Fanfold the dirty linen (i.e., drawsheet and the bottom sheet) toward the center of the bed as close to and under the patient as possible ❷. **Rationale:** *Doing this leaves the near half of the bed free to be changed.*

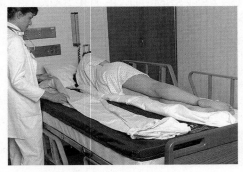

Source: Ronald May/Pearson Education, Inc.

❷ Moving soiled linen as close to the patient as possible to make room for clean sheet.

- Place the new bottom sheet on the bed, and vertically fanfold the half to be used on the far side of the bed as close to the patient as possible ❸. Tuck the sheet under the near half of the bed and miter the corner if a contour sheet is not being used.

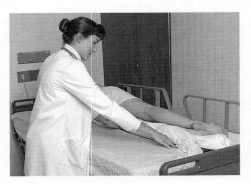

Source: Ronald May/Pearson Education, Inc.

❸ Smooth and tighten new bottom sheet on half of the bed.

- Place the clean drawsheet on the bed with the center fold at the center of the bed. Fanfold the uppermost half vertically at the center of the bed and tuck the near side edge under the side of the mattress ❹.

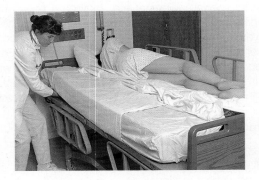

❹ Placing a clean drawsheet on the bed.

SKILL 2.2 Bedmaking: Occupied, Unoccupied (*continued*)

- When stripping and making a bed, conserve time and energy by stripping and making up one side as much as possible before working on the other side.
- Assist the patient to roll over toward you, maintaining good body alignment, over the fanfolded bed linens at the center of the bed, onto the clean side of the bed ❺.
- Move the pillows to the clean side for the patient's use. Raise the side rail before leaving the side of the bed.

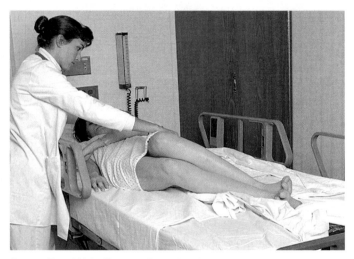

Source: Ronald May/Pearson Education, Inc.

❺ Assist patient to roll over to side of bed toward you onto clean linen.

- Move to the other side of the bed and lower the side rail.
- Remove the used linen and place it in the portable hamper or tucked into a pillowcase at the end of the bed before it is gathered up for disposal.
- Unfold the fanfolded bottom sheet from the center of the bed.
- Facing the side of the bed, use both hands to pull the bottom sheet so that it is smooth and tuck the excess under the side of the mattress.
- Unfold the drawsheet fanfolded at the center of the bed and pull it tightly with both hands (see ❹). Pull the sheet in three divisions: (a) Face the side of the bed to pull the middle division, (b) face the far top corner to pull the bottom division, and (c) face the far bottom corner to pull the top division.
- Tuck the excess drawsheet under the side of the mattress.

6. Reposition the patient in the center of the bed.
    - Reposition the pillows at the center of the bed.
    - Assist the patient to the center of the bed. Determine what position the patient requires or prefers and assist the patient to that position.
7. Apply or complete the top bedding.
    - Spread the top sheet over the patient and either ask the patient to hold the top edge of the sheet or tuck it under the shoulders. The sheet should remain over the patient when the bath blanket or used sheet is removed.
    - Complete the top of the bed (see page 108).

CAUTION! Most patients can safely stay in bed without side rails being raised. Follow facility policy regarding having the top of bed side rails raised. If side rails are used, the nurse must assess the patient's physical and mental status and closely monitor high-risk (frail, older, or confused) patients to avoid entrapment, injuries, and deaths (FDA, 2014).

8. Ensure continued safety of the patient.
    - Raise the side rails. Place the bed in the low position before leaving the bedside.
    - Attach the call light to the bed linen within the patient's reach.
    - Put items used by the patient within easy reach.
    - Perform hand hygiene. Leave the patient safe and comfortable.
9. Complete documentation using forms, checklists, or electronic dropdown lists supplemented by nurse's notes or additional comments as appropriate. Many agencies use a checklist that indicates if bed linens were changed.

UNOCCUPIED BED

Procedure

1. If the patient is in bed, prior to performing the procedure, introduce self and verify the patient's identity using two identifiers. Explain to the patient what you are going to do, why it is necessary, and how the patient can participate.
2. Perform hand hygiene and observe other appropriate infection control procedures (e.g., clean gloves).
3. Provide for patient privacy.
4. Place the fresh linen on the patient's chair or overbed table; do not use another patient's bed. **Rationale:** *This prevents cross-contamination (the movement of microorganisms from one patient to another) via soiled linen.*
5. Assess and assist the patient out of bed using assistive devices (e.g., cane, walker, safety belt) as appropriate. **Rationale:** *This ensures patient safety.*
    - Make sure that this is an appropriate and convenient time for the patient to be out of bed.
    - Assist the patient to a comfortable chair.
6. Raise the bed to a comfortable working height and use good body mechanics to prevent injuries.
7. Apply clean gloves if linens and equipment have been soiled with secretions and/or excretions.
8. Strip the bed (i.e., remove bed linens).
    - Check bed linens for any items belonging to the patient, and detach the call bell or any drainage tubes from the bed linen.
    - Loosen all bedding systematically, starting at the head of the bed on the far side and moving around the bed up to the head of the bed on the near side. **Rationale:** *Moving around the bed systematically prevents stretching and reaching and possible muscle strain.*
    - Remove the pillowcases, if soiled, and place the pillows on the bedside chair near the foot of the bed.
    - Fold reusable linens, such as the bedspread and top sheet on the bed, into fourths ❻. First, fold the linen in

(*continued on next page*)

SKILL 2.2 Bedmaking: Occupied, Unoccupied *(continued)*

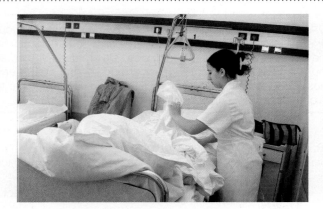

Source: LADA/Clinique Montmartre/Science Source

6 Fold reusable linens into fourths when removing them from the bed.

> half by bringing the top edge even with the bottom edge, and then grasp it at the center of the middle fold and bottom edges. **Rationale:** *Folding linens saves time and energy when reapplying the linens on the bed and keeps them clean.*
> - Remove the incontinent pad and discard it if soiled.
> - Roll all soiled linen inside the bottom sheet, hold it away from your uniform, and place it directly into the linen hamper, not on the floor **7**. **Rationale:** *These actions are essential to prevent the transmission of microorganisms to the nurse and others.*

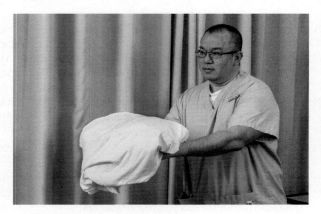

Source: Rick Brady/Pearson Education, Inc.

7 Roll soiled linen inside the bottom sheet and hold away from the body.

- Wipe the mattress with disinfectant if soiled.
- Grasp the mattress securely, using the lugs if present, and move the mattress up to the head of the bed.
- Remove and discard gloves if used. Perform hand hygiene.
9. Apply the bottom sheet and drawsheet.
- Place the folded bottom sheet with its center fold on the center of the bed **8**. Make sure the sheet is hem-side down for a smooth foundation. Spread the sheet out over the mattress, and allow a sufficient amount of

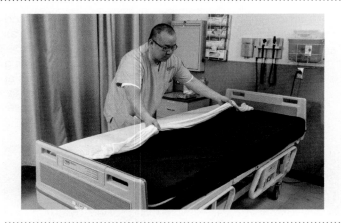

8 Placing the bottom sheet on the bed.

sheet at the top to tuck under the mattress. **Rationale:** *The top of the sheet needs to be well tucked under to remain securely in place, especially when the head of the bed is elevated.* Place the sheet along the edge of the mattress at the foot of the bed and do not tuck it in (unless it is a contour or fitted sheet).
- Miter the sheet at the top corner on the near side **9**, **10** and tuck the sheet under the mattress, working from the head of the bed to the foot.

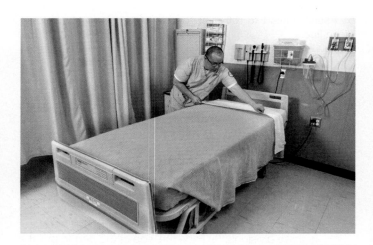

9 Mitered corners at foot of bed help keep bed linens secure.

- If a drawsheet is used, place it over the bottom sheet so that the centerfold is at the centerline of the bed and the top and bottom edges extend from the middle of where the patient's back would be on the bed to the area where the midthigh or knee would be **11**. Fanfold the uppermost half of the folded drawsheet at the center or far edge of the bed and tuck in the near edge.
- *Optional:* Before moving to the other side of the bed, place the top linens on the bed hem-side up, unfold them, tuck them in, and miter the bottom corners. **Rationale:** *Completing one entire side of the bed at a time saves time and energy.*

SKILL 2.2 Bedmaking: Occupied, Unoccupied (*continued*)

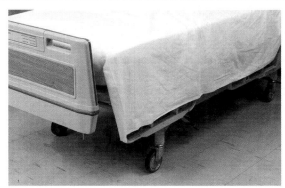

A

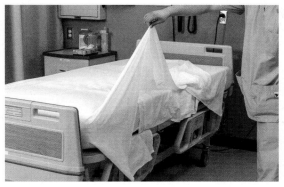

B

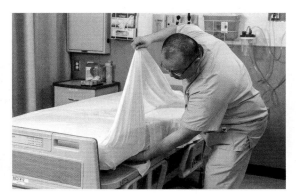

C

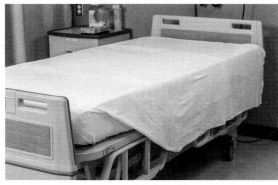

D

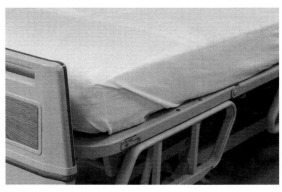

E

🔟 Mitering the corner of a bed: *A,* Tuck in the bedcover (sheet, blanket, and/or spread) firmly under the mattress at the bottom or top of the bed. *B,* Lift the bed cover so that it forms a triangle with the side edge of the bed and the edge of the bedcover is parallel to the end of the bed. *C,* Tuck the part of the cover that hangs below the mattress under the mattress while holding the triangle up or against the bed. *D,* Bring the tip of the triangle down toward the floor while the other hand holds the fold of the cover against the side of the mattress. *E,* Remove the hand and tuck the remainder of the cover under the mattress, if appropriate. The sides of the top sheet, blanket, and bedspread may be left hanging freely rather than tucked in, if desired.

10. Move to the other side and secure the bottom linen.
    - Tuck in the bottom sheet under the head of the mattress, pull the sheet firmly, and miter the corner of the sheet.
    - Pull the remainder of the sheet firmly so that there are no wrinkles. **Rationale:** *Wrinkles can cause discomfort for the patient and breakdown of skin. Tuck the sheet in at the side.*
    - Tuck in the drawsheet, if appropriate.
11. Apply or complete the top sheet, blanket, and spread.
    - Place the top sheet, hem-side up, on the bed so that its center fold is at the center of the bed and the top edge is even with the top edge of the mattress.
    - Unfold the sheet over the bed.

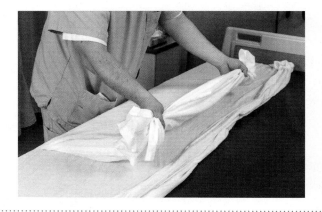

🔟🔟 Placing a clean drawsheet on the bed.

(*continued on next page*)

SKILL 2.2 Bedmaking: Occupied, Unoccupied (*continued*)

- *Optional:* Make a vertical or a horizontal toe pleat in the sheet. A toe pleat provides additional room for the patient's feet and helps prevent foot drop.
  a. *Vertical toe pleat:* Make a fold in the sheet 5–10 cm (2–4 in.) perpendicular to the foot of the bed ⑫.

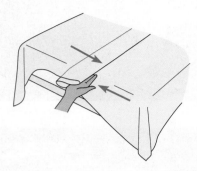

⑫ A vertical toe pleat.

  b. *Horizontal toe pleat:* Make a fold in the sheet 5–10 cm (2–4 in.) across the bed near the foot ⑬.

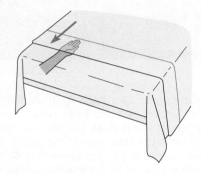

⑬ A horizontal toe pleat: Make a fold in the sheet 5 to 10 cm (2 to 4 in.) across the bed near the foot.

- Loosening the top covers around the feet after the patient is in bed is another way to provide additional space ⑭.

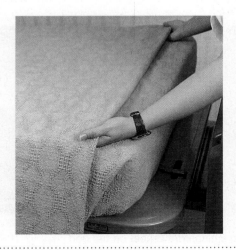

⑭ Pleat top linen to allow space for feet.

- Follow the same procedure for the blanket and the spread, but place the top edges about 15 cm (6 in.) from the head of the bed to allow a cuff of sheet to be folded over them.
- Tuck in the sheet, blanket, and spread at the foot of the bed, and miter the corner, using all three layers of linen. Leave the sides of the top sheet, blanket, and spread hanging freely unless toe pleats were provided.
- Fold the top of the top sheet down over the spread, providing a cuff ⑮. **Rationale:** *The cuff of sheet makes it easier for the patient to pull the covers up.*
- Move to the other side of the bed and secure the top bedding in the same manner.

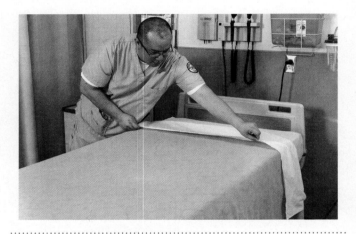

⑮ Making a cuff of the top linens.

12. Put clean pillowcases on the pillows as required.
   - Grasp the closed end of the pillowcase at the center with one hand.
   - Gather up the sides of the pillowcase and place them over the hand grasping the case. Then grasp the center of one short side of the pillow through the pillowcase ⑯.
   - With the free hand, pull the pillowcase over the pillow.
   - Adjust the pillowcase so that the pillow fits into the corners of the case and the seams are straight. **Rationale:** *A smoothly fitting pillowcase is more comfortable than a wrinkled one.*
   - Place the pillows appropriately at the head of the bed.

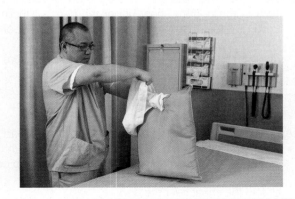

⑯ Method for putting a clean pillowcase on a pillow.

SKILL 2.2 Bedmaking: Occupied, Unoccupied (*continued*)

13. Provide for patient comfort and safety.
    - Attach the call light so that the patient can conveniently reach it. Some call lights have clamps that attach to the sheet or pillowcase. Others are attached by a safety pin. Most beds now have a call light button on the side rail.
    - If the bed is currently being used by a patient, either fold back the top covers at one side or fanfold them down to the end of the bed. **Rationale:** *This makes it easier for the patient to get into the bed.*
    - Place the bedside cabinet and the overbed table so that they are available to the patient.
    - Leave the bed in the high position if the patient is returning by stretcher, or place in the low position if the patient is returning to bed after being up ambulating or sitting in a chair.
14. Complete documentation using forms, checklists, or electronic dropdown lists supplemented by nurse's notes or additional comments as appropriate.
    - Many agencies use a checklist that indicates if bed linens were changed.
    - Record any nursing assessments, such as the patient's physical status and pulse and respiratory rates before and after being out of bed, as indicated.

SURGICAL BED

A **surgical bed** is used for the patient who is having surgery and will return to bed for the postoperative phase. When making a surgical bed, the linens are horizontally fanfolded to facilitate transfer of the patient into the bed. In some agencies, the patient is brought back to the unit on a stretcher and transferred to the bed in the room. In other agencies, the patient's bed is brought to the surgery suite and the patient is transferred there. In the latter situation, the bed needs to be made with clean linens as soon as the patient goes to surgery so that it can be taken to the operating room when needed.

- Strip the bed.
- Place and leave the pillows on the bedside chair. **Rationale:** *Pillows are left on a chair to facilitate transferring the patient into the bed.*
- Apply the bottom linens as for an unoccupied bed. Place a bath blanket on the foundation of the bed if this is facility practice. **Rationale:** *A flannel bath blanket provides additional warmth.*
- Place the top covers (sheet, blanket, and bedspread) on the bed as you would for an unoccupied bed. Do not tuck them in, miter the corners, or make a toe pleat.
- Make a cuff at the top of the bed as you would for an unoccupied bed. In the same way, fold linens up from the bottom.
- On the side of the bed where the patient will be transferred, fold up the two outer corners of the top linens so they meet in the middle of the bed forming a triangle ⑰.
- Pick up the apex or point of the triangle and fanfold the top linens lengthwise to the side of the bed opposite from where the patient will enter the bed ⑱. **Rationale:** *This facilitates the patient's transfer into the bed.*
- Leave the bed in high position with the side rails down. **Rationale:** *The high position facilitates the transfer of the patient.*

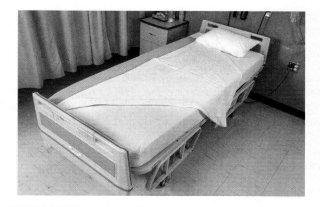

⑰ Fold up the two outer corners of the top linens, forming a triangle.

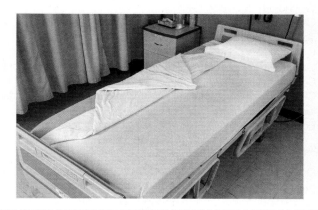

⑱ Surgical bed. The linens are horizontally fanfolded to one side of the bed to facilitate transfer of the patient into the bed.

- Lock the wheels of the bed if the bed is not to be moved. **Rationale:** *Locking the wheels keeps the bed from rolling when the patient is transferred from the stretcher to the bed.*

SAMPLE DOCUMENTATION

[date] 0700 Up to shower without assistance, bed linen changed, call bell repositioned at HOB, upper left side rail up. *M. Grassland*

Lifespan Considerations
CHILDREN

- Check if the child has a favorite blanket and if it was brought from home. If so, make sure you replace it on the bed after changing the bed linens.

OLDER ADULTS

- Because the older adult's skin can be thin, tender, and fragile, be sure to check that the linens are dry and free of wrinkles and be especially careful when pulling linens underneath the older patient.

SKILL 2.3 Eyes and Contact Lenses: Caring for

Promotes cleanliness and supports the patient's vision to remove crusting at the inner and outer canthus.

Delegation or Assignment

Assisting the patient with eye care can be delegated or assigned to the UAP. Remind the UAP to notify the nurse of anything that looks out of the ordinary. The nurse remains responsible for the assessment, interpretation of abnormal findings, and determination of appropriate responses. Note that state laws for UAPs vary, so this task might be assigned to the UAP rather than delegated.

Equipment

- Small basin
- Sterile water or normal saline solution
- Washcloth or cotton balls
- Clean gloves
- Towel
- Contact lens container (contact lens only)
- Commercially prepared cleaning solution (contact lens only)
- Commercially prepared disinfecting solution (contact lens only)
- Commercially prepared rinsing and storing solution (contact lens only)
- Enzymatic agent (protein remover) (contact lens only)

Preparation

- Determine patient's eye care needs, and obtain healthcare provider's order if needed.
- Explain necessity for and method of eye care to patient. Discuss how patient can assist you.
- Collect necessary equipment.

EYE CARE

Procedure

1. Introduce self to patient and verify the patient's identity using two identifiers. Explain to the patient what you are going to do, why it is necessary, and how the patient can participate. Discuss how the results will be used in planning further care or treatments.
2. Perform hand hygiene and observe appropriate infection control procedures.
3. Don gloves. Provide for patient privacy.
4. Use water or saline solution at room temperature.
5. Using the washcloth or cotton balls moistened in water or saline, gently wipe each eye from the inner to outer canthus. Use separate cotton ball or corner of washcloth for each eye. **Rationale:** *This prevents cross-contamination from one eye to the other.*
6. If crusting is present, gently place a warm, wet compress over eye(s) until crusting is loosened.
7. Dispose of used supplies and return basin to appropriate area.
8. Remove and discard gloves.
9. Perform hand hygiene. Leave patient safe and comfortable.
10. Complete documentation using forms, checklists, or electronic dropdown lists supplemented by nurse's notes or additional comments as appropriate.

For a comatose patient

- Use a dropper to instill a sterile ophthalmic solution (liquid tears, saline, methylcellulose) every 3–4 hr as ordered by the healthcare provider. **Rationale:** *This helps to prevent corneal drying and ulceration.*
- Keep patient's eyes closed if blink reflex is absent. If eye pads or patches are used, explain their purpose to patient's family. Do not tape eyes shut. **Rationale:** *Corneal abrasions and drying occur when eyes lose blink reflex.*
- Remove gloves and perform hand hygiene.
- Remove patch and evaluate condition of eye every 4 hours. Keep patient safe and comfortable.

CONTACT LENS CARE

Procedure

1. Place patient in semi-Fowler's position, and place a towel under the patient's chin.
2. Perform hand hygiene and don gloves.
3. Place the tip of your thumb across the lower lid below its margin.
4. Place the tip of the forefinger of the same hand on the upper lid above its margin.
5. Spread eyelids apart as wide as possible and locate outer edges of soft lens which should appear as a rim around outer edge of iris.
6. With other hand, place thumb and forefinger directly on soft lens.
7. Gently remove soft lens from surface of eyeball by squeezing lens between thumb and fingertip. To remove rigid lens, place thumb on lower eyelid and index finger on upper lid. Press gently against eyeball to release suction; lens is released as eyelids meet lens edge. Catch lens in your hand. **Rationale:** *Corneas are avascular and the use of contact lenses interrupts flow of oxygen into cornea. Removing lenses for a period of time allows oxygen to reach the cornea, thus preventing corneal complications.*
   Note: A suction cup can be placed gently against lens for easy removal of lens. Squeeze suction cup with dominant hand, place on lens, open finger slightly to create suction between lens and cup. Rock lens gently to remove it.
8. Release eyelids.
9. Place lens in palm of hand or place disposable lenses in trash. Disposable lenses are not to be cleaned or reused. Lens cleaners are not available for these lenses.
10. Place 2–3 drops of cleaning solution on lens.
11. Clean lens thoroughly by rubbing between fingertip and palm of hand for 20–30 seconds.
12. Rinse lens thoroughly with sterile saline solution or rinsing solution. Use only lens cleaning system recommended by ophthalmologist. Do not interchange cleaning solution systems.
13. Place lens in disinfecting solution according to healthcare provider directions. Time varies from hours to 1 full day. **Rationale:** *This destroys microorganisms on lenses.*
14. Rinse lens thoroughly with rinsing solution.
15. Repeat procedure on second lens.

SKILL 2.3 Eyes and Contact Lenses: Caring for (continued)

16. Use enzyme tablet or solution according to healthcare provider orders, usually weekly. **Rationale:** *This removes stubborn protein and lipids.*
17. Clean lens container daily and leave open to dry. Replace as directed by healthcare provider, either weekly or monthly.
18. Remove gloves and perform hand hygiene. Leave patient safe and comfortable.
19. Complete documentation using forms, checklists, or electronic dropdown lists supplemented by nurse's notes or additional comments as appropriate.

SAMPLE DOCUMENTATION

[date] 1545 Washcloth moistened with sterile normal saline, each eye wiped from inner to outer canthus using different areas of washcloth, no crustation noted either eye, denies tenderness of eye area or blurring of vision, tolerated procedure without incidence. *W. Gomez*

Patient Teaching

Instruct the patient in the following safety issues for contact lens:

- Notify healthcare provider immediately if eyes are red, uncomfortable, or you can't see clearly.
- Use only rinsing solution, not saliva, to wet lenses.
- Use only commercially prepared saline solution or rinsing solution to cleanse lenses.
- Do not interchange types of lens cleaning systems.
- Maintain lens care regimen prescribed by healthcare provider.
- Put on makeup before inserting lens.
- Use appropriate type of lenses for their intended use. Do not use daily-wear lenses at night or disposable lenses more than once.
- Do not allow soft lenses to dry out.
- Contact lens wearers should be instructed to carry appropriate identification on type and care for specific lens worn.

SKILL 2.4 Feet: Caring for

Many aspects of health and well-being are negatively impacted with foot problems if they compromise mobility and the ability to move about as desired in daily living. Maintaining foot health can have a positive effect on general health and well-being.

Delegation or Assignment

Foot care for the *nondiabetic* patient can be delegated or assigned to the UAP. Remind the UAP to notify the nurse of anything that looks out of the ordinary. Review with the UAP the facility policy about cutting or trimming nails. The nurse remains responsible for the assessment, interpretation of abnormal findings, and determination of appropriate responses. Note that state laws for UAPs vary, so this task might be assigned to the UAP rather than delegated.

Equipment

- Wash basin containing warm water
- Pillow
- Moisture-resistant disposable pad
- Towels
- Soap
- Washcloth
- Toenail cleaning and trimming equipment, if facility policy permits
- Lotion or foot powder

Preparation

Assemble all of the necessary equipment and supplies if nails need trimming and facility policy permits.

Procedure

1. Prior to performing the procedure, introduce self and verify the patient's identity using two identifiers. Explain to the patient what you are going to do, why it is necessary, and how the patient can participate.
2. Perform hand hygiene and observe other appropriate infection control procedures (e.g., clean gloves).
3. Provide for patient privacy by drawing the curtains around the bed or closing the door to the room. Some agencies provide signs indicating the need for privacy. **Rationale:** *Hygiene is a personal matter.*
4. Prepare the equipment and the patient.
   - Fill the washbasin with warm water at about 40°C–43°C (105°F–110°F). **Rationale:** *Warm water promotes circulation, and it comforts and refreshes.*
   - Assist the ambulatory patient to a sitting position in a chair, or the bed-bound patient to a supine or semi-Fowler's position.
   - Place a pillow under the bed patient's knees, if not contraindicated. **Rationale:** *This provides support and prevents muscle fatigue.*
   - Place the washbasin on the moisture-resistant pad at the foot of the bed for a bed patient or on the floor in front of the chair for an ambulatory patient ❶.
   - For a bed patient, pad the rim of the washbasin with a towel. **Rationale:** *The towel prevents undue pressure on the skin.*
5. Wash the foot.
   - Place one of the patient's feet in the basin and wash it with soap, paying particular attention to the interdigital areas. Prolonged soaking is generally not recommended for patients with diabetes or individuals with peripheral vascular disease. **Rationale:** *Prolonged soaking may remove natural skin oils, thus drying the skin and making it more susceptible to cracking and injury.*

(continued on next page)

SKILL 2.4 Feet: Caring for (*continued*)

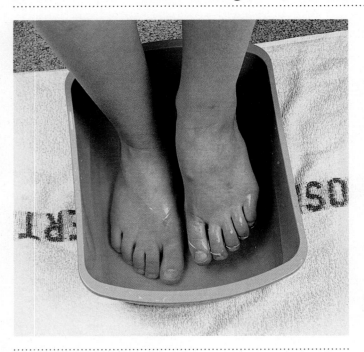

1 Place towel on floor in front of patient and place feet in basin for soaking.

- Rinse the foot well to remove soap. **Rationale:** *Soap irritates the skin if not completely removed.*
- Rub calloused areas of the foot with the washcloth. **Rationale:** *This helps remove dead skin layers.*
- If the nails are brittle or thick and require trimming, replace the water and allow the foot to soak for 10–20 min. **Rationale:** *Soaking softens the nails and loosens debris under them.*
- Clean the nails as required with a manicure tool such as an orange stick. **Rationale:** *This removes excess debris that harbors microorganisms.*
- Remove the foot from the basin and place it on the towel.
6. Dry the foot thoroughly and apply lotion or foot powder.
   - Blot the foot gently with the towel to dry it thoroughly, particularly between the toes. **Rationale:** *Harsh rubbing can damage the skin. Thorough drying reduces the risk of infection.*
   - Apply lotion or lanolin cream to the foot but not between the toes. **Rationale:** *This lubricates dry skin and keeps the area between the toes dry.*
   or
   - Apply a foot powder containing a nonirritating deodorant if the feet tend to perspire excessively. **Rationale:** *Foot powders have greater absorbent properties than regular bath powders; some also contain menthol, which makes the feet feel cool.*
7. If facility policy permits, trim the nails of the first foot while the second foot is soaking.
   - See the information on nail care below for the appropriate method to use for trimming nails. Note that in many agencies, toenail trimming requires a healthcare pro-

vider's order or is contraindicated for patients with diabetes mellitus, toe infections, and peripheral vascular disease, unless performed by a podiatrist, general practice healthcare provider, or advanced practice nurse.
8. When the procedure is complete, perform hand hygiene. Leave patient safe and comfortable.
9. Complete documentation using forms, checklists, or electronic dropdown lists supplemented by nurse's notes or additional comments as indicated below. Document any foot problems observed.
   - Follow facility policy. Foot care is not generally recorded unless problems are noted.
   - Record any signs of inflammation, infection, breaks in the skin, corns, troublesome calluses, bunions, and pressure areas. This is of particular importance for patients with peripheral vascular disease and diabetes.

SAMPLE DOCUMENTATION

[date] 0900 Foot care provided after bath, toenails are thick, yellow, hard, and curling over nail ends. Unable to cut toenails. Denies any pain of toe ends, but states cannot really feel as well as he could in the past. Unable to assess capillary refill due to hardness and discoloration of toenails, able to move toes and has decreased touch sensation. Dr. Johnson notified of toenails status. *P. Kimberly*

Nail Care

- Check the facility's policy regarding nail care. Often, podiatrists must be consulted for patients with diabetes.
- To provide nail care, you need a nail cutter or sharp scissors, a nail file, an orange stick to push back the cuticle, hand lotion or mineral oil to lubricate any dry tissue around the nails, and a basin of water to soak the nails if they are particularly thick or hard.
- If needed, soak and then dry one hand or foot. Then cut the nail or file it straight across beyond the end of the finger or toe. Avoid trimming or digging into nails at the lateral corners. **Rationale:** *Trimming toes at the corners predisposes the patient to ingrown toenails.*
- In patients who have diabetes or circulatory problems, file rather than cut the nails. Inadvertent injury to tissues can occur if scissors are used.
- After the initial cut or filing, file to round the corners of the nail and clean under the nail.
- Gently push back the cuticle, taking care not to injure it.
- Care for each finger or toe in the same manner.
- Record and report any abnormalities, such as an infected cuticle or inflammation of the tissue around the nail.
- If eyesight, fine motor control, or cognition prevents the patient from safely trimming the nails at home, refer the patient to a podiatrist or manicurist.

SKILL 2.4 Feet: Caring for *(continued)*

Patient Teaching

- Wash the feet daily, and dry them well, especially between the toes.
- When washing, inspect the skin of the feet for breaks or red or swollen areas. Use a mirror if needed to visualize all areas.
- To prevent burns, check the water temperature before immersing the feet.
- Cover the feet, except between the toes, with creams or lotions to moisten the skin. Lotion will also soften calluses. A lotion that reduces dryness effectively is a mixture of lanolin and mineral oil.
- To prevent or control an unpleasant odor due to excessive foot perspiration, wash the feet frequently and change socks and shoes at least daily. Special deodorant sprays or absorbent foot powders are also helpful.
- File the toenails rather than cutting them to avoid skin injury. File the nails straight across the ends of the toes. If the nails are too thick or misshapen to file, consult a podiatrist.
- Wear clean stockings or socks daily. Avoid socks with holes or darns that can cause pressure areas.
- Wear comfortable, well-fitting shoes that neither restrict the foot nor rub on any area; rubbing can cause corns and calluses. Check worn shoes for rough spots in the lining. Break in new shoes gradually by increasing the wearing time 30 to 60 minutes each day.

- Avoid walking barefoot, because injury and infection may result. Wear slippers in public showers and in change areas to avoid contracting athlete's foot or other infections.
- Several times each day exercise the feet to promote circulation. Point the feet upward, point them downward, and move them in circles.
- Avoid wearing constricting garments such as knee-high elastic stockings, and avoid sitting with the legs crossed at the knees, which may decrease circulation.
- When the feet are cold, use extra blankets and wear warm socks rather than using heating pads or hot water bottles, which may cause burns. Test bathwater before stepping into it.
- Wash any cut on the foot thoroughly, apply a mild antiseptic, and notify the healthcare provider.
- Avoid self-treatment for corns or calluses. Pumice stones and some callus and corn applications can injure the skin. Do not cut calluses or corns. Consult a podiatrist or healthcare provider first.
- Notify the healthcare provider about any abnormal sores or drainage, pain, or changes in temperature, color, and sensation of the foot.

SKILL 2.5 Hair: Caring for

The appearance of the hair often reflects a person's feelings of self-concept and sociocultural well-being. Becoming familiar with hair care needs and practices that may be different from our own is an important aspect of providing competent nursing care to all patients. People who feel ill may not groom their hair as before. A dirty scalp and hair are itchy and uncomfortable, and can have an odor. The hair may also reflect state of health (e.g., excessive coarseness and dryness may be associated with endocrine disorders such as hypothyroidism).

Delegation or Assignment

Brushing and combing hair, shampooing hair, and shaving facial hair can be delegated or assigned to the UAP unless the patient has a condition in which the procedure would be contraindicated (e.g., cervical spinal injury or trauma). The nurse needs to assess the UAP's knowledge and experience of hair care for patients of other cultures, if appropriate. The nurse remains responsible for the assessment, interpretation of abnormal finds, and determination of appropriate actions. Note that state laws for UAPs vary, so this task might be assigned to the UAP rather than delegated.

Equipment

- Clean brush and comb (A wide-toothed comb may be preferred by some individuals because finer combs pull the hair into knots and may also break the hair.)
- Two bath towels

- Hair oil preparation or other hair care products, as requested by patient

For Shampooing Hair
- Shampoo
- Conditioner, if desired
- Hair dryer, if allowed by hospital

For Disposable System
- Package containing shampoo cap ① ②

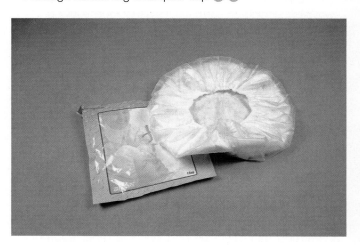

① Shampoo system activated by microwave.

(continued on next page)

SKILL 2.5 Hair: Caring for (continued)

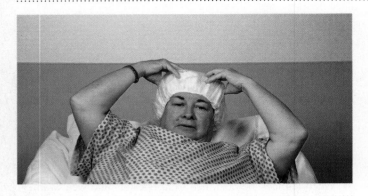

2 Disposable shampoo cap can be used for patients on bed rest.

Note: Ensure that electrical equipment is checked by maintenance department before using. **Rationale:** *This confirms that equipment is grounded and mechanically safe.*

Preparation

- Determine patient's hair care needs. Each person has particular ways of caring for hair. Many people oil their hair daily because it tends to be dry; others have oily hair that may lead to an itchy scalp. Some people brush their hair vigorously before retiring; others comb their hair infrequently.
- Collect and assemble equipment.
- Help patient into a comfortable position to perform hair care.

Safety Considerations

If the patient is an older adult, do not press the neck down on the edge of the sink—this position can diminish circulation to the brain and has been reported to be a possible cause of strokes.

- Shampooing the hair can be accomplished in a variety of ways depending on the patient's usual routine and physical condition. In many institutions, a healthcare provider's order is necessary before shampooing a patient's hair.
- If possible, the easiest way to shampoo is to assist the patient in the shower. Caution should be taken to prevent the patient from becoming overly tired or weak while in the shower. (Use shower chair if necessary.)

HAIR CARE

Procedure

1. Prior to performing the procedure, introduce self and verify the patient's identity using two identifiers. Explain to the patient what you are going to do, why it is necessary, and how the patient can participate.
2. Perform hand hygiene and observe other appropriate infection control procedures (e.g., clean gloves).
3. Provide for patient privacy by drawing the curtains around the bed or closing the door to the room. Some agencies

provide signs indicating the need for privacy. **Rationale:** *Hygiene is a personal matter.*
4. Position and prepare the patient appropriately.
   - Assist the patient who can sit to move to a chair. **Rationale:** *Hair is more easily brushed and combed when the patient is in a sitting position.* If health permits, assist a patient confined to a bed to a sitting position by raising the head of the bed. Otherwise, assist the patient to alternate side-lying positions, and do one side of the head at a time.
   - If the patient remains in bed, place a clean towel over the pillow and the patient's shoulders. Place it over the sitting patient's shoulders. **Rationale:** *The towel collects any removed hair, dirt, and scaly material.*
   - Remove any pins or ribbons in the hair.
5. Remove any mats or tangles gradually.
   - Separate the hair into sections to untangle mats using one's fingers to pull them apart or work them out with repeated brushings to help prevent hair breakage and discomfort.
   - If the hair is very tangled, rub alcohol or an oil, such as mineral oil, on the strands to help loosen the tangles. Use a large open-toothed comb to untangle hair in sections as needed.
   - Dampen the hair with water or use a leave-in conditioner to help stop hair from tangling.
   - Comb out tangles in a small section of hair toward the ends. Stabilize the hair with one hand and comb toward the ends of the hair with the other hand. **Rationale:** *This avoids scalp trauma.*
6. Brush and comb the hair.
   - For short hair, brush and comb one side at a time. Divide long hair into two sections by parting it down the middle from the front to the back. If the hair is very thick, divide each section into front and back subsections or into several layers.
7. Arrange the hair as neatly and attractively as possible, according to the individual's desires.
   - Ask if the patient would like the hair braided. **Rationale:** *Braiding will decrease tangling; however, the choice is the patient's.*
8. When procedure is complete, perform hand hygiene. Leave patient safe and comfortable.
9. Complete documentation using forms, checklists, or electronic dropdown lists supplemented by nurse's notes or additional comments as appropriate. Document assessments and special nursing interventions. Daily combing and brushing of the hair are not normally recorded.

SHAMPOOING HAIR

Procedure

For Routine Hair Care

1. Have all hair care items within reach.
2. Drape towel over patient's shoulders.
3. Brush or comb patient's hair from scalp to hair ends, using gentle, even strokes.

SKILL 2.5 Hair: Caring for (*continued*)

- *Tangled hair:* Use short gentle strokes. Work from end of hair shaft toward scalp. May use conditioner to make combing easier.
- *Curly hair:* Use wet comb on wet hair (water or oil) for ease of combing.

4. Style hair in a manner suitable to patient.
5. Replace hair care items in appropriate place and clean items as needed.
6. Perform hand hygiene.

For Patient on a Stretcher

1. Have shampoo items readily available.
2. Position stretcher with head end at sink.
3. Lock wheels on stretcher. **Rationale:** *This prevents the gurney from moving away from the sink.*
4. Pad the edge of the sink with a towel or bath blanket.
5. Move the patient's head just beyond the edge of the stretcher. **Rationale:** *This allows water to run off more easily.*
6. Put a pillow or a rolled blanket under the patient's shoulders. **Rationale:** *This helps elevate and extend the head.*
7. Drape one towel over patient's shoulders and around neck. Place another towel within reach.
8. Use a washcloth to protect patient's eyes. Wet hair and gently make lather with shampoo.
9. Rinse thoroughly and repeat if necessary.
10. Towel dry, add conditioner if desired, and rinse again.
11. Using a dry towel, pat hair dry, and wrap turban style to transport back to room.
12. Use hair dryer if available.
13. Style as desired.
14. Replace equipment.
15. Perform hand hygiene.

For Patient Using Disposable System

1. Heat shampoo package in microwave for no more than 30 seconds.
2. Perform hand hygiene.
3. Open package and check temperature. **Rationale:** *Patients react to heat at different temperatures; therefore, check the cap temperature with patient before placing on patient's head.*
4. Place cap on head. Ensure that all hair is contained within the cap. For longer hair, place cap on top of head and then tuck all hair up inside cap.
5. Gently massage cap with hands, 1–2 min for short hair and 2–3 min for longer hair. **Rationale:** *This will assist in saturating the hair with the solution. There is no need to rinse hair after using solution.*

***

CAUTION! If hair is tangled, the cap may need to stay on for a longer period of time in order to saturate hair. If blood or other secretions are present on hair, they may need to be removed using the washcloths from the disposable bath system before attempting to shampoo the hair.

***

6. Remove cap and place in appropriate receptacle.
7. Towel dry hair.

8. Complete hair care according to patient's needs and desires.
9. Perform hand hygiene.
   Note: Disposable hair care systems provide a quick and easy way to freshen patient's hair with minimal patient movement.

***

Health Promotion: Head Lice and Nits Infestation

Head lice are tiny wingless insects that can live on the human scalp and feed exclusively on human blood 3 to 4 times a day. They don't fly, jump or hop, but they crawl. They can live up to 30 days, and their eggs can live about two weeks. They are spread by close contact with another person who has lice, touching clothing or bedding, or sharing hats, towels, brushes, or combs. They easily spread in overcrowded living conditions or among school children. Lice are more active at night in the dark, resulting in many people experiencing a crawling sensation on their scalp. Head lice cause intense itching of the scalp. Because people scratch vigorously, they can develop scratch marks on their scalp which can lead to infection. Head lice do not carry or spread diseases, but they are a nuisance. There is a stigma that people with head lice are dirty and unkempt, but the reality is lice just want human blood. There are other varieties of lice that can infest the human body.

Sometimes people with head lice infestation will have small, red bumps on their scalp, neck, and shoulders which may have drainage and become crusty. The eggs, or nits, are tiny white, yellow, or tan specks that cling to the bottom of the hair shaft. Head lice are very hard to see without the help of a good bright light and possibly a magnifying glass. To protect yourself while you are assessing the scalp, wear clean gloves and do not touch the patient's clothing while observing the scalp area.

There are assessment kits that include a fine-toothed comb to make parts in the hair for better visualization of the scalp and hair shafts ❸. Look for tiny bugs and white specks at the base of hair shafts. Examine the whole scalp, neck, and around the ears. If lice and white specs on hair shafts are noted, ask another nurse to inspect the patient's scalp to verify your assessment. The patient needs to be told about the lice infestation of the scalp in a calm and therapeutic manner. Let the patient know the healthcare provider will be notified

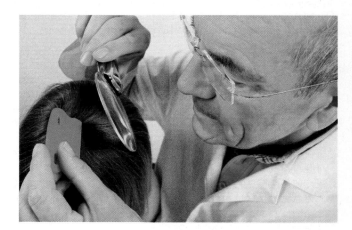

Source: Westend61/GmbH/Alamy Stock Photo

❸ **Use magnifying glass when inspecting for head lice.**

(*continued on next page*)

SKILL 2.5 Hair: Caring for (continued)

and will order appropriate treatment. There are many treatments including lotions and shampoos that contain pesticides/insecticides that can help rid the scalp of the lice and nits. Determine if the patient is allergic to ragweed or chrysanthemums. **Rationale:** *Pyrethrin is obtained from these plants and cannot be used to treat lice if patient has an allergic reaction to them.* A fine-toothed comb or special lice comb is necessary in this process.

In the healthcare facility, patients infested with lice and nits are moved to a private room, and contact isolation personal protective equipment (PPE) is recommended. Depending on how long the patient will be hospitalized, the treatment can be initiated while in the hospital and then continued at home. The patient's clothing will need to be put

in tightly closed bags and given to family members to take home and wash in hot water and soap. The family also needs to take care of the home environment to prevent transmission to other family members and prepare the home for the patient's return. Many times, family members will undergo the treatment of their scalp, also.

Sources: Data from Centers for Disease Control and Prevention (CDC). (2015). *Parasites – Lice – Head Lice.* Retrieved from http://www.cdc.gov/parasites/lice/head/treatment.html

American Academy of Dermatology (AAD). (2015). *Head lice: Overview, Symptoms, Causes, Treatment, Tips.* Retrieved from https://www.aad.org/public/diseases/contagious-skin-diseases/head-lice

SKILL 2.6 Hearing Aid: Removing, Cleaning, and Inserting

This skill provides patients assistance with the maintenance and care of assistive hearing device.

Delegation or Assignment

A nurse can delegate or assign the task of caring for a hearing aid to the UAP. It is important, however, for the nurse to first determine that the UAP knows the correct way to care for a hearing aid. Inform the UAP to report the presence of ear inflammation, discomfort, excess wax, or drainage to the RN. The nurse remains responsible for the assessment, interpretation of abnormal finds, and determination of appropriate actions. Note that state laws for UAPs vary, so this task might be assigned to the UAP rather than delegated.

Equipment

- Patient's hearing aid
- Soap, water, and towels or a damp cloth
- Pipe cleaner or toothpick (optional)
- New battery (if needed)

Preparation

- Speak facing the patient for improved communication.
- Place a towel on the bedside table so that all the hearing aid parts can be in clear view to avoid losing a part or mistakenly dropping a part.

Procedure

1. Prior to performing the procedure, introduce self and verify the patient's identity using two identifiers. Explain to the patient what you are going to do, why it is necessary, and how the patient can participate.
2. Perform hand hygiene and observe other appropriate infection control procedures (e.g., clean gloves).
3. Provide for patient privacy by drawing the curtains around the bed or closing the door to the room. Some agencies provide signs indicating the need for privacy. **Rationale:** *Hygiene is a personal matter.*
4. Remove the hearing aid.
   - Turn the hearing aid off and lower the volume. The on/off switch may be labeled "O" (off), "M" (microphone), "T" (telephone), or "TM" (telephone/microphone).

Rationale: *The batteries continue to run if the hearing aid is not turned off.*
   - Remove the earmold by rotating it slightly forward and pulling it outward.
   - If the hearing aid is not to be used for several days, remove the battery. **Rationale:** *Removal prevents corrosion of the hearing aid from battery leakage.*
   - Store the hearing aid in a safe place and label with patient's name. Avoid exposure to heat and moisture. **Rationale:** *Proper storage prevents loss or damage.*
5. Clean the earmold.
   - Detach the earmold if possible. Disconnect the earmold from the *receiver of a body* hearing aid or from the hearing aid case of behind-the-ear and eyeglass hearing aids where the tubing meets the hook of the case. Do not remove the earmold if it is glued or secured by a small metal ring. **Rationale:** *Removal facilitates cleaning and prevents inadvertent damage to the other parts.*
   - If the earmold is detachable, soak it in a mild soapy solution. Rinse and dry it well. Do not use isopropyl alcohol. **Rationale:** *Alcohol can damage the hearing aid.*
   - If the earmold is not detachable or is for an in-the-ear aid, wipe the earmold with a damp cloth.
   - Check that the earmold opening is patent. Blow any excess moisture through the opening or remove debris (e.g., earwax) with a pipe cleaner or toothpick.
   - Reattach the earmold if it was detached from the rest of the hearing aid.
6. Insert the hearing aid.
   - Determine from the patient if the earmold is for the left or the right ear.
   - Check that the battery is inserted in the hearing aid. Confirm that the hearing aid is off, and make sure the volume is turned all the way down. **Rationale:** *A volume that is too loud is distressing.*
   - Inspect the earmold to identify the ear canal portion. Some ear molds are fitted for only the ear canal and concha; others are fitted for all the contours of the ear. The canal portion, common to all, can be used as a guide for correct insertion.
   - Line up the parts of the earmold with the corresponding parts of the patient's ear.

SKILL 2.6 Hearing Aid: Removing, Cleaning, and Inserting (continued)

- Rotate the earmold slightly forward, and insert the ear canal portion.
- Gently press the earmold into the ear while rotating it backward.
- Check that the earmold fits snugly by asking the patient if it feels secure and comfortable.
- Adjust the other components of a behind-the-ear or body hearing aid.
- Turn the hearing aid on, and adjust the volume according to the patient's needs.

7. Correct problems associated with improper functioning.
- If the sound is weak or there is no sound:
  a. Ensure that the volume is turned high enough.
  b. Ensure that the earmold opening is not clogged.
  c. Check the battery by turning the hearing aid on, turning up the volume, cupping your hand over the earmold, and listening. A constant whistling sound indicates the battery is functioning. If necessary, replace the battery. Be sure that the negative (–) and positive (+) signs on the battery match those where indicated on the hearing aid.
  d. Ensure that the ear canal is not blocked with wax, which can obstruct sound waves.
- If the patient reports a whistling sound or squeal after insertion:
  a. Turn the volume down.
  b. Ensure that the earmold is properly attached to the receiver.
  c. Reinsert the earmold.

8. When the procedure is complete, perform hand hygiene. Leave patient safe and comfortable.
9. Complete documentation using forms, checklists, or electronic dropdown lists supplemented by nurse's notes or additional comments as appropriate. Document pertinent data as indicated below.
- Routine removal, cleaning, and insertion of a hearing aid are not normally recorded.
- However, it is important to report and record any problems the patient has with the hearing aid.

Patient Teaching

- It is important to tell the patient who has just purchased a hearing aid that it often takes weeks or even months to adjust to it. At first, sounds will seem shrill as patients start hearing high-frequency sounds that had been forgotten. Remind them that it is a hearing aid, not a hearing cure. Encourage them not to give up.
- The patient needs to adjust to the hearing aid gradually by increasing the amount of time each day until the aid can be worn for a full day.
- Encourage patients to purchase their hearing aids from a company that has a minimum warranty of a 30-day return policy.
- Emphasize the importance of maintaining the hearing aid, that is, having it cleaned and checked regularly.

SKILL 2.7 Mouth: Regular and Unconscious or Debilitated Patient, Caring for

Oral care is important to maintain healthy teeth, gums, and tongue. It can help prevent bad breath, dry mouth, cold sores, tooth decay, or thrush. Good oral hygiene includes daily stimulation of the gums, mechanical brushing and flossing of the teeth, flushing of the mouth, and regular checkups by a dentist. The nurse is often in a position to help people maintain oral hygiene by helping or teaching them to clean their teeth and oral cavity, by inspecting whether patients (especially children) have done so, or by actually providing mouth care to patients who are ill or incapacitated.

Delegation or Assignment

A nurse can delegate or assign the task of providing or assisting the patient with oral hygiene to the UAP. It is important, however, for the nurse to determine first that the UAP knows the correct way to provide oral care. Tell the UAP to report the presence of inflammation, discomfort, tenderness, or drainage to the RN. The nurse remains responsible for the assessment, interpretation of abnormal finds, and determination of appropriate actions. Note that state laws for UAPs vary, so this task might be assigned to the UAP rather than delegated.

Equipment

- Disposable cleansing cloth system or towels, washcloth, basin with water and soap
- Dental care items (i.e., toothbrush, toothpaste, dental floss, denture cup, denture cleaner, or clean washcloth)
- Mouthwash
- Emesis basin, water cup
- Clean gloves

For Unconscious or Debilitated Patient Only

- Bite-block to hold the mouth open and teeth apart (optional)
- Tissue or piece of gauze to remove dentures (optional)
- Rubber-tipped bulb syringe
- Suction catheter with suction apparatus when aspiration is a concern
- Foam swabs and cleaning solution for cleaning the mucous membranes
- Water-soluble lip moisturizer

(continued on next page)

SKILL 2.7 Mouth: Regular and Unconscious or Debilitated Patient, Caring for (continued)

Preparation

- Adjust the bed to a comfortable working height, and assist the patient into a comfortable position.
- The patient with a nasogastric tube or who is receiving oxygen is likely to develop dry oral mucous membranes, especially if the patient breathes through the mouth. More frequent oral hygiene will be needed.
- Oral care can be done as often as needed for the unconscious patient to prevent oral complications.
- Always have oral suction ready to use when providing oral care to the unconscious patient to prevent aspiration.

ORAL HYGIENE

Procedure

1. Introduce self to patient (and parent of child) and verify the patient's identity using two identifiers. Explain to the patient (and parent of child) what you are going to do, why it is necessary, and how the patient can participate. Discuss how the results will be used in planning further care or treatments.
2. Perform hand hygiene and observe appropriate infection control procedures.
3. Provide for patient privacy.
4. Place a towel under the patient's chin.
5. Apply clean gloves.
6. Moisten the bristles of the toothbrush with tepid water and apply toothpaste to it.
7. Use a soft toothbrush (a small one for a child) and the patient's choice of toothpaste.
8. For the patient who must remain in bed, place or hold the curved basin under the patient's chin, fitting the small curve around the chin or neck.
9. Inspect the mouth and teeth.
10. Hand the toothbrush to the patient, or brush the patient's teeth as follows:
    a. Hold the brush against the teeth with the bristles at a 45-degree angle. The tips of the outer bristles should rest against and penetrate under the gingival sulcus ❶. The brush will clean under the sulcus of two or three teeth at one time. **Rationale:** *This sulcular technique removes plaque and cleans under the gingival margins.*
    b. Move the bristles up and down gently in short strokes from the sulcus to the crowns of the teeth ❷.

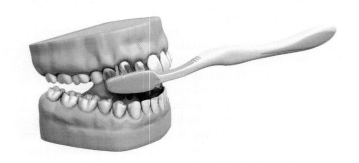

❷ Brushing from the sulcus to the crowns of the teeth.

    c. Repeat until all outer and inner surfaces of the teeth and sulci of the gums have been cleaned.
    d. Clean the biting surfaces by moving the brush back and forth over them in short strokes ❸.

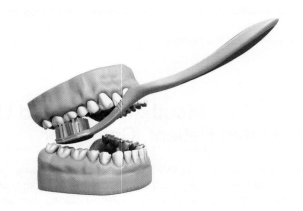

❸ Brushing the biting surfaces.

    e. Brush the tongue gently with the toothbrush. **Rationale:** *Brushing removes bacteria and freshens breath. A coated tongue may be caused by poor oral hygiene, low fluid intake, and side effects of medications. Brushing gently and carefully helps prevent gagging or vomiting.*
11. Hand the patient the water cup or mouthwash to rinse the mouth vigorously. Then ask the patient to spit the water and excess toothpaste into the basin. Some agencies supply a standard mouthwash. Alternatively, a mouth rinse of normal saline can be an effective cleaner and moisturizer. **Rationale:** *Vigorous rinsing loosens food particles and washes out already loosened particles.*
12. Repeat the preceding step until the mouth is free of toothpaste and food particles.

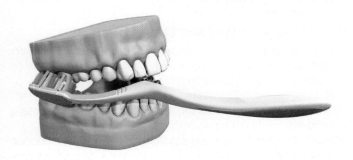

❶ The sulcular technique: Place the bristles at a 45-degree angle with the tops of the outer bristles under the gingival margins.

SKILL 2.7 Mouth: Regular and Unconscious or Debilitated Patient, Caring for *(continued)*

13. Remove the curved basin and help the patient wipe the mouth.
14. Assist the patient to floss independently, or floss the teeth of an alert and cooperative patient as follows. Waxed floss is less likely to fray than unwaxed floss; particles between the teeth attach more readily to unwaxed floss than to waxed floss.
    a. Wrap one end of the floss around the third finger of each hand ④.

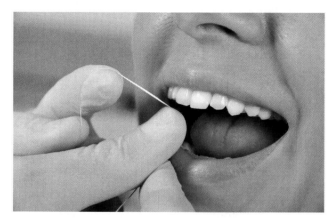

Source: Vetkit/Fotolia

④ Stretching the floss between the fingers of each hand.

    b. To floss the upper teeth, use your thumb and index finger to stretch the floss ⑤. Move the floss up and down between the teeth. When the floss reaches the gum line, gently slide the floss into the space between the gum and the tooth. Gently move the floss away from the gum with up and down motions (American Dental Association, 2016), Cleaning your teeth). Start at the back on the right side and work around to the back of the left side, or work from the center teeth to the back of the jaw on either side.

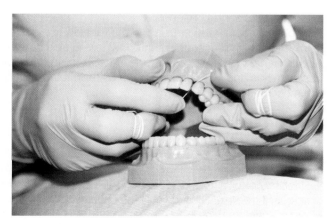

Source: Hannah Gal/Science Source

⑤ Flossing the teeth, using the fingers to stretch the floss.

    c. To floss the lower teeth, use your index fingers to stretch the floss.
15. Give the patient tepid water or mouthwash to rinse the mouth and a curved basin in which to spit the water.
16. Assist the patient in wiping the mouth.
17. Remove and clean the curved basin.
18. Remove and discard gloves. Perform hand hygiene. Leave patient safe and comfortable.
19. Complete documentation using forms, checklists, or electronic dropdown lists supplemented by nurse's notes or additional comments as appropriate.

ARTIFICIAL DENTURES

- Remove the dentures.
  - Perform hand hygiene. Apply gloves. **Rationale:** *Wearing gloves decreases the likelihood of spreading infection.*
  - If the patient cannot remove the dentures, using the tissue or gauze, grasp the upper plate at the front teeth with your thumb and second finger, and move the denture up and down slightly ⑥. **Rationale:** *The slight movement breaks the suction that holds the plate on the roof of the mouth.*

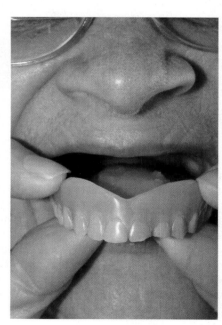

Source: Sdominick/E+/Getty Images

⑥ Removing the top dentures by first breaking the suction.

  - Lower the upper plate, move it out of the mouth, and place it in the denture container.
  - Lift the lower plate, turning it so that the left side, for example, is slightly lower than the right, to remove the plate from the mouth without stretching the lips. Place the lower plate in the denture container.

(continued on next page)

SKILL 2.7 Mouth: Regular and Unconscious or Debilitated Patient, Caring for (continued)

- Remove a partial denture by exerting equal pressure on the border of each side of the denture, not on the clasps, which can bend or break.
- Clean the dentures.
  - When cleaning dentures, hold them firmly and take care not to drop them ❼. Place a washcloth under them if using a sink. **Rationale:** *A washcloth prevents damage if the dentures are dropped against a hard surface.*

Note: If patients perform self-cleaning of dentures, ensure that dentures are placed in the appropriate container ❽. **Rationale:** *Many older adult patients leave dentures on food trays and risk losing them when food trays are removed. Replacement dentures may not be covered by Medicare.*

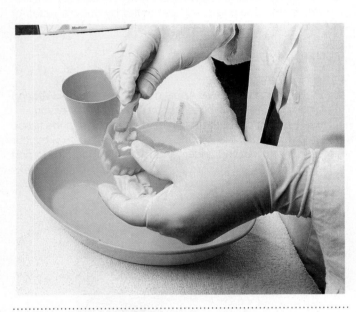

❼ Cleaning the dentures.

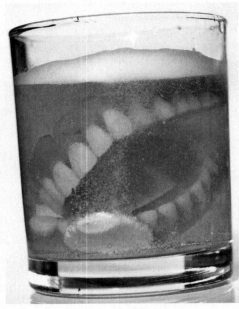

Source: Carsten Rademacher/mauritius images GmbH/Alamy Stock Photo

❽ Dentures soaking in solution prior to patient self-cleaning.

- Using a toothbrush or special stiff-bristled brush, scrub the dentures with the cleaning agent and tepid water. Rinse the dentures with tepid running water. **Rationale:** *Rinsing removes the cleaning agent and food particles.* If the dentures are stained, soak them in a commercial cleaner. Be sure to follow the manufacturer's directions. To prevent corrosion, dentures with metal parts should not be soaked overnight
- Inspect the dentures and the mouth.
  - Observe the dentures for any rough, sharp, or worn areas that could irritate the tongue or mucous membranes of the mouth, lips, and gums.
  - Inspect the mouth for any redness, irritated areas, or indications of infection.
  - Assess the fit of the dentures. People who have them should see a dentist at least once a year to check the fit and the presence of any irritation to the soft tissues of the mouth. Patients who need repairs to their dentures or new dentures may need a referral for financial assistance.
- Return the dentures to the mouth.
  - Offer some mouthwash and a curved basin to rinse the mouth. If the patient cannot insert the dentures independently, insert the plates one at a time. To avoid injuring the lips, hold each plate at a slight angle while inserting it.

- Assist the patient as needed.
  - Wipe the patient's hands and mouth with the towel.
  - If the patient does not want to or cannot wear the dentures, store them in a denture container with water. Label the container with the patient's name and identification number. (Do not place the container on the food tray.)
- Remove and discard gloves. Perform hand hygiene. Leave the patient safe and comfortable.
- Complete documentation using forms, checklists, or electronic dropdown lists supplemented by the nurse's notes or additional comments as appropriate and include all assessments and any problems such as an irritated area on the mucous membrane.

CARE FOR THE UNCONSCIOUS OR DEBILITATED PATIENT

Procedure

1. Prior to performing the procedure, if the patient is conscious, introduce self and verify the patient's identity using two identifiers. Explain to the patient and the family what you are going to do and why it is necessary.
2. Perform hand hygiene and observe other appropriate infection control procedures (e.g., clean gloves).

SKILL 2.7 Mouth: Regular and Unconscious or Debilitated Patient, Caring for (*continued*)

3. Provide for patient privacy by drawing the curtains around the bed or closing the door to the room. Some agencies provide signs indicating the need for privacy. **Rationale:** *Hygiene is a personal matter.*
4. Position the unconscious patient in a side-lying position, with the head of the bed lowered. **Rationale:** *In this position, the saliva automatically runs out by gravity rather than being aspirated into the lung. This position also allows for suctioning, if needed.* This position is chosen for the unconscious patient receiving mouth care. If the patient's head cannot be lowered, turn it to one side. **Rationale:** *The fluid will readily run out of the mouth or pool in the side of the mouth, where it can be suctioned.*

CAUTION! Oral suctioning is done using a Yankauer suction tip (or suction catheter) connected to a suction device. See Skill 11.14 for oral suctioning procedure and photo of a Yankauer suction tip.

---

5. Place the towel under the patient's chin.
6. Place the curved basin against the patient's chin and lower cheek to receive the fluid from the mouth ❾.

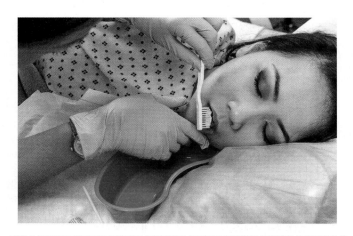

❾ Position of patient and placement of curved basin when providing special mouth care.

7. Apply gloves.
8. Clean the teeth and rinse the mouth.
9. If the patient has natural teeth, brush the teeth as described above in this skill. Brush gently and carefully to avoid injuring the gums. If the patient has artificial teeth, clean them as described above in this skill.
10. Rinse the patient's mouth by drawing about 10 mL of water or alcohol-free mouthwash into the syringe and injecting it gently into each side of the mouth. **Rationale:** *If the solution is injected with force, some of it may flow down the patient's throat and be aspirated into the lungs.*
11. Watch carefully to make sure that all of the rinsing solution has run out of the mouth into the basin. If not, suction the

fluid from the mouth. **Rationale:** *Fluid remaining in the mouth may be aspirated into the lungs.*
12. Repeat rinsing until the mouth is free of toothpaste, if used.
13. If the tissues appear dry or unclean, clean them with the foam swabs or gauze and cleaning solution following facility policy.
14. Picking up a moistened foam swab, wipe the mucous membrane of one cheek. Discard the swab in a waste container; use a fresh one to clean the next area. **Rationale:** *Using separate applicators for each area of the mouth prevents the transfer of microorganisms from one area to another.*
15. Clean all mouth tissues in an orderly progression, using separate applicators: the cheeks, roof of the mouth, base of the mouth, and tongue.
16. Observe the oral tissues closely for inflammation, dryness, or lesions.
17. Rinse the patient's mouth as described.
18. Remove the basin, and dry around the patient's mouth with the towel. Replace artificial dentures, if indicated.
19. Lubricate the patient's lips with water-soluble moisturizer. **Rationale:** *Lubrication prevents cracking and subsequent infection.*
20. Remove and discard gloves. Perform hand hygiene.
21. Complete documentation using forms, checklists, or electronic dropdown lists supplemented by the nurse's notes or additional comments as appropriate. Document assessment of the teeth, tongue, gums, and oral mucosa. Include any problems such as sores or inflammation and swelling of the gums.

SAMPLE DOCUMENTATION

[date] 1730 Small amount of salivary secretions suctioned from mouth, turned to right side, teeth brushed and gums swabbed, toothpaste and saliva suctioned from mouth, triggered swallowing for about 10 seconds, remains unresponsive to verbal stimuli, tolerated procedure without incidence. *K. Thigpen*

Lifespan Considerations

NEWBORNS AND INFANTS

▪ Most dentists recommend that dental hygiene should begin when the first tooth erupts and be practiced after each feeding. Cleaning can be accomplished by using a wet washcloth or small gauze moistened with water.

CHILDREN

▪ Beginning at about 18 months of age, brush the child's teeth with a soft toothbrush. Use only a toothbrush moistened with water. Introduce toothpaste later and use one that contains fluoride.

(*continued on next page*)

SKILL 2.7 Mouth: Regular and Unconscious or Debilitated Patient, Caring for *(continued)*

■ Frequent snacking on products containing sugar increases the child's risk for developing cavities.

OLDER ADULTS

■ Oral care is often difficult for certain older adults to perform if there are problems with dexterity or cognitive problems with dementia.

■ Dryness of the oral mucosa is a common finding in older adults. Because this can lead to tooth decay, advise patients to discuss it with their dentist or healthcare provider.

■ Decay of the tooth root is common among older adults. When the gums recede, the tooth root is more vulnerable to decay.

■ Promoting good oral hygiene can have a positive effect on older adults' ability to eat.

SKILL 2.8 Perineal-Genital Area: Caring for

Perineal-genital care is also referred to as perineal care or peri-care. Perineal care as part of the bed bath is embarrassing for many patients. Most patients who require a bed bath from the nurse are able to clean their own perineal area with minimal assistance. The nurse may need to hand a moistened washcloth and soap to the patient, rinse the washcloth, and provide a towel. When needed, the nurse provides perineal care efficiently and in a matter-of-fact manner.

Delegation or Assignment

Perineal-genital care can be delegated or assigned to the UAP; however, if the patient has recently had perineal, rectal, or genital surgery, the nurse needs to assess if it is appropriate for the UAP to perform perineal-genital care. The nurse remains responsible for the assessment, interpretation of abnormal finds, and determination of appropriate actions. Note that state laws for UAPs vary, so this task might be assigned to the UAP rather than delegated.

Equipment

■ Bath towel
■ Bath blanket
■ Clean gloves
■ Bath basin with warm water at 43°C–46°C (110°F–115°F)
■ Soap
■ Washcloth

Additional Care

■ Solution bottle, pitcher, or container filled with warm water or a prescribed solution
■ Bedpan to receive rinse water
■ Perineal pad

Preparation

■ Determine whether the patient is experiencing any discomfort in the perineal-genital area.
■ Obtain and prepare the necessary equipment and supplies.
■ Most patients understand what is meant if the nurse simply says, "I'll give you a washcloth to finish your bath." Older patients may be familiar with the term private parts. Whatever expression the nurse uses, it needs to be one that the patient understands and one that is comfortable for the nurse to use.

Procedure

1. Prior to performing the procedure, introduce self and verify the patient's identity using two identifiers. Explain to the patient what you are going to do, why it is necessary, and how the patient can participate, being particularly sensitive to any embarrassment felt by the patient.
2. Perform hand hygiene and observe other appropriate infection control procedures (e.g., clean gloves).
3. Provide for patient privacy by drawing the curtains around the bed or closing the door to the room. Some agencies provide signs indicating the need for privacy. **Rationale:** *Hygiene is a personal matter.*
4. Prepare the patient:
   ● Fold the top bed linen to the foot of the bed and fold the gown up to expose the genital area.
   ● Place a bath towel under the patient's hips. **Rationale:** *The bath towel prevents the bed from becoming soiled.*
5. Position and drape the patient and clean the upper inner thighs.
   ● Cover the body and legs with the bath blanket positioned so a corner is at the head, the opposite corner at the feet, and the other two on the sides. Drape the legs by tucking the bottom corners of the bath blanket under and then over the inner sides of the legs ❶. **Rationale:** *Minimum exposure lessens embarrassment and helps to provide warmth.* Bring the middle portion of the base of the blanket up and then over the pubic area.

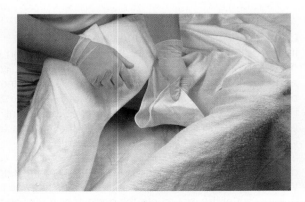

❶ Draping the patient for perineal-genital care.

SKILL 2.8 Perineal-Genital Area: Caring for (continued)

- Position the female in a dorsal recumbent position (back-lying position with the knees flexed and spread well apart).
- Position the male patient in a supine position with knees slightly flexed and hips slightly externally rotated.
- Apply gloves. Wash and dry the upper inner thighs using long strokes from knees upward toward the perineal area.

6. Inspect the perineal area.
   - Note particular areas of inflammation, excoriation, or swelling, especially between the labia in females and the scrotal folds in males.
   - Also note excessive discharge or secretions from the orifices and the presence of odors.

7. Wash and dry the perineal-genital area.

Female
- Clean the labia majora. Then spread the labia to wash the folds between the labia majora and the labia minora ❷. **Rationale:** Secretions that tend to collect around the labia minora facilitate bacterial growth.

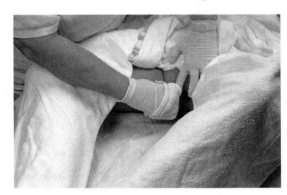

❷ Cleaning the labia.

- Use separate quarters of the washcloth for each stroke, and wipe from the pubis to the rectum. For menstruating women and patients with indwelling catheters, use clean wipes. Use a clean wipe for each stroke. **Rationale:** *Using separate quarters of the washcloth or new wipes prevents the transmission of microorganisms from one area to the other. Wipe from the area of least contamination (the pubis) to that of greatest (the rectum).*
- Rinse the area well. You may place the patient on a bedpan and use a peri-wash or a solution bottle to pour warm water over the area. Dry the perineum thoroughly, paying particular attention to the folds between the labia. **Rationale:** *Moisture supports the growth of many microorganisms.*
- For post-delivery or menstruating females, apply a perineal pad as needed from front to back. **Rationale:** *This prevents contamination of the vagina and urethra from the anal area.*

Male
- Wash and dry the penis, using firm strokes.
- If the patient is uncircumcised, retract the prepuce (foreskin) to expose the glans penis (the tip of the penis) for cleaning. Replace the foreskin after cleaning and drying the glans penis ❸. **Rationale:** *Retracting the foreskin is*

necessary to remove the smegma (thick, cheesy secretion) that collects under the foreskin and facilitates bacterial growth. Replacing the foreskin prevents constriction of the penis, which may cause edema.

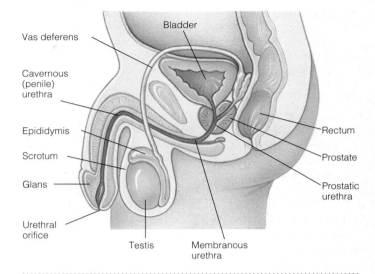

❸ Male genitals.

- Wash and dry the scrotum. The posterior folds of the scrotum may need to be cleaned when the buttocks are cleaned. **Rationale:** *The scrotum tends to be more soiled than the penis because of its proximity to the rectum; thus it is usually cleaned after the penis.*

8. Inspect perineal orifices for intactness.
   - Inspect particularly around the urethra in patients with indwelling catheters. **Rationale:** *A catheter may cause excoriation around the urethra.*

9. Clean the natal cleft (between the gluteal folds) and the entire buttocks.
   - Assist the patient to turn onto the side facing away from you.
   - Pay particular attention to the anal area and posterior folds of the scrotum in males. Clean the anus with toilet tissue if necessary before washing it.
   - Dry the area well.

10. Remove and discard gloves. Perform hand hygiene. Leave patient safe and comfortable.

11. Complete documentation using forms, checklists, or electronic dropdown lists supplemented by nurse's notes or additional comments as appropriate. Document any unusual findings such as redness, excoriation, skin breakdown, discharge or drainage, and any localized areas of tenderness.

SAMPLE DOCUMENTATION

[date] 0645 Perineal care provided with washing and then 4 ounces warm water via peri-bottle, no discharge noted; labia tissue intact; denies any tenderness to area; perineum dried; procedure tolerated with no incident. *C. Keys*

SKILL 2.9 Shaving: Male Patient

Delegation or Assignment

Shaving a male patient can be delegated or assigned to the UAP. Remind the UAP to notify the nurse of anything that looks out of the ordinary. Review with the UAP the facility safety policy about using an electric shaver brought in from home. The nurse remains responsible for the assessment, interpretation of abnormal findings, and determination of appropriate responses. Note that state laws for UAPs vary, so this task might be assigned to the UAP rather than delegated.

Equipment

- Safety or electric razor, specific to patient's needs or wishes
- Shaving cream
- Aftershave lotion (optional)
- Two towels
- Basin of warm water

Preparation

- Determine how the patient usually shaves (i.e., use of safety edge or electric razor; special products).
- Check to see if the patient has excessive bleeding tendencies due to pathological conditions (hemophilia) or the use of specific medications (anticoagulants or large doses of aspirin). **Rationale:** *If patient is accidentally cut, it could lead to some loss of blood.*

CAUTION!

- According to the hospital policy, be sure to have the electric razor checked for safety aspects. Some hospitals do not allow patients to use their own electric razors.
- A beard or a mustache should not be shaved off without the patient's consent.

Procedure

1. Introduce self to patient and verify the patient's identity using two identifiers. Explain to the patient what you are going to do, why it is necessary, and how the patient can participate. Discuss how the results will be used in planning further care or treatments.
2. Perform hand hygiene and observe appropriate infection control procedures.
3. Provide for patient privacy.
4. Place patient in sitting position.
5. Place towel over chest and under chin.
6. Put up mirror on overbed table.
7. *With safety edge razor*:
   - Don gloves and apply a warm, moist towel to soften the hair.
   - Apply a thick layer of soap or shaving cream to the shaving area.
   - Holding skin taut, use firm but small strokes in the direction of hair growth.
   - Gently remove soap or lather with a warm, damp towel. Inspect for areas you may have missed.

   With electric razor:
   - Use rotating motion of razor and start from lateral aspect of face and move toward chin and upper lip area.
   - Clean razor with brush, or remove razor head and clean facial hair from head of razor.
8. Apply aftershave lotion as desired.
9. Reposition patient for comfort if needed.
10. Remove gloves and replace equipment.
11. Perform hand hygiene. Leave the patient safe and comfortable.

» Medication Administration Systems

Expected Outcomes

1. Medication Administration Records (MARs) are kept current with healthcare provider's orders.
2. Rationales for medication administration are clear.
3. Medications are administered according to the "rights of medication administration."
4. Medications remain controlled and safe.
5. Documentation for medications is accurate and complete.

SKILL 2.10 Automated Dispensing System: Using

Automated dispensing systems allow medications to be stored and dispensed near the point of care while controlling, tracking, and documenting medication distribution. Medications can be efficiently distributed to improve patient safety.

Delegation or Assignment

Using an automated dispensing system involves knowledge and medication administration skills. Therefore, this skill is not delegated or assigned to the UAP. In some states, a trained UAP may administer certain medications to stable patients in long-term care settings. Assessment and evaluation of effectiveness of the medication remain the responsibility of the nurse.

SKILL 2.10 Automated Dispensing System: Using (*continued*)

Equipment

- Automated dispensing system (e.g., PYXIS)
- Patient's electronic Medication Administration Record (MAR) ❶

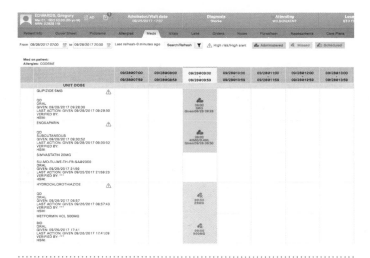

❶ Example of a medication administration record.

Procedure

1. Touch the screen to activate the system.
2. Enter your ID code number and user password or scanned fingerprint. **Rationale:** *This process controls access to medications.*
3. From the main menu, select command on medication management station (e.g., *remove, waste, return*).
4. Select patient's room number, medication, and name and additional identifiers (e.g., *birth date, hospital number*).
5. Touch/select medication desired from the patient's displayed list of ordered medications.
6. Validate that patient's medication record matches selected medication and dose on monitor screen ❷.

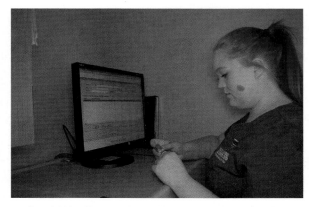

Source: Ronald May/Pearson Education, Inc.

❷ Check healthcare provider's order against medication administration record (MAR).

CAUTION! The usual checks and balances between nurses and pharmacists may be bypassed with automated dispensing systems, increasing the potential for medication errors.

7. Type in quantity (#) of doses desired if indicated by a range of possible doses ordered.
8. Enter a witness ID/scan (by another nurse) to validate wasted medication (if partial dose is needed).
9. Remove the medication from the automated delivery system ❸.

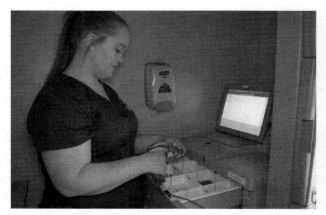

Source: Ronald May/Pearson Education, Inc.

❸ Locate medications in patient's drawer. Retrieve medication to be given and inspect label.

10. Close drawer/storage door, and exit the system.
11. Check and prepare medication and administer according to route ❹.
    Note: Certain medications (e.g., cough syrup and other patient-specific multiple-dose medications) may be dispensed by pharmacy and placed in the patient's medication drawer rather than being accessed through the automated system.

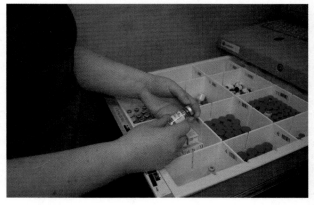

Source: Ronald May/Pearson Education, Inc.

❹ Check individually wrapped medication against patient's MAR.

(*continued on next page*)

SKILL 2.10 Automated Dispensing System: Using (continued)

Safety Consideration

- No technology system eliminates the risk for error.
- Never become complacent about what technology can do to support safe practice.
- No computer has your ability to think critically, to understand whether an ordered drug is appropriate for your patient.
- Technology (e.g., barcode use) increases the amount of time spent administering medications, but does reduce time spent in documentation.

EVIDENCE-BASED PRACTICE

Safety of Medication Management and Administration

Problem

An ongoing clinical and economic challenge for healthcare facilities continues to be the frequency of adverse drug events (ADEs). The economic impact reflects longer stays in a healthcare facility, additional treatments, increased insurance costs, and costs related to lawsuits. Facilities want to improve patient safety, so they are motivated to seek solutions. One process solution is called the "closed-loop medication management system" which has the connectivity to support drug management and administration processes from end to end.

Evidence

In one study, the system begins with the electronic medical record (EMR). Then computer healthcare provider-order entries are entered and sent to the pharmacy. The EMR is available to all departments to view and to add additional patient information for everyone's convenience. Use of this automated medication management system at one hospital reduced the number of steps for medication administration from 17 to 5 and led to a reduction of ADEs from 3.5 per 1000 patients to 0.52 per 1000 patients. In another study, use of an

A Closed-Loop Medication Management System

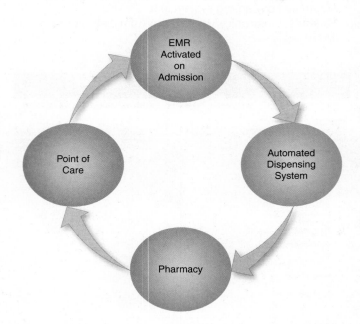

automated packaging and dispensing system resulted in a 40% reduction in missed doses and a decrease in cart fill-time of 71%.

Implications

The automation of medication-specific processes eliminates many steps in the process, decreasing opportunities for human error. Implementation of automated medication management systems were shown to improve patient safety, increase efficiency of medication dispensing, and increase cost savings.

Source: Based on Grosch, S. (2015). *Improving Patient Safety and Cutting Costs with Healthcare Automation*. Swisslog Healthcare Solutions. Retrieved from http://docplayer.net/3496160-Improving-patient-safety-and-cutting-costs-with-health-care-automation.html

---

SKILL 2.11 Medication: Preparing and Administering

There are several systems involved with medication preparation and administration. Nurses are an important part of the human and system processes that collectively work to prevent errors when prescribing, dispensing, preparing, and administering medications.

Delegation or Assignment

General medication preparation and administration involves knowledge and medication administration skills. Therefore, this skill is not delegated or assigned to the UAP. In some states, a trained UAP may administer certain medications to stable patients in long-term care settings. Assessment and evaluation of effectiveness of the medication remain the responsibility of the nurse.

Equipment

- Reference resources (e.g., *Physicians' Desk Reference*, pharmacology textbook, drug handbook)

- Calculator, as needed
- Medication Administration Record (MAR)
- Patient's chart
- Automated Dispensing Device (medication cart or cabinet)
- Prepared medication (administration only)
- Gloves (if indicated)
- Stethoscope and sphygmomanometer, if indicated (administration only)

MEDICATION PREPARATION

Procedure

1. Check healthcare provider's orders and patient's MAR for medications patient is to receive (drug, dosage, route of administration, time intervals).
2. Identify any unfamiliar drugs.

SKILL 2.11 Medication: Preparing and Administering (*continued*)

3. Research unfamiliar drugs using appropriate reference:
   a. Generic and trade name
   b. Drug classification and major uses
   c. Pharmacologic actions
   d. Safe dosage, route, and time of administration
   e. Side effects; adverse reactions
   f. Nursing implications
   g. Patient teaching points
4. Review patient's record for allergies, pertinent lab results, any factors that contraindicate administration of medications, such as an NPO status or scheduled procedure.
5. Check patient's daily MAR with previous day's MAR every 24 hours for each drug's dosage, route, and time to be given. **Rationale:** *Pharmacy produces each daily MAR sheet. Any new medication, discontinued medication, or altered dosage must be identified and verified with the healthcare provider's orders.*
6. Validate carefully that the MAR is consistent with the healthcare provider's most recent order for each medication. **Rationale:** *Some medication dosages are adjusted on a daily basis. Errors in transmission of intentions may occur between healthcare provider, pharmacy, and patient's MAR.*

CAUTION! Sometimes patients will have more than one healthcare provider writing medication orders.

Remember to check all recent order sheets when reconciling medications on the MAR.

---

7. Perform hand hygiene.
8. Take medication cart to patient's room or go to the medication device or cabinet.
9. Open medication cart; take out patient's medication drawer.
10. Starting at the top of the MAR, check each medication in order against the medication packages in the drawer. Alternately, remove patient's medication from the automated dispensing system and place in a medicine cup (also see Skill 2.10).
11. Retrieve medication(s) to be given and compare drug label with MAR. **Rationale:** *This is a safety check to ensure the right medication is given.*
12. Inspect label for expiration date, and ensure that medication is indicated for ordered route of administration. **Rationale:** *Different preparations of the same medication are used for different routes of administration.*
13. Determine if any preparation is necessary to prepare the correct dosage.
14. Determine if any calculation is necessary to prepare the correct dosage.
15. Calculate patient's dosage based on strength of medication, if indicated. Have another nurse double check your calculations for high-alert medications. (Also see Skill 2.14 for formulas.)
16. Prepare medication as indicated, checking drug label before, during, and after preparation.

MEDICATION ADMINISTRATION

Procedure

1. Check patient's name and room number against the MAR and lock the medication cart, if cart is used, before leaving it to enter the patient's room ❶. **Rationale:** *Locking the cart is a safety measure.*

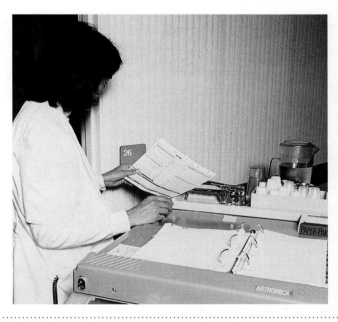

❶ Check patient's name and room number against medication record.

2. Check patient's identity with two identifiers ❷.

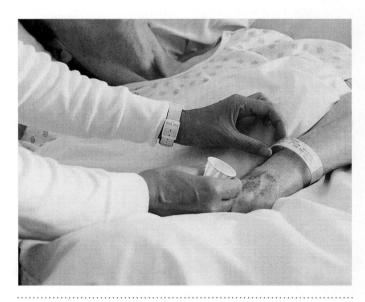

❷ Check patient's identification band and ask patient to state name and birth date.

(*continued on next page*)

SKILL 2.11 Medication: Preparing and Administering (continued)

CAUTION! Use at least two patient identifiers other than room number when administering medications or providing treatments (e.g., stated name, birth date, or hospital number, posted picture of patient, family member who can identify patient, or another nurse who can validate patient's identity).

3. Provide for patient privacy.
4. Explain procedure and purpose of medication to patient.
5. Perform hand hygiene and assist patient to appropriate position for medication administration.
6. Check patient's vital signs if indicated before administering medication. **Rationale:** *A medication's effects may cause hemodynamic instability if patient's vital signs are at the high or low extreme of normal.*
7. Don gloves if indicated. **Rationale:** *Parenteral and enteral medication administration may require the use of gloves.*
8. Administer medication at the right time and adhere to the "rights" of medication administration (see **Table 2–2 》**).
9. Dispose of equipment appropriately; then remove gloves, if used, and perform hand hygiene.
10. Complete documentation using forms, checklists, or electronic dropdown lists supplemented by nurse's notes or additional comments as appropriate. Record administered medications on patient's MAR; the time, medication given, dosage, and route (including site of injection); and any relevant assessment findings.

The Rights of Medication Administration

In the past, there were a standard "5 Rights of Medication Administration: right patient, right drug, right route, right time, and right dose." Nursing practices have changed to include a few more rights for safe medication administration.

- **Right medication.** Compare medication container label to the MAR three times (when obtaining the medication, when preparing the medication, and after preparation). Note medication expiration date. Know action, dosage, and method of administration. Know side effects of the medication and any allergies the patient might have.
- **Right patient.** Check the room and bed number and patient's identity band. Validate correct patient with two identifiers other than room number (e.g., stated name and date of birth).

TABLE 2–2 Schedule Example of Medication Times

q am	0800
q day	0900
bid	1000, 1800
tid	1000, 1400, 1800
qid	1000, 1400, 1800, 2000
ac, hs	0730, 1130, 1630, 2200
q 4 hr	0400, 0800, 1200, 1600, 2000, 2400
q 6 hr	0200, 0800, 1400, 2000
q 8 hr	0200, 1000, 1800
q12 hr	1000, 2200

- **Right time.** Medication given 30 to 60 minutes before or after time ordered may be acceptable. Follow facility policy.
- **Right route.** If a change in route is indicated, request new orders from healthcare provider.
- **Right dose.** Validate calculations of divided doses with another nurse. Have another nurse double check your preparation of insulin, potassium chloride, morphine, hydromorphone HCl, heparin, and warfarin sodium (Joint Commission high-alert drugs). Know the usual dose and question any dose outside safe range.
- **Right documentation.** After administration, documentation may be considered to be the sixth right. The nurse should document the name of the drug, the dose and route, time administered, and the patient's response to the medication administered.
- **Right patient education.** Patient is informed of side-effects of the medications to receive. Inform patient to tell the nurse if unwanted reaction to the medication occurs.
- **Right assessment.** Vital signs may need to be checked before giving a medication that may change the pulse, blood pressure, or respirations. Laboratory results may indicate an ordered medication may not be safe to give, so it warrants checking with the healthcare provider first.
- **Right reason.** Confirm the rationale for the ordered medication including why is the patient taking this medication.
- **Right response.** Verify the drug given to the patient results in the desired effect.
- **Right reactions.** Confirm medication allergies of the patient are checked before administering the medication.
- **Right to refuse.** Does the patient refuse the medication ordered?

Safety Considerations

Bar Code Medication Administration is an electronic system to prevent medication errors by improving accuracy of medication inventory control and recordkeeping. A handheld device is used to scan the barcode on the patient and the medication label ❸ ❹. It can then recognize the original five rights of medication administration: The right patient is getting the right medication in the right amount by the right route and at the right time.

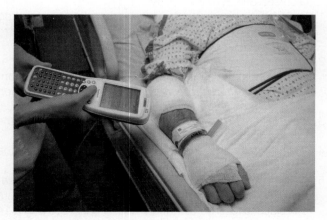

Source: Celina Burkhart/Pearson Education, Inc.

❸ Scan the barcode on the patient's ID band.

SKILL 2.11 Medication: Preparing and Administering (*continued*)

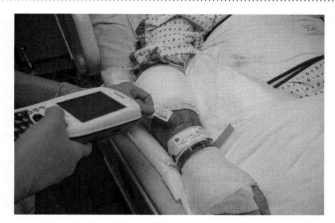

Source: Celina Burkhart/Pearson Education, Inc.

④ Scan the barcode on the unopened medication packaging to confirm matching.

Medication Safety Measures

- Accurately and completely reconcile the patient's medications across the continuum of care.
- Keep all medicines in locked carts or cabinets.
- Limit access to and use special safeguards with "high-alert" drugs (those causing significant patient harm if used in error; e.g., hypoglycemic, anticoagulant, anesthetic agents, narcotics, paralytic agents, chemotherapy drugs, certain cardiac drugs). This list is periodically updated by the Institute for Safe Medication Practices (ISMP).
- Keep narcotics in double-locked cabinets or PYXIS. Count all narcotics with oncoming staff at the end of each shift.
- Separate topical medications from parenteral or oral medications.
- Clearly label all prepared medication containers (syringes, medicine cups, solutions). Check with another nurse (1) mathematical calculations for dosages and (2) dispensed/prepared "high-alert" drugs and those for high-risk patients (e.g., insulin, anticoagulants, concentrated electrolytes, digoxin, and hemodynamic agents if not premixed).
- Do not leave any medication at patient's bedside unless there is a specific healthcare provider's order to do so.
- Report any errors in drug administration to charge nurse and patient's healthcare provider immediately. Monitor the patient closely for adverse effects. Document the drug given, and complete a written variance report.
- Provide complete instructions to patients regarding medication to be used at home.

Parts of Medication Orders

- Patient's name and date of birth
- Date and time medication was ordered
- Name of medication (generic and/or brand)
- Medication dosage
  - For pediatric patients, usually the dose is weight-based excluding medications which do not have a weight-based dosing.
- Route of administration and any special instruction for administration

- Frequency (quantity, such as one time only) and/or intervals, such as every 8 hours
- Duration of therapy as appropriate
- If ordered as a "prn" medication, needs to include reason for use (for example, morphine 4 mg IV q 4 hr prn for pain)
- Signature of individual ordering the drug

Common communication breakdowns leading to medication errors include:

- Unapproved or unclear abbreviations
- Illegible writing
- Misplaced or unnoticed decimals (e.g., .2 rather than 0.2)
- "Verbal orders"
- Incomplete orders

  See **Table 2–3 》** for abbreviations.

The Joint Commission (TJC) (2015) has identified certain abbreviations that are associated with frequent errors in medication administration. The website for TJC keeps a list of abbreviations that should not be used. For example, the word "unit" should always be spelled

TABLE 2–3 List of Common Abbreviations/ Symbols Related to Medication Administration

aa	of each	NPO	nothing by mouth
a.c.	before meals	oz	ounce
ad lib.	freely, as desired	p.c.	after meals
BID	twice each day	per	by, through
c̄	with	PO	by mouth
C	carbon	prn, *or* PRN	whenever necessary
Ca	calcium	q.h.	every hour
Cl	chlorine	q.i.d.	four times each day
dr *or* Z	dram	q.s.	as much as required, quantity sufficient
et	and		
GI	gastrointestinal	q2h	every 2 hours
gt *or* gtt	drop(s)	q3h	every 3 hours
HS	hour of sleep	q4h	every 4 hours
H₂O	water	RX	treatment, "take thou"
H₂O₂	hydrogen peroxide		
IM	intramuscular	s̄	without
K	potassium	STAT	immediately
kg	kilogram	TID	three times each day
lb *or* #	pound	tsp	teaspoon
m	meter	°	degree
mcg	microgram	–	minus, negative, alkaline reaction
mEq	milliequivalent		
mg	milligram	+	plus, positive, acid reaction
mL or ml	milliliter	%	percent
mmol	millimole	v	Roman numeral 5
Na	sodium	vii	Roman numeral 7
NA	not applicable	ix	Roman numeral 9
NG	nasogastric	xiii	Roman numeral 13

(*continued on next page*)

SKILL 2.11 Medication: Preparing and Administering *(continued)*

out, because its abbreviations (u, U) can be misread. The abbreviations Q.D. (every day) and Q.O.D. (every other day) are often mistaken for each other. Therefore, TJC recommends writing out "daily" or "every other day." "MS" can mean morphine sulfate or magnesium sulfate. The Joint Commission recommends writing out morphine sulfate or magnesium sulfate.

Orders with zero should be written with special care. For a full unit (e.g., 1 mg), avoid the "trailing zero" (**do not write** 1.0 mg). If the trailing zero is used and the decimal point is not seen, 10 mg might be administered instead of 1 mg.

If the ordered amount of medication is less than one unit (e.g., seven-tenths of a milligram), it is important to include a zero before the decimal (0.7 mg). Otherwise, the amount may be read as 7 mg, resulting in administration of 10 times the ordered dose.

Safety Considerations
REPORTING ACTUAL OR POTENTIAL ERROR

Report any actual or potential error (e.g., sound-alike/look-alike drug names, confusion over abbreviations) to the ISMP website. All communications are kept confidential. The ISMP publicizes warnings and notices in response to submitted information to help alert other professionals to potentially dangerous medication pitfalls.

NATIONAL PATIENT SAFETY GOALS

All Joint Commission–accredited agencies must have protocols developed for documenting and reconciling medications across the continuum of patient care (admission, transfer, discharge). A list of the patient's home medications is compared with the admitting medication orders. Upon transfer, medications being taken are compared with orders in the new unit. Upon discharge, medications taken in the hospital are compared to the discharge medication orders. Verification, clarification, and reconciliation of discrepancies help prevent adverse drug events throughout the patient's hospitalization.

The Joint Commission's Hospital National Patient Safety Goals guideline for 2017 identifies specific safety goals related to medication administration.

One priority preventive action is to make sure all medications, solutions, and their containers (includes syringes, medicine cups, and basins) are appropriately labeled in all patient-care settings. Another focus on medication safety is to prevent errors during anticoagulant therapy, including the healthcare provider's order, accurate medication preparation, and correct administration to the right patient. A final measure to improve medication safety is accuracy in communicating about a patient's medications to other appropriate care providers, like during a hand-off report, shift report, or transfer report of patient to another appropriate nurse, unit, or facility.

SKILL 2.12 Narcotic Control System: Using

Safety Note! *During scheduled clinical time, nursing students may have a learning opportunity to observe or assist with this skill only with faculty permission and with direct supervision from faculty or another RN.*

Delegation or Assignment

Using the narcotic control system involves knowledge and medication administration skills. Therefore, this skill is not delegated or assigned to the UAP. UAPs may be asked by the nurse to report any change in patient status or vital signs. Assessment and evaluation of effectiveness of the medication remain the responsibility of the nurse.

Equipment

- MAR
- Narcotic sign-out sheet or electronic footprint
- Controlled medication

Procedure

For Patient Administration

1. Check patient's MAR for narcotic order.
2. Check dose and time last narcotic was administered.

CAUTION! If the narcotic depresses breathing, note patient's level of sedation and respiratory rate before administering, document assessment before administering the narcotic, and continue to monitor the patient's level of sedation and respiratory rate for change.

3. Unlock and open narcotics drawer, and find appropriate narcotic container ❶.

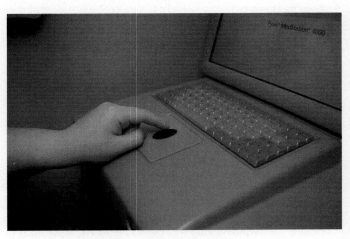

Source: Ronald May/Pearson Education, Inc.

❶ Unlock the narcotics drawer. Some units have a User ID and password for scanned fingerprint control access to medication.

4. Count the number of pills, ampules, or prefilled cartridges in container.
5. Check the narcotics sign-out sheet, and check that the number of narcotics in the drawer matches the number on the specific narcotics sign-out sheet. **Rationale:** *Federal laws on controlled substances require careful monitoring of narcotics.*

SKILL 2.12 Narcotic Control System: Using (*continued*)

6. Correct any discrepancy before proceeding with narcotic administration.
7. Sign out the narcotic on the narcotics sheet after taking the narcotic out of the drawer.
8. Lock drawer after removing medication ❷.

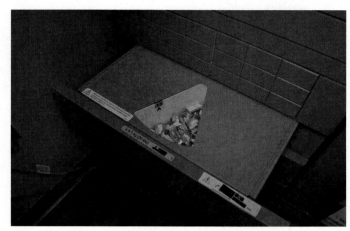

Source: Ronald May/Pearson Education, Inc.

❷ Lock narcotics drawer after removing medication. Keep the key with you at all times.

9. Administer medication according to specific oral or parenteral procedure.
10. Document narcotic on patient's MAR according to usual procedure. Include patient's pain rating (e.g., 8/10) and sedation level before and after narcotic administration according to facility policy.

For Unit Narcotics Stock

11. Check narcotics counts every change of shift. One off-going and one on-coming *licensed* nurse must check the narcotics together. The number on each narcotics sign-out sheet must match the number of that particular narcotic remaining in the drawer.
12. Explore any discrepancy in stock and recorded dispensed narcotics numbers. **Rationale:** *Counts must balance. It is the nurse's responsibility to account for all controlled substances dispensed.*
13. Licensed nurses cosign the narcotics record if the count is accurate.

Patient Teaching

- Carry a complete list of all prescriptions, over-the-counter (OTC) medications, and home remedies at all times. Learn the names of the medications as well as their actions and possible adverse effects.
- Keep all medications out of reach of children and pets.
- Take medications only as prescribed. Know which medications need to be taken on an empty stomach and which can be taken with food/meals.
- Immediately consult the nurse, pharmacist, or primary care provider about any problems with the medication.
- Always check the medication label to make sure the correct medication is being taken.
- Request labels printed with larger type on medication containers if there is difficulty reading the label.
- Check the expiration date and discard outdated medications. Previously, most people discarded old medicines by flushing them down the toilet. The Environmental Protection Agency (EPA) no longer recommends this. Inform patients to check with their local government. Many cities and towns have household hazardous waste facilities where old medicines can be disposed. Expired medications may be placed in the trash if the following precautions are used: Keep the medication in the original container and mark out the person's name. Add a nontoxic but bad-tasting product (e.g., cayenne pepper, mustard) to the container to keep individuals or animals from eating it. Place in a sturdy container, tape the container shut, and have this container be the last thing put in the garbage can.
- Ask the pharmacist to substitute childproof caps with ones that are more easily opened, as necessary.
- If a dose or more is missed, do not take two or more doses; ask the pharmacist or primary care provider for directions.
- Do not crush or cut a tablet or capsule without first checking with the primary care provider or pharmacist. Doing so may affect the medication's absorption.
- Never stop taking a prescribed medication without first discussing it with the primary care provider.
- Always check with the pharmacist before taking any non-prescription medications or herbs. Some OTC medications or herbs can interact with the prescribed medication. Additionally, the nurse can set up a medication plan to assist patients and family members to remember a schedule. Weekly pill containers (available at pharmacies) or a written plan may be helpful.

❯❯ Medication Preparation

Expected Outcomes

1. Dosage calculations are accurate.
2. Medications are prepared using safe procedures.
3. Medications are accurately labeled and safely administered.
4. Complications and errors of medication administration are prevented.

SKILL 2.13 Ampule Medication: Removing

Ampules are commonly used to package solutions. The medication is only in contact with glass, and the packaging is 100% tamperproof.

Delegation or Assignment

Preparing medications from ampules involves knowledge and use of sterile technique. Therefore, these skills are not delegated or assigned to the UAP. The nurse can request the UAP to report patient observations to the nurse for follow-up. In some states, a trained UAP may administer certain medications to stable patients in long-term care settings. Assessment and evaluation of effectiveness of the medication remain the responsibility of the nurse.

Equipment

- Patient's MAR (hard copy or electronic)
- Ampule of sterile medication
- File (if ampule is not scored) and small gauze square or plastic ampule opener
- Antiseptic swabs
- Syringe, appropriate size for amount being drawn out of ampule
- Needle appropriate size for administering the medication
- Filter needle for withdrawing medication from the ampule (safety action)

Preparation

- Check the MAR.
- Check the label on the ampule carefully against the MAR to verify that the correct medication and dosage are being prepared.
- Follow the three label checks for administering medications. Read the label on the medication (1) when it is taken from the medication cart, (2) before withdrawing the medication, and (3) after withdrawing the medication.
- Organize the equipment.

Procedure

1. Perform hand hygiene and observe other appropriate infection control procedures (e.g., clean gloves).
2. Prepare the medication ampule for drug withdrawal.
   - Flick the upper stem of the ampule several times with a fingernail. **Rationale:** *This will bring all medication down to the main portion of the ampule.*
   - Use an ampule opener, or place a piece of gauze or an unopened alcohol wipe between your thumb and the ampule neck or around the ampule neck, and break off the top by bending it toward you to ensure the ampule is broken away from yourself and others ❶. **Rationale:** *The gauze protects the fingers from the broken glass, and any glass fragments will spray away from the nurse.*
   - Dispose of the top of the ampule in the sharps container.

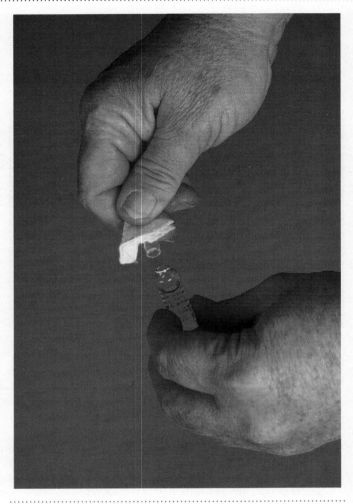

❶ Breaking the neck of an ampule using an unopened alcohol wipe.

CAUTION! Small fragments of glass can be released when the ampule is broken open. Use an ampule opener when possible. This device covers the section of the ampule that is broken and prevents small pieces of glass from being scattered.

3. Withdraw the medication.
   - Place the ampule on a flat surface.
   - Attach the filter needle or straw to the syringe. **Rationale:** *The filter needle prevents glass particles from being withdrawn with the medication.*
   - Remove the cap from the filter needle and insert the needle into the center of the ampule.
   - Hold the ampule slightly on its side, if necessary, to obtain all of the medication ❷.
   - After removing syringe from ampule, tap syringe barrel below air bubbles to dislodge them to hub of syringe.
   - Eject air with syringe in an upright position. If amount of solution is overdrawn, invert syringe and remove

SKILL 2.13 Ampule Medication: Removing *(continued)*

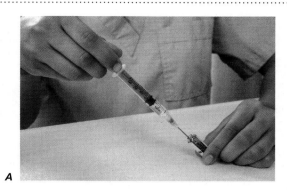

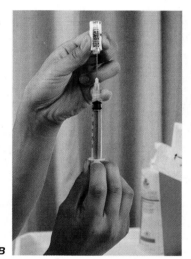

Source: Rick Brady/Pearson Education, Inc.

❷ Withdrawing medication: **A,** from an ampule on a flat surface; **B,** from an inverted ampule.

excess solution to the medical waste (black box) receptacle. **Rationale:** *Appropriate waste disposal is mandated by the Environmental Protection Agency (EPA).*

● Dispose of the filter needle or straw by placing it in a sharps container ❸.

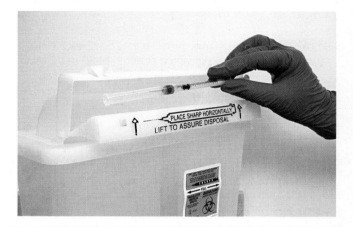

❸ Discard syringe in biohazard container following use.

● Replace the filter needle or straw with a regular needle, tighten the cap at the hub of the needle, and push solution into the needle, to the prescribed amount.

● Label the syringe with medication name and dosage drawn up in the syringe. **Rationale:** *This can be used to do a last medication check for accuracy before administering the medication to the patient.*

SKILL 2.14 Calculating Dosages

Delegation or Assignment

Doing medication calculations involve knowledge and skills of medication administration. Therefore, these skills are not delegated or assigned to the UAP. The nurse can request the UAP to report patient observations to the nurse for follow-up. In some states, a trained UAP may administer certain medications to stable patients in long-term care settings and will thus calculate dosage. Assessment and evaluation of effectiveness of the medication remain the responsibility of the nurse.

Equipment

- Orders for dosage of medication needed
- Dosage of medication on hand

Procedure

1. To calculate oral dosages, use the following formula, noting that *D* and *H* must be in same unit of measure:

$$\frac{D}{H} = X$$

where
D = dose desired
H = dose on hand
X = dose to be administered.

Example: Give 500 mg of ampicillin sodium when the dose on hand is in capsules containing 250 mg.

$$\frac{500 \text{ mg}}{250 \text{ mg}} = 2 \text{ capsules}$$

2. To calculate dose when in liquid form, use the following formula:

$$\frac{D}{H} \times Q = X$$

where
D = dose desired
H = dose on hand
Q = quantity
X = amount to be administered.

(continued on next page)

SKILL 2.14 Calculating Dosages (*continued*)

Example: Give 375 mg of ampicillin when it is supplied as 250 mg/5 mL.

$$\frac{375 \text{ mg}}{250 \text{ mg}} \times 5$$
$$1.5 \times 5 = 7.5 \text{ mL}$$

3. To calculate parenteral dosages, use the following formula:

$$\frac{D}{H} \times Q = X$$

Example: Give patient 40 mg gentamicin C complex sulfate. On hand is a multidose vial with a strength of 80 mg/2 mL.

$$\frac{40}{80} \times 2 = 1 \text{ mL}$$

4. To calculate dosages for newborns, infants, and children using body surface area (BSA), use the following formula:

$$\frac{\text{BSA}}{1.7 \times \text{adult dose}} = \text{pediatric dose}$$

5. To calculate dosages for newborns, infants, and children using Clark's weight rule:

$$\text{Child's dose} = \frac{\text{child's wt. in lbs.}}{150} \times \text{adult dose}$$

6. To calculate dosages for newborns, infants, and children using pediatric dosage-strength medications:

Child's dose = child's wt. in kg. × dosage strength (mg/kg).

Safe calculations include total dosage amount and frequency/24 hr.

SKILL 2.15 Mixing Medications in One Syringe

Safety Note! *During scheduled clinical time, nursing students may have a learning opportunity to observe or assist with this skill only with faculty permission and with direct supervision from faculty or another RN.*

Delegation or Assignment

Mixing medications in one syringe involves knowledge and use of aseptic technique. Therefore, this procedure is not delegated or assigned to the UAP. The nurse can request the UAP to report patient observations to the nurse for follow-up. In some states, a trained UAP may administer certain medications to stable patients in long-term care settings. Assessment and evaluation of effectiveness of the medication remain the responsibility of the nurse.

Equipment

- Patient's MAR, hard copy or electronic
- Two vials of medication; one vial and one ampule; two ampules; or one vial or ampule and one cartridge
- Antiseptic swabs
- Sterile syringe (appropriate size for volume of medication) and safety needle or insulin syringe and needle (specific for insulin injection)
- Additional sterile subcutaneous or intramuscular safety needle as needed

Preparation

- Check the MAR.
- Check the label on the medications carefully against the MAR to make sure that the correct medication is being prepared.
- Follow the three label checks for administering medications. Read the label on the medication (1) when it is taken from the medication cart, (2) before withdrawing the medication, and (3) after withdrawing the medication.

- Before preparing and combining the medications, ensure that the total volume of the injection is appropriate for the injection site.
- Organize the equipment.

CAUTION! Check appropriate text or consult facility pharmacist to ensure compatibility of medications before combining in a syringe for injection.

Procedure

1. Perform hand hygiene and observe other appropriate infection control procedures (e.g., clean gloves).
2. Prepare the medication ampule or vial for drug withdrawal.
   - Inspect the appearance of the medication for clarity. Note, however, that some medications are cloudy after mixing the vial, ampule, or cartridge. **Rationale:** *Preparations that have changed in appearance should be discarded.*
   - If using insulin, thoroughly mix the solution in each vial prior to administration by rotating the vials between the palms of the hands. **Rationale:** *Mixing ensures an adequate concentration and thus an accurate dose. Shaking insulin vials can make the medication frothy, making precise measurement difficult.*
   - Clean the tops of the vials with antiseptic swabs.
3. Withdraw the appropriate dosage of medications.

MIXING MEDICATIONS FROM TWO VIALS

- Take the syringe and draw up a volume of air equal to the volume of medications to be withdrawn from both vials A and B.
- Inject a volume of air equal to the volume of medication to be withdrawn into vial A. Make sure the needle does not touch the solution ❶. **Rationale:** *This prevents cross-contamination of the medications.*

SKILL 2.15 Mixing Medications in One Syringe *(continued)*

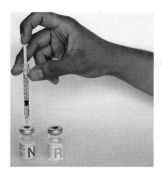

Source: Patrick Watson/Pearson Education, Inc.

① Mixing two vials of different types of insulin.

▪ Withdraw the needle from vial A and inject the remaining air into vial B **②**.

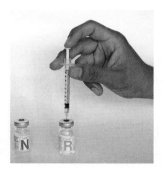

Source: Patrick Watson/Pearson Education, Inc.

②

▪ Withdraw the required amount of medication from vial B **③**. **Rationale:** *The same needle is used to inject air into and withdraw medication from the second vial. It must not be contaminated with the medication in vial A.*

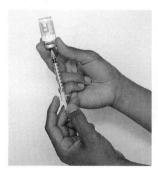

Source: Patrick Watson/Pearson Education, Inc.

③

▪ Using a newly attached sterile needle (unless, like an insulin syringe, the prepackaged syringe has a fixed needle), withdraw the required amount of medication from vial A **④**. Avoid pushing the plunger because that will introduce medication B into vial A. If using a syringe with a fused needle, withdraw the medication from vial A. The syringe now contains a mixture of medications from vials A and B. **Rationale:** *With this method,*

neither vial is contaminated by microorganisms or by medication from the other vial. Be careful to withdraw only the ordered amount and not to create air bubbles. Rationale: The syringe now contains two medications, and an excess amount cannot be returned to the vial.

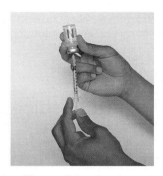

Source: Patrick Watson/Pearson Education, Inc.

④

MIXING MEDICATIONS FROM ONE VIAL AND ONE AMPULE

▪ First prepare and withdraw the medication from the vial. **Rationale:** *The ampule does not require the addition of air prior to withdrawal of the drug because it is an open container.*

▪ Then withdraw the required amount of medication from the ampule.

MIXING MEDICATIONS FROM ONE CARTRIDGE AND ONE VIAL OR AMPULE

▪ First ensure that the correct dose of the medication is in the cartridge. Discard any excess medication and air.

▪ Draw up the required medication from the vial or ampule into the cartridge. Note that when withdrawing medication from a vial, an equal amount of air must first be injected into the vial.

▪ If the total volume to be injected exceeds the capacity of the cartridge, use a syringe with sufficient capacity to withdraw the desired amount of medication from the vial or ampule, and transfer the required amount from the cartridge to the syringe.

Alternative Method for Combining Medications

▪ Draw up ordered dose from each vial or ampule into two separate syringes. First syringe must be able to hold entire volume of combined medications.

▪ Remove needle from first syringe.

▪ Pull back plunger of first syringe to allow space for volume of second medication to be added.

▪ Insert needle of second syringe into hub of first syringe.

▪ Slowly inject medication of second syringe through first syringe hub, then withdraw needle.

▪ Attach new needle to first syringe.

▪ Discard needles and second syringe.

(continued on next page)

SKILL 2.15 Mixing Medications in One Syringe (*continued*)

For Preparing Prefilled Medication Cartridge Syringe

- Hold barrel of cartridge syringe (e.g., Tubex) in one hand and pull back on plunger with other hand.
- Insert prefilled medication cartridge, needle first, into cartridge barrel.
- Twist cartridge syringe flange clockwise until it is secure.
- Screw plunger rod onto screw at bottom of medication cartridge until it fits firmly and tightly into rubber stopper.

- Remove needle guard and any air bubbles.
- Determine if dosage in cartridge is greater than required amount. If so, invert Tubex and gently expel excess medication, being careful to maintain sterility of needle. **Rationale:** *If permanent needle is contaminated, the cartridge becomes contaminated and must be discarded.*
- Replace needle guard, using scoop method.

SKILL 2.16 Vial Medication: Removing

Delegation or Assignment

Preparing medications from vials involves knowledge and use of sterile technique. Therefore, these techniques are not delegated or assigned to the UAP. The nurse can request the UAP to report patient observations to the nurse for follow-up. In some states, a trained UAP may administer certain medications to stable patients in long-term care settings. Assessment and evaluation of effectiveness of the medication remain the responsibility of the nurse.

Equipment

- Patient's MAR (hard copy or electronic)
- Vial of sterile medication
- Antiseptic swabs
- Safety needle and syringe
- Filter needle (check facility policy)
- Sterile water or normal saline, if drug is in powdered form

Procedure

1. Perform hand hygiene and observe other appropriate infection control procedures (e.g., clean gloves).
2. Prepare the medication vial for drug withdrawal.
   - Mix the solution, if necessary, by rotating the vial between the palms of the hands, not by shaking. **Rationale:** *Some vials contain aqueous suspensions, which settle when they stand. In some instances, shaking is contraindicated because it may cause the mixture to foam.*
   - Remove the protective cap, or clean the rubber cap of a previously opened vial with an antiseptic wipe by rubbing in a circular motion. **Rationale:** *The antiseptic cleans the rubber cap and reduces the number of microorganisms.*
3. Withdraw the medication.
   - Attach a filter needle, as facility practice dictates, to draw up premixed liquid medications from multidose vials. **Rationale:** *Using the filter needle prevents any solid particles from being drawn up through the needle.*
   - Ensure that the needle is firmly attached to the syringe.
   - Remove the cap from the needle, then draw up into the syringe the amount of air equal to the volume of the medication to be withdrawn.

- Carefully insert the needle into the upright vial through the center of the rubber cap, maintaining the sterility of the needle.
- Inject the air into the vial, keeping the bevel of the needle above the surface of the medication ➊. **Rationale:** *The air will allow the medication to be drawn out easily because negative pressure will not be created inside the vial. The bevel is kept above the medication to avoid creating bubbles in the medication.*

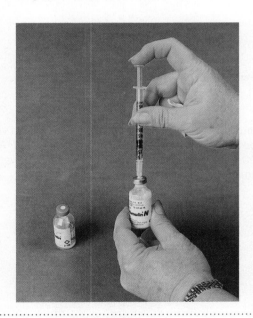

➊ Injecting air into a vial.

- Withdraw the prescribed amount of medication using either of the following methods:
  a. Hold the vial down (i.e., with the base lower than the top), move the needle tip so that it is below the fluid level, and withdraw the medication ➋.

  or

  b. Invert the vial, ensure the needle tip is below the fluid level, and gradually withdraw the medication ➌. **Rationale:** *Keeping the tip of the needle below the fluid level prevents air from being drawn into the syringe.*

SKILL 2.16 Vial Medication: Removing (*continued*)

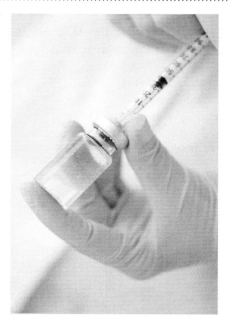

Source: Milena Boniek/PhotoAlto/Alamy Stock Photo

② Withdrawing a medication from a vial that is held with the base down.

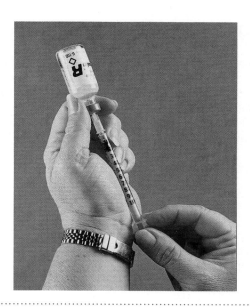

③ Withdrawing a medication from an inverted vial.

- Hold the syringe and vial at eye level to determine that the correct dosage of drug has been drawn into the syringe. Eject air remaining at the top of the syringe into the vial.
- When the correct volume of medication is obtained, withdraw the needle from the vial, and replace the cap over the needle using the one-hand scoop method, thus maintaining its sterility and preventing possible needlestick injuries **④**.

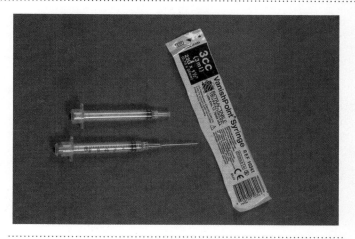

④ Healthcare facilities must use safety needles to conform to needlestick safety legislation.

- If necessary, gently tap the syringe barrel with a finger or pen while holding the syringe with the needle end pointing up to dislodge any air bubbles present in the syringe. Carefully and slowly expel the air and any excess medication from the syringe, maintaining the "needle up" position. **Rationale:** *The tapping motion will cause the air bubbles to rise to the top of the syringe where they can be ejected out of the syringe. Sometimes when ejecting the air bubbles, the resulting amount of medication is less than ordered. Drawing up a little extra medication, as in the previous step, helps avoid this.*
- If giving an injection, replace the filter needle, if used, with a regular or safety needle of the correct gauge and length. Eject air from the new needle.
- Label the syringe with the medication name and dosage drawn up in the syringe. **Rationale:** *This can be used to do a last medication check for accuracy before administering the medication to the patient.*

CAUTION! Change the needle after withdrawing medication from ampule or vial.

Federal needlestick safety legislation **requires** healthcare facilities to implement devices that protect against accidental needlesticks.

USING MULTIDOSE VIALS

- Read the manufacturer's directions.
- Withdraw an equivalent amount of air from the vial before adding the diluent, unless otherwise indicated by the directions.
- Add the amount of sterile water or saline indicated in the directions.
- If a multidose vial is reconstituted, label the vial with the date and time it was prepared, the amount of drug contained in each milliliter of solution, and your initials. **Rationale:** *Time*

(*continued on next page*)

SKILL 2.16 Vial Medication: Removing (*continued*)

is an important factor to consider in the expiration of these medications.

■ Once the medication is reconstituted, store it in a refrigerator or as recommended by the manufacturer.

CAUTION! If multiple-use vials are opened, they should be marked with the date and time the container is entered and nurse's initials. Consult the product label or package insert to determine if refrigeration is necessary. Unless contamination is suspected, the Centers for Disease Control and Prevention (CDC) recommends that the vial be discarded either when empty or on the expiration date set by the manufacturer.

Reconstituting Powdered Medication

■ Insert needle into upright powdered medication vial.

■ Remove the amount of air equal to desired quantity of diluent; this provides space for the diluent.

■ Inject diluent into upright powdered medication vial.

■ Remove needle and cover with guard.

■ Rotate powdered medication vial with diluent between palms. Do not shake vial because shaking creates air bubbles and may cause difficulty withdrawing medication dose.

■ Withdraw medication from vial.

≫ Medication Routes

Expected Outcomes

1. Patient is given medication without difficulty.
2. Desired effects of medication occur without side effects.
3. Patient self-administers medication according to instructions.
4. Documentation on the MAR is accurate and current.
5. Medication's therapeutic effect is achieved.

SKILL 2.17 Ear Medication: Administering

Otic medications are used to treat infection, soften cerumen (earwax), and relieve pain. Sterile drops and irrigation solutions are used even though the ear canal is not considered sterile because nonsterile medications and solutions could introduce an infection.

Delegation or Assignment

Due to the need for assessment, interpretation of patient status, and use of sterile technique, otic medication administration is not delegated or assigned to the UAP. The nurse can request the UAP to report patient observations to the nurse for follow-up. In some states, a trained UAP may administer certain medications to stable patients in long-term care settings. Assessment and evaluation of effectiveness of the medication remain the responsibility of the nurse.

Equipment

■ Clean gloves
■ Cotton-tipped applicator
■ Correct medication bottle with a dropper
■ Flexible rubber tip (optional) for the end of the dropper, which prevents injury from sudden motion, for example, by a disoriented patient
■ Cotton fluff

For Irrigation Only

■ Moisture-resistant towel
■ Basin (e.g., emesis basin)

■ Irrigating solution at 37°C (98.6°F) temperature, about 500 mL (16 oz) or as ordered. **Rationale:** *A solution that is not at body temperature may induce dizziness from caloric stimulation.*
■ Container for the irrigating solution
■ Irrigating bulb syringe

Preparation

■ Check healthcare provider's orders if the MAR is unclear or pertinent information is missing.
■ Check the MAR.
■ Check for the drug name, strength, number of drops, and prescribed frequency.
■ Check patient allergy status.
■ Report any discrepancies to the charge nurse or primary care provider, as facility policy dictates.
■ Know the reason why the patient is receiving the medication, the drug classification, contraindications, usual dose range, side effects, and nursing considerations for administering and evaluating the intended outcomes of the medication.

EAR DROPS

Procedure

1. Compare the label on the medication container with the MAR and check the expiration date. **Rationale:** *Outdated medications are not safe to administer.*

SKILL 2.17 Ear Medication: Administering (*continued*)

2. If necessary, calculate the medication dosage.
3. Introduce self and explain to the patient what you are going to do, why it is necessary, and how the patient can participate. The administration of an otic medication is not usually painful. Discuss how the results will be used in planning further care or treatments.
4. Perform hand hygiene and observe other appropriate infection control procedures (e.g., clean gloves).
5. Provide for patient privacy.
6. Prepare the patient.
   * Prior to performing the procedure, verify the patient's identity using two identifiers or follow facility protocol. **Rationale:** *This ensures that the right patient receives the right medication.*
   * Assist the patient to a comfortable position for eardrop administration, usually lying with the ear being treated uppermost.
7. Clean the pinna of the ear and the meatus of the ear canal.
   * Apply gloves if infection is suspected.
   * Use cotton-tipped applicators and solution to wipe the pinna and auditory meatus. **Rationale:** *This removes any discharge present before the instillation so that it won't be washed into the ear canal.* Ensure that applicator does *not* go into the ear canal. **Rationale:** *This avoids damage to tympanic membrane or wax becoming impacted within the canal.*
8. Administer the ear medication.
   * Warm the medication container in your hand, or place it in warm water for a short time. **Rationale:** *This promotes patient comfort and prevents nerve stimulation and dizziness.*
   * Partially fill the ear dropper with medication.
   * Straighten the auditory canal. Pull the pinna upward and backward for patients 3 years and older; pull down and back for patients younger than 3 years old ❶. **Rationale:** *The auditory canal is straightened so that the solution can flow the entire length of the canal.*

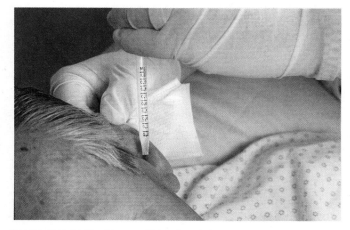

Source: Ronald May/Pearson Education, Inc.

❶ Lift pinna upward and backward to instill eardrops in an adult. For a child under 3 years, pull the pinna gently down and back before instilling drops.

* Instill the correct number of drops along the side of the ear canal.
* Press gently but firmly a few times on the tragus of the ear (the cartilaginous projection in front of the exterior meatus of the ear). **Rationale:** *Pressing on the tragus assists the flow of medication into the ear canal.*
* Ask the patient to remain in the side-lying position for about 5 minutes. **Rationale:** *This prevents the drops from escaping and allows the medication to reach all sides of the canal cavity.*
* Insert a small piece of cotton fluff loosely at the meatus of the auditory canal for 15–20 min. Do not press it into the canal. **Rationale:** *The cotton helps retain the medication when the patient is vertical. If pressed tightly into the canal, the cotton would interfere with the action of the drug and the outward movement of normal secretions.*
* If wearing gloves, remove them. Perform hand hygiene. Leave patient safe and comfortable.
* Complete documentation using forms, checklists, or electronic dropdown lists supplemented by nurse's notes or additional comments as appropriate.

EAR IRRIGATION

▪ Explain that the patient may experience a feeling of fullness, warmth, and occasionally discomfort when the fluid comes in contact with the tympanic membrane.
▪ Assist the patient to a sitting or lying position with head tilted toward the affected ear. **Rationale:** *The solution can then flow from the ear canal to a basin.*
▪ Place the moisture-resistant towel around the patient's shoulder under the ear to be irrigated, and place the basin under the ear to be irrigated.
▪ Fill the syringe with solution.
or
▪ Hang up the irrigating container, and run solution through the tubing and the nozzle. **Rationale:** *Solution is run through to remove air from the tubing and nozzle.*
▪ Straighten the ear canal.
▪ Insert the tip of the syringe into the auditory meatus, and direct the solution gently upward against the top of the canal. **Rationale:** *The solution will flow around the entire canal and out at the bottom. The solution is instilled gently because strong pressure from the fluid can cause discomfort and damage the tympanic membrane.*
▪ Continue instilling the fluid until all the solution is used or until the canal is cleaned, depending on the purpose of the irrigation. Take care not to block the outward flow of the solution with the syringe.
▪ Place a cotton fluff in the auditory meatus to absorb the excess fluid.
▪ Assist the patient to a side-lying position on the affected side. **Rationale:** *Lying with the affected side down helps drain the excess fluid by gravity.*
▪ Remove and discard gloves. Perform hand hygiene.
▪ Assess the patient's response and the character and amount of discharge, appearance of the canal, discomfort,

(*continued on next page*)

SKILL 2.17 Ear Medication: Administering (*continued*)

and so on, immediately after the instillation and again when the medication is expected to act. Inspect the cotton ball for any drainage. Leave patient safe and comfortable.

- Document all nursing assessments and interventions relative to the procedure. Include the name of the drug or irrigating solution, the strength, the number of drops if a liquid medication, the time, and the response of the patient.

SAMPLE DOCUMENTATION

[date] 0900 Ear canal red, with small amount of purulent drainage; 0.25 mL of ciprofloxacin 0.2% otic drops instilled in left ear canal, cotton applied for 15 minutes; tolerated well without incident. *R. Bailey*

SKILL 2.18 Enteral Tube Medication: Administering

Safety Note! *During scheduled clinical time, nursing students may have a learning opportunity to observe or assist with this skill only with faculty permission and with direct supervision from faculty or another RN.*

Enteral tube feedings help all ages of individuals who cannot eat sufficient quantities of food to meet nutritional needs. There are various tube feeding formulas on the market to meet individual patient needs. A liquid form is the preferred drug preparation for enteral tube. If the drug is not available as a liquid, tablets can be crushed into a powder and capsules can be opened up. There are certain medications that should not be given by enteral tube such as enteric coated, chewable, or sustained/controlled release medications. Medications should not be mixed with formula to make them liquids, to avoid interactions of the combination.

Delegation or Assignment

The administration of medications through an enteral tube is performed by the nurse and is not delegated or assigned to the UAP. The nurse can inform the UAP of the intended therapeutic effects and/or specific side effects of the medication and request the UAP to report specific patient observations to the nurse for follow-up. Assessment and evaluation of effectiveness of the medication remain the responsibility of the nurse.

Equipment

- Medication to be administered
- Disposable medication cups: small paper or plastic calibrated medication cups for liquids
- 60-mL syringe with catheter tip for large-bore tube or Luer-Lok tip for small-bore tube
- Pill crusher for medications that can be and need to be crushed
- Tongue blade or straw to stir dissolved medication
- pH test strip
- Warm water to dissolve crushed medications
- Tap water (room temperature) or sterile water or normal saline for flushing tube (check facility policy)
- Emesis basin
- Clean gloves
- MAR (hard copy or electronic)

Preparation

- Know the reason why the patient is receiving the medication, the drug classification, contraindications, usual dosage range, side effects, and nursing considerations for administering and evaluating the intended outcomes for the medication.
- Check healthcare provider's orders and the MAR.
- Check the MAR for the drug name, dosage, frequency, route of administration, and expiration date for administration of the medication, if appropriate. **Rationale:** *Orders for certain medications (e.g., narcotics, antibiotics) expire after a specified time frame and need to be reordered by the primary care provider.*
- If the MAR is unclear or pertinent information is missing, compare the MAR with the prescriber's most recent written order.
- Report any discrepancies to the charge nurse or the prescriber, as facility policy dictates.
- Organize the supplies. **Rationale:** *Organization of supplies saves time and reduces the chance of error.*
- Gather medications on the MAR for each patient so that medications can be prepared for one patient at a time.

Procedure

1. Introduce self and verify the patient's identity using two identifiers. **Rationale:** *This ensures that the right patient receives the medication.*
2. Perform hand hygiene and observe other appropriate infection control procedures (e.g., clean gloves).
3. Provide for patient privacy.
4. Prepare the patient.
   - Assist the patient to a Fowler's position in bed or a sitting position in a chair. If a sitting position is contraindicated, a slightly elevated right side-lying position is acceptable. **Rationale:** *These positions enhance gravitational flow and prevent aspiration of fluid into the lungs.*
   - If not previously assessed, take the required assessment measures, such as pulse and respiratory rates or blood pressure. Take the apical pulse rate before administering digitalis preparations. Take blood pressure before giving antihypertensive drugs. Take the respiratory rate prior to administering narcotics. **Rationale:** *Narcotics depress the respiratory center.* If any of the findings are above or below the

SKILL 2.18 Enteral Tube Medication: Administering (*continued*)

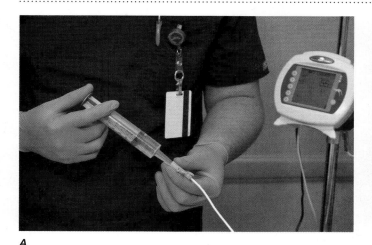

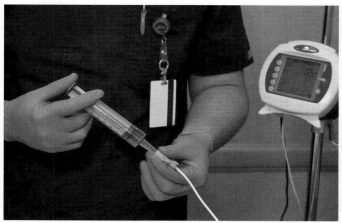

A

B

Sources: (Left and Right) Ronald May/Pearson Education, Inc.

❶ **A,** Flush with 15 mL water before administering any medication. **B,** Give each medication separately, allowing it to flow through the tube by gravity. Between and after medications, flush tube again with 15 mL water. Record the total amount of liquid on the intake and output (I&O) sheet.

predetermined parameters, consult the primary care provider before administering the medication.

5. Prepare medications for appropriate administration by enteral tube (e.g., use liquids or crush and dissolve tablets). Calculate medication dosage accurately.

6. Explain the purpose of the medication and how it will help, using language that the patient can understand. Include relevant information about effects; for example, tell the patient receiving an analgesic to expect a decrease in pain. **Rationale:** *Information can facilitate acceptance of and compliance with the therapy.*

7. Apply clean gloves.

8. If patient is receiving a continuous tube feeding, press the "Hold" button on the enteric feeding pump. **Rationale:** *Pausing or holding the pump temporarily stops the administration of the tube feeding.*

9. Disconnect tubing that is being used for suction or feeding from gastric tube. Place cap on end of tubing. **Rationale:** *Putting a cap on the end of the tubing prevents contamination.*

10. Assess tube placement (review Skill 10.11 for methods).

11. Assess for residual gastric content.
    - Pinch or fold over the gastric tube. **Rationale:** *Pinching or folding over the tubing prevents gastric contents from flowing out of the tube.*
    - Gently aspirate all the stomach contents when patient is not receiving continuous feeding and measure the residual volume.
    - Return residual back to stomach. **Rationale:** *Returning the residual prevents loss of fluids and electrolytes.* Pinch or fold over the gastric tube and remove the syringe.
    - Check facility policy if residual volume is greater than 100 mL.

12. Administer the medication(s).
    - Remove the plunger from the syringe and connect the syringe to a pinched or folded over tube.

Rationale: *Pinching or folding over the tube prevents excess air from entering the stomach and causing distention.*

- Put 15 mL of water into the syringe barrel to flush the tube before administering the first medication ❶. Raise or lower the barrel of the syringe to adjust the flow as needed. Pinch or clamp the tubing before all of the water is instilled. **Rationale:** *This prevents excess air from entering the stomach.*
- Pour liquid or dissolved medication into syringe barrel and allow to flow by gravity into enteral tube.
- If administering more than one medication, flush with 15 mL of water between each medication.
- After administering the last medication, flush the tube with 15 mL of water. **Rationale:** *Flushing clears the tube and helps prevent clogging of the tube.*
- Pinch or fold over the gastric tube and reconnect to tubing for continuous tube feeding. If the patient was previously connected to suction, keep the gastric tube clamped for 20–30 min after giving the medication. **Rationale:** *Keeping the tube clamped for that time will help ensure that the medication is absorbed before restarting the suction.*
- Remove and discard gloves. Perform hand hygiene.

13. Document each medication given.
    - Record the medication given, dosage, time, any complaints or assessments of the patient, and your signature.
    - If medication was refused or omitted, record this fact on the appropriate record; document the reason, when possible, and the nurse's actions according to facility policy.
    - Record fluid intake accurately if patient is on intake and output.

(*continued on next page*)

SKILL 2.18 Enteral Tube Medication: Administering (*continued*)

14. Dispose of all supplies appropriately.
    - Replenish stock (e.g., medication cups) and return cart to the appropriate place.
    - Discard used disposable supplies.

CAUTION! Consult with pharmacist before deciding to alter the form of *any* medication. Have pharmacist substitute liquid form of medication if available, or substitute a short-acting formulation that can be safely crushed for administration. Contact the healthcare provider for a substitute medication if formulation alternatives are unavailable.

SAMPLE DOCUMENTATION

[date] 1000 Nasogastric (NG) tube suction turned off for tube placement check with 20 mL of air pushed in, air swish heard over gastric area left upper quadrant (LUQ) abdomen with stethoscope, had residual 15 mL gastric contents, replaced back in stomach, acetaminophen 325 mg tablets × 2 crushed, instilled 15 mL water prior to and after medication and 15 mL in-between; no clumping in tube noted; NG tube remains secured at right nares; intermittent suction off × 30 minutes; tolerated without incident. *B. Poppins*

SKILL 2.19 Eye Medication: Administering

There is a wide variety of ophthalmic medications available, such as antivirals, anti-inflammatories, antibiotics, and antiallergy medications. Eye conditions and disorders treated with these medications include ocular hypertension, cataracts, eye infections, glaucoma, and macular degeneration. Most eye medications are in the form of drops or an ointment.

Delegation or Assignment

Due to the need for assessment, interpretation of patient status, and use of sterile technique, ophthalmic medication administration is not delegated or assigned to the UAP. The nurse can request the UAP to report patient observations to the nurse for follow-up. In some states, a trained UAP may administer certain medications to stable patients in long-term care settings. Assessment and evaluation of effectiveness of the medication remain the responsibility of the nurse.

Equipment

- Clean gloves
- Sterile absorbent sponges soaked in sterile normal saline
- Medication
- Sterile eye dressing (pad) as needed and paper tape to secure it

Eye Irrigation Only

- Irrigating solution (e.g., normal saline) and irrigating syringe or tubing
- Dry sterile absorbent sponges
- Moisture-resistant towel
- Basin (e.g., emesis basin)

Preparation

- Verify healthcare provider's orders and check the medication administration record (MAR).
- Check for the drug name, dose, and strength. Also confirm the prescribed frequency of the instillation and which eye (or both eyes) to be treated.
- Check patient allergy status.
- If the MAR is unclear or pertinent information is missing, compare it with the most recent primary care provider's written order.
- Report any discrepancies to the charge nurse or primary care provider, as facility policy dictates.
- Know the reason why the patient is receiving the medication, the drug classification, contraindications, usual dose range, side effects, and nursing considerations for administering and evaluating the intended outcomes of the medication.

APPLYING MEDICATION

Procedure

1. Compare the label on the medication tube or bottle with the MAR and check the expiration date. **Rationale:** *Outdated medications are not safe to administer.*
2. If necessary, calculate the medication dosage.
3. Introduce self and verify the patient's identity using two identifiers or follow facility policy. **Rationale:** *This ensures that the right patient receives the right medication.* Explain to the patient what you are going to do, why it is necessary, and how the patient can participate. The administration of an ophthalmic medication is not usually painful. Ointments are often soothing to the eye, but some liquid preparations may sting initially. Discuss how the results will be used in planning further care or treatments.
4. Perform hand hygiene and observe other appropriate infection control procedures (e.g., clean gloves).
5. Provide for patient privacy.
6. Assist the patient to a comfortable position, usually lying.
7. Clean the eyelid and the eyelashes.
    - Apply clean gloves.
    - Use sterile cotton balls moistened with sterile irrigating solution or sterile normal saline, and wipe from the inner canthus to the outer canthus. **Rationale:** *If not removed, material on the eyelid and lashes can be washed into the*

SKILL 2.19 Eye Medication: Administering (*continued*)

eye. *Cleaning toward the outer canthus prevents contamination of the other eye and the lacrimal duct.*

8. Administer the eye medication.
   - Check the ophthalmic preparation for the name, strength, and number of drops if a liquid is used. **Rationale:** *Checking medication data is essential to prevent a medication error.* Draw the correct number of drops into the shaft of the dropper if a dropper is used. If ointment is used, discard the first bead. **Rationale:** *The first bead of ointment from a tube is considered to be contaminated.*
   - Instruct the patient to look up to the ceiling. Give the patient a dry sterile absorbent sponge. **Rationale:** *The person is less likely to blink if looking up. While the patient looks up, the cornea is partially protected by the upper eyelid. A sponge is needed to press on the nasolacrimal duct after a liquid instillation to prevent systemic absorption or to wipe excess ointment from the eyelashes after an ointment is instilled.*
   - Expose the lower conjunctival sac by placing the thumb or fingers of your nondominant hand on the patient's cheekbone just below the eye and gently drawing down the skin on the cheek. If the tissues are edematous, handle the tissues carefully to avoid damaging them. **Rationale:** *Placing the fingers on the cheekbone minimizes the possibility of touching the cornea, avoids putting any pressure on the eyeball, and prevents the person from blinking or squinting.*
   - Holding the medication in the dominant hand, place hand on patient's forehead to stabilize hand. Approach the eye from the side and instill the correct number of drops onto the outer third of the lower conjunctival sac. Hold the dropper 1–2 cm (0.4–0.8 in.) above the sac ❶. **Rationale:** *The patient is less likely to blink if a side approach is used. When instilled into the conjunctival sac, drops will not harm the cornea as they might if dropped directly on it. The dropper must not touch the sac or the cornea.*

   or
   - Holding the tube above the lower conjunctival sac, squeeze 2 cm (0.8 in.) of ointment from the tube into the lower conjunctival sac from the inner canthus outward.

❶ Instilling eye drops into the lower conjunctival sac.

- Instruct the patient to close the eyelids but not to squeeze them shut. **Rationale:** *Closing the eye spreads the medication over the eyeball. Squeezing can injure the eye and push out the medication.*
- For liquid medications, press firmly or have the patient press firmly on the nasolacrimal duct for at least 30 seconds ❷. **Rationale:** *Pressing on the nasolacrimal duct prevents the medication from running out of the eye and down the duct, preventing systemic absorption.*

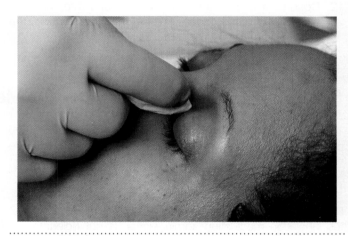

❷ Pressing on the eye's nasolacrimal duct.

EYE IRRIGATION

- Place absorbent pads under the head, neck, and shoulders. Place an emesis basin next to the eye to catch drainage. Some eye medications cause systemic reactions such as confusion or a decrease in heart rate and blood pressure if the eye drops go down the nasolacrimal duct and get into the systemic circulation.
- Expose the lower conjunctival sac. Or, to irrigate in stages, first hold the lower lid down, then hold the upper lid up. Exert pressure on the bony prominences of the cheekbone and beneath the eyebrow when holding the eyelids. **Rationale:** *Separating the lids prevents reflex blinking. Exerting pressure on the bony prominences minimizes the possibility of pressing the eyeball and causing discomfort.*
- Fill and hold the eye irrigator about 2.5 cm (1 in.) above the eye. **Rationale:** *At this height the pressure of the solution will not damage the eye tissue, and the irrigator will not touch the eye.*
- Irrigate the eye, directing the solution onto the lower conjunctival sac from the inner canthus to the outer canthus. **Rationale:** *Directing the solution in this way prevents possible injury to the cornea and prevents fluid and contaminants from flowing down the nasolacrimal duct.*
- Irrigate until the solution leaving the eye is clear (no discharge is present) or until all the solution has been used.
- Instruct the patient to close and move the eye periodically. **Rationale:** *Eye closure and movement help to move secretions from the upper to the lower conjunctival sac.*

(*continued on next page*)

SKILL 2.19 Eye Medication: Administering (continued)

- Clean and dry the eyelids as needed. Wipe the eyelids gently from the inner to the outer canthus to collect excess medication.

9. Remove and discard gloves. Perform hand hygiene.
10. Apply an eye pad if needed, and secure it with paper eye tape.
11. Assess the patient's response immediately after the instillation or irrigation and again after the medication should have acted.
12. Document all relevant assessments and interventions. Include the name of the drug or irrigating solution, the strength, the number of drops if a liquid medication, the time, and the response of the patient.

> **SAMPLE DOCUMENTATION**
>
> [date] 1300 Left eye area cleaned with warm saline and dried; one drop ketorolac tromethamine 0.5% ophthalmic solution instilled left eye; closed eye for 2 minutes; denies pain of the left eye at this time; tolerated without incident. *C. Gibbs*

SKILL 2.20 Inhaler, Dry Powder Medication: Administering

This hand-held inhaler delivers medication in the form of a dry powder to the lungs as the patient inhales through it. There are no propellants or other ingredients involved.

Delegation or Assignment

Due to the need for assessment and interpretation of patient status inhalation medication administration is not delegated or assigned to the UAP. The nurse can request the UAP to report patient observations to the nurse for follow-up. In some states, a trained UAP may administer certain medications to stable patients in long-term care settings. Assessment and evaluation of effectiveness of the medication remain the responsibility of the nurse.

Equipment

- Dry powder capsule intended for oral inhalation
- Medication package insert (instructions)
- Handheld inhalation device intended for medication to be given

Preparation

- Check the healthcare provider's orders and the MAR.
- Check for the drug name, strength, and prescribed frequency.
- Check patient allergy status.
  - If the MAR is unclear or pertinent information is missing, compare it with the most recent primary care provider's written order.
  - Report any discrepancies to the charge nurse or primary care provider, as facility policy dictates.
  - Know the reason why the patient is receiving the medication, the drug classification, contraindications, usual dose range, side effects, and nursing considerations for administering and evaluating the intended outcomes of the medication.
- Review medication package insert instructions.

Procedure

1. Prior to performing the procedure, introduce self and verify the patient's identity using two identifiers or follow facility policy. Explain to the patient what you are going to do, why it is necessary, and how the patient can participate. Discuss how the results will be used in planning further care or treatments.
2. Take dry powder capsule package and inhalation device to patient's room.
3. Perform hand hygiene and observe other appropriate infection control procedures.
4. Provide for patient privacy.
5. Assist patient to a sitting position.
6. Remove capsule from package, peeling back foil cover to expose only one capsule. **Rationale:** *Capsules should be used immediately; unused capsules exposed to air may lose effectiveness.*
7. Open the outer cap of inhaler device (pull cap upward).
8. Open the mouthpiece.
9. Insert the capsule into the center of the chamber of the inhalation device ①.

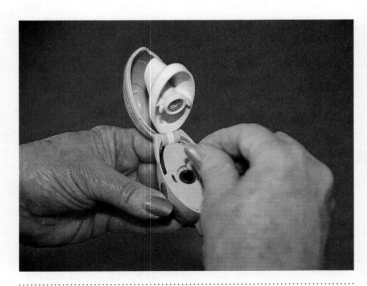

① **Insert capsule into center of chamber of the inhalation device.**

SKILL 2.20 Inhaler, Dry Powder Medication: Administering (continued)

10. Hold the device upright, and, leaving the outer cap open, close mouthpiece/lid firmly until a click is heard. Leave the outer cap open.
11. Press the side-mounted piercing button in completely, then release. **Rationale:** *The piercing button punctures the capsule, allowing medication to be released upon inhalation.*
12. Have the patient breathe out completely.
13. Have the patient keep the head in an upright position and place lips tightly around the mouthpiece.
14. Have patient breathe slowly and deeply with sufficient energy to hear the medication capsule vibrate. **Rationale:** *As long as the capsule rattles, the patient's inhalation is fast enough.*
    Note: Some dry powder inhalers (DPIs) require a fast initial inhalation to activate the medication distribution.
15. Have the patient hold the deep breath as long as comfortable, then return to normal breathing.
16. Have patient repeat steps 12 through 15 if indicated in medication package insert. **Rationale:** *Repeating the steps may be necessary to get the full dose of medication.*
17. Open mouthpiece and discard remaining capsule.
18. Close mouthpiece and outer cap and store at patient's bedside.
19. Clean unit only as necessary, using warm water and allowing device to air dry thoroughly before next use. **Rationale:** *No cleaning agents should be used and the device should not be wet when used.*
20. When procedure is complete, perform hand hygiene. Leave patient safe and comfortable.
21. Complete documentation using forms, checklists, or electronic dropdown lists supplemented by nurse's notes or additional comments as appropriate.

SAMPLE DOCUMENTATION

[date] 0500 C/o trouble catching his breath; P-88, R-22, O_2 sat. 94% on room air. Small wheezing heard on expiration bilaterally lower lung fields. DPI inhaler brought to room and prepared for patient to use. After one prolonged inspiration with DPI inhaler, patient less anxious and states he is breathing easier; after 6 minutes, P-82, R-18, O_2 sat. 96 % on room air, skin dry, no respiratory distress noted. *T. Wertz*

SKILL 2.21 Inhaler, Metered-Dose Medication: Administering

A metered dose inhaler delivers a specific amount of medication in an aerosol form, instead of a tablet or capsule. This hand-held device has a pressurized canister inside a plastic case with a mouthpiece attached. It uses a chemical propellant to push the medication out of the inhaler. As the device is pressed, inhalation takes the medication directly into the lungs.

Delegation or Assignment

Due to the need for assessment and interpretation of patient status, inhaled medication administration is not delegated or assigned to the UAP. The nurse can request the UAP to report patient observations to the nurse for follow-up. In some states, a trained UAP may administer certain medications to stable patients in long-term care settings. Assessment and evaluation of effectiveness of the medication remain the responsibility of the nurse.

Equipment

Metered-dose nebulizer with medication canister and extender if indicated

Preparation

- Check the healthcare provider's orders and the MAR.
- Check for the drug name, strength, and prescribed frequency.
- Check patient allergy status.
  - If the MAR is unclear or pertinent information is missing, compare it with the most recent primary care provider's written order.
  - Report any discrepancies to the charge nurse or primary care provider, as facility policy dictates.
  - Know the reason why the patient is receiving the medication, the drug classification, contraindications, usual dose range, side effects, and nursing considerations for administering and evaluating the intended outcomes of the medication.

Procedure

1. Compare the label on the medication container with the MAR and check the expiration date. **Rationale:** *Outdated medications are not safe to administer.*
2. Introduce self and verify the patient's identity with two identifiers or follow facility policy. **Rationale:** *This ensures that the right patient receives the right medication.* Explain to the patient what you are going to do, why it is necessary, and how the patient can participate. Discuss how the results will be used in planning further care or treatments.
3. Perform hand hygiene and observe other appropriate infection control procedures (e.g., clean gloves).
4. Provide for patient privacy.

(continued on next page)

SKILL 2.21 Inhaler, Metered-Dose Medication: Administering *(continued)*

5. Explain to the patient that this nebulizer delivers a measured dose of drug with each push of the medication canister, which fits into the top of the nebulizer.
6. Instruct the patient to use the metered-dose nebulizer as follows:

Metered-dose Inhaler (MDI)

- Ensure that the canister is firmly and fully inserted into the inhaler.
- Remove the mouthpiece cap. Holding the MDI upright, shake the inhaler vigorously for 3 to 5 seconds to mix the medication evenly.
- Exhale comfortably (as in a normal full breath).
- Hold the inhaler with the canister on top and the mouthpiece at the bottom.
  - a. Hold the MDI 2–4 cm (1–2 in.) from the open mouth.

  or
  - b. Put the mouthpiece far enough into the mouth with its opening toward the throat such that the lips can tightly close around the mouthpiece.

Metered-dose Inhaler with Spacer

- Insert the MDI mouthpiece into the spacer.
- Holding the inhaler and spacer, shake vigorously for 3 to 5 seconds to mix the medication evenly.
- An MDI with a spacer or extender is always placed in the mouth.

7. Administer the medication.
- Press down *once* on the MDI canister (which releases the dose) and inhale slowly (for 3–5 seconds) and deeply through the mouth ❶.
- Hold your breath for 10 seconds or as long as possible. **Rationale:** *This allows the aerosol to reach deeper airways.*

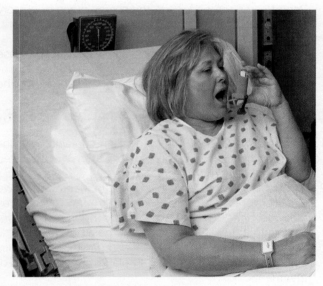

Source: Ronald May/Pearson Education, Inc.

❶ Depress inhalation device while inhaling slowly (3–5 sec) and deeply through mouth.

- Remove the inhaler from or away from the mouth.
- Exhale slowly through *pursed* lips. **Rationale:** *Controlled exhalation keeps the small airways open during exhalation.*

8. Repeat the inhalation if ordered. Wait 1–2 min between inhalations of bronchodilator medications. **Rationale:** *The first inhalation has a chance to work and the subsequent dose reaches deeper into the lungs.*
- Many MDIs contain steroids for an anti-inflammatory effect. Prolonged use increases the risk of fungal infections in the mouth, indicating a need for attentive mouth care.
- Following use of the inhaler, rinse mouth with water and spit it out to remove residual medication in the mouth.
- Clean the MDI mouthpiece, and spacer if appropriate, daily. Use mild soap and water, rinse it, and let it air dry before reusing.
- Store the canister at room temperature. Avoid extremes of temperature.
- Report adverse reactions such as restlessness, palpitations, nervousness, or rash to the primary care provider.

9. Perform hand hygiene. Leave patient safe and comfortable.
10. Document all nursing assessments and interventions relative to the procedure. Include the name of the drug, the strength, the time, and the response of the patient.

SAMPLE DOCUMENTATION

[date] 0200 C/o trouble catching his breath, P-92, R-26, O_2 sat. on room air 95%, wheezing heard on expiration bilaterally lower lung fields. MDI inhaler brought to room and prepared for patient to use. After two prolonged inspirations with MDI inhaler, patient states he is breathing easier and feels he is getting enough air, after 10 minutes, P-84, R-20, O_2 sat. on room air 97%, skin dry, no respiratory distress noted. *T. Barn*

Safety Considerations

- If two inhalers are to be used, the bronchodilator medication (which opens the airways) should be given prior to other medications. A mnemonic to help remember this is B before C (i.e., bronchodilator before corticosteroid).

- Check inhaler medication label for number of actuations (propellant-driven medication doses, e.g., 200). Have patient maintain a record of actuations and discard after the number indicated. Final puffs may be nothing but propellant, which would not dilate airways in an emergency situation.

- Inhaled steroids may not be correctly used by patients because they do not associate these medications with immediate symptom relief. The bronchodilators act to open the airways in the short term. However, it is the inhaled steroids that act as "chemical Band-Aids" to keep airway inflammation under control.

SKILL 2.22 Nasal Medication: Administering

Most nasal medications are delivered locally as a decongestant spray or liquid for allergy and cold symptoms or treatment of infected sinuses with antibiotics. Some systemic medications are available in a spray form to treat nicotine replacement and migraines.

Delegation or Assignment

Due to the need for assessment and interpretation of patient status, nasal medication administration is not delegated or assigned to the UAP. The nurse can request the UAP to report patient observations to the nurse for follow-up. In some states, a trained UAP may administer certain medications to stable patients in long-term care settings. Assessment and evaluation of effectiveness of the medication remain the responsibility of the nurse.

Equipment

- Tissues
- Clean gloves
- Correct medication bottle with a dropper or spray nozzle

Preparation

- Check the healthcare provider's orders and the MAR.
- Check for the drug name, strength, and number of drops. Also confirm the prescribed frequency of the instillation and which side of the nose is to be treated.
- Check patient allergy status.
- If the MAR is unclear or pertinent information is missing, compare it with the most recent primary care provider's written order.
- Report any discrepancies to the charge nurse or primary care provider, as facility policy dictates.
- Know the reason why the patient is receiving the medication, the drug classification, contraindications, usual dose range, side effects, and nursing considerations for administering and evaluating the intended outcomes of the medication.

Procedure

1. Compare the label on the medication container with the medication record and check the expiration date. **Rationale:** *Outdated medications are not safe to administer.*
2. If necessary, calculate the medication dosage.
3. Introduce self and verify the patient's identity with two identifiers or follow facility policy. **Rationale:** *This ensures that the right patient receives the right medication.* Explain to the patient what you are going to do, why it is necessary, and how the patient can participate. The administration of nasal medication is not usually painful. Discuss how the results will be used in planning further care or treatments.
4. Perform hand hygiene and observe other appropriate infection control procedures (e.g., clean gloves).
5. Provide for patient privacy.

6. Assist the patient to a comfortable position.
   - To treat the opening of the eustachian tube, have the patient assume a back-lying position ❶ ❷. **Rationale:** *The drops will flow into the nasopharynx, where the eustachian tube opens.*

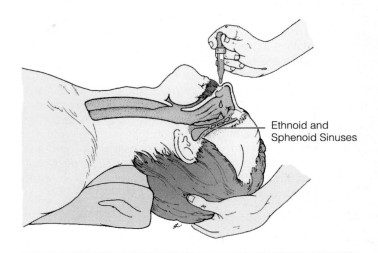

Ethnoid and Sphenoid Sinuses

❶ Instruct patient to tilt head backward and place dropper inside nares when instilling nose drops.

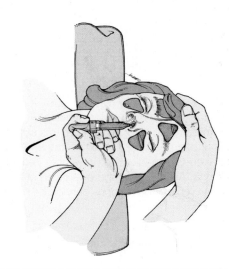

❷ Tilt patient's head back for nose drops to reach maxillary and frontal sinuses.

- To treat the ethmoid and sphenoid sinuses, have the patient assume a back-lying position with the head over the edge of the bed or a pillow under the shoulders so that the head is tipped backward.
- To treat the maxillary and frontal sinuses, have the patient assume the same back-lying position, with the head turned toward the side to be treated. If only one side is to be treated, be sure the patient is positioned so that the correct side is accessible. If the patient's head

(continued on next page)

SKILL 2.22 Nasal Medication: Administering (*continued*)

is over the edge of the bed, support it with your hand so that the neck muscles are not strained.

7. Administer the medication.
   - Apply clean gloves.
   - Draw up the required amount of solution into the dropper.
   - Hold the tip of the dropper just above the nostril, and direct the solution laterally toward the midline of the superior concha of the ethmoid bone as the patient breathes through the mouth. Do not touch the mucous membrane of the nares. **Rationale:** *If the solution is directed toward the base of the nasal cavity, it will run down the eustachian tube. Touching the mucous membrane with the dropper could contaminate the dropper, damage the membrane, and cause the patient to sneeze.*
   - Repeat for the other nostril if indicated.
   - Ask the patient to remain in the position for 5 minutes. **Rationale:** *The patient remains in the same position to help the solution come in contact with all of the nasal surface or flow into the desired area.*
   - Discard any remaining solution in the dropper, and dispose of soiled supplies appropriately.
   - Remove and discard gloves. Perform hand hygiene.

8. Document all nursing assessments and interventions relative to the procedure. Include the name of the drug or irrigating solution, the strength, the number of drops if a liquid medication, the time, and the response of the patient.

SAMPLE DOCUMENTATION

[date] 0900 Nasal congestion noted both nares, mouth breathing, bulb syringe used to suction both nares, mucoid thin secretions removed, no acute distress noted, but fussy, P-104, R-24, O_2 sat. room air 97%, breath sounds congested both sides, Fluticasone sprayed – I spray each nares as ordered. *T. Handy*

SKILL 2.23 Nebulized Medication, Non-pressurized Aerosol (NPA): Administering

Aerosol nebulizers deliver respiratory medications rapidly and directly into the airways with each inhalation by the patient where it can be absorbed. The medication is solid or liquid particles suspended in a gas that is dispensed in a cloud or mist via facemask, T-piece, or mouthpiece.

Delegation or Assignment

Administering medications by nebulizer involves knowledge and medication administration skills. Therefore, this skill is not delegated or assigned to the UAP. In some states, a trained UAP may administer certain medications to stable patients in long-term care settings. Assessment and evaluation of effectiveness of the medication remain the responsibility of the nurse.

Equipment

- Nebulizer medication chamber
- T-piece, mouthpiece, or mask
- Corrugated tubing
- Airflow tubing
- Prescribed medication (e.g., bronchodilator)
- Prescribed diluent (normal saline)
- Wall source (or other source) for compressed air, or oxygen with flowmeter

Preparation

- Review medication preparation protocol.
- Perform hand hygiene.
- Dilute medication as ordered and place in nebulizer chamber.
- Attach one end of tubing to compressed air source.
- Attach other end of tubing to nozzle at side or bottom of nebulizer.
- Keep nebulizer chamber vertical, and connect top of chamber to mask or T-piece sidearm.
- Hold mouthpiece in its protective cover, and attach to one end of T-piece.
- Attach corrugated tubing to other end of T-piece.

Procedure

1. Prior to performing the procedure, introduce self and verify the patient's identity using two identifiers. Explain to the patient what you are going to do, why it is necessary, and how the patient can participate. Discuss how the results will be used in planning further care or treatments.
2. Perform hand hygiene and observe other appropriate infection control procedures.
3. Provide for patient privacy.
4. Assess patient's respiratory rate, effort, and breath sounds prior to breathing treatment as time allows.
5. Turn on air or oxygen (6–8 liters/min) source, and observe for mist flow.
   - If the patient is receiving 3 liters/min or less of oxygen therapy, deliver aerosolized medications with compressed air (yellow wall outlet).
   - If the patient is receiving 4 liters/min or more of oxygen therapy, deliver the aerosol medication with the oxygen flowmeter (green wall outlet) set at 6–8 liters/min.
6. Have patient place mouthpiece in mouth and close lips ❶.
7. Instruct patient to breathe normally in and out of mouthpiece or mask.
8. Have patient take a deep breath and hold for several seconds, then exhale slowly every 3 to 5 breaths. (Treatment is complete when all medication is used and no mist is seen.)

SKILL 2.23 Nebulized Medication, Non-pressurized Aerosol (NPA): Administering (*continued*)

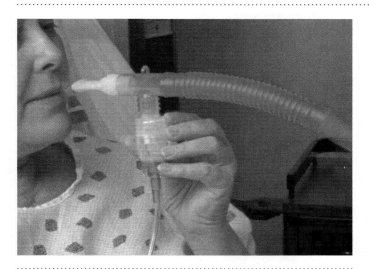

1. Nonpressurized aerosol (NPA) treatment in progress.

9. Turn power (air or O_2 flow) off, and unplug compressor (if used), or reset prescribed O_2 flow rate.
10. Reassess patient's respiratory rate, effort, and breath sounds post breathing treatment.
11. Clean mouthpiece, and place equipment in plastic bag at bedside. (Dispose of and replace components according to facility policy.)
12. Perform hand hygiene. Leave patient safe and comfortable.

13. Complete documentation using forms, checklists, or electronic dropdown lists supplemented by nurse's notes or additional comments as appropriate.

SAMPLE DOCUMENTATION

[date] 1530 Shortness of breath (SOB) noted with moderate amount of distress post walking to bathroom and returning to bed; P-92, R-28, B/P 168/96, O_2 sat. 1 liters per minute (LPM) oxygen via nasal cannula 90%; breath sounds demonstrate rhonchi, gurgles, and wheezing throughout lung fields; albuterol jet nebulizer treatment with face mask implemented. *T. Green*

1550 Remains SOB without distress; P-88, R-24, O_2 sat. 1 LPM oxygen via nasal cannula 91%; breath sounds remain with rhonchi, gurgles, and wheezing throughout; skin warm and moist. Dr. Randolph notified and is coming. *T. Green*

CAUTION! The plastic containers with respiratory medications for nebulizers are similar to the plastic containers for single-dose eye drops. Both products have the drug name molded into the plastic, but it is difficult to see.

SKILL 2.24 Oral Medication: Administering

Administering oral medications involves more than just giving medication to patients. It also includes awareness of how the medications are absorbed and distributed throughout the body, the effects of the medications, and potential adverse reactions that may occur. Forms of oral medicines include tablets, capsules, solutions, elixirs, or other liquids. Adequate water, approximately 30–120 mL, should be swallowed with the medications to dissolve solid medications or dilute the liquids. Some medicines are absorbed while in the mouth such as buccal and sublingual ones. Always check the oral cavity for retained medicine particles. Physiological rhythms, use of alcohol, and stress may either inhibit or accelerate drug biodynamics. The concomitant use of herbs and other OTC preparations can also alter the patient's response to drug therapy.

Delegation or Assignment

In acute care settings, administration of oral/enteral medications is performed by the nurse and is not delegated or assigned to the UAP. The nurse can inform the UAP of the intended therapeutic effects and/or specific side effects of the medication and request the UAP to report specific patient observations to the nurse for follow-up. In some states, a trained UAP may administer certain medications to stable patients in long-term care settings. It is important, however, for the nurse to remember that the medication knowledge of the UAP is limited and assessment and evaluation of the effectiveness of the medication remain the responsibility of the nurse.

Equipment

- Medication dispensing system
- Disposable medication cups: small paper or plastic cups for tablets and capsules, waxed or plastic calibrated medication cups for liquids
- MAR (hard copy or electronic)
- Pill crusher/cutter
- Straws to administer medications that may discolor the teeth or to facilitate the ingestion of liquid medication for certain patients
- Drinking glass and water or juice
- Soft foods such as applesauce or pudding to use for crushed medications for patients who may choke on liquids

Preparation

- Know the reason why the patient is receiving the medication, the drug classification, contraindications, usual dosage range,

(*continued on next page*)

SKILL 2.24 Oral Medication: Administering *(continued)*

side effects, and nursing considerations for administering and evaluating the intended outcomes for the medication.

■ Check the healthcare provider's orders and the MAR.

■ Check for the drug name, dosage, frequency, route of administration, and expiration date for administering the medication, if appropriate. **Rationale:** *Orders for certain medications (e.g., narcotics, antibiotics) expire after a specified time frame and need to be reordered by the healthcare provider.*

■ If the MAR is unclear or pertinent information is missing, compare the MAR with the prescriber's most recent written order.

■ Report any discrepancies to the charge nurse or the prescriber, as facility policy dictates.

■ Check the patient's allergy status.

■ Verify the patient's ability to take medication orally.

■ Determine whether the patient can swallow, is NPO, is nauseated or vomiting, has gastric suction, or has diminished or absent bowel sounds.

■ Organize the supplies. **Rationale:** *Organization of supplies saves time and reduces the chance of error.*

■ Gather medications on MAR for each patient so medications can be prepared and administered for one patient at a time.

■ Cultural and genetic factors can affect how a patient reacts to medications. Cultural acceptance factors include values and beliefs, educational level, previous experiences, family influence, and healthcare provider–patient relationship.

Safety Considerations

2016 NATIONAL PATIENT SAFETY GOAL (NPSG) FOR USING MEDICINES SAFELY

The Joint Commission's process for using medicines safely is as follows:

■ *Before a procedure,* label medicines that are not labeled, such as medicines in syringes, cups, and basins. Do this in the area where medicines and supplies are set up.

■ Take extra care with patients who take anticoagulant medicines.

■ Record and pass along correct information about a patient's medicines. Find out what medicines the patient is taking. Compare those medicines to new medicines given to the patient. Make sure the patient knows which medicines to take when at home. Remind the patient it is important to have an up-to-date list of medicines to give the healthcare provider at every appointment.

Procedure

1. Introduce self to patient (parent as appropriate) and verify the patient's identity using two identifiers. Explain to the patient (or parent as appropriate) what you are going to do, why it is necessary, and how the patient can participate. Discuss how the results will be used in planning further care or treatments.

2. Perform hand hygiene and observe appropriate infection control procedures.

3. Provide for patient privacy.

4. Unlock the dispensing system.

5. Obtain appropriate medication following rights of medication administration.
   ● Read the MAR and take the appropriate medication from the shelf, drawer, or refrigerator. The medication may be dispensed in a bottle, box, or unit-dose package.
   ● Compare the label of the medication container or unit-dose package against the order on the MAR (hard copy or electronic). ❶. **Rationale:** *This is a safety check to ensure that the right medication is given.*

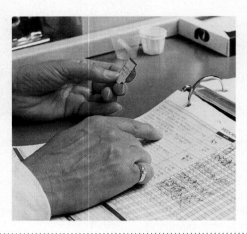

❶ Compare the medication label to the MAR.

   ● Check the expiration date of the medication. Return expired medications to the pharmacy. **Rationale:** *Outdated medications are not safe to administer.*
   ● Use only medications that have clear, legible labels. **Rationale:** *This ensures accuracy.*

6. Prepare the medication.
   ● Calculate the medication dosage accurately.
   ● Prepare the correct amount of medication for the required dose, without contaminating the medication. **Rationale:** *Aseptic technique maintains drug cleanliness.*
   ● While preparing the medication, recheck each prepared drug and container with the MAR again. **Rationale:** *This second safety check reduces the chance of error.*

Tablets or Capsules

   ● Place packaged unit-dose capsules or tablets directly into the medicine cup. Do not remove the medication from the package until at the bedside. **Rationale:** *The wrapper keeps the medication clean. Not removing the medication facilitates identification of the medication in the event the patient refuses the drug or assessment data indicate to hold the medication. Unopened unit-dose packages can usually be returned to the medication cart.*
   ● If using a stock container, pour the required number into the bottle cap, and then transfer the medication to the disposable cup without touching the tablets.
   ● Keep narcotics and medications that require specific assessments, such as pulse measurements, respiratory rate or depth, or blood pressure, separate from the others. **Rationale:** *This reminds the nurse to complete the*

SKILL 2.24 Oral Medication: Administering *(continued)*

needed assessment(s) in order to decide whether to give the medication or to withhold the medication if indicated.

- Break only scored tablets if necessary to obtain the correct dosage. Use a cutting or splitting device if needed ❷. Check facility policy as to whether unused portions of a medication are to be discarded.

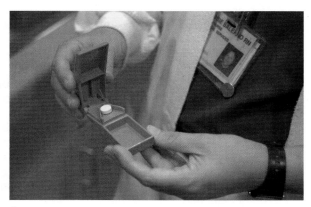

A

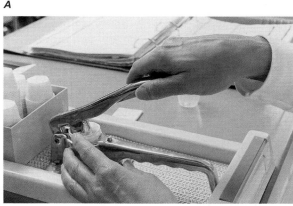

B

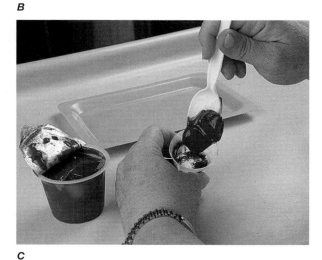

C

❷ **A**, If partial dose is ordered, place tablet in pill cutter to be cut in half. **B**, Place pill in crusher to crush tablet, or pulverize/crush pill in unit-dose container. **C**, Mix pulverized medication (or powder from opened capsule) carefully in small amount of soft food (pudding, jelly, applesauce).

- If the patient has difficulty swallowing, check if the medication can be crushed. If it is safe to do so, crush the tablet to a fine powder with a pill crusher or between two medication cups. Then, mix the powder with a small amount of soft food (e.g., custard, applesauce). (See ❷ *B* and *C*.) Some drug handbooks have an appendix listing "Do Not Crush" medications. The Institute for Safe Medication Practices (2015) website provides an updated list of medications that should not be crushed, including time-released and enteric-coated medications. Oxycodone (OxyContin), a long-acting narcotic that normally lasts 12 hours after administration, is an example of tablets that should not be crushed. Crushing these tablets may cause a potentially fatal overdose of oxycodone.

CAUTION! Check with the pharmacy before crushing tablets. Extended release, irritant (I), enteric-coated (EC), orally disintegrating tablets (ODT), effervescent tablet (EVT), slow-release (SR), or sublingual tablets should not be crushed.

Liquid Medication

- Thoroughly mix the medication before pouring. Discard any medication that has changed color or turned cloudy. Remove the cap and place it upside down on the countertop. **Rationale:** *This avoids contaminating the inside of the cap.*
- Hold the bottle so the label is next to the palm of the hand and pour the medication away from the label at eye level to read dose correctly ❸. **Rationale:** *This prevents the label from becoming soiled and illegible as a result of spilled liquids.*

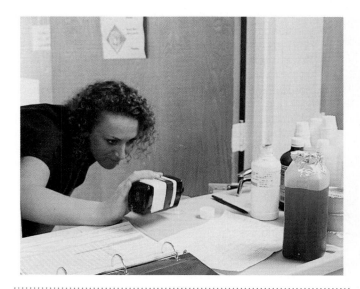

❸ Pour liquid medication at eye level to read dose correctly.

- Place the medication cup on a flat surface at eye level and fill it to the desired level, using the *bottom* of the

(continued on next page)

SKILL 2.24 Oral Medication: Administering (continued)

meniscus (crescent-shaped upper surface of a column of liquid) to align with the container scale ❹. **Rationale:** *This method ensures accuracy of measurement.*

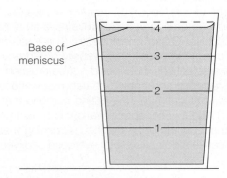

Base of meniscus

❹ The bottom of the curved meniscus is the measuring guide.

- Before capping the bottle, wipe the lip with a paper towel. **Rationale:** *This prevents the cap from sticking.*
- When giving small amounts of liquids (e.g., less than 5 mL), prepare the medication in a sterile syringe without the needle or in a specially designed oral syringe. Label the syringe with the name of the medication and the route (PO). **Rationale:** *Any oral solution removed from the original container and placed into a syringe should be labeled to avoid medications being given by the wrong route (e.g., IV). This practice facilitates patient safety and avoids tragic errors.*
- Keep unit-dose liquids in their package and open them at the bedside.

Oral Narcotics

- If a facility uses a manual recording system for controlled substances, check the narcotic record for the previous drug count and compare it with the supply available. Some medications, including narcotics, are kept in plastic containers that are sectioned and numbered.
- Remove the next available tablet and drop it in the medicine cup.
- After removing a tablet, record the necessary information on the appropriate narcotic control record and sign it. A co-signer may be required.
Note: Computer-controlled dispensing systems allow access only to the selected drug and automatically record its use.

All Medications

- Place the prepared medication and MAR together on the medication cart.
- Recheck the label on the container before returning the bottle, box, or envelope to its storage place. **Rationale:** *This third check further reduces the risk of error.*
- Never leave prepared medications unattended. **Rationale:** *This precaution prevents potential mishandling errors.*
- Lock the medication cart before entering the patient's room. **Rationale:** *This is a safety measure because*

medication carts must not be left open when unattended.
- Check the room number against the MAR if facility policy does not allow the MAR to be removed from the medication cart. **Rationale:** *This is another safety measure to ensure that the nurse is entering the correct patient room.*

7. Introduce self and verify the patient's identity using two identifiers. **Rationale:** *This ensures that the right patient receives the medication.*
8. Provide for patient privacy.
9. Prepare the patient.
   - Assist the patient to a sitting position or, if not possible, to a side-lying position. **Rationale:** *These positions facilitate swallowing and prevent aspiration.*
   - If not previously assessed, take the required assessment measures, such as pulse and respiratory rates or blood pressure. Take the apical pulse rate before administering digitalis preparations. Take blood pressure before giving antihypertensive drugs. Take the respiratory rate prior to administering narcotics. **Rationale:** *Narcotics depress the respiratory center.* If any of the findings are above or below the predetermined parameters, consult the primary care provider before administering the medication.
10. Explain the purpose of the medication and how it will help, using language that the patient can understand. Include relevant information about effects; for example, tell the patient receiving a diuretic to expect an increase in urine output. **Rationale:** *Information can facilitate acceptance of and compliance with the therapy.*
11. Administer the medication at the correct time.
    - Take the medication to the patient within 30 minutes before or after the scheduled time or follow facility policy (some facilities allow 60 minutes before or after the scheduled time).
    - Give the patient sufficient water or preferred juice to swallow the medication. Before using juice, check for any food and medication incompatibilities. **Rationale:** *Fluids ease swallowing and facilitate absorption from the gastrointestinal tract.* Liquid medications other than antacids or cough preparations may be diluted with 15 mL (½ oz) of water to facilitate absorption.
    - If the patient is unable to hold the pill cup, use the pill cup to introduce the medication into the patient's mouth, and only give one tablet or capsule at a time. **Rationale:** *Putting the cup to the patient's mouth maintains the cleanliness of the nurse's hands. Giving one medication at a time eases swallowing.*
    - If an older child or adult has difficulty swallowing, ask the patient to place the medication on the back of the tongue before taking the water. **Rationale:** *Stimulation of the back of the tongue produces the swallowing reflex.*
    - If the medication has an objectionable taste, ask the patient to suck a few ice chips beforehand, or give the medication with juice, applesauce, or bread if there are no contraindications. **Rationale:** *The cold temperature of*

SKILL 2.24 Oral Medication: Administering (*continued*)

the ice chips will desensitize the taste buds, and juices or bread can mask the taste of the medication.

- If the patient says that the medication you are about to give is different from what the patient has been receiving, do not give the medication without first checking the original order. **Rationale:** *Most patients are familiar with the appearance of medications taken previously. Unfamiliar medications may signal a possible error.*
- Stay with the patient until all medications have been swallowed. **Rationale:** *The nurse must see the patient swallow the medication before the drug administration can be recorded.* The nurse may need to check the patient's mouth to ensure that the medication was swallowed and not hidden inside the cheek. A healthcare provider's order or facility policy is required for medications left at the bedside.

12. When the procedure is complete, perform hand hygiene. Leave the patient safe and comfortable.

13. Document each medication given.
    - Record the medication given, dosage, time, any complaints or assessments of the patient, and your signature on the MAR.
    - If medication was refused or omitted, record this fact on the appropriate record; document the reason, when possible, and the nurse's actions according to facility policy.

14. Dispose of all supplies appropriately.
    - Replenish stock (e.g., medication cups) and return the cart to the appropriate place.
    - Discard used disposable supplies.

SAMPLE DOCUMENTATION

[date] 0800 Awake and alert; explained reason for digoxin tablet; apical P-78 beats/min and irregular; digoxin 0.25 mg given PO with water. Tolerated without complaint. *R. Gathers*

SKILL 2.25 Rectal Medication: Administering

Safety Note! *During scheduled clinical time, nursing students may have a learning opportunity to observe or assist with this skill only with faculty permission and with direct supervision from faculty or another RN.*

Medications prepared specifically to be inserted into the rectum include liquid solutions given by enema, creams, lotions, ointments inserted internally using an applicator, and suppositories (a mixture of medicine and a wax-like substance to form a semi-solid, bullet-shaped form that melts from body heat after insertion into the rectum). Rectal medications should not be used for patients with a recent history of rectal, bowel, or prostate gland surgery or rectal bleeding.

Delegation or Assignment

Due to the need for assessment and interpretation of patient status, rectal medication administration is not delegated or assigned to the UAP. The nurse can request the UAP to report patient observations to the nurse for follow-up. In some states, a trained UAP may administer certain medications to stable patients in long-term care settings. Assessment and evaluation of effectiveness of the medication remain the responsibility of the nurse.

Equipment

- Correct suppository
- Clean glove
- Water-soluble lubricant

Preparation

- Check the healthcare provider's orders and the MAR.
- Check patient allergy status.

- Check for the drug name, strength, and prescribed frequency.
    - If the MAR is unclear or pertinent information is missing, compare it with the most recent primary care provider's written order.
    - Report any discrepancies to the charge nurse or primary care provider, as facility policy dictates.
    - Know the reason why the patient is receiving the medication, the drug classification, contraindications, usual dose range, side effects, and nursing considerations for administering and evaluating the intended outcomes of the medication.
- Be sensitive about any embarrassment with this invasive procedure the patient may express. Provide support and treat procedure with normalcy as the nurse.

Procedure

1. Compare the label on the medication container with the medication record and check the expiration date. **Rationale:** *Outdated medications are not safe to administer.*
2. Introduce self and identify patient using two identifiers or follow facility policy. **Rationale:** *This ensures that the right patient receives the right medication.* Explain to the patient what you are going to do, why it is necessary, and how the patient can participate. Discuss how the results will be used in planning further care or treatments.
3. Perform hand hygiene and observe other appropriate infection control procedures (e.g., clean gloves).
4. Provide for patient privacy.
5. Prepare the patient.
    - Assist the patient to a left lateral or left Sims position, with the upper leg acutely flexed. **Rationale:** *The left*

(continued on next page)

SKILL 2.25 Rectal Medication: Administering *(continued)*

lateral Sims position is preferred because it positions the sigmoid colon downward, which allows gravity to help retain the suppository.

- Fold back the top bedclothes to expose only the buttocks.

6. Prepare the equipment.
   - Unwrap the suppository, and leave it on the opened wrapper.
   - Apply gloves before inserting the suppository. **Rationale:** *The gloves prevent contamination of the nurse's hands by rectal microorganisms and feces.*
   - Lubricate the smooth, rounded end of the suppository, or follow the manufacturer's instructions. **Rationale:** *The smooth, rounded end is inserted first. Water-soluble lubrication prevents anal friction and tissue damage on insertion.*
   - Lubricate the gloved index finger.

7. Insert the suppository.
   - Ask the patient to breathe through the mouth. **Rationale:** *This usually relaxes the external anal sphincter.*
   - Insert the suppository gently into the anus, rounded end first (or according to the manufacturer's instructions) and along the wall of the rectum with the gloved index finger ❶. For an adult, insert the suppository 10 cm (4 in.) or after passing the sphincter. **Rationale:** *The rounded end facilitates insertion. The suppository needs to be placed along the wall of the rectum, rather than amid feces, in order to be absorbed effectively.*

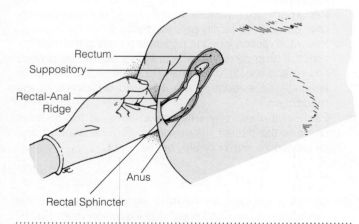

Rectum
Suppository
Rectal-Anal Ridge
Anus
Rectal Sphincter

❶ Insert rectal suppository beyond the anal rectal ridge to ensure it is retained.

- Withdraw the finger. Press the patient's buttocks together for a few minutes. **Rationale:** *This helps minimize any urge to expel the suppository.*
- Remove the glove by turning it inside out and discard. **Rationale:** *Turning the glove inside out contains the rectal microorganisms and prevents their spread.*
- Perform hand hygiene.
- Ask the patient to remain flat or in the left lateral position for at least 5 minutes. **Rationale:** *This helps prevent expulsion of the suppository. The suppository should be retained at least 30–40 min or according to manufacturer's instructions.*
- If the patient has been given a laxative suppository, place the call light within easy reach to summon assistance for the bedpan or toilet.

8. Leave the patient safe and comfortable.

9. Document all nursing assessments and interventions relative to the procedure. Include the type of suppository given/name of the drug, the time it was given, the amount of time it was retained if it was expelled, the results or effects, and the response of the patient.

SAMPLE DOCUMENTATION

[date] 2130 Vomited small amount gastric secretions, states she is feeling nauseated, Phenergan 25 mg suppository inserted rectally per order. *W. Baker*

2230 States she is not nauseated now, no more vomiting noted, resting quietly at this time. *W. Baker*

Lifespan Considerations
NEWBORNS, INFANTS, AND CHILDREN

- Obtain assistance to immobilize a newborn, infant, or young child. **Rationale:** *This prevents accidental injury due to sudden movement during the procedure.*

- For a child under 3 years, the nurse should use the gloved fifth finger for insertion. After this age, a gloved index finger can commonly be used.

- For a child, newborn, or infant, insert a suppository 5 cm (2 in.) or less.

SKILL 2.26 Sublingual Medication: Administering

Sublingual medications are given under the tongue for rapid absorption through the mucous membranes and directly into the bloodstream. These medications can come in the form of tablets, films, or sprays. For best therapeutic results, tablets should not be swallowed, chewed, or crushed. Examples of medications that are administered sublingually are cardiovascular drugs, vitamins, enzymes, steroids,

certain barbiturates, and some medications for mental health concerns.

Delegation or Assignment

Due to the need for assessment and interpretation of patient status, sublingual medication administration is not delegated

SKILL 2.26 Sublingual Medication: Administering (*continued*)

or assigned to the UAP. The nurse can request the UAP to report patient observations to the nurse for follow-up. In some states, a trained UAP may administer certain medications to stable patients in long-term care settings. Assessment and evaluation of effectiveness of the medication remain the responsibility of the nurse.

Equipment

- Correct medication
- Clean gloves as needed

Preparation

- Check healthcare provider's orders and the MAR.
- Check for the drug name, strength, and instructions for giving to patient.
- Check patient allergy status.
- If the MAR is unclear or pertinent information is missing, compare it with the most recent primary care provider's written order.
- Report any discrepancies to the charge nurse or primary care provider, as facility policy dictates.
- Know the reason why the patient is receiving the medication, the drug classification, contraindications, usual dose range, side effects, and nursing considerations for administering and evaluating the intended outcomes of the medication.

Procedure

1. Compare the label on the medication container with the medication record and check the expiration date. **Rationale:** *Outdated medications are not safe to administer.*
2. Introduce self and verify the patient's identity with two identifiers. **Rationale:** *This ensures that the right patient receives the right medication.* Explain to the patient what you are going to do, why it is necessary, and how the patient can participate. Discuss how the results will be used in planning further care or treatments.
3. Perform hand hygiene and observe other appropriate infection control procedures (e.g., clean gloves).
4. Provide for patient privacy.
5. Place patient in a sitting position.
6. Explain that the patient must not swallow drug or eat, smoke, or drink until medication is completely absorbed.
7. Ask patient to place tablet under the tongue or to hold tongue up so tablet can be placed under tongue ❶. **Rationale:** *This ensures that absorption will be rapid and complete due to the vast network of capillaries in this area.* If patient is unable to place tablet under the tongue, don a clean glove before holding medicine cup to mouth and tap tablet under the tongue.
   - *Alternate:* Hold medication spray canister vertically with spray opening as close to mouth as possible. Deliver 1 or 2 metered sprays onto or under tongue, then have patient close mouth immediately. Tell patient not to inhale medication.
8. Evaluate patient for drug action and possible side effects. Monitor vital signs.

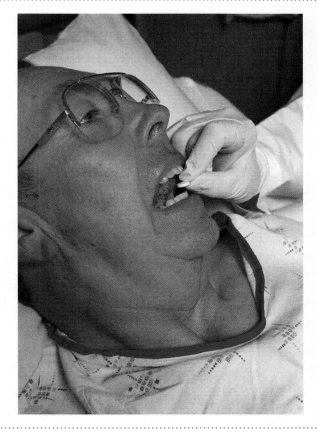

❶ Sublingual medication is placed under patient's tongue for rapid absorption.

9. When procedure is complete, remove glove and perform hand hygiene. Leave patient safe and comfortable.
10. Complete documentation using forms, checklists, or electronic dropdown lists supplemented by nurse's notes or additional comments as appropriate.

SAMPLE DOCUMENTATION

[date] 1510 C/o chest discomfort after walking down hallway and returning to room, wants a nitroglycerin tablet for his angina pain; P-88, R-20, B/P 126/84 mmHg; assisted back to bed in semi-Fowler's position; nitroglycerine tablets 0.4 mg sublingual retrieved from patient's bedside cabinet drawer. One tablet placed under tongue; encouraged patient to sit quietly, slow breathing down, and let the medication work. *T. Daniels*

EVIDENCE-BASED PRACTICE

Guidelines—Nitroglycerin Tablets

The National Library of Medicine at the National Institutes of Health advises patients who have been previously prescribed nitroglycerin to

(*continued on next page*)

SKILL 2.26 Sublingual Medication: Administering *(continued)*

follow the prescriber's instructions carefully. In the event of chest discomfort/pain, common guidelines are as follows:

■ Sit down and take one dose of nitroglycerin when an attack begins. Do not chew or swallow nitroglycerin tablets. Instead, place the tablet under the tongue or between the cheek and gum and wait for it to dissolve. The tablet may cause burning or tingling as it dissolves for some patients. This is common, but the tablet works even if there is no burning or tingling. The affect it has on the chest pain needs to be monitored.

■ If symptoms do not improve much or if they worsen, take a second dose after 5 minutes have passed and a third dose 5 minutes after the second dose. Call for emergency medical help right away if chest pain has not gone away completely 5 minutes after you take the third dose. (Some care providers will instruct patients to call for emergency help if symptoms are not relieved or if they worsen after the first dose.)

Source: Data from U.S. National Library of Medicine (NLM). (2014). DailyMed. Nitrostat – nitroglycerin tablet. Retrieved from https://dailymed.nlm.nih.gov/dailymed/drugInfo.cfm?setid=79ba021e-183c-4b4d-822e-4ff5ef54ca61.

SKILL 2.27 Topical Medication: Applying

Forms of topical medication for this skill include creams, ointments, lotions, and powders. It is essential *always* to wear gloves and maintain standard precautions when applying topical medications to skin, tissue, or mucous membranes. There is a potential for you to absorb any medications that directly come in contact with your own skin or mucous membranes.

Delegation or Assignment

Due to the need for assessment and interpretation of patient status, topical medication administration is not delegated or assigned to the UAP. The nurse can request the UAP to report patient observations to the nurse for follow-up. In some states, a trained UAP may administer certain medications to stable patients in long-term care settings. Assessment and evaluation of effectiveness of the medication remain the responsibility of the nurse.

Equipment

■ Medication container (tube or jar)
■ Soap and water to cleanse skin
■ Clean gloves
■ Tongue blade
■ Gauze or transparent dressing (as indicated)
■ Clear plastic or silk medical tape
■ Pen (to label dressing, if indicated)

Preparation

■ Check healthcare provider's orders and the MAR.
■ Check for the drug name, strength, and application instructions.
■ Check patient allergy status.
■ If the MAR is unclear or pertinent information is missing, compare it with the most recent primary care provider's written order.
■ Report any discrepancies to the charge nurse or primary care provider, as facility policy dictates.
■ Know the reason why the patient is receiving the medication, the drug classification, contraindications, usual dose range, side effects, and nursing considerations for administering and evaluating the intended outcomes of the medication.

Procedure

1. Take medication container and dressing supplies to patient's room.

2. Compare the label on the medication container with the MAR and check the expiration date. **Rationale:** *Outdated medications are not safe to administer.*

3. Introduce self and verify the patient's identity with two identifiers or follow facility policy. **Rationale:** *This ensures that the right patient receives the right medication.* Explain to the patient what you are going to do, why it is necessary, and how the patient can participate. Discuss how the results will be used in planning further care or treatments.

4. Perform hand hygiene and observe other appropriate infection control procedures (e.g., clean gloves).

5. Provide for patient privacy.

6. Complete necessary focused assessments or vital signs and document on MAR.

7. Cleanse affected skin area with prescribed cleanser to remove previous topical medications; dry thoroughly.

8. Remove gloves, perform hand hygiene, and don clean gloves.

9. Squeeze medication from tube or use a tongue blade to take cream/ointment from medication container.

10. Spread small quantity of medication smoothly and evenly with gloved hand or tongue blade over patient's skin following direction of hair follicles. **Rationale:** *Gloves facilitate smooth application.*

11. Apply dressing if indicated ❶. **Rationale:** *Dressing may ensure that medication is not rubbed off.*

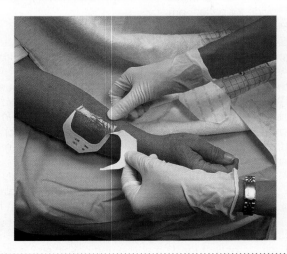

❶ Apply dressing; then label with date, time, and initials.

SKILL 2.27 Topical Medication: Applying (*continued*)

12. Label dressing with date, time, and your initials.
13. Remove gloves and perform hand hygiene.
14. Check that the patient is safe and comfortable. Return medication container to storage area.
15. Complete documentation using forms, checklists, or electronic dropdown lists supplemented by nurse's notes or additional comments as appropriate.

CAUTION! Systemic absorption of topical medication from open lesions can result in toxic reactions.

SAMPLE DOCUMENTATION

[date] 1015 Burn area right lower arm washed with soap and water; blisters of area intact, skin remains reddened and dry, small amount of clear weeping noted, no signs or symptoms S&S infection noted; silver sulfadiazine 1% cream applied in thin layer to burn area with sterile tongue blade; sterile fluff dressing applied to area, wrapped with 3" gauze wrap and secured with tape. Tolerated dressing change without complications. *D. White*

SKILL 2.28 Transdermal Patch Medication: Applying

A transdermal patch medication is a variety of topical medication. It is essential *always* to wear gloves and maintain standard precautions when applying transdermal patch medications to skin. There is a potential for you to absorb some of the patch medication if it comes in direct contact with your skin.

Delegation or Assignment

Due to the need for assessment and interpretation of patient status, applying a transdermal medication patch is not delegated or assigned to the UAP. The nurse can request the UAP to report patient observations to the nurse for follow-up. In some states, a trained UAP may administer certain medications to stable patients in long-term care settings. Assessment and evaluation of effectiveness of the medication remain the responsibility of the nurse.

Equipment

- Medication patch or tube
- Gloves
- Premeasured medication administration paper
- Soap and water
- Clear plastic wrap (optional)
- Tape and pen for labeling dressing

Preparation

- Check healthcare provider's orders and the MAR.
- Check for the drug name, strength, and application instructions.
- Check patient allergy status.
- If the MAR is unclear or pertinent information is missing, compare it with the most recent primary care provider's written order.
- Report any discrepancies to the charge nurse or primary care provider, as facility policy dictates.
- Know the reason why the patient is receiving the medication, the drug classification, contraindications, usual dose range, side effects, and nursing considerations for administering and evaluating the intended outcomes of the medication.

- Obtain transdermal patch or premeasured paper that accompanies medication tube.
- Carefully read the manufacturer's directions for application. **Rationale:** *Directions as well as application areas of the body differ.*

Safety Considerations

- Never cut a transdermal patch. Doing so releases the entire dose of medication at once to the patient. Overdose and accidental death may occur.

- Manufacturers' directions for application of transdermal agents differ significantly. Body temperature and blood flow to different regions influence the suggested application site. Always adhere to the manufacturer's specific guidelines and precautions when administering these systems.

Procedure

1. Compare the label on the medication container with the MAR and check the expiration date. **Rationale:** *Outdated medications are not safe to administer.*
2. Introduce self and verify the patient's identity with two identifiers. **Rationale:** *This ensures that the right patient receives the right medication.* Explain to the patient what you are going to do, why it is necessary, and how the patient can participate. Discuss how the results will be used in planning further care or treatments.
3. Perform hand hygiene, don clean gloves ❶, and observe other appropriate infection control procedures.
4. Provide for patient privacy.
5. Alternate areas with each dose of medication to prevent skin irritation.
6. Remove previous medicated paper/patch, fold patch in half with sticky side in, and discard in biohazard box.

CAUTION! Always remove old medicated paper/patch to avoid over-dosing patient absorbing medication from the old and new papers/patches.

(*continued on next page*)

SKILL 2.28 Transdermal Patch Medication: Applying (*continued*)

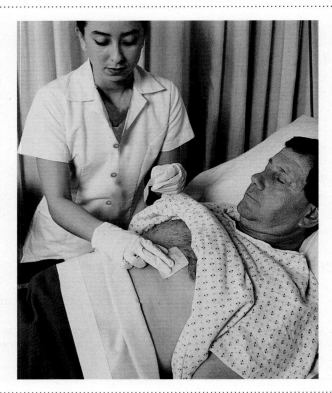

① Wear gloves to prevent drug absorption through fingertips.

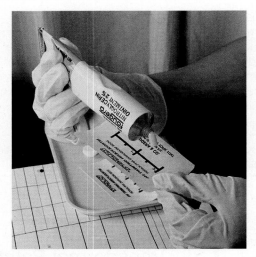

Source: Ronald May/Pearson Education, Inc.

② Use premeasured paper to measure medication dosage.

7. Cleanse area before applying new dose patch or paper at another site.
8. Place prescribed medication directly on paper ② (usually 1.25- to 2.5-cm [½- to 1-in.] strip).
9. Apply medicated paper to clean, dry, hairless, intact skin.
10. Use paper to spread medication paste over a 5-cm (2-in.) area. Secure paper with tape or cover medicated area with plastic wrap and tape.
11. For patch, remove protective covering and immediately apply patch to clean, dry, hairless, intact skin.
12. Press patch with palm for 30 seconds to attain a good seal.
13. Remove gloves and perform hand hygiene.
14. Label patch or paper with date, time, and your initials. Dispose of waste appropriately.
15. Leave patient safe and comfortable. Return medication tube to appropriate storage area.
16. Complete documentation using forms, checklists, or electronic dropdown lists supplemented by nurse's notes or additional comments as appropriate.

> **SAMPLE DOCUMENTATION**
>
> [date] 2300 States lower back pain keeping her from sleeping, wants something for the pain; P-84, R-18, B/P 122/82; denies this is a new problem, states "I've had this pain for years now." Last Fentanyl patch at 1315. Old patch removed, skin washed and dried. PRN Fentanyl 25 mcg/h transdermal patch applied to right scapular area of back. Tolerated procedure without incident. *L. Henry*

Safety Considerations

The use of heating pads or hot tubs can increase the absorption rate of transdermal medications. The no-adhesive backing of some drug patches contains metal that may not be visible. These may become heated during an MRI and can cause second-degree burns. Warnings may be missing from patch labels. Patches should be removed before an MRI. Self-improvement patches purporting to deliver herbs or other substances (marketed on TV or the internet) are not FDA regulated. Counterfeit patches also endanger patients. Refer patients to the FDA website for more information.

Dispose of used transdermal patch by folding sticky sides together and discarding in medical waste receptacle to protect others from exposure to medication. Do not flush used patches down the toilet because trace amounts of the drug may appear in treated water.

SKILL 2.29 Vaginal Medication: Administering

Safety Note! *During scheduled clinical time, nursing students may have a learning opportunity to observe or assist with this skill only with faculty permission and with direct supervision from faculty or another RN.*

Vaginal medications are given to relieve vaginal discomfort, reduce inflammation, prevent or treat infection, as hormone replacement therapy, and for contraception. Forms of vaginal medications include foams, creams, jellies, and suppositories. Creams, foams, and jellies can be administered with an

SKILL 2.29 Vaginal Medication: Administering *(continued)*

applicator. Suppositories can be administered with an applicator or gloved finger. An irrigation, or douche, can be used to wash or clean the inside of the vagina.

Delegation or Assignment

Due to the need for assessments and interpretation of patient status, vaginal medication administration is not delegated or assigned to the UAP. The nurse can request the UAP to report patient observations to the nurse for follow-up. In some states, a trained UAP may administer certain medications to stable patients in long-term care settings. Assessment and evaluation of effectiveness of the medication remain the responsibility of the nurse.

Equipment

- Drape
- Correct medication
- Applicator for medication as appropriate
- Clean gloves
- Water-soluble lubricant (if inserting a suppository)
- Disposable towel
- Clean perineal pad

For Irrigation Only

- Moisture-proof pad
- Vaginal irrigation set (these are often disposable) containing a nozzle, tubing, clamp, and a container for the solution
- Irrigating solution (the solution should be warmed to a temperature of 37.8C–43.3°C [100°F–110°F] if not specified, to minimize discomfort caused by cooler solutions.)

Preparation

- Check the healthcare provider's orders and the MAR.
- Check for the drug name, strength, and prescribed frequency.
- Check patient allergy status.
- If the MAR is unclear or pertinent information is missing, compare it with the most recent primary care provider's written order.
- Report any discrepancies to the charge nurse or primary care provider, as facility policy dictates.
- Know the reason why the patient is receiving the medication, the drug classification, contraindications, usual dose range, side effects, and nursing considerations for administering and evaluating the intended outcomes of the medication.

Procedure

1. Compare the label on the medication container with the medication record and check the expiration date. **Rationale:** *Outdated medications are not safe to administer.*
2. If necessary, calculate the medication dosage.
3. Introduce self and verify identification of the patient using two identifiers. **Rationale:** *This ensures that the right patient receives the right medication.* Explain to the patient what you are going to do, why it is necessary, and how she can participate. Explain to the patient that a vaginal instillation is normally a painless procedure, and in fact may bring relief from itching and burning if an infection is present. Many people feel embarrassed about this procedure, and some may prefer to perform the procedure

themselves if instruction is provided. Discuss how the results will be used in planning further care or treatments.
4. Perform hand hygiene and observe other appropriate infection control procedures (e.g., clean gloves).
5. Provide for patient privacy.
6. Prepare the patient.
   - Ask the patient to void. **Rationale:** *If the bladder is empty, the patient will have less discomfort during the treatment, and the possibility of injuring the vaginal lining is decreased.*
   - Assist the patient to a back-lying position with the knees flexed and the hips rotated laterally.
   - Drape the patient appropriately so that only the perineal area is exposed.
7. Prepare the equipment.
   - Unwrap the suppository, and put it on the opened wrapper.
   or
   - Fill the applicator with the prescribed cream, jelly, or foam. Directions are provided with the manufacturer's applicator.
8. Assess and clean the perineal area.
   - Apply gloves. **Rationale:** *Gloves prevent contamination of the nurse's hands from vaginal and perineal microorganisms.*
   - Inspect the vaginal orifice, note any odor or discharge from the vagina, and ask about any vaginal discomfort.
   - Provide perineal care to remove microorganisms. **Rationale:** *This decreases the chance of moving microorganisms into the vagina.*
9. Administer the cream, foam, jelly, vaginal suppository, or irrigation (see below).

Vaginal Suppository

- Lubricate the rounded (smooth) end of the suppository, which is inserted first. **Rationale:** *Lubrication facilitates insertion.*
- Lubricate your gloved index finger.
- Expose the vaginal orifice by separating the labia with your nondominant hand.
- Insert the suppository about 5–10 cm (2–4 in.) along the posterior wall of the vagina ①, or as far as it will go. **Rationale:** *The posterior wall of the vagina is about 2.5*

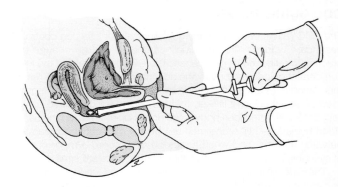

① Insert vaginal suppository at least 5 cm (2 in.) into vaginal canal using applicator as shown.

(continued on next page)

SKILL 2.29 Vaginal Medication: Administering *(continued)*

cm (1 in.) longer than the anterior wall because the cervix protrudes into the uppermost portion of the anterior wall.

- Ask the patient to remain lying in the supine position for 5–10 min following insertion. The hips may also be elevated on a pillow. **Rationale:** *This position allows the medication to flow into the posterior fornix after it has melted.*

Vaginal Cream, Jelly, or Foam

- Gently insert the applicator about 5–10 cm (2–4 in.).
- Slowly push the plunger until the applicator is empty.
- Remove the applicator and place it on the towel. **Rationale:** *The applicator is put on the towel to prevent the spread of microorganisms.*
- Discard the applicator if disposable or clean it according to the manufacturer's directions.
- Ask the patient to remain lying in the supine position for 5–10 min following the insertion.

Vaginal Irrigation

- Place the patient on a bedpan.
- Clamp the tubing. Hold the irrigating container about 30 cm (12 in.) above the vagina. **Rationale:** *At this height, the pressure of the solution should not be great enough to injure the vaginal lining.*
- Run fluid through the tubing and nozzle into the bedpan. **Rationale:** *Fluid is run through the tubing to remove air and to moisten the nozzle.*
- Insert the nozzle carefully into the vagina. Direct the nozzle toward the sacrum, following the direction of the vagina.

- Insert the nozzle about 7–10 cm (3–4 in.), start the flow, and rotate the nozzle several times. **Rationale:** *Rotating the nozzle irrigates all parts of the vagina.*
- Use all of the irrigating solution, permitting it to flow out freely into the bedpan.
- Remove the nozzle from the vagina.
- Assist the patient to a sitting position on the bedpan. **Rationale:** *Sitting on the bedpan will help drain the remaining fluid by gravity.*

10. Ensure patient comfort.
    - Dry the perineum with tissues as required.
    - Apply a clean perineal pad if there is excessive drainage.
11. Remove and discard gloves. Perform hand hygiene. Leave patient safe and comfortable.
12. Document all nursing assessments and interventions relative to the skill. Include the name of the drug or irrigating solution, the strength, the time, and the response of the patient.

SAMPLE DOCUMENTATION

[date] 0800 Peri care completed by patient, states vaginal discharge has lessened; helped to a dorsal recumbent position; clindamycin phosphate 100 mg suppository instilled in vagina using an applicator. Patient asked to remain in supine position for 10 minutes. Tolerated without incident. *C. Ramona*

≫ Parenteral Routes

Expected Outcomes

1. Safe technique prevents self-harm when administering parenteral injections.
2. Injection is as painless as possible for the patient.
3. Injection is administered without complications.
4. Medication is infused safely over appropriate time span.
5. IV piggyback medication is safely compatible with IV solution.

Safety Considerations

CDC GUIDELINES

The CDC (2015) provides many guidelines about infection control for healthcare workers. These guidelines should and do change best practice to reflect current evidence. The CDC has modified the infection control guidelines for vaccine administration. The current recommendation is that the person administering a vaccine is not required to wear gloves unless it is likely that the person will come into contact with potentially infectious body fluids or has open areas on the hands. Hand hygiene is still recommended before medication preparation, between patients, and when hands become soiled. Proper disposal of syringes, needles, and medication containers is still stressed.

The CDC guidelines changed based on the Occupational Safety and Health Administration (OSHA 2015) regulations on bloodborne pathogens. One of the standards in these regulations focuses on when to wear protective gloves. The standard states that gloves need to be worn when the employee can reasonably anticipate contact with blood, other potentially infectious materials, mucous membranes,

or nonintact skin when accessing the vascular system and when coming in contact with contaminated items or surfaces.

Healthcare facilities are now making decisions about policies and procedures concerning how much protection is needed when giving intramuscular, subcutaneous, and intradermal medication injections. Sometimes nurses can predict when they will have exposure from direct or indirect contact with blood or body fluids (such as when obtaining a drop of blood from a patient to put in a glucometer). However, they cannot always predict such events as a leak back of blood from an injection, a complication from administering a routine injection, or microscopic skin breakdown on their own hands. Wearing gloves as a reasonable preventive precaution provides a higher level of safety for both patients and nurses.

Source: Data from Centers for Disease Control and Prevention (CDC). (2015). *Epidemiology and prevention of vaccine-preventable diseases.* Retrieved from http://www.cdc.gov/vaccines/pubs/pinkbook/vac-admin.html; Occupational Safety and Health Administration (OSHA). (2015). *U.S. Department of Labor, Regulations (Standards – 29-CFR). Part Title: Occupational Safety and Health Standards. Title: Bloodborne Pathogens.* Retrieved from https://www.osha.gov/pls/oshaweb/owadisp.show_document?p_table=FEDERAL_REGISTER&p_id=16265

TECHNIQUES TO MINIMIZE PAIN WHEN ADMINISTERING INTRADERMAL, INTRAMUSCULAR, AND SUBCUTANEOUS INJECTIONS:

- Encourage patient to relax the injection area.
- Use a new needle and syringe for each injection.
- Avoid injecting into sensitive or hardened tissue.
- Prevent antiseptic from clinging to needle during insertion by waiting until prepped skin area is completely air dried.
- Reduce puncture pain by "darting" needle quickly into tissue.
- Use as small a gauge needle as appropriate (see **Table 2–4 >>**).
- Inject medication slowly and evenly.
- Maintain grasp on syringe; do not move needle once inserted.
- Withdraw needle quickly after injection.
- Inject medication at room temperature.
- Make sure no air bubbles remain in the syringe before the injection.
- Don't change the direction of the needle during insertion or withdrawal.

TABLE 2–4 Sites for Injections

Older Child and Adult

Route	Sites	Needle Angle (Degrees)	Needle Length (in.) Needle Gauge (G) ❶	Maximum Volume	Syringe Size ❷,❸
Intramuscular (IM)	■ Deltoid muscle	90	$5/8$–1 23–25	1 mL	1 mL or 3 mL
	■ Vastus lateralis muscle	90	1–1 $1/2$ 19–23	3 mL*	3 mL or 5 mL
	■ Ventrogluteal site (preferred site)	90	1– 1 $1/2$ (up to 3 for large adult) 19–23	3 mL*	3 mL or 5 mL
Intradermal (ID)	■ Inner aspect of forearm ■ Scapular area of back ■ Upper chest ■ Medial thigh	10–15	$3/8$–$1/2$ 25–27	0.1 mL	Tuberculin syringe 1 mL
Subcutaneous (Sub-Q)	■ Fatty tissue of abdomen ■ Lateral/posterior upper arm or thigh ■ Scapular area of back ■ Upper ventrodorsal gluteal areas	45–90	$1/2$–$5/8$ 25–27	1.5 mL	1 mL or 3 Ml

Newborn, Infant, and Small Child

Intramuscular (IM) Route	Sites	Needle Angle (Degrees)	Needle Length (in.) Needle Gauge (G)
Newborn, Infant/Small Child (less than 2 years old)	Vastus lateralis muscle (in anterolateral aspect of middle or upper thigh)	90	$5/8$–1 23–25
Walking Child (greater than 2 years old)	Deltoid muscle Ventrogluteal site Vastus lateralis muscle	90	$5/8$–1 $1/4$ 23–25

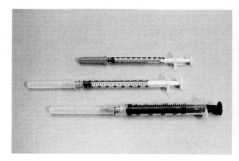

Source: Ronald May/Pearson Education, Inc.

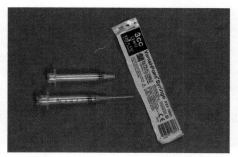

Source: Ronald May/Pearson Education, Inc.

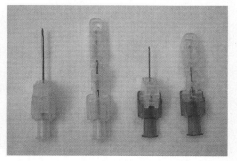

Source: Ronald May/Pearson Education, Inc.

❶ Three types of syringes: insulin, tuberculin, and 3 mL. The type of syringe should be close in capacity to the amount of medication ordered.

❷ Healthcare facilities must use safety needles to conform to needlestick safety legislation.

❸ Safety needles with retractable needles.

* If volume of medication is more than 5 mL for adult, 3 mL for child, or 1 mL for newborn or infant, divide dose into two syringes and give in separate sites

Patient Teaching

The above techniques can be taught to a patient diagnosed with diabetes learning to self-administer insulin injections to help minimize pain.

- For intramuscular injections only.
  - Positioning
    - Place patient on side with upper knee flexed for ventrogluteal injection.

- Have patient place hand on hip to relax deltoid muscle.
- Ensure that needle length reaches muscle for IM injection.
- Use Z-track technique if ordered (also see Skill 2.34).
- EMLA cream, a topical anesthetic containing lidocaine and prilocaine, that requires a healthcare provider's order, may be applied 30–40 min prior to injection.

SKILL 2.30 Injection, Intradermal: Administering

This route of medication administration is commonly used for an allergy-skin test, tuberculin skin test, or injection of a local anesthetic as part of a treatment procedure. Nurses mostly use a tuberculin syringe with a small-gauge short needle inserted at a 15-degree angle for injection into the dermal layer of the skin.

Delegation or Assignment

Administering intradermal injections involves knowledge and medication administration skills. Therefore, this skill is not delegated or assigned to the UAP. In some states, a trained UAP may administer certain medications to stable patients in long-term care settings. Assessment and evaluation of effectiveness of the medication remain the responsibility of the nurse.

Equipment

- Medication (e.g., 0.1 mL purified protein derivative antigen for tuberculin testing)
- Unit dose (1-mL) tuberculin syringe with a ⅜- to ½-in., 25- to 27-gauge needle
- Antimicrobial wipes
- Gauze pads
- Clean gloves
- Pen to mark injection site (provide location of injection site in documentation)

Preparation

- Check healthcare provider's orders and the MAR.
- Check for the drug name, strength, and application instructions.
- Check patient allergy status.
- If the MAR is unclear or pertinent information is missing, compare it with the most recent primary care provider's written order.
- Report any discrepancies to the charge nurse or primary care provider, as facility policy dictates.
- Know the reason why the patient is receiving the medication, the drug classification, contraindications, usual dose range, side effects, and nursing considerations for administering and evaluating the intended outcomes of the medication.

Procedure

1. Compare the label on the medication container with the MAR and check the expiration date. **Rationale:** *Outdated medications are not safe to administer.*

2. If necessary, calculate the medication dosage.
3. Introduce self and verify the patient's identity with two identifiers or follow facility policy. **Rationale:** *This ensures that the right patient receives the right medication.* Explain to the patient what you are going to do, why it is necessary, and how the patient can participate. Discuss how the results will be used in planning further care or treatments.
4. Perform hand hygiene and observe other appropriate infection control procedures (e.g., clean gloves).
5. Don clean gloves.
6. Provide for patient privacy.
7. Select lesion-free injection site on undersurface, upper third of forearm for skin testing.
8. Cleanse area with antimicrobial wipe and allow to dry.
9. Remove needle guard.
10. Grasp the patient's dorsal forearm to pull the skin taut gently on ventral forearm.
11. Holding the syringe almost parallel to skin, insert needle at a 10- to 15-degree angle with bevel facing up, about ⅛ in. ❶. Needle point should be visible under skin. DO NOT ASPIRATE.
12. Inject medication slowly, observing for a wheal (blister) ❷ formation and blanching at the site. **Rationale:** *This indicates that the medication was injected within the dermis. If no wheal develops, injection was given too deeply.*
13. Withdraw needle at same angle as inserted. Pat area gently with dry gauze pad but DO NOT MASSAGE. **Rationale:** *Massaging could disperse medication.*
14. Activate needle safety feature and discard syringe unit in puncture proof container.
15. Mark injection site with pen for future assessment.

CAUTION! For tuberculin testing, instruct patient to return and have the site checked by the healthcare provider in 48–72 hr.

---

16. Return patient to safe, comfortable position.
17. Dispose of gloves and perform hand hygiene.
18. Complete documentation using MAR, forms, checklists, or electronic dropdown lists supplemented by nurse's notes or additional comments as appropriate, include site and antigen.

SKILL 2.30 Injection, Intradermal: Administering (*continued*)

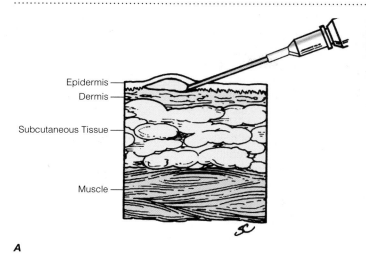

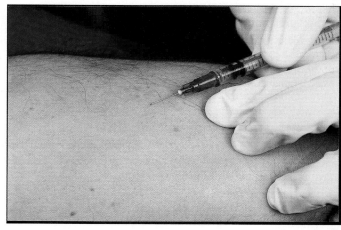

A   **B**

1 *A,* Insert needle at a 15-degree angle just under the epidermis for intradermal injection. *B,* Insert needle with bevel up for intradermal injection.

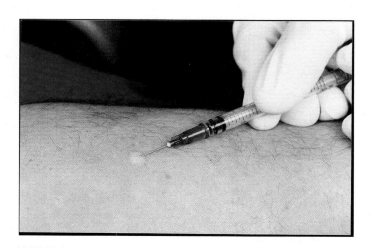

2 Inject solution to form wheal on skin.

EVIDENCE-BASED PRACTICE

Should Nurses Aspirate Before Injection?

Problem

Healthcare facilities have had policies and procedures stating nurses needed to aspirate for all intramuscular (IM) and subcutaneous injections except for anticoagulants and insulin. Originally, aspiration (pulling back on the syringe plunger after the needle has been inserted and before injection) was considered a safety action, so nurses were taught to aspirate before injecting medication. The CDCs Advisory Committee on Immunization Practices (ACIP) now recommends not to aspirate prior to injection of vaccines or toxoids because there are anatomically no large blood vessels at the recommended IM injection sites—ventrogluteal, vastus lateralis, and deltoid muscles.

Evidence

The practice of aspiration before injecting medications has not been evaluated scientifically, so there is no evidence that supports this procedure is necessary. A literature search demonstrated a lack of data regarding aspiration practice, either in confirming correct needle placement or in being able to eliminate incidence of injecting medication into a subcutaneous blood vessel. There is a potential to reduce injection duration time for the patient and the nurse.

There are no reports of any patient being injured because of failure to aspirate. Aspiration during an IM or subcutaneous injection at recommended sites is not necessary because the veins and arteries within reach of a needle at these sites are too small to allow an intravenous push of vaccine without blowing out the vessel. The recommended time to aspirate (5–10 seconds) to confirm no blood return is usually not done.

In one study over a 4-year period, 36,000 allergy injections were administered using aspiration for blood return before administration, with no blood aspirated during any of the injections.

Implications

Nationally, healthcare facilities and nursing programs are currently reviewing policies and procedures for safe injection of IM and subcutaneous medication administration and making decisions based on the CDC recommendations.

Sources: Data from National Nursing Practice Network. (2013). Hettinger, D., & Jurkovich, P. *Featured EBP Project–June 2013. Evidence-based Injection Practice: To Aspirate or Not.* Retrieved from http://www.nnpnetwork.org/staff-nurses/latestnews/newsitem?nid=52; Centers for Disease Control and Prevention (CDC). (2015). *Epidemiology and prevention of vaccine-preventable diseases. The Pink Book. Vaccine Administration.* Retrieved from http://www.cdc.gov/vaccines/pubs/pinkbook/vac-admin.html

SKILL 2.31 Injection, Intramuscular: Administering

This route of medication administration is used when others are not recommended, such as when the medication is irritating to veins (rules out using intravenous route), destroyed by the digestive system (rules out oral route), or needs to be absorbed faster than subcutaneous injection. Muscle tissue is very vascular and can hold a large volume of medication.

Delegation or Assignment

Administering intramuscular (IM) injections involves knowledge and medication administration skills. Therefore, this skill is not delegated or assigned to the UAP. In some states, a trained UAP may administer certain medications to stable patients in long-term care settings. Assessment and evaluation of effectiveness of the medication remain the responsibility of the nurse.

Equipment

- Medication vial, ampule, or prefilled syringe
- 3-mL syringe 1.5- to 3.8-cm (⅝- to 1½ -in.) long, 19- to 25-gauge needle, depending on the muscle site and fat thickness (may need up to 7.5-cm [3-in.] length needle for large adult)
- Antimicrobial swab
- Gauze pad
- Clean gloves

Preparation

- Check healthcare provider's orders and the MAR.
- Check for the drug name, strength, and application instructions.
- Check patient allergy status.
- If the MAR is unclear or pertinent information is missing, compare it with the most recent primary care provider's written order.
- Report any discrepancies to the charge nurse or primary care provider, as facility policy dictates.
- Know the reason why the patient is receiving the medication, the drug classification, contraindications, usual dose range, side effects, and nursing considerations for administering and evaluating the intended outcomes of the medication.

Procedure

1. Compare the label on the medication container with the MAR and check the expiration date. **Rationale:** *Outdated medications are not safe to administer.*
2. Check patient's MAR for sites of previous IM injections. **Rationale:** *IM injections should be rotated to prevent local post-injection complications.*
3. If necessary, calculate the medication dosage.
4. Take prepared injection to patient's room.
5. Introduce self and verify the patient's identity with two identifiers or follow facility policy. **Rationale:** *This ensures that the right patient receives the right medication.* Explain to the patient what you are going to do, why it is necessary, and how the patient can participate. Discuss how the results will be used in planning further care or treatments.
6. Provide for patient privacy. Perform hand hygiene and don gloves.

7. Select injection site, identifying bony landmarks. Consider patient's size, amount, and viscosity of medications being injected. Alternate sites each time injections are given.
8. Cleanse area with antimicrobial swab and allow to air dry.
9. Spread skin taut between thumb and forefinger (grasping muscle is acceptable in pediatric and geriatric patients with less fatty tissue) to ensure needle placement in muscle belly.
10. Insert needle at a 90-degree angle to the muscle, using a quick, darting motion ❶. **Rationale:** *This angle facilitates medication reaching muscle.*

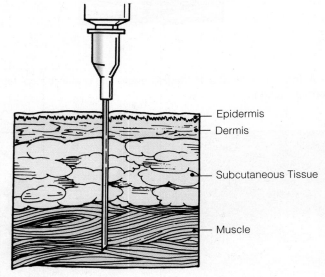

❶ Insert needle at 90-degree angle for IM injections into muscle.

11. Inject medication slowly. **Rationale:** *This allows time for medication to disperse through tissue.*
12. Hold needle in place for 10 seconds to prevent leak back. Then withdraw needle and massage area with dry gauze sponge.
13. Activate needle safety feature.
14. Dispose of syringe and needle unit in puncture-proof container.
15. Return patient to safe and comfortable position.
16. Discard gloves and perform hand hygiene.
17. Complete documentation using MAR, forms, checklists, or electronic dropdown lists supplemented by nurse's notes or additional comments as appropriate. Chart medication and site of injection.

SAMPLE DOCUMENTATION

[date] 1200 ampicillin 250 mg IM given per healthcare provider's order in right ventrogluteal site without incident; tolerated with no complaints. *D. Trever*

SKILL 2.31 Injection, Intramuscular: Administering (continued)

VENTROGLUTEAL INJECTION SITE ②

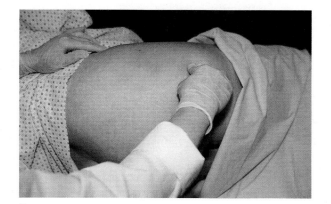

Anterior superior iliac spine

Injection site
Iliac crest

Greater trochanter of femur

A

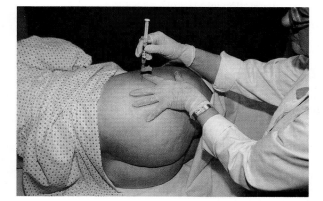

B

C

VASTUS LATERALIS INJECTION SITE ③

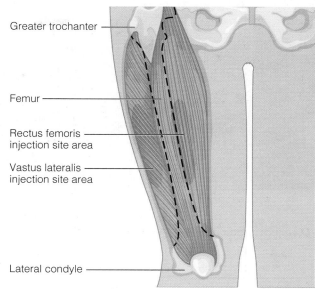

Greater trochanter

Femur

Rectus femoris injection site area

Vastus lateralis injection site area

Lateral condyle

A

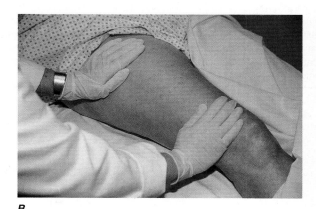

B

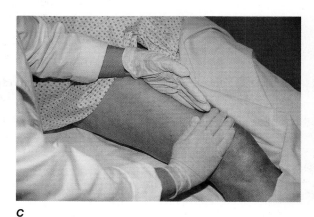

C

② *A,* Overlay of hand shows area of injection into ventrogluteal site for IM injections (patient's right side). *B,* Locate greater trochanter and anterior superior iliac spine. *C,* Place palm at trochanter and index finger at anterior superior iliac spine; fan remaining fingers posteriorly.

③ *A,* Shaded area indicates site location for vastus lateralis injection. *B,* Select site 1 hand-breadth below greater trochanter and 1 hand-breadth above knee for vastus lateralis injection. *C,* Site is middle third and anterior lateral aspect of thigh.

(continued on next page)

SKILL 2.31 Injection, Intramuscular: Administering (*continued*)

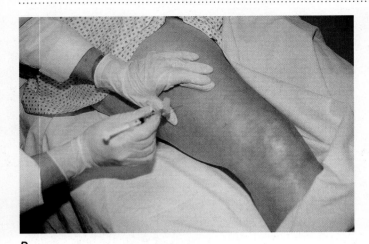

D

❸ D, Inject medications at 90-degree angle directly into muscle.

Safety Considerations

During intramuscular injections, the child patient should be restrained by the parent or assistant. Alternatively, the child's arm closest to the adult can be wrapped around the adult's waist, leaving just the other arm in front to immobilize. The leg not used for the injection is securely located between the adult's legs. Be certain that the child can breathe freely during restraining procedures.

DELTOID IM INJECTION SITE ❹

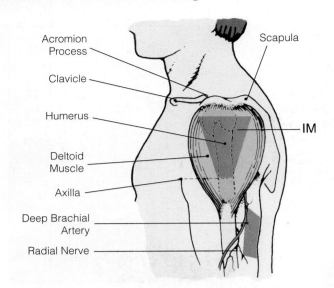

A

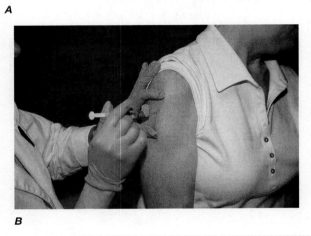

B

❹ A, Locate deltoid site on outer lateral aspect of upper arm. **B,** Inject medication into deltoid area site.

SKILL 2.32 Injection, Subcutaneous: Administering

In this route, the medication is injected into the fatty tissue layer between the skin and the muscle. The absorption rate is very slow, sometimes over a period of 24 hours, because the tissue is less vascular.

Delegation or Assignment

Administering subcutaneous injections involves knowledge and medication administration skills. Therefore, this skill is not delegated or assigned to the UAP. In some states, a trained UAP may administer certain medications to stable patients in long-term care settings. Assessment and evaluation of effectiveness of the medication remain the responsibility of the nurse.

Equipment

- Nonirritating medication
- 3-mL syringe with needle length 1.25–1.5 cm (½–⅝ in.) and usually 25- to 27-gauge
- Antimicrobial wipes
- Gauze pads
- Clean gloves

Preparation

- Check healthcare provider's orders and the MAR.
- Check for the drug name, strength, and application instructions.

SKILL 2.32 Injection, Subcutaneous: Administering (*continued*)

- Check patient allergy status.
- If the MAR is unclear or pertinent information is missing, compare it with the most recent primary care provider's written order.
- Report any discrepancies to the charge nurse or primary care provider, as facility policy dictates.
- Know the reason why the patient is receiving the medication, the drug classification, contraindications, usual dose range, side effects, and nursing considerations for administering and evaluating the intended outcomes of the medication.

Procedure

1. Compare the label on the medication container with the MAR and check the expiration date. **Rationale:** *Outdated medications are not safe to administer.*
2. If necessary, calculate the medication dosage.
3. Introduce self and verify the patient's identity with two identifiers or follow facility policy. **Rationale:** *This ensures that the right patient receives the right medication.* Explain to the patient what you are going to do, why it is necessary, and how the patient can participate. Discuss how the results will be used in planning further care or treatments.
4. Perform hand hygiene and observe other appropriate infection control procedures (e.g., clean gloves).
5. Don clean gloves. Provide for patient privacy.
6. Select fatty site for injection (e.g., abdomen, avoiding a 5-cm [2-in.] radius around umbilicus), alternating sites for each injection ❶. **Rationale:** *This prevents repeated trauma to tissue.*
7. Cleanse area with antimicrobial wipe and let dry. Remove needle guard.

8. Use thumb and forefinger and gently grasp loose area ("pinch an inch") of fatty tissue on appropriate site (e.g., posterior-lateral aspect, middle third of arm) ❷. **Rationale:** *This ensures insertion of medication within subcutaneous tissue, not muscle.*
   Note: This action is not necessary when there is substantial fatty tissue.

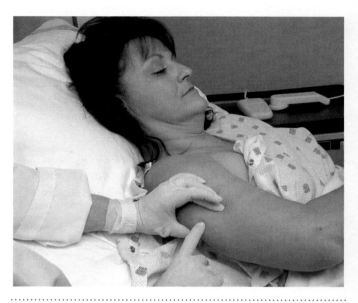

❷ Select site on lateral aspect of mid-upper arm for subcutaneous injection.

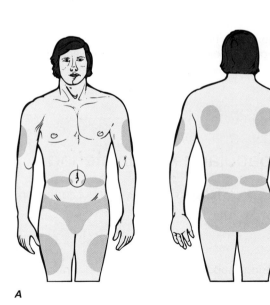

A

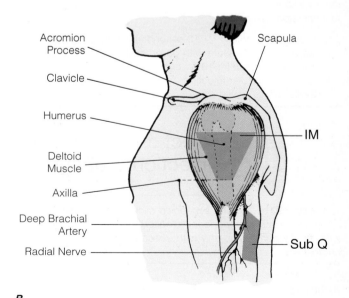

B

❶ *A*, Sites for subcutaneous injections given routinely. (Avoid umbilicus area.) Abdomen site preferred for insulin injection because absorption is more predictable. *B*, Use upper shaded triangle for IM injection in upper arm; use lower shaded area for subcutaneous injection.

(continued on next page)

SKILL 2.32 Injection, Subcutaneous: Administering (continued)

9. Hold syringe like a dart between the thumb and forefinger.
10. Insert needle at a 45- or 90-degree angle. A 90-degree angle is used more commonly due to short needles on prepackaged syringes ❸. **Rationale:** *Angle varies with the amount of subcutaneous tissue, selected site, and needle length.*
11. Inject medication slowly, 10 sec/mL.
12. Wait 10 seconds to prevent leak back, then withdraw needle quickly and activate needle safety feature.
13. Release tissue and massage area with dry gauze sponge (if indicated). **Rationale:** *Massaging area aids absorption.*
14. Discard needle/syringe unit in puncture-proof container.
15. Return patient to position of comfort.
16. Discard gloves and perform hand hygiene.
17. Complete documentation using MAR, forms, checklists, or electronic dropdown lists supplemented by nurse's notes or additional comments as appropriate. Record medication and site used.

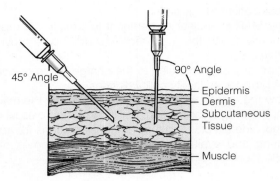

A

SAMPLE DOCUMENTATION

[date] 0730 Regular insulin 8 units subcutaneous right arm following sliding scale protocol ordered, tolerated without incident. *R. White*

Safety Considerations

After given a subcutaneous or intramuscular injection, you may see a drop of blood or medication at the site of the injection. This is called a leak back. When it is blood, a capillary may have been nicked just below the skin surface and blood has followed the needle track to the skin surface. If it is medication, the medication has followed the needle track to the skin surface. Here are three commonly used options that can stop leak backs:

1. Leave the needle in for 10 seconds after injecting medication.
2. Apply gentle pressure with gauze pad (never massage action) over injection site for 10 seconds.
3. For intramuscular injection, use the Z-track method (also see Skill 2.34).

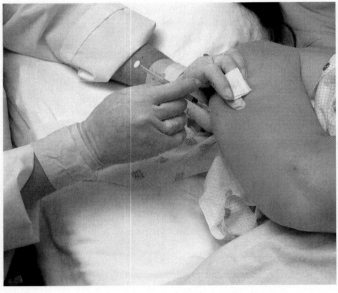

B

❸ *A,* Insert needle at 45- or 90-degree angle into tissue for subcutaneous injection. *B,* Insert needle at 45- or 90-degree angle, using short needle for subcutaneous injection.

SKILL 2.33 Injection, Subcutaneous Anticoagulant: Administering

Safety Note! *During scheduled clinical time, nursing students may have a learning opportunity to observe or assist with this skill only with faculty permission and with direct supervision from faculty or another RN.*

Anticoagulants prevent blood from clotting. Sometimes clots form in the deep veins of the legs from prolonged immobility and block the flow of blood. The clots may also break off and block blood supply in other areas of the body such as the heart or brain leading to a heart attack or brain attack. Anticoagulants are also called blood thinners

because they are used to prevent this clot formation process in deep veins.

Delegation or Assignment

Administering subcutaneous injectable anticoagulants involves knowledge and medication administration skills. Therefore, this skill is not delegated or assigned to the UAP. In some states, a trained UAP may administer certain medications to stable patients in long-term care settings. Assessment and evaluation of effectiveness of the medication remain the responsibility of the nurse.

SKILL 2.33 Injection, Subcutaneous Anticoagulant: Administering *(continued)*

Equipment

- Medication container, vial, or prefilled syringe *(carefully note some anticoagulants are measured in units per milliliter and others in milligrams per milliliter)*
- 1-mL tuberculin syringe or unit-dose syringe with a 1.25- to 1.5-cm (½- to ⅝-in.) long, 25- to 27-gauge needle

or

- Tubex or carpuject injector for prefilled syringe
- Antimicrobial swabs
- Dry gauze sponge
- Clean gloves

Preparation

- Check healthcare provider's orders and the MAR.
- Check for the drug name, strength, and application instructions.
- Check patient allergy status.
- If the MAR is unclear or pertinent information is missing, compare it with the most recent primary care provider's written order.
- Report any discrepancies to the charge nurse or primary care provider, as facility policy dictates.
- Know the reason why the patient is receiving the medication, the drug classification, contraindications, usual dose range, side effects, and nursing considerations for administering and evaluating the intended outcomes of the medication.
- Review process for providing injections.
- Perform hand hygiene.
  Note: To avoid loss of drug, do not clear prefilled syringe needle of air before injecting medication such as with low molecular weight heparin (LMWH) or fondaparinux sodium (Arixtra).

Procedure

1. Check patient's MAR for site of previous injection. **Rationale:** *Injections should be rotated to prevent local post-injection complications.*
2. Take prepared injection to patient's room.
3. Compare the label on the medication container with the MAR and check the expiration date ❶. **Rationale:** *Outdated medications are not safe to administer.*

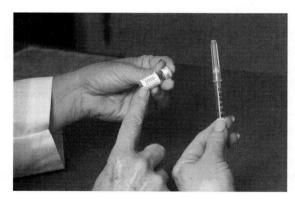

Source: Barbara C. Martin

❶ Low-molecular-weight heparin and needle.

4. Recheck calculated medication dosage.
5. Introduce self and verify the patient's identity with two identifiers. **Rationale:** *This ensures that the right patient receives the right medication.* Explain to the patient what you are going to do, why it is necessary, and how the patient can participate. Discuss how the results will be used in planning further care or treatments.
6. Perform hand hygiene and observe other appropriate infection control procedures (e.g., clean gloves).
7. Don clean gloves.
8. Provide for patient privacy.
9. Assist patient to supine position.
10. Select site on patient's lower abdomen (at least two fingerbreadths from umbilicus) or select area of fatty tissue above iliac crest. **Rationale:** *Anticoagulants should not be administered IM or in the extremities.*
11. Avoid ecchymotic area or lesions.
12. Cleanse site gently with antimicrobial swab, and allow to air dry.
13. Gently pinch an inch of subcutaneous tissue (fat roll) between thumb and forefinger of nondominant hand and hold fat pad throughout injection.
14. Hold syringe between thumb and forefinger of dominant hand and insert full length of needle into skinfold at a 90-degree angle.
15. Inject medication slowly without aspirating first. Press prefilled syringe plunger rod firmly as far as it will go. **Rationale:** *Aspiration can rupture small vessels and increase risk of bleeding into tissue.*
16. Wait 10 seconds before gently withdrawing needle at same angle in which it entered skin. **Rationale:** *This allows medication to absorb into tissue and minimizes bruising.*
    Note: Release of fondaparinux sodium (Arixtra) plunger will cause needle to retract into the security sleeve as it automatically withdraws from the skin.
17. Press and hold dry gauze sponge over injection site. **Rationale:** *This prevents back-tracking of medication.*
18. Do not massage area ❷. **Rationale:** *This may cause tissue damage and bruising.*

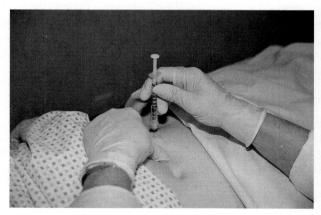

Source: Barbara C. Martin

❷ To prevent tissue damage and bruising, do not aspirate or massage anticoagulant injections.

(continued on next page)

SKILL 2.33 Injection, Subcutaneous Anticoagulant: Administering (*continued*)

19. Activate needle safety feature and discard syringe in puncture-proof container ❸.

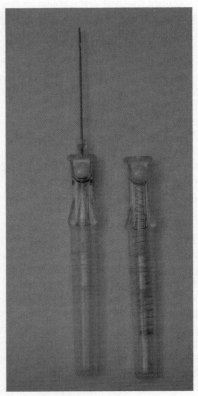

Source: Barbara C. Martin

❸ Activate needle safety feature; then, dispose of syringe in sharps container.

20. Return patient to a safe and comfortable position.
21. Remove gloves and perform hand hygiene.
22. Complete documentation using MAR, forms, checklists, or electronic dropdown lists supplemented by nurse's notes or additional comments as appropriate.

Safety Considerations

- Heparin is available in a variety of strengths (e.g., vials of 1000, 2500, 5000, 10,000, and 25,000 units/mL). *Carefully* check vial units per milliliter before drawing into syringe and have another nurse double check your calculations and prepared injection.

- Heparin is considered a high-risk medication and requires close monitoring. Bleeding is the most common side effect. Monitor for bruises, epistaxis, gum bleeding, hemoptysis, hematuria, and hemorrhage.

- Protamine sulfate is the antidote for heparin. It neutralizes the anticoagulant effects by binding to it.

- Laboratory monitoring typically includes measurements of coagulations, such as activated partial thromboplastin time (aPTT), prothrombin time (PT), plasma heparin concentration (antifactor UFH Xa), whole blood clotting time, activated clotting time, plus a complete blood count (CBC) to monitor platelets and assess for bleeding. The aPTT is most commonly used as a global measure of a patient's overall anticoagulation.

SKILL 2.34 Injection, Z-Track Method: Using

The Z-track method prevents medication from leaking into the "track" of the needle; it is recommended for administering intramuscular medications into the ventrogluteal, deltoid, or vastus lateralis sites.

Delegation or Assignment

Using the Z-track method involves knowledge and medication administration skills. Therefore, this skill is not delegated or assigned to the UAP. In some states, a trained UAP may administer certain medications to stable patients in long-term care settings. Assessment and evaluation of effectiveness of the medication remain the responsibility of the nurse.

Equipment

- Syringe
- 5-cm (2-in.) needle for injection
- Medication

- Antimicrobial swabs
- Dry gauze sponge
- Clean gloves

Preparation

- Check healthcare provider's orders and the MAR.
- Check for the drug name, strength, and application instructions.
- Check patient allergy status.
- If the MAR is unclear or pertinent information is missing, compare it with the most recent primary care provider's written order.
- Report any discrepancies to the charge nurse or primary care provider, as facility policy dictates.
- Know the reason why the patient is receiving the medication, the drug classification, contraindications, usual dose range, side effects, and nursing considerations for

SKILL 2.34 Injection, Z-Track Method: Using (continued)

administering and evaluating the intended outcomes of the medication.

- Use filter needle to draw up prescribed medication into syringe as needed.
- Attach new 5-cm (2-in.) sterile needle to syringe. **Rationale:** *A new needle prevents introducing medication that could be irritating to tissue. A long needle allows medication to go deep into the muscle.*

Safety Considerations

Medications that cause irritation or necrosis to the tissue, such as Vistaril or steroids, must be administered using the Z-track method to avoid leak backs from intramuscular injections. Some medications like iron are dark colored and can cause staining of the skin with leak backs. Such medications should be administered deep intramuscularly using the Z-track method. For obese patients a longer needle, such as a 5- or 7.5-cm (2-in. or 3-in.) needle, should be used so that the medication is absorbed into muscle (not fat) tissue and blood level of drug is achieved.

Procedure

1. Take medication to the patient's room.
2. Compare the label on the medication container with the MAR and check the expiration date. **Rationale:** *Outdated medications are not safe to administer.*
3. If necessary, calculate the medication dosage.
4. Introduce self and verify the patient's identity with two identifiers or follow facility policy. **Rationale:** *This ensures that the right patient receives the right medication.* Explain to the patient what you are going to do, why it is necessary, and how the patient can participate. Discuss how the results will be used in planning further care or treatments.
5. Perform hand hygiene and observe other appropriate infection control procedures (e.g., clean gloves).
6. Don clean gloves.
7. Provide for patient privacy.
8. Position patient for ventrogluteal or vastus lateralis injection.
9. Cleanse site with antimicrobial swab and allow to dry.
10. Pull skin 2.5–3.8 cm (1–1½ in.) laterally away from the injection site. **Rationale:** *This tissue displacement creates a track that keeps medication from seeping into subcutaneous tissue.*
11. Maintain displacement and insert needle at a 90-degree angle ❶. Aspirate for blood return (if facility policy).
12. Inject medication slowly (10 sec/mL) and wait 10 seconds to prevent backflow, keeping skin taut. **Rationale:** *Permits muscle relaxation and absorption of medication.*
13. Withdraw needle and release retracted skin ❷. **Rationale:** *Lateral tissue displacement interrupts needle track and seals medication in the muscle when the tissue is released.*

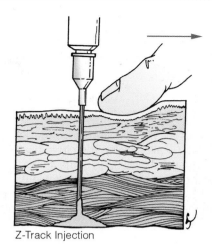

Z-Track Injection

❶ Z-track injection: Maintaining displacement, insert needle at 90-degree angle. Aspirate by pulling back on plunger, checking to see if needle is in blood vessel (if facility policy). If blood is aspirated, discard and prepare new injection.

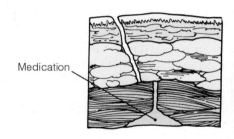

Medication

❷ Z-track injection, after displacement released. Method is used to prevent backflow of medications into subcutaneous tissue.

14. Apply light pressure with dry gauze sponge. Do not massage. **Rationale:** *Massage may disperse medication into subcutaneous tissue and cause tissue irritation.*
15. Activate needle safety feature.
16. Return patient to a position of comfort and safety.
17. Discard gloves and equipment in appropriate area.
18. Perform hand hygiene.
19. Complete documentation using MAR, forms, checklists, or electronic dropdown lists supplemented by nurse's notes or additional comments as appropriate.

SAMPLE DOCUMENTATION

[date] 0400 Moderate amount vomitus noted in emesis basin, states she has been feeling nauseated; hydroxyzine (Vistaril) 25 mg IM left ventrogluteal with Z-track injection, tolerated without complaint. *P. Diaz*

SKILL 2.35 Insulin Injection: Using a Syringe, Pen, or Pump

Safety Note! *During scheduled clinical time, nursing students may have a learning opportunity to observe or assist with this skill only with faculty permission and with direct supervision from faculty or another RN.*

Delegation or Assignment

Administration of insulin injections involves knowledge and medication administration skills. Therefore, this skill is not delegated or assigned to the UAP. In some states, a trained UAP may administer certain medications to stable patients in long-term care settings. Assessment and evaluation of effectiveness of the medication remain the responsibility of the nurse.

Equipment

Insulin Vials

- Patient's Medication Administration Record (MAR), hard copy or electronic
- Insulin vials
  - Unopened vials of insulin should be stored in a refrigerator.
  - An opened vial of insulin may be refrigerated or kept at room temperature; recommend discard after 28 days (when a vial of insulin is first used, the date it is opened and the nurse's initials should be added to the label).
- Insulin should not be exposed to light or to temperatures over 27°C (80°F).
- Do not use insulin that exhibits clumping, frosting, or precipitation.
- Insulin syringe, available in ³/₁₀-, ½-, and 1-mL sizes (the standard U100 syringe is used with U100 insulin)
- Needles, 29- to 31-gauge short needles
- Antiseptic swabs
- Dry gauze sponge
- Clean gloves

Preparation

- Check healthcare provider's orders with MAR. Check MAR for last injection site.
- Obtain patient's blood glucose level before preparation to determine appropriate administration of insulin.
- Check patient allergy status.
- If the MAR is unclear or pertinent information is missing, compare it with the most recent primary care provider's written order.
- Report any discrepancies to the charge nurse or primary care provider, as facility policy dictates.
- Know the reason why the patient is receiving the medication, the drug classification, contraindications, usual dose range, side effects, and nursing considerations for administering and evaluating the intended outcomes of the medication.
- Follow the three label checks for administering medications. Read the label on the medication (1) when it is taken from the medication cart, (2) before withdrawing the medication, and (3) after withdrawing the medication.
- Organize the equipment.

For a Newly Diagnosed Diabetic Patient

- Explain to the patient that the dose of short-acting insulin must be adjusted according to blood glucose test results.
- Explain that there is a variation in levels—the lowest blood glucose level is before meals and the highest is 1–2 hr after meals.
- Explain that the goal of treatment is to eliminate wide swings in glucose levels.

Preparation for One-insulin Solution

1. Check healthcare provider's orders and the MAR (**Table 2–5 ≫**).
2. Perform hand hygiene.
3. Turn intermediate or long-acting (cloudy) insulin vial top to bottom 10 times. **Rationale:** *This brings cloudy insulin solution into suspension. Clear insulins do not require this.*

CAUTION! Do not shake insulin vials, as this destroys insulin potency. Rolling the vial fails to bring insulin into suspension. Turning the vial top to bottom several times brings the solution into suspension without destroying potency.

4. Wipe top of insulin bottle with antimicrobial swab.
5. Remove needle guard and place on tray.
6. Pull plunger of syringe down to desired amount of medication (e.g., 12 units). Inject amount of air into air space, not into insulin solution. **Rationale:** *Injecting air directly into insulin solution causes bubbles.*
7. Withdraw ordered amount of insulin into syringe.
8. Validate MAR, insulin bottle, and prepared syringe. **Rationale:** *Checking insulin helps safeguard against errors.*
9. Remove needle from vial and expel air from syringe.
10. Replace needle guard.
11. Double check dosage amount with another nurse.
12. Take medication to patient's room.

Preparation for Two-insulin Solutions

1. Check healthcare provider's orders and the MAR (Table 2–5).
2. Perform hand hygiene.
3. Turn vial A (cloudy) intermediate insulin top to bottom 8–10 times. **Rationale:** *This brings cloudy solution into suspension.*
4. Wipe top of both insulin bottles with alcohol.
5. Take needle guard off and place on tray.
6. Pull plunger of syringe down to desired total units of insulin.
7. Step 1: Insert needle and inject prescribed amount of air into vial A (cloudy) insulin ❶. Withdraw needle.
8. Step 2: Insert needle and inject remaining air in syringe into vial B (clear) insulin.
9. Step 3: Invert and withdraw medication while needle remains in vial B (clear). **Rationale:** *Withdrawing clear insulin first prevents inadvertent injection of intermediate-acting insulin into rapid- or short-acting insulin bottle, which would slow its rapid action.*

SKILL 2.35 Insulin Injection: Using a Syringe, Pen, or Pump (continued)

TABLE 2–5 Insulin Types and Therapeutic Action (in min or hr*)

Types	Injection Time	Onset	Peak	Duration
Very Rapid Acting (clear solution)				
lispro (Humalog)	Within 15 min AC or immediately PC	5–15 min	30–90 min	3–5 hr
aspart (NovoLog)	Within 5–10 min AC			
glulisine (Apidra)	15 min AC or within 20 min after *starting* a meal			
Short Acting (clear solution)				
insulin regular (Novolin R)	Per order	0.5–1 hr	2–4 hr	5–7 hr
insulin regular (Humulin R)	Within 30–60 min AC			
Intermediate Acting (cloudy solution)				
insulin isophane (Humulin N [NPH])	Per order	1–2 hr	6–10 hr	16–24 hr
human insulin isophane suspension (Novolin N [NPH])	Per order	1–3 hr	8 hr	12–16 hr
Mixtures (cloudy solution)				
Novolin 70/30 (70% NPH, 30% Regular)	Per order	30 min	Varies	10–16 hr
Humulin 70/30 (70% NPH, 30% Regular)	Within 30–60 min AC	30 min		
Humulin 50/50 (50% NPH, 50% Regular)	Within 30–60 min AC	30 min		
Humalog 75/25 *(75% lispro protamine suspension, 25% insulin lispro)*	Within 15 min AC	10–15 min		
Humalog 50/50 *(50% lispro protamine suspension, 50% insulin lispro)*	Within 15 min AC	10–15 min		
NovoLog 70/30 *(70% aspart protamine suspension, 30% insulin aspart)*	Within 15 min AC	5–15 min		
Long Acting				
glargine (Lantus) *(clear solution)*	Daily	4–6 hr	No peak	24 hr
detemir (Levemir) *(clear solution)*				

*The time of insulin action may vary significantly in different patients and in the same patient at different times.

**AC = before meals; PC = after meals.

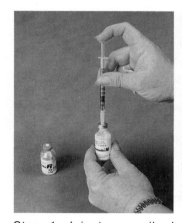 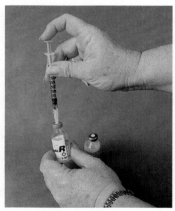 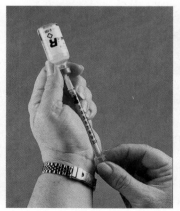 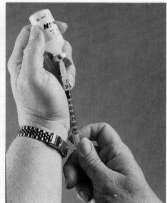

Step 1: Inject prescribed amount of air into intermediate-acting (cloudy) insulin vial—withdraw needle without needle touching solution.

Step 2: Inject prescribed amount of air into rapid- or short-acting (clear) insulin vial. Do not withdraw needle.

Step 3: Invert vial of rapid- or short-acting insulin; withdraw prescribed amount of medication and withdraw needle from vial.

Step 4: Invert intermediate-acting insulin vial and withdraw exact amount without injecting insulin into bottle.

① Steps for two-insulin preparation for routine subcutaneous injection. Avoid umbilicus area. Abdomen is preferred site for insulin injection as absorption is more predictable.

(continued on next page)

SKILL 2.35 Insulin Injection: Using a Syringe, Pen, or Pump (*continued*)

10. Step 4: Withdraw needle and insert it into vial A (cloudy) to withdraw the required amount of medication. Avoid pushing the plunger because that will introduce medication B (clear) into vial A (cloudy). If using a syringe with a fused needle, withdraw the medication from vial A (cloudy). The syringe now contains a mixture of medications from vials A (cloudy) and B (clear). **Rationale:** *With this method, neither vial is contaminated by microorganisms or by medication from the other vial.* Be careful to withdraw only the ordered amount and not to create air bubbles. **Rationale:** *The syringe now contains two medications, and an excess amount cannot be returned to the vial.*

11. Double check your preparations with another nurse ❷. Take medication to the patient's room.

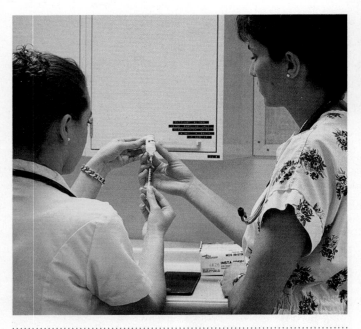

❷ Double check insulin dose with a second nurse to help prevent errors in preparation.

Procedure

1. In the patient's room, compare the label(s) on the medication container(s) with the MAR and check the expiration date. **Rationale:** *Outdated medications are not safe to administer.*
2. Recheck the medication dosage.
3. Introduce self and verify the patient's identity with two identifiers or follow facility policy. **Rationale:** *This ensures that the right patient receives the right medication.* Explain to the patient what you are going to do, why it is necessary, and how the patient can participate. Discuss how the results will be used in planning further care or treatments.

4. Perform hand hygiene and observe other appropriate infection control procedures (e.g., clean gloves). Don gloves.
5. Select appropriate site on lateral aspect of mid-upper arm for insulin subcutaneous injection ❸ (if possible, use routine sites patient uses at home to inject insulin; for a new diabetic, use abdomen, avoiding a 5-cm (2-in.) radius around umbilicus), alternating sites for each injection. **Rationale:** *This prevents repeated trauma to tissue.*

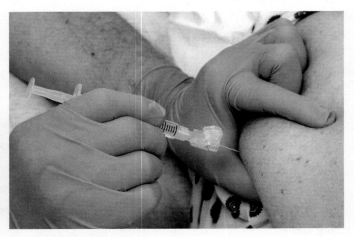

Source: Rick Brady/Pearson Education, Inc.

❸ Administering a subcutaneous injection into pinched tissue.

6. Cleanse area with antimicrobial wipe and let dry. Remove needle guard.
7. Use thumb and forefinger and gently grasp loose area of fatty tissue on appropriate site. **Rationale:** *This ensures insertion of medication within subcutaneous tissue, not muscle.*
8. Hold syringe like a dart between the thumb and forefinger.
9. Insert needle at a 90-degree angle and administer injection.
10. Inject medication slowly, 10 sec/mL.
11. Wait 10 seconds to prevent leak back, then withdraw needle quickly and activate needle safety feature.
12. Release tissue and apply pressure with dry gauze sponge (if indicated).
13. Discard needle/syringe unit in puncture-proof container.
14. Return patient to position of comfort.
15. Discard gloves and perform hand hygiene.
16. Complete documentation using MAR, forms, checklists, or electronic dropdown lists supplemented by nurse's notes or additional comments as appropriate. Record medication and site used.

SAMPLE DOCUMENTATION

[date] 0730 Regular insulin 6 units given subcutaneously left abdomen per order for 0720 blood glucose 138; tolerated without incident. *G. Patty*

SKILL 2.35 Insulin Injection: Using a Syringe, Pen, or Pump (*continued*)

EVIDENCE-BASED PRACTICE

Double Checking Drug Doses

Double checks of medications have sometimes been considered a "weak" intervention because even when done, many medication errors still occur. Vague reminders to use critical thinking when double checking medications have little positive impact on reducing errors. A new systematic review showed there is not enough evidence to draw conclusions about double checking medication administration. Certain factors have been linked to ongoing medication errors:

- The expectation that someone else will make sure a mistake is not made
- The lack of focus that comes attempting to do math while the "double checking" nurse is watching (This produces ambiguity about who is doing the calculation and who is approving it.)
- Lack of time
- The tendency not to check the order again after a distraction has occurred.

Further research into the value of double checks is advised. Current recommendations for the double-checking process include the following:

- Eliminate language such as "That's right, isn't it?" and substitute language that suggests independent calculation, such as "What dose did you get?"
- Perform an audit for processes that require double checks and determine how often audits are being done correctly.
- Learn from errors discovered after a double check process.
- Limit double checks to high alert medications, such as insulin.

Source: Based on Institute for Safe Medication Practices, 2013. *Acute Care Medication Safety Alert, Independent Double Checks: Undervalued and Misused: Selective Use of This Strategy Can Play an Important Role in Medication Safety.* Retrieved from https://www.ismp.org/newsletters/acutecare/showarticle.aspx?id=51

Safety Considerations

Do not massage site following injection of certain drugs such as insulin or heparin because this hastens absorption and drug action and may cause tissue irritation.

Hypoglycemia (blood sugar less than 60 mg/dL) is the most common adverse effect of insulins. Patient should wear a medical alert bracelet/ID to alert others. The patient should be instructed to carry at least 15 g of fast-acting sugar (e.g., glucose tablet, 1 Tbsp sugar, jelly, honey, or tube of cake frosting) to be taken in the event of a hypoglycemic reaction.

The IV route is superior for administering sliding-scale insulin to a patient who is obese. Adipose tissue slows onset of insulin action.

Long-acting insulin, glargine (Lantus), is a clear solution. It is not to be mixed with any other type of insulin or solution. It is given subcutaneously and is not intended for IV use.

EXAMPLE OF MIXING INSULINS

The following is an example of mixing 10 units of regular insulin and 30 units of NPH insulin, which contains protamine.

- Check healthcare provider's orders and the MAR.
- Perform hand hygiene.
- Wipe top of both insulin bottles with alcohol. Gently rotate NPH vial to mix contents.

- Pull plunger of syringe down to 40 total units of insulin (10 units of regular and 30 units of NPH insulin).
- Inject 30 units of air into the NPH vial and withdraw the needle. (There should be no insulin in the needle.) The needle should not touch the insulin.
- Inject 10 units of air into the regular insulin vial and immediately withdraw 10 units of regular insulin. Always withdraw the regular insulin first. **Rationale:** *This minimizes the possibility of the regular insulin becoming contaminated with the additional protein in the NPH.*
- Reinsert the needle into the NPH insulin vial and withdraw 30 units of NPH insulin. (The air was previously injected into the vial.) Be careful to withdraw only the ordered amount and not to create air bubbles. If excess medication has been drawn up, discard the syringe and begin the procedure over again. **Rationale:** *The syringe now contains two medications, and an excess amount cannot be returned to the vial because the syringe contains regular insulin, which, if returned to the NPH vial, would dilute the NPH with regular insulin. The NPH vial would not provide accurate future dosages of NPH insulin.*

By using this method, you avoid adding NPH insulin to the regular insulin.

CAUTION! One way to determine which insulin to withdraw first is to remember the saying "Clear to cloudy." (Regular insulin is clear, and NPH is cloudy due to the proteins in the insulin.)

Patient Teaching

Self-Administration of Insulin

1. Perform hand hygiene.
2. Have a vial of insulin, the insulin syringe with needle, and alcohol pads ready to use.
3. Remove the cover from the needle.
4. Fill the syringe with an amount of air equal to the number of units of insulin, and insert the needle into the vial.
5. Push air into the vial, invert the vial, and withdraw the prescribed units of insulin.
6. Either carefully replace the cover over the needle or set the syringe down carefully so that the needle does not touch anything.
7. Wipe the selected skin site with alcohol. The injection is less likely to be painful if the alcohol is allowed to dry.
8. Pinch up a fold of skin, and insert the needle into the tissue at the recommended angle.
9. Insert the insulin.
10. Withdraw the needle. Do not rub the injection site. If bleeding occurs, apply light pressure to the injection site with a cotton ball or gauze pad.
11. Do not recap the needle. Dispose of the needle in an appropriate sharps container. Reuse of needles is not recommended.
12. Perform hand hygiene.

(*continued on next page*)

SKILL 2.35 Insulin Injection: Using a Syringe, Pen, or Pump (continued)

USING AN INSULIN PEN

Equipment

- Insulin delivery device labeled with patient's name
- Prefilled pen or cartridge with correct insulin type with instructions for use
- Device-compatible needle
- Antimicrobial swab

Safety Considerations

Insulin injection "Dial-A-Dose" pens contain a prefilled multidose cartridge available with various types of insulin.

- The pen is intended for single-patient use.
- Do not aspirate contents out of the pen cartridge with a needle because pen calibration will no longer be accurate.
- A sterile disposable needle is attached for each injection.
- An "air shot" primes the needle before the appropriate dose (units) of insulin is dialed for injection.

After initial use, device may be kept for 28 days. Most devices should not be stored in the refrigerator or exposed to excessive heat.

Preparation

- Check healthcare provider's order with MAR. Perform hand hygiene.
- Identify patient by checking the patient's identity band and asking patient to state name and birth date.
- Review device instructions with the patient.
- Have patient perform hand hygiene.
- Instruct patient to perform steps below.

Procedure

1. Remove pen cap and insert insulin cartridge if indicated. Check insulin for type, expiration date, and appearance.
2. Turn pen upside down at least 10 times. **Rationale:** *This creates suspension of cloudy insulin*.
3. Remove needle cap and attach sterile needle immediately before injecting.
4. Prime insulin pen by pulling dose knob out in direction of arrow until a "0" appears in the dose window. **Rationale:** *A dose cannot be dialed until the dose knob is pulled out*.
5. Dial 2 units by turning the dose knob. Point the pen up and tap the cartridge holder to collect air at the top. Then push the plunger and repeat until a drop of insulin appears at the tip of the needle ❹. **Rationale:** *This removes air and ensures proper dosing. This may require six "air shots" for some pens (e.g., the InnoLet, an easy-to-use doser that has a large, easy-to-read dial)*.
6. Turn the dose knob to the required number of insulin units to be injected. Don gloves.
7. Use an antiseptic wipe to swab the injection site.
8. Pinch up skin, insert needle, and release skin before injection. Using the thumb on the dose knob and the palm of your hand grasping the pen, inject the insulin until the dose in the window is 0.

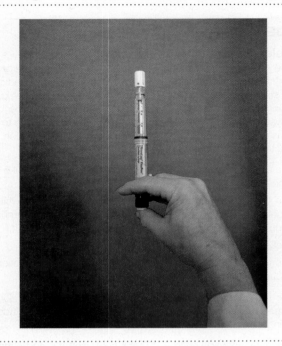

❹ Air shot clears cartridge and needle of air and primes needle for injection.

9. Press device "push button" completely and keep depressed for 10 seconds before removing needle from skin ❺.

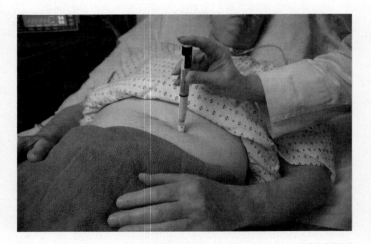

❺ Press pen firmly on patient's abdomen to engage needle; inject dialed units and hold 10 seconds before releasing. Remove needle, dispose in sharps receptacle. Recap and return pen to storage area for future use.

10. Do not massage the area.
11. Carefully remove the needle from the device and dispose of it in the sharps container.
12. Replace device cap and store according to directions.
13. Complete documentation using MAR, forms, checklists, or electronic dropdown lists supplemented by nurse's notes or additional comments as appropriate. Record medication and site used.

SKILL 2.35 Insulin Injection: Using a Syringe, Pen, or Pump (*continued*)

USING AN INSULIN PUMP

- Continuous subcutaneous insulin infusion (CSII) is a form of intensive insulin therapy utilized as an alternative to multiple daily injections in an attempt to achieve optimal glycemic control and decrease risk of long-term complications of diabetes. Insulin pumps are manufactured by a number of companies that provide 24-hr emergency and clinical specialists to assist patients with the start-up of their pumps. All models consist of a battery-powered pump with insulin reservoir, an infusion catheter, and microcomputer that allows programming to deliver basal and bolus doses according to the healthcare provider's orders ❻. Only rapid-acting or short-acting insulin is used.

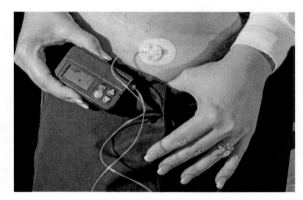

Source: Marmaduke St. John/Alamy Stock Photo

❻ Insulin pump attached to infusion set. Abdominal site is preferred because insulin absorption is faster and most predictable.

- CSII more closely mimics release of insulin by the pancreas with continuous-delivery basal and bolus insulin infusion.
- Basal rate(s) is the amount of insulin delivered (units per hour) to keep blood glucose levels in target range between meals and overnight.
- Bolus is the additional amount of insulin delivered immediately before meals or for episodes of hyperglycemia, the greatest risk associated with insulin pump therapy.

- The patient should be referred to a certified diabetes educator before the start of pump use. Insulin boluses will be based on blood glucose readings and carbohydrate grams intake.
- The patient performs frequent fingerstick blood glucose checks: before adjusting any insulin dose, fasting, before meals, 2 hours after eating, at bedtime, and at 3 a.m. weekly.
- Lifestyle advantages: flexibility; insulin needs can be tailored to changes in schedule (mealtime, exercise, or sleep).

Safety Considerations

Insulin pump management and education should be done by a certified diabetes educator who is also a certified insulin pump trainer.

If insulin must be discontinued (e.g., for MRI, CT scan), the pump should be disconnected. Blood glucose level should be checked before disconnecting and upon reconnecting. Ketoacidosis can occur within 2 hours if insulin delivery is interrupted.

- Mixtures of rapid-acting (Humalog) and intermediate or long-acting insulin should be administered within 10 minutes before a meal.
- Mixtures of NPH and regular (short-acting) insulin should be administered 20–30 min prior to a meal.
- Mixtures may be stored in a refrigerator for up to 30 days and should be gently resuspended prior to injection.
- Insulin type and brand should remain consistent for an individual patient.

Patient Teaching

- Always keep an extra vial of insulin available.
- Always have a vial of regular insulin available for emergencies.
- Ensure patient and family members can recognize signs of hypoglycemia and hyperglycemia.
- Always keep a candy or sugar source available to treat hypoglycemia if it occurs.
- Ensure that the patient knows to eat within 15 minutes of injecting rapid-acting insulins.
- Ensure that the patient can demonstrate safe self-administration of insulin injections before discharge.

SKILL 2.36 Intravenous Medication: Adding to Fluid Container

This method provides a fast and efficient continuous flow of medication to the patient based on the rate of intravenous (IV) fluid flow. Some IV fluid containers come prefilled with a medication such as lidocaine HCl, or pharmacy departments at healthcare facilities are responsible for adding medications to IV fluid containers.

Delegation or Assignment

Adding medications to IV fluid containers involves the application of nursing knowledge and critical thinking. The nurse does not delegate or assign this procedure to the UAP. However,

the nurse can inform the UAP of the intended therapeutic effects and/or specific side effects of the medication(s) in the IV and direct the UAP to report specific patient observations to the nurse for follow-up. The nurse remains responsible for the assessment, interpretation of abnormal findings, and determination of appropriate responses.

Equipment

- Patient's MAR, hard copy or electronic
- Correct sterile medication

(*continued on next page*)

SKILL 2.36 Intravenous Medication: Adding to Fluid Container (*continued*)

- Diluent for medication in powdered form (see manufacturer's instructions)
- Correct IV solution container, if a new one is to be attached
- Antiseptic swabs
- Sterile syringe of appropriate size (e.g., 5 or 10 mL) and a 2.5- to 3.8-cm (1- to 1½-in.) long, 20- or 21-gauge sterile safety needle if not using a needleless system
- IV additive label

Preparation

- Check healthcare provider's order and the MAR.
- Check the label on the medication carefully against the MAR to make sure that the correct medication is being prepared.
- Check for the drug name, strength, and application instructions.
- Check patient allergy status.
- Follow the three safety label checks for administering medications. Read the label on the medication (1) when it is taken from the medication cart, (2) before withdrawing the medication, and (3) after withdrawing the medication.
- Confirm that the dosage and route are correct.
- Verify which IV solution is to be used with the medication.
- Consult a pharmacist, if required, to confirm compatibility of the drugs and solutions being mixed.
- Organize the equipment.

Procedure

1. Perform hand hygiene and observe other appropriate infection control procedures (e.g., clean gloves).
2. Prepare the medication ampule or vial for drug withdrawal. Check the facility's practice for using a filter needle to withdraw premixed liquid medications from multidose vials or ampules.
3. Add the medication to the IV container.
4. Apply a colored preprinted *Medication Added* label ❶ providing the following information: patient name, room, date, drug, time, amount, added by, use before, and storage.

MEDICATION ADDED

PATIENT   RM.

DRUG

AMOUNT

ADDED BY

DATE   TIME

START TIME _____ FLOW RATE _____

EXP. DATE

❶ Colored, preprinted *Medication Added* label.

CAUTION! As a safety action, a *Medication Added* label must be applied to the IV fluid container immediately after adding the medication to alert others that a medication has been added because many medications added to IV fluid containers are clear.

5. Introduce self to patient (parent) and verify the patient's identity using two identifiers. **Rationale:** *This ensures that the right patient receives the right medication.* Explain to the patient (parent) what you are going to do, why it is necessary, and how the patient can participate. Discuss how the results will be used in planning further care or treatments.
6. Perform hand hygiene and observe appropriate infection control procedures.

To a New IV Container

- Locate the injection port. Clean the port with the antiseptic or alcohol swab. **Rationale:** *This reduces the risk of introducing microorganisms into the container when the needle is inserted.*
- Remove the needle cap from the syringe, insert the needle through the center of the injection port, and inject the medication into the bag. Activate the needle safety device. Mix the medication and solution by gently rotating or slowly inverting the bag or bottle several times. **Rationale:** *This should disperse the medication throughout the solution.*
- Complete the IV additive label with the patient's name and room number (if appropriate), name and dose of medication, date, time, and nurse's initials. Attach it on the bag or bottle. **Rationale:** *This documents that medication has been added to the solution. The label should be easy to read when the bag is hanging.*
- Clamp the IV tubing. Remove the spike from the current IV container, taking care not to touch anything with the exposed spike. Place the used IV container in a sink or basin temporarily while attaching the new IV container. Spike the bag or bottle with IV tubing and hang the IV. If no IV infusion was running, be sure to fully flush the IV solution through the new tubing and verify that no air bubbles are present in the tubing prior to connecting to the IV access. **Rationale:** *Clamping prevents rapid infusion of the solution.*
- Regulate infusion rate as ordered. Often a controller device such as an IV pump is used to ensure accurate rate of infusion.

To an Existing Infusion

- Determine that the IV solution in the container is sufficient for adding the medication. **Rationale:** *Sufficient volume is necessary to dilute the medication adequately.*
- Confirm the desired dilution of the medication, that is, the amount of medication per milliliter of solution.
- Close the infusion clamp. **Rationale:** *This prevents the medication from infusing directly into the patient as it is injected into the bag or bottle.*
- Wipe the medication port with the alcohol or disinfectant swab. **Rationale:** *This reduces the risk of introducing microorganisms into the container when the needle is inserted.*

7. Remove the needle cover from the medication syringe.

- While supporting and stabilizing the bag with your thumb and forefinger, carefully insert the syringe needle through the port and inject the medication. **Rationale:**

SKILL 2.36 Intravenous Medication: Adding to Fluid Container (*continued*)

The bag is supported during the injection of the medication to avoid punctures. If the bag is too high to reach easily, lower it from the IV pole. Activate the needle safety device.

- Remove the bag from the pole and gently rotate or invert the bag. **Rationale:** *This will mix the medication and solution.* Rehang the container and regulate the flow rate, making sure that no air has entered the tubing during the procedure. **Rationale:** *This establishes the correct flow rate.*
- Complete the medication label and apply to the IV fluid container. Recheck controller device if used.

8. Dispose of the equipment and supplies according to facility practice. **Rationale:** *This prevents inadvertent injury to others and the spread of microorganisms.*
9. Complete documentation using MAR, forms, checklists, or electronic dropdown lists supplemented by nurse's notes or additional comments as appropriate.

SAMPLE DOCUMENTATION
[date] 1330 NS 1000 mL bag of IV fluids with 1 ampule MVI added, hung at 100 mL/hr, infusing without incident. *R. Greenly*

SKILL 2.37 Intravenous Medication, Intermittent: Using a Secondary Set

Intermittent intravenous (IV) medications are given at scheduled times. Medications are mixed in a small bag of IV fluid and then connected to the primary IV infusion line to be administered to the patient. If the patient is receiving continuous IV fluids, safety of compatibility is a major consideration.

Delegation or Assignment

The administration of intermittent IV medications involves the application of nursing knowledge and critical thinking. Check the state's nurse practice act to verify the scope of practice for the LPN/LVN as it relates to IV medication administration. Facility policy also must be checked and followed. This skill is not delegated or assigned to the UAP. The nurse, however, can inform the UAP of the intended therapeutic effects and/or specific side effects of the medication and direct the UAP to report specific patient observations to the nurse for follow-up. The nurse remains responsible for the assessment, interpretation of abnormal finds, and determination of appropriate actions.

Equipment

- Patient's MAR (hard copy or electronic)
- 50- to 250-mL infusion bag with medication (most medication infusion bags are prepared by the pharmacist)
- Secondary administration set
- Antiseptic swabs
- Sterile needle if system is not needleless
- Tape
- Sterile needle or needleless adapter, syringe, and saline if medication is incompatible with the primary infusion

Preparation

- Check healthcare provider's orders and the MAR.
  - Check the additive label on the medication carefully against the MAR to make sure that the correct medication is being prepared.

- Confirm that the dosage is correct.
- Ensure medication compatibility with primary infusion solution.
- Consult a pharmacist, if required, to confirm compatibility of the drugs and IV solutions being mixed.
- Organize the equipment.
- Remove medication bag from the refrigerator 30 minutes before administration, if appropriate.

Procedure

1. Perform hand hygiene and observe other appropriate infection control procedures (e.g., clean gloves).
2. Provide for patient privacy.
3. Prepare the patient.
   - Prior to performing the procedure, introduce self and verify the patient's identity using facility protocol. **Rationale:** *This ensures that the right patient receives the right medication.*
   - If not previously assessed, take the appropriate assessment measures necessary for the medication.
4. Explain the purpose of the medication and how it will help, using language that the patient can understand. Include relevant information about the effects of the medication. **Rationale:** *Information can facilitate acceptance of and compliance with the therapy.*
5. Assemble the secondary infusion:
   - Close clamp on secondary infusion tubing and spike the secondary medication infusion bag.
   - Insert the secondary tubing needleless cannula into the distal primary tubing port located above the infusion pump ❶.
   - Hang the secondary container above the level of the primary bag ❷. Use the extension hook to lower the primary bag if a piggyback setup is required. Some infusion pumps do not require this.

(*continued on next page*)

SKILL 2.37 Intravenous Medication, Intermittent: Using a Secondary Set (*continued*)

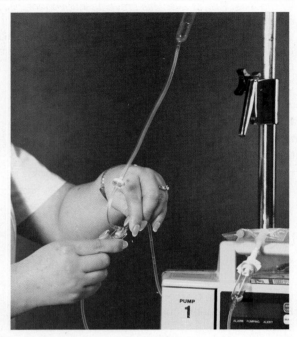

Source: Ronald May/Pearson Education, Inc.

❶ Insert needleless cannula of secondary tubing into distal primary tubing port located above the infusion pump.

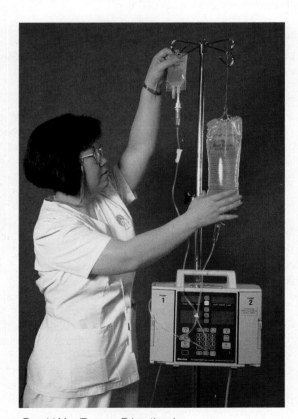

Source: Ronald May/Pearson Education, Inc.

❷ Hang secondary bag on IV pole; lower primary bag.

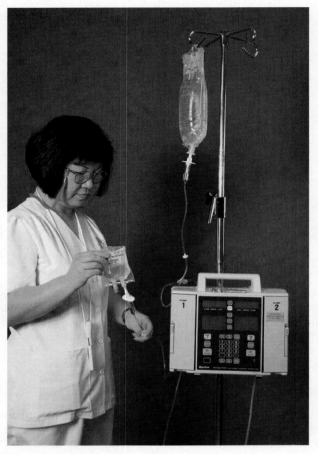

Source: Ronald May/Pearson Education, Inc.

❸ Lower medication bag to clear tubing and back-prime tubing.

- Lower medication bag to clear tubing and back-prime tubing ❸. **Rationale:** *This method of priming the secondary tubing allows for no loss of medication.*
- Attach appropriate label to the secondary tubing. *Secondary tubing is usually changed every 24–48 hr. Check facility policy.*
- If the secondary tubing remains from a prior medication administration, attach a new needleless cannula. **Rationale:** *Changing the needleless cannula will reduce the risk of transmission of microorganisms.*

CAUTION! Each IV medication bag requires its own secondary tubing. Medication from the IV infusion bag remains in the tubing. It is important, when hanging subsequent IV infusion bags, to hang the same medication on the same secondary tubing to avoid mixing incompatible medications. Because secondary lines create a means for micro-organisms to enter the primary line, repeated changes should be avoided. Secondary tubing should be "backflushed" and used for the length of time allowed by agency policy.

SKILL 2.37 Intravenous Medication, Intermittent: Using a Secondary Set (*continued*)

6. If the medication is *not* compatible with the primary infusion, temporarily discontinue the primary infusion. Flush the primary line with a sterile saline solution before attaching the secondary set. To flush the line, wipe the port with an antiseptic swab, clamp the primary line, and, using a sterile syringe and needleless adapter, instill sufficient sterile saline solution through the port to flush any primary fluid out of the infusion tubing.

7. Program the IV pump for the infusion rate of the IV medication bag.

8. Unclamp the secondary IV tubing and check that the secondary solution is infusing.

9. After infusion of secondary IV medication bag, regulate the rate of the primary solution by adjusting the clamp or IV pump infusion rate. Some infusion pumps will do this automatically. If the medication is not compatible with the primary infusion, after infusing the secondary IV medication bag, flush the primary line with a sterile saline solution as in step 6 above before beginning the primary infusion.

10. Leave the secondary bag and tubing in place for future administration or discard as appropriate.

11. When the procedure is complete, perform hand hygiene, and leave the patient safe and comfortable.

12. Document relevant data.
    - Record the date, time, medication, dose, route, and solution; assessment of the IV site, if appropriate; and the patient's response.
    - Record the volume of fluid of the medication infusion bag on the patient's intake and output record.

USING A SALINE LOCK

Intermittent infusion devices may be attached to an intravenous catheter to allow medications to be administered intravenously without requiring a continuous intravenous infusion. The device may also have a port at one end of the lock and a needleless injection cap at the other end with the extension tubing between the two ends.

- Prepare two, normal saline prefilled syringes (3 mL each).
- Spike the medication bag with minidrip (60 gtt/mL) IV tubing.
- Attach the needleless adapter to the tubing, prime the tubing, and close the clamp.
- Clean the needleless injection port of the saline lock with an antiseptic swab. Open the saline lock clamp, if appropriate.
- Insert the first saline syringe into the port and gently aspirate to check for patency. Flush slowly with 1–3 mL (depending on facility policy), noting any resistance, swelling, pain, or burning. **Rationale:** *This ensures placement of IV in vein.*
- After connecting the IV tubing to the injection port of the lock, administer the medication regulating the drip rate to allow medication to infuse for appropriate time period. Macrodrip (10–20 gtt/mL) tubing may also be used if using an IV pump to regulate the flow.
- When the medication has been infused, disconnect the IV tubing, maintaining sterility of the end of the IV tubing. Insert the second saline syringe into the port and gently flush the saline lock with 1–3 mL (depending on facility policy).

Rationale: *This clears the tubing and maintains patency.* Clamp the saline lock after flushing, if appropriate.
- Dispose of syringes in the appropriate container.

ADDING MEDICATION TO A VOLUME-CONTROL INFUSION

- Withdraw the required dose of the medication into a syringe.
- Ensure that there is sufficient fluid in the volume-control fluid chamber to dilute the medication. Generally, at least 50 mL of fluid is used. Check the directions from the drug manufacturer or consult the pharmacist.
- Close the inflow to the fluid chamber by adjusting the upper roller or slide clamp above the fluid chamber; also ensure that the clamp on the air vent of the chamber is open.
- Clean the medication port on the volume-control fluid chamber with an antiseptic swab ❹.

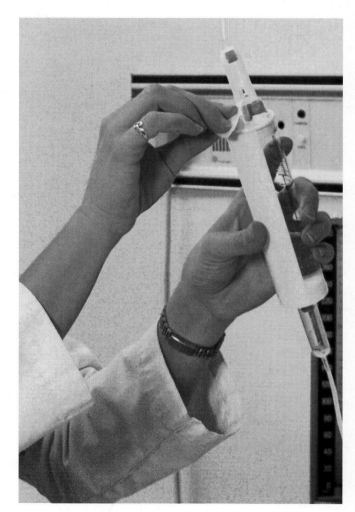

Source: Ronald May/Pearson Education, Inc.

❹ Swab injection port before infusing medication.

(*continued on next page*)

SKILL 2.37 Intravenous Medication, Intermittent: Using a Secondary Set (continued)

- Inject the medication into the port of the appropriately filled volume-control set (i.e., the ordered amount of solution).
- Gently rotate the fluid chamber until the fluid is well mixed **5**.
- Regulate the flow by adjusting the lower roller clamp below the fluid chamber.
- Attach a medication label to the volume-control fluid chamber.
- Document relevant data and monitor the patient and the infusion.

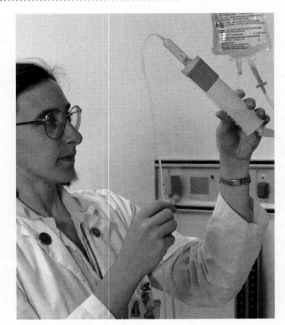

Source: Ronald May/Pearson Education, Inc.

5 After instilling medication, gently mix with solution in volume control chamber.

SAMPLE DOCUMENTATION
[date] 2000 ampicillin 250 mg IV piggyback given; no immediate reaction noted. *W. Blitz*

SKILL 2.38 Intravenous Medication, IV Push: Administering

Safety Note! *During scheduled clinical time, nursing students may have a learning opportunity to observe or assist with this skill only with faculty permission and with direct supervision from faculty or another RN.*

An IV push medication is literally pushed into the patient in a short amount of time by the nurse using a syringe. This is usually done as close to the IV site as possible. Some facilities may use a mini-infuser pump as an alternative means of infusing a medication over a short amount of time.

Delegation or Assignment

The administration of intravenous medication via IV push involves the application of nursing knowledge and critical thinking. This procedure is not delegated or assigned to the UAP. The nurse, however, can inform the UAP of the intended therapeutic effects and/or specific side effects of the medication and direct the UAP to report specific patient observations to the nurse for follow-up.

Note: Administration of IV push medications varies by state nurse practice acts. For example, some states may allow the RN to delegate certain medications to be given by an LPN/LVN, whereas other states may allow only the RN to administer IV push medications. Nurses need to know their scope of practice according to their state's nurse practice act and facility policies.

Equipment

- Patient's MAR (hard copy or electronic)
- Medication in a prefilled syringe, vial, or ampule
- Sterile syringe (3–5 mL) (to prepare the medication)
- Sterile needles, 2.5 cm (1 in.), 21–25 gauge (needle is not needed if using a needleless system)
- Antiseptic swabs
- Watch with a digital readout or second hand
- Clean gloves

IV Push for an IV Lock Also Needs

- Sterile syringe (3 mL) (for the saline or heparin flush)
- Vial of preservative-free normal saline to flush the IV catheter or vial of heparin flush solution or both depending on facility practice. **Rationale:** *These maintain the patency of the IV lock. Saline is frequently used for peripheral locks.*
- Sterile needles (21 gauge) (needle is not needed if using a needleless system)

Preparation

- Check healthcare provider's orders with the MAR.
- Check the label on the medication carefully against the MAR to make sure that the correct medication is being prepared.
- Follow the three safety label checks for correct medication and dose. Read the label on the medication (1) when it is

SKILL 2.38 Intravenous Medication, IV Push: Administering (*continued*)

taken from the medication cart, (2) before withdrawing the medication, and (3) after withdrawing the medication.
- Calculate medication dosage accurately and the recommended delivery rate (e.g., 20 mg over 1 minute).
- Confirm that the route is correct. Check patient allergies.
- Organize the equipment.

Procedure

1. Introduce self to patient (parent) and verify the patient's identity using two identifiers. **Rationale:** *This ensures that the right patient receives the right medication.* Explain to the patient (parent) what you are going to do, why it is necessary, and how the patient can participate. Discuss how the results will be used in planning further care or treatments.
2. Perform hand hygiene and observe appropriate infection control procedures (e.g., clean gloves).
3. Provide for patient privacy.
4. Prepare the medication.

Existing Line

- Prepare the medication according to the manufacturer's direction. **Rationale:** *It is important to have the correct dose and the correct dilution.*

IV Lock

- If flushing with saline:
   a. Prepare two normal saline prefilled syringes (3 mL each).
- If flushing with heparin (if indicated by facility policy) and saline:
   a. Prepare one syringe with 1 mL of heparin flush solution (if indicated by facility policy).
   b. Prepare two normal saline prefilled syringes (3 mL each).
   c. Draw up the medication into a syringe.
5. Put a small-gauge needle on the syringe if using a needle system.
6. Perform hand hygiene and apply clean gloves. **Rationale:** *This reduces the transmission of microorganisms and reduces the likelihood of the nurse's hands contacting the patient's blood.*
7. If not previously assessed, take the appropriate assessment measures necessary for the medication. If any of the findings are above or below the predetermined parameters, consult the healthcare provider before administering the medication.
8. Clean the injection port with the antiseptic swab. **Rationale:** *This prevents microorganisms from entering the circulatory system during needle insertion.*

   - If using an IV lock with needle, insert the needle of the syringe containing normal saline through the center of the injection port (or for a needleless system, attach the syringe to the injection port), and aspirate for blood. **Rationale:** *The presence of blood confirms that the catheter or needle is in the vein. In some situations, blood will not return even though the lock is patent.*

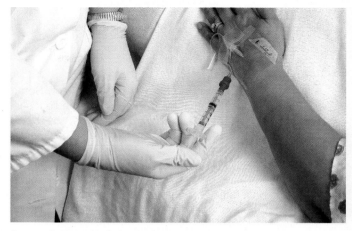

Source: Ronald May/Pearson Education, Inc.

❶ Flush the lock by injecting saline using the push-pause method.

   Flush the lock by injecting 2–3 mL saline using the push-pause method ❶ (a rapid succession of push-pause-push-pause movements exerted on the plunger of the syringe barrel).
9. Administer the medication by IV push.

IV Lock with Needle

- Remove the needle and syringe. Activate the needle safety device.
- Clean the lock's injection port with an antiseptic swab. **Rationale:** *This prevents the transfer of microorganisms.*
- Insert the needle of the syringe containing the prepared medication through the center of the injection port.
- Inject the medication slowly at the recommended rate of infusion. Use a watch or digital readout to time the injection. Observe the patient closely for adverse reactions. Remove the needle and syringe when all medication has been administered. **Rationale:** *Injecting the drug too rapidly can have a serious untoward reaction.*
- Activate the needle safety device.
- Clean the injection port of the lock.
- Attach the second saline syringe, and inject 2–3 mL of saline (depending on facility policy). **Rationale:** *The saline injection flushes the medication through the catheter and prepares the lock for heparin if this medication is used. Heparin is incompatible with many medications.*
- If heparin is to be used, insert the heparin syringe and inject the heparin slowly into the lock.

IV Lock with Needleless System

- Remove the syringe.
- Insert the syringe containing the medication into the port.
- Inject the medication following the precautions described previously.

(*continued on next page*)

SKILL 2.38 Intravenous Medication, IV Push: Administering (continued)

- Withdraw the syringe.
- Repeat injection of 2–3 mL of saline (depending on facility policy).

Existing Line

- Identify the injection port closest to the patient. Some ports have a circle indicating the site for needle insertion. **Rationale:** *An injection port must be used because it is self-sealing. Any puncture to the plastic tubing will cause a leak.*
- Clean the port with an antiseptic swab.
- Stop the IV flow by closing the clamp or pinching the tubing above the injection port.
- Connect the syringe to the IV system.
  a. Needle system:
    - Hold the port steady.
    - Insert the needle of the syringe that contains the medication through the center of the port. **Rationale:** *This prevents damage to the IV line and to the diaphragm of the port.*
  b. Needleless system:
    - Remove the cap from the needleless syringe. Connect the tip of the syringe directly to the port.
    - Inject the medication at the ordered rate. Use the watch or digital readout to time the medication administration. **Rationale:** *This ensures safe drug administration because a too-rapid injection could be dangerous.*
- After injecting the medication, withdraw the needle and activate the needle safety device. For a needleless system, detach the syringe and attach a new sterile cap to the port.
- Release the clamp or tubing. Resume IV flow as ordered.

10. Dispose of equipment according to facility practice. **Rationale:** *This reduces needlestick injuries and the spread of microorganisms.*
11. Remove and dispose of gloves. Perform hand hygiene.
12. Observe the patient closely for adverse reactions.
13. Determine facility policy about recommended times for changing the IV lock. Some agencies advocate a change every 48–72 hr for peripheral IV devices.
14. Document all relevant information.
    - Record the date, time, drug, dose, and route; patient response; and assessments of infusion or heparin lock site if appropriate.

SAMPLE DOCUMENTATION

[date] 1100 C/o left flank pain × 20 minutes, states "Feels like the stone is moving." Skin warm and dry P-98, R-22, B/P 134/90 morphine sulfate 2 mg IV push given as ordered. *V. Carlton*

POSITIONING A CHILD FOR INJECTIONS OR INTRAVENOUS ACCESS

Preparation

- Determine if the parent wants to be present during an uncomfortable procedure or to be available after the procedure to comfort the child.
- When the parent wishes to be present, discuss the parent's role (e.g., holding the child or providing distraction or comfort during the procedure).
- Make sure the person positioning and holding the child (parent or other assistant) clearly understands what body parts must be held still and how to do this safely.

Procedure

Supine Position

1. Place the child in a supine position on a bed or stretcher. **Rationale:** *This position allows the child to see what is happening so that some of the child's fear is reduced.*
2. Have the parent, a nurse, or an assistant lean over the child to restrain the child's body and extend the extremity to be used for access or injection. **Rationale:** *The nurse's body provides a source of human contact as well as securing the child so that the procedure can be done quickly.*

Sitting Position

1. Have the child sit on the parent's or assistant's lap with the legs held firmly between the assistant's legs.
2. The child's arm closest to the adult can be wrapped around the back of the parent's or assistant's waist.
3. Have the parent or assistant hold the child firmly against the chest, wrapping arms around the child's upper body. Hold firmly but gently, ensuring that the child has chest expansion allowing for normal breathing. **Rationale:** *This hugging position adds comfort as well as security so the procedure can be done quickly.*

» Critical Thinking Options for Unexpected Outcomes

Not all unexpected outcomes require further nursing intervention; however, many times they do. When the patient demonstrates a change in signs/symptoms indicating an emerging problem, the nurse should immediately assess and troubleshoot what is happening. The assessment data must be processed quickly to formulate a hypothesis so the nurse can make a clinical judgment. The nurse then decides how best to resolve the problem and improve the patient's situation for a better outcome.

EXPECTED OUTCOME	UNEXPECTED OUTCOME	POSSIBLE INTERVENTIONS
Beds and Activities of Daily Living Bed remains clean, dry, and free of wrinkles.	Patient refuses to have bed made.	▪ Assess reason for refusal. Patient may be in pain or does not want to be disturbed. ▪ Offer to make the bed at a later time. ▪ Change only the pillowcase and drawsheet, if patient allows. ▪ Beds do not need to be changed unless soiled or damp, so allow patient's independence, if possible.
Transmission of pathogenic microorganisms is prevented with universal precautions.	Cross-contamination occurs from improper linen disposal.	▪ Follow facility exposure policy and follow up with Employee Health. ▪ Provide adequate linen hampers for the nursing personnel. ▪ Attend education programs on infection control.
Patient's skin, hair, and nails are clean, odor free, and without irritation.	Patient's skin becomes irritated from linen or begins to break down.	▪ Obtain hypoallergenic linen. ▪ Place therapeutic mattress under patient. ▪ Provide skin care with appropriate lotion.
Bathing and hygiene care are completed without complications.	Even with increased oral hygiene, patient still has odorous breath.	▪ Use antiseptic mouthwash between oral hygiene care. ▪ Notify the healthcare provider, as this could be a symptom of systemic disease. ▪ Obtain dental consultation to check for presence of dental caries or gum disease. ▪ Examine patient's nutritional intake. Absent nutrients or imbalanced intake of fats, protein, or carbohydrates can result in bad breath.
Patient is comfortable.	Patient complains of extreme oral mucosal irritation or sensitivity.	Request healthcare provider's order for one of the following solutions: ▪ Saline solutions: for soothing, cleansing rinses ▪ Anesthetic solutions: to dull extreme pain in the oral cavity ▪ Effervescent solutions (e.g., hydrogen peroxide or ginger ale) to loosen and remove debris from the mouth ▪ Coating solutions (e.g., Maalox) to protect irritated surfaces ▪ Antibacterial–antifungal rinses (e.g., nystatin [Mycostatin]) to prevent the spread of organisms that cause thrush.
Bathing and hygiene care are completed without complications.	Patient needs care after oral surgery or oral trauma.	▪ Oral care following surgery or trauma is always ordered by the healthcare provider. ▪ No oral hygiene care should be attempted until healthcare provider has clearly defined the specific care. ▪ Suctioning equipment should always be present. ▪ Assessment of patient's head, face, neck, and general status is critical at this time.
	Patient is unwilling to accept a complete bed bath.	▪ Respect patient's wishes and use other opportunities for assessment. ▪ Have patient wash hands, face, and genitals. You should wash back and give back care. Re-explain the purpose of the bath to the patient and request patient participation.
Patient's skin, hair, and nails are clean, odor free, and without irritation.	Patient has foul odor even after perineal care.	▪ Obtain order for sitz bath. ▪ Request order for medicated solution. ▪ Request culture of discharge so the appropriate treatment can be instituted.
Patient is comfortable.	Shaving is difficult and painful for the patient.	▪ Place warm towels on area to be shaved for 15 minutes. ▪ Apply more shaving cream. ▪ Ensure that razor is sharp.
Eyes and surrounding area are clean and free from crusting.	Eyelids become crusted from exudate.	▪ Place warm, moist washcloth across eyes and leave in place for several minutes. ▪ Moisten cotton applicator stick with sterile saline and gently twist the applicator stick over crusted surface to assist in removing crust.
Medication Administration Rationale for medication administration is clear.	Medication or dosage on MAR does not fit patient's clinical picture.	▪ Compare new MAR with previous MAR. ▪ Compare new MAR with recent healthcare provider's orders. ▪ Discuss concerns with facility protocol. ▪ Contact healthcare provider for clarification.
Sign-out documentation for medications is accurate.	Medication sign-out sheet does not correspond to remaining stock.	▪ Check with other nurses who may have dispensed stock medication. ▪ Check MARs for unclaimed stock that may have been administered. ▪ Complete discrepancy report if sign-out sheets and stock cannot be reconciled.

(continued on next page)

EXPECTED OUTCOME	UNEXPECTED OUTCOME	POSSIBLE INTERVENTIONS
Medication is administered according to the "six rights."	Patient receives wrong medication.	■ Document the medication administered on patient's MAR. ■ Monitor patient closely for potential undesired effects, and document findings. ■ Notify patient's healthcare provider, and document. ■ Complete anonymous variance report according to facility policy. ■ Always check two patient identifiers before administering medication.
Medication Preparation Dosage calculations are accurate.	Nurse is unsure of dosage calculation.	■ Utilize helpful calculation formulas. ■ Use a calculator. ■ Request that another nurse check calculation or conversion. ■ Seek facility pharmacist's assistance.
Complications of medication administration are prevented.	Patient has an allergic or anaphylactic response to medication.	■ Immediately stop or hold medication. ■ Notify healthcare provider at once; prepare to administer epinephrine to dilate bronchi and support blood pressure. If reaction is severe: ■ Keep patient flat in bed with head elevated. ■ Take vital signs every 10–15 min; stay with patient. ■ Assess for hypotension or respiratory distress. ■ Establish airway, if necessary. ■ Have emergency equipment available. ■ Provide psychological support to patient to alleviate fears. ■ Record type and progression of reactions.
Patient takes medication without difficulty.	Patient has difficulty swallowing medication.	■ Offer water before administering oral medication. ■ Crush medications if appropriate and administer mixed with food such as applesauce, pudding, or jelly. ■ Consult pharmacist to dispense same medication in liquid form. ■ If difficulty continues, consult healthcare provider for altered route of medication delivery (rectal, parenteral). ■ Request swallow study.
	Patient is nauseated and oral medications have not been taken.	■ Hold medication. ■ Notify healthcare provider for antiemetic medication order and alternate route for administering necessary medications. ■ Administer antiemetic if ordered, then administer medication when patient's nausea is relieved.
Medication therapeutic effect is achieved.	Patient's discomfort is not relieved with sublingual nitroglycerin.	■ Check bottle for expiration date—potency is lost 3 months after opening bottle. ■ Administer second tablet in 5 min. If discomfort continues, administer opiate analgesic, call rapid response team, notify healthcare provider, and obtain stat ECG. ■ Administer no more than three tablets/sprays in a 15-min period. ■ Monitor for blood pressure effect. Hold medication if systolic BP is less than 90 mmHg. ■ Consult with healthcare provider for blood test for possible myocardial injury and need for continuous cardiac monitoring.
	Patient fails to have BM after laxative suppository administration.	■ Reassess abdomen and check patient for rectal fecal impaction. ■ Consult with healthcare provider to order oil-retention enema or cleansing enema. ■ Teach patient ways to prevent constipation.
Desired local effect of medication is achieved without undesired side effects.	Patient states that breathing has not improved after using inhaler.	■ Place patient in Fowler's position. ■ Validate that MDI/spacer/NPA device is functioning properly (e.g., canister shaken before use). ■ Check number of actuations left in MDI canister. ■ Validate that patient's lips have tight fit around MDI mouthpiece so mist is inhaled. ■ Instruct patient to hold breath 10 sec after MDI use and to wait 2 min between puffs.
	Patient using MDI reports painful white patches in mouth.	■ Instruct patient to use spacer with MDI steroid medication. ■ Instruct patient to rinse mouth with water and expectorate after administering MDI steroid. ■ Notify healthcare provider of findings.

EXPECTED OUTCOME	UNEXPECTED OUTCOME	POSSIBLE INTERVENTIONS
Parenteral Routes Injection is administered without complications.	Ecchymosis occurs following heparin injection.	■ Rotate injection site. ■ Do not inject medication into ecchymotic area. ■ Do not aspirate before injection or massage site following needle withdrawal. ■ Do not pinch tightly when forming fat pad in preparation for injection site. ■ Apply ice to area before injecting heparin.
	Medication is administered using wrong parenteral route.	■ Notify healthcare provider; medications may need to be administered to reverse the action of the medication. ■ Monitor patient's response closely and report adverse findings immediately. ■ Medication administered IM or IV rather than subcutaneous route leads to faster absorption rates; therefore an assessment must be done to determine effects. (IV administration has immediate action.) ■ Complete unusual occurrence report according to facility policy.
	Patient has allergic or anaphylactic response to medication.	■ Call rapid response team immediately. ■ Maintain a patent airway and follow airway, breathing, circulation (ABCs) of emergency care. ■ Notify patient's healthcare provider. ■ Document incident; place allergy alert bracelet on patient. ■ Complete unusual occurrence report according to facility policy.
Injection is as painless as possible.	Patient experiences pain with IM injection.	■ Use Z-track method for ventrogluteal or vastus lateralis sites to prevent medication from leaking into subcutaneous tissue. ■ Use new needle for injection. ■ Inject medication slowly (10 sec/mL) to allow medication to diffuse. ■ Hold needle in place for 10 seconds after injection. ■ Use a dry gauze sponge to apply pressure to site after withdrawing needle.
IV piggyback medication is compatible with IV solution.	Solution in primary IV tubing is incompatible with medication to be administered via secondary piggyback solution.	■ Turn primary infusion off. ■ Before administering medication, flush primary tubing with solution compatible with medication (e.g., normal saline). ■ Hang a separate solution compatible with medication and run through line to flush during drug administration.

REVIEW Questions

1. A client having a knee replacement is returning to the care area. Which technique should the nurse use when making this client's bed?
   1. Move the pillows to the clean side of the bed.
   2. Fanfold the dirty linen toward the center of the bed.
   3. Create a triangle and fanfold the top linens to one side of the bed.
   4. Make a fold in the sheet 5–10 cm (2–4 in.) perpendicular to the foot of the bed.

2. The nurse instructs a client with diabetes on conducting foot care at home. Which client statement indicates teaching has been effective?
   1. "I should file my toe nails."
   2. "I should wash my feet when necessary."
   3. "I should wear shoes when out of doors."
   4. "I should use a heating pad to warm my feet."

3. The nurse prepares to provide mouth care to a 20-month-old client. What action should the nurse take when completing this care?
   1. Lower the head of the bed.
   2. Place the client in a side-lying position.
   3. Use a soft-bristled brush moistened with water.
   4. Use a syringe to apply mouthwash to the oral cavity.

4. The nurse asks the team leader to check a medication before providing it to a client. Which medication is the nurse most likely preparing to administer?
   1. Insulin
   2. Digoxin
   3. Penicillin
   4. Furosemide

5. The nurse prepares to administer an oral dose of medication to an adult. Which information does the nurse need to calculate the amount of medication to give to this client?
   1. Quantity
   2. Dose desired
   3. Weight in pounds
   4. Body surface area

6. The nurse prepares an injection from two vials of medication. If following the traditional method, what should the nurse do after withdrawing the required amount of medication from the second vial?
   1. Insert the required amount of air into the first vial.
   2. Remove the needle and attach a new sterile needle to the syringe.
   3. Draw the prescribed amount of medication from the first vial into a separate syringe.
   4. Pull back the syringe plunger to allow space for volume of second medication to be added.

7. A client with a gastrostomy tube needs to receive three medications at 1000 hours. How many milliliters of water should the nurse have available to provide these medications correctly?
   1. 30 mL
   2. 45 mL
   3. 60 mL
   4. 90 mL

8. The nurse evaluates a client's ability to use a metered-dose inhaler with a spacer. Which observation indicates that additional teaching is required?
   1. Inhales deeply for 5 seconds
   2. Holds the breath for 2 seconds
   3. Presses down once on the canister
   4. Exhales slowly through pursed lips

9. The nurse prepares to apply a transdermal patch medication to a client. Which approach should the nurse take when applying this medication?
   1. Select a skin area that is clean, dry, hairless, and intact.
   2. Apply the patch on the same skin area as the previous patch.
   3. Remove the previous patch and cleanse the skin with alcohol.
   4. Apply the medication to the skin and cover with the patch paper.

10. The nurse notes that leak-back occurred after providing a subcutaneous injection of heparin to a client. Which action should the nurse take at this time?
    1. Massage the site with a gauze pad.
    2. Prepare another dose of the medication.
    3. Apply a pressure dressing to be removed after 30 minutes.
    4. Apply pressure to the injection site for 10 seconds with a gauze pad.

11. The manager observes as a new graduate provides an intramuscular injection using the Z-track method to a client. For which action should the manager intervene?
    1. Displaces tissue laterally
    2. Angles the syringe at 45 degrees
    3. Applies pressure to the site with a gauze pad
    4. Waits 10 seconds before removing the needle

12. The nurse prepares to administer an intravenous push medication to a client. Which action should the nurse make first after injecting the medication through the injection port?
    1. Aspirate for a blood return.
    2. Remove the needle and syringe.
    3. Flush the injection port with heparin.
    4. Cleanse the injection port with an antiseptic swab.

Note: For answers and rationales for the review questions, go to Appendix A or your Pearson MyLab Nursing and eText.

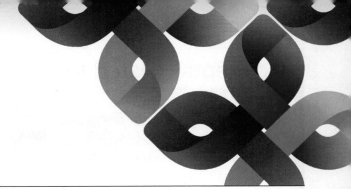

Chapter 3
Comfort

Chapter at a Glance

❶ Nursing students may observe or assist with the following skills only with faculty permission and while under direct supervision of faculty or another RN.

≫ The Concept of Comfort

To comfort someone implies intentional offering of self to bring solace or ease of distress and pain; providing comfort is a characteristic action of nurses. Comfort can also mean a feeling of ease or relief from distress and pain, which is an intention of nursing interventions. A patient's distress or pain may be physical, psychological, spiritual, environmental, or sociocultural. It may be an acute condition or a chronic one. Comfort needs of patients can be measured by a variety of pain scales available for assessing pain in infants, children, and adults.

Comfort is provided to patients and their families through interventions called comfort measures, such as teaching relaxation strategies, providing distractions, teaching controlled breathing, scheduled repositioning, applying localized heat or cold, promoting exercise, and counseling. End-of-life care measures support quality of life for the patient and also help the patient die with dignity. These measures include maintaining pain relief, keeping the patient clean and dry, using skin lotion and lip balm for comfort, scheduled repositioning, and using therapeutic touch. Comfort care builds rapport and trust in the nurse-patient relationship.

Learning Outcomes

3.1 Discuss six priority assessment questions to ask the patient about pain being experienced.

3.2 Explain how to do a pain assessment on a child who is crying and complaining of hurting.

3.3 Discuss the advantages of using a pain scale when doing a pain assessment.

3.4 Differentiate priority safety considerations for the patient receiving application of dry heat and dry cold measures.

3.5 List four safety priorities for the patient using a patient-controlled analgesia (PCA) pump.

3.6 Describe five nonpharmaceutical strategies the patient might use for pain relief.

3.7 Discuss consideration for the customs, beliefs, and rituals of the patient and family when providing end-of-life nursing care.

3.8 Explain five essential nursing interventions for the patient who is dying.

The following feature links some, but not all, of the concepts related to assessment. They are presented in alphabetical order.

Concepts Related to
Comfort

CONCEPT	RELATIONSHIP TO COMFORT	NURSING IMPLICATIONS
Caring Interventions	Implement appropriate interventions for the patient in pain	■ Monitor patient for pain relief ■ Implement a variety of nonpharmaceutical measures and administer medications ordered to relieve patient's pain
Collaboration	Collaborate with the healthcare provider for appropriate comfort measures.	■ Advocate for changes in medications ordered if pain relief is not obtained by patient ■ Make recommendations to the healthcare provider about pain relief options using clinical judgment
Ethics	Implement comfort measures for all individuals.	■ Provide consistent comfort measures to all patients in distress or pain at all ages
Grief and Loss	Emotional distress and anticipatory grief	■ Provide support and encouragement, use active listening, use therapeutic communication, and offer referral to support group or counseling
Mobility	Maintenance of functional movement	■ Provide patient encouragement and assistance in completing self-care, support activities of movement
Stress and Coping	Mental fatigue of caring for a dying loved one and then adjusting to the loss	■ Provide respite care information to family, explain expected behaviors of a dying patient, provide support in helping family cope with loss

>> Acute/Chronic Pain Management

Expected Outcomes

1. Pain is controlled through an integrative approach of complementary and conventional health therapies.
2. Patient is satisfied with level of pain control.
3. Patient receives adequate pain management; pain level does not interfere with ambulation (mobility) or activities of daily living and care.

4. Patient's anxiety level is lowered in relation to pain.
5. Patient is able to identify and alleviate discomfort caused by psychological distress.

SKILL 3.1 Pain in Newborn, Infant, Child, Adult: Assessing

Appropriate assessment of pain for patients of all ages is essential for proper pain treatment. To manage pain successfully, nurses need to do periodic pain assessments, including before and after pain relief interventions. A comprehensive pain history can help identify the patient's previous experiences with pain, interventions the patient uses to relieve pain, and the expectations of pain management. There is an assortment of pain assessment tools available to assist the nurse doing an assessment of pain for all ages.

Delegation or Assignment

The nurse is responsible for the initial assessment and regular reassessment of pain. It may be that unlicensed assistive personnel (UAP) most frequently assess patients for pain if responsible

for vital signs. After the assessment and in collaboration with the patient, the nurse can discuss and delegate or assign the performance of appropriate comfort measures to the UAP. For example, the UAP may reposition the patient at regular intervals, give the patient a back massage, or provide rest periods. Emphasize to the UAP the importance of reporting any changes in the patient's pain to the nurse. Note that state laws for UAPs vary, so this task might be assigned to the UAP rather than delegated.

Equipment

■ Pain management flow sheet ❶
■ Pain rating scale appropriate for age
  ● Neonatal Infant Pain Scale (NIPS) (newborn, infant less than six weeks old) **(Table 3–1 >>)**

SKILL 3.1 Pain in Newborn, Infant, Child, Adult: Assessing (*continued*)

Pain Management Flow Sheet

Patient's stated pain level goal: _____

Arousal Score
0 = Alert	1 = Medically sedated/ETT
2 = Drowsy	3 = Somnolent
	4 = Asleep

Nonpharmacologic interventions
C = Cold	P = Pacifier
D = Distraction	PO = Positioning
H = Heat	R = Relaxation
HO = Holding	RO = Rocking
I = Imagery	S = Security object
M = Massage	T = TENS unit
MU = Music	0 = Other

Analgesia Order
1 = Increase in dosage/rate
2 = Decrease in dosage/rate
3 = Extra bolus
4 = PRN medication for break-through pain
5 = Discontinue

Reason for Analgesia Order
1 = Unrelieved pain
2 = Decreased arousal/neuroscore
3 = Side effects (see below)
4 = Discontinue therapy/change to oral route
5 = Adverse drug reactions
(Document all adverse drug reactions.)

Side Effects
A = Anxiety	N = Nausea	0 = None
C = Confused	R = Respiratory depression	
Co = Constipation	U = Urinary retention	
I = Itching	V = Vomiting	

Sensory Function: Epidural Only
0 = Moves all extremities well
1 = Unable to move all extremities well

Motor Function: Epidural Only
0 = Able to feel tactile pressure
1 = Unable to feel tactile pressure

Neuro Score: Epidural Only
0 = No numbness, no weakness
1 = Medically sedated/ETT
2 = Numbness without weakness
3 = Numbness and weakness

Catheter Site: Epidural Only
1 = No redness, drainage, inflammation or swelling
2 = Red, inflamed
3 = Visible clear drainage
4 = Visible purulent drainage
5 = Visible serosanguinous/sanguinous drainage
6 = Swelling

Catheter Integrity Upon Removal: Epidural Only
1 = Catheter tip visually intact
2 = Catheter NOT visually intact

Flow Sheet Rows
Date
Time
Initials
Mode of admin
Level of pain
Location of pain
Frequency of pain
Type of pain
Arousal score
Nonpharmacologic intervention
Analgesia order
Reason for order
Side effects
Adverse effects (Y/N)
Sensory function: Epidural only
Motor function: Epidural only
Neuro score: Epidural only
Catheter site: Epidural only
Cath integrity: Epidural only
O2 saturation
Respirations
Pulse
Blood pressure

Signature | **Initials**

Patient Identification Label

Mode of Administration
A-PO opioid and nonopioid medications
B-PCA infuser basal with patient control
C-Continuous infusion
D-Epidural infuser continuous basal only
E-Epidural infuser basal & patient control
F-Intermittent IV/IM injection
G-Transdermal opioids
H-On-Q-pump
I-Per rectum

Level of Pain Assessment Scales
Wong-Baker FACES Pain Rating Scale
0 NO HURT	1 HURTS LITTLE BIT	2 HURTS LITTLE MORE	3 HURTS EVEN MORE	4 HURTS WHOLE LOT	5 HURTS WORST

0-10 Pain Scale
0 ---------- 10
No pain or pain relieved — Worst pain imaginable

0-10 Sum Scale

A. Vocal
0 = Positive/ETT
1 = Whimpers
2 = Crying
3 = Screaming

C. Facial
0 = Smiling
1 = Neutral
2 = Frown/grimace
3 = Clenched teeth

B. Body Movement
0 = Moves easily
1 = Neutral shifting
2 = Tense/flailing limbs

D. Touching (localizing)
0 = No touching
1 = Reaching/patting
2 = Grabbing

Location of Pain
Right   Left   Left   Right

A = No pain
B-Z = Use letters to mark location of pain on graph

Frequency of Pain
0 = Occasional   F = Frequent   C = Constant

Type of Pain
A = Burning	D = Sharp	G = Isolated
B = Stabbing	E = Shooting	H = Other
C = Radiating	F = Dull	

Source: From Pain Management Flow Chart. Published by Sunrise Hospital and Medical Center.

1 Pain management flow sheet. Children's Hospital.

SKILL 3.1 Pain in Newborn, Infant, Child, Adult: Assessing (continued)

TABLE 3–1 Neonatal Infant Pain Scale (NIPS)

Characteristic	Scoring Criteria
Facial expression	
0 = Relaxed muscles	■ Restful face with neutral expression
1 = Grimace	■ Tight facial muscles; furrowed brow, chin, and jaw (*Note:* At low gestational ages, newborns may have no facial expression.)
Cry	
0 = No cry	■ Quiet, not crying
1 = Whimper	■ Mild moaning, intermittent cry
2 = Vigorous cry	■ Loud screaming, rising, shrill, and continuous (*Note:* Silent cry may be scored if newborn is intubated, as indicated by obvious facial movements.)
Breathing patterns	
0 = Relaxed	■ Relaxed, usual breathing pattern maintained
1 = Change in breathing	■ Change in breathing, irregular, faster than usual, gagging, or holding breath
Arm movements	
0 = Relaxed/restrained	■ Relaxed, no muscle rigidity, occasional random (with soft restraints) movements of the arms
1 = Flexed/extended	■ Tense, straight arms; (or) rigid; (or) rapid extension and flexion
Leg movements	
0 = Relaxed/restrained	■ Relaxed, no muscle rigidity, occasional random (with soft restraints) movements of legs
1 = Flexed/extended	■ Tense, straight legs; rigid or rapid extension and flexion
State of arousal	
0 = Sleeping/awake	■ Quiet, peaceful, sleeping; alert and settled
1 = Fussy	■ Alert and restless or thrashing; fussy

Source: Data from Lawrence, J., Alcock, D., McGrath, P., Kay, J., MacMurray, S. B., & Dulberg, C. (1993). The development of a tool to assess neonatal pain. *Neonatal Network, 12*(6), 59–66; Morrow, C. (2010). Reducing neonatal pain during routine heel lance procedures. *American Journal of Maternal Child Nursing, 35*(6), 346–354.

- FLACC Pain Scale (infant, small child less than 3 years old)
- Oucher Scale (child between 3–7 years old) ❷
- FACES Rating Scale (child greater than 3 years old, adult) ❸
- Numeric Pain Rating Scale (child greater than 4 years old, adult) ❹
- Stethoscope, pulse oximeter

FLACC AND REVISED FLACC (R-FLACC) PAIN SCALE

The FLACC Pain Scale is designed to measure acute pain in infants and small children less than 3 years old by observing designated behaviors in nonverbal or preverbal patients who are unable to verbalize their level of pain. Behaviors are observed while the patient is sleeping or awake to determine a postoperative pain level. The r-FLACC Pain Scale uses additional descriptors to validate pain intensity in small children with developmental disability or cognitive impairment who are unable to self-report their level of acute pain.

FLACC is an acronym for the five categories of behaviors that are assessed: **F**ace, **L**egs, **A**ctivity, **C**ry, and **C**onsolability. The patient's body and legs are observed uncovered for up to five minutes. Parents can be instructed about these categories and include their input on individual child behaviors.

The patient is numerically rated in each of the five categories using a 0–2 scale. The category scores are then totaled for a possible score of 0–10. The total score is then interpreted to determine the intensity of pain present, with 0 being comfort with no pain and 10 being severe pain or discomfort. This scale can be used until the child is able to self-report pain using another pain scale.

Preparation

- Identify those factors that may cause the patient to be in pain. For example, does the patient have a prior history of low back pain or diabetic neuropathy? Has the patient had a major surgical procedure? Has the patient experienced recent trauma? Noticing the child's diet and behavior can provide cues about pain. For example, in the infant or child, eating new foods can upset the stomach or drinking less fluid can cause constipation which may result in abdominal pain. Children pull at their ears when they have an ear infection and become quieter when not feeling well. Note the patient's baseline vital signs.
- Identify the patient's preferred method of communication. Make necessary arrangements if translators are needed. Use therapeutic play communication with children.
- Expressions of pain vary from culture to culture and may vary from person to person within a culture.
  - Use a standard measure when asking about pain.
  - Accept the patient's beliefs about pain.
  - Identify and support the patient's methods of coping with pain, whether that is spiritual (offering up suffering in prayer), social (having multiple family members participate in care), or stoic (quietly accepting the pain).
  - Regularly evaluate the effect of treatment on the pain and on the patient's overall well-being.

SKILL 3.1 Pain in Newborn, Infant, Child, Adult: Assessing (continued)

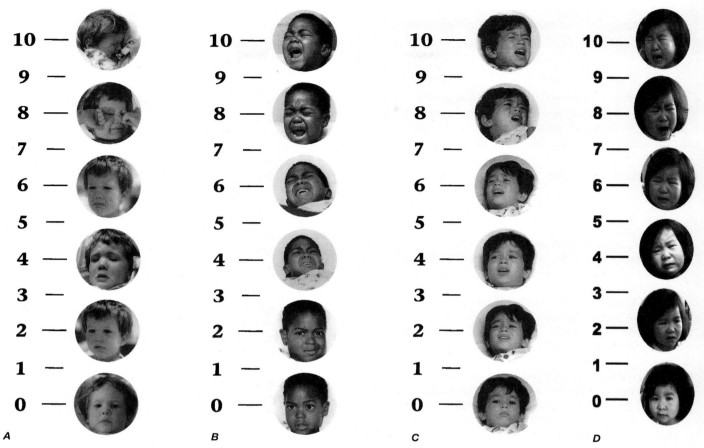

A   B   C   D

Source: Oucher Scale from Oucher. Copyright © by Pain Associates in Nursing. Used by permission of Pain Associates in Nursing.

Note: In the form presented in this book, the Oucher is for educational purposes only and cannot be used for patient care. **A,** The Caucasian version of the Oucher, developed and copyrighted by Judith E. Beyer, RN, PhD, 1983. **B,** The African American version of the Oucher, developed and copyrighted by Mary J. Denyes, RN, PhD, and Antonio M. Villarruel, RN, PhD, 1990. Cornelia P. Porter, RN, PhD, and Charlotta Marshall, RN, MSN, contributed to the development of the scale. **C,** The Hispanic version of the Oucher, developed and copyrighted by Antonio M. Villarruel, RN, PhD, and Mary J. Denyes, RN, PhD, 1990. **D,** The Asian version of the Oucher, developed and copyrighted by C. H. Yeh, RN, PhD, and C. H. Wang, BNS, 2003. http://www.oucher.org.

❷ Oucher Scale 3–7 years.

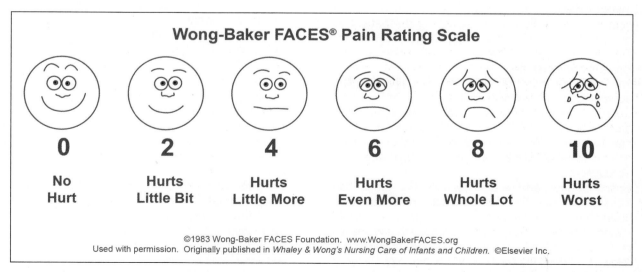

Source: © 1983 Wong-Baker FACES Foundation. www.WongBakerFACES.org. Used with permission. Originally published in Whaley & Wong's Nursing Care of Infants and Children. © Elsevier Inc.

❸ The FACES rating scale.

(continued on next page)

SKILL 3.1 Pain in Newborn, Infant, Child, Adult: Assessing *(continued)*

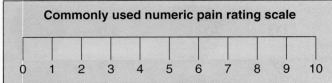

Commonly used numeric pain rating scale

| 0 | 1 | 2 | 3 | 4 | 5 | 6 | 7 | 8 | 9 | 10 |

"On a scale of 0 to 10 with 0 meaning you are having no pain, and 10 meaning you are having the worst possible pain you can imagine, where would you rate your pain?"

④ Numeric pain rating scale.

Procedure

1. Prior to performing the procedure, introduce self and verify the patient's identity using two identifiers. Explain to the patient (and parent as appropriate) what you are going to do, why it is necessary, and how the patient can participate. Discuss how the results will be used in planning further care or treatments.
2. Perform hand hygiene and observe other appropriate infection control procedures.
3. Provide for patient privacy.
4. Assess the patient's perception of pain. For patients experiencing acute or severe pain, the nurse may focus on the first three aspects of the assessment below—determining location, intensity, and quality—and quickly follow with an intervention. Patients with less severe or chronic pain can usually provide a more detailed description, and the nurse can obtain a comprehensive pain assessment.
   - *Location:* Ask the patient to place a mark on the figure on the pain assessment flow sheet or form, if appropriate. If there is more than one area of pain, use letters (e.g., A, B, C) to differentiate among the various sites. If the patient is unable or unwilling to mark the figure, ask the patient to tell you where the pain is located. Follow up by asking the patient to point to the painful site with one finger. **Rationale:** *This will help verify if the verbal description and the location are the same.*
   - *Intensity:* Ask the patient to rate the pain using the appropriate scale per facility policy.
   - *Quality:* Ask the patient, "What words would you use to describe your pain?" **Rationale:** *Although this question may be difficult for the patient to answer, the assessment is most accurate when the patient provides the description.*
   - *Onset, duration, and recurrence:* This assessment can include such questions as "How long have you been having pain?" "Have you noticed any activity (e.g., swallowing, eating, stress, urinating, exertion) that increases or decreases the pain?" "How long does the pain last?" "How often does the pain occur?" "Is the pain better or worse at certain times of the day or night?"
   - *Manner of expressing pain:* Observe for behavioral cues such as grimacing, crying, or a change in body posture

(see ③). **Rationale:** *Learning how a patient expresses pain is particularly important for the patient who cannot communicate, is very young, very old, or unable to hear, or has learned not to express pain because of a belief that it is a sign of weakness.*
   - *Precipitating factors:* Ask what causes or increases the pain. **Rationale:** *Knowledge of those activities can both help prevent the pain from occurring and sometimes help determine the cause.*
   - *Alleviating factors:* Ask questions such as "What makes the pain go away or lessen?" "What methods of relief have you tried?" "How long did you use them?" "How effective were they?" **Rationale:** *Asking these questions can assist the nurse and the patient to determine if some of the methods (such as listening to music or relaxation) can continue to be used while at the healthcare facility.*
   - *Associated symptoms:* Ask if there are any other symptoms (e.g., nausea, vomiting, dizziness) that occur prior to, with, or after the pain. **Rationale:** *These symptoms may relate to the onset of the pain or may result from the presence of the pain.*
   - *Effects of pain:* Explore the patient's feelings and the effect the pain has on the patient's life. This is particularly important for the patient with chronic pain. **Rationale:** *Assessing the areas of sleep, appetite, physical activity, relationships, emotions, and concentration provides the nurse with information about the level of the patient's functioning on a daily basis.*
   - *Other comments:* Ask if there is any other information that would be helpful for the healthcare providers and nurses to know. Emphasize that you want to work with the patient and family to get the safest control of the pain.

CAUTION! Perception is an individual's reality. The patient's self-report of pain is what must be used to determine pain intensity. The nurse is obligated to record the pain intensity as reported by the patient. If the nurse challenges the believability of the patient's report, it undermines the therapeutic relationship and prevents the nurse from being an advocate for the person with pain.

5. Assess physiological response to pain. Note blood pressure, pulse rate, respiratory rate, skin color, and presence of diaphoresis. **Rationale:** *Signs of sympathetic nervous system stimulation (fight or flight) may be present with acute pain; however, patients with chronic pain may not have physical signs because of CNS adaptation.*
6. Do a focused assessment on the affected body part, if appropriate. **Rationale:** *Additional assessment may provide information about the pain and possible intervention.*
7. Document findings of the pain assessment and include the intervention(s) and the patient's response to the intervention(s). **Rationale:** *Thorough assessment and documentation assists the nurse to gain insights into the nature and pattern of the patient's pain and ensures*

SKILL 3.1 Pain in Newborn, Infant, Child, Adult: Assessing *(continued)*

continuity of care. Maintaining a pain management flow sheet (see ❶*) will clarify and communicate each patient's pain experience to enhance effective pain relief efforts. In settings where a pain management flow sheet is not used, complete documentation using forms, checklists, or electronic dropdown lists supplemented by nurse's notes or additional comments as appropriate.*

SAMPLE DOCUMENTATION

[date] 0900 Admitted for elective foot surgery; c/o dull, throbbing, continuous pain in right cheek and jaw area radiating to right shoulder. Rates pain at 6/10. States pain began 6 months ago. Holding jaw throughout interview, became tearful when describing negative effects on sleep, mood, and daily functioning. Associates onset with stress at work, and states she has been clenching her teeth throughout the day and grinding her teeth during sleep. States pain seems worse today with anxiety about surgery. Reports that acetaminophen and heating pad relieve pain temporarily. Given moist heat pack to use now and relaxation breathing demonstrated with patient participation. *M. Blaszko*

0930 Rates pain at 1/10. Referrals to TMJ specialist and counseling made per order. Discussed maintaining a daily pain diary to identify patterns and to share with healthcare provider. *M. Blaszko*

PAIN RATING SCALES

The goal of pain assessment is to provide accurate information about the location and intensity of pain and its effects on the patient's functioning. Various pain scales have been developed to assess pain in the newborn, infant, child, and adult. Some pain assessment scales rely on the nurse's observation of the patient's behavior if the patient is nonverbal. Other scales depend on the patient's report of pain intensity.

Neonatal Infant Pain Scale (NIPS) (see Table 3–1)

- Use in preterm and term babies up to 6 weeks after birth.
- Observe the baby's facial expression, cry quality, breathing pattern, arm and leg position, and state of arousal.

FLACC Pain Scale

- This scale is designed to measure acute pain in infants and small children less than 3 years old following surgery or while sleeping.
- FLACC is an acronym for the five categories that are assessed: face, legs, activity, cry, and consolability.
- Use until the child is able to self-report pain with another pain scale.

Oucher Scale (see 2)

- Use in children between 3–7 years of age. Select the scale that matches the child's ethnic background—Caucasian, African American, or Hispanic.
- The child selects the face that matches his or her level of pain. The older child can select a number between 0 and 10.

FACES Rating Scale (see 3)

- Use in children over 3 years old and adults who are unable to understand or respond to the number rating scale.
- Patient is asked to point to the face that best describes how the pain makes them feel. The number under the face is recorded.

Numeric Pain Rating Scale (see 4)

- Designed for children over 4 years old and adults.
- Patient is asked to self-report the intensity of pain on a scale of 0 to 10, with 0 meaning having no pain and 10 meaning having the worse possible pain imaginable.

Health Promotion
DAILY PAIN DIARY

For patients who experience chronic pain, a daily diary may illuminate pain patterns and factors that exacerbate or mediate the pain experience. Trends in pain relief can be monitored by the healthcare provider. They support pain management decisions about quality of life and improvements in level of wellness. In home care, the family or other caregiver can be taught to complete the diary. The record can include:

- Time or onset of pain and activity or situation preceding pain
- Relevant data (e.g., weather conditions the patient deems significant)
- Physical pain character (quality) and intensity level (0–10)
- Emotions experienced and intensity level (0–10)
- Use of analgesics or other relief measures
- Duration of pain
- Time spent in relief activities and effectiveness of these activities

Lifespan Considerations
NEWBORN AND INFANT

- Giving a newborn or infant, particularly a very-low-birth-weight newborn or infant, a water and sucrose solution administered through a pacifier is effective in reducing pain during procedures that may be painful, but should not replace anesthetic or analgesic medications when indicated.

CHILD

- Distract the child with toys, books, or pictures.
- Hold the child to console and promote comfort.
- Explore misconceptions about pain and correct in understandable "concrete" terms. Be aware of how your explanations may be misunderstood. For example, telling a child that surgery will not hurt because the child will be "put to sleep" will be very upsetting to a child who knows of an animal that was "put to sleep."

(continued on next page)

SKILL 3.1 Pain in Newborn, Infant, Child, Adult: Assessing *(continued)*

- Children can use their imagination during guided imagery. To use the "pain switch," ask the child to imagine a pain switch (even give it a color) and tell them to visualize turning the switch off in the area where there is pain. A "magic glove" or "magic blanket" is an imaginary object that the child applies on areas of the body (e.g., hand, thigh, back, hip) to lessen discomfort.

OLDER ADULT

- Promote the patient's use of pain control measures that have worked in the past for the patient.

- Spend time with the patient and listen carefully.
- Clarify questions about medications prescribed. Evaluate patient's physical dexterity to take analgesic medications when at home, ability to renew prescriptions or over-the-counter medications at the pharmacy, and warning signs to report to healthcare provider.
- Carefully review the treatment plan to avoid drug–drug, food–drug, or disease–drug interactions.

SKILL 3.2 Pain Relief: Back Massage

Back massage is a comfort measure that can aid relaxation, promote circulation of blood and lymph, and decrease muscle tension. It may ease anxiety because the physical contact communicates caring. By increasing superficial circulation as well as neurologic distraction, pain intensity can be directly reduced as a result of massage. The use of creams or lotions may amplify therapeutic potential. Massage is contraindicated in areas of skin breakdown, suspected clots, or infections.

Delegation or Assignment

The nurse can delegate or assign this skill to the UAP; however, the nurse should first assess for the UAP's comfort and ability, any contraindications, and patient willingness to participate. The nurse remains responsible for assessment, interpretation of abnormal findings, and determination of appropriate responses. Note that state laws for UAPs vary, so this task might be assigned to the UAP rather than delegated.

Equipment

- Lotion
- Towel for excess lotion

Preparation

- Determine (1) previous assessments of the skin, (2) special lotions to be used, and (3) positions contraindicated for the patient.
- Arrange for a quiet environment with no interruptions to promote maximum effect of the back massage.

Procedure

1. Prior to performing the procedure, introduce self and verify the patient's identity using two identifiers. Explain to the patient what you are going to do, why it is necessary, and how the patient can participate. Encourage the patient to give you feedback as to the amount of pressure you are using during the back rub.
2. Perform hand hygiene and observe other appropriate infection control procedures.
3. Provide for patient privacy.

4. Prepare the patient.
   - Assist the patient to move to the near side of the bed within your reach and adjust the bed to a comfortable working height. **Rationale:** *This prevents back strain.*
   - Establish which position the patient prefers. The prone position is recommended for a back rub. The side-lying position can be used if a patient cannot assume the prone position.
   - Expose the back from the shoulders to the inferior sacral area. Cover the remainder of the body. **Rationale:** *This prevents chilling and minimizes exposure.*
5. Massage the back ❶.
   - Pour a small amount of lotion onto the palms of your hands and hold it for a minute. The lotion bottle can also be placed in a bath basin filled with warm water. **Rationale:** *Back rub preparations tend to feel uncomfortably cold to people. Warming the solution facilitates patient comfort.*
   - Using your palm, begin in the sacral area using smooth, circular strokes.

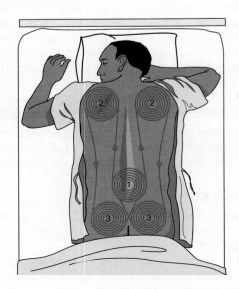

❶ One suggested pattern for a back massage.

SKILL 3.2 Pain Relief: Back Massage (*continued*)

- Move your hands up the center of the back and then over both scapulae.
- Massage in a circular motion over the scapulae.
- Move your hands down the sides of the back.
- Massage the areas over the right and left iliac crests. Massage the back in an orderly pattern using a variety of strokes and appropriate pressure.
- Apply firm, continuous pressure without breaking contact with the patient's skin.
- Repeat above for 3–5 min, obtaining more lotion as necessary.
- While massaging the back, assess for skin redness, areas of decreased circulation, and patient comfort.
- Pat dry any excess lotion with a towel.
6. When the procedure is complete, perform hand hygiene and leave patient safe and comfortable.
7. Complete documentation using forms, checklists, or electronic dropdown lists supplemented by nurse's notes or additional comments as appropriate. Document that a back massage was performed and the patient's response. Record any unusual findings.

SAMPLE DOCUMENTATION

[date] 1400 Reports aching, intermittent back pain; wincing and grimacing when attempting to move in bed; rates pain at 4–5 on 0–10 scale; states uses massage to help relieve pain when at home. Back massaged; stated the massage helped him to relax. Lights dimmed and door to room closed. *M. Black*

1430 Rates pain at 1–2/10. States feels "much more comfortable." Moving in bed with ease. *M. Black*

SKILL 3.3 Pain Relief: Complementary Health Approaches

To help meet physical needs of patients in pain, many nurses integrate interventions beyond pain medication to help patients relax and ease their discomfort. The complementary therapies in this skill to support pain relief are controlled breathing, progressive muscle relaxation, and guided imagery relaxation techniques. These techniques are especially helpful for patients suffering from pain due to musculoskeletal conditions.

Delegation or Assignment

The nurse is responsible for assessing the patient's willingness to participate in complementary relaxation exercises for pain management in addition to their medical treatments. The nurse teaches the patient about the techniques of controlled breathing for relaxation, progressive muscle relaxation, and guided imagery. Noninvasive pain management relaxation techniques can then be delegated or assigned to the UAP if experienced with using the techniques and if comfortable helping the patient practice them. The nurse instructs the UAP to report patient observations to the nurse for follow-up. Assessment and evaluation of effectiveness of the exercise remain the responsibility of the nurse. Note that state laws for UAPs vary, so this task might be assigned to the UAP rather than delegated.

Equipment

- No equipment is required for controlled breathing and guided imagery relaxation

Progressive Muscle Relaxation Only
- A printed relaxation script that an individual can read until the patient learns the technique. Many are available online and through stress management resource books and tapes.
- CD player or smart phone (optional). Machine could be used to provide the script for the exercise or for the playing of background music.

Preparation

- Allow 10–15 min of uninterrupted time for the session. Ensure that the environment is private, quiet, comfortable, and at a temperature that suits the patient. The patient should have an empty bladder. **Rationale:** *Interruptions or distractions interfere with the patient's ability to achieve full relaxation. Once patients learn how to use this technique, they will be able to do it in less than 5 minutes as part of self-care and ongoing stress management.*
- If you are motivated to learn complementary health relaxation techniques to help patients manage their pain, numerous classes are available. To implement certain complementary health therapies such as therapeutic touch, acupressure, or acupuncture, you will need specialized classes/training.

Procedure

1. Introduce self to patient (parent) and verify the patient's identity using two identifiers. Explain to the patient (parent) what you are going to do, why it is necessary, and how the patient can participate. Discuss how the results will be used in planning further care or treatments. Explain the rationale and benefits of complementary

(*continued on next page*)

SKILL 3.3 Pain Relief: Complementary Health Approaches (*continued*)

health approaches. Ask the patient about the goals for the session. This type of therapy can provide relaxation and feelings of empowerment, lead to creative problem solving, and facilitate healing. The content used can vary depending on the patient's goals. Many books, tapes, and CDs are available for those who want to learn more about these powerful techniques. **Rationale:** *The patient is an active participant in an exercise and can offer direction for the session.*

2. Perform hand hygiene and observe appropriate infection control procedures.
3. Provide for patient privacy.

CONTROLLED BREATHING

4. Instruct patient to sit so that his or her back is well supported, with spine straight but not rigid ❶.

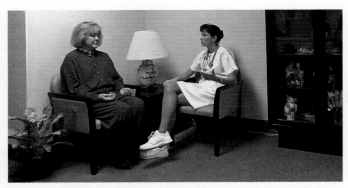

Source: Ronald May/Pearson Education, Inc.

❶ Find a quiet room to teach the relaxation process.

5. Have patient place feet flat on floor and place hands on legs.
6. If patient is lying down, have the patient place hands at sides.
7. Suggest patient find a comfortable position, close eyes, and take a deep, slow breath through nostrils.
8. Continue giving the patient the following instructions using this sample script:
   • Extend your abdominal muscles.
   • Hold your breath for the count of four. Then very slowly release the air through slightly parted lips, making a whoosh sound.
   • When you think that all the air is out, hold your stomach in to push out even more air.
   • Repeat this breathing pattern several times so that your body relaxes.
   • Breathe in through your nostrils to the count of four—1-2-3-4. Hold it—1-2-3-4—and slowly expel the breath all the way out, slowly releasing the air through your mouth.
   • As the air goes out, feel all of the tension drain out with it.
   • Now double the count, and breathe in slowly, filling your lungs all the way to the top to the count of eight—1-2-3-4-5-6-7-8. Hold it—1-2-3-4—and now slowly release the breath—5-6-7-8.

   • Again breathe in slowly to the count of 10 and count for the patient—1-2-3-4-5-6-7-8-9-10. Hold it to the count of eight—1-2-3-4-5-6-7-8—and slowly release the air through your mouth to the count of 10—1-2-3-4-5-6-7-8-9-10. Pause.
   • Continue with your regular breathing pattern, letting your lungs breathe for you.
9. Stop the process by having the patient open his or her eyes. Proceed to step 10 below.

PROGRESSIVE MUSCLE RELAXATION

4. Prepare the patient by doing the following:
   • Tell the patient how progressive muscle relaxation works.
   • Provide a rationale for the procedure. **Rationale:** *It has been noted that muscular tension accompanies most stress states. By aiming to reduce muscle tension, the negative effects of stress on the mind–body can be lessened.*
   • Ask the patient to identify the stressors operating in the patient's life and the reactions to these stressors. **Rationale:** *Awareness is important as the patient learns how to cope effectively.*
   • Demonstrate the method of tensing and relaxing groups of muscles and have the patient do it with you. It is easy to start with making fists—tensing the muscles with 100% effort the first time, and then with only 50% effort the second time. **Rationale:** *Demonstration and initial practice enables the patient to understand the progression of muscle relaxation more clearly.*
   • Assist the patient to a comfortable position.
5. If music is to be used, select music that is instrumental, calming, neutral, and unfamiliar to the patient. **Rationale:** *Music should not be recognizable and should not intentionally elicit memories or emotion. In this way, the music will enhance relaxation. Classical music can sometimes be too "busy" and may evoke memories and emotion that could be distracting for the patient.*
   • Ensure that all body parts are supported and the joints slightly flexed with no strain or pull on the muscles (e.g., arms and legs should not be crossed). **Rationale:** *Assuming a position of comfort facilitates relaxation.*
6. Encourage the patient to begin slow, deep diaphragmatic or abdominal breathing to rest the mind and begin relaxing the body. Inhaling through the nose and exhaling through the mouth (pursed lips are best) slows down the breath and enhances relaxation.
7. Instruct the patient to tense and then relax each group of muscles starting from the head and moving down the body. Use a tone of voice throughout the exercise that invites participation rather than directs.
   • The following script suggestions are one way of doing the technique.
     a. Take in a deep breath, and close eyes tightly shut, furrowing your brows and wrinkling your forehead.

SKILL 3.3 Pain Relief: Complementary Health Approaches *(continued)*

Hold this contraction with the most effort you can, and then release as you exhale slowly. Again, take a breath and contract these same muscles with half the effort you used last time. Hold, hold, and now release with your breath, feeling the tension leave your body as a soothing wave of relaxation flows over your head and face. . . . You could keep your eyes softly closed throughout this exercise. . . .

b. You might want to clench your jaw as you breathe in, feeling the muscles in your cheeks and throat and base of your tongue tightening as you hold, hold, and then release. You could repeat this contraction as you inhale, and hold with less tension this time, and then release as you exhale, allowing all of these muscles to soften, allowing your teeth to rest just slightly apart.

c. Next, pull your shoulders up toward your ears as you take a full and gentle breath in and hold as tightly as you can. Now relax and release your shoulders with your breath, allowing a soothing wave of relaxation to flow into your neck and shoulder area. This time hunch your shoulders up with only half the effort you used last time . . . hold it . . . and release, allowing any tension to run down your arms and through your hands and out the tips of your fingers. . . .

d. Next, you could inhale and make tight fists of both hands and hold these fists as strongly as you can. Release your fists and your breath. Take another breath in and make fists again, this time with less effort . . . hold . . . and release, allowing tension to leave your hands, being replaced with softness.

e. Now we can focus on the arms. As you breathe in, think about contracting the muscles of the arms, perhaps making fists again, and feeling the entire length of your arms tightening and flexing. Hold, hold, and release, feeling the tension leaving your arms and flowing out through your hands and fingertips. This time breathe in and tighten your arms with less effort, and then release with your breath, feeling a sense of comfort and peace as the tension leaves you now.

f. You could focus on your abdominal muscles, and pull them in tightly as if to button your navel onto the front of your spine. You may even notice tension in your back muscles. Hold this as tightly as you can. Exhale and release all of these muscles, feeling as if a band of tightness around your midsection is being released. Breathe in and tense this abdominal and low back band of muscles again. Hold more gently this time and then release, exhaling slowly. Enjoy the feelings as your muscles become relaxed and loose.

g. You could inhale deeply and flex your hip and buttock muscles, feeling yourself lift as the muscles contract. Hold, and then release as you exhale. This time, flex these muscles a bit more gently, aware of

the peace that is flowing throughout your body as you continue to relax.

h. You could inhale and flex your heels away from your body as you pull your toes hard, hard toward your face. Hold this, feeling your calf and thigh muscles flexing as well, and then release as you exhale. Inhale again and this time press your toes away from your face and feel the tension throughout the entire length of your leg once again. You can repeat this with less effort, and feel the whole body relax and release.

- Encourage the patient to breathe slowly and deeply during the entire procedure. **Rationale:** *Quiet, full, slow breathing with an emphasis on prolonged exhalation elicits a parasympathetic response that is the opposite of the fight-or-flight response.*
- Speak in a calm voice that encourages relaxation and coach the patient to mentally focus on each muscle group being addressed. **Rationale:** *By suggesting rather than directing throughout the process, you avoid triggering any underlying control issues in the patient.*

8. Ask the patient to state whether any tension remains after all muscle groups have been tensed and relaxed.
   - Repeat the procedure for muscle groups that are not relaxed.

9. Terminate the relaxation exercise slowly by counting from 1–3, suggesting that the patient will feel calm and alert.
   - Ask the patient to move the body slowly: first the hands and feet, then arms and legs, and finally the head and neck.
   - Remind the patient that this technique can be used any time the patient needs to release tension or wants to feel more relaxed. Proceed to step 10 below.

GUIDED IMAGERY

4. Assist the patient to a reclining position and ask the patient to close the eyes. **Rationale:** *A position of comfort can enhance the patient's focus during the imagery exercise.*

5. Implement actions to induce relaxation.
   - Speak clearly in a calming and neutral tone of voice. **Rationale:** *Positive voice coaching can enhance the effect of imagery. A shrill or loud voice can distract the patient from the image.*
   - Ask the patient to take slow, full diaphragmatic/abdominal breaths and to relax all muscles. Use progressive muscle relaxation exercises as needed to assist the patient to achieve total relaxation.
   - Guide patients through relaxation breathing and then through muscle relaxation. Then begin to guide them toward a most beautiful or peaceful place. Patients may have been to this place before or may be imagining this place. Do *not* impose your own suggestions as to where the place might be. Patients know where they want and need to go! Slowly guide them to approach

(continued on next page)

SKILL 3.3 Pain Relief: Complementary Health Approaches (continued)

and then finally enter the place. Prompt them to use all of their senses as they look around the place, listen to the sounds of the place, feel the air, feel what's underfoot, and smell the fragrances of the place. Have them find and move toward a safe spot where they can rest for a short amount of time.

- While patients are in their safe spot, you can assist them to do some work. For example, if they need stress management or pain relief, they can picture themselves (from the safety of their very safe spot) in a potentially tense situation. Then have them inhale and exhale slowly three times, saying to themselves "relax, relax, relax" with each exhalation. For internal healing work, encourage the patient to focus on a meaningful image of power and use it to control the specific problem. Or, the patient can be educated beforehand to use anatomical and physiological imagery for her own healing. These kinds of goals are facilitated with some prior preparation on the part of the nurse and patient, and many resources exist to prepare people for this work. Ask the patient to use all the senses when practicing imagery. **Rationale:** *Using all the senses enhances the patient's benefit from imagery. Patients may be asked to assign a color to their pain, and then identify a color signifying "no pain." Then they can use imagery to change the color of their pain to the "no-pain color."*

6. Take the patient out of the image by suggesting that it is time for the patient to leave this most beautiful and safe place. Suggest that the patient can return at any time desired and that slow breathing will lead the way.
   - Slowly count from 1–3, suggesting that it is time for the patient to leave this most beautiful and safe place. Suggest that the patient come back into the here and now.

Tell the patient that feelings of being rested and refreshed occur on the count of 3.

7. Remain until the patient is alert. If the patient remains in a trancelike state, simply repeat that the patient will wake up on the number 3 and count to three again. No harm will occur if the patient stays "asleep." You can allow the patient to remain so, or gently touch the patient to facilitate awakening.

8. Following the experience, ask the patient to describe the physical and emotional feelings elicited by the imagery session. The meanings images have for the individual patient can be very helpful in the therapeutic process. Direct the patient to explore the response to images because this enables the patient to modify the imagery for future sessions.

9. Encourage the patient to practice the imagery technique.
   - Imagery is a technique that can be done independently by the patient once the patient knows how.

10. When the procedure is complete, perform hand hygiene and leave the patient safe and comfortable.

11. Complete documentation using forms, checklists, or electronic dropdown lists supplemented by nurse's notes or additional comments as appropriate.

SAMPLE DOCUMENTATION

[date] 2300 Reports "mild" headache, 1–2/10 on pain scale; Also expressing anxiety about recent diagnosis, having difficulty falling asleep; Progressive muscle relaxation taught using relaxation music as a background; Participated fully, stated "headache is gone;" Asleep when nurse returned with sleep med; Sleep med. held. B. Montgomery

---

SKILL 3.4 Pain Relief: Transcutaneous Electrical Nerve Stimulation (TENS) Unit, Using

Safety Note! *During scheduled clinical time, nursing students may have a learning opportunity to observe or assist with this skill only with faculty permission and with direct supervision from faculty or another RN.*

The TENS unit is a noninvasive mechanical device used for nerve-related acute and chronic pain conditions. It sends stimulating pulses across the skin surface and along nerve tracts to help prevent pain signals from reaching the brain. These devices also can help stimulate the body to produce higher levels of endorphins, which are the body's own natural pain relievers.

Delegation or Assignment

The assessment for and application of a transcutaneous electrical nerve stimulation (TENS) unit requires specialized knowledge and problem solving. It is important for the nurse to understand how this method of pain management works. In an acute care health setting, the nurse would not delegate or assign the skill of managing a TENS unit to the UAP. A TENS unit is often ordered for home use and the nurse is responsible for teaching the patient or caregiver how to safely and effectively use the device.

SKILL 3.4 Pain Relief: Transcutaneous Electrical Nerve Stimulation (TENS) Unit, Using *(continued)*

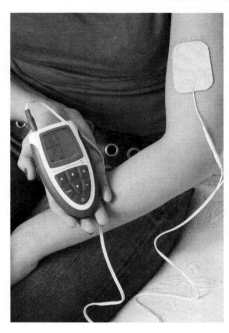

Source: Hilary Morgan/Alamy Stock Photo

1 A transcutaneous electrical nerve stimulator (TENS) unit.

Equipment

- TENS unit **1**
- Bath basin with warm water
- Soap
- Washcloth
- Towel
- Conduction cream, gel, or water (see manufacturer's instructions)
- Hypoallergenic tape

Procedure

1. Prior to performing the procedure, check the healthcare provider's order, introduce self and verify the patient's identity using two identifiers. Explain to the patient what you are going to do, why it is necessary, and how the patient can participate. The TENS unit may not completely eliminate pain but should reduce pain to a level that allows the patient to rest more comfortably and/or carry out everyday activities.
2. Perform hand hygiene and observe other appropriate infection control procedures.
3. Provide for patient privacy.
4. Prepare the equipment.
   - Insert the battery into the TENS unit to test its functioning.
   - With the TENS unit off, plug the lead wires into the battery-operated unit at one end, leaving the electrodes at the other end.
5. Clean the application area.
   - Wash, rinse, and dry the designated area with soap and water. **Rationale:** *This reduces skin irritation and facilitates adhesion of the electrodes to the skin for a longer period of time.*
6. Apply the electrodes to the patient.
   - If the electrodes are not pre-gelled, moisten them with a small amount of water or apply conducting gel. (Consult the manufacturer's instructions.) **Rationale:** *This facilitates electrical conduction.*
   - Place the electrodes on a clean, unbroken area of skin around the site of pain. Choose the area according to the location, nature, and origin of the pain.
   - Ensure that the electrodes make full surface contact with the skin. Tape all sides evenly with hypoallergenic tape. **Rationale:** *This prevents an accidental burn.*
7. Turn the unit on.
   - Ascertain that the amplitude control is set at level 0.
   - Slowly increase the intensity of the stimulus (amplitude) until the patient notes a slight increase in discomfort.
   - When the patient notes discomfort, slowly decrease the amplitude until the patient notes a pleasant sensation. Once this has been achieved, keep the TENS unit set at this level to maintain blockage of the pain sensation. Most patients select frequencies between 60–100 Hz.
8. Monitor the patient.
   - If the patient complains of itching, pricking, or burning, explore the following options:
     a. Turn the pulse-width dial down.
     b. Check that the entire electrode surface is in contact with the skin.
     c. Increase the distance between the electrodes.
     d. Select another type of electrode suitable for the model of TENS unit in use.
     e. Discontinue the TENS and consider the possibility of another brand of TENS.
   - If the sensation of the stimulus is unpleasant, too intense, or distracting, turn down both the amplitude and pulse-width dial.
   - If the patient complains of headache or nausea during application or use, turn down both the amplitude and the pulse-width dial. Repositioning of the electrodes may also be helpful.
   - If further troubleshooting is not effective, discontinue use of the TENS unit and notify the healthcare provider.
9. After the treatment:
   - Turn off the controls and unplug the lead wires from the control box.
   - Clean the electrodes according to the manufacturer's instructions. Clean the patient's skin with soap and water.

(continued on next page)

SKILL 3.4 Pain Relief: Transcutaneous Electrical Nerve Stimulation (TENS) Unit, Using (*continued*)

- Replace the used battery pack with a charged battery. Begin recharging the used battery.
- If continuous therapy is used, remove the electrode patches and inspect the skin at least once daily.

10. Provide patient teaching.
    - Review instructions for use with the patient and verify that the patient understands.
    - Have the patient demonstrate the use of the TENS unit and verbalize ways to troubleshoot if headache, nausea, or unpleasant sensations occur.
    - Instruct the patient not to submerge the unit in water but instead to remove and reapply it after bathing.

11. When the procedure is complete, perform hand hygiene and leave patient safe and comfortable.

12. Complete documentation using forms, checklists, or electronic dropdown lists supplemented by nurse's notes or additional comments as appropriate. Record the date and time TENS therapy was initiated, the location of electrode placement and status of skin in that area, the character and quality of the pain, settings of TENS unit used, side effects experienced, and the patient's response.

SAMPLE DOCUMENTATION

[date] 1100 Reports sharp pain in right hip that radiates down back of right leg; Rates pain at 3/10, and achieves some relief with positional changes that take weight off of hip; TENS applied over lateral aspect of right hip at 70 Hertz. *M. Johnstone*

1110 Reports nausea; Frequency reduced to 60 Hertz; nausea resolved. *M. Johnstone*

1140 TENS discontinued; Rates pain at 0–1/10; No c/o nausea; Skin intact. *M. Johnstone*

Patient Teaching

TENS units are frequently ordered for home use to relieve chronic pain. Instruct the patient or caregiver on the following:

- How to use and care for the TENS equipment
- How to troubleshoot if side effects or problems occur and whom to call if the equipment malfunctions
- Where and how to obtain supplies needed for the TENS unit
- How to remove the electrodes daily and check for skin breakdown at the electrode sites
- How to keep a pain diary to monitor pain onset, activity before pain, pain intensity, use of analgesics or other relief measures, and so on

- When to contact a healthcare professional if planned pain control measures are ineffective
- What preferred and selected nonpharmacological techniques and complementary therapies to use, such as relaxation, guided imagery, distraction, music therapy, massage, and so on (**Table 3–2 ≫**)
- What pain control measures to use before the pain becomes severe
- What effects untreated pain can have
- How to access community resources, home care agencies, and associations that offer self-help groups and educational materials.

TABLE 3–2 Nonpharmacological Approaches to Pain

Physical Methods	Advantages
TENS—stimulating skin with mild electric current—provides pain relief by blocking pain impulses to the brain	Noninvasive method
	Higher level of activity
	Reported to have greater effect for postoperative pain
	Gives staff confidence they can assist patient with pain
	Choice for chronic pain
Acupuncture—traditional Chinese form of treating diseases and pain through insertion and manipulation of needles at specific points on the body	Insertion of thin needles not painful to the patient
	Pain-relieving capacity lasting beyond actual procedure
	May provide relief when no other method works
Biofeedback—electric monitoring device that feeds back effect of behavior so patient can control internal processes (e.g., heartbeat)	Noninvasive method
	Completely controlled by patient
	Promotes stress reduction as well as pain relief
	After mastery, instruments not needed to achieve result

SKILL 3.4 Pain Relief: Transcutaneous Electrical Nerve Stimulation (TENS) Unit, Using (*continued*)

TABLE 3–2 Nonpharmacological Approaches to Pain (*continued*)

Physical Methods	Advantages
Vibration or massage—hands-on manipulation of muscles or electrical form of massage (vibration)	Noninvasive method—electrically alleviates pain by numbness or paresthesia or through touch Increases circulation and endorphins to area Relaxes muscles and reduces tension on nerves and promotes relaxation Useful only for light to moderate pain
Cold therapy—cold wraps, gel packs, cold therapy, ice massage; not used on irradiated tissue or when patients have peripheral vascular disease	Relieves pain faster than heat therapy Numbs nerves and decreases inflammation and spasms Effective for nerve, abdominal, and lower back pain Alters pain threshold Decreases tissue injury response
Heat therapy—heat wraps, dry heat, moist heat; not used on irradiated tissue or tumors	Noninvasive method Decreases pain by reducing inflammation Promotes relaxation of muscles Increases vasodilation and blood flow to area Facilitates clearance of tissue toxins and fluids
Counterirritants—mentholated ointments or lotions (Ben-Gay or Icy Hot)	May contain salicylates (reduces inflammation) but dangerous if patient has potential bleeding problems May be irritating to the skin—potential skin breakdown
Acupressure—a form of touch therapy using the thumbs or fingertips to apply pressure to the same body points used in acupuncture; derived from Shiatsu and traditional Chinese medicine	Noninvasive method Redirects energy flow through pressure on meridian points Reduces pain and increases endorphins
Chiropractic adjustment	Manipulates muscles and realigns spinal column nerve function Restores structural integrity and balance
Cognitive–Behavioral Methods	**Advantages**
Relaxation—body relaxation of muscles used with imagery, therapist instruction	Relaxes tense muscles and reduces stress Effective in reducing pain Easy to learn and implement techniques for self-mastery Reduces fear and anxiety connected to pain
Imagery—visualization technique of forming sensory images, or seeing in the "mind's eye" an image that distracts from the sensation of pain	Effective in reducing pain Patient control of use and timing of technique Reduces high-level anxiety connected to pain
Deep breathing—techniques using breath to control pain	Effective in reinforcing body relaxation and visualization Reduces pain through breath control; increases oxygen utilization
Hypnosis—creating a state of altered consciousness so that patient is susceptible to instruction	Effective with a patient who is suggestive and who experiences tension and anxiety accompanying pain

SKILL 3.5 Patient-Controlled Analgesia (PCA) Pump: Using

Safety Note! *During scheduled clinical time, nursing students may have the learning opportunity to observe or assist with this skill only with faculty permission and with direct supervision from faculty or another RN.*

The computer-controlled PCA pump delivers a specific amount of pain medication intravenously to the patient at set intervals or can be programmed so the patient can self-administer a preset dose of pain medication at controlled time intervals when the patient pushes a button. PCA pumps have been used for adult patients and pediatric patients as young as 5–6 years old. There are safety features that prevent anyone from overriding the pump's programmed settings. Also, the

(*continued on next page*)

SKILL 3.5 Patient Controlled Analgesia (PCA) Pump: Using *(continued)*

medication is locked into place so it cannot be removed from the pump without the key or keypad code.

Delegation or Assignment

Initiating and maintaining a PCA pump requires application of nursing knowledge, aseptic technique, critical thinking, and administration of a controlled substance and, therefore, is not delegated or assigned to the UAP. The nurse can inform the UAP of the intended therapeutic effects and specific side effects of the medication and direct the UAP to report specific patient observations (e.g., unrelieved pain) to the nurse for follow-up. The UAP must not administer a dose (push the button) for the patient.

Equipment

- PCA pump and appropriate tubing ❶
- Keypad code or key for locking mechanism
- Operational manual for specific pump to be used
- Alcohol swab

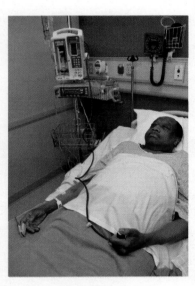

Source: Ronald May/Pearson Education, Inc.

❶ Continuous IV narcotic drip for pain-control.

Preparation

- Before initiating PCA therapy, determine factors that may contraindicate use (e.g., impaired mental status, impaired respiratory status), the amount of narcotic specified by the order, bolus and continuous infusion dosage parameters, and type of primary fluid.
- Calculate:
  - The initial bolus dose based on the number of milligrams of drug per milliliter of fluid
  - The dose per intermittent bolus delivery
  - The 4-hour lockout drug limit.
- Check for patient allergies.
- Check the healthcare provider's orders and medication administration record (MAR).
- Check the label on the medication carefully against the MAR to make sure that the correct medication is being prepared.

- Know the reason why the patient is receiving the medication, the drug classification, contraindications, usual dose range, side effects, and nursing considerations for administering and evaluating the intended outcomes of the medication.
- Organize the equipment.

Safety Considerations

Patient-controlled analgesia is one way to deliver a small constant flow of pain medication. Medications to relieve pain may be given orally for mild to moderate pain, intramuscularly for longer duration of relief, and intravenously for acute, severe pain. They can also be titrated intravenously. Other routes include sublingual, rectal, transdermal, and spinal. The type of medication prescribed by the healthcare provider may be decided upon based on the intensity of pain and length of time required to have pain relief. These medications include over-the-counter nonopioid drugs, NSAIDS, opioids, and combinations of these drugs and dosages. Epidural pain management is often used to relieve pain during labor (also see Skill 14.8 for more information).

Procedure

1. Prior to performing the procedure, check healthcare provider's order, introduce self, and verify the patient's identity using two identifiers. Explain to the patient the purpose and operation of the PCA, why it is necessary, and how the patient can participate.
2. Perform hand hygiene and observe other appropriate infection control procedures.
3. Provide for patient privacy.
4. If not previously assessed, take baseline vital signs. If any of the findings are above or below the predetermined parameters, consult the healthcare provider before administering the medication.
5. Set up the PCA infusion line according to the manufacturer's instructions.
   - Attach needleless adapter to end of PCA tubing.
   - Prime the PCA tubing.
   - Clamp the tubing. **Rationale:** *This prevents accidental administration of a bolus dose and flushing of the primary line with the narcotic.*
   - Place the medication syringe in the PCA machine according to the operational instructions.
   - Two nurses should each verify patient's identification, the IV tubing set-up and medication/amount to infuse, and the PCA pump settings before starting PCA therapy.
6. Connect the PCA infusion line to the primary fluid line.
   - Cleanse injection port of primary IV with alcohol swab.
   - Connect the PCA tubing to the primary fluid line at the injection port closest to the patient.
7. Deliver the loading dose, as prescribed.
   - Set the pump for a lockout time of zero minutes.
   - Set the volume to be delivered based on calculated dosage volume for the loading dose.
   - Unclamp the tubing and inject the loading dose by pressing the loading dose control button.
8. Set the safety parameters for the infusion on the PCA pump according to the manufacturer's instructions. For example:
   - Dose volume limits. **Rationale:** *This will limit the amount of drug that the patient can receive when the patient pushes the control button.*

SKILL 3.5 Patient Controlled Analgesia (PCA) Pump: Using *(continued)*

- Lockout interval between each dose. The lockout interval is generally between 5–15 min. **Rationale:** *This sets the minimum time that must elapse before the patient can receive another dose of the drug. Lockout time is based on the usual onset of the IV narcotic and the assessment of the patient.*
- Dosage limit. Set the dosage limit (usually 1 or 4 hours) as specified on the orders. **Rationale:** *This is an additional safety feature to limit the amount of medication delivered.*

9. Lock the machine.
   - Close the door on the pump.
   - Look for any digital cues or alarms that may indicate the machine is not set, and make corrections as needed.
   - Lock the machine with the key or keypad code.
10. Begin the infusion.
    - Place the patient control button within reach.

CAUTION! The antidote naloxone (Narcan) is indicated for signs of opioid analgesic overdose, including pinpoint pupils, respiratory depression, bradycardia, and unresponsiveness.

---

11. Perform hand hygiene and leave the patient safe and comfortable.

12. Monitor the status of the patient every 2 hours during the first 24–36 hr of infusion and regularly thereafter, depending on the patient's health and facility protocol.
13. Monitor the infusion.
    - Observe the IV site for signs of infiltration and phlebitis.
    - Inspect the tubing for kinks that may occlude the line.
    - Note the total number of doses and milligrams received.
14. Complete documentation using forms, checklists, or electronic dropdown lists supplemented by nurse's notes or additional comments as appropriate. Record the initiation of PCA, the dose setting, the doses received, pain intensity, and all assessments. See facility protocol for specific guidelines.

SAMPLE DOCUMENTATION

[date] 0100 P-88, R-18, B/P 128/84; morphine 4 mg IV bolus loading dose by PCA pump as ordered, then PCA pump set for morphine drip of 2 mg/mL, patient's bolus dose—on demand, 2 mg every 20 min, lockout period—10 min, 4-hour limit—30 mg; will continue to monitor vital signs and pain scale self-report. *E. Knowles*

SKILL 3.6 Sleep Promotion: Assisting

Sleep is the body's time to refresh, restore, and prepare for the next day of activities. Adequate sleep time is important to mental and physical well-being and helps the brain to process information, learn, and remember. It can improve an individual's ability to tolerate pain by decreasing pain sensitivity. People with chronic and acute pain often lose sleep time, which can affect their daily routines. Helping patients in pain get a good night's sleep is important to their health and quality of life.

Delegation or Assignment

The nurse is responsible for assessing the patient's readiness to make changes in health behaviors to promote improved health and well-being. The nurse teaches, or coaches, the patient about integrative healthcare strategies focused on sleep-promoting relaxation. The UAP can then assist the patient in these activities to help the patient be comfortable and prepare for sleep. The nurse instructs the UAP to report patient observations to the nurse for follow-up. Assessment and evaluation of effectiveness of the exercise remain the responsibility of the nurse. Note that state laws for UAPs vary, so this task might be assigned to the UAP rather than delegated.

Equipment

- No equipment is required for sleep promotional relaxation activities.

Preparation

- Discuss sleep promotional relaxation activities with the patient during the day so patient will be ready to put them to practice at bedtime.

- At bedtime, allow 15–30 min to prepare the patient and environment to support sleep. Ensure that the environment is private, quiet, comfortable, dimly lit, and at a temperature that suits the patient. Ensure that the patient has an empty bladder. **Rationale:** *Interruptions or distractions interfere with the patient's ability to achieve full relaxation. Once patients learn how to use this technique, they will be able to do it in less than 5 minutes as part of self-care and ongoing stress management.*

Procedure

1. Introduce self to the patient and verify the patient's identity using two identifiers. Explain to the patient what you are going to do and how the patient can participate. Discuss how the results will be used in planning further care or treatments.
2. Perform hand hygiene and observe appropriate infection control procedures.
3. Provide for patient privacy.
4. Assist the patient to find a comfortable position.
5. Proceed with a teaching, or coaching, discussion with the patient about individual health promotion and wellness strategies including the importance of adequate sleep duration and quality to the mind and body.
6. When the discussion is completed, perform hand hygiene and leave the patient safe and comfortable.
7. Complete documentation using forms, checklists, or electronic dropdown lists supplemented by nurse's notes or additional comments as appropriate.

(continued on next page)

SKILL 3.6 Sleep Promotion: Assisting (*continued*)

Patient Teaching

To promote sleep, teach the patient to:

- Establish a regular bedtime and wake-up time for all days of the week to enhance biological rhythm. (A short daytime nap (e.g., 15–30 min), particularly among older adults, can be restorative and not interfere with nighttime sleep. A younger person with insomnia should not nap.)
- Establish a regular, relaxing bedtime routine before sleep such as reading, listening to soft music, taking a warm bath, or doing some other quiet activity you enjoy.
- Avoid dealing with office work or family problems before bedtime.
- Get adequate exercise during the day to reduce stress, but avoid excessive physical exertion at least 3 hours before bedtime.
- Use the bed for sleep or sexual activity, so that you associate it with sleep. Take work material, computers, and TVs out of the bedroom. Lying awake, tossing and turning, will strengthen the association between wakefulness and lying in bed (many people with insomnia report falling asleep in a chair or in front of the TV but having trouble falling asleep in bed).

- If unable to sleep, get out of bed, go into another room, and pursue some relaxing activity until you feel drowsy.
- Create an environment that is dark, quiet, comfortable, and cool. Keep noise to a minimum; block out extraneous noise as necessary with white noise from a fan, air conditioner, or white noise machine. Music is not recommended as studies have shown that music promotes wakefulness because it is interesting and people will pay attention to it.
- Sleep on a comfortable mattress and pillows.
- Avoid heavy meals 2–3 hours before bedtime.
- Avoid alcohol and caffeine-containing foods and beverages (e.g., coffee, tea, chocolate) at least 4 hours before bedtime. Caffeine can interfere with sleep. Both caffeine and alcohol act as diuretics, creating the need to void during sleep time.
- Use sleeping medications only as a last resort. Use OTC medications sparingly because many contain antihistamines that cause daytime drowsiness.
- Take analgesics before bedtime to relieve aches and pains.
- Consult healthcare provider about adjusting other medications that may cause insomnia.

SAMPLE DOCUMENTATION

[date] 2200 States unable to get to sleep because cast on right arm prevents him from lying on his side like he usually does; denies pain of right arm; right hand fingers pink, brisk capillary refill, able to move all fingers, denies tingling or numbness; positioned on left side with right arm supported with pillows; lights dimmed; door closed. *R. Smith*

2245 Deep breathing audible; remains on left side with right arm on pillows; sleeping at this time. *R. Smith*

EVIDENCE-BASED PRACTICE

Sleep Quality

Problem

Sleep loss because of acute and chronic pain affects millions of Americans. Pain interferes with how long people sleep and the quality of their sleep. Pain is a stressor that can lead to poor health. Sleep debt, or sleep deficit, occurs when someone does not get enough sleep. A large sleep deficit can lead to mental or physical fatigue. People without pain generally do not experience a sleep deficit.

Evidence

Results of a survey done by the National Sleep Foundation in 2015 showed that 21% reported chronic pain and 36% acute pain, for a total of 57% of Americans experiencing some form of pain; 43% reported being pain free. Of those with no pain, 65% reported good sleep quality, while only 45% of those with acute pain and 37% of those with chronic pain reported the same.

Sleep problems were reported to interfere with work by more than half the people with chronic pain, and only 23% of people without

pain. Those with pain also reported that lack of sleep interfered with mood, activities, relationships, and enjoyment of life, overall. Nearly 1 in 4 people with chronic pain reported being diagnosed with a sleep disorder by a healthcare provider, compared with 6% of all others.

Implications

Sleep quality and duration can be strong indicators of overall health and quality of life. A higher motivation to make getting enough sleep a priority was associated with longer sleep durations and better quality of sleep, even for those with pain. Having pain can result in sleeplessness, poor quality of sleep, and frequent awakenings during sleep. Insomnia can develop. The recommendation to promote sleep duration and improve the quality of sleep is to practice good sleep hygiene, such as limiting caffeine consumption, limiting alcohol intake, using sleep aid medications under supervision of a healthcare provider, and practicing relaxation techniques.

Source: Based on National Sleep Foundation. (2016). *Sleep Disorders Problems. Pain and Sleep*. Retrieved from https://sleepfoundation.org/sleep-disorders-problems/pain-and-sleep

Lifespan Considerations

CHILDREN

Learning to sleep alone without the parent's help is a skill that all children need to master. Regular bedtime routines and rituals such as reading a book help children learn this skill and can prevent sleep disturbance. Some sleep disturbances seen in children include the following:

- *Trained night feeder:* Infants who are fed during the night and fed until they fall asleep and then put into bed, or infants who have a bottle left with them in their bed learn to expect and demand middle-of-the-night feedings. Infants who are growing well do not need night feeding after about 4 months of age. Infants who are failing to thrive may need feeding at night.

SKILL 3.6 Sleep Promotion: Assisting (*continued*)

- *Sleep refusal:* Many toddlers and young children are resistant to settling down to sleep. This sleep refusal may be due to not being tired, anxiety about separation from the parent, stress (e.g., a recent move), lack of a regular sleep routine, the child's temperament, or changes in sleep arrangements (e.g., move from a crib to a "big" bed).

- *Night terrors:* Night terrors are partial awakenings from non-REM, stage III or IV sleep. They are usually seen in children 3–6 years of age. The child may sleepwalk or may sit up in bed screaming and thrashing about. They usually cannot be wakened, but they should be protected from injury, helped back to bed, and soothed back to sleep. Babysitters should be alerted to the possibility of a night terror occurring. Children do not remember the incident the next day, and there is no indication of a neurological or emotional problem. Excessive fatigue and a full bladder may contribute to the problem. Having the child take an afternoon nap and empty the bladder before going to sleep at night may be helpful.

ADULTS

- New jobs, pregnancy, and babies are common examples of situations that often disrupt the sleep of a young adult.

- The sleep patterns of middle-aged adults can be disrupted if they are taking care of older parents and/or chronically ill partners in the home.

OLDER ADULTS

The quality of sleep is often diminished in older adults. Some of the leading factors that often are influential in sleep disturbances include the following:

- Side effects of medications
- Gastroesophageal reflux disease
- Respiratory and circulatory disorders, which may cause breathing problems or discomfort
- Pain from arthritis, increased stiffness, or impaired immobility
- Nocturia
- Depression
- Loss of life partner and/or close friends
- Confusion related to delirium or dementia

>> Heat and Cold Application

Expected Outcomes

1. Bleeding and edema formation are minimized.
2. Patient reports decrease in pain.
3. Inflammatory response is enhanced.
4. Target core body temperature is achieved.
5. Patient has no adverse responses to therapy (arrhythmias, bleeding, shivering, after drop, or rebound hyperthermia).

Heat and cold are applied to the body to promote comfort and the repair and healing of tissues. The form of thermal application generally depends on its purpose. Cold applied to a body part draws heat from the area; heat, of course, warms the area. The application of heat or cold produces physiological changes in the temperature of the tissues, size of the blood vessels, capillary blood pressure, capillary surface area for exchange of fluids and electrolytes, and tissue metabolism. The duration of the application also affects the response. See **Table 3–3** for a summary of the physiological effects of heat and cold, **Table 3–4** >> for selected indications for the use of heat and cold, and **Table 3–5** >> for correct temperatures for heat and cold applications.

Variables Affecting Physiological Tolerance to Heat and Cold

- *Body part location:* The back of the hand and foot are not very temperature sensitive. In contrast, the inner aspect of the wrist and forearm, the neck, and the perineal area are temperature sensitive.

- *Size of the exposed body part:* The larger the area exposed to heat and cold is, the lower is the tolerance.

- *Individual tolerance:* The very young and the very old generally have the lowest tolerance. Individuals who have neurosensory impairments may have a high tolerance, but the risk of injury is greater.

- *Length of exposure:* People feel hot and cold applications most while the temperature is changing. After a period of time, tolerance increases.

- *Intactness of skin:* Injured skin areas are more sensitive to temperature variations.

Contraindications to the Use of Heat and Cold Therapies

Determine the presence of any conditions contraindicating the use of heat.

- *The first 24 hours after traumatic injury:* Heat increases bleeding and swelling.

TABLE 3–3 Physiological Effects of Heat and Cold

Heat	Cold
Vasodilation	Vasoconstriction
Increases capillary permeability	Decreases capillary permeability
Increases cellular metabolism	Decreases cellular metabolism
Increases inflammation	Slows bacterial growth, decreases inflammation
Sedative effect	Local anesthetic effect

- *Active hemorrhage:* Heat causes vasodilation and increases bleeding.
- *Noninflammatory edema:* Heat increases capillary permeability and edema.
- *Localized malignant tumor:* Because heat accelerates cell metabolism and cell growth and increases circulation, it may accelerate metastases (secondary tumors).
- *Skin disorder that causes redness or blisters:* Heat can burn or cause further damage to the skin.

Determine the presence of any conditions contraindicating the use of cold.

- *Open wounds:* Cold can increase tissue damage by decreasing blood flow to an open wound.
- *Impaired circulation:* Cold can further impair nourishment of the tissues and cause tissue damage. In patients with Raynaud disease, cold increases arterial spasm.
- *Allergy or hypersensitivity to cold:* Some patients have an allergy to cold that may be manifested by an inflammatory response, for example, erythema, hives, swelling, joint pain,

and occasional muscle spasm. Some react with a sudden increase in blood pressure, which can be hazardous if the person is hypertensive.

Determine the presence of any conditions indicating the need for special precautions during heat and cold therapy.

- *Neurosensory impairment:* Individuals with sensory impairments are unable to perceive that heat is damaging the tissues and are at risk for burns, or they are unable to perceive discomfort from cold and are unable to prevent tissue injury.
- *Impaired mental status:* Individuals who are confused or have an altered level of consciousness need monitoring and supervision during applications to ensure safe therapy.
- *Impaired circulation:* Individuals with peripheral vascular disease, diabetes, or congestive heart failure lack the normal ability to dissipate heat via the blood circulation, which puts them at risk for tissue damage with heat applications. Cold applications are contraindicated for these people.
- *Open wounds:* Tissues around an open wound are more sensitive to heat and cold.

TABLE 3–4 Selected Indications for the Use of Heat and Cold

Indication	Effect of Heat	Effect of Cold
Muscle spasm	Relaxes muscles and increases their contractility	Relaxes muscles and decreases their contractility
Inflammation	Increases blood flow, softens exudates	Decreases capillary permeability and blood flow through vasoconstriction, slows cellular metabolism
Pain	Relieves pain, possibly by promoting muscle relaxation, increasing circulation, and promoting psychological relaxation and a feeling of comfort; acts as a counterirritant	Decreases pain by slowing nerve conduction rate and blocking nerve impulses; produces numbness, acts as a counterirritant, increases pain threshold
Joint contracture	Reduces contracture and increases joint range of motion by allowing greater distention of muscles and connective tissue	
Joint stiffness	Reduces joint stiffness by decreasing viscosity of synovial fluid and increasing tissue's capability of being distended or stretched	
Traumatic injury		Decreases bleeding by constricting blood vessels; decreases edema by reducing capillary permeability

TABLE 3–5 Temperatures for Hot and Cold Applications

Description	Temperature	Application
Very cold	Below 15°C (59°F)	Ice bags
Cold	15°C–18.3°C (59°F–65°F)	Cold pack
Cool	18.3°C–26.7°C (65°F–80°F)	Cold compresses
Tepid	26.7°C–36.7°C (80°F–98°F)	Alcohol sponge bath
Warm	36.7°C–40°C (98°F–104°F)	Warm bath, aquathermia pads
Hot	40°C–46.1°C (104°F–115°F)	Hot soak, irrigations, hot compresses
Very hot	Above 46.1°C (above 115°F)	Hot water bags for adults

SKILL 3.7 Cooling Blanket: Applying

A cooling blanket lowers body temperature by cold transferring from the blanket to the patient. (The blanket temperature can be changed to raise or lower the patient's temperature.) There are many uses for a cooling blanket related to reversing hyperthermia. They can be used to lower the patient's body temperature as a comfort measure when patients have a prolonged high fever from infection. They can also be used to

treat high temperature side effects of malignant hyperthermia, from anesthesia.

Delegation or Assignment

Setting up the cooling blanket can be delegated or assigned to the UAP. The nurse gives the UAP any instructions specific to the patient or procedure. When the cooling blanket is ready,

SKILL 3.7 Cooling Blanket: Applying (continued)

the nurse will verify the temperature setting and assign the UAP time intervals to monitor the patient's vital signs. The nurse remains responsible for the assessment, interpretation of abnormal findings, and determination of appropriate responses. Note that state laws for UAPs vary, so this task might be assigned to the UAP rather than delegated.

Equipment

- Thermal (heating/cooling) unit
- Sterile or distilled water
- Low-reading (below 34.4°C [94°F]) thermometer: rectal probe and lubricant, esophageal probe, urinary retention catheter, or pulmonary artery catheter with cable and module for continuous core temperature monitoring, depending on thermometer used
- Clean gloves
- Disposable thermal (cooling) blanket
- One sheet or thin blanket
- Covering for patient
- Four towels to wrap patient's lower arms and legs
- Tape
- Lower extremity (or foot) compression wraps
- Sphygmomanometer and stethoscope or automated BP monitoring equipment
- Continuous ECG monitoring (if indicated)
- Supplemental oxygen therapy as healthcare provider orders

Preparation

- Check healthcare provider's orders for desired patient temperature.
- Identify medications patient has received (narcotic, sedative).
- Gather equipment and take to patient's room.
- Connect power cord to grounded outlet.
- Ensure that reservoir (sterile or distilled water) level is adequate.
- Obtain baseline vital signs.

Procedure

1. Introduce self to patient and verify the patient's identity using two identifiers. Explain to the patient what you are going to do, why it is necessary, and how the patient can participate. Discuss how the results will be used in planning further care or treatments.
2. Perform hand hygiene and observe appropriate infection control procedures.
3. Provide for patient privacy.
4. Place the cooling blanket on the bed ❶, and connect it to the temperature control unit machine. **Rationale:** *The cooling blanket increases heat transfer from the patient and reduces body temperature by conduction.*
   - Push the tubing tab to insert male tubing connector of the cooling pad into inlet opening. Release the tab.
   - Repeat connection using the outlet opening.
   - Turn the unit ON by pushing the power switch ❷.
   - Enter patient's target temperature set point.
5. Place a sheet or a thin bath blanket over the cooling blanket.
6. Place patient on the cooling blanket.

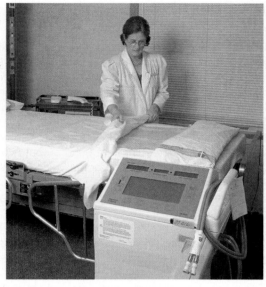

Source: Ronald May/Pearson Education, Inc.

❶ Disposable cooling blanket is covered by a sheet to protect the patient's skin.

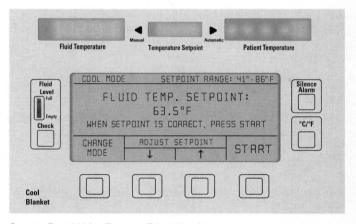

Source: Ronald May/Pearson Education, Inc.

❷ Set fluid temperature to ordered set point, and press START.

7. Apply leg or foot compression wraps. **Rationale:** *This helps to prevent thrombus formation and reduces edema.*
8. Wrap the patient's lower arms and hands and lower legs and feet (and scrotum if indicated) in towels and tape to secure. **Rationale:** *This prevents stimulation of skin thermoreceptors that initiate shivering.*
9. Establish continuous core temperature monitoring.
10. Set the master temperature control to either automatic or manual operation. **Rationale:** *There are two separate temperature controls, one for automatic and one for manual operation.*

(continued on next page)

SKILL 3.7 Cooling Blanket: Applying (continued)

AUTOMATIC CONTROL

- Don clean gloves.
- If using rectal thermometer probe, digitally examine patient's rectum to determine it is empty of stool. **Rationale:** *Rectal temperature probe must make contact with mucosa.*
- Insert lubricated temperature probe into patient's rectum 5 cm (2 in.).
- If using bladder retention catheter with integrated temperature probe, determine that urine output is at least 20 mL/hr. **Rationale:** *Probe actually measures urine temperature.*
- Set temperature control at the desired temperature (fluid temperature set point).
- Turn automatic mode light on and press "START." **Rationale:** *The pad fluid temperature will adjust automatically to bring patient's temperature to a selected set point.*
- Check that the pad temperature limits are set as ordered and proceed to step 11 below.

or

MANUAL CONTROL

- Observe that the *manual* mode light is on.
- Monitor the fluid set point, which indicates the temperature of pad. **Rationale:** *This ensures pad temperature is maintained at desired level.*

11. Set the temperature control to 37°C (98.6°F), and begin lowering temperature 1°C (1.8°F) every 30 minutes to 1 hour as tolerated to prevent shivering, until 33°C or 34°C (91.4°F or 93.2°F) or set temperature is reached. **Rationale:** *Blanket will cool patient to set temperature independent of patient's temperature. Gradual cooling helps prevent shivering.*
12. Monitor patient's temperature. **Rationale:** *This prevents excessive cooling.*
13. Assess patient every 15 minutes for early signs of shivering: ECG muscle tremor artifact, jaw line "hum," or trapezius muscle tension.
14. If early signs of shivering occur, discontinue therapy and notify healthcare provider or refer to facility hypothermia protocol. **Rationale:** *Shivering causes an increase in core temperature, thus defeating the purpose of treatment. Shivering imposes a heavy metabolic burden and increases oxygen demand.*

Mild	32°C–37°C	(89.6°F–98.6°F)
Moderate	28°C–32°C	(82.4°F–89.6°F)
Severe	20°C–28°C	(68°F–82.4°F)

15. Monitor vital signs every 15–30 min during therapy. **Rationale:** *Bradycardia may occur. Blood pressure usually remains elevated due to vasoconstriction.*
16. Monitor ECG for possible arrhythmias. **Rationale:** *Potassium shifts into cells with induced hypothermia.*
17. Monitor patient's serum glucose. **Rationale:** *Insulin levels are decreased with induced hypothermia. Glucose levels may rise with shivering.* An insulin drip may be necessary to maintain glucose at 80–130 mg/dL.
18. Turn and deep-breathe patient every 1–2 hr. **Rationale:** *Hypothermia reduces carbon dioxide production with possible resultant hypoventilation.*
19. Monitor patient's skin condition and bony prominences every 2 hours. **Rationale:** *Patient is at risk for pressure ulcers when skin temperature is lowered.*
20. Turn off unit when patient's temperature is 1°C–3°C (1.8F–5.4°F) above desired temperature. **Rationale:** *Cooling will continue upon discontinuation of therapy.*
21. Monitor vital signs every 15 minutes during rewarming.
22. Observe for edema. **Rationale:** *Hypothermia causes fluid shift into the interstitium.*
23. Clean and return reusable equipment to appropriate area and dispose of blanket.
24. Monitor patient's vital signs frequently after discontinuation of treatment. **Rationale:** *Overshoot hypothermia may occur.*
25. Keep patient safe and comfortable.
26. When the procedure is complete, perform hand hygiene and leave patient safe and comfortable.
27. Complete documentation using forms, checklists, or electronic dropdown lists supplemented by nurse's notes or additional comments as appropriate.

SAMPLE DOCUMENTATION

[date] 1325 67-year-old female admitted with hyperthermia, T-40.2°C (104.3°F) (R), P-92, R – 20, B/P 164/92; confused to identify time and place, mumbling, thrashing arms about; skin hot to touch and dry; placed on insulated cooling blanket set at 37°C (98.6°F), rectal probe positioned without incident. *T. Jetta*

SKILL 3.8 Dry Cold: Applying

Application of cold therapy slows circulation which slows down blood flow to an injury resulting in less pain and swelling of the area. Intermittent cold application also reduces local inflammation, muscle spasm, and pain. Cold can be applied with an ice pack, gel pack, or disposable cold pack. The cold device should be covered with a washcloth or thin towel and never be applied directly to skin.

Delegation or Assignment

Application of certain cold measures (e.g., cooling baths) may be delegated or assigned to the UAP. The nurse gives the UAP any instructions specific to the patient or procedure. Assessment of the patient and the determination that the measure is safe to employ are the responsibility of the nurse. The UAP may observe

SKILL 3.8 Dry Cold: Applying (*continued*)

the area being treated during usual care and must report abnormal findings to the nurse. Abnormal findings must be validated and interpreted by the nurse. Note that state laws for UAPs vary, so this task might be assigned to the UAP rather than delegated.

Equipment

- Ice bag, collar, glove, or cold pack ❶
- Ice chips
- Protective covering
- Roller gauze, a binder or a towel, and tape
- Countdown timer device

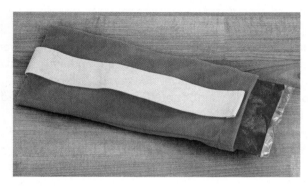

Source: Sasimoto/Shutterstock.

❶ A commercial chemical cold pack.

Preparation

- Check healthcare provider's orders for cold therapy.
- Test all equipment for proper functioning and integrity (lack of leaks) before taking it to the patient if possible.
- Know the reason why the patient is receiving cold therapy, contraindications, usual response, complications, and nursing considerations for applying the cold therapy.
- Gather equipment and supplies and go to patient's room.

Procedure

1. Prior to performing the procedure, introduce self and verify the patient's identity using two identifiers. Explain to the patient what you are going to do, why it is necessary, and how the patient can participate. Discuss how the results will be used in planning further care or treatments.
2. Perform hand hygiene and observe other appropriate infection control procedures.
3. Provide for patient privacy. Expose only the area to be treated, and provide warmth to avoid chilling.
4. Assist the patient to a comfortable position, and support the body part requiring the application.
5. Set the countdown timer for amount of time for cold application. Apply the cold measure.

ICE BAG, COLLAR, OR GLOVE

- Fill the device one half to two thirds full of crushed ice. **Rationale:** *Partial filling makes the device more pliable so that it can be molded to a body part.*

- Remove excess air by bending or twisting the device. **Rationale:** *Air inflates the device so that it cannot be molded to the body part.*
- Insert the stopper securely into an ice bag or collar, or tie a knot at the open end of a glove. **Rationale:** *This prevents leakage of fluid when the ice melts.*
- Hold the device upside down, and check it for leaks.
- Cover the device with a soft cloth cover, if it is not already equipped with one. **Rationale:** *The cover absorbs moisture that condenses on the outside of the device. It is also more comfortable for the patient.*
- Hold the device in place with roller gauze, ties, a binder, or a towel. Secure with tape as necessary. ❷

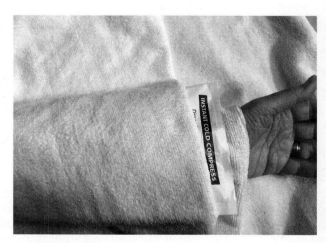

Source: Ronald May/Pearson Education, Inc.

❷ Wrap towel or gauze roll around cold pack to secure it.

Safety Considerations

Never apply a fully cooled reusable cold pack directly to the skin; also, do not over-insulate the area.

Bony areas (knee, ankle, elbow) usually require half the treatment time that fatty areas require. Superficial nerves at these joint sites are especially vulnerable to cold-induced neuropathy, especially if cold is combined with compression.

Crushable chemical packs should be used as the last resort because they are not as cold nor do they last as long as crushed ice.

Do not apply an instant chemical pack to the face and never use pins to secure pack. Leakage of chemical contents can cause serious injury. If skin is exposed to contents, immediately flush skin with copious amounts of water and notify healthcare provider.

- Frozen gel packs and crushed ice packs using ice frozen in a refrigerator or freezer (−16.1°C to −18.8°C [3°F to −2°F]) should not be applied directly to the skin.
- Packs with ice from an ice machine (−1.1°C [30°F]) do not require insulation.
- During cryotherapy, erythema will occur.
- The patient will experience four stages of cold progression: cold/stinging/burning/numbness.
- Discontinue therapy upon numbness and proceed to step 9 below.

(*continued on next page*)

SKILL 3.8 Dry Cold: Applying (continued)

or

DISPOSABLE COLD PACK

- Strike, squeeze, or knead the cold pack according to the manufacturer's instructions (see ①). **Rationale:** *The action activates the chemical reaction that produces the cold.*
- Cover with a soft cloth cover if the pack does not have a cover. Most commercially prepared cold packs have soft outer coverings to permit application directly to the body part.

6. Instruct the patient as follows:
   - Remain in position for the duration of the treatment.
   - Call the nurse if discomfort is felt.
7. Monitor the patient during the application.
   - Assess the patient in terms of comfort and skin reaction (e.g., pallor, mottled appearance) as frequently as necessary for the patient's safety (e.g., every 5–10 min). Check more often if patient has had previous negative responses to applications and or patient has difficulty reporting problems.
   - Report untoward reactions and remove the application.

8. Leave the cold in place for only the designated period of time using the countdown timer device. **Rationale:** *Avoid the rebound phenomenon and the harmful effects of prolonged cold.*
9. Remove the cold measure and assist patient to comfortable position. Clean area, empty water and ice from cold devices.
10. Perform hand hygiene. Leave patient safe and comfortable.
11. Complete documentation using forms, checklists, or electronic dropdown lists supplemented by nurse's notes or additional comments as appropriate, including the application of the cold measure and the patient's response.

SAMPLE DOCUMENTATION

[date] 2245 Right foot and ankle swollen toes to lower calf; Reports pain is 7/10; Moves toes and ankle, pedal pulses present. Skin warm, no bruising (skin discoloration) or wounds noted. Padded ice pack applied ×10 minutes. Reports pain 5/10. *P. Wilder*

SKILL 3.9 Dry Heat: Applying

Application of heat therapy increases circulation which opens up blood vessels that can reduce pain in joints and relax muscles, ligaments, and tendons. Intermittent heat application also reduces muscle spasm and can increase ease of movement. Heat can be applied with a heating pad, gel pack, or disposable heat pack. The heat device should be covered with a washcloth or thin towel and never be applied directly to skin.

Delegation or Assignment

Application of certain heat measures (e.g., baths) may be delegated or assigned to the UAP. Assessment of the patient and the determination that the measure is safe to employ are the responsibility of the nurse. The UAP may observe the area being treated during usual care and must report abnormal findings to the nurse. Abnormal findings must be validated and interpreted by the nurse. Note that state laws for UAPs vary, so this task might be assigned to the UAP rather than delegated.

Equipment

- Hot water bottle (bag) ①
  - Hot water bottle with a stopper
  - Cover
- Electric heating pad
  - Electric pad and control
  - Cover (waterproof if there will be moisture under the pad when it is applied)
  - Gauze ties (optional)
- Aquathermia pad ②
  - Pad
  - Distilled water
  - Control unit

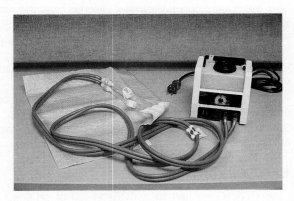

① Hot water bottle and cloth covers.

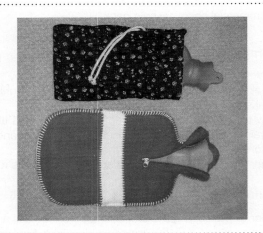

② An aquathermia heating unit and pad.

SKILL 3.9 Dry Heat: Applying (*continued*)

- Cover
- Gauze ties or tape (optional)
- One or two commercially prepared disposable hot packs
- Countdown timer

Preparation

- Check healthcare provider's orders about heat treatment.
- Test all equipment if possible for proper functioning and integrity (lack of leaks) before taking it to the patient.
- Know the reason why the patient is receiving heat therapy, contraindications, usual response, complications, and nursing considerations for applying the heat therapy.
- Gather equipment and supplies and go to patient's room.

Procedure

1. Prior to performing the procedure, introduce self and verify the patient's identity using two identifiers. Explain to the patient what you are going to do, why it is necessary, and how the patient can participate. Discuss how the results will be used in planning further care or treatments.
2. Perform hand hygiene and observe other appropriate infection control procedures.
3. Provide for patient privacy.
   - Expose only the area to be treated.
4. Set the countdown timer for amount of time for heat application. Apply the heat device.

HOT WATER BOTTLE

(Most commonly used in the home setting)

- Follow recommended practice for the appropriate temperature of the water.
- Fill the hot water bottle about two thirds full.
- Expel the air from the bottle. **Rationale:** *Air remaining in the bottle prevents it from molding to the body part being treated.*
- Secure the stopper tightly.
- Hold the bottle upside down, and check for leaks.
- Dry the bottle.
- Wrap the bottle in a towel or hot water bottle cover (see ❶).
- Apply the bottle to the body part using pillows to support it if necessary and proceed to step 5 below.

ELECTRIC HEATING PAD

(Most commonly used in the home setting)

- Ensure that the body area is dry. **Rationale:** *Electricity in the presence of moisture can conduct a shock.*
- Check that the electric pad is functioning properly. The cord should be free from cracks, wires should be intact, heating components should not be exposed, and temperature distribution over the pad should be even.
- Place the cover on the pad. Some models have waterproof covers to be used when the pad is placed over a moist dressing. **Rationale:** *Moisture could cause the pad to short circuit and burn or shock the patient.*
- Plug the pad into the electric socket.
- Set the control dial for the correct temperature.
- After the pad has heated, place the pad over the body part to which heat is being applied.

- Use gauze ties instead of safety pins to hold the pad in place, if needed, and proceed to step 5 below. **Rationale:** *A pin might strike a wire, damaging the pad and giving an electric shock to the patient.*

AQUATHERMIA PAD (ALSO CALLED A K-PAD)

- Fill the unit with distilled water until it is two thirds full (see ❷). The unit will warm the water, which circulates through the pad.
- Secure the lid.
- Regulate the temperature with the key if it has not been preset. Normal temperature is 40°C–46.1°C (104°F–115°F). Check the manufacturer's instructions.
- Cover the pad with a towel or pillowcase.
- Plug in the unit.
- Check for any leak or malfunctions of the pad before use.
- Use tape or gauze ties to hold the pad in place. Never use safety pins. They can cause leakage. Proceed to step 5 below.
- If unusual redness or pain occurs at this point, discontinue the treatment, and report the patient's reaction.

DISPOSABLE HOT PACK

- Microwave, strike, squeeze, or knead the pack according to the manufacturer's directions.
- Note the manufacturer's instructions about the length of time that heat is produced.
- Depending on the type of pack, wrap in a towel or enclose in a cover prior to application.
5. Give the patient the following instructions:
   - Do not insert any sharp, pointed object (e.g., a pin) into the bottle, pack, or pad.
   - Do not lie directly on the bottle or pad. **Rationale:** *The surface below the object promotes heat absorption instead of normal heat dissipation.*
   - To prevent injury, avoid adjusting the heat higher than specified. **Rationale:** *The degree of heat felt shortly after application will decrease, because the body's temperature receptors quickly adapt to the temperature. This adaptive mechanism can lead to tissue injury if the temperature is adjusted higher.*
   - Call the nurse if any discomfort is felt.
6. Leave the heat in place for only the designated time to avoid the rebound phenomenon, usually 30 minutes using the countdown timer device. Check the application and skin area after 5–10 min to be sure the skin is intact.
7. When the procedure is complete, perform hand hygiene and leave the patient safe and comfortable.
8. Complete documentation using forms, checklists, or electronic dropdown lists supplemented by nurse's notes or additional comments as appropriate.

SAMPLE DOCUMENTATION

[date] 1400 Insulated K-pad placed over left forearm at 40°C (104°F) for 15 minutes per order; states the heat feels good on her arm; tolerated without incident. *M. Goodman*

(*continued on next page*)

SKILL 3.9 Dry Heat: Applying (*continued*)

Safety Considerations

Heat transfers more quickly than cold therapy. Do not allow the patient to lie on a "constant heat source" such as a heating pad or aquathermia pad.

Contraindications to heat therapies include acute injury or inflammation, recent or potential hemorrhage, deep venous thrombophle-bitis, impaired circulation, impaired sensation, and impaired mentation.

When treating an area where skin is not intact, cover the lesion with sterile gauze and insulating barrier before applying heat.

Do not apply heat to an edematous area until the reason for edema has been determined.

SKILL 3.10 Moist Pack and Tepid Sponges: Applying

Moist packs can be cold or warm temperature depending on the reason for the moist pack. Dry heat therapy is easy and convenient to use, but it may dry the skin. Moist heat penetrates more deeply and is better for patients with aging or dry skin. Cold compresses, evaporating lotion, and ice to suck on are types of moist cold. Some types of moist heat are warm soaks and warm compresses. Tepid hydrotherapy uses water for pain relief and treatment such as a whirlpool bath, a soak, or underwater massage.

Delegation or Assignment

Application of unsterile compresses or packs may be delegated or assigned to the UAP. Assessment of the patient and the determination that the measure is safe to employ are the responsibility of the nurse. The UAP may observe the area being treated during usual care and must report abnormal findings to the nurse. Abnormal findings must be validated and interpreted by the nurse. Note that state laws for UAPs vary, so this task might be assigned to the UAP rather than delegated.

Equipment

Use sterile equipment and supplies for an open wound.
 Clean gloves (sterile gloves as appropriate)

Compress

- Disposable gloves or sterile gloves (for an open wound)
- Solution at the strength and temperature specified by the healthcare provider or the facility
- Container for the solution
- Thermometer
- Gauze squares
- Cotton applicator sticks
- Petroleum jelly
- Insulating towel
- Plastic wrap
- Ties (e.g., roller gauze or masking tape)
- Hot water bottle or aquathermia pad (optional)

or

- Ice bag (optional)
- Sterile dressing, if required

Moist Pack

- Clean gloves
- Flannel pieces or towel packs
- Hot-pack machine for heating the packs

or

- Basin of water with some ice chips
- Cotton applicator sticks
- Petroleum jelly
- Insulating material (e.g., flannel or towels)
- Plastic wrap
- Hot water bottle (optional)

or

- Ice bag (optional)
- Sterile dressing, if required

Tepid Sponges

- Water or other coolant at prescribed temperature
- Basin or tub
- Washcloth and towels
- Bath blanket
- Electric fan
- Automated blood pressure unit
- Core temperature thermometer, cable, and module to monitor

Preparation

- Check healthcare provider's orders for type of cold or heat application.
- If possible, perform care so that the application of the compress, pack, or tepid sponges will not need to be interrupted for other activities such as toileting.
- Know the reason why the patient is receiving the cold or heat therapy, contraindications, usual response, complications, and nursing considerations for its application.
- Gather equipment and supplies and go to patient's room.

Procedure

1. Prior to performing the procedure, introduce self and verify the patient's identity using two identifiers. Explain to the patient what you are going to do, why it is necessary, and how the patient can participate. Discuss how the results will be used in planning further care or treatments.
2. Perform hand hygiene and observe other appropriate infection control procedures.
3. Provide for patient privacy.
   - Expose only the area to be treated.

SKILL 3.10 Moist Pack and Tepid Sponges: Applying (*continued*)

MOIST PACKS

4. Assist the patient to a comfortable position.
5. Expose the area for the compress or pack.
6. Provide support for the body part requiring the compress or pack.
   - If indicated, apply clean gloves, and remove the wound dressing. Remove and discard gloves. Perform hand hygiene. Don gloves.
7. Moisten the compress or the pack.
   - Place the gauze in the solution and proceed to step 8 below.
   or
   - Heat the flannel or towel in a steamer, or chill it in the basin of water and ice chips.
8. Protect the surrounding skin as indicated.
9. If a wound is exposed, using a cotton applicator stick apply petroleum jelly to the skin surrounding the wound, not on the wound or open areas of the skin. **Rationale:** *Jelly protects the skin from possible burns, maceration, and the irritating effects of some solutions.*
10. Apply the moist compress or pack. Set the countdown timer for amount of time for application.
    - Wring out the gauze compress so that the solution does not drip from it. For a sterile compress, use sterile forceps or sterile gloves to wring out the gauze.
    - Apply the gauze lightly and gradually to the designated area and, if tolerated by the patient, mold the compress close to the body then proceed to step 8 below. **Rationale:** *Air is a poor conductor of cold or heat, and molding excludes air.*
    or
    - Wring out the flannel (for a sterile pack, use sterile gloves).
    - Apply the flannel to the body area, molding it closely to the body part.
11. Immediately insulate and secure the application.
12. Cover the gauze or flannel quickly with a dry towel ❶ and a piece of plastic wrap. **Rationale:** *This step helps maintain the temperature of the application and thus its effectiveness.*

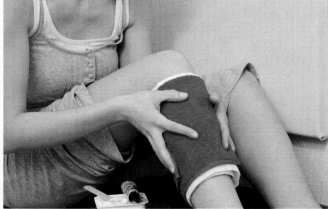

Source: Allesalltag/Alamy Stock Photo

❶ A towel wrapped around moist compress.

13. Secure the compress or pack in place with gauze ties or tape.
14. *Optional:* Apply a hot water bottle, aquathermia pad, or ice bag over the plastic wrap to maintain the heat or cold.
15. Monitor the patient.
    - Assess the patient for discomfort at 5- to 10-minute intervals. If the patient feels any discomfort, assess the area for erythema, numbness, maceration, or blistering.
    - For applications to large areas of the body, note any change in the pulse, respirations, and blood pressure.
    - In the event of unexpected reactions, terminate the treatment and report to the nurse in charge.
16. Remove the compress or pack at the specified time using the countdown timer device.
    - Compresses and packs with an external heat or cold source on top may remain in place 1–2 hr. Without external heat or cold, they need to be changed every few minutes.
    - Apply a sterile dressing if one is required. Proceed to step 17 below.

TEPID SPONGES, SOAKS

Procedure

4. Establish continuous core monitoring (rectal, esophageal, bladder, or pulmonary artery), if indicated.
5. Establish ongoing blood pressure and cardiac monitoring.
6. Monitor skin color and vital signs every 15–30 min during cooling. Immerse washcloths or material for sponging in ordered solution, generally 21.1°C–27.2°C (70°F–81°F). **Rationale:** *Cool application reduces heat by conduction.*
7. Wring out excess solution and place cloths on neck, axillae, groin. **Rationale:** *The vascularity of these areas promotes cooling.*
8. Depending on type of bath, change cloths every 5 minutes. **Rationale:** *This prevents cloths from warming and losing effectiveness.*

CAUTION! Do not immerse the patient in cold or ice slush. Resulting peripheral vasoconstriction will impair body cooling and induce shivering, which produces heat.

---

9. Cool the ambient temperature to 20°C–22.2°C (68°F–72°F). **Rationale:** *This enhances therapy by convection and evaporation.*
10. Direct a warm fan onto patient to promote evaporation. **Rationale:** *This enhances cooling by evaporation.*
11. Assess patient for early signs of shivering (ECG tremor artifact, palpable jaw line "hum," or trapezius muscle tension).
12. Stop treatment if patient has early signs of shivering and notify healthcare provider. **Rationale:** *Shivering raises core temperature, defeating purpose of cooling intervention.* The healthcare provider may order a narcotic or benzodiazepine for sedation.

(*continued on next page*)

SKILL 3.10 Moist Pack and Tepid Sponges: Applying (*continued*)

13. Monitor patient's temperature frequently. When temperature has decreased to the desired level, dry skin and replace light covering over patient; reposition for comfort. **Rationale:** *A thin patient will cool faster than one with more subcutaneous fat.*
14. Continue to monitor vital signs, cardiac rhythm, I&O, and electrolytes.
15. Provide fluids and a high-calorie diet. **Rationale:** *Increased temperatures increase metabolic rate.*
16. Place clothes in linen hamper and return equipment to utility or storage area.
17. When the procedure is complete, perform hand hygiene and leave patient safe and comfortable.
18. Complete documentation using forms, checklists, or electronic dropdown lists supplemented by nurse's notes or additional comments as appropriate, including the compress or pack and the patient's response.

SAMPLE DOCUMENTATION

[date] 0430 T-39°C (102.2°F) (O), P-92 bpm, R-22/min, B/P 142/88 mmHg; awake and alert, skin flushed, warm and dry; states he feels hot; bedspread removed, sheet left in place, thermostat lowered; cool washcloths placed on neck, axillae, and groin, refreshed in cool water every 15 minutes; vital signs monitored and sensorium. Tolerating cool compresses without complaint. *P. Hayes*

0530 T-38.6°C (O), P-88 bpm, R-20/min, B/P 136/84 mmHg. *P. Hayes*

SKILL 3.11 Neonatal Incubator and Infant Radiant Warmer: Using

Newborns can sometimes have trouble maintaining their temperatures in the normal range. Incubators and radiant warmers are used to maintain the body temperature of newborns resulting in less heat lost by the baby during cellular metabolic reactions. Skin temperature as well as air temperature can be controlled to maintain the baby's body temperature and lessen body heat loss.

Delegation or Assignment

Setting up the neonatal incubator/infant radiant warmer can be delegated or assigned to the UAP. The nurse gives the UAP any instructions specific to the patient or procedure. When the incubator or warmer is ready, the nurse will verify temperature settings. The nurse can request the UAP to report patient observations to the nurse for follow-up. The nurse remains responsible for the assessment, interpretation of abnormal findings, and determination of appropriate responses.

Equipment

- Radiant warmer with skin probe and temperature gel patch to secure probe to newborn's skin ① ②
- Bedding and positioning aids appropriate for bed and newborn

Preparation

- Check healthcare provider's order. Follow manufacturer's operating instructions for safety. (Several different radiant warmers/infant care centers are available.)
- Check caster locks to make certain that each is in locked position.
- Adjust bed to desired position.
- Plug cord into three-prong receptacle.
- Turn power switch on; bed will take approximately 30 seconds to power up.

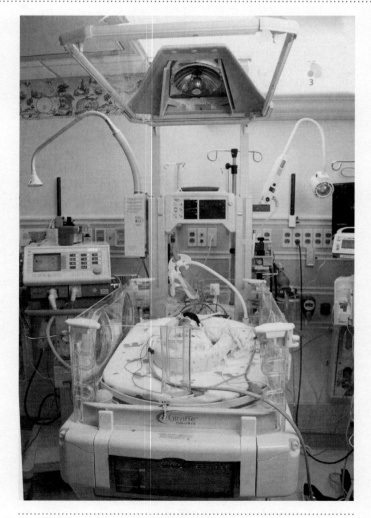

① Giraffe bed in radiant warmer mode, offering quick and easy access to the critically ill neonate.

SKILL 3.11 Neonatal Incubator and Infant Radiant Warmer: Using *(continued)*

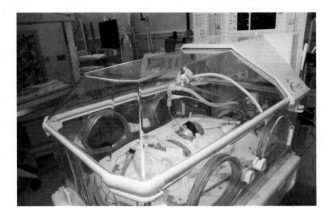

❷ Giraffe bed in incubator mode, offering a quiet, neutral thermal environment.

- Set bed to manual control mode for desired temperature. **Rationale:** *This allows bed to warm up prior to placing baby on bed.*

Procedure

1. Introduce self to parent if present and verify the patient's identity using two identifiers. Explain to the parent if present what you are going to do, why it is necessary, and how the patient can participate. Discuss how the results will be used in planning further care or treatments.
2. Perform hand hygiene and observe appropriate infection control procedures.
3. Plug temperature probe into bed. **Rationale:** *To obtain a digital recording of the baby's skin temperature.*
4. Place newborn on bed, then set bed to skin control mode.
5. Attach skin probe with polished surface over a location of fatty tissue on baby's body, avoiding any bony prominence.

6. Attach temperature gel patch to secure probe to newborn's skin; do not use adhesive tape. **Rationale:** *To prevent skin irritation. The baby's skin is very thin and fragile.*
7. Allow 3–5 min for probe to reach newborn's temperature.

CAUTION! For safety, protect the newborn's eyes with eye covers to prevent harm from prolonged exposure to the light from the lamp in the warmer unit.

---

8. Monitor placement of skin probe:
   - Validate appropriate skin temperature reading. **Rationale:** *If reading is not at desired temperature, probe may need to be repositioned.*
   - Inspect newborn's skin under probe at regular intervals. **Rationale:** *A baby's skin is delicate and irritates easily.*
   - Change probe location if irritation begins to appear.
9. Maintain safety and comfort measures for the patient.
10. Perform hand hygiene.
11. Complete documentation using forms, checklists, or electronic dropdown lists supplemented by nurse's notes or additional comments as appropriate.

SAMPLE DOCUMENTATION

[date] 2100 Radiant warmer turned on to pre-warm linen and mattress. T-36°C (96.8°F) (R), P-168 bpm, R-38/min; warmer temperature setting on medium per order; newborn placed supine in warmer, temperature skin probe applied right upper abdomen; cap, top, and socks applied. *G. Potter*

SKILL 3.12 Sitz Bath: Assisting

A sitz bath, or hip bath, is a warm shallow bath the patient sits in to ease pain, soreness, burning, or inflammation of the anus or vaginal areas caused by hemorrhoids, prostate, or vaginal infections, or uterine cramps.

Delegation or Assignment

Providing a sitz bath can be delegated or assigned to the UAP. The nurse remains responsible for assessment, interpretation of abnormal findings, and determination of appropriate responses.

Equipment

- Disposable sitz bath with tubing and bag ❶
- Warm water (40°C–42.7°C [104°F–109°F]) *Note:* Cold temperature may be indicated for patient's situation.
- Towels for drying
- Clean gloves
- Countdown timer device

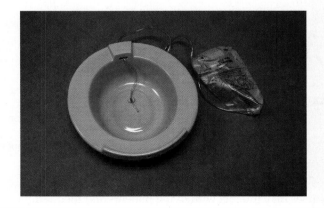

❶ Individual disposable sitz bath units are used for infection control purposes.

(continued on next page)

SKILL 3.12 Sitz Bath: Assisting (*continued*)

Preparation

- Verify healthcare provider's order for sitz bath, duration, and frequency of treatments.
- Raise toilet seat and place sitz bath basin with "FRONT" facing the front of the toilet bowl.
- Fill basin with warm water (40°C–42.7°C [104°F–109°F]) one half to two thirds full.
- Close flow tubing clamp.
- Open top of plastic bag and fill with hot water (40°C–42.7°C [104°F–109°F]).
- Hang bag at a level higher than the sitz basin so that fluid will flow by gravity.
- Insert tubing through front or rear entry hole in sitz bath, then snap or secure tubing into channel or "eye" in bottom of basin.

Procedure

1. Introduce self to patient and verify the patient's identity using two identifiers. Explain to the patient what you are going to do, why it is necessary, and how the patient can participate. Discuss how the results will be used in planning further care or treatments.
2. Perform hand hygiene and observe appropriate infection control procedures.
3. Assist patient to treatment area with accessible call bell.
4. Provide privacy by placing sign on door.
5. Check to ensure that temperature of thermotherapy water is 40.5°C–43.3°C (105°F–110°F). *Note:* Most hospitals control water temperature so that it will not exceed 43.3°C (110°F).
6. Assist patient to sit in sitz bath for 15–20 min using a countdown timer device.
7. Maintain water temperature by continually adding water of appropriate temperature to bag. *Note:* Overflow will drain into toilet through openings in back of basin.
8. Upon completion, assist patient to dry the area and allow patient to sit briefly to allow normalization of blood pressure and to prevent hypotension upon standing. **Rationale:** *Due to vasodilation, orthostatic hypotension may occur with rapid position change following warm sitz bath.*

9. Don clean gloves, empty and rinse patient's sitz basin, and store in convenient location for future use. Discard soiled linen.
10. Discard soiled gloves and perform hand hygiene.
11. When the procedure is complete, perform hand hygiene and leave patient safe and comfortable.
12. Complete documentation using forms, checklists, or electronic dropdown lists supplemented by nurse's notes or additional comments as appropriate.

SAMPLE DOCUMENTATION

[date] 0825 Sitz bath with warm water for 20 minutes; states hemorrhoid pain is relieved at this time; assisted back to bed; tolerated without incident. *T. Hope*

Lifespan Considerations

INFANTS/CHILDREN

- The temperature of water in a hot water bottle should be 40.5°C–46.1°C (105°F–115°F) for a child under 2 years of age.

OLDER ADULTS

Older adult patients may be more susceptible to injury from heat and cold therapy as a result of physiological changes or medical conditions.

- The epidermal cells are replaced more slowly in older adults.
- Skin in older adults is thin and contains less moisture.
- Older adults have a reduced sensitivity to pain, and therefore may not feel untoward effects of heat and cold treatment.
- Temperature should be reduced when using heat therapy because older adult patient's skin burns more easily.
- Peripheral circulation may be compromised due to atherosclerosis or microvascular disease.
- Sensation in distal extremities may be impaired in older adult patients with neuropathy due to diabetes.
- Serious infections may not elicit a febrile response.
- Living conditions and financial limitations may not afford adequate environmental temperature control.

» End-of-Life Care

Expected Outcomes

1. Patient is able to progress through stages of grief with support of family and nursing staff.
2. Patient's beliefs about death and dying are considered throughout the dying process.
3. Patient's dignity is maintained while completing postmortem care.
4. Patient's relatives are supported by staff during grief process.
5. Appropriate procedures are carried out for organ donations.

Nurses may interact with dying patients and their families or caregivers in a variety of settings, from fetal demise (death of an unborn child), to the adolescent victim of an accident, to the older adult patient who finally succumbs to a chronic illness. Death can be viewed as a person's final opportunity to experience life in ways that bring significance and fulfillment. The nurse's role is to manage physical, emotional, and spiritual nursing care of the dying patient and the patient's family.

Caring for the dying and the bereaved (those individuals mourning the dead) is one of the nurse's most complex and challenging responsibilities, bringing into play all skills needed for holistic physiological and psychosocial care. This skill emphasizes physical care. It is beyond the scope of this skill to address in detail theoretical concepts such as grief and grieving or legal aspects such as the process of organ donation and living wills.

CAUTION! The goal of care for the dying patient changes from curative to palliative care. Helping the patient achieve a measure of comfort and knowing that family members and significant others are being supported during this process is a comfort for the patient.

SKILL 3.13 Physiological Needs of the Dying Patient: Managing

For the patient who is dying, comfort care is an essential part of medical care to prevent or relieve suffering as much as possible while respecting the dying patient's wishes. Family members may become overwhelmed as caregivers, so they need support, encouragement, and respite time. Comfort measures should be initiated for the following common physiological needs of the patient: pain, problems breathing, feeling tired, feeling more sensitive to cold temperatures, decrease in movement, and lack of appetite or unwillingness to drink liquids.

Delegation or Assignment

Comfort measures and supportive care strategies for care of patients at the end of life are often delegated or assigned to the UAP. The nurse reviews with the UAP those measures and strategies needed for a specific patient. The UAP must inform the nurse if the patient appears in unanticipated or unrelieved distress. The nurse remains responsible for assessment, interpretation of abnormal finds, and determination of appropriate actions. Note that state laws for UAPs vary, so this task might be assigned to the UAP rather than delegated.

Equipment

Needed equipment depends on the specific comfort measures being provided. Items may include medications, linens, and hygiene supplies.

Preparation

- Review healthcare provider's orders for end-of-life care and resuscitative measures to be done in an emergency.
- There may be customs, beliefs, and rituals surrounding dying and death for consideration by the nurse planning end-of-life care for the patient and support for the family. There are multiple resources available for the nurse to gain an understanding of the different cultural or religious approaches to dying and death. The dying person may be best to let the nurse know of needs or requests at this time in life. Family can contribute input or guidance about care during this time as religious practices, rituals, and beliefs may have a significant importance to the patient and or family. As appropriate and practical, the nurse should try to support the patient and family requests.
- The physiological needs of people who are dying are related to a slowing of body processes and to homeostatic imbalances. Interventions include: providing personal hygiene measures; controlling pain; relieving respiratory difficulties; assisting with movement, nutrition, hydration, and elimination; and providing measures related to sensory changes.

Clinical Manifestations of Impending Clinical Death

- Loss of muscle tone
  - Relaxation of the facial muscles (e.g., the jaw may sag)
  - Difficulty speaking
  - Difficulty swallowing and gradual loss of the gag reflex
  - Decreased activity of the gastrointestinal tract, with subsequent nausea, accumulation of flatus, abdominal distention, and retention of feces, especially if narcotics or tranquilizers are being administered
  - Possible urinary and rectal incontinence due to decreased sphincter control
  - Diminished body movement
- Slowing of the circulation
  - Diminished sensation
  - Mottling and cyanosis of the extremities
  - Cold skin, first in the feet and later in the hands, ears, and nose (the patient, however, may feel warm if there is a fever)
  - Slower and weaker pulse
  - Decreased blood pressure
- Changes in respirations
  - Rapid, shallow, irregular, or abnormally slow respirations
  - Noisy breathing, referred to as the death rattle, due to collecting of mucus in the throat
  - Mouth breathing, dry oral mucous membranes
- Sensory impairment
  - Blurred vision
  - Impaired senses of taste and smell
  - Various consciousness levels may exist just before death. Some patients are alert, whereas others are drowsy, stuporous, or comatose. Hearing is thought to be the last sense lost.

Procedure

1. Prior to performing the procedure, introduce self and verify the patient's identity using two identifiers. Explain to the patient and family what you are going to do, why it is necessary, and how the patient can participate.
2. Perform hand hygiene and observe other appropriate infection control procedures.
3. Provide for patient privacy depending on the specific interventions.
4. Perform bathing/hygiene.
   - Provide frequent baths and linen changes if diaphoretic, incontinent, or need for odor control. **Rationale:** *Dying individuals may have wounds, fever, or loss of sphincter control, which can be both uncomfortable when substances are left on the skin and cause distressing smells.*
   - Give mouth care as needed for dry mouth, to remove secretions, and to provide comfort.
   - Apply moisturizing creams, lip balm, and lotions for dry skin, and moisture-barrier skin preparations for incontinent patients.
   - Cleanse skin areas around wounds or areas that collect wound drainage.

(continued on next page)

SKILL 3.13 Physiological Needs of the Dying Patient: Managing *(continued)*

- When the dying patient's systems begin to dysfunction and stop working, a strong sweet pungent musky odor begins to permeate the air around them. The breath and body fluids from the skin and the mouth may smell like acetone. Bowel and bladder muscle control will diminish and the smell of stool and urine will be noted.

5. Provide pain control.
   - Pain control is essential to enable patients to maintain some quality in their life and their daily activities, including eating, moving, and sleeping. There are a variety of medications used to control the pain associated with terminal illness, such as narcotics and nonnarcotic analgesics, antianxiety, and antidepressant drugs.
   - Usually the healthcare provider determines the dosage, but the patient's opinion should be considered; the patient is the one ultimately aware of personal pain tolerance and fluctuations of internal states. Because healthcare providers usually prescribe a range for the dosage of pain medication, nurses use their own judgment as to the specific amount and frequency of pain medication needed to provide patient relief.
   - Because of decreased blood circulation, if analgesics cannot be administered orally, they are given by intravenous infusion, sublingually, or rectally, rather than subcutaneously or intramuscularly. **Rationale:** *Subcutaneous or intramuscular injections given to patients with impaired circulation will not reach the desired receptors and, thus, will be ineffective.*
   - Patients on narcotic pain medications also require implementation of a protocol to treat opioid-induced constipation.
   - Under periods of stress, the brain releases endorphins, morphine-like substances that modulate pain perception. Although studied primarily in animal models and in near-death experiences, some scientists believe that large amounts of endorphins may be released at the time of death. This could explain the seemingly peaceful sense of dissociation from the reality of pain, floating outside the body, seeing a tunnel, or moving toward the light that is expressed by some individuals.

6. Provide respiratory support.
   - For patients with difficulty clearing their own airway, place in Fowler's position if conscious, lateral position if unconscious. **Rationale:** *Fowler's position makes breathing easier. The lateral position allows secretions to drain out rather than entering the patient's airway.*
   - Perform oral throat suctioning as needed, especially for conscious patients who express discomfort.
   - Apply nasal oxygen for hypoxic patients as ordered. **Rationale:** *Supplemental oxygen may relieve the signs and symptoms of oxygen deprivation such as confusion.*
   - Anticholinergic medications (e.g., atropine, hyoscine hydrobromide) as ordered may be indicated to help dry secretions. Note that noisy respirations, sometimes referred to as the *death rattle*, are believed to be more distressing to those who have to listen to the sounds than the condition is for the dying patient.
   - For patients who have air hunger (the sensation of needing to breathe), open windows or use a fan to circulate air. Morphine may be indicated as ordered in an acute episode.

7. Assist with movement.
   - Assist patient out of bed periodically, as patient is able.
   - Regularly change patient's position.
   - Support patient's position with pillows, blanket rolls, or towels as needed.
   - Elevate patient's legs when sitting up.
   - Implement pressure ulcer prevention program and use pressure-relieving surfaces as indicated.

8. Provide nutrition and hydration as indicated.
   - Administer antiemetics to treat nausea as ordered.
   - Encourage favorite foods as tolerated.
   - Support family members who may be very concerned that their loved one is not eating or drinking sufficiently or who believe that failure to push nutrition signifies giving up and failure.
   - In some states, a feeding tube cannot be removed from a person in a persistent vegetative state (PVS) without a prior directive from the patient, but in other states the removal is allowed at the family's request or with a healthcare provider's order.
   - Teach family that patients with dehydration and alterations in electrolytes at the end of life may not be experiencing discomfort. In addition, dehydration actually reduces secretions and the need for elimination.

9. Assist with elimination.
   - For constipation, provide dietary fiber as tolerated or stool softeners or laxatives as needed.
   - Perform meticulous skin care in response to incontinence of urine or feces.
   - Keep the bedpan, urinal, or commode chair within easy reach and the call light within reach for assistance with elimination.
   - Use absorbent pads under incontinent patients; change linen as often as needed.
   - Urinary catheterization may be performed, if necessary.
   - Keep the room as clean and odor free as possible.

10. Be aware of sensory changes.
    - Check the patient's preference for a light or dark room. Position so that patient can view the television, favorite items or photos, or a window as desired.
    - Hearing is not diminished; speak clearly and do not whisper. Use music as desired.
    - Touch sensation is diminished, but patient will feel pressure of touch.
    - Provide gown, clothing, and bedding that feels and looks as the patient prefers.
    - Facilitate patient interaction with others as desired. This may require flexing facility rules regarding visiting hours or presence of pets. Advocate for the patient as much as possible about these.
    - Implement a pain management protocol if indicated; medicate for other sensory alterations such as itching as ordered.

11. Family members should be encouraged to participate in the physical care of the dying person as much as they wish to and are able. The nurse can suggest they assist with bathing, speak or read to the patient, and hold hands. The nurse

SKILL 3.13 Physiological Needs of the Dying Patient: Managing (*continued*)

must not, however, have specific expectations for family members' participation. Those who feel unable to care for or be with the dying person also require support from the nurse and from other family members. They should be shown an appropriate waiting area if they wish to remain nearby.

12. Consider how routine care should be modified based on the dying patient. Often vital signs are measured less frequently, blood and other laboratory tests are no longer performed, and active, invasive, or expensive treatment measures (such as antibiotics for infection) are suspended. Caring for dying patients who have agreed to organ donation can also be complex in terms of determining which medications, treatments, or equipment must be continued until the time for organ procurement has arrived.

13. When the procedure is complete, perform hand hygiene and leave patient safe and comfortable.

14. Complete documentation using forms, checklists, or electronic dropdown lists supplemented by nurse's notes or additional comments as appropriate, including all patient care, especially the effectiveness of symptom management activities.

SAMPLE DOCUMENTATION

[date] 23:30

S "I am so tired. Please don't make me turn right now. Could you give me some ice chips?"

O Lotion and massage to reachable back and extremities. Repositioned slightly to shift weight off bony prominences. Ice chips given and placed within reach.

A Care modified to support dying patient autonomy.

P Turn q3h instead of q2h as the patient prefers. Reinforce need to assess and treat dependent skin areas. Assess need for analgesics before each turn. Request pressure-reducing mattress. *S. Amber*

Patient Teaching

Caregivers of a dying person need ongoing support and ongoing teaching as the patient's condition changes. Some of these teaching needs include:

- Ways to feed the patient when swallowing becomes difficult
- Ways to transfer and reposition the patient safely
- Ways to communicate if verbalization becomes more difficult
- Nonpharmacological methods of pain control
- Comfort measures, such as frequent oral care and frequent repositioning
- Person to contact for different sources of support (e.g., respite care, pharmacies that deliver to the home, information about interpreting changes in the patient's condition).

Safety Considerations

People facing death may need help accepting that they have to depend on others. Some dying patients require only minimal care; others need continuous attention and services. People need help, well in advance of death, in planning for the period of dependence. They need to consider what will happen and how and where they would like to die.

A major factor in determining whether a person will die in a healthcare facility or at home is the availability of willing and able caregivers. If the dying person wishes to be at home, and family or others can provide care to maintain symptom control, the nurse should facilitate a referral to outpatient hospice services. Hospice staff and nurses will then conduct a full assessment of the home and care providers' skills.

Although the original hospice was a freestanding facility, according to the National Hospice and Palliative Care Organization, in 2014, approximately 1.6–1.7 million patients received services from hospice. The hospice concept is also implemented in hospice centers (31.8% of cases), palliative care areas in acute care hospitals (9.3% of cases), and at patient's place of residence (58.9% of cases). Most insurance policies, including Medicare, cover hospice services.

Source: Based on National Hospice and Palliative Care Organization (NHPCO). (2015). *NHPCO's Facts and Figures Hospice Care in America 2015 Edition.* Retrieved from https://webcache.googleusercontent.com/search?q=cache:t9KFylfsg3kJ; https://www.nhpco.org/sites/default/files/public/Statistics_Research/2015_Facts_Figures.pdf+&cd=1&hl=en&ct=clnk&gl=us

SKILL 3.14 Postmortem Care: Providing

Postmortem care is the care provided to a patient immediately after death. It is done to prepare the patient's body for viewing by the family and ensure proper identification of the patient prior to transport to the funeral home or morgue. This is a time to provide appropriate disposition of the patient's belongings.

Delegation or Assignment

Postmortem care can be delegated or assigned to the UAP after the activities described above have been completed so that the UAP knows what tubes or other medical devices can be removed or other special care provided. Note that state laws for UAPs vary, so this task might be assigned to the UAP rather than delegated.

Equipment

- Shroud kit ❶ or other linens used by the healthcare facility to wrap the body
- Washcloths, towels
- Absorbent pads
- Clean gloves and any other personal protective equipment as indicated by the patient's condition
- Patient gown (if the family will be viewing the body)
- Bags for personal belongings and the medical record document used to record transfer of the belongings and valuables

(*continued on next page*)

SKILL 3.14 Postmortem Care: Providing (*continued*)

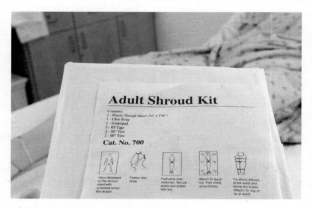

Source: Rick Brady/Pearson Education, Inc.

❶ Shroud contents.

Preparation

■ Consider whether more than one person is needed to perform the postmortem care since turning the body is involved. For caregivers who are performing postmortem care for the first time, it is especially advised that at least two caregivers work together to provide the care.

■ Postmortem care can be time consuming. Arrange for someone to cover the caregiver's other patients during this time.

■ There may be customs, beliefs, and rituals surrounding the deceased patient's body care. There are multiple resources available for the nurse to gain an understanding of the different cultural or religious approaches for care of the deceased patient's body. The dying person may have already let the nurse know of any requests about this and family can contribute input or guidance. As appropriate and practical, the nurse should try to support the patient and family requests.

Procedure

1. Observe appropriate infection control procedures. Apply clean gloves.
2. Because the deceased person's family often wants to view the body immediately after death, and because it is important that the deceased appear natural and comfortable, nurses need to position the body, place dentures in the mouth, and close the eyes and mouth before rigor mortis sets in.
   - Normally the body is placed in a supine position with the arms either at the sides, palms down, or across the abdomen.
   - After blood circulation has ceased, the red blood cells break down, releasing hemoglobin, which discolors the surrounding tissues. This discoloration, referred to as **livor mortis**, appears in the lowermost or dependent areas of the body. One pillow is placed under the head and shoulders to prevent blood from discoloring the face by settling in it.
   - Close the eyelids and hold in place for a few seconds so they remain closed.
   - Dentures are usually inserted to help give the face a natural appearance. The mouth is then closed.

- If the body will be viewed in the hospital:
  - Place a clean gown on the patient, and comb the hair.
  - Adjust the top bed linens neatly to cover the patient to the shoulders.
  - Provide tissues, soft lighting, and chairs for the family.
  - Remove all equipment, soiled linen, and supplies from the bedside.
3. Some agencies require that all tubes in the body remain in place; in other agencies, tubes may be cut to within 2.5 cm (1 in.) of the skin and taped in place; in others, all tubes may be removed. In some cases, if a central IV line is in place, it may be left to assist with the process of preserving the body (embalming). Use the same careful handling you would use with a living body. **Rationale:** *As the body cools, the skin loses its elasticity and can easily be broken when removing dressings and adhesive tape.*
4. Soiled areas of the body are washed; however, a complete bath is not necessary, because the body will be washed by the mortician (also referred to as an undertaker), a person trained in the care of the dead.
5. Absorbent pads are placed under the buttocks to take up any feces and urine released because of relaxation of the sphincter muscles.
6. Remove all jewelry, except a wedding band in some instances, which is taped to the finger.
7. The deceased's wrist identification tag is left on. After the body has been viewed by the family, additional identification tags are applied. **Rationale:** *Mislabeling can create legal problems if the body is inappropriately identified and prepared incorrectly for burial or a funeral.*
8. Wrap the body in a **shroud**, a large piece of plastic or cotton material used to enclose a body after death (see ❶). Apply identification to the outside of the shroud ❷.

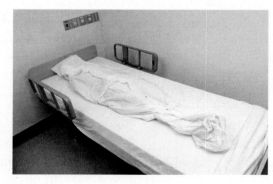

Source: Rick Brady/Pearson Education, Inc.

❷ A body wrapped in a shroud.

- If the dentures were placed in the mouth for the viewing, secure the jaw with a strap or remove them so they do not fall out as the mouth muscles relax.
- Remove and discard gloves. Perform hand hygiene.
9. Take the body to the morgue if arrangements have not been made to have a mortician pick it up from the patient's room. Nurses have a duty to handle the deceased with dignity and to label the body appropriately. **Rationale:** *Mishandling can cause emotional distress to survivors.*

SKILL 3.14 Postmortem Care: Providing (*continued*)

10. Complete documentation using forms, checklists, or electronic dropdown lists supplemented by nurse's notes or additional comments as appropriate. Include postmortem care completed, what items were removed from the body, whether the body was viewed by the family, and whether the body was taken to the morgue (and by whom) or picked up by the funeral home from the room.

SAMPLE DOCUMENTATION

[date] 0245 Postmortem care given to deceased patient. Body of patient cleaned, wrapped, and prepared for morgue; identification tags applied; personal clothing put in plastic bag for family; no jewelry found on body of patient. *E. Vest*

0319 Body to morgue by A. Mendez via stretcher. *E. Vest*

Safety Considerations

- State laws vary about what to do in coroner cases (for example, sudden death occurring in a person without a known natural cause, suspicious circumstances, unknown cause of death, and deaths caused by violence). Check your state's policies for guidelines on postmortem care of body and tubes, clothing, and so forth, when forensic evidence is present that must be preserved.

- Inform the funeral home if the patient has tuberculosis or any other infectious disease so appropriate care can be taken to prevent contamination of the environment.

- If the family will take more than an hour to get to the healthcare facility to view the body, the decision to have the body moved from the hospital morgue to the funeral home before the family arrives may need to be made. The process of rigor mortis begins at the time of death. Approximately 12 hours later all of the muscles are affected resulting in rigidity of the body. Rigidity remains approximately for 24–36 hr after death at which time the muscles become flaccid.

Lifespan Considerations
CHILDREN

- Children's responses to death or loss depend on the messages they get from adults and others around them as well as their understanding of death. When adults are able to cope effectively with a death, they are more likely to be able to support children through the process.

- Comprehension of death evolves as the person develops.

- *From infancy to 5 years:* Children do not understand the concept of death. An infant's sense of separation forms the basis for later understanding of loss and death. They believe death is reversible, a temporary departure, or sleep.

- *Ages 5–9 years:* Child understands that death is final. Believes own death can be avoided. Associates death with aggression or violence. Believes wishes or unrelated actions can be responsible for death.

- *Ages 9–12 years:* Child understands death as the inevitable end of life. Begins to understand own mortality, expressed as interest in afterlife or as fear of death.

- *Ages 12–18 years:* Adolescent fears a lingering death. May fantasize that death can be defied, acting out defiance through reckless behaviors (e.g., dangerous driving, substance abuse). Seldom thinks about death, but views it in religious and philosophic terms. May seem to reach "adult" perception of death but be emotionally unable to accept it. May still hold concepts from previous developmental stages.

- It is a challenging situation to provide competent comfort care to meet the needs of a dying child. Providing comfort care for parents who are experiencing the death of a child can be sad and stressful. Parents will likely feel shock, disbelief, and a mix of many other emotions. The nurse supports the parents by giving objective and specific information about the child's condition, arranging for the parents to be close to the child as often as they desire, and facilitating parent participation in the child's care.

OLDER ADULTS

- Older adults who are dying often may have a need to know that their lives had meaning. An excellent way to assure them of this is to make audiotapes or videotapes of them telling stories of their lives. This gives the patient a sense of value and worth and also lets the patient know that family members and friends will also benefit from it. Doing this with children and grandchildren often eases communication and support during this difficult time.

- Older adults may fear prolonged illness and see death as having multiple meanings (e.g., freedom from pain, or reunion with already deceased family members).

- Older adults may see death as an end of suffering and loneliness.

- Death is usually not feared if the person has lived a long and fulfilled life, having completed all developmental tasks.

- Spiritual beliefs or philosophy of life are important.

≫ Critical Thinking Options for Unexpected Outcomes

Not all unexpected outcomes require further nursing intervention; however, many times they do. When the patient demonstrates a change in signs/symptoms indicating an emerging problem, the nurse should immediately assess and troubleshoot what is happening. The assessment data must be processed quickly to formulate a hypothesis so the nurse can make a clinical judgment. The nurse then decides how best to resolve the problem and improve the patient's situation for a better outcome.

EXPECTED OUTCOME	UNEXPECTED OUTCOME	POSSIBLE INTERVENTIONS
Acute/Chronic Pain Management Patient is able to identify and alleviate stress caused by mental concerns.	Patient moves into the stage of exhaustion, and stress becomes dangerous to health.	■ Immediately take measures to remove stressors through medication, complete rest, and so forth. ■ Implement specific stress-reducing measures, such as relaxation processes, visualization, and biofeedback.
Pain is controlled through nonpharmacological methods such as massage, complementary health therapy, or TENS.	Patient cannot focus on a relaxation technique.	■ Explore other options of relaxation techniques with patient that have worked with other patients. ■ Ask the patient about diversional activities done at home to relax.
Patient is satisfied with level of pain control.	Patient experiences pain, asks about alternative measures for relief.	■ Cold therapy may be an option, or heat/cold alternating therapy as counterirritants; these therapies alter nerve transmission. ■ Assess if application is too hot. ■ Ensure that temperature is not over 43.3°C (110°F) if heating pad is used. ■ Explore complementary health options with patient.
Heat and Cold Application Noninflammatory edema is reduced.	Swelling is not reduced with heat therapy.	■ Ensure that acute inflammation is not present, because heat therapy will not reduce swelling (exudate) due to acute tissue injury. ■ Support venous return by elevating the part.
Patient reports decrease in pain.	Patient complains pain from local edema is increasing.	■ Elevate extremity above level of heart. ■ Ensure that body surface is sufficiently covered with cold application to cause vasoconstriction. ■ Check that area is not over-insulated.
Bleeding and edema formation are minimized.	Bleeding/bruising continues in spite of local cold applications.	■ Reassess area for possible "bleeders," which may require cautery or ligation by the healthcare provider. ■ Apply pressure to site to stop bleeding. ■ Assess pulse distal to bleed.
Patient has no adverse responses to therapy (arrhythmias, bleeding, shivering, afterdrop or rebound hyperthermia).	Patient begins to shiver.	■ Stop the procedure or warm the solution a few degrees (or both). ■ Monitor temperature because shivering causes an increase in the metabolic rate, leading to an increase in heat production. ■ Monitor temperature every 15 minutes to detect additional temperature decrease. ■ Contact healthcare provider for medication order (narcotic or sedative agent). ■ Provide supplemental oxygen therapy.
Target core body temperature is achieved.	Cooling blanket does not function properly.	■ Check that plug is connected to the outlet. ■ Check that the fluid level is sufficient and that unit freezing has not occurred. ■ Check that the thermistor probe is properly connected. ■ Check that the cool limit on the pad is not set too high.
End-of-Life Care Postmortem care is completed, maintaining patient's dignity.	Patient is not identified properly when sent to the morgue.	■ Check patient's identity band and shroud label before releasing patient to mortician. ■ Request another nurse to check labels.
Appropriate procedures are carried out for organ donations.	Donated organs are needed.	■ Provide support to family members and an opportunity to ask questions. ■ Obtain signatures for consent form. (Kidneys should be removed within 1 hour after death. Eyes should be removed within 6–24 hr after death.) ■ Examine reverse side of driver's license, or remind the charge nurse to call mortician if burial plans have been made previously, to check on permission for organ donation through a living will.

REVIEW Questions

1. The nurse delegates a client's back massage to an unlicensed assistive personnel (UAP). While observing the UAP perform the massage, at what action by the UAP should the nurse intervene?
   1. Begins massaging at the sacrum
   2. Applies lotion directly to the skin
   3. Applies pressure without breaking skin contact
   4. Massages in a circular motion over the scapulae

2. The nurse coaches a client to breathe deeply and slowly while performing progressive relaxation. At the conclusion of this exercise, which assessment finding indicates that this respiratory pattern has been effective?
   1. Heart rate 64 and regular
   2. Respiratory rate 24/min
   3. Blood pressure 168/90 mmHg
   4. Pulse oximetry 88% on room air

3. A client asks how an "electric box" is going to stop leg pain. How should the nurse respond when explaining a TENS unit to the client?
   1. "It is an electrical form of a massage."
   2. "It is based on an ancient method that uses specific points located on meridians throughout the body."
   3. "It stimulates the skin with a mild electric current and relieves pain by blocking pain impulses to the brain."
   4. "It is an electric monitoring device that provides information about your behavior so you can control internal processes."

4. Unlicensed assistive personnel (UAP) report that a client with patient-controlled analgesia (PCA) is complaining of pain. What action should the nurse take first?
   1. Change the dose volume limit on the pump.
   2. Direct the UAP to push the button on the pump.
   3. Assess for the amount of medication remaining in the pump.
   4. Ask when the client delivered the last dose through the pump.

5. The healthcare provider prescribes an ice pack to be applied to a client's knee for 10 minutes every 4 hours. Two minutes into the first application, the client complains of stinging. What should the nurse do?
   1. Remove the pack.
   2. Remove the protective wrap around the pack.
   3. Document that the client refused to use the pack.
   4. Encourage the client to keep the pack on the site.

6. During a home visit a client asks why, after using a heating pad as prescribed, the area being treated feels more painful. What assessed information would explain the client's issue?
   1. Cover on the pad intact
   2. Applied to the area for an hour
   3. Control set on prescribed temperature
   4. Used gauze ties to secure the pad in place

7. The nurse notes that the temperature of an infant in a radiant warmer is below the prescribed setting. Which observation could explain this assessment finding?
   1. Bed set to skin control mode
   2. Gel patch applied over skin probe
   3. Skin probe applied over infant's elbow
   4. Temperature probe plugged into the bed

8. A client who is dying is prescribed pain medication that can be administered via the subcutaneous, intramuscular, or intravenous route. What assessment finding should the nurse use to select the route to administer the medication?
   1. Mouth open
   2. Cyanotic forearms
   3. Abdominal distention
   4. Dry oral mucous membranes

Note: For answers and rationales for the review questions, go to Appendix A or your Pearson MyLab Nursing and eText.

Chapter 4
Elimination

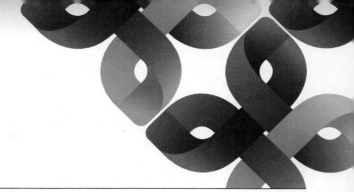

Chapter at a Glance

Assessment: Collecting Specimens

❶ Nursing students may observe or assist with the following skills only with faculty permission and while under direct supervision of faculty or another RN.

» The Concept of Elimination

Elimination is the management of waste product removal from the body. The main organs involved are the skin, lungs, kidneys, and intestinal tract. Toxic substances are filtered through the liver. If the body does not remove waste products, they build up in the body and become life-threatening. Nurses will encounter patients of all ages with bladder and bowel elimination issues in all areas of care. Being familiar with bladder complications such as retention, kidney stones, incontinence, and infection and bowel complications such as constipation, diarrhea, incontinence, and obstruction will enable nurses to support and provide appropriate interventions for their patients.

Learning Outcomes

4.1 Summarize the sequence of steps in obtaining a urine specimen from a urinary closed drainage system.

4.2 Explain safety considerations when assisting a patient to use a bedside commode.

4.3 Show the actions in sequence for administering a warm water enema to an older adult.

4.4 Give examples of priority assessment data to collect when changing a fecal ostomy pouch.

4.5 Explain peritoneal dialysis for the removal of body fluids and body wastes.

4.6 Support the rationale for teaching patients undergoing peritoneal dialysis the signs of peritonitis, fever, nausea or vomiting, and redness or pain around the exit site.

4.7 Give examples of four safety precautions for a fistula or graft to teach a patient that undergoes hemodialysis.

4.8 Summarize ways to maintain sterile technique when performing urinary catheterization.

The following feature links some, but not all, of the concepts related to assessment. They are presented in alphabetical order.

Concepts Related to
Elimination

CONCEPT	RELATIONSHIP TO ELIMINATION	NURSING IMPLICATIONS
Fluids and Electrolytes	Fluid intake balanced with fluid output	▪ Monitor patient's intake and output ▪ Encourage fluids for dehydration as appropriate
Infection	Hygiene of perineal and anal areas to prevent cross transference of contaminates	▪ Encourage female patients to wipe from front to back after urination and defecation ▪ Assist in peritoneal care as patient needs
Perioperative Care	Post-surgical care of urinary ostomy or fecal ostomy wounds and drainage	▪ Assess ostomy site with dressing changes ▪ Apply pouch to ostomy when time is appropriate ▪ Monitor ostomy site for complications
Teaching and Learning	Bowel and bladder incontinence	▪ Support patient during bowel or bladder training ▪ Discuss available products to help protect skin from dribbling ▪ Demonstrate care techniques to patient adapting to bowel or bladder alterations
Tissue Integrity	Preventing tissue impairment at perineal and anal areas	▪ Protect perineal and anal tissues from irritation by urine or feces incontinence

» Assessment: Collecting Specimens

Expected Outcomes

1. Patient understands purpose of test.
2. Patient is able to follow procedure of collection when appropriate.
3. Specimen collected is adequate for testing.

SKILL 4.1 Bladder Scanner: Using

Safety Note! *During scheduled clinical time, nursing students may have a learning opportunity to observe or assist with this skill only with faculty permission and with direct supervision from faculty or another RN.*

This portable, hand-held ultrasound device can quickly and easily perform a noninvasive scan of the bladder. The scanner uses an ultrasound probe and transducer to reflect sound waves from the patient's bladder to the scanner. It can be used to assess patients for post-void residual volume and other situations to determine if the bladder is emptying appropriately. Healthcare facilities only allow nurses trained and competent in using a bladder scanner to do a bladder scan on patients for safety precautions. The bladder scanner is considered specialized equipment.

Delegation or Assignment

Performing a bladder scan is not delegated or assigned to the UAP. The nurse can request the UAP to report patient observations to the nurse for follow-up. Assessment and evaluation remain the responsibility of the nurse.

Equipment

▪ Ultrasound bladder scanning device
▪ Ultrasound conducting gel
▪ Tissues

Preparation

▪ Check healthcare provider's order to do a bladder scan (some facilities do not require a healthcare provider's order for the nurse to do a bladder scan, but all facilities require nurses to be trained in using a bladder scanner for safety and competency before using it independently).
▪ If patient is female, ask if she has had a hysterectomy or is pregnant. **Rationale:** *If a hysterectomy is not documented and settings are not adjusted appropriately, results may be inaccurate. Scanner is not indicated for pregnant patients.*
▪ Determine time and amount of last void or assist patient to empty bladder if residual volume is to be evaluated.

SKILL 4.1 Bladder Scanner: Using (*continued*)

- Determine that patient does not have an indwelling catheter. **Rationale:** *Scanner reflects off the catheter bulb, giving an echo reading.*
- Gather needed equipment and supplies and go to patient's room.

Procedure

1. Introduce self to patient and verify the patient's identity using two identifiers. Explain to the patient what you are going to do, why it is necessary, and how the patient can participate. Discuss how the results will be used in planning further care or treatments.
2. Perform hand hygiene and observe appropriate infection control procedures.
3. Provide for patient privacy.
4. Place patient flat and supine, and palpate patient's bladder to locate appropriate site.
5. Turn the device on and press "SCAN."
6. Apply conducting gel to scanner head.
7. Select MALE or FEMALE mode on scan unit. Select *MALE MODE* if female patient has had a hysterectomy.
8. Fanfold linens to expose patient's suprapubic area.
9. Place head of scanner 2.5 cm (1 in.) above patient's symphysis pubis, directed toward the bladder, and align the icon ❶.
10. Press scan head button and hold scanner still until a beep is heard.
11. Scan until bladder image is lined up on cross-hairs.
12. Take several scans at different angles and press "DONE" when finished.
13. Press "PRINT" for a printout of patient's bladder volume in milliliters.
14. Wipe gel from patient's skin.
15. Reposition patient for comfort.
16. Wipe ultrasound probe with antiseptic solution.
17. Perform hand hygiene and leave patient safe and comfortable.

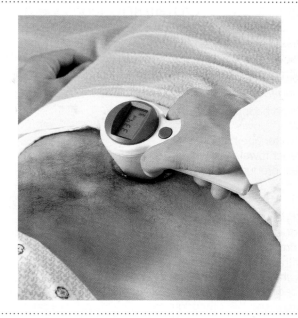

❶ Handheld portable ultrasound bladder scanner.

18. Complete documentation using forms, checklists, or electronic dropdown lists supplemented by nurse's notes or additional comments as appropriate, including procedure results.

SAMPLE DOCUMENTATION

[date] 1430 C/o feeling like she needs to void but only voided small amount of urine since 1000 this morning. Small amount distention with tenderness lower abd. noted. Bladder scan done, reads 130 mL urine in bladder. Dr. Cross notified. *T. Klein*

SKILL 4.2 Stool Specimen, Routine, Culture, Ova, Parasites: Obtaining

Stool testing may be done to help diagnose certain conditions affecting the digestive tract such as bacteria, viruses, ova and parasites, or antigen tests to identify specific microbes such as *Clostridium difficile*. Stool tests can also help diagnose nutrition absorption problems and identify colorectal cancer.

Delegation or Assignment

The UAP may obtain and collect stool specimen(s). The nurse, however, needs to consider the collection process before delegating or assigning this task. For example, a random stool specimen collected in a specimen container may be delegated or assigned, but a stool culture requiring a sterile swab in a test tube should be done by the nurse. Use of an incorrect collection technique can cause inaccurate test results.

The task of obtaining and testing a stool specimen for occult blood may be performed by the UAP. The nurse should instruct the UAP to tell the nurse if blood is detected or if the test is positive. Also, the stool specimen should be saved to allow the nurse to repeat the test. Note that state laws for UAPs vary, so this task might be assigned to the UAP rather than delegated.

Equipment

Collecting a Stool Specimen

- Clean bedpan or bedside commode
- Clean gloves
- Cardboard or plastic specimen container (labeled) with a lid or, for stool culture, a sterile swab in a test tube, as policy dictates

(*continued on next page*)

SKILL 4.2 Stool Specimen, Routine, Culture, Ova, Parasites: Obtaining (continued)

- Two tongue blades
- Paper towel
- Completed laboratory requisition and label for container

Testing the Stool for Occult Blood

- Clean bedpan or bedside commode
- Clean gloves
- Two tongue blades
- Paper towel
- Test product

Preparation

- Check healthcare provider's orders.
- For a newborn or infant, the stool specimen is scraped from the diaper, being careful not to contaminate the stool with urine.
- A child who is toilet trained should be able to provide a fecal specimen, but may prefer being assisted by a parent. When explaining the procedure to the child, ask the parent what words the family normally uses to describe a bowel movement, and use those words.
- Older adults may need assistance if serial stool specimens are required.
- Assemble the needed equipment. Post a sign in the patient's bathroom if a timed specimen is required (e.g., "Save All Stools").

Procedure

1. Prior to performing the procedure, introduce self and verify the patient's identity using two identifiers. Explain to the patient the purpose of the stool specimen and how the patient can assist in collecting it. Discuss how the results will be used in planning further care or treatments. Give ambulatory patients the following information and instructions:
   - Defecate in a clean bedpan or bedside commode.
   - Do not contaminate the specimen with urine or menstrual discharge, if possible. (Void before giving the specimen collection.)
   - Do not place toilet tissue in the bedpan after defecation, because contents of the paper can affect the laboratory analysis.
   - Notify the nurse as soon as possible after defecation, particularly for specimens that need to be sent to the laboratory immediately after collection.
2. Perform hand hygiene and observe other appropriate infection control procedures.
   - Don clean gloves and follow medical aseptic technique meticulously when obtaining stool samples (i.e., when handling the patient's bedpan, when transferring the stool sample to a specimen container, and when disposing of the bedpan contents).
3. Provide for patient privacy.
4. Assist patients who need help.
   - Assist the patient to a bedside commode or a bedpan placed on a bedside chair or under the toilet seat in the bathroom.

- Don clean gloves to prevent hand contamination, and clean the patient as required. Inspect the skin around the anus for any irritation, especially if the patient defecates frequently and has liquid stools.
5. Transfer the required amount of stool to the stool specimen container.
   - Use one or two tongue blades to transfer some or all of the stool to the specimen container, taking care not to contaminate the outside of the container. The amount of stool to be sent depends on the purpose for which the specimen is collected. Usually, 2.5 cm (1 in.) of formed stool or 15 to 30 mL of liquid stool is adequate. For some timed specimens, however, the entire stool passed may need to be sent. Visible pus, mucus, or blood should be included in the sample.
   - For a culture, dip a sterile swab into the specimen, preferably where purulent fecal matter is present in the feces. Place the swab in a sterile test tube using sterile technique.
   - For a fecal occult blood test (FOBT) using the traditional Hemoccult test, see below.
   - Wrap the used tongue blades in a paper towel before disposing of them in a waste container. **Rationale:** *These measures help prevent the spread of microorganisms through contact with other articles.*
   - Place the lid on the container as soon as the specimen is in the container and proceed to step 6 below. **Rationale:** *Putting the lid on immediately prevents the spread of microorganisms.*

HEMOCCULT TEST (FOBT)

- Don clean gloves.
- Follow the manufacturer's directions. For example:
  - For a Hemoccult slide, smear a thin layer of feces over the circle inside the envelope, and drop reagent solution onto the smear ❶.
  - Note the reaction. For all tests, a blue color indicates a positive result, that is, the presence of occult blood. Proceed to step 6 below.

FOR BACTERIAL CULTURE

- Don clean gloves before collecting stool specimen.
- Collect exudate, mucus, and blood with all specimens.
- Place a small amount of feces in a waxed cardboard container (if entire specimen is not needed). Proceed to step 6 below.

FOR OVA AND PARASITES

- Collect exudate, mucus, and blood with all specimens ❷.
  - Place stool into container (with a preservative fluid).
  - Mash the specimen in the container until mixed well with preservative. **Rationale:** *Parasites thrive in this type of medium.*
  - Replace and tighten cup. Shake the contents until mixed well.

SKILL 4.2 Stool Specimen, Routine, Culture, Ova, Parasites: Obtaining (*continued*)

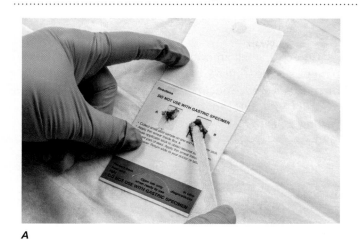

A

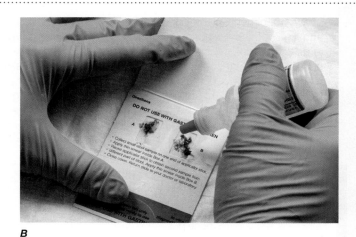

B

❶ *A,* Opening the front cover of a Hemoccult slide and applying a thin smear of feces on the slide; *B,* Opening the flap on the back of the slide and applying two drops of developing fluid over each smear.

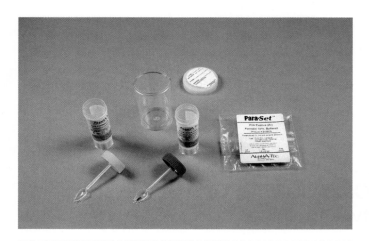

❷ Equipment necessary for collecting ova and/or parasite specimen.

■ Keep loose fluid specimens at body temperature to be examined within 30 minutes. **Rationale:** *Organisms must be seen in their active stages. Loose, fluid stools are likely to contain trophozoites or intestinal amoebas and flagellates. Well-formed or semiformed stool specimens do not usually need to be maintained at body temperature or be examined quickly even though they may contain ova or a cystic form of parasites.*

■ Collect complete stools after purgative medications are administered. **Rationale:** *When the presence of tapeworms is suspected, all stools must be examined in their entirety in order to find the head of the parasite.* Do not give barium, oil, and laxatives containing heavy metals that interfere with the extraction process for 7 days before stool examination. **Rationale:** *Ova or cysts are not revealed in the presence of these materials.* Use only normal saline solution or tap water if an enema must be

administered to collect specimens. Do not use soap suds or other substances.

■ Do not contaminate the specimen with urine because it kills amoeba.

■ Collect three random, normally passed stool specimens to ensure accurate test results.

6. Ensure patient safety and comfort.
   ● Empty and clean the bedpan or commode, and return it to its place.
   ● Remove and discard the gloves. Perform hand hygiene.

7. Label and send the specimen to the laboratory.
   ● Ensure that the specimen label and the laboratory requisition have the correct information on them and are securely attached on the specimen container. **Rationale:** *Inappropriate identification of the specimen can lead to errors of diagnosis or therapy for the patient.*
   ● Ensure that specimens are placed in appropriate biohazard containers or specimen bags.
   ● Send entire specimen for bacterial culture to the laboratory immediately after collection. If there is any delay, the specimen must be iced.
   ● Specimens to be cultured or tested for parasites need to be sent immediately. If this is not possible, follow the directions on the specimen container. In some instances, refrigeration is indicated because bacteriological changes take place in stool specimens left at room temperature. Never place a stool specimen in a refrigerator that contains food or medication. **Rationale:** *This prevents contamination of "clean" items with "dirty" items. It also follows OSHA standards for biohazard materials.*

8. Complete documentation using forms, checklists, or electronic dropdown lists supplemented by nurse's notes or additional comments as appropriate. Record the collection

(*continued on next page*)

SKILL 4.2 Stool Specimen, Routine, Culture, Ova, Parasites:
Obtaining (*continued*)

of the specimen on the patient's chart. Include the date and time of the collection and all nursing assessments (e.g., color, odor, consistency, and amount of feces); presence of abnormal constituents, such as blood or mucus; results of test for occult blood if obtained; discomfort during or after defecation; status of perianal skin; any bleeding from the anus after defecation. For an FOBT, record the type of test product used and the reaction.

SAMPLE DOCUMENTATION

[date] 0630 Small amount stool collected from patient's bedpan, dark brown, formed, no blood or mucus noted. Specimen to lab for stool analysis as ordered; tolerated without incident; in bed resting. *E. Dover*

Patient Teaching

Testing for Pinworms at Home

Note: This test is rarely done or seen in hospital settings, so if pinworms are suspected, the parents can be taught how to obtain a specimen at home. The specimen container with paddle to collect the specimen can be obtained from the patient's healthcare provider's office.

1. Wear clean gloves.
2. Collect a stool specimen from the child upon arising in the morning before bathing or cleansing the child, and before the child passes a bowel movement.

   Note: For very active children, specimens may be collected a few hours after going to bed, while the child is sleepy and more cooperative. **Rationale:** *Pinworms, when present, migrate out of the anus to lay eggs during sleep.*

3. Remove cap in which is inserted a plastic paddle with one side coated with a nontoxic, adhesive material. This side is marked "sticky side." Do not touch this side with fingers.
4. Separate buttocks and press the sticky side against several areas around anus using moderate pressure.
5. Replace the paddle in tube. Be sure there is no stool on paddle.
6. Label container with patient's full name, address, and date.
7. Keep specimen at room temperature until all specimens are collected (on consecutive days). Return all tubes to the healthcare provider's office.

CAUTION! After treatment (drug of choice is mebendazole) and to prevent reinfection, use meticulous cleaning practices and teach parents of the child to do the same.

SKILL 4.3 Urine Specimen, Clean-Catch, Closed Drainage System
for Culture and Sensitivity: Obtaining

A urine culture is performed to determine the presence of bacteria and other pathogens that may be causing a urinary tract or kidney infection. Bladder urine is normally sterile but bacteria can enter the urethra and cause an infection. Sensitivity, or susceptibility testing, is done to determine which antibiotics will be most effective in treating the patient's infection.

Delegation or Assignment

The UAP may be delegated or assigned the collection of a clean-catch or midstream urine specimen. It is important, however, that the nurse inform the UAP how to instruct the patient in the correct process for obtaining the specimen. Proper cleansing of the urethra should be emphasized to avoid contaminating the urine specimen. Note that state laws for UAPs vary, so this task might be assigned to the UAP rather than delegated.

Equipment

Equipment used varies from facility to facility. Some agencies use commercially prepared disposable clean-catch kits.

Others use facility-prepared sterile trays. Both prepared trays and kits generally contain the following items:

- Clean gloves
- Antiseptic towelettes
- Sterile specimen container
- Specimen identification label

   In addition, the nurse needs to obtain the following:

- Completed laboratory requisition form and container label
- Urine receptacle, if the patient is not ambulatory
- Basin of warm water, soap, washcloth, and towel for the nonambulatory patient

Preparation

- Review the healthcare provider's orders.
- Collect the necessary equipment needed for the collection of the specimen.
- Use visual aids, if available, to assist the patient to understand the midstream collection technique.
- For a clean-catch urine specimen, an older adult may have difficulty controlling the stream of urine.

SKILL 4.3 Urine Specimen, Clean-Catch, Closed Drainage System for Culture and Sensitivity: Obtaining (*continued*)

- An older female adult with arthritis may have difficulty holding the labia apart during the collection of a clean-catch urine specimen.

Procedure

1. Prior to performing the procedure, introduce self and verify the patient's identity using two identifiers. Explain to the patient that a urine specimen is required, give the reason, and explain the method to be used to collect it. Discuss how the results will be used in planning further care or treatments.
2. Perform hand hygiene and observe other appropriate infection control procedures.
3. Provide for patient privacy.
4. For an ambulatory patient who is able to follow directions, instruct the patient on how to collect the specimen.

CLEAN-CATCH

- Direct or assist the patient to the bathroom.
- Ask the patient to wash and dry the genitals and perineal area with soap and water. **Rationale:** *Washing the perineal area reduces the number of skin and transient bacteria, decreasing the risk of contaminating the urine specimen.*
- Ask the patient if sensitive to any antiseptic or cleansing agents. **Rationale:** *This will avoid unnecessary irritation of the genitals or perineum.*
- Instruct the patient on how to clean the urinary meatus with antiseptic towelettes. **Rationale:** *The antiseptic further reduces bacterial contamination of the urinary meatus and the risk of contaminating the specimen.*

For Female Patients

- Use each towelette only once. Clean the perineal area from front to back and discard the towelette ❶. Use all towelettes provided (usually two or three). **Rationale:** *Cleaning from front to back cleans the area of least contamination to the area of greatest contamination.*

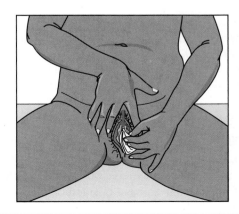

❶ Cleansing the female urinary meatus. Spread the labia minora with one hand and with the other hand, cleanse perineal area from front to back.

For Male Patients

- If uncircumcised, retract the foreskin slightly to expose the urinary meatus.
- Using a circular motion, clean the urinary meatus and the distal portion of the penis ❷. Use each towelette only once, then discard. Clean several inches down the shaft of the penis. **Rationale:** *This cleans from the area of least contamination to the area of greatest contamination.*

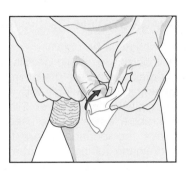

❷ Cleansing the male urinary meatus. Retract the foreskin if needed. Using a towelette, cleanse the urinary meatus by moving in a circular motion from center of the urethral opening around the glans and down the distal portion of the shaft of the penis.

5. For a patient who requires assistance, prepare the patient and equipment.
   - Apply clean gloves.
   - Wash the perineal area with soap and water, rinse, and dry.
   - Assist the patient onto a clean commode or bedpan. If using a bedpan or urinal, position the patient as upright as allowed or tolerated. **Rationale:** *Assuming a normal anatomical position for voiding facilitates urination.*
   - Remove and discard gloves. Perform hand hygiene.
   - Open the clean-catch kit, taking care not to contaminate the inside of the specimen container or lid. Place the lid in the upright position. **Rationale:** *It is important to maintain sterility of the specimen container to prevent contamination of the specimen.*
   - Apply clean gloves.
   - Clean the urinary meatus and perineal area as described in step 4.
6. Collect the specimen from a nonambulatory patient or instruct an ambulatory patient on how to collect it.
   - Instruct the patient to start voiding. **Rationale:** *Bacteria in the distal urethra and at the urinary meatus are cleared by the first few milliliters of urine expelled.*
   - Place the specimen container into the midstream of urine and collect the specimen, taking care not to touch the container to the perineum or penis. **Rationale:** *It is important to avoid contaminating the interior of the specimen container and the specimen itself.*

(*continued on next page*)

SKILL 4.3 Urine Specimen, Clean-Catch, Closed Drainage System for Culture and Sensitivity: Obtaining (*continued*)

- Collect urine in the container.
- Cap the container tightly, touching only the outside of the container and the cap. **Rationale:** *This prevents contamination or spilling of the specimen.*
- If necessary, clean the outside of the specimen container with disinfectant. **Rationale:** *This prevents transfer of microorganisms to others.*
- Remove and discard gloves. Perform hand hygiene and proceed to step 7 below.

CLOSED DRAINAGE SYSTEM

Sterile urine specimens can be obtained from closed drainage systems by inserting a sterile needle attached to a syringe through a drainage port in the tubing. Aspiration of urine from catheters can be done only with self-sealing rubber catheters—not plastic, silicone, or Silastic catheters. When self-sealing rubber catheters are used, the needle is inserted just above the location where the catheter is attached to the drainage tubing. The area from which to obtain urine may be marked by a patch on the catheter. Closed drainage urinary systems now have needleless ports, which avoids use of a needle to obtain a sample ❸. This protects the nurse from a needlestick injury and maintains the integrity and sterility of the catheter system by eliminating the need to puncture the tubing.

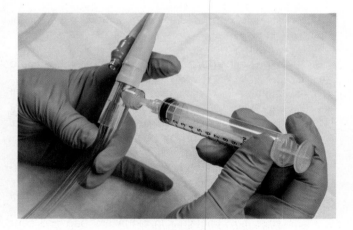

❸ Obtaining a urine specimen from a retention catheter using a needleless port.

The needleless port accepts a Luer-Lok syringe. Position the syringe perpendicular to the center of the port and insert, twist, and lock into the port. When the specimen is obtained and the syringe removed, the port seals itself.

To collect a specimen from a Foley (retention) catheter or a drainage tube, follow these steps:

- Apply clean gloves.
- If there is no urine in the catheter, clamp the drainage tubing at least 8 cm (3 in.) below the sampling port for about

30 minutes. **Rationale:** *This allows fresh urine to collect in the catheter.*
- Wipe the area where the needle or Luer-Lok syringe will be inserted with a disinfectant swab. The site should be distal to the tube leading to the balloon to avoid puncturing this tube. **Rationale:** *Disinfecting the needle insertion site removes any microorganisms on the surface of the catheter, thereby avoiding contamination of the needle and the entrance of microorganisms into the catheter.*
- Insert the needle at a 30- to 45-degree angle. This angle of entrance facilitates self-sealing of the rubber. Insert the Luer-Lok syringe at a 90-degree angle for the needleless port.
- Withdraw the required amount of urine, for example, 3 mL for a urine culture or 10 mL for a routine urinalysis.
- Unclamp the catheter.
- Transfer the urine to the specimen container. If a sterile culture tube is used, make sure the needle or syringe (depending on the system) does not touch the outside of the container.
- Discard the syringe and needle (depending on the system) in an appropriate sharps container.
- Cap the container.
- Remove and discard gloves. Perform hand hygiene.

7. Leave patient safe and comfortable. Label the specimen and transport it to the laboratory.
   - Ensure that the specimen label is attached to the specimen cup, not the lid, and that the laboratory requisition provides the correct information. Place the specimen in a plastic bag that has a biohazard label on it. Attach the requisition securely to the bag. **Rationale:** *Inaccurate identification or information on the specimen container can result in errors of diagnosis or therapy.*
   - Arrange for the specimen to be sent to the laboratory immediately. **Rationale:** *Bacterial cultures must be started immediately before any contaminating organisms can grow, multiply, and produce false results.*
8. Complete documentation using forms, checklists, or electronic dropdown lists supplemented by nurse's notes or additional comments as appropriate.
   - Record collection of the specimen, any pertinent observations of the urine such as color, odor, or consistency, and any difficulty in voiding that the patient experienced.
   - Indicate on the lab slip if the patient is taking any current antibiotic therapy or if the patient is menstruating.

SAMPLE DOCUMENTATION

[date] 0800 Informed of need for clean-catch urine for C&S. Instructed how to perform. Stated she understood. Urine specimen cloudy, deep amber. States she continues to have burning on urination. Urine specimen sent to lab. Antibiotic started per orders. *T. Sanchez*

SKILL 4.4 Urine Specimen, Ileal Conduit: Obtaining

An ileal conduit, or ileostomy, uses a short segment of the ileum that has been removed from the rest of the small intestines to redirect urine so it flows out of the body and drains into a bag located on the abdomen. Indications for an ileal conduit include removal of the bladder for severe trauma, malignancy, congenital defect of the urinary tract, or neurogenic nonfunctioning bladder.

Equipment

- Sterile catheter kit
- Sterile gloves (extra pair)
- Prep solution
- Sterile saline or water
- Underpad
- New urinary pouch
- Supplies necessary to apply new pouch
- Bath blanket, towels
- Clean gloves
- Soap and water
- Pitcher of water and glass
- Biohazard bag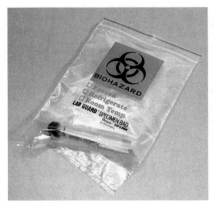

Source: Ronald May/Pearson Education, Inc.

❶ Biohazard bag for transportation of specimens.

Preparation

- Review healthcare provider's orders and patient care plan.
- Gather equipment.

Procedure

1. Introduce self to patient and verify the patient's identity using two identifiers. Explain to the patient what you are going to do, why it is necessary, and how the patient can participate. Discuss how the results will be used in planning further care or treatments.
2. Perform hand hygiene and observe appropriate infection control procedures.
3. Provide for patient privacy and don gloves.

4. Place bath blanket over patient's chest and position top covers over lower abdomen.
5. Place towels around stoma. **Rationale:** *Urine will leak around catheter.*
6. Open sterile packages.
7. Remove pouch or pouch and wafer/flange.
   Note: Do not use pouch contents to obtain urine specimen.
8. Remove and discard gloves. Perform hand hygiene and don sterile gloves.
9. Place sterile drape over stoma.
10. Remove lid from specimen container, and place end of catheter into container.
11. Apply lubricant to catheter.
12. Use forceps to pick up cotton ball and prep stoma with solution and rinse with sterile saline or water.
13. Insert tip of catheter into stoma approximately 4 cm (1.5 in.) ❷.

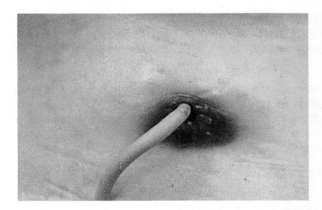

❷ A catheter is used to obtain a specimen from an ileal conduit.

14. When urine specimen is obtained (usually not more than 5–25 mL), remove catheter. If no urine is obtained, have patient drink water.
15. Return lid to specimen container and apply label.
16. If wafer is removed, wash and dry peristomal area.
17. Replace pouch or apply new pouch.
18. Remove and discard gloves. Perform hand hygiene and leave patient safe and comfortable.
19. Place specimen container in biohazard bag and send specimen to lab immediately or refrigerate.
20. Complete documentation using forms, checklists, or electronic dropdown lists supplemented by nurse's notes or additional comments as appropriate.

SAMPLE DOCUMENTATION

[date] 1325 Urine specimen for C&S obtained; 55 mL of cloudy amber urine withdrawn with sterile catheter inserted into ileostomy stoma; new pouch applied to stoma, area pink and intact; tolerated without complaint. *D. Handler*

SKILL 4.5 Urine Specimen, Routine, 24-Hour: Obtaining

A routine urinalysis evaluates a sample of urine to detect and assess its appearance, concentration, and content for urinary tract infection, kidney disease, and diabetes. A 24-hour urine is used to assess kidney functioning problems by measuring the amounts of urea (made when protein breaks down) and creatinine (formed from muscle breakdown).

Delegation or Assignment

The UAP may be assigned to collect a routine urine specimen. Provide the UAP with clear directions on how to instruct the patient to collect his or her own urine specimen or how to collect the specimen correctly for the patient who may need to use a bedpan or urinal.

Equipment

- Clean gloves as needed
- Clean bedpan, urinal, or commode for patients who are unable to void directly into the specimen container
- Wide-mouthed specimen container or newborn or infant urine specimen collection bag
- Completed laboratory requisition and label for container

For 24-Hour Urine Collection Only

- Appropriate specimen containers with or without preservative in accordance with the specific test
- Sign on or near the bed indicating the specific times for urine collection
- Ice-filled container in patient's room (bathroom)

Preparation

- Review healthcare provider's orders.
- Obtain needed equipment.
- Obtain a specimen container with preservative (if indicated) from the laboratory. Label the container with identifying information for the patient, the test to be performed, time started, and time of completion.
- For a newborn or infant, a specimen bag is used to collect the urine specimen. The specimen bag has an adhesive backing that attaches to the skin ❶. After the newborn or

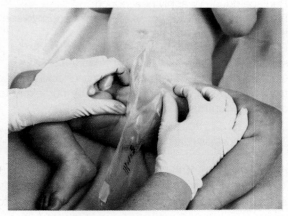

Source: Bindler/Pearson Education, Inc.

❶ Remove adhesive backing from urine collection bag and place securely over penis.

infant has voided a desired amount, gently remove the bag from the skin.

CAUTION! When applying the urine bag on girls, begin by placing the bag between the anus and the vagina and then allow it to adhere to the labia. For boys, be sure the bag adheres to the scrotum and that the scrotum is not inside the bag's opening.

- Provide a clean receptacle for collecting urine (bedpan, commode, or toilet collection device).
- Post signs in the patient's chart, room, and bathroom alerting personnel to save all urine during the specified time.
- Determine if the patient requires supervision or assistance in the bathroom. Patients who are seriously ill, physically incapacitated, or disoriented may need to use a bedpan or urinal in bed. A fracture bedpan may be needed for a patient with a hip fracture.

For 24-Hour Urine Collection Only

- Obtain a specimen container with preservative (if indicated) from the laboratory. Label the container with identifying information for the patient, the test to be performed, time started, and time of completion.
- Provide a clean receptacle for collecting urine (bedpan, commode, or toilet collection device).
- Some biochemical testing of urine is performed using dry reagent strips, or dipsticks at certain agencies. The dipstick contains dried reagents needed for a specific test. The person performing the test dips the strip into the urine, lets it sit for a specified amount of time, and compares the color change to a standard chart. For some examples of urine biochemical tests, see **Table 4–1 ≫**.
- Post signs in the patient's chart, room, and bathroom alerting personnel to save all urine during the specified time.

ROUTINE URINE SPECIMEN

Procedure

1. Prior to performing the procedure, introduce self and verify the patient's identity using facility protocol. Explain the purpose of the urine specimen and how the patient can assist.
   - Explain that all specimens must be free of fecal contamination, so voiding needs to occur at a different time from defecation and the patient needs to discard the toilet tissue in the toilet or in a waste bag rather than in the bedpan. **Rationale:** *Tissue in the specimen makes laboratory analysis more difficult.*
   - Discuss how the results will be used in planning further care or treatments. Give ambulatory patients the following information and instructions:
2. Perform hand hygiene and observe other appropriate infection control procedures such as using gloves when handling specimen containers.
   - Give the patient the specimen container, and direct the patient to the bathroom to void into it.
3. Provide for patient privacy.

SKILL 4.5 Urine Specimen, Routine, 24-Hour: Obtaining *(continued)*

TABLE 4–1 Quick-Result Urine Tests

Note: Always use a fresh urine sample and follow manufacturer's instructions.

Urine Test	Equipment	Procedure
For specific gravity	Clean gloves, multiple-test dipstick that has a separate reagent area for specific gravity	▪ Don clean gloves and place dipstick into the urine specimen. ▪ Observe the color and compare it to a standardized color chart on the bottle.
For pH	Clean gloves, dipstick or litmus paper (red or blue)	▪ Don a glove and dip a strip of either red or blue litmus paper into the urine specimen. ▪ Observe the color of the litmus paper and compare it to a standardized color chart on the bottle. The blue litmus paper, more commonly used, remains blue if the urine is alkaline and turns red if it is acidic. The red litmus paper remains red in the presence of acidic urine and turns blue if the urine is alkaline. Whichever litmus strip is used, red always indicates acidic urine and blue always indicates alkaline urine.
For glucose	Clean gloves, reagent tablet or reagent test strip, appropriate color chart, clean test tube and a dropper, if a tablet is used	▪ Don gloves. Most agencies require a second-voided specimen: Ask the patient to void, and in 30 minutes to void again, providing a specimen for the test this time. ▪ If Clinitest tablets are used, be careful not to touch the bottom of the test tube because it becomes extremely hot when the tablet boils in the presence of urine and water.
For ketone bodies ❷	Clean gloves, reagent tablet or dipstick	▪ Don a glove and place one or two drops of urine on a reagent tablet (e.g., an Acetest tablet) or dip a reagent test strip (e.g., Ketostix) into the urine. ▪ Observe and compare the results with the appropriate color chart to determine the quantity of ketones present.

Source: Ronald May/Pearson Education, Inc.

❷ Ketone strips are checked against the chart for ketone bodies.

Urine Test	Equipment	Procedure
For occult blood	Clean gloves, reagent strip	▪ Don a glove, and dip the reagent strip (e.g., Hemastix) into a sample of urine. ▪ Compare the color change with a color chart in the same manner as with other reagent strips.

4. Assist patients who are seriously ill, physically incapacitated, or disoriented. Provide required assistance in the bathroom, or help the patient to use a bedpan or urinal in bed. Direct patient to void in the container.

5. Ensure that the specimen is sealed and the container clean.
   - Put the lid tightly on the container. **Rationale:** *This prevents spillage of the urine and contamination of other objects.*
   - If the outside of the container has been contaminated by urine, apply clean gloves and clean it with soap and water. **Rationale:** *This prevents the spread of microorganisms.*
   - Remove and discard gloves. Perform hand hygiene and leave patient safe and comfortable. Proceed to step 6 below.

24-HOUR URINE SPECIMEN

1. Determine the patient's ability to understand instructions and to provide urine samples independently. Are there any fluid or dietary requirements associated with the test? Are there any medication restrictions or requirements for the test?

2. Tell the patient the purpose of the test and how the patient can assist. Then provide the following information and instructions:
   - State when the specimen collection will begin and end. (For example, a 24-hour urine test commonly begins at 0700 hours and ends at the same hour the next day.)
   - All urine must be saved and placed in the specimen containers once the test starts.

(continued on next page)

SKILL 4.5 Urine Specimen, Routine, 24-Hour: Obtaining (*continued*)

- Urine must be free of fecal contamination and toilet tissue.
- Each specimen must be given to the nursing staff immediately so that it can be placed in the appropriate specimen bottle.

3. Start the collection period.
   - Ask the patient to void in the toilet or bedpan or urinal. *Discard* this urine (check facility procedure), and document the time the test starts with this discarded specimen. **Rationale:** *The patient voids before the timed test begins to empty the bladder. The discarded urine may have been collecting in the bladder for many hours. For accuracy of the urine content and quantity, the timed collection period must begin at the time the patient empties the bladder.* Collect all subsequent urine specimens, including the one collected at the end of the period.
   - Ask the patient to ingest the required amount of liquid for certain tests or to restrict fluid intake. Follow the test directions.
   - Intake and output should be implemented and documented.
   - Instruct the patient to void all subsequent urine into the bedpan or urinal and to notify the nursing staff when each specimen is provided. Some tests require voiding at specified times.
   - Label the specimen containers sequentially (e.g., first specimen, second specimen, third specimen) if separate specimens are required.

4. Collect all of the required specimens.
   - Place each specimen into the appropriately labeled container. For some tests, each specimen is not kept separately but is poured into a large bottle.
     Note: All urine specimens must be collected for timed collections. If one voiding is missed, the timed urine collection may need to be restarted and the lab notified.
   - If the outside of the specimen container is contaminated with urine, apply gloves and clean it with soap and water. **Rationale:** *Cleaning prevents the transfer of microorganisms to others.*

5. Ensure that each specimen is refrigerated throughout the timed collection period. If not refrigerated, specimens are often kept on ice. Preservative may be used. **Rationale:** *Refrigeration or another form of cooling prevents bacterial decomposition of the urine.*

- Measure the amount of each urine specimen if required.
- Ask the patient to provide the last specimen 5–10 min before the end of the collection period.
- Inform the patient that the test is completed.
- Remove the signs and the specimen equipment from the patient's unit and bathroom.
- Remove and discard gloves. Perform hand hygiene and leave patient safe and comfortable.

CAUTION! Note any dietary restrictions or medication precautions in preparation for 24-hour urine collection.

---

6. Label and transport the specimen to the laboratory, using appropriate biohazard specimen bags or containers.
   - Ensure that the specimen label and the laboratory requisition have the correct information on them. Attach them securely to the specimen container. **Rationale:** *Inappropriate identification of the specimen can lead to errors of diagnosis or therapy for the patient.*
   - Arrange for the specimen to be taken immediately to the laboratory or placed in a refrigerator. **Rationale:** *When left at room temperature, urine deteriorates relatively rapidly from bacterial contamination; specimens should be analyzed immediately after collection. If the urine specimen is delayed from reaching the lab by more than 1 hour, a new specimen may be needed.*
   - For the 24-hour urine collection, record the starting time of the test, the name of the test, and completion of the specimen collection on the patient's chart. Include the date and specific time. In addition, if indicated for the specific test, note the time each urine specimen was collected, the volume of each specimen, the appearance of the urine, and other relevant data such as fluid intake or restrictions.

7. Document the collection of the specimen on the patient's chart. Include the date and time of collection and the appearance and odor of the urine.

SAMPLE DOCUMENTATION

[date] 1125 Urine specimen for routine urinalysis obtained; 35 mL of clear light amber urine sent; tolerated without complaint. *D. Handy*

≫ Bladder Interventions

Expected Outcomes

1. Patient voids 200 to 500 mL of urine without discomfort or difficulty.
2. Skin irritation does not occur with condom catheter use.
3. Suprapubic catheter remains intact.
4. Patient remains free of urinary tract infection.
5. Patient demonstrates self-care skills.
6. Peristomal skin remains intact and healthy.

SKILL 4.6 Bedpan: Assisting

Two types of bedpans are commonly used for toileting of a bedridden patient. The regular bedpan requires patients to raise their hips or roll on their side for correct placement. A fracture pan is designed for patients in casts or those who had hip surgery that cannot raise their hips up or roll on the regular bedpan.

Delegation or Assignment

The UAP commonly assists patients with bedpans. The nurse must determine if the specific patient has unique needs that require special training. Ensure that personnel are aware of any specimens that need to be collected. Abnormal findings must be validated and interpreted by the nurse. Note that state laws for UAPs vary, so this task might be assigned to the UAP rather than delegated.

Equipment

- Clean bedpan ❶ and cover
- Toilet tissue
- Basin of water, soap, washcloth, and towel
- Equipment for a specimen if required
- Clean gloves
- Disposable absorbent pad

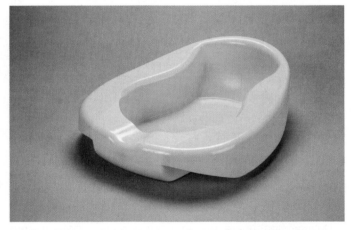

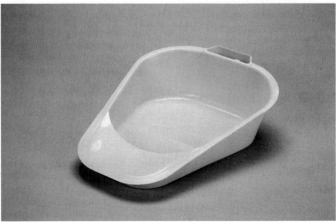

Sources: (Top and Bottom) Ronald May/Pearson Education, Inc.

❶ A bedpan and fracture pan used for patients in bed.

Preparation

- Adjust the bed to a height appropriate to prevent back strain.
- Elevate the rail on the opposite side of the bed. **Rationale:** *This prevents the patient from falling and provides a hand grasp for the patient if needed.*
- Evaluate the need for assistance in performing this skill.

Procedure

1. Prior to performing the procedure, introduce self to the patient and verify the patient's identity using two identifiers. Explain to the patient what you are going to do, why it is necessary, and how the patient can participate.
2. Perform hand hygiene and observe other appropriate infection control procedures.
3. Apply clean gloves.
4. Provide for patient privacy.
5. Prepare the patient.

CAUTION! Individuals (especially children) may use very different terms for a bowel movement. The nurse may need to try several different common words before finding one the patient understands.

- For patients who can assist by raising their buttocks, fold down the top bed linen on the near side to expose the hip, and adjust the gown so that it will not fall into the bedpan. **Rationale:** *A pie fold of the top bed linens exposes the patient minimally and facilitates placement of the bedpan.*
- For patients who cannot raise their buttocks onto and off a bedpan, fold the top bed linens down to the hips.
6. Place patient on the bedpan.
    - For patients who can lift their buttocks:
      a. Ask patients to flex the knees, rest their weight on the back and the heels, and then raise the buttocks. Patients can use a trapeze, if present, or grasp the side rail for support. Assist patients to lift the buttocks by placing the hand nearest the person's head palm up under the lower back, resting the elbow on the mattress, and using the forearm as a lever. **Rationale:** *Use of appropriate body mechanics by patient and nurse prevents unnecessary muscle strain and exertion.*
      b. Place the absorbent pad on the bed where the bedpan will be located. Position a regular bedpan under the buttocks with the narrow end toward the foot of the bed and the buttocks resting on the smooth, rounded rim. Place a slipper (fracture) pan with the flat end under the patient's buttocks. **Rationale:** *Improper placement of the bedpan can cause skin abrasion to the sacral area and spillage of the bedpan's contents.*
    - For patients who cannot lift their buttocks:
      a. Assist the patient to a side-lying position.
      b. Place the bedpan against the buttocks with the open rim toward the foot of the bed.
      c. Smoothly roll the patient onto the bedpan while holding the bedpan against the buttocks.

(continued on next page)

SKILL 4.6 Bedpan: Assisting *(continued)*

7. Elevate the head of the bed to a semi-Fowler position. **Rationale:** *This position relieves strain on the patient's back and permits a more normal position for elimination.* Recheck the position of the bedpan because it may have been repositioned while the head of the bed was being raised.
   - If the person is unable to assume a semi-Fowler position, place a small pillow under the back, or help the patient to another comfortable position.
8. Replace the top bed linen.
9. Provide the patient with toilet tissue, raise the side rail, lower the bed height, and ensure that the call light is readily accessible. Ask the patient to signal when finished. Leave only when, in your judgment, it is safe to do so. **Rationale:** *Having necessary items within reach prevents falls.*

Removing a Bedpan

10. Return the bed to the position used when giving the bedpan.
    - Hold the bedpan steady to prevent spillage of its contents.
    - Cover the bedpan, and place it on an adjacent chair with a pad or towel under it. **Rationale:** *Covering the bedpan reduces offensive odors and reduces the patient's embarrassment.*
11. Assist the patient with any needed hygienic measures.
    - Wrap toilet tissue several times around the gloved hand, and wipe the person from the pubic area to the anal area, using one stroke for each piece of tissue. **Rationale:** *Cleaning in this direction—from the less soiled area to the more soiled area—helps prevent the spread of microorganisms.*
    - Place the soiled tissue in the bedpan.

- Wash the anal area with soap and water as indicated, and thoroughly dry the area. **Rationale:** *Adequate washing and drying prevents skin abrasion and excessive accumulation of microorganisms.*
- Remove the disposable absorbent pad or replace the drawsheet if it is soiled.
- Offer the patient materials to wash and dry the hands. **Rationale:** *Hand washing following elimination is a practice that helps prevent the spread of microorganisms.*
12. Attend to any unpleasant odors in the environment with a nonaerosol deodorizer. **Rationale:** *Elimination odor can be embarrassing to patients and visitors alike. However, sprays may be harmful to people with respiratory problems, and some perfume sprays are offensive to some people.*
13. Attend to the used bedpan.
    - Acquire a specimen and measure output if required. Place it in the appropriately labeled container.
    - Empty and clean the bedpan. Provide a clean bedpan cover, if necessary, before returning it to the patient's unit.
    - Remove and discard gloves. Perform hand hygiene and leave the patient safe and comfortable.
14. Complete documentation using forms, checklists, or electronic dropdown lists supplemented by nurse's notes or additional comments as appropriate, including color, odor, amount, and consistency of feces.

SAMPLE DOCUMENTATION

[date] 1725 Had small amount of soft, light brown stool; tolerated without complaint. *D. Tandy*

SKILL 4.7 Bladder Irrigation: Continuous

Safety Note! *During scheduled clinical time, nursing students may have a learning opportunity to observe or assist with this skill only with faculty permission and with direct supervision from faculty or another RN.*

Delegation or Assignment

Due to the need for special skills and knowledge, urinary irrigation is generally not delegated or assigned to the UAP. If the patient has continuous irrigation, the UAP may care for the patient and note abnormal findings. These must be validated and interpreted by the nurse.

Equipment

- Irrigating solution (2000 mL sterile normal saline, or less than drainage bag volume) as prescribed
- IV tubing with roller clamp
- IV pole
- Antiseptic swabs
- Clean gloves

Preparation

- Review healthcare provider's orders and patient care plan.
- Note if patient has triple lumen indwelling catheter and drainage bag ❶.

Procedure

1. Introduce self to patient and verify the patient's identity using two identifiers. Explain to the patient what you are going to do, why it is necessary, and how the patient can participate. Discuss how the results will be used in planning further care or treatments.
2. Perform hand hygiene and observe appropriate infection control procedures.
3. Provide for patient privacy.
4. Don clean gloves.
5. Remove protective covering from spike on tubing, and insert spike into insertion port of solution container. Use aseptic technique.

SKILL 4.7 Bladder Irrigation: Continuous (*continued*)

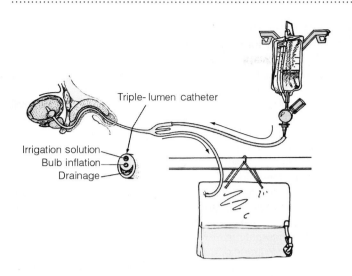

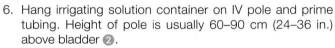

① Maintain continuous bladder irrigation by using a triple-lumen catheter for procedure.

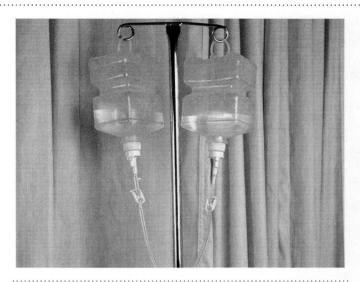

② Hang irrigating solution on IV pole at height of 60–90 cm (24–36 in.) above bladder.

6. Hang irrigating solution container on IV pole and prime tubing. Height of pole is usually 60–90 cm (24–36 in.) above bladder **②**.
   - Remove protective cover from end of tubing using aseptic technique.
   - Open roller clamp, and allow irrigating solution to run through tubing until all air is expelled. **Rationale:** *This prevents air from entering bladder and causing discomfort.*
   - Close roller clamp.
7. Connect tubing to catheter irrigating (indwelling) lumen using aseptic technique.
8. Check for patency of catheter; ensure there are no clots or foreign bodies that may obstruct catheter.
9. Remove and discard gloves. Perform hand hygiene and don new gloves.
10. Adjust drip rate of irrigating solution by adjusting the clamp on the tubing to increase or decrease based on urine outflow color.
    - Infuse continuously to keep urine drainage pink to clear.
    - When drainage is dark red or contains tissue or blood clots, increase drip rate. **Rationale:** *Increased drip rate will clear the drainage and flush out debris and clots.*
    - Change irrigation solution bottle using aseptic technique.
11. Check for bladder distention or abdominal pain. Note urine color.
12. Monitor urine output at least every hour to observe patency of system.
13. Empty drainage bag as needed. Subtract amount of irrigant infused from total output to obtain urine output and record.
14. Maintain catheter traction if taped to thigh. **Rationale:** *This promotes venous hemostasis.*
15. Remove and discard gloves. Perform hand hygiene and leave patient safe and comfortable.
16. Complete documentation using forms, checklists, or electronic dropdown lists supplemented by nurse's notes or additional comments as appropriate.

CAUTION! Procedure is done to flush clots and debris from bladder after prostatic surgery, to prevent catheter obstruction, and to promote patency. Immediately report bright red urine outflow because this indicates an arterial bleed.

SKILL 4.8 Bladder Irrigation: Providing

Safety Note! *During scheduled clinical time, nursing students may have a learning opportunity to observe or assist with this skill only with faculty permission and with direct supervision from faculty or another RN.*

Produces a washing out of the urinary bladder with specified solution to flush blood clots and debris (such as unwanted sediment, mucous, bacteria, tiny calculi) out of the bladder, restore patency of a urinary catheter, or instill medication to the bladder lining. This procedure is commonly done after a trans urethral resection of prostate (TURP) and for adults and children who do not have the capability to squeeze out urine or empty to completion due to disease or medical conditions.

(*continued on next page*)

SKILL 4.8 Bladder Irrigation: Providing *(continued)*

Delegation or Assignment

Due to the need for sterile technique, urinary irrigation is generally not delegated or assigned to the UAP. If the patient has continuous irrigation, the UAP may care for the patient and note abnormal findings. These must be validated and interpreted by the nurse.

Equipment

- Clean gloves, two pairs
- Retention catheter in place
- Drainage tubing and bag (if not in place)
- Drainage tubing clamp
- Antiseptic swabs
- Sterile receptacle
- Infusion tubing
- IV pole

For Open Irrigation Using a Two-way Indwelling Catheter Only

- Use an irrigation set ❶ or assemble individual items, including the following items:
  - Disposable water-resistant towel
  - Sterile irrigating solution
  - Sterile basin
  - Sterile 30- to 50-mL irrigating syringe
  - Sterile protective cap for drainage tubing

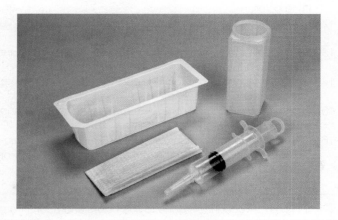

❶ An irrigation set.

Preparation

- Review healthcare provider's orders.
  - Before irrigating a catheter or bladder, check (1) the **reason** for the irrigation; (2) the **order** authorizing the continuous or intermittent irrigation (in most agencies, a primary care provider's order is required); (3) the type of sterile **solution**, the amount, and strength to be used, and the rate (if continuous); and (4) the type of **catheter** in place. If these are not specified on the patient's chart, check facility protocol.
- Sterile irrigating solution warmed or at room temperature (Label the irrigant clearly with the words *Bladder Irrigation,* including the information about any medications that have been added to the original solution, and the date, time, and nurse's initials.)

Procedure

1. Prior to performing the procedure, introduce self and verify the patient's identity using two identifiers. Explain to the patient what you are going to do, why it is necessary, and how the patient can participate. The irrigation should not be painful or uncomfortable. Discuss how the results will be used in planning further care or treatments.
2. Perform hand hygiene and observe other appropriate infection control procedures.
3. Provide for patient privacy.
4. Apply clean gloves.
5. Empty, measure, and record the amount and appearance of urine present in the drainage bag. Discard urine and gloves. **Rationale:** *Emptying the drainage bag allows more accurate measurement of urinary output after the irrigation is in place or completed. Assessing the character of the urine provides baseline data for later comparison.*
6. Prepare the equipment.
   - Perform hand hygiene.
   - Connect the irrigation infusion tubing to the irrigating solution and flush the tubing with solution, keeping the tip sterile. **Rationale:** *Flushing the tubing removes air and prevents it from being instilled into the bladder.*
   - Apply clean gloves and cleanse the port with antiseptic swabs.
   - Connect the irrigation tubing to the input port of the three-way catheter.
   - Connect the drainage bag and tubing to the urinary drainage port if not already in place.
   - Remove and discard gloves. Perform hand hygiene.
7. Irrigate the bladder.
   - For closed continuous bladder irrigation using a three-way catheter, open the clamp on the urinary drainage tubing (if present) ❷. **Rationale:** *This allows the irrigating solution to flow out of the bladder continuously.*

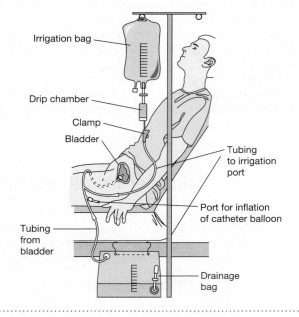

❷ A continuous bladder irrigation (CBI) setup.

SKILL 4.8 Bladder Irrigation: Providing (*continued*)

a. Apply clean gloves.
b. Open the regulating clamp on the irrigating fluid infusion tubing and adjust the flow rate as prescribed by the primary care provider or to 40–60 drops/min if not specified.
c. Assess the drainage for amount, color, and clarity. The amount of drainage should equal the amount of irrigant entering the bladder plus expected urine output. Empty the bag frequently so that it does not exceed half full.

- For closed intermittent irrigation, determine whether the solution is to remain in the bladder for a specified time.
  a. If the solution is to remain in the bladder (a bladder irrigation or instillation), close the clamp to the urinary drainage tubing. **Rationale:** *Closing the flow clamp allows the solution to be retained in the bladder and in contact with bladder walls.*
  b. If the solution is being instilled to irrigate the catheter, open the flow clamp on the urinary drainage tubing. **Rationale:** *Irrigating solution will flow through the urinary drainage port and tubing, removing mucous shreds or clots.*
  c. If a three-way catheter is used, open the flow clamp to the irrigating fluid infusion tubing, allowing the specified amount of solution to infuse. Then close the clamp on the infusion tubing.

  or

  a. If a two-way catheter is used, connect an irrigating syringe with a needleless adapter to the injection port on the drainage tubing and instill the solution.
  b. After the specified period the solution is to be retained has passed, open the drainage tubing flow clamp and allow the bladder to empty.
  c. Assess the drainage for amount, color, and clarity. The amount of drainage should equal the amount of irrigant entering the bladder plus expected urine output.
- Remove and discard gloves. Perform hand hygiene and proceed to step 8 below.

CAUTION! Opening a closed urinary drainage system is indicated as a last resort to reestablish catheter patency. Manual irrigation should be done carefully for a patient with transurethral resection of a bladder tumor due to risk of bladder rupture.

OPEN IRRIGATION USING A TWO-WAY INDWELLING CATHETER

- Prepare the equipment.
  - Perform hand hygiene.
  - Using aseptic technique, open supplies and pour the irrigating solution into the sterile basin or receptacle. **Rationale:** *Aseptic technique is vital to reduce the risk of instilling microorganisms into the urinary tract during the irrigation.*
  - Place the disposable water-resistant towel under the catheter.
  - Apply clean gloves.
  - Disconnect catheter from drainage tubing and place the catheter end in the sterile basin. Place the sterile protective cap over the end of the drainage tubing. **Rationale:** *The end of the drainage tubing will be considered contaminated if it touches bed linens or skin surfaces.*
  - Draw the prescribed amount of irrigating solution into the syringe, maintaining the sterility of the syringe and solution.
- Irrigate the bladder.
  - Insert the tip of the syringe into the catheter opening.
  - Gently and slowly inject the solution into the catheter at approximately 3 mL per second. In adults, about 30–40 mL generally is instilled for catheter irrigations; 100–200 mL may be instilled for bladder irrigation or instillation. **Rationale:** *Gentle instillation reduces the risks of injury to bladder mucosa and of bladder spasms.*
  - Remove the syringe and allow the solution to drain back into the basin.
  - Continue to irrigate the patient's bladder until the total amount to be instilled has been injected or when fluid returns are clear and/or clots are removed.
  - Remove protective cap from drainage tube and wipe with antiseptic swab.
  - Reconnect catheter to drainage tubing.
  - Remove and discard gloves. Perform hand hygiene.
  - Assess the drainage for amount, color, and clarity. The amount of drainage should equal at least the amount of irrigant entering the bladder plus any urine that may have been dwelling in the bladder.
8. Assess the patient's comfort and the urinary output.
   - Apply clean gloves.
   - Empty the drainage bag and measure the contents. Subtract the amount of irrigant instilled from the total volume of drainage to obtain the volume of urine output.
   - Remove and discard gloves. Perform hand hygiene and leave the patient safe and comfortable.
9. Complete documentation using forms, checklists, or electronic dropdown lists supplemented by nurse's notes or additional comments as appropriate.
   - Note any abnormal constituents such as blood clots, pus, or mucous shreds.

SAMPLE DOCUMENTATION

[date] 0810 Closed continuous bladder irrigation with sterile normal saline infusing at 50 gtts/min.; few red stringy clots noted in tubing and faint pink-tinged coloring noted at bottom of drainage bag; Denies pain at this time, states ready for breakfast. *P. Hanger*

SKILL 4.9 Commode: Assisting

A bedside commode is a movable toilet that does not have running water. It looks like a chair with a toilet seat and has a bucket underneath. The bucket can be removed for cleaning after the commode is used. It can be placed beside the bed if the patient cannot get to the bathroom.

Delegation or Assignment

Assisting the patient to a commode chair may be delegated or assigned to the UAP. The nurse gives the UAP any instructions specific to the patient or procedure and remains responsible for assessing, interpreting abnormal findings, and determining, appropriate responses. Note that state laws for UAPs vary, so this task might be assigned to the UAP rather than delegated.

Equipment

- Commode with locking wheels or rubber-tipped legs
- Toilet tissue
- Nurse's call button
- Slippers
- Bath blanket

Preparation

- Have commode chair positioned next to the bed.
- Some cultures incorporate the participation of family members to provide personal care, particularly assistance with using a bedpan or bedside commode, to maintain modesty.

Procedure

1. Introduce self to patient and verify the patient's identity using two identifiers. Explain to the patient what you are going to do, why it is necessary, and how the patient can participate. Discuss how the results will be used in planning further care or treatments.
2. Perform hand hygiene and observe appropriate infection control procedures.
3. Provide for patient privacy.
4. Place commode at foot of bed. Be sure to lock wheels on commode if needed.
5. Place slippers on patient.
6. Raise head of bed to facilitate moving patient to edge of bed.
7. Move patient to edge of bed and assist to a sitting position at edge of bed. Instruct patient to place feet flat on floor.
8. Stand directly in front of patient, blocking patient's toes with your feet and patient's knees with your knees. *Rationale: Prevents patient from buckling knees.*
9. Flex your knees.
10. Place your arms securely around patient's waist, use transfer belt, or follow facility policy for moving device. *Rationale: This helps stabilize the patient for transfer.*
11. When starting to transfer, avoid bending at the waist. *Rationale: This prevents back strain.*
12. Instruct patient to push self off bed and support his or her own weight.
13. Straighten your knees and hips as you raise patient to standing position.

14. Pivot patient in front of commode ①. Instruct patient to grasp arm rest on farthest side.

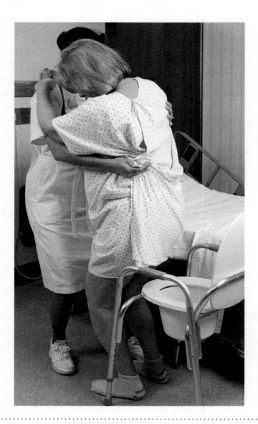

① Pivot with patient and bend knees when seating patient.

15. Lower patient onto commode, using correct body mechanics (flexing your hip and knees but not your back) to ensure patient is securely positioned on commode.
16. Place toilet tissue within easy reach.
17. Cover patient with bath blanket for warmth and privacy.
18. Place call bell within easy access of patient.
19. Provide privacy by closing curtains and shutting door.
20. Perform hand hygiene.
21. Assist patient back to bed.
22. Empty and clean commode. Measure output as needed.
23. Perform hand hygiene and leave the patient safe and comfortable.
24. Complete documentation using forms, checklists, or electronic dropdown lists supplemented by nurse's notes or additional comments as appropriate, including the amount, color, appearance, and odor of urine or stool and type of support needed for transfer to commode.

SAMPLE DOCUMENTATION

[date] 2200 Up to commode chair with assistance; voided 120 mL of clear light amber urine; back to bed with no complaints. *W. Murphy*

SKILL 4.10 Urinal: Assisting

A male patient uses a urinal to void into when unable to walk to the commode or bathroom or when bedridden.

Delegation or Assignment

Assisting the patient with a urinal is often delegated or assigned to the UAP. Ensure that the UAP is aware of any specimens to be collected. The nurse must validate and interpret abnormal findings. Note that state laws for UAPs vary, so this task might be assigned to the UAP rather than delegated.

Equipment

- Clean urinal ❶ ❷
- Toilet tissue
- Equipment for specimen if required
- Clean gloves

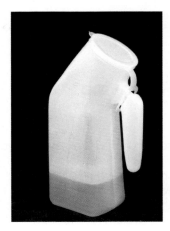

Source: James E. Knopf/Shutterstock

❶ Male urinal.

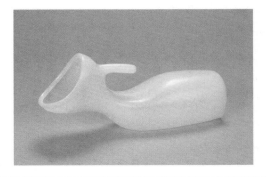

❷ Female urinal.

Preparation

- Assist the patient to an appropriate position.
- Males confined to bed may prefer a semi-Fowler position, or the male may prefer a standing position at the side of the bed if health permits.
- Determine if there are any restrictions in positioning the patient. Inquire whether the patient has used a urinal previously. If so, determine if the patient has any unique needs related to the use of the urinal. Locate the patient's urinal.

Procedure

1. Prior to performing the procedure, introduce self and verify the patient's identity using two identifiers. Explain to the patient how to use a urinal if needed.
2. Perform hand hygiene and observe other appropriate infection control procedures.
3. Provide for patient privacy. Don gloves.
4. Assist the patient with using the urinal:
   - Offer the urinal so that the patient can position it independently.
   or
   - Place the urinal between the patient's legs with the handle uppermost so that urine will flow into it.
   - Leave the signal cord within reach of the person. **Rationale:** *The patient can then call for assistance if required.*
   - Perform hand hygiene. Leave for 2–3 min or until the patient signals.
   or
   - Remain if the patient needs support to stand at the bedside or other assistance.
5. Assist the patient with removing the urinal as needed.
   - Apply clean gloves. Remove the urinal.
   - If wet, wipe the area around the urethral orifice with a tissue. Dry the perineum.
   - If wet, change the linens or pad under the patient.
   - Provide the patient with hand wipes, a dampened washcloth, or water, soap, and a towel to wash and dry hands.
6. Attend to the urine as required.
   - Measure the urine if the patient is on monitored intake and output, and transfer a specimen to the appropriate container if required.
   - Empty and rinse out the urinal, and return it to the bedside unit. If the male patient prefers, the urinal may be hung on the side rail by its handle for easy access.
   - Remove and discard gloves. Perform hand hygiene and leave the patient safe and comfortable.
7. Complete documentation using forms, checklists, or electronic dropdown lists supplemented by nurse's notes or additional comments as appropriate. Record the amount of urine, if it was measured, and all assessment data (e.g., cloudy urine, reddened perineum).

SAMPLE DOCUMENTATION

[date] 1320 Assisted with use of urinal due to arm in cast. Voided 450 mL dark yellow, clear, odorless urine. Specimen to lab for UA. Encouraged to drink more fluids; ice water and juice placed at bedside. Patient verbalizes agreement to increase intake. Tolerated without incident. *K. Clark*

(continued on next page)

SKILL 4.10 Urinal: Assisting (*continued*)

Lifespan Considerations

NEWBORNS AND INFANTS

- Newborns and infants have no conscious control, and the urine is released after a small amount accumulates in the bladder.

CHILDREN

- In children, 50–200 mL stimulates stretch receptors in the bladder.
- Urinary control usually takes place between 2–4½ years of age. Boys can be slower than girls in developing this control.
- Teaching proper perineal hygiene can reduce infection. Girls should learn to wipe from front to back and wear cotton underwear. **Rationale:** *Wiping from front to back prevents stool or vaginal secretions from contaminating the urethral meatus. Wearing cotton underwear is recommended over nylon because it "breathes" and is less likely to support bacterial growth.*
- Teach children and parents that children should go to the bathroom as soon as the sensation to void is felt and not try to hold the urine in.

OLDER ADULTS

- Bladder capacity decreases in older adults, as does ability to completely empty the bladder.
- Decreased muscle tone may lead to nocturia, frequency, and increased residual.
- Altered cognition may lead to incontinence since it prevents the person from understanding the need to urinate and the actions needed to perform the activity.
- Many older men have enlarged prostate glands, which can inhibit complete emptying of the bladder. This often results in urinary retention and urgency, which sometimes causes incontinence.
- Women past menopause have decreased estrogen, which results in a decrease in perineal tone and support of bladder, vagina, and pelvic tissues. This often results in urgency and stress incontinence and can even increase the incidence of urinary tract infections (UTIs).
- Increased stiffness and pain in joints, previous joint surgery, and neuromuscular problems can impair mobility and often make it difficult to get to the bathroom.

SKILL 4.11 Urinary Catheter: Caring for and Removing

Urinary catheter care helps reduce the risk of infection. The skin around the catheter and the proximal catheter area needs to be kept as clean as possible using soap and water daily. Hand hygiene before and after handling a catheter and maintaining a "closed" drainage system will also help prevent introduction of bacteria into the bladder.

Delegation or Assignment

Routine care of the patient with an indwelling catheter may be delegated or assigned to the UAP. Abnormal findings must be validated and interpreted by the nurse. Removal of an indwelling catheter may be performed by the UAP according to facility policy, if they have been thoroughly trained and are aware of conditions that could arise that require the assistance of a nurse. Note that state laws for UAPs vary, so this task might be assigned to the UAP rather than delegated.

Equipment

- Clean gloves, three pairs
- Washcloth, soap, and towels
- Graduated container to measure urine

For Catheter Removal Only

- Paper towel or waste receptacle
- Luer-Lok or slip-tip syringe at least as large as the size of the retention balloon (printed on the inflation port)

Preparation

- Review healthcare provider's orders.
- Determine an appropriate time for catheter care or removal, and patient's knowledge and need for teaching.

Procedure

1. Introduce self and verify the patient's identity using two identifiers. Explain to the patient what you are going to do, why it is necessary, and how the patient can participate. Discuss how the results will be used in planning further care or treatments.
2. Perform hand hygiene and observe other appropriate infection control procedures.
3. Provide for patient privacy and don gloves.
4. Prepare the patient.
   - Position the patient in a supine position.
   - Drape the patient, exposing only the perineal area.

Perform Catheter Care

- Apply clean gloves.
- Wash the urinary meatus and the proximal catheter area with soap and water, being careful not to pull on the catheter. Dry gently.
- Remove and discard gloves. Perform hand hygiene and proceed to step 5 below.

Remove the Catheter

- Place a towel or receptacle between the patient's legs.
- Detach the catheter from where it has been secured to the patient's skin.
- Don clean gloves.
- Insert the hub of the syringe into the inflation tube of the catheter.
- Withdraw all the fluid from the balloon ❶ ❷ **Rationale:** *This will permit the balloon to deflate.* If not all fluid can be removed, report this fact to the nurse in charge before proceeding. *Do not pull* the catheter while the balloon is inflated. **Rationale:** *The urethra may be injured if the inflated balloon is pulled through it.*

SKILL 4.11 Urinary Catheter: Caring for and Removing (*continued*)

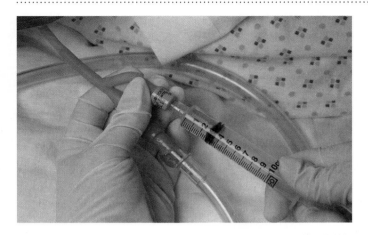

❶ Insert syringe hub into balloon port and withdraw fluid from retention catheter balloon.

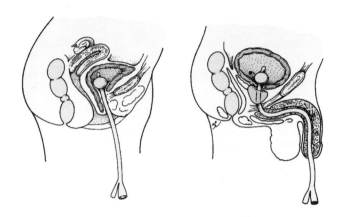

❷ To prevent damage to urethra, balloon must be deflated before removing.

- Gently withdraw the catheter, observe for intactness of tip, and place in the towel or waste receptacle. **Rationale:** *If the catheter is not intact, parts may remain in the bladder. Report this immediately to the nurse in charge or primary care provider.*
- Wash and dry the perineal area. Remove gloves and perform hand hygiene. Proceed to step 5.

CAUTION! Do not aspirate balloon vigorously. Doing so may collapse inflation lumen and prevent balloon deflation.

---

5. Empty the urine collection bag.
   - Apply clean gloves.
   - Obtain the graduated container used for measuring urine for that patient.
   - Place a paper towel on the floor below the bag.
   - Remove the end of the drainage tube from its protective housing on the collection bag without touching the end.
   - Point the tube into the graduated container and release the clamp.
   - After the bag is completely emptied, cleanse the end of the tube according to facility policy (e.g., with an alcohol swab), clamp the tube, and replace it into the protective housing.
   - Note the volume and characteristics of the urine. Empty the container into the toilet if the urine does not need to be saved.
   - Rinse the graduated container and return it to its storage location.
6. Discard all used supplies in appropriate receptacles.
7. Remove and discard gloves. Perform hand hygiene and leave the patient safe and comfortable.
8. Complete documentation using forms, checklists, or electronic dropdown lists supplemented by nurse's notes or additional comments as appropriate.
   - *For catheter removal procedure only,* record the time the catheter was removed; the intactness of the catheter; the amount, color, and clarity of the urine; and how patient tolerated the procedure.
9. *For catheter removal procedure only,* determine time of first voiding and the amount voided over the first 8 hours. Compare this with the fluid intake. **Rationale:** *When the fluid output is considerably less than the fluid intake, the bladder may be retaining urine.* If urine retention is suspected, scan or palpate the bladder for fullness. Use noninvasive methods to encourage voiding such as allowing the patient to hear running water or placing the patient's hand in water. Notify the primary care provider if the patient has not voided in 8 hours (or another interval specified by policy) because the patient may need to be recatheterized. Record the voiding or other action taken.

SAMPLE DOCUMENTATION

[date] 1015 Foley removed intact after aspirating balloon for 10 mL fluid without difficulty. Moderate amount white sediment noted around catheter tip. Peri care provided. Skin intact and without lesions. Taught to continue goal intake of fluids of 150 mL/hour. Verbalized agreement. Tolerated without complaint. *S. Brown*

[date] 1645 Up to BR. Voided 600 mL amber urine. C/o slight burning at start of urination. States will continue fluid intake. Dr. Wertz notified of burning on urination. *S. Brown*

SKILL 4.12 Urinary Catheterization: Performing

A routine medical procedure of inserting a urinary catheter into the patient's bladder via the urethra allows the patient's urine to drain freely from the bladder. This procedure is performed for both diagnostic and therapeutic purposes.

Delegation or Assignment

Due to the need for sterile technique and detailed knowledge of anatomy, insertion of a urinary catheter is not always delegated or assigned to the UAP. In some states, a trained UAP may perform a urinary catheterization. Assessment and evaluation of effectiveness of the procedure remain the responsibility of the nurse. Note that state laws for UAPs vary, so this task might be assigned to the UAP rather than delegated.

Equipment

- Sterile catheter of appropriate size (An extra catheter should also be at hand.)

CAUTION! Recommended urinary catheter sizes for children:

> Newborn: 3.5–5 French umbilical catheter
>
> Infant: 5–6 French
>
> Toddler and preschooler: 6–10 French
>
> School-age child: 10–12 French
>
> Adolescent: 12–14 French

Catheterization Kit ❶ *or Individual Sterile Items*
- Sterile gloves
- Waterproof drape(s)
- Antiseptic solution
- Cleansing balls
- Forceps
- Water-soluble lubricant
- Urine receptacle
- Specimen container

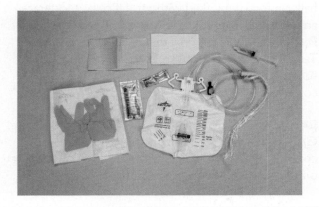

❶ Indwelling catheter insertion kit for catheterization.

For an Indwelling Catheter
- Syringe prefilled with sterile water in amount specified by catheter manufacturer ❷
- Collection bag and tubing
- 5–10 mL 2% Xylocaine gel or water-soluble lubricant for urethral injection (if facility permits)

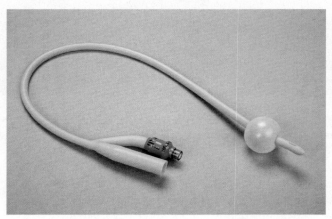

A

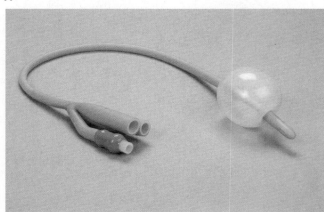

B

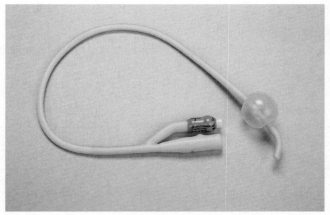

C

❷ *A,* A retention (Foley) catheter with the balloon inflated; *B,* Three-way Foley catheter, often used for continuous bladder irrigation; *C,* Coudé catheter tip.

SKILL 4.12 Urinary Catheterization: Performing (*continued*)

- Clean gloves
- Supplies for performing perineal cleansing
- Bath blanket or sheet for draping the patient
- Adequate lighting (obtain a flashlight or lamp if necessary.)

Preparation

- Review healthcare provider's orders.
- If using a catheterization kit, read the label carefully to ensure that all necessary items are included.
- Allow adequate time to perform the catheterization. Although the entire procedure can require as little as 15 minutes, several sources of difficulty could result in a much longer time period. If possible, this procedure should not be performed just prior to or after the patient eats.
- Some patients may feel uncomfortable being catheterized by nurses of the opposite gender. If this is the case, obtain the patient's permission. Also consider whether facility policy requires or encourages having a person of the patient's same gender present for the procedure.

Procedure

1. Prior to performing the procedure, check healthcare provider's order, introduce self and verify the patient's identity using two identifiers. Explain to the patient what you are going to do, why it is necessary, and how the patient can participate.
2. Perform hand hygiene and observe other appropriate infection control procedures.
3. Provide for patient privacy.
   - Apply clean gloves and perform routine perineal care to cleanse the meatus from gross contamination. For women, use this time to locate the urinary meatus relative to surrounding structures.
   - Remove and discard gloves. Perform hand hygiene.
4. Place the patient in the appropriate position and drape all areas except the perineum.
   - *Female:* supine with knees flexed, feet about ½ m (2 ft) apart, and hips slightly externally rotated, if possible
   - *Male:* supine, thighs slightly abducted or apart
5. Establish adequate lighting. Stand on the patient's right if you are right-handed, on the patient's left if you are left-handed.
6. If using a collecting bag and it is not contained within the catheterization kit, open the drainage package and place the end of the tubing within reach. **Rationale:** *Because one hand is needed to hold the catheter once it is in place, open the package while two hands are still available.*
7. Remove and discard gloves. Perform hand hygiene.
8. Open the catheterization kit ❸. Place a waterproof drape under the buttocks (female) or penis (male) without contaminating the center of the drape with your hands.
9. Apply sterile gloves ❹.
10. Organize the remaining supplies:
    - Saturate the cleansing balls with the antiseptic solution.
    - Open the lubricant package.
    - Remove the specimen container and place it nearby with the lid loosely on top.

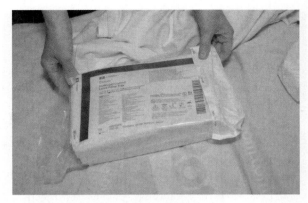

Source: Ronald May/Pearson Education, Inc.

❸ Open the sterile package by tearing it along the lined edge of the plastic wrap.

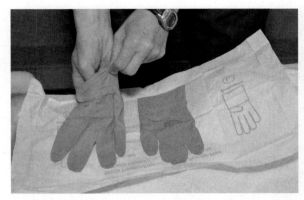

Source: Ronald May/Pearson Education, Inc.

❹ Don sterile gloves, being careful not to contaminate the sterile field.

11. Attach the prefilled syringe to the indwelling catheter inflation hub ❺, ❻, ❼. Follow facility policy regarding pretesting of the balloon.
    Note: Silicone catheter balloons should *not* be pretested.

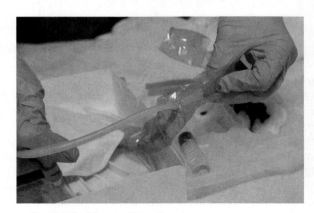

Source: Ronald May/Pearson Education, Inc.

❺ Remove Foley from protective sleeve.

(*continued on next page*)

SKILL 4.12 Urinary Catheterization: Performing *(continued)*

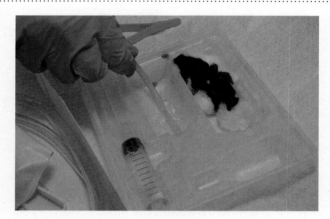

Source: Ronald May/Pearson Education, Inc.

⑥ Lubricate tip of catheter to facilitate insertion without trauma.

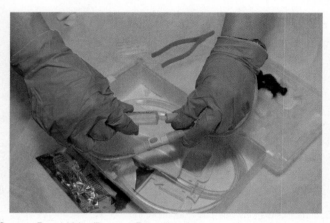

Source: Ronald May/Pearson Education, Inc.

⑦ Insert the tip of the prefilled sterile water syringe into the catheter side arm to inflate the balloon after the catheter is inserted.

12. Lubricate the catheter 2.5–5 cm (1–2 in.) for females, 15–17.5 cm (6–7 in.) for males and place it with the drainage end inside the collection container.
13. If desired, place the fenestrated drape over the perineum, exposing the urinary meatus.
14. Cleanse the meatus.
    Note: The nondominant hand is considered contaminated once it touches the patient's skin.

For Female Patients

■ Use your nondominant hand to spread the labia so the meatus is visible. Establish firm but gentle pressure on the labia. The antiseptic may make the tissues slippery, but the labia must not be allowed to return over the cleaned meatus. (*Note:* Location of the urethral meatus is best identified during the cleansing process.) Pick up a cleansing ball with the forceps in your dominant hand and wipe one side of the labia majora in an anteroposterior direction ⑧. Use great care that wiping the patient does not contaminate this sterile hand. Use a new ball for the opposite side. Repeat for the labia minora. Use the last ball to cleanse directly over the meatus.

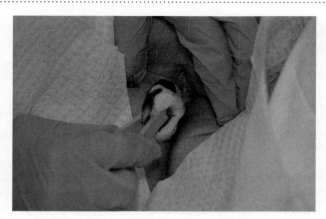

Source: Ronald May/Pearson Education, Inc.

⑧ Cleanse meatus by using one downward stroke per cotton ball to wipe each side and directly over meatus.

For Male Patients

■ Use your nondominant hand to grasp the penis just below the glans. If necessary, retract the foreskin. Hold the penis firmly upright, with slight tension. **Rationale:** *Lifting the penis in this manner helps straighten the urethra.* Pick up a cleansing ball with the forceps in your dominant hand and wipe from the center of the meatus in a circular motion around the glans to the base. Use great care that wiping the patient does not contaminate this sterile hand. Using a new ball each time, repeat this action three more times. The antiseptic may make the tissues slippery but the foreskin must not be allowed to return over the cleaned meatus and the penis must not be dropped.

15. Insert the catheter ⑨.
    • Grasp the catheter firmly 5–7.5 cm (2–3 in.) from the tip. Ask the patient to take a slow deep breath and insert the catheter as the patient exhales. Slight resistance is expected as the catheter passes through the sphincters. If necessary, twist the catheter or hold pressure on the catheter until the sphincter relaxes.

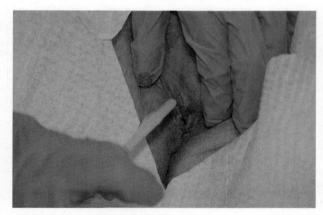

Source: Ronald May/Pearson Education, Inc.

⑨ Insert catheter gently into meatus until urine begins to flow; then advance another 2.5–5 cm (1–2 in.).

SKILL 4.12 Urinary Catheterization: Performing (*continued*)

- Advance the catheter 5 cm (2 in.) farther after the urine begins to flow through it. **Rationale:** *This is to be sure it is fully in the bladder, will not easily fall out, and balloon is completely in the bladder.*
- If the catheter accidentally contacts the labia or slips into the vagina, it is considered contaminated and a new, sterile catheter must be used. The contaminated catheter may be left in the vagina until the new catheter is inserted to help avoid mistaking the vaginal opening for the urinary meatus.

16. Hold the catheter with the nondominant hand.
17. For an indwelling catheter, inflate the retention balloon with the designated volume ⑩.
    - Without releasing the catheter (and, for females, without releasing the labia), hold the inflation valve between two fingers of your nondominant hand while you attach the syringe (if not left attached earlier when testing the balloon) and inflate with your dominant hand. If the patient complains of discomfort, immediately withdraw the instilled fluid, advance the catheter further, and attempt to inflate the balloon again.
    - Pull gently on the catheter until resistance is felt to ensure that the balloon has inflated and to place it in the trigone of the bladder.

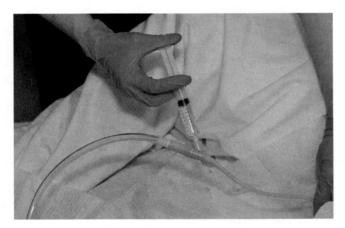

Source: Ronald May/Pearson Education, Inc.

⑩ Inject water from prefilled syringe into catheter balloon after inserting catheter.

CAUTION! Catheter-associated urinary tract infection (CAUTI) is the most common type of healthcare-associated infection. Chronic irritation and inflammation of bladder mucosa due to long-term (over 8 months) presence of an indwelling catheter (urethral or suprapubic) is associated with an increased risk for bladder cancer.

---

18. Collect a urine specimen if needed. For a straight catheter, allow 20–30 mL to flow into the bottle without touching the catheter to the bottle. For an indwelling catheter preattached to a drainage bag, a specimen may be taken from the bag this initial time only.

19. Allow the straight catheter to continue draining into the urine receptacle ⑪. If necessary (e.g., an open system), attach the drainage end of an indwelling catheter to the collecting tubing and bag.

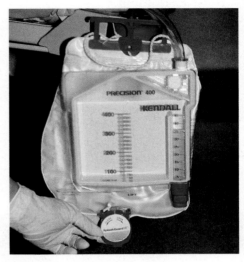

Source: Ronald May/Pearson Education, Inc.

⑪ Attach urine collection bag to nonmovable part of bed. Do not allow tubing to hang below collection bag.

20. Examine and measure the urine. In some cases, only 750–1000 mL of urine are to be drained from the bladder at one time. Check facility policy for further instructions if this should occur.
21. Remove the straight catheter when urine flow stops. For an indwelling catheter, secure the catheter tubing to the thigh for female patients and the upper thigh or lower abdomen for male patients with enough slack to allow usual movement ⑫. A manufactured catheter-securing device can be used to secure the catheter tubing to the patient. **Rationale:** *This prevents unnecessary trauma to the urethra.* Next hang the bag below the level of bladder. No tubing should fall below the top of the bag nor touch the floor.
22. Wipe any remaining antiseptic or lubricant from the perineal area. Replace the foreskin if retracted earlier. Return the patient to a comfortable position. Instruct the

SAMPLE DOCUMENTATION
2/24/15 0530 Patient agreed to insertion of indwelling catheter for pre-op as per orders. #16 Foley with balloon inflated with 10 mL sterile saline inserted without difficulty, secured to thigh, connected to straight drainage. Immediate return of 100 mL pale, clear yellow urine. Tolerated with no complaints of discomfort. *G. Hampton*

(*continued on next page*)

SKILL 4.12 Urinary Catheterization: Performing *(continued)*

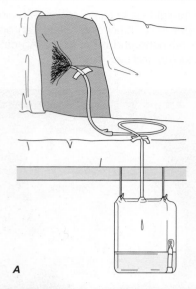

A

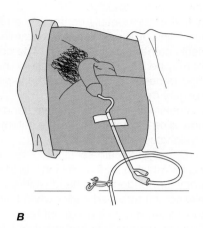

B

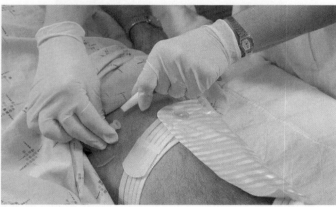

C

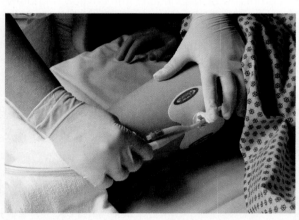

D

⑫ Tape the catheter to the *A,* inside of a female's thigh or *B,* thigh or abdomen of a male patient; *C,* A Velcro catheter securement device; *D,* A dissolvable, adhesive device with a swivel clamp to hold the urinary catheter in place.

patient on positioning and moving with the catheter in place.

23. Discard all used supplies in appropriate receptacles.

24. Remove and discard gloves. Perform hand hygiene and leave the patient safe and comfortable.

25. Complete documentation using forms, checklists, or electronic dropdown lists supplemented by nurse's notes or additional comments as appropriate, including the catheterization procedure, catheter size, and results.

Patient Teaching

Teach the patient going home with an indwelling catheter to:

- Never pull on the catheter.
- Keep the catheter tubing attached to the leg using a catheter securing device.
- Ensure that there are no kinks or twists in the tubing.
- Keep the urine drainage bag below the level of the bladder.
- Report signs and symptoms of a urinary tract infection (UTI) including burning, urgency, abdominal pain, cloudy urine; in older adults, confusion may be an early sign.

- Maintain adequate oral intake of fluids.
- Know catheter and bag changes are the responsibility of the nurse and are usually performed once a month, although facility policy may differ.
- Discuss with the nurse any issues of sexuality related to having an indwelling catheter. Nurses who are not familiar or comfortable with providing the patient this information must request another healthcare provider to assume this responsibility.

SKILL 4.12 Urinary Catheterization: Performing (*continued*)

INTERMITTENT SELF-CATHETERIZATION AT HOME USING CLEAN TECHNIQUE

Many home care patients who require assistance with emptying their bladders are usually placed on intermittent clean catheterization protocols rather than having an indwelling catheter. If spontaneous voiding returns, frequency of catheterizations can be extended to every 12 hours and discontinued when the residual urine is consistently less than 100 mL in 24 hours. Teach the patient to:

- Keep necessary equipment and supplies available at home
  - Straight catheters in clean container, plastic bag, or wrapped in aluminum foil
  - Washcloth, soap, water
  - Water-soluble lubricant (e.g., K-Y, Surgilube)
  - Plastic bags
  - Basin or container
  - Mirror
- Attempt to urinate and if unable to do so, follow these steps:
  - Perform hand hygiene and gather equipment. (Keep equipment in one large container.)
  - Assume a sitting position on bed or commode. (Place plastic under towel if bed is used.)
  - Insert the catheter.

For female patients
- Separate labia with one hand while cleaning with soap and water front to back with other hand.
- Position mirror to visualize urinary meatus.
- Remove catheter from container (plastic bag or aluminum foil).
- Lubricate end of catheter with water-soluble lubricant and place other end in container to catch urine.
- While holding labia apart with one hand, insert catheter about 8 cm (3 in.) or until urine flows.

For male patients
- Retract the foreskin, if present, and wash tip of penis with soap and water.

- Remove catheter from container (plastic bag or aluminum foil).
- Lubricate the first 18–25 cm (7–10 in.) of catheter with water-soluble lubricant. Place other end in container to catch urine.
- Hold penis at right angle to body, keeping foreskin retracted. Insert catheter about 18–25 cm (7–10 in.) into penis or until urine begins to flow. Then insert catheter about 2.5 cm (1 in.) farther.

- Press down with abdominal muscles to promote bladder emptying.
- Pinch off catheter after all urine has drained and withdraw gently, holding tip of catheter upright.
- Wash and dry perineal area.
- Wash catheter in warm, soapy water.
- Rinse with clear water and dry outside with paper towel.
- Place in plastic bag for storage.
- Use catheters for 2–4 weeks and then discard.
- Perform hand hygiene.

Lifespan Considerations

NEWBORNS, INFANTS, AND CHILDREN

- Adapt the size of the catheter for pediatric patients.
- Ask a family member to assist in holding the child during catheterization, if appropriate.

OLDER ADULTS

- Obtaining consent and cooperation from older adults may take longer than with younger patients.
- When catheterizing older adults, be very attentive to problems of limited movement, especially in the hips. Arthritis, or previous hip or knee surgery, may limit the movement of older adults and cause discomfort. Modify the position (e.g., side-lying) as needed to perform the procedure safely and comfortably. For women, obtain the assistance of another nurse to flex and hold the patient's knees and hips as necessary or place her in a modified Sims position.

SKILL 4.13 Urinary Diversion Pouch: Applying

Safety Note! *During scheduled clinical time, nursing students may have a learning opportunity to observe or assist with this skill only with faculty permission and with direct supervision from faculty or another RN.*

Urinary diversion reroutes the normal flow of urine out of the body. This can be a permanent or temporary condition depending on why it is done. The external pouch collects the urine and needs to be periodically emptied.

Delegation or Assignment

Due to the complexity of the procedure, the need for assessment skills, and use of aseptic technique, applying a urinary diversion pouch is not delegated or assigned to the UAP. However, aspects of ostomy function are observed during usual care

and may be recorded by individuals other than the nurse. Abnormal findings must be validated and interpreted by the nurse.

Equipment

- One- or two-piece urinary pouch with skin barrier, flange, and spigot at bottom of pouch to empty urine
- Items to clean stoma (e.g., soft cloth or gauze sponges) and warm water
- Plastic bag for disposal of used equipment
- Gauze for drying skin and for wicking stoma
- Underpad to protect bedding
- Scissors if indicated
- Protective barriers such as skin prep, skin gel, or protective barrier film if necessary

(*continued on next page*)

SKILL 4.13 Urinary Diversion Pouch: Applying *(continued)*

- Stoma measuring guide
- Clean gloves

Preparation

- Review healthcare provider's order and patient care plan. Pouch should be changed every 3–7 days.
- Gather equipment.

Procedure

1. Introduce self to patient and verify the patient's identity using two identifiers. Explain to the patient what you are going to do, why it is necessary, and how the patient can participate. Discuss how the results will be used in planning further care or treatments.
2. Perform hand hygiene and observe appropriate infection control procedures.
3. Provide for patient privacy, don gloves, and prepare the patient.
   - Assist the patient to a comfortable position.
   - Place protective pad under patient.
   - Drape the patient with a bath blanket over patient's chest and position top covers over lower abdomen.
4. Empty, then remove entire ostomy appliance by pushing the skin gently away from the appliance and peeling the appliance downward. Discard in plastic bag.
5. Wash stoma and peristomal skin with warm water and soap if needed, rinse well, and pat skin dry. **Rationale:** *Chemical or perfumed wipes can irritate skin or may interfere with pouch seal.*
   Note: Stoma may bleed slightly when wiped.
6. Check stoma for healing; it should be bright but not dark red and moist, and raised 1.3–2.5 cm (½–1 in.) above skin surface (or may be flush). Check for mucocutaneous separation ulceration, encrustation, and signs of infection, skin sensitivities, or allergies.
7. Check skin surrounding stoma to ensure urine has not been draining under the wafer, causing skin irritation.
8. Prepare new urinary pouch ❶. Place gauze over stoma to prevent urine from oozing onto skin. A wick can be placed in stoma, if needed. **Rationale:** *To keep urine from contact with skin during pouch change.* Measure stoma site with measuring guide, unless pouch has precut opening.

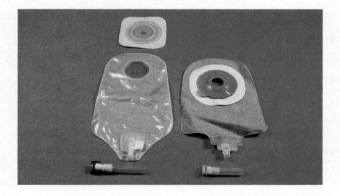

❶ One-piece and two-piece urinary diversion pouches.

9. Trace size of stoma on wafer and cut 0.2–0.3 cm (1/16–1/8 in.) larger ❷. **Rationale:** *This small opening prevents leakage of effluent onto skin; however, the size is large enough to prevent pressure on the stoma from the wafer rubbing on skin.*

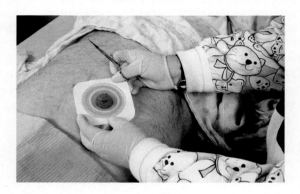

❷ Cut wafer opening slightly larger than stoma.

10. Apply protective barrier (only if indicated) to skin surrounding stoma or to wafer ❸. Do not use lotion. **Rationale:** *Protective barriers contain alcohol and cause burning, and may interfere with seal.* In addition, barrier must be removed with adhesive remover.

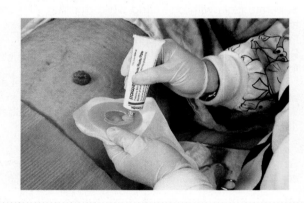

❸ Apply protective barrier paste to wafer only if indicated.

11. Let site dry thoroughly ❹.

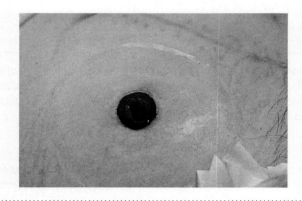

❹ Cleanse stoma and peristomal skin; allow it to dry thoroughly.

SKILL 4.13 Urinary Diversion Pouch: Applying *(continued)*

12. Remove paper from adhesive on wafer of one- or two-piece appliance.
13. Remove wick and center wafer over stoma; apply to dry skin, starting at bottom, and working up around stoma. Press wafer on skin for 3 minutes ⑤. **Rationale:** *To promote adherence to skin.* If two-piece pouch, attach pouch to wafer flange.

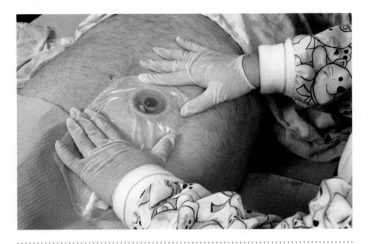

⑤ Apply pouch and press firmly to facilitate seal.

14. Remove air from clean pouch and close spout. Attach pouch to gravity drainage bag only while patient is in bed. Empty pouch when one third full.
15. Discard equipment in appropriate receptacle.
16. Remove and discard gloves. Perform hand hygiene and leave the patient safe and comfortable.
17. Complete documentation using forms, checklists, or electronic dropdown lists supplemented by nurse's notes or additional comments as appropriate.

CAUTION! Thin plastic tubes (stents) may be placed in each ureter during surgery. These remain in place for up to 10 days. They serve to maintain patency until swelling has subsided at ureteroileal anastomosis site (6–10 days). Their presence and length of exposure should be documented. The surgeon should be notified when they wash out into collection pouch.

SAMPLE DOCUMENTATION

[date] 1345 Old pouch emptied of 145 mL light-amber-colored clear urine. Pouch removed. Stoma red and intact. Area cleaned with soap and water then dried. Wafer opening cut to size and pouch applied. Tolerated procedure without complaint. *M. Varner*

SKILL 4.14 Urinary External Device: Applying

Safety Note! *During scheduled clinical time, nursing students may have a learning opportunity to observe or assist with this skill only with faculty permission and with direct supervision from faculty or another RN.*

A condom catheter is a male urinary incontinence device that consists of a flexible sheath that fits over the penis just like a condom and is then attached to a tube. Urine drains through the tube into a drainage bag. There are leg bags, which hold a small amount of urine and attach to the patient's leg, and there are larger urine collection bags.

Delegation or Assignment

Applying a condom catheter may be delegated or assigned to the UAP. However, the nurse must determine if the patient has unique needs such as impaired circulation or latex allergy that would require special training in the use of the condom catheter. Abnormal findings must be validated and interpreted by the nurse. Note that state laws for UAPs vary, so this task might be assigned to the UAP rather than delegated.

Equipment

- Condom sheath of appropriate size: small, medium, large, extra-large (Use the manufacturer's size guide as indicated.

Use latex-free silicone for patients with latex allergies. Use self-adhering condoms, or those with Velcro, or other external securing device.) ①
- Leg drainage bag if ambulatory or urinary drainage bag with tubing
- Clean gloves
- Basin of warm water and soap
- Washcloth and towel

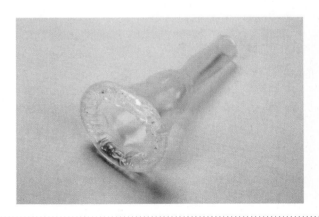

① An external or condom catheter.

(continued on next page)

SKILL 4.14 Urinary External Device: Applying (*continued*)

Preparation

- Review healthcare provider's orders.
- Verify any patient allergies, including a latex allergy.
- Determine if the patient has had an external catheter previously and any difficulties with it.
- Perform any procedures that are best completed without the catheter in place; for example, weighing the patient would be easier without the tubing and bag.
- Assemble the leg drainage bag or urinary drainage bag for attachment to the condom sheath.
- If the condom supplied is not rolled onto itself, roll the condom outward onto itself to facilitate easier application. On some models, an inner flap will be exposed. This flap is applied around the urinary meatus to prevent the reflux of urine.

CAUTION! Urinary tract infection (UTI) can occur with indwelling catheters. An external urine collection system is recommended for incontinent men without urine retention because they are comfortable and there is less chance of a UTI.

Procedure

1. Prior to performing the procedure, introduce self and verify the patient's identity using two identifiers. Explain to the patient what you are going to do, why it is necessary, and how he can participate.
2. Perform hand hygiene and observe other appropriate infection control procedures.
3. Provide for patient privacy. Position the patient in either a supine or a sitting position.
   - Drape the patient appropriately with the bath blanket, exposing only the penis.
4. Apply clean gloves.
5. Inspect and clean the penis.
   - Clean the genital area and dry it thoroughly. **Rationale:** *This minimizes skin irritation and excoriation after the condom is applied.*
6. Apply and secure the condom.
   - Roll the condom smoothly over the penis, leaving 2.5 cm (1 in.) between the end of the penis and the rubber or plastic connecting tube ❷. **Rationale:** *This space*

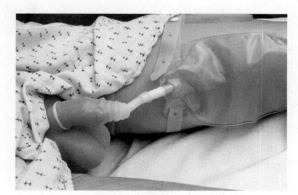

Source: George Draper/Pearson Education, Inc.

❷ The condom rolled over the penis.

prevents irritation of the tip of the penis and provides for full drainage of urine.
   - Secure the condom firmly, but not too tightly, to the penis. Avoid catching pubic hair if possible. Some condoms have an adhesive inside the proximal end that adheres to the skin of the base of the penis. Many condoms are packaged with special fixation material. If neither is present, use a strip of flexible self-adhesive tape or Velcro around the base of the penis over the condom. Ordinary tape is contraindicated because it is not flexible and can stop blood flow.
7. Securely attach the urinary drainage system.
   - Make sure that the tip of the penis is not touching the condom and that the condom is not twisted. **Rationale:** *A twisted condom could obstruct the flow of urine.*
   - Attach the urinary drainage system to the condom.
   - Remove and discard gloves. Perform hand hygiene.
   - If the patient is to remain in bed, attach the urinary drainage bag to the bed frame.
   - If the patient is ambulatory, attach the bag to the patient's leg ❸. **Rationale:** *Attaching the drainage bag to the leg helps control the movement of the tubing and prevents twisting of the thin material of the condom appliance at the tip of the penis.*

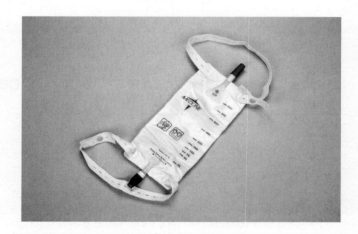

❸ Urinary drainage leg bag.

8. Teach the patient about the drainage system.
   - Instruct the patient to keep the drainage bag below the level of the condom and to avoid loops or kinks in the tubing. Instruct the patient to report to healthcare personnel any pain, irritation, swelling, or wetness/leaking around the penis.
9. Inspect the penis 30 minutes following the condom application and at least every 4 hours. Check for urine flow.
   - Assess the penis for swelling and discoloration. **Rationale:** *This indicates that the condom is too tight.*
   - Assess urine flow if the patient has voided. Normally, some urine is present in the tube if the flow is not obstructed.

SKILL 4.14 Urinary External Device: Applying (*continued*)

10. Change the condom as indicated and provide skin care. In most settings, the condom is changed daily.
    - Remove the flexible tape or Velcro strip, apply clean gloves, and roll off the condom.
    - Wash the penis with soapy water, rinse, and dry it thoroughly.
    - Assess the foreskin for signs of irritation, swelling, and discoloration.
    - Apply a new condom.
    - Remove and discard gloves. Perform hand hygiene.
11. Complete documentation using forms, checklists, or electronic dropdown lists supplemented by nurse's notes or additional comments as appropriate. Record the application of the condom, the time, and pertinent observations such as irritated areas on the penis.

SAMPLE DOCUMENTATION

[date] 2245 Condom catheter applied for the night per patient request. Glans clean, skin intact. Catheter attached to bedside collection bag. Instructed to notify staff if pain, irritation, swelling, or wetness/leaking occurs. Verbalized that he would. *L. Chan*

SKILL 4.15 Urinary Ostomy: Caring for

Safety Note! *During scheduled clinical time, nursing students may have a learning opportunity to observe or assist with this skill only with faculty permission and with direct supervision from faculty or another RN.*

A urostomy channels urine to the outside of the patient's abdomen instead of going to the bladder. The opening to the abdomen is called a stoma which must be kept clean to prevent infection of the surrounding skin and kidneys.

Delegation or Assignment

Due to the complexity of the procedure, the need for assessment skills, and use of aseptic technique, changing a urostomy device is not delegated or assigned to the UAP. However, aspects of urostomy function are observed during usual care and may be recorded by individuals other than the nurse. Abnormal findings must be validated and interpreted by the nurse.

Equipment

- One-piece ❶ or two-piece urinary pouch
- Tail closure clamp
- Clean gloves
- Cleaning materials, including tissues, warm water, mild soap (optional), cotton balls, washcloth or gauze pads, towel
- Skin barrier/prep (gel, liquid, powder, or film)
- Stoma measuring guide
- Pen or pencil and scissors
- Deodorant liquid drops (optional)
- Bedpan or graduated cylinder

Preparation

- Review healthcare provider's orders.
- Review the patient's record to determine the type of urinary diversion. Determine when the device was last changed and any pertinent findings at that time.
- Determine the need for an appliance change.
- Assess the used appliance for leakage of urine. **Rationale:** *Urine irritates the peristomal skin.*

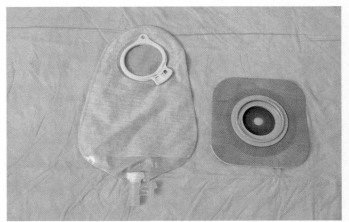

A

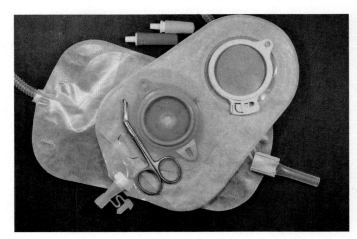

B

*Sources: **A**, Kenneth Sponsler/123RF.com; **B**, Mariola Anna S/ Shutterstock*

---

❶ **A,** One-piece urostomy system; **B,** Urostomy supplies.

(continued on next page)

SKILL 4.15 Urinary Ostomy: Caring for (continued)

■ Ask the patient about any discomfort at or around the stoma. **Rationale:** *A burning sensation may indicate breakdown beneath the faceplate of the pouch.*

■ Assess the fullness of the pouch. **Rationale:** The weight of an overly full bag may loosen the faceplate and separate it from the skin, causing the urine to leak and irritate the peristomal skin.

■ If there is pouch leakage or discomfort at or around the stoma, change the appliance.

■ Select an appropriate time to change the appliance. Avoid times close to meals or visiting hours. **Rationale:** *Ostomy odor may reduce appetite or embarrass the patient.*

Procedure

1. Prior to performing the procedure, introduce self and verify the patient's identity using two identifiers. Explain to the patient what you are going to do, why it is necessary, and how the patient can participate. Discuss how the results will be used in planning further care or treatments. Changing an ostomy appliance should not cause discomfort, but it may be distasteful to the patient. Communicate acceptance and support to the patient. It is important to change the appliance competently and quickly. Include support individuals as appropriate.

2. Perform hand hygiene and observe other appropriate infection control procedures.

3. Provide for patient privacy.

4. Assist the patient to a comfortable sitting or lying position in bed or a sitting or standing position in the bathroom. **Rationale:** *Lying or standing positions may facilitate smoother pouch application.*

5. Empty and remove the ostomy appliance.
   Note: Because urine flows continuously, if the stoma can be measured for the new appliance with the appliance in place, perform step 8 first. This can usually be accomplished if the pouch is thin or transparent enough to fit the measuring guide snugly over the stoma while it is in place.
   ● Apply clean gloves.
   ● Empty the pouch through the bottom opening into a bedpan or graduated cylinder. **Rationale:** *Emptying before removing the pouch prevents spillage of urine onto the patient's skin.*
   ● Peel the bag off slowly while holding the patient's skin taut. **Rationale:** *Holding the skin taut minimizes patient discomfort and prevents abrasion of the skin.*
   ● Place tissue or gauze pad over the stoma, and change as needed. **Rationale:** *This absorbs urine seepage from the stoma.*

6. Clean and dry the peristomal skin and stoma.
   ● Use warm water, mild soap (optional), and damp cotton balls, gauze, or a washcloth and towel to clean the skin and stoma. Check facility practice on the use of soap. **Rationale:** *Soap is sometimes not advised because it can be irritating to the skin.*
   ● Dry the area thoroughly by patting with a towel or cotton balls. **Rationale:** *Excess rubbing can abrade the skin.*

7. Assess the stoma and peristomal skin.
   ● Inspect the stoma for color, size, shape, and bleeding.
   ● Inspect the peristomal skin for any redness, ulceration, or irritation. Transient redness after removal of adhesive is normal.

8. Prepare and apply the new pouch.
   ● Use the guide to measure the size of the stoma.
   ● On the backing of the skin barrier, trace a circle the same size as the stomal opening.
   ● Cut out the traced stoma pattern to make an opening in the skin barrier. Make the opening no more than 0.3 cm (⅛ in.) larger than the stoma. **Rationale:** *This allows space for the stoma to expand slightly when functioning and minimizes the risk of urine contacting peristomal skin.*
   ● Remove the backing to expose the sticky adhesive side of the barrier. The backing can be saved and used as a pattern when making an opening for future skin barriers.
   ● Apply the peristomal skin barrier to the faceplate of the ostomy appliance or around the stoma depending on the manufacturer's recommendations. Skin barrier powder may be used on irritated skin, but Skin-Prep liquid may not be applied to irritated skin.
   ● Center the faceplate over the stoma, and gently press it onto the patient's skin, smoothing out any wrinkles or bubbles. Hold in place for about 30 seconds. **Rationale:** *The heat and pressure help activate the adhesives in the skin barrier.*
   ● Remove the air from the pouch. **Rationale:** *Removing the air helps the pouch lie flat against the abdomen.*
   ● *Optional:* Place approximately 10 drops of deodorant in the pouch.
   ● Close the pouch by turning up the bottom a few times, fanfolding its end lengthwise, and securing it with a tail closure clamp or replacing the drainage outlet cap (see ❶).
   ● Discard all used supplies in appropriate receptacles.
   ● Remove and discard gloves, perform hand hygiene, and leave the patient safe and comfortable.

9. Complete documentation using forms, checklists, or electronic dropdown lists supplemented by nurse's notes or additional comments as appropriate.

SAMPLE DOCUMENTATION

[date] 0900 Urostomy bag changed due to slight leakage. Had been in place for 6 days. No redness or irritation around stoma. Stoma pink, bled a few drops when washed. Patient states home care RN changes the appliance when home. Tolerated without incident. *M. Earl*

SKILL 4.16 Urinary Suprapubic Catheter: Caring for

Safety Note! *During scheduled clinical time, nursing students may have a learning opportunity to observe or assist with this skill only with faculty permission and with direct supervision from faculty or another RN.*

A suprapubic catheter is inserted into the patient's bladder through a small opening in his or her abdomen to drain urine from the bladder. The catheter is connected to a drainage bag outside the body, which needs to be emptied every few hours.

Delegation or Assignment

Due to the complexity of the procedure, the need for assessment skills, and use of aseptic technique, this procedure is not delegated or assigned to the UAP. However, aspects of function are observed during usual care and may be recorded by individuals other than the nurse. Abnormal findings must be validated and interpreted by the nurse.

Equipment

- Closed drainage system, including Foley catheter tubing and bag
- Catheter clamp and plug
- Dry sterile dressing and tape if ordered
- Cleansing solution
- Clean gloves
- Sterile gloves

Preparation

- Review healthcare provider's orders and patient care plan.
- Gather equipment and supplies.

Procedure

1. Introduce self to patient and verify the patient's identity using two identifiers. Explain to the patient what you are going to do, why it is necessary, and how the patient can participate. Explain the purpose of the catheter and describe the procedure for continuous or intermittent urinary drainage. Discuss how the results will be used in planning further care or treatments.
2. Perform hand hygiene and observe appropriate infection control procedures.
3. Provide for patient privacy.
4. Observe catheter for patency. **Rationale:** *The most common problem with suprapubic catheters is occlusion with sediment or clots.*
   - *First 24 hours:* Check the catheter every hour to detect possible obstruction. Urine output should be in excess of 30 mL/hr.
   - *Day 2:* Check the catheter every 8 hours.
   - *Day 3:* Check the catheter when the catheter is unclamped.
5. Maintain a closed drainage system. Do not open system to irrigate or obtain urine sample.
6. Observe for signs of urinary tract infection (color, odor, presence of sediment).

7. Keep the dressing dry around site of insertion. Apply a new dressing, maintaining sterile technique, every morning and as necessary.
   - Place bed in high position.
   - Perform hand hygiene and don clean gloves.
   - Remove old dressing, discard gloves, and dispose in appropriate container.
   - Perform hand hygiene and open sterile supplies.
   - Open cleansing solution and pour over sterile gauze.
   - Don sterile gloves.
   - Assess skin surrounding suprapubic catheter.
   - Cleanse area with cleansing solution. Allow to dry.
   - Apply sterile dressing and secure with tape 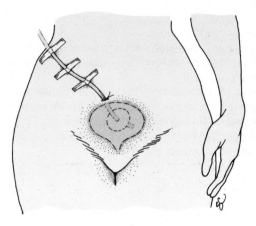.
   - Remove gloves and supplies and discard in appropriate container.
   - Perform hand hygiene.
   - Replace bed in low position.

1 Tape catheter and connect to a closed system.

8. Perform clamping protocol according to healthcare provider orders for intermittent urinary drainage.
   - Explain the clamping procedure and ask patient to help monitor the clamping.
   - Instruct patient to report if there are feelings of fullness in the bladder during clamping.
   - Don clean gloves.
   - Clamp the catheter.
9. Empty the drainage bag or remove drainage tubing from catheter, maintaining aseptic technique.
   - Place drainage tubing in sterile package to maintain sterility.
   - Place catheter plug in catheter end.
   - Remove and discard gloves. Perform hand hygiene.
   - Record urine output on intake and output (I&O) record.
   - Leave the catheter clamped or plugged for 3–4 hr depending on patient's level of comfort and healthcare provider's orders.
10. At 3- to 4-hour intervals, or when patient feels bladder fullness, ask patient to void normally. Perform hand hygiene

(continued on next page)

SKILL 4.16 Urinary Suprapubic Catheter: Caring for (continued)

and don clean gloves to measure the urine and record output on I&O bedside record.

11. Immediately after patient voids, unclamp catheter and leave unclamped for 5 minutes, collecting the residual urine.
    - Measure the residual urine following unclamping of the catheter.
    - Reclamp catheter.
    - Remove gloves and perform hand hygiene.
    - If ordered, send a urine specimen to laboratory after the first clamping. **Rationale:** This *specimen is used to check for presence of microorganisms.*

12. Repeat clamping protocol every 3–4 hr according to healthcare provider orders. The catheter may be open to drainage from bedtime until 6 a.m.

13. When the patient is voiding normally, clamp the catheter throughout the night in preparation for its removal.

14. When the patient's residual urine output is less than 100 mL or retains less than 20% of residual urine on two successive checks, notify the healthcare provider for removal of the catheter.

15. Cleanse insertion area with antimicrobial swab.

16. Deflate balloon and remove catheter, if order written for nurse to remove.

17. Perform hand hygiene and don clean gloves.

18. Apply a 2 × 2 sterile dressing over the insertion site.

19. Dispose of the catheter in biohazard bag.

20. Remove gloves, perform hand hygiene, and leave the patient safe and comfortable.

21. If the patient is discharged from the hospital with the catheter, provide the following teaching for home care:
    - Instruct the patient to drink one glass of fluid every hour while awake.
    - Instruct patient to follow clamping procedure when awake or as instructed by healthcare provider.
    - Instruct the patient to leave the catheter open to the drainage system at night. (Drainage system may be urinary tubing and bag or leg bag.)
    - Tell patient to notify healthcare provider if dysuria occurs when voiding or if urine becomes cloudy, odorous, or has sediment.

22. Complete documentation using forms, checklists, or electronic dropdown lists supplemented by nurse's notes or additional comments as appropriate. Document time catheter clamped; length of time clamped; patient's ability to void spontaneously; patient's feelings of fullness; time specimen sent to laboratory; color, amount, and odor of urine obtained; and color, amount, and odor of residual urine.

SAMPLE DOCUMENTATION

[date] 1645 Catheter clamped 1230 today (4 hr 15 min). Patient tried to urinate unsuccessfully. Denies urge to urinate or feeling of fullness. Urine emptied from bag, 80 mL clear amber urine obtained and sent to lab. Healthcare provider notified of urine output. *R. Byrd*

Patient Teaching

Teach the patient with a suprapubic catheter how to do self-care at home.

- Keep necessary equipment and supplies available at home.
    - Catheter plug and clamp
    - Closed drainage system
    - Sterile dressings if necessary
    - Clean gloves
    - Receptacle to drain urine from drainage bag
    - Normal saline solution or mild soap and water
    - White vinegar
    - Applicator sticks
    - 4 × 4 gauze pads
    - Paper tape
- Clean the catheter site and empty the drainage bag.
    - Wash hands and put on some gloves.
    - Clean around catheter site with normal saline solution or mild soap and water. Use applicator sticks to remove material from around catheter opening.
    - Ensure catheter is not pulling on exit site. Tape catheter to skin so a gentle curve is present to prevent tugging on catheter.
    - Empty catheter bag or leg bag into a container and then dispose of contents in toilet or, if removing bag, empty directly into toilet.
    - Clean drainage bag with warm water and soap every day or two. Place one teaspoon of vinegar in rinse water to reduce odor.
    - Replace catheter bag on catheter.
    - Remove and discard gloves. Wash hands.
- Do bladder testing for residual urine.
    - Wash hands and catheter connections with soap and water.
    - Clamp the suprapubic tube so it does not drain. Use catheter plug or clamp.
    - Attempt to void when you feel the urge to urinate. Measure amount of urine.
    - Unclamp the suprapubic tube immediately after voiding; empty urine into container and measure residual urine amount.
    - Keep a log of each voiding and residual amount.
    - Call healthcare provider with findings when residual amount is less than 20% voided amount. Usually, this amount is about 60 mL. Usually, the suprapubic tube is removed when patient is able to urinate without complications.
- Monitor carefully for signs of urinary tract infection and notify your healthcare provider immediately. Check for bladder pain, confusion, bleeding, temperature over 37.8°C (100°F), chills, cloudy urine, drainage or edema around the suprapubic tube.

» Bowel Interventions

Expected Outcomes

1. Patients experience increased comfort and relief from abdominal distention.
2. Enema administered without difficulty.
3. Relief obtained from fecal impaction or constipation.
4. Ostomy pouch remains intact without leakage for 3–5 days.
5. Pouching system provides maximal skin protection.
6. Patient gradually assumes an active role in applying the ostomy pouch.
7. Patient's skin remains free of erythema, excoriation, and infection.

SKILL 4.17 Bowel Routine, Develop Regular: Assisting

A bowel routine is a scheduled practice to prevent or relieve constipation, or maintain regular bowel movements. Bowel training reestablishes the bowel's normal reflexes by repeating a routine until it becomes a habit. The practice can include behaviors or medicines to move the bowels. Constipation can come from several situations, but being constipated can be uncomfortable and make a patient feel unhealthy.

Delegation or Assignment

Teaching and coaching a patient in developing a regular bowel routine or habit is done by the nurse and not delegated or assigned to the UAP. However, the UAP can make observations during usual care which can be recorded by individuals other than the nurse. Abnormal findings must be validated and interpreted by the nurse.

Equipment

- Clean gloves, 1 or 2 pairs
- Lubricant
- Bedpan or commode
- Absorbent pad
- Specific enema if ordered
- Washcloth and towel

Preparation

- Review healthcare provider's orders and patient care plan.
- Review patient's allergies.
- Identify daily pattern and time of day patient usually evacuates bowels.
- Evaluate diet, exercise, and former use of medications for bowel evacuation.
- Administer the following drugs as ordered:
  a. Stool softener such as Colace, Dialose, Coloxyl—daily
  b. Bulk former such as Metamucil or FiberCon—usually daily to three times a day (tid)
  c. Mild laxative such as Senokot, Doxidan, Dulcolax—8 hr before program
  d. Suppository such as glycerin or Dulcolax just before digital stimulation.
- Gather necessary equipment or supplies.

Procedure

1. Introduce self to patient and verify the patient's identity using two identifiers. Explain to the patient what you are going to do, why it is necessary, and how the patient can participate. Discuss how the results will be used in planning further care or treatments.
2. Perform hand hygiene and observe appropriate infection control procedures.
3. Provide for patient privacy.
4. Don gloves. You may want to double-glove to prevent contamination if glove tears.
5. Perform digital stimulation or other maneuver one half hour after dinner or breakfast or according to patient's time schedule for evacuation (per healthcare provider's order). **Rationale:** *Food stimulates bowel activity.*

CAUTION! When performing digital stimulation there is the potential risk of stimulating the vagus nerve which can result in bradycardia (pulse rate less than 60 bpm) or shortness of breath. Observe for faintness, pallor, nausea, chest discomfort, or diaphoresis. If any of these signs/symptoms occur, stop the procedure immediately, remove the enema tube, stay with the patient, and call for help.

---

6. Place patient on toilet or commode. (Use bedpan if patient is on bed rest.) **Rationale:** *Assuming normal posture for bowel movement facilitates evacuation.*
7. Encourage patient to contract abdominal muscles or bend forward while bearing down. **Rationale:** *Increases abdominal pressure and helps evacuate the bowel.*
8. Remove and discard gloves. Perform hand hygiene.
9. Provide privacy and sufficient time for evacuation.
10. Don gloves.
11. Wash and dry perineal area if patient is unable to do so.
12. Remove and discard gloves.
13. Place patient in wheelchair or bed and position for comfort.
14. Perform hand hygiene and leave the patient safe and comfortable.

SAMPLE DOCUMENTATION

[date] 0750 Demonstrated and coached to massage anal area while wearing glove to stimulate bowel movement. Had a successful bowel movement of small amount formed brown stool without pain or straining. Tolerated procedure without complaint. *O. Diaz*

(continued on next page)

SKILL 4.17 Bowel Routine, Develop Regular: Assisting *(continued)*

15. Complete documentation using forms, checklists, or electronic dropdown lists supplemented by nurse's notes or additional comments as appropriate.
16. Wean patient away from suppositories and laxatives when spontaneous bowel movements occur with digital stimulation or other routine maneuver.

Patient Teaching

Good bowel training programs include:

- Initiation of defecation on demand with digital stimulation and abdominal massage
- Evacuation at same time each day; best time is 20–40 min after a meal
- Proper diet, increased fiber and fluids
- Daily physical exercise regimen
- Patient and family education

Lifespan Considerations

Preventing Constipation

OLDER ADULTS

- Assess constipation by obtaining the patient's history, including information regarding the amount of fluid intake, food ingested, and dietary fiber.
- Review medications associated with an increased risk of developing constipation; screen for polypharmacy.
- Identify bowel patterns using a bowel diary.
- Increase fluids to 1500–2000 mL/day as appropriate; minimize caffeine and alcohol intake.
- Promote regular consistent toileting.
- Tailor physical activity to patient's physical abilities.

EVIDENCE-BASED PRACTICE

Management of Constipation in Older Adults

Constipation is a very common disorder, and its prevalence increases with age, as reported by 26% of women and 16% of men ages 65 years and older. In people over age 84, the incidence increases to 34% and 26%, respectively.

There are three types of constipation, and treatment may vary by type.

- Functional constipation is the term used when patients experience small, hard stools that are difficult to pass. There may be abdominal pain or discomfort that is relieved with evacuation. Intestinal transit times and pelvic function studies are normal.
- Pelvic floor constipation—difficult or inadequate expulsion of stool—is due to faulty coordination of the abdominal and pelvic floor muscles, altered perineal descent, or structural abnormalities.
- Slow transit constipation (colonoparesis) involves some degree of partial paralysis in the colon resulting from dysfunction of the colonic nerves, smooth muscle, or both.

Effective management can occur with (1) education about diet and exercise and (2) use of certain techniques, such as timing of evacuation, breathing, and positioning on the toilet. Fiber supplements in water may improve consistency and weight of stool in some patients, but in others (such as patients with severe pelvic floor dysfunction), high-fiber supplements may have a negative effect. Therefore, knowing the primary cause of constipation is an important factor in establishing effective treatment.

Sources: Data from Global Business Media. (2014). HFA Healthcare. Managing Constipation in the Elderly. Special Report. Retrieved from https://issuu.com/globalbusinessmedia.org/docs/special_report_25_-_managing_consti Health Communities.com. (2014). *Constipation in older adults.* Retrieved from http://www.healthcommunities.com/constipation/older-adults-elderly-constipation.shtml Schuster, B., Kosar, L., & Kamrul, R. (2015). *Constipation in older adults: Stepwise approach to keep things moving.* Retrieved from http://www.cfp.ca/content/61/2/152.full

SKILL 4.18 Bowel Diversion Ostomy Appliance: Changing

Safety Note! *During scheduled clinical time, nursing students may have a learning opportunity to observe or assist with this skill only with faculty permission and with direct supervision from faculty or another RN.*

A bowel diversion ostomy is done after damaged portions of the intestines are removed. Stool is diverted to the outside of the abdomen via bowel and exits the body through the stoma. An ostomy appliance is attached to the stoma to collect the stool.

Delegation or Assignment

Care of a *new* ostomy is not delegated or assigned to the UAP. However, aspects of ostomy function are observed during usual care and may be recorded by individuals other than the nurse. Abnormal findings must be validated and interpreted by the nurse. In some agencies, the UAP may remove and replace well-established ostomy appliances.

Equipment

- Clean gloves
- Bedpan
- Moisture-proof bag (for disposable pouches)
- Cleaning materials, including warm water, mild soap (optional), washcloth, towel
- Tissue or gauze pad
- Skin barrier (optional)
- Stoma measuring guide
- Pen or pencil and scissors
- New ostomy pouch ❶ ❷ with optional belt ❸

SKILL 4.18 Bowel Diversion Ostomy Appliance: Changing (*continued*)

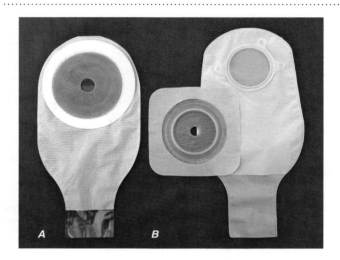

① *A,* One-piece ostomy appliance of pouching system; *B,* two-piece ostomy or pouching system.

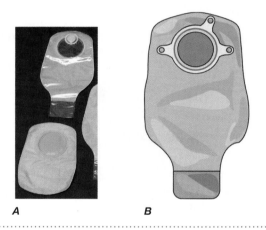

A	*B*

② *A,* Closed pouch; *B,* drainable pouch.

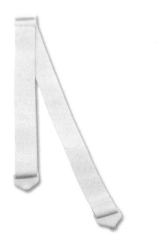

Source: Hollister, Inc.

③ Adjustable ostomy belt.

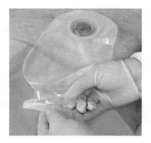

④ Applying a pouch clamp.

- Tail closure clamp **④**
- Deodorant for pouch (optional)

Preparation

- Review healthcare provider's orders.
- Determine the need for an appliance change.
- Assess the used appliance for leakage of stool. **Rationale:** *Stool can irritate the peristomal skin.*
- Ask the patient about any discomfort at or around the stoma. **Rationale:** *A burning sensation may indicate breakdown beneath the faceplate of the pouch.*
- Assess the fullness of the pouch. **Rationale:** *The weight of an overly full bag may loosen the skin barrier and separate it from the skin, causing the stool to leak and irritate the peristomal skin.*
- If there is pouch leakage or discomfort at or around the stoma, the appliance needs to be changed.
- Select an appropriate time to change the appliance.
  - Avoid times close to mealtimes or visiting hours. **Rationale:** *Ostomy odor and stool may reduce appetite or embarrass the patient.*
  - Avoid times immediately after meals or the administration of any medications that may stimulate bowel evacuation. **Rationale:** *It is best to change the pouch when drainage is least likely to occur.*

Procedure

1. Introduce self and verify the patient's identity using two identifiers. Explain to the patient what you are going to do, why it is necessary, and how the patient can participate. Discuss how the results will be used in planning further care or treatments. Changing an ostomy appliance should not cause discomfort, but it may be distasteful to the patient. Communicate acceptance and support to the patient. It is important to change the appliance competently and quickly. Include support individuals as appropriate.
2. Perform hand hygiene and observe other appropriate infection control procedures.
3. Don clean gloves.
4. Provide for patient privacy preferably in the bathroom, where patients can learn to deal with the ostomy as they would at home.

(*continued on next page*)

SKILL 4.18 Bowel Diversion Ostomy Appliance: Changing (*continued*)

5. Assist the patient to a comfortable sitting or lying position in bed or preferably a sitting or standing position in the bathroom. **Rationale:** *Lying or standing positions may facilitate smoother pouch application (i.e., avoid wrinkles).*

6. Unfasten the belt if the patient is wearing one.

7. Empty the pouch and remove the ostomy skin barrier.
   - Empty the contents of a drainable pouch through the bottom opening into a bedpan or toilet. **Rationale:** *Emptying before removing the pouch prevents spillage of stool onto the patient's skin.*
   - If the pouch uses a clamp, do not throw it away because it can be reused.
   - Assess the consistency, color, and amount of stool.
   - Peel the skin barrier off slowly, beginning at the top and working downward, while holding the patient's skin taut. **Rationale:** *Holding the skin taut minimizes patient discomfort and prevents abrasion of the skin.*
   - Discard the disposable pouch in a moisture-proof bag.

8. Clean and dry the peristomal skin and stoma.
   - Use toilet tissue to remove excess stool.
   - Use warm water, mild soap (optional), and a washcloth to clean the skin and stoma. Check facility practice on the use of soap. **Rationale:** *Soap is sometimes not advised because it can be irritating to the skin.* If soap is allowed, do not use deodorant or moisturizing soaps. **Rationale:** *They may interfere with the adhesives in the skin barrier.*
   - Dry the area thoroughly by patting with a towel. **Rationale:** *Excess rubbing can abrade the skin.*

9. Assess the stoma and peristomal skin.
   - Inspect the stoma for color, size, shape, and bleeding.
   - Inspect the peristomal skin for any redness, ulceration, or irritation. Transient redness after the removal of adhesive is normal.

10. Place a piece of tissue or gauze over the stoma, and change it as needed. **Rationale:** *This absorbs any seepage from the stoma while the ostomy appliance is being changed.*

11. Prepare and apply the skin barrier (peristomal seal).
    - Use the guide to measure the size of the stoma ❺.
    - On the backing of the skin barrier, trace a circle the same size as the stomal opening.
    - Cut out the traced stoma pattern to make an opening in the skin barrier ❻. Make the opening no more than 0.3–0.6 cm (⅛–¼ in.) larger than the stoma. **Rationale:** *This allows space for the stoma to expand slightly when functioning and minimizes the risk of stool contacting peristomal skin.*

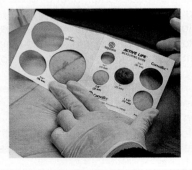

❺ A guide for measuring the stoma.

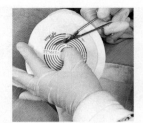

❻ The nurse is making a stoma opening on a disposable one-piece pouch.

- Remove the backing to expose the sticky adhesive side. The backing can be saved and used as a pattern when making an opening for future skin barriers.
- Remove the tissue or gauze placed over the stoma before applying the pouch.

For a One-Piece Pouching System

- Center the one-piece skin barrier and pouch over the stoma, and gently press it onto the patient's skin for 30 seconds (check with the facility about using a stoma paste barrier product) ❼ ❽. **Rationale:** *The heat and pressure help activate the adhesives in the skin barrier.*

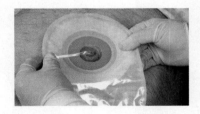

❼ Centering the skin barrier over the stoma.

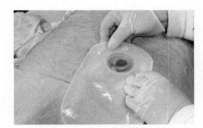

❽ Pressing the skin barrier of a disposable one-piece pouch for 30 seconds to activate the adhesives in the skin barrier.

For a Two-Piece Pouching System

- Center the skin barrier over the stoma and gently press it onto the patient's skin for 30 seconds.
- Snap the pouch onto the flange or skin barrier wafer.
- For drainable pouches, close the pouch according to the manufacturer's directions.
- Remove and discard gloves. Perform hand hygiene, leave the patient safe and comfortable, and then proceed to step 12 below.

SKILL 4.18 Bowel Diversion Ostomy Appliance: Changing (*continued*)

EMPTYING A DRAINABLE POUCH

- Empty the pouch when it is one third to one half full of stool or gas. **Rationale:** *Emptying the pouch before it is overfull helps avoid breaking the seal with the skin, resulting in stool coming in contact with the skin.*
- While wearing gloves, hold the pouch outlet over a bedpan or toilet. Lift the lower edge up.
- Unclamp or unseal the pouch.
- Drain the pouch. Loosen feces from the sides by moving fingers down the pouch.
- Clean the inside of the tail of the pouch with a tissue or a premoistened towelette.
- Apply the clamp or seal the pouch.
- Dispose of used supplies.
- Remove and discard gloves. Perform hand hygiene and leave the patient safe and comfortable.

12. Complete documentation using forms, checklists, or electronic dropdown lists supplemented by nurse's notes or additional comments as appropriate. Report and record pertinent assessments and interventions. Report any increase in stoma size, change in color indicative of circulatory impairment, and presence of skin irritation or erosion. Record on the patient's chart discoloration of the stoma, the appearance of the peristomal skin, the amount and type of drainage, the patient's reaction to the procedure, the patient's experience with the ostomy, and skills learned by the patient.

> ### SAMPLE DOCUMENTATION
>
> [date] 0900 Colostomy bag changed. Moderate to large amount of semi-formed brown stool. Stoma reddish color. No redness or irritation around stoma. Patient looked at stoma today and started asking questions about how she will be able to change the pouch when she is home. Asked if she would like to do the next pouch change. Stated "yes." Tolerated bag change without incident. *G. Hsu*

SKILL 4.19 Colostomy: Irrigating

Safety Note! *During scheduled clinical time, nursing students may have a learning opportunity to observe or assist with this skill only with faculty permission and with direct supervision from faculty or another RN.*

A colostomy is a surgical procedure that brings one end of the large intestines out through an opening, or stoma, made in the abdominal wall. Stools moving through the intestine are diverted through the stoma into a collection bag attached to the abdomen.

Delegation or Assignment

Care of a *new* colostomy is not delegated or assigned to the UAP. However, aspects of colostomy function are observed during usual care and may be recorded by individuals other than the nurse. Abnormal findings must be validated and interpreted by the nurse. In some agencies, UAP may remove and replace well-established ostomy appliances.

Equipment

- Solution container with 500–1000 mL warm water ❶
- Irrigating tubing connected to colon catheter or stoma cone
- Clean gloves, 3 pairs
- Irrigating sleeve cut long enough to reach water level in toilet
- Items to clean skin and stoma (e.g., washcloths or gauze sponges)
- Plastic bag for disposal of used pouch
- Clean pouch and closure device
- Skin barriers
- Water-soluble lubricant
- Hook near toilet or IV pole

Preparation

- Review healthcare provider's orders.
- Determine the need for an appliance change.
- Assess the used appliance for leakage of stool. **Rationale:** *Stool can irritate the peristomal skin.*
- Ask the patient about any discomfort at or around the stoma. **Rationale:** *A burning sensation may indicate breakdown beneath the faceplate of the pouch.*
- Assess the fullness of the pouch. **Rationale:** *The weight of an overly full bag may loosen the skin barrier and separate it from the skin, causing the stool to leak and irritate the peristomal skin.*
- If there is pouch leakage or discomfort at or around the stoma, the appliance needs to be changed.
- Select an appropriate time to change the appliance.
  - Avoid times close to mealtimes or visiting hours. **Rationale:** *Ostomy odor and stool may reduce appetite or embarrass the patient.*
  - Avoid times immediately after meals or the administration of any medications that may stimulate bowel evacuation. **Rationale:** *It is best to change the pouch when drainage is least likely to occur.*

Procedure

1. Introduce self to patient and verify the patient's identity using two identifiers. Explain to the patient what you are going to do, why it is necessary, and how the patient can participate. Discuss how the results will be used in planning further care or treatments.

(*continued on next page*)

SKILL 4.19 Colostomy: Irrigating (*continued*)

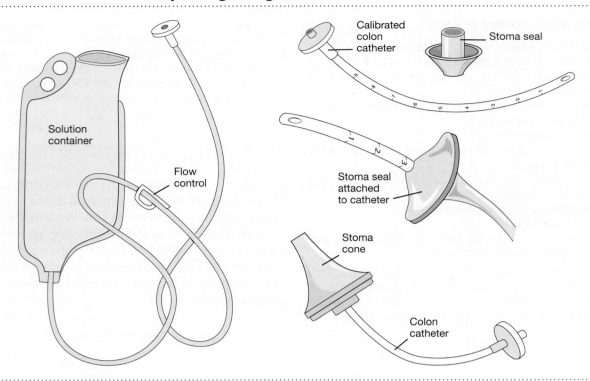

Solution container

Flow control

Calibrated colon catheter

Stoma seal

Stoma seal attached to catheter

Stoma cone

Colon catheter

❶ Colostomy irrigation equipment.

2. Perform hand hygiene and observe appropriate infection control procedures.
3. Provide for patient privacy and don gloves.
4. Fill the solution bag with 500 mL of warm (body temperature) tap water or other solution as ordered.
5. Hang the solution bag on an IV pole so that the bottom of the container is at the level of the patient's shoulder, or 30–45 cm (12–18 in.) above the stoma.
6. Attach the colon catheter securely to the tubing.
7. Open the regulator clamp, and run fluid through the tubing to expel air from it. Close the clamp until ready for the irrigation.
8. Assist the patient who must remain in bed to a side-lying position. Place a disposable pad on the bed in front of the patient, and place the bedpan on top of the disposable pad, beneath the stoma. Assist an ambulatory patient to sit on the toilet or on a commode in the bathroom.
9. Remove the colostomy bag and dispose of used pouch in a plastic bag.
10. Center the irrigation drainage sleeve over the stoma and attach it snugly. Direct the lower, open end of the drainage sleeve into the bedpan or between the patient's legs into the toilet.
11. Lubricate the tip of the stoma cone or colon catheter with a water-soluble lubricant.
12. Using a rotating motion, insert the catheter or stoma cone through the opening in the top of the irrigation drainage sleeve and gently through the stoma. Insert a catheter only 7 cm (3 in.); insert a stoma cone just until it fits snugly. **Rationale:** *Use of a stoma cone avoids the risk of perforating the bowel.*

13. Open the tubing clamp, and allow the fluid to flow into the bowel. If cramping occurs, stop the flow until the cramps subside and then resume the flow.
14. After all the fluid is instilled, remove the catheter or cone and allow the colon to empty, usually 10–15 min.
15. Cleanse the base of the irrigation drainage sleeve, and seal the bottom with a drainage clamp, following the manufacturer's instructions.
16. Encourage an ambulatory patient to move around for about 30 minutes to completely empty the colon.
17. Empty and remove the irrigation sleeve.
18. Clean the area around the stoma, and dry it thoroughly.
19. Apply skin barrier and colostomy appliance as needed.
20. When procedure is complete, perform hand hygiene and leave patient safe and comfortable.
21. Complete documentation using forms, checklists, or electronic dropdown lists supplemented by nurse's notes or additional comments as appropriate.

SAMPLE DOCUMENTATION

[date] 1420 550 mL warm water via cone catheter inserted into stoma 7.5 cm (3 in.). Post 15 minutes, moderate amount of brown formed stool returned. Stoma and surrounding skin cleaned with warm water and dried—remain intact with no signs of infection. New collection pouch applied over stoma. Tolerated procedure without complaint. *M. Lopez*

SKILL 4.19 Colostomy: Irrigating (*continued*)

Patient Teaching

Irrigating a Colostomy

Teach the patient going home how to irrigate his or her colostomy.

- Keep necessary equipment and supplies available at home
  - Solution container with 1000 mL warm water
  - Irrigating tubing with cone
  - Clean gloves, three pairs
  - Irrigating sleeve cut long enough to reach water level in toilet
  - Items to clean skin and stoma (e.g., washcloths or gauze sponges)
  - Plastic bag for disposal of used pouch
  - Clean pouch and closure device
  - Skin barriers
  - Water-soluble lubricant
  - Hook near toilet
- Take periodic deep breaths and try to relax while following these steps:
  - Wash hands and put on clean gloves.
  - Remove and dispose of used pouch in plastic bag.
  - Clean stoma and skin with warm water and soft cloth. Assess skin for signs of irritation or breakdown.
  - Apply irrigation sleeve to peristomal skin, and place belt around waist.
  - Fill container with 1000 mL lukewarm water (500 mL for first irrigation). **Rationale:** *Lukewarm water temperature is 40°C–43°C (105°F–110°F). This temperature prevents injury from hot solutions and cramping from cold solutions.*
  - Suspend container on bathroom hook at level of your shoulders (no higher than 46 cm [18 in.] above stoma).
  - Open roller clamp and allow solution to run through tubing; close clamp. **Rationale:** *This removes air from tubing and prevents discomfort for patient.*
- Sit on toilet or on chair in front of toilet.
- Place sleeve between your thighs and direct end into toilet.
- Lubricate cone tip with water-soluble lubricant.
- Position cone in sleeve by placing through top opening. If cone cannot be inserted easily, do not force it.
- Hold cone snugly against stoma. **Rationale:** *This prevents backflow of solution.*
- Open roller clamp on tubing and allow water to run through cone while inserting cone into stoma.
- Instill solution (750–1000 mL) slowly. **Rationale:** *The container height and rate of water flow affects results obtained. If you begin feeling light-headed or have dizziness stop instillation.* **Rationale:** *These are symptoms of a vagal response.*
- Clamp tubing briefly if cramping occurs.
- Remove cone and close off or fold over top of sleeve.
- Remain seated until most stool and solution return, usually 10–15 min.
- Remove gloves and discard.
- Rinse sleeve with water, dry bottom of sleeve, and close end of sleeve.
- Wear the sleeve in this manner for 30–60 min while proceeding with other activities. **Rationale:** *This allows time for expelling solution or feces and prevents accidental evacuation.* Then remove, clean, and store sleeve.
- Cleanse skin and stoma with warm water and dry thoroughly. Apply skin barriers and clean pouch.
- Place discarded supplies in trash. Remove gloves and wash your hands.

Going Home with a Colostomy

- Keep the names and phone numbers of a wound ostomy continence nurse, supply vendor, and other resource people to contact when needed. Use internet resources for information and support.
- Look for signs that may indicate a problem that needs to be reported to a healthcare provider, such as peristomal redness, skin breakdown, and changes in stomal color.
- Care for the ostomy and appliance when traveling.
- Use infection control precautions, including proper disposal of used pouches since these cannot be flushed down a toilet.
- Identify ways to help children handle concerns about odor and appearance. Provide information about ostomy care and community support groups. A visit from someone who has had an ostomy under similar circumstances may be helpful.

SKILL 4.20 Enema and Retention Enema: Administering

An enema instills fluid into the lower bowel via the rectum most commonly to cleanse the bowel before a medical examination or procedure or to relieve constipation.

Delegation or Assignment

Administration of some enemas may be delegated or assigned to the UAP. However, the nurse must ensure the personnel are competent in the use of standard precautions. Abnormal findings such as inability to insert the rectal tip, patient inability to retain the solution, or unusual return from the enema must be validated and interpreted by the nurse. Note that state laws for UAPs vary, so this task might be assigned to the UAP rather than delegated.

Equipment

- Disposable linen-saver pad
- Bath blanket
- Bedpan or commode
- Clean gloves
- Water-soluble lubricant if tubing not prelubricated
- Paper towel

Large-Volume Enema

- Solution container with tubing of correct size and tubing clamp
- Correct solution, amount ❶, and temperature

(*continued on next page*)

SKILL 4.20 Enema and Retention Enema: Administering (*continued*)

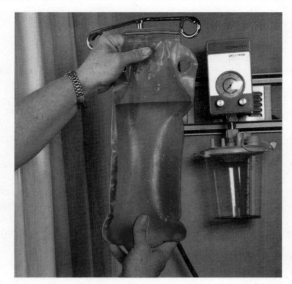

Source: Ronald May/Pearson Education, Inc.

① Fill bag to 750–1000 mL with tepid solution.

Small-Volume Enema

■ Prepackaged container of enema solution with lubricated tip

Retention Enema

■ Commercially prepared disposable oil retention enema (adult: 150–200 mL oil; child: 75–100 mL oil)
■ Skin care items (e.g., soap, water, towels)

Preparation

■ Review healthcare provider's orders.
■ Run some solution **②** through the connecting tubing of a large-volume enema set and the rectal tube to expel any air

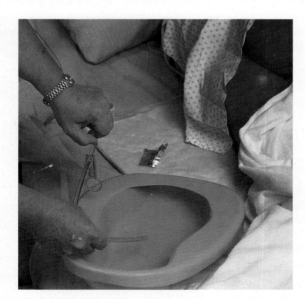

Source: Ronald May/Pearson Education, Inc.

② Allow solution to run through tubing to expel air.

in the tubing, then close the clamp. **Rationale:** *Air instilled into the rectum, although not harmful, causes unnecessary distention.*

■ Lubricate **③** about 5 cm (2 in.) of the rectal tube (some commercially prepared enema sets already have lubricated nozzles). **Rationale:** *Lubrication facilitates insertion through the sphincter and minimizes trauma.*

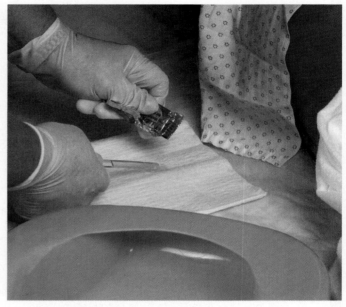

Source: Ronald May/Pearson Education, Inc.

③ Lubricate tip of tubing to prevent rectal injury.

Procedure

1. Prior to performing the procedure, introduce self and verify the patient's identity using two identifiers. Explain to the patient what you are going to do, why it is necessary, and how the patient can participate. Discuss how the results will be used in planning further care or treatments. Indicate that the patient may experience a feeling of fullness while the solution is being administered. Explain the need to hold the solution as long as possible.
2. Perform hand hygiene and observe other appropriate infection control procedures.
3. Don clean gloves.
4. Provide for patient privacy.
5. Prepare the enema solution ordered for the patient. Use warm water, or warm the prepared enema container with solution. **Rationale:** *Warming the enema solution to body temperature is beneficial to stimulate the rectal mucosa. Cold solutions should be avoided as they may cause cramping.*
6. Assist the adult patient to a left lateral position, with the right leg as acutely flexed as possible and the linen-saver pad under the buttocks. Place bedpan or commode within reach. **Rationale:** *This position facilitates the flow of solution by gravity into the sigmoid and descending colon, which are on the left side. Having the*

SKILL 4.20 Enema and Retention Enema: Administering *(continued)*

right leg acutely flexed provides for adequate exposure of the anus.

7. Expose anal opening, and gently insert the enema tube.
   - For patients in the left lateral position, lift the upper buttock. **Rationale:** *This ensures good visualization of the anus.*
   - Insert the tube smoothly and slowly into the rectum, directing it toward the umbilicus. **Rationale:** *The angle follows the normal contour of the rectum. Slow insertion prevents spasm of the sphincter.*
   - Insert the tube 7–10 cm (3–4 in.). **Rationale:** *Because the anal canal is about 2.5–5 cm (1–2 in.) long in the adult, insertion to this point places the tip of the tube beyond the anal sphincter into the rectum.*
   - If resistance is encountered at the internal sphincter, ask the patient to take a deep breath and let it out slowly, then run a small amount of solution through the tube. **Rationale:** *This relaxes the internal anal sphincter.*
   - Never force tube or solution entry. If instilling a small amount of solution does not permit the tube to be advanced or the solution to flow freely, withdraw the tube. Check for any stool that may have blocked the tube during insertion. If present, flush it and retry the procedure. You may also need to perform a digital rectal examination (check with facility policy) to determine if there is an impaction or other mechanical blockage. If resistance persists, end the procedure and report the resistance to the healthcare provider and nurse in charge.

8. Slowly administer the enema solution.
   - Raise the solution container, and open the clamp to allow fluid flow.

   or

   - Compress a pliable commercially prepared enema container by hand.
   - During most low enemas, hold or hang the solution container no higher than 30 cm (12 in.) above the rectum. **Rationale:** *The higher the solution container is held above the rectum, the faster the flow and the greater the force (pressure) in the rectum.* During a high enema, ❹ hang the solution container about 45 cm (18 in.) above the rectum. **Rationale:** *The fluid must be instilled farther to clean the entire bowel.* See facility protocol.
   - Administer the fluid slowly. If the patient complains of fullness or pain, lower the container or use the clamp to stop the flow for 30 seconds, and then restart the flow at a slower rate. **Rationale:** *Administering the enema slowly and stopping the flow momentarily decreases the likelihood of intestinal spasm and premature ejection of the solution.*

CAUTION! When administering an enema to the patient there is the potential risk of stimulating the vagus nerve which can result in bradycardia (pulse rate less than 60 bpm) or shortness of breath. Observe for faintness, pallor, nausea, chest discomfort, or diaphoresis. If any of these signs/symptoms occur, stop the procedure immediately, remove the enema tube, stay with the patient, and call for help.

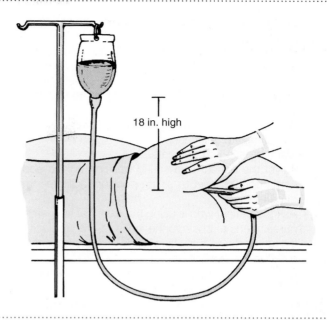

18 in. high

❹ Place enema solution container no more than 45 cm (18 in.) above rectum for safety.

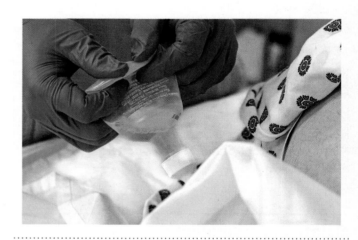

❺ Rolling up a commercial enema container.

- If you are using a plastic commercial container, roll it up as the fluid is instilled. This prevents subsequent suctioning of the solution ❺. After all the solution has been instilled or when the patient cannot hold any more and feels the desire to defecate (the urge to defecate usually indicates that sufficient fluid has been administered), close the clamp and remove the enema tube from the anus.
- Place the enema tube in a disposable towel as you withdraw it. Clean and dispose of equipment.

9. Encourage the patient to retain the enema.
   - Ask the patient to remain lying down. **Rationale:** *It is easier for the patient to retain the enema when lying*

(continued on next page)

SKILL 4.20 Enema and Retention Enema: Administering (*continued*)

down than when sitting or standing, because gravity promotes drainage and peristalsis.

- Request that the patient retain the solution for the appropriate amount of time, for example, 5–10 min for a cleansing enema or 30–60 min for a retention enema. **Rationale:** The *purpose of an enema is to soften stool.*
  - A cleansing enema may need to be given to remove oil and stimulate defecation.
10. Assist the patient to defecate.
    - Assist the patient to a sitting position on the bedpan, commode, or toilet. A sitting position facilitates the act of defecation.
    - Ask the patient who is using the toilet not to flush it. The nurse needs to observe the feces.
    - If a specimen of feces is required, ask the patient to use a bedpan or commode.
    - Don gloves and provide hygienic care if needed. Discard washcloth and towel in laundry.
11. Remove and discard gloves. Perform hand hygiene and leave the patient safe and comfortable.
12. Complete documentation using forms, checklists, or electronic dropdown lists supplemented by nurse's notes or additional comments as appropriate. Document the type and volume of enema given. Describe the results and patient response.

SAMPLE DOCUMENTATION

[date] 1000. States last BM five days ago. Abdomen distended and firm. Bowel sounds hypoactive. Fleet's enema given per order resulting in large amount of firm brown stool. States he "feels better." M. Lopez

---

Safety Considerations

Occasionally a nurse needs to administer an enema to a patient who is unable to control the external sphincter muscle and thus cannot retain the enema solution for even a few minutes. In that case, after the rectal tube is inserted, the patient assumes a supine position on a bedpan. The head of the bed can be elevated slightly, to 30 degrees if necessary for easier breathing, and pillows support the patient's head and back.

Lifespan Considerations
NEWBORNS, INFANTS, AND CHILDREN

- Provide a careful explanation to the parents and child before the procedure. An enema is an intrusive procedure and therefore may cause the patient or parent to become anxious.
- The enema solution should be isotonic (usually normal saline). Some hypertonic commercial solutions (e.g., Fleet phosphate enema) can lead to hypovolemia and electrolyte imbalances. In addition, the osmotic effect of the enema may produce diarrhea and subsequent metabolic acidosis.
- Newborns, infants, and small children do not exhibit sphincter control and need to be assisted in retaining the enema. The nurse administers the enema while the newborn, infant, or child is lying with the buttocks over the bedpan, and the nurse firmly presses the buttocks together to prevent the immediate expulsion of the solution. Older children can usually hold the solution if they understand what to do and are not required to hold it for too long a period. It may be necessary to ensure that the bathroom is available for an ambulatory child before starting the procedure or to have a bedpan or portable commode at the bed ready.
- The enema solution needs to be warmed before giving to the child.
- Large-volume enemas consist of 50–200 mL in children less than 18 months old; 200–300 mL in children 18 months to 5 years; and 300–500 mL in children 5–12 years old.
- Careful explanation is especially important for the preschool child.
- For newborns, infants, and small children, the dorsal recumbent position is frequently used. Position them on a small padded bedpan with support for the back and head. Secure the legs by placing a diaper under the bedpan and then over and around the thighs. Place the underpad under the patient's buttocks to protect the bed linen, and drape the patient with the bath blanket.
- Insert the tube 5–7.5 cm (2–3 in.) in a child and only 2.5 cm (1 in.) in a newborn or infant.
- For children, lower the height of the solution container appropriately for the age of the child. See facility protocol.
- To assist a small child in retaining the solution, apply firm pressure over the anus with tissue wipes, or firmly press the buttocks together.

OLDER ADULTS

- Older adults may fatigue easily.
- Older adults may be more susceptible to fluid and electrolyte imbalances. Use tap water enemas with great caution.
- Monitor the patient's tolerance during the procedure, watching for vagal episodes (e.g., slow pulse) and dysrhythmias.
- Protect older adults' skin from prolonged exposure to moisture.
- Assist older patients with perineal care as indicated.

SKILL 4.21 Fecal Impaction: Removing

Safety Note! *During scheduled clinical time, nursing students may have a learning opportunity to observe or assist with this skill only with faculty permission and with direct supervision from faculty or another RN.*

A fecal impaction is a large solid, dry, hard stool stuck in the rectum as a result of untreated chronic constipation or overuse of laxatives. Treatment can be an enema, stool softeners, glycerin suppositories, or digital removal.

Bowel Interventions **271**

SKILL 4.21 Fecal Impaction: Removing (*continued*)

Delegation or Assignment

Due to the potential results of stimulation of the vagus nerve during the procedure, digital removal of an impaction is generally not delegated or assigned to the UAP. However, signs and symptoms of problems may be observed during usual care and may be recorded by individuals other than the nurse. Abnormal findings must be validated and interpreted by the nurse.

Equipment

- Bath blanket
- Disposable absorbent pad
- Bedpan and cover
- Toilet tissue
- Clean gloves
- Lubricant
- Soap, water, and towel
- Topical lidocaine (follow facility policy)

Preparation

- Review the healthcare provider's orders. Check the facility policy to determine if a healthcare provider's order is required. **Rationale:** *Rectal manipulation can cause stimulation of the vagus nerve, resulting in a slowing of the heart rate.*
- Review patient's allergies.
- If the facility permits the use of the topical anesthetic lidocaine, 1–2 mL should be inserted into the anal canal 5 minutes prior to the procedure. **Rationale:** *This will numb the anal and rectal areas, reducing the pain of the procedure.*

Procedure

1. Prior to performing the procedure, introduce self and verify the patient's identity using two identifiers. Explain to the patient what you are going to do, why it is necessary, and how the patient can participate. Discuss how the results will be used in planning further care or treatments. This procedure is distressing, tiring, and uncomfortable, so the person may desire the presence of another nurse or support person.
2. Perform hand hygiene and observe other appropriate infection control procedures.
3. Don clean gloves (double gloving may be a consideration).
4. Provide for patient privacy.
5. Assist the patient to a right or left lateral or Sims position with the back toward you. **Rationale:** *When the person lies on the right side, the sigmoid colon is uppermost; thus, gravity can aid removal of the feces. Positioning on the left side allows easier access to the sigmoid colon.*
6. Place a disposable absorbent pad under the patient's hips, and arrange the top bed linen to ensure that it falls obliquely over the hips, exposing only the buttocks.

7. Place the bedpan and toilet tissue nearby on the bed or a bedside chair.
8. Lubricate the gloved index finger. **Rationale:** *Lubricant reduces resistance by the anal sphincter as the finger is inserted.*
9. Remove the impaction. Have the patient take slow, deep breaths during the procedure. Ensure the patient does not hold the breath. **Rationale:** *Holding the breath can stimulate a vagal response.*
   - Gently insert the index finger into the rectum, moving toward the umbilicus.
   - Gently massage around the stool. **Rationale:** *Gentle action prevents damage to the rectal mucosa. A circular motion around the rectum dislodges the stool, stimulates peristalsis, and relaxes the anal sphincter.*
   - Work the finger into the hardened mass of stool to break it up ❶. If you cannot break up the impaction with one finger, insert two fingers and try to break up the impaction scissor style.
   - Work the stool down to the anus, remove it in small pieces, and place them in the bedpan. Carefully continue to remove as much fecal material as possible.

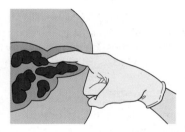

❶ Digital removal of fecal impaction.

CAUTION! When removing an impaction there is the potential risk of stimulating the vagus nerve which can result in bradycardia (pulse rate less than 60 bpm) or shortness of breath. Observe for faintness, pallor, nausea, chest discomfort, or diaphoresis. If any of these signs/symptoms occur, stop the procedure immediately, stay with the patient, and call for help.

   - Assist the patient to a position on a clean bedpan, commode, or toilet. **Rationale:** *Digital stimulation of the rectum may induce the urge to defecate.*
10. Assist the patient with hygienic measures as needed.
    - Wash the rectal area with soap and water and dry gently.
    - Remove and discard gloves. Perform hand hygiene and leave the patient safe and comfortable.
11. Complete documentation using forms, checklists, or electronic dropdown lists supplemented by nurse's notes or additional comments as appropriate.

(continued on next page)

SKILL 4.21 Fecal Impaction: Removing (*continued*)

[date] 2120 C/o not being able to have a bowel movement, last bowel movement 3 days ago. Hard, dry, stool noted just inside anal sphincter. Digital removal of impacted stool per Dr. Raymond's order. Returned moderate amount hard, dry, dark brown stool. Pulse rate 82–86 throughout procedure, skin warm and dry. States feeling better now. *R. Chou*

Lifespan Considerations
OLDER ADULTS

■ Fecal impaction is not uncommon with older adult patients due to decreased mobility and exercise, dietary habits, or tendency to overuse enemas and laxatives.

■ Encourage patients to decrease use of laxatives and enemas, increase fluid intake and fiber in diet, and increase exercise. Dehydration resulting from inadequate fluid intake leads to constipation and fecal impaction.

SKILL 4.22 Fecal Ostomy Pouch: Applying

Safety Note! *During scheduled clinical time, nursing students may have a learning opportunity to observe or assist with this skill only with faculty permission and with direct supervision from faculty or another RN.*

The pouch is a bag-like device that is applied to the ostomy to collect the fecal material. It adheres to the body and cannot be seen through clothing. It must be emptied every few hours and can be replaced as needed.

Delegation or Assignment

Due to the complexity of the procedure, the need for assessment skills, and use of aseptic technique, this procedure is not delegated or assigned to the UAP. In some states, a trained UAP may change ostomy pouches on well-established stomas. Abnormal findings must be validated and interpreted by the nurse.

Equipment

■ One- or two-piece transparent ostomy pouch with adhesive wafer
■ Warm water and mild soap
■ Soft cloths
■ Bath blanket
■ Plastic bag for pouch disposal
■ Tail closure or night adapter for pouch
■ Clean gloves
■ Graduate or bedpan
■ Measuring guide
■ Tissues
■ Ostomy scissors and dark marking pen

Preparation

■ Review healthcare provider's orders and review patient care plan.
■ Determine exact supplies patient uses ❶ **A–D**.
■ Gather equipment.

Procedure

1. Introduce self to patient and verify the patient's identity using two identifiers. Explain to the patient what you are going to do, why it is necessary, and how the patient can participate. Discuss how the results will be used in planning further care or treatments.
2. Perform hand hygiene and observe appropriate infection control procedures.
3. Provide for patient privacy and don gloves.
4. Raise bed to high position.
5. Place bath blanket over patient. Place absorbent pad or towels under patient. **Rationale:** *This protects the bed from spillage.*
6. Observe placement of stoma. **Rationale:** *This determines normal amount of output and consistency.* (Immediately after surgery, all stomas will have very liquid stool and high flatus output.)

CAUTION! To promote the patient's self-esteem and body image, be aware of your own body language. Even subtle changes in the way you look at the stoma could indicate disgust or disapproval and an altered self-esteem could result.

7. Empty old pouch into graduated container, bedpan, or toilet.
8. Remove old pouch by pushing against skin as you pull backing from skin and discard in plastic bag. Save tail closure on bottom of pouch.
9. Measure output, if ordered.
10. Clean skin and stoma gently with warm water and soft cloth. **Rationale:** *Oily substances can interfere with pouch adhesive. If adhesive doesn't come off, leave it on the skin. If you pick at it, the peristomal skin can be damaged.*
11. Dry skin well with soft cloth. Keep tissues available if stoma functions while pouch is off.
12. Observe skin; it should be free of erythema or excoriation. The stoma is assessed for changes in size, ulceration, and

SKILL 4.22 Fecal Ostomy Pouch: Applying (*continued*)

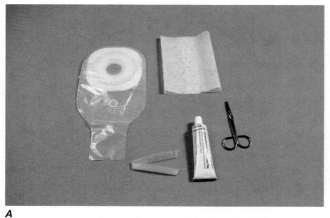

A

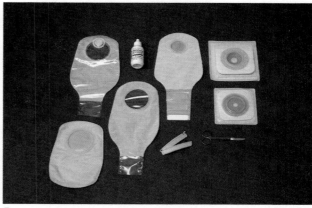

B

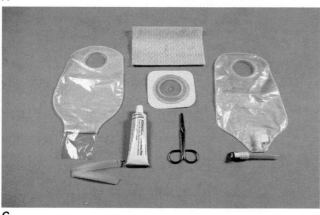

C

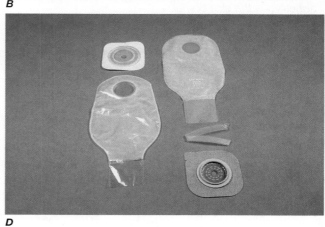

D

Sources: **A–D,** Ronald May/Pearson Education, Inc.

❶ **A,** Supplies needed to change one-piece pouches; **B,** fabric pouches, convexity faceplates, pouch with filter; **C,** supplies needed to change two-piece pouches; **D,** two-piece fecal pouches.

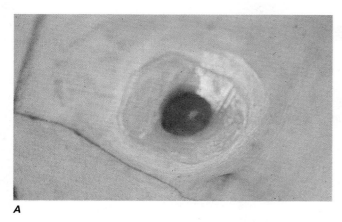

A

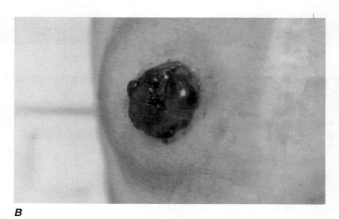

B

Sources: **A,** and **B,** Ronald May/Pearson Education, Inc.

❷ **A,** Viable stoma; **B,** nonviable parastomal hernia.

color (stoma should be moist, pink, or beefy red) ❷. Notify the healthcare provider if stoma is black, blue, or purple. This indicates a nonviable stoma.
13. Measure stoma at the base with measuring guide.
14. Trace measured pattern on pouch.

15. Cut pouch to pattern, making sure opening is large enough (at least 0.3 cm [⅛ in.]) to encircle stoma without pushing on edges. **Rationale:** *No skin should appear between the pouch edge and the stoma.*

(*continued on next page*)

SKILL 4.22 Fecal Ostomy Pouch: Applying (*continued*)

16. If using a two-piece pouch, snap the wafer and pouch together.
17. Remove paper from skin barrier on pouch and save it. **Rationale:** *This may be used as a pattern for next pouch change.*
18. Apply a ring of skin barrier paste to opening on pouch.
19. Apply Stomahesive powder to denuded skin only.
20. Remove paper from outer ring.
21. Center and apply pouch to clean and dry skin. Smooth edges of adhesive to skin. **Rationale:** *If adhesive is wrinkled, it may result in leakage from pouch.* To promote optimum wear of the pouch, warm the adhesive by placing your gloved hand over the adhesive and gently hold it over the site for ½–1 min. **Rationale:** *This will activate the adhesive in the skin barrier.*
22. Pouches can be applied over an incision. **Rationale:** *Incisions are sealed within 24 hours of surgery.*
23. Close and secure end of pouch with tail closure.
    - Ensure bowed end is next to body. **Rationale:** *This provides a better fit to body, and prevents outpouching of clamp through clothing.*
    - Lay hook on top of bag and fold bag 2.5 cm (1 in.) over end of pouch.
    - Squeeze clamp together to close.

24. Remove soiled pouch and tissues from bedside.
25. Remove and discard gloves. Perform hand hygiene.
26. Position patient for safety and comfort. Return bed to low position.
27. Put away supplies and reorder as necessary.
28. Complete documentation using forms, checklists, or electronic dropdown lists supplemented by nurse's notes or additional comments as appropriate.

CAUTION! Patients with ostomies will need a nutritional consult and a written dietary guide. They need to limit the amount of hard-to-digest foods for at least the first 2 to 3 weeks postop. Also, limiting gas-producing foods will prevent gas-forming odors.

Changing One-Piece Fecal Ostomy Pouch ❸

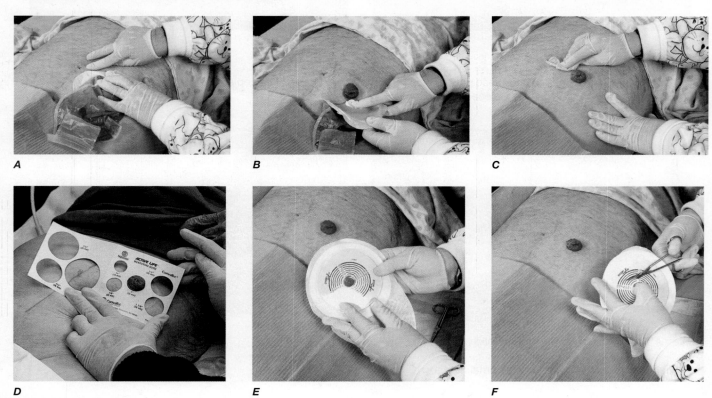

A   *B*   *C*

D   *E*   *F*

Sources: *A–F,* Ronald May/Pearson Education, Inc.

❸ *A,* Starting at upper corner, remove old pouch; *B,* As you remove old pouch, push against skin while pulling down on pouch; *C,* Clean skin with warm water and dry well; *D,* Measure stoma size; *E,* Remove plastic covering from one-piece pouch; *F,* Cut pouch opening to encircle stoma without pushing on its edges.

SKILL 4.22 Fecal Ostomy Pouch: Applying *(continued)*

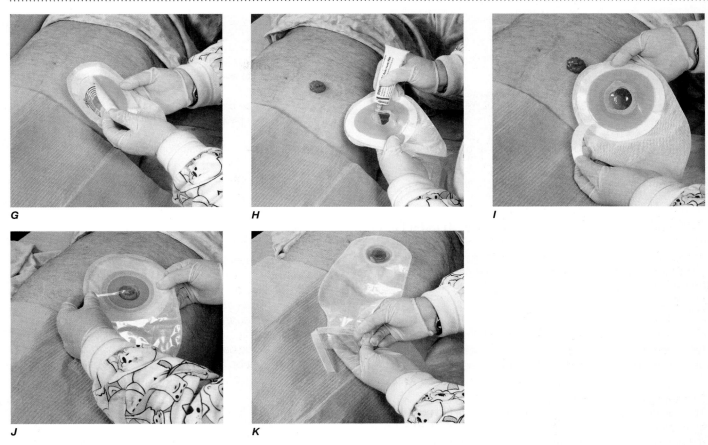

G   H   I

J   K

*Sources: **G–K,** Ronald May/Pearson Education, Inc.*

❸ *(continued)* **G,** Remove paper from inner wafer and save pattern for future pouch changes; **H,** Apply ring of paste to opening on pouch; **I,** Remove paper from outer adhesive ring of pouch; **J,** Center and apply pouch to clean, dry skin; **K,** After applying one-piece pouch, clamp bottom of pouch.

Loop Colostomy with Rod/Rod Removed ❹

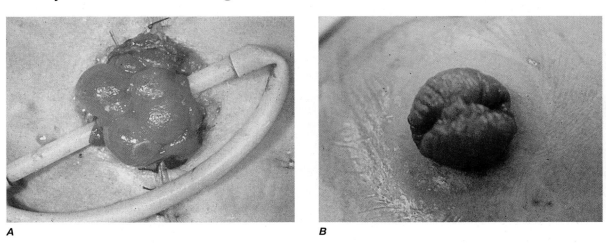

A   B

*Sources: **A,** and **B,** Ronald May/Pearson Education, Inc.*

❹ **A,** Loop of bowel is brought onto the abdomen and is supported by a plastic rod; **B,** The plastic rod is removed. Two openings are made in the colostomy. Proximal loop is functional and discharges fecal material. Distal end is nonfunctional and discharges only mucus.

(continued on next page)

SKILL 4.22 Fecal Ostomy Pouch: Applying (*continued*)

Patient Teaching

- Empty pouch when it's one third full of stool or flatus.
  a. Empty into toilet.
  b. Pouch should last for 3–4 days.
- Rinse pouch using room temperature water and a rubber ear syringe (squirt into pouch).
- Use pouch deodorant if desired.
- Empty each morning and last thing at night, even if not one third full.

- Check seal on daily basis for tight fit; change if needed.
- Instruct patient to always carry a supply of ostomy equipment for emergency use.
- Instruct patient on emptying and cleaning pouch, opening and closing clamp, observing and cleaning peristomal area, and changing pouch.
- Have patient return demonstration until able to perform activities correctly.

SKILL 4.23 Rectal Tube: Inserting

Safety Note! *During scheduled clinical time, nursing students may have a learning opportunity to observe or assist with this skill only with faculty permission and with direct supervision from faculty or another RN.*

A long slender tube is inserted into the rectum in order to relieve flatulence and allow flatus to pass more easily. It can also be used to remove diarrhea fecal matter in some situations.

Delegation or Assignment

The nurse first determines that the UAP knows the correct way to insert a rectal tube and monitor the patient. Placement of a rectal tube can be delegated or assigned to the UAP in some states when trained to do this procedure. Signs and symptoms of problems may be observed during usual care and recorded by UAP. Abnormal findings must be validated and interpreted by the nurse. Note that state laws for UAPs vary, so this task might be assigned to the UAP rather than delegated.

Equipment

- Rectal tube: size 22–24 straight (French) for adults and size 12–18 French for children
- Small plastic bag or stool specimen container
- Hypoallergenic paper tape
- Water-soluble lubricant
- Bed protector
- Clean gloves, 2 pairs
- Washcloth and towel

Preparation

- Review healthcare provider's orders and patient plan of care.
- Gather needed equipment and supplies.

Procedure

1. Introduce self to patient and verify the patient's identity using two identifiers. Explain to the patient what you are going to do, why it is necessary, and how the patient can participate. Discuss how the results will be used in planning further care or treatments.
2. Perform hand hygiene and observe appropriate infection control procedures.

3. Provide for patient privacy.
4. Don gloves.
5. Place patient on left side in a recumbent position and drape. **Rationale:** *This position facilitates insertion of tube following the normal curve of rectum and sigmoid colon.*
6. Place bed protector under patient.
7. Tape the plastic bag around the distal end of the rectal tube or insert the tube into the stool specimen container.
8. Vent the upper side of the plastic bag to prevent inflation.
9. Lubricate the proximal end of the rectal tube with water-soluble lubricant.
10. Gently separate buttocks, and ask the patient to take in a deep breath and let it out slowly. **Rationale:** *Taking a deep breath relaxes the anal sphincter and prevents tissue trauma during tube insertion.* Gently insert the tube into the patient's rectum, past the external and internal anal sphincters (5–10 cm [2–4 in.]) in adults; 2.5–7.5 cm [1–3 in.] in children). Do not force the rectal tube ❶.
11. With adults, gently tape the tube in place, using hypoallergenic paper tape. With children, hold the tube in place manually.

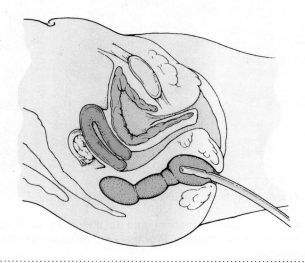

❶ Insert rectal tube past the external and internal anal sphincters.

SKILL 4.23 Rectal Tube: Inserting (continued)

12. Remove and discard gloves. Perform hand hygiene.
13. Take patient's pulse.

CAUTION! With rectal tube placement, there is the potential risk of stimulating the vagus nerve which can result in bradycardia (pulse rate less than 60 bpm) or shortness of breath. Observe for faintness, pallor, nausea, chest discomfort, or diaphoresis. If any of these signs or symptoms occur, stop the procedure immediately, remove the rectal tube, stay with the patient, and call for help.

---

14. Leave the tube in place no longer than 20 minutes. **Rationale:** *Prolonged stimulation of the anal sphincter may result in a loss of the neuromuscular response. The prolonged presence of a catheter may cause pressure necrosis of the mucosal surface.*
15. Don gloves.
16. Remove the tube and provide perianal care.
17. Help the patient assume a comfortable position.
18. Clean the tubing, and place in bathroom if it is to be reused. Remove and discard the plastic bag.

19. Instruct the patient that chewing gum, sucking on candy, drinking liquids through a straw, carbonated beverages, and smoking tend to promote the swallowing of air and increase abdominal distention.
20. Remove and discard gloves. Perform hand hygiene and leave the patient safe and comfortable.
21. Complete documentation using forms, checklists, or electronic dropdown lists supplemented by nurse's notes or additional comments as appropriate.

SAMPLE DOCUMENTATION

[date] 1815 C/o cramping throughout abdomen. Last bowel movement earlier in day and normal. Abdomen distended, hyperactive bowel sounds. States it "feels like a lot of gas." Rectal tube inserted with instant flatus expelled. Tube left in for 5 minutes with large amount of flatus expelled. Rectal tube removed, states, "feels so much better now." Tolerated without complication. *T. Bynes*

≫ Dialysis

Expected Outcomes

1. Dialysis proceeds without complication (excess fluids and wastes removed from blood).
2. Vascular access site remains patent.
3. Patient demonstrates self-care after teaching.

SKILL 4.24 Dialysis, Peritoneal: Catheter Insertion, Assisting

Safety Note! *During scheduled clinical time, nursing students may have a learning opportunity to observe or assist with this skill only with faculty permission and with direct supervision from faculty or another RN.*

Catheters used for peritoneal dialysis can be inserted into the abdomen percutaneously, using a local anesthetic at the bedside, or during a laparoscopy or surgical incision procedure using general anesthesia in a surgical suite. Peritoneal dialysis eliminates waste from the blood when the kidneys fail or cannot function effectively.

Delegation or Assignment

Assisting with peritoneal catheter insertion is a sterile procedure and is not delegated or assigned to the UAP. The nurse can request a UAP to report patient observations to the nurse for follow-up. Assessment and evaluation remain the nurse's responsibility.

Equipment

- Sterile gloves, masks, caps, goggles, and gowns for healthcare provider, nurse, and anyone assisting; mask for patient

- Dialysis solution
- Sterile peritoneal dialysis set:
  - Peritoneal catheter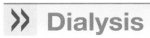
  - Local anesthetic (e.g., lidocaine), 25-gauge 1.8-cm (⅝-in.) needle, and 3-mL syringe
  - Alcohol sponges
  - Scalpel with a blade
  - Precut gauze to place around the catheter
  - Drape
  - Transfer set
  - Protective transfer set cap
  - Sutures, needles, and needle driver
  - Trocar (the sharp, needle-like instrument used to make a hole in body tissues)
  - Connector
  - 4 × 4 gauze square
  - Specimen container
  - Antiseptic ointment (e.g., povidone-iodine or mupirocin)
- 10-mL syringe and 3.8-cm (1.5-in.) needle
- Scissors

(continued on next page)

SKILL 4.24 Dialysis, Peritoneal: Catheter Insertion, Assisting (continued)

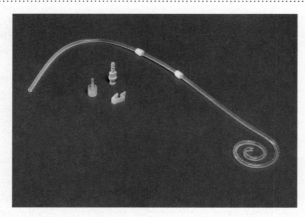

Source: Dover, Kendall, Monoject, Shirley, Aqua-Seal, Kangaroo and Argyle are trademarks of a Covidien company. Images provided courtesy of Covidien. © 2014 Covidien.

❶ An Argyle double-cuff curl catheter. This multiple side-hole catheter has two or three cuffs, a removable hub, and a screw cap.

- Skin preparation/dressing set:
  - Chlorhexidine gluconate 2%, povidone-iodine, or other disinfecting solution
  - Razor and blade or scissors
  - Gauze sponges
  - Hypo-allergenic tape

Preparation

- Verify signed informed consent form in patient's record.
- Although the primary care provider will have already done initial patient and family teaching, the nurse can reinforce key elements.
  - Review the technique of peritoneal dialysis and its purpose with the patient and family.
  - Explain that since the kidneys are not functioning properly, this procedure will rid the blood and body of excess wastes and fluid that are normally excreted by the kidneys.
  - Explain that inserting the trocar (which is the primary care provider's responsibility) may be uncomfortable. The discomfort can be reduced by the patient tensing the abdominal muscles as if for a bowel movement.
  - Explain that the purpose of the masks, gowns, gloves, and caps is to reduce the possibility of contaminating the site during insertion. Then explain that the patient will also need to wear a mask for the same reason.
- Review healthcare provider's orders and gather necessary equipment and supplies.
- Review patient's allergies.

Procedure

1. Prior to performing the procedure, introduce self and verify the patient's identity using two identifiers. Explain to the patient what your role will be, why it is necessary, and how the patient can participate. Remind the patient that additional teaching will be done at the time of the actual peritoneal dialysis treatment.

2. Perform hand hygiene and observe other appropriate infection control procedures throughout the various phases of the procedure. Assist the patient with use of the mask.
3. Provide for patient privacy.
4. Prepare the patient.
   - Ask the patient to urinate before the procedure. In some cases, bowel cleansing is also done prior to catheter insertion. **Rationale:** *Emptying the bladder and bowels moves them away from the peritoneal wall and lessens the danger that they will be punctured by the trocar.*
   - Administer analgesics and prophylactic antibiotics as ordered.
   - Assist the patient to a supine position, and arrange the bedding to expose the area around the umbilicus. **Rationale:** *The insertion site is usually in the midline just below the umbilicus.*
5. Prepare the solution and the tubing.
6. Implement surgical aseptic practices and body fluid precautions according to facility protocol.
   - Apply masks. **Rationale:** *Applying masks prior to breaking the seals on the packages reduces the chance of contamination.*
   - Apply cap, gown, and goggles.
   - Open the dialysis set and any sterile supplies not part of the set.
   - Apply sterile gloves.
7. Assist the healthcare provider as needed during and after the catheter insertion.
   - Ensure that the transfer set that has been connected to the catheter is securely capped.
   - Cover the catheter site with antiseptic ointment and pre-cut sterile gauze, and tape the occlusive dressing in place.
   - Remove and discard gloves. Perform hand hygiene.
8. Administer prophylactic antibiotics as ordered.
9. Recheck vital signs. Report to the healthcare provider if significantly different from baseline.
10. Clean up procedure area.
11. Perform hand hygiene and leave the patient safe and comfortable.
12. Complete documentation using forms, checklists, or electronic dropdown lists supplemented by nurse's notes or additional comments as appropriate. Record the procedure, patient's response, and appearance of exit site and dressing.

SAMPLE DOCUMENTATION

[date] 1430 Double-cuff coiled Tenckhoff peritoneal catheter inserted in right lower quadrant by Dr. Novar under local anesthesia using sterile technique throughout. Post-insertion VS consistent with baseline. Catheter taped to abdominal skin. Dry, sterile, occlusive dressing applied to exit site. Tolerated with small amount of tenderness stated but resting quietly now. *U. Schmidt*

SKILL 4.25 Dialysis, Peritoneal: Procedures, Assisting

Safety Note! *During scheduled clinical time, nursing students may have a learning opportunity to observe or assist with this skill only with faculty permission and with direct supervision from faculty or another RN.*

Delegation or Assignment

Conducting peritoneal dialysis procedures is not delegated or assigned to the UAP. However, the patient's status is observed during usual care and may be recorded by individuals other than the nurse. Abnormal findings must be validated and interpreted by the nurse.

Equipment

For Infusing the Dialysate

- Container of peritoneal solution at body temperature, of the amount and kind ordered by the healthcare provider (Bags range in size from 1–3 liters.)
- IV pole
- Sterile peritoneal dialysis administration set (separate or combined pieces):
  - Y connector
  - IV-type tubing for dialysate
  - Drainage bag with tubing
- Sterile transfer set cap
- Dialysis log or flow sheet
- Clean gloves
- Mask and goggles
- Povidone-iodine swabs or other antiseptic per facility protocol. (Some agencies recommend a sterile bowl and antiseptic for soaking the transfer set tubing.)

For Changing the Catheter Site Dressing

- Sterile gloves and masks (gowns and goggles as needed)
- Sterile cotton-tipped applicators
- Chlorhexidine gluconate, povidone-iodine solution, or soap and water as specified by facility protocol
- Povidone-iodine ointment
- Precut sterile 2 × 2 gauze or slit transparent occlusive dressing
- Hypoallergenic tape

Preparation

- Review healthcare provider's orders and patient's plan of care.
- Review patient's allergies.
- Determine when the last dressing change was performed. Following initial catheter insertion, the dressing is not changed for several days to allow for stabilization of the catheter exit site. Subsequently, the dressing should be changed when wet, soiled, loose, or at intervals specified by facility policy.
- Gather equipment and supplies.

Procedure

1. Introduce self and verify the patient's identity using two identifiers. Explain to the patient what you are going to do, why it is necessary, and how the patient can participate. Discuss how the results will be used in planning further care or treatments.

2. Perform hand hygiene and observe other appropriate infection control procedures.
3. Provide for patient privacy.
4. Prepare the solution and the tubing.
   - Examine the label on the container and the expiration date. Examine the dialysate solution. It should be clear and the seals unbroken.
   - Warm the dialysate using an approved warmer (not a microwave oven) to at least body temperature. **Rationale:** *Warmed solution enhances exchange and is more comfortable for the patient.*
   - Following facility policy for the required technique, add any prescribed medication to the dialysate solution. This may require soaking the injection port of the bag in antiseptic solution. Heparin is sometimes added. **Rationale:** *This prevents the accumulation of fibrin in the catheter.*
   - Apply a mask and spike the solution container. Close the clamp, and hang the container on the IV pole.
   - Prime the tubing: Remove the protective cap and hold the tubing over a cup or basin. Maintain the sterility of the end of the tubing and the cap. Open the clamp and let the fluid run through the tubing, removing all bubbles. Close the tubing clamp. **Rationale:** *This rids the tubing of air that could enter the peritoneal cavity, causing discomfort and preventing free drainage outflow.*
5. Connect the solution to the catheter ❶.
   - Apply clean gloves, mask, and goggles.
   - Free the catheter end from the dressing if necessary.
   - Cleanse or soak the transfer set that connects to the Y connector with povidone-iodine or other specified disinfectant for the time listed in the facility protocol (usually 5 minutes). If tubing is not already attached, remove the cap from the transfer set and attach the Y connector and end of the tubing from the solution to the catheter.
   - Connect the drainage receptacle to the outflow tubing if not preattached. Close the outflow tubing clamp.

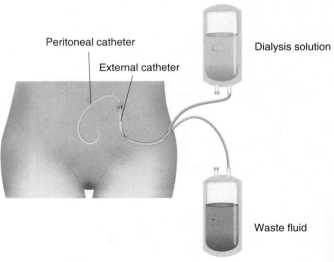

Peritoneal catheter

External catheter

Dialysis solution

Waste fluid

Source: Grei/Shutterstock

❶ Peritoneal dialysis system.

(continued on next page)

SKILL 4.25 Dialysis, Peritoneal: Procedures, Assisting (*continued*)

- If necessary, cover the catheter site with the precut sterile gauze, and tape the dressing in place. Minimize handling of the catheter.
- Remove and discard gloves. Perform hand hygiene.

6. Infuse the peritoneal dialysate.
   - Open the clamp on the inflow tubing so that the dialysate can flow into the peritoneal cavity for the time specified by the order. If no rate is specified, the patient can usually tolerate a steady open flow.
   - Observe the patient for any signs of discomfort, particularly respiratory distress or abdominal pain.
   - After the fluid has infused, clamp the inflow tubing. **Rationale:** *With the tubing clamped, air will not enter the peritoneal cavity.*
   - Leave the fluid in the cavity for the designated time.

7. Ensure patient comfort and safety.
   - Assist the patient into a comfortable position.
   - Monitor the patient's vital signs.
   - Periodically assess the patient's comfort during the dwell time.

8. Remove the fluid.
   - Unclamp the outflow tubing, and permit the fluid to drain into the drainage bag by gravity for about 30 minutes.
   - If the fluid does not drain freely, assist the patient to change position, or raise the head of the bed. If specified, drain only the amount ordered.

9. Assess the outflow fluid.
   - Observe the appearance of the outflow fluid. **Rationale:** *A cloudy pink-tinged or blood-tinged return may indicate peritonitis (infection/inflammation of the peritoneal cavity).* During the first two to four exchanges following insertion of the peritoneal dialysis catheter, the return may be blood tinged but should quickly progress to a straw-color return.
   - Apply clean gloves.
   - Measure the amount of outflow fluid, and discard the fluid and used supplies in an appropriate area.

10. Calculate the fluid balance for each exchange.
    - Compare the amount of outflow fluid with the amount of solution infused for each exchange.
    - If more fluid was infused than removed, the patient's fluid balance is positive (+); if more fluid was removed than infused, the fluid balance is negative (–).

    Example:
    + 2000 mL dialysate solution infused
    – 1500 mL fluid returned in drainage bag
    = 500 mL balance for this exchange

    - Repeat steps for each exchange.

11. Calculate the cumulative fluid balance at least every 24 hours. The cumulative fluid balance should be negative.
    - Add the balance from each exchange (from step 10) to the total exchange balance:

    Example:

Previous cumulative exchange balance	+500 mL
Present exchange balance	–700 mL
Cumulative exchange balance	–200 mL

12. Check the dressing at the catheter site if present.
    - Assess the dryness or wetness of the dressing. **Rationale:** *The dressing should remain dry during dialysis.*
    - To change the catheter site dressing, use the equipment listed above and follow correct technique for assessing and changing the dressing. Do not forcibly remove crusts or scabs. **Rationale:** *This may irritate skin and increase the risk of exit site infection.* Dressings may not be necessary for well-healed insertion sites.

13. If another bag is not to be infused at this time, or after the infusion of the new bag, disconnect the catheter from the tubing, and cover the end of the catheter with a new sterile cap. **Rationale:** *This allows the catheter to remain in place between each of the exchanges without contamination of the catheter.*

14. Remove and discard gloves. Perform hand hygiene.

15. Complete documentation using forms, checklists, or electronic dropdown lists supplemented by nurse's notes or additional comments as appropriate. Include the time during which the fluid infused, the exchange number, dialysate and additives used, details of the exchange balance, color of outflow solution from patient, patient's response, appearance of the catheter exit site and dressing, and patient's weight before and after the set of exchanges (daily).

SAMPLE DOCUMENTATION

[date] 0830 First I L dialysate infused over 20 minutes thru PD catheter. VS unchanged, no complaints of discomfort. Insertion site dressing clean and dry. S. Everley

1330 VS stable, dressing dry & intact. 950 mL pink-tinged fluid returned from PD catheter by gravity flow over 20 minutes. PD bag #2, I L, infused in I5 minutes. Ambulated in hall independently without complaint, sitting in chair now quietly. S. Everley

---

Patient Teaching

Most patients undergoing peritoneal dialysis perform these procedures themselves at home. The nurse performs the initial teaching and documents that the patient and family are knowledgeable and able to demonstrate the techniques involved. In addition, the nurse assists with arrangements for all equipment and supplies that the patient requires for home care.

For patients using continuous ambulatory peritoneal dialysis (CAPD), the empty dialysate solution bag can be left attached to the catheter during dwelling and is then used as the drainage bag. A special belt ❷ that stabilizes the catheter and holds the administration set between uses is available.

SKILL 4.25 Dialysis, Peritoneal: Procedures, Assisting (*continued*)

Teach the patient and family the following steps:

- Store supplies in a clean, cool, dry place.
- Examine the solution for any signs of contamination before using it.
- Warm the dialysate for about 1 hour using a heating pad that has been checked for appropriate temperature.
- Hang the dialysate bag at approximately shoulder height for infusion. Assist the patient with obtaining an IV pole or other hanging device.
- Perform thorough hand hygiene and wear a surgical mask when changing tubing.
- Record weight and dialysis fluid balance daily or as ordered. Weight should be measured after draining the dialysate, and on the same scale, at the same time of day, and wearing similar clothing each time.
- Report any signs of peritonitis, for example:
  - Fever
  - Nausea or vomiting
  - Redness or pain around the exit site.

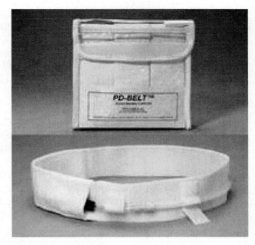

Source: Kelly Trakalo/Pearson Education, Inc.

❷ Peritoneal dialysis belt with tubing pouch stored in place.

Continuous Ambulatory Peritoneal Dialysis (CAPD) at Home

CAPD is a type of peritoneal dialysis that some patients use at home because it allows them to move around and do activities while fluid is in the peritoneal cavity.

- Necessary equipment and supplies at home
  - Sterile dialysate solution, 1 to 2 bags, warmed
  - Heating pad
  - Transfer set, either Y-set tubing or straight, and cap
  - Disconnect cap (e.g., FlexiCap or MiniCap)
  - Hook on wall of room used for dialysis or portable IV pole
  - Clamp
  - Paper towels
  - Low stool or table
  - Intake and output record
  - Sterile gloves, 2 pairs
  - Mask
  - Antibacterial soap
  - Cleansing solution for catheter
  - Medication, as ordered
- Equipment for dressing change
  - Dressing materials
  - Antimicrobial swabs or sterile 4 × 4 dressings and povidone-iodine (Betadine) solution
  - Tape
  - Sterile gloves, 2 pairs
  - Forceps (optional)
  - Povidone iodine ointment
  - 4 × 4 gauze pads and precut drain dressings
  - Warm soapy water, if needed
- For draining fluid (to be done four times daily)
  - Don gloves and uncap catheter maintaining aseptic technique.
  - Attach sterile bag and transfer set to catheter for draining dialysate.
  - Place bag on low stool or table below level of patient's abdomen. **Rationale:** *This position allows fluid to drain by gravity from patient's peritoneal cavity.*

- Unclamp tubing. Allow fluid to drain into bag from abdomen until flow ceases, approximately 10–20 min.
- Reclamp tubing.
- Examine drainage for discoloration or cloudiness. **Rationale:** *Change in color may indicate presence of infection; the presence of a white gelatin-like material indicates shredding of the peritoneal lining's old skin; an increase in this fibrin indicates potential peritonitis.*
- Disconnect tubing from drainage bag while maintaining aseptic technique. Unscrew catheter from tubing and attach disconnect cap, according to facility's instruction. **Rationale:** *The glucose in the dialysate solution predisposes the patient to infections.*
- Weigh drainage bag on scale. Effluent should weigh at least 2 kg (4.5 lb). This is equal to 2 L of fluid. **Rationale:** *This ensures all fluid is drained from the abdomen.*
- Dispose of effluent into toilet.
- Double bag tubing and drainage bag. Place biohazardous label on bag. Discard by placing in biohazardous container. Tubing is usually disposed of following each exchange.
- Remove and discard gloves and mask. Perform hand hygiene.
- Check blood pressure and pulse. **Rationale:** *Rapid fluid shift may cause hypotension.*
- For infusing dialysate
  - Warm dialysate. The bag can be encased in a heating pad for 1 hour. DO NOT PLACE IN MICROWAVE. **Rationale:** *Microwave heating will produce uneven heating and can cause burning in the patient.*
  - Perform hand hygiene for 3 minutes with antibacterial soap. **Rationale:** *This prevents contamination.*
  - Gather equipment. Don gloves.
  - Open plastic wrap on dialysate solution and inspect solution bag for expiration date and color and consistency of dialysate. Assess bag for possible leaks.
  - Add medications as ordered. Maintain sterile technique during this step. **Rationale:** *Some patients add routine drugs to dialysate, such as insulin.*
  - Connect tubing to dialysate bag by removing protective cover from port and spiking into dialysate bag. Maintain

(*continued on next page*)

SKILL 4.25 Dialysis, Peritoneal: Procedures, Assisting (*continued*)

sterility throughout this step. Each manufacturer has a slightly different mechanism for connecting the tubing and bag. Follow manufacturer's directions.
- Hang new dialysate bag on hook, which is positioned above patient at shoulder height.
- Open clamp and adjust height to ensure inflow of solution by gravity over a 10- to 20-minute period.
- Clamp tubing.
- Discard empty dialysate bag or place in a holding pouch at patient's waist, according to type of transfer set being used.
- Allow fluid to remain in peritoneal cavity approximately 4 hours.
- Remove and discard gloves. Perform hand hygiene.
- Repeat procedure 4 times daily, the last time at bedtime, allowing fluid to remain in peritoneal cavity overnight.
- Ensure that patient and caregiver are knowledgeable in strict aseptic technique.
- Notify healthcare provider if there is evidence of infection.

■ For dressing change
- Perform hand hygiene.
- Don sterile gloves.
- Remove old dressing with sterile gloves.
- Remove any dried blood or drainage with warm, soapy water.
- Saturate 4 × 4 dressings with povidone-iodine (Betadine) solution or use swabs and clean skin around catheter, moving in concentric circles from the catheter site outward. Remove crusted material, if present.
- Inspect site for infection (erythema, edema, warmth, exudate).
- Apply povidone-iodine ointment to catheter site using sterile dressings.
- Change gloves.
- Place two precut drain dressings over catheter site, and tape dressing. **Rationale:** *Dressings are secured to prevent infection at site.*
- Remove and discard gloves. Perform hand hygiene.

SKILL 4.26 Hemodialysis: Central Venous Dual-Lumen Catheter, Caring for

Safety Note! *During scheduled clinical time, nursing students may have a learning opportunity to observe or assist with this skill only with faculty permission and with direct supervision from faculty or another RN.*

The large bore double lumen catheter provides central venous dialysis access for short-term hemodialysis until peripheral extremity vessels can be used for a more durable internal arteriovenous (AV) fistula.

Delegation or Assignment

Due to the complexity of the procedure, the need for assessment skills, and use of aseptic technique, this procedure is not delegated or assigned to the UAP. However, aspects of function are observed during usual care and may be recorded by individuals other than the nurse. Abnormal findings must be validated and interpreted by the nurse.

Equipment

- Heparin, 1000 units/mL
- Sterile normal saline for injection
- Betadine spray
- Sterile 4 × 4 gauze pads
- Sterile transparent occlusive dressings if indicated
- Tape
- Luer-Lok catheter caps
- Nonsterile drape
- Two 3-mL syringes
- Two 20-mL syringes
- Clean gloves
- Two masks
- Sterile gloves

Preparation

- Review healthcare provider's orders and patient's plan of care.
- Gather all equipment and supplies.

Procedure

1. Introduce self to patient and verify the patient's identity using two identifiers. Explain to the patient what you are going to do, why it is necessary, and how the patient can participate. Discuss how the results will be used in planning further care or treatments.
2. Perform hand hygiene and observe appropriate infection control procedures.
3. Provide for patient privacy.
4. Fill two 20-mL syringes with 20 mL each of normal saline, and two 3-mL syringes with 3 mL of 1000 units/mL heparin.
5. Mask patient and self, and don clean gloves.
6. Place drape under catheter lumens.
7. Remove gauze wrap from lumens, if present, and discard in appropriate receptacle.
8. Remove and discard gloves. Perform hand hygiene.
9. Open sterile supplies.
10. Holding corner of 4 × 4 gauze, place under catheter lumens.
11. Spray lumens with povidone-iodine (Betadine) and allow to dry.
12. Don sterile gloves.
13. Remove old lumen caps.
14. Use 4 × 4 gauze to pick up new caps and place on lumens.
15. Unclamp and inject 20 mL of saline solution into each lumen using positive pressure technique.
16. Inject 3 mL of heparin into each catheter using positive pressure technique.

SKILL 4.26 Hemodialysis: Central Venous Dual-Lumen Catheter, Caring for (*continued*)

17. Reclamp lumens.
18. Remove old dressing, and discard in biohazard receptacle ❶.

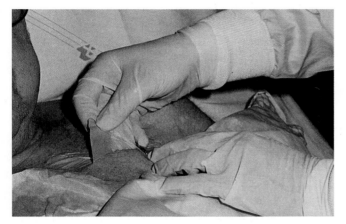

Source: Ronald May/Pearson Education, Inc.

❶ Maintain sterility while carefully removing dressing from dual-lumen catheter.

19. Cleanse area surrounding catheter with antimicrobial swabs ❷.

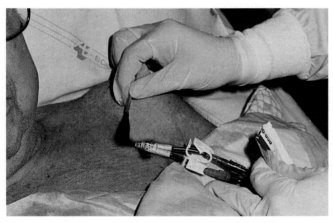

Source: Ronald May/Pearson Education, Inc.

❷ Cleanse catheter insertion site with antimicrobial swabs.

20. Place sterile transparent dressing over catheter insertion site.
    Note: Provide catheter site care after each dialysis treatment. Dressing is not required after permanent catheter site epithelializes around catheter (about 2 weeks).
21. If desired, wrap lumens in gauze and tape. **Rationale:** *This prevents skin irritation from lumen clamps.*
22. Dispose of equipment in biohazard receptacle.
23. Remove and discard gloves and mask. Perform hand hygiene and leave the patient safe and comfortable.
24. Complete documentation using forms, checklists, or electronic dropdown lists supplemented by nurse's notes or additional comments as appropriate.
25. Monitor patient daily and document signs of infection, bleeding, or displacement of catheters ❸.

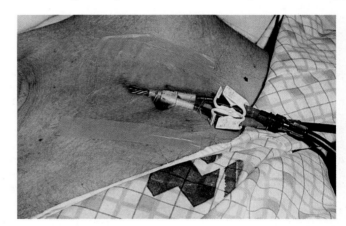

Source: Ronald May/Pearson Education, Inc.

❸ Monitor frequently for signs of infection, bleeding, or catheter displacement.

CAUTION! Central venous dual-lumen dialysis catheter (DLC) maintenance (heparin "pack" and site dressing) is performed *only* by the nephrology nurse after a dialysis treatment. These catheters are not maintained the way central venous access devices (CVADs) are. Instead, they are "packed" with undiluted heparin after dialysis, then "unpacked" (3 mL blood withdrawn from catheter) before the next dialysis treatment.

SKILL 4.27 Hemodialysis: Procedures, Caring for, Assisting

Safety Note! *During scheduled clinical time, nursing students may have a learning opportunity to observe or assist with this skill only with faculty permission and with direct supervision from faculty or another RN.*

In hemodialysis, a dialysis machine filters wastes, salts, and fluid from blood when kidneys are not healthy enough to do this sufficiently.

Delegation or Assignment

Due to the complexity of the procedure, the need for assessment skills, and use of aseptic technique, this procedure is not delegated or assigned to the UAP. However, aspects of function are observed during usual care and may be recorded by individuals other than the nurse. Abnormal findings must be validated and interpreted by the nurse.

(*continued on next page*)

SKILL 4.27 Hemodialysis: Procedures, Caring for, Assisting (continued)

Equipment

- Dialyzer (types are hollow fiber or cellulose acetate)
- 1000-mL bag of 0.9% normal saline IV solution
- Machine blood lines
- Fistula needles, $^{15}/_{16}$ gauge, 2.5–5 cm (1–1.5 in.) in length
- Sterile gauze pads, alcohol swabs, and povidone-iodine or ChloraPrep swabs
- Two 3-mL syringes
- Two 20-mL syringes
- Drape
- Patient mask
- Hemostats, cannula clamps
- Tape
- Sterile gloves and clean gloves
- Gown
- Protective goggles and face mask or visor shield
- 12-mL syringe
- Heparin solution 1000 units/mL
- Hemastix
- Nonsterile gauze pads

Preparation

- Review healthcare provider's orders and patient's plan of care.
- Obtain dialysate bath composition as ordered.
- Set up 1000-mL IV of normal saline using IV tubing in blood line set.
- Load heparin pump (e.g., 8 mL of heparin) per manufacturer's instructions. **Rationale:** *Heparin is added to the system just before blood enters the dialyzer to prevent clotting. The clotting mechanism is activated when blood moves outside body and is in contact with foreign substances.*
- Check location of nearest emergency power outlet. **Rationale:** *It is important to maintain electric current if routine power fails.*
- Test dialysis machine ❶ for presence of bleach with Hemastix. **Rationale:** *This detects the presence of caustic agents that could result in patient complications.*
- Prime dialyzer and arterial and venous blood lines with saline.

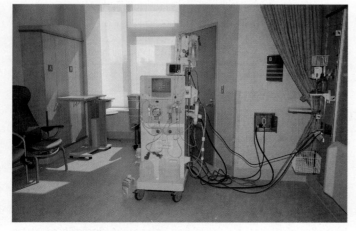

Source: Rick Brady/Pearson Education, Inc.

❶ Hemodialysis unit used to treat renal failure patients.

- Hang additional IV solution of saline. **Rationale:** *Saline infusions must be available immediately for rapid reversal of hypotension or discontinuation of dialysis.*
- Connect pressure monitor lines to both arterial and venous drip chambers. **Rationale:** *This monitors the amount of hydrostatic pressure exerted on blood in the ultrafiltration process used to extract fluid throughout dialysis treatment.*
- Set the alarm pressures, both high and low.
- Connect air leak detector to venous drip chamber.
- Test all machine alarms: venous and arterial pressure, air detector, and blood leak detector.
- Connect arterial and venous lines for recirculation with adapter, and turn blood pump to 200 mL/min.
- Document alarm checks in dialysis log.
- When a hemodialysis patient is hospitalized:
  - Place an identifying bracelet on access arm
  - Post safety precautions at head of bed (e.g., "Do not use access arm for blood pressure or venipuncture" and "Fluid restriction specified")
  - Notify dialysis specialty nurse of patient's admission to hospital

---

CAUTION! Cultural Variances Related to Renal Function

- African Americans have a more rapid decline in glomerular filtration rate than do Caucasians.
- Hypertensive African Americans have decreased renal excretion of sodium, making sodium restriction an important factor in treatment.
- Hypertension, diabetes, and end-stage renal disease (ESRD) are three to four times more common in African Americans and American Indians than in Caucasians.

Source: Data from the National Kidney Foundation website. 2016. *African Americans and Kidney Disease,* https://www.kidney.org/news/newsroom/factsheets/African-Americans-and-CKD

Procedure

FOR ARTERIOVENOUS (AV) FISTULA OR GRAFT

1. Place blood line at the same level as the bed.
2. Don mask and gown. Put on goggles, and perform hand hygiene.
3. Don clean gloves, and remove dressing, if used. Remove and discard gloves and perform hand hygiene.
4. Don sterile gloves.
5. Clean access site using ChloraPrep or alcohol swab, then povidone–iodine swab. Using a circular motion, cleanse from needle insertion site outward. Allow to dry. **Rationale:** *Cleansing occurs from cleanest to dirtiest area preventing contamination of the site.*
6. Insert needles into fistula or graft ❷. Tape securely to extremity.
7. Obtain blood for predialysis blood samples as ordered by the healthcare provider. (Usually electrolytes, hematocrit, clotting time, etc.)
8. After blood is drawn for lab work, heparin bolus should be given to the patient according to healthcare provider's order—start heparin pump at ordered rate.

SKILL 4.27 Hemodialysis: Procedures, Caring for, Assisting *(continued)*

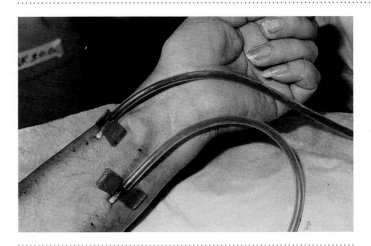

2 Arterial and venous needles placed in graft for hemodialysis.

9. Prime the extracorporeal circuit with blood.
   - Connect arterial tubing of the blood line to the patient's arterial site.
   - Connect venous tubing.
   - Unclamp venous blood line.
   - Unclamp arterial blood line.
   - Clamp saline infusion line. Remove gloves and perform hand hygiene.
10. Note time of dialysis initiation.
11. Tape all connections securely; secure blood tubing to the patient's extremity.
12. Set alarm pressures, both high and low.
13. Establish blood flow rate (usually 200–400 mL/min) and the dialysate rate of 500 mL/hr. **Rationale:** *These flow rates allow the imbalances in fluids and electrolytes to be corrected rapidly (3–4 hr per run and 2–3 times/week).*
14. Ensure that access connections are visible.
15. Check patient's blood pressure and pulse once dialysis has been initiated, then every 30 minutes unless otherwise indicated.
16. Assess patient at least every 30 minutes for vital signs and potential complications.
17. Administer any ordered medication through the venous line. **Rationale:** *Medication infuses into patient, not machine.*
18. Turn heparin infusion off during the last 30–60 min or as ordered.
19. Perform hand hygiene and leave the patient safe and comfortable.
20. Complete documentation using forms, checklists, or electronic dropdown lists supplemented by nurse's notes or additional comments as appropriate.

ONGOING CARE OF A HEMODIALYSIS PATIENT

1. Limit fluid intake to prescribed amount (e.g., 1500 mL/day).
2. Maintain individualized diet as prescribed: high-quality protein 1.1 g/kg ideal body wt/day; sodium 70 mEq/day; potassium, average 70 mEq/day.
3. Check blood pressure for hypertension/hypotension; check temperature for possible infection.

4. Auscultate heart and lung sounds for signs of fluid overload (pulmonary edema and pericarditis).
5. Provide access site care.
6. Observe mental status—indicative of fluid and electrolyte imbalance.
7. Administer Epogen, if ordered, to improve hemoglobin level (given at time of dialysis).
8. Encourage regular rest periods.
9. Weigh daily to assess fluid accumulation.
10. Use antibacterial soap and lotion to bathe. **Rationale:** *This decreases the risk of staphylococcal infections.*
11. Determine that the patient understands when and how to take medications (e.g., Tums with meals).
12. Provide continued emotional support.
    - Allow for expression of feelings about change in body image and role performance.
    - Encourage expression of fears.
    - Encourage caregiver support.
    - Give support for required change in lifestyle.
13. Instruct patient to prevent obstruction to blood flow on fistula arm.
14. Document care and patient response.

Note: Dialysis adequacy is improved with increased prescription, conversion of catheters to grafts or fistulas, and by not shortening treatments.

TERMINATING HEMODIALYSIS SESSION

1. Don gloves, gown, goggles, and protective mask.
2. Remove tape and dressing to visualize needle insertion site.
3. Place pads under connectors.
4. Open IV of normal saline to return blood on the arterial side of tubing.
5. Start blood pump at 200 mL/min.
6. Return venous blood via the return site to reinfuse the blood.
7. Clamp lines.
8. Remove needles according to unit protocol and apply pressure to sites for 5–10 min ❸ ❹ ❺.

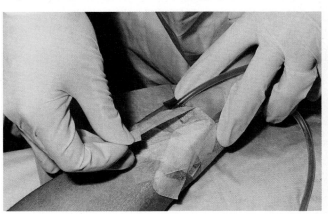

Source: Ronald May/Pearson Education, Inc.

❸ Carefully remove tape from needle sites when terminating dialysis.

(continued on next page)

SKILL 4.27 Hemodialysis: Procedures, Caring for, Assisting (*continued*)

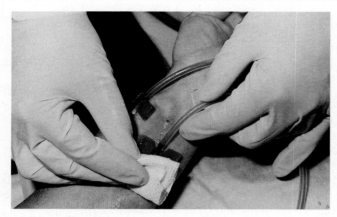

Source: Ronald May/Pearson Education, Inc.

④ Remove arterial and venous needles, using needle safety shields.

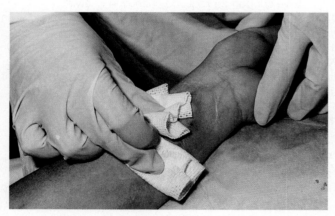

Source: Ronald May/Pearson Education, Inc.

⑤ Apply pressure over needle site for 5–10 min.

9. Apply sterile dressing to needle sites, maintaining aseptic technique. **Rationale:** *For acute renal failure patients, sepsis is the primary cause of patient death.*
10. Remove and discard protective gear. Perform hand hygiene.
11. Measure and document postdialysis vital signs and weight.

SAMPLE DOCUMENTATION

[date] 1600 Returned from hemodialysis unit. B/P 142/86, P-82, R-18, T- 37.1°C (98.8°F). AV fistula dressing dry and intact left arm. States ready to take a short nap now. *T. May*

The Hemodialysis Process

Hemodialysis works by removing blood from the patient's arterial access site (graft, fistula, or catheter). It travels through a blood pump and an arterial pressure monitor to a dialyzer (filter). In the dialyzer, the blood is separated from the dialysate by a synthetic semipermeable membrane. The dialysate (bath) runs against the blood flowing on the opposite side of the semipermeable membrane leading to osmosis, diffusion, and ultrafiltration. Fluid, electrolytes, and toxins are removed from the blood. The blood then flows from the dialyzer through a tubing system to the patient's venous access site. Fluid is removed through the use of hydrostatic pressure applied to the blood and a negative hydrostatic pressure applied to the dialysate bath. The difference between these two pressures is termed *transmembrane pressure,* and this results in the process of ultrafiltration.

Blood Flow for Dialysis

An adequate vascular access should permit blood flow to the dialyzer of 200–400 mL/min. Optimal blood access and blood flow to the dialyzer influences dialysis efficiency.

Safety Precautions for Fistula or Graft

- Feel for vibration (thrill) over access site regularly.
- Do not measure blood pressure on extremity.
- Do not perform venipuncture in extremity.
- Counsel patient not to wear constrictive clothing on extremity.
- Counsel patient to avoid lying on extremity.
- Avoid carrying heavy loads with access extremity.
- Immediately report swelling, discoloration, drainage, or coldness, numbness, or weakness of hand.

Assessing Arteriovenous (AV) Fistula

- Perform hand hygiene.
- Position patient's arm so fistula is easily accessed.
- Palpate the area to feel for thrill (vibration). This indicates arterial to venous blood flow and fistula patency.
- Auscultate with a stethoscope to detect a bruit (swishing noise). This indicates a patent fistula.
- Palpate pulses distal to fistula to check circulation.
- Observe capillary refill in extremity digits.
- Assess for numbness, tingling, coldness, pallor, or alternation in sensation in digits of fistula extremity.
- Assess for signs and symptoms of infection: redness, edema, soreness, warmth, or increased temperature.

Note: Vascular access promotes more efficient removal and replacement of blood during dialysis, resulting in fewer complications. Vascular access should be prepared weeks or months before using it for dialysis. This will stabilize the graft site and ensure adequate blood flow when used for dialysis.

⟫ Critical Thinking Options for Unexpected Outcomes

Not all unexpected outcomes require further nursing intervention; however, many times they do. When the patient demonstrates a change in signs or symptoms indicating an emerging problem, the nurse should immediately assess and troubleshoot what is happening. The assessment data must be processed quickly to formulate a hypothesis so the nurse can make a clinical judgment. The nurse then decides how best to resolve the problem and improve the patient's situation for a better outcome.

EXPECTED OUTCOME	UNEXPECTED OUTCOME	POSSIBLE INTERVENTIONS
Collecting a Specimen Patient is able to follow procedure of collection when appropriate.	Patient is embarrassed by having to give stool specimen.	▪ Place a bedpan or other collection device under the toilet seat in the bathroom to obtain specimen. ▪ If patient is confined to bed, pull sheets over patient's legs and draw curtains around the bed until procedure is completed. ▪ If odor occurs from passage of stool, place a non-aerosol air freshener in room.
Specimen collected is adequate for test.	Patient passes liquid stools.	▪ Determine if part or entire specimen is required for test. ▪ Obtain a plastic container with a cover and several large cotton swabs. ▪ Dip cotton swabs into the liquid stool. Place swabs in plastic container. ▪ After procedure, pay close attention to skin care. A protective ointment may be necessary to protect skin from liquid stools.
Bladder Interventions Patient voids 200–500 mL of urine without discomfort or difficulty.	Unable to void on bedpan	▪ Run water in sink. ▪ Massage the lower abdomen. ▪ Place a hot washcloth on the abdomen. ▪ Pour warm water over the perineum with patient positioned on toilet or bedpan. ▪ Give patient a sitz bath after obtaining an order.
	Catheter cannot be inserted into male patient.	Obtain new catheter kit and follow these actions: ▪ Hold penis vertical to patient's body; insert lidocaine gel. ▪ Insert catheter while applying slight traction by gently pulling upward on the shaft of the penis. ▪ If resistance is encountered, rotate catheter, increase traction, and lower angle of penis. ▪ Ask patient to cough. ▪ Try using a Coudé or 12 Fr catheter (some facilities require a healthcare provider's order for this type of catheter).
Skin irritation does not occur with condom catheter use.	Penis becomes reddened with condom catheter use.	▪ Remove condom. ▪ Notify the healthcare provider for topical medication prescription. ▪ Apply adult brief and change frequently until problem resolves. ▪ Make sure penis is clean and dry and protective coating is applied before condom application. ▪ Clip rolled portion of condom to prevent constriction at base of penis.
Suprapubic catheter remains intact.	Suprapubic catheter becomes dislodged.	▪ Place sterile dressing over catheter insertion site; do not attempt to replace catheter. ▪ Notify healthcare provider. ▪ Obtain new catheter to prepare for insertion by healthcare provider.

(continued on next page)

EXPECTED OUTCOME	UNEXPECTED OUTCOME	POSSIBLE INTERVENTIONS
Patient remains free of urinary tract infection.	Patient develops urinary tract infection.	■ Note signs and symptoms of UTI: cloudy malodorous urine with sediment, bladder discomfort/spasms, elevated temperature. ■ Notify healthcare provider to obtain order for urinalysis, culture and sensitivity, and antimicrobial therapy. ■ Increase fluid intake to at least 2–3 L/day (unless contraindicated). ■ Maintain continuous urine drainage per suprapubic catheter.
Pouching system does not leak.	Pouching system leaks.	■ Check area for crease or dip in skin, which allows urine to pool and leak out. ■ Fill in dip area with skin barrier to prevent pooling. ■ Apply belt to improve fit. ■ Apply another type of pouch (e.g., convex). ■ Change more frequently if leak is due to dissolving of skin barrier—or use different barrier. ■ Advise patient to avoid using soaps or wipes to clean area because they interfere with pouch adhesion.
Patient demonstrates self-care skills.	Patient is unable to manage own urinary diversion.	■ Simplify pouch procedure if possible. ■ Provide detailed instruction in more simplified manner. ■ Include caregiver in teaching to assist and support patient. ■ Refer patient to home health facility for follow-up care.
Bowel Interventions Relief is obtained from fecal impaction or constipation.	When digital stimulation is performed, patient exhibits reflex spasm that prevents stool expulsion.	■ Apply local anesthetic around rectum and anus, if ordered. ■ Wait for spasm to relax, and then proceed with stimulation.
	Patient exhibits signs and symptoms of vagal response during removal of fecal impaction.	■ Immediately discontinue procedure. ■ Place patient in supine position with legs elevated. ■ Monitor vital signs every 5–15 min until condition is stable. ■ Notify healthcare provider of findings and request medication order for antispasmodic, such as atropine. ■ Be prepared for emergency situation, even though it is not likely to occur.
Relief is obtained from fecal impaction or constipation.	Fecal impaction is not relieved.	■ Check orders for oil retention enema. ■ Check catheter size needed. ■ Obtain order for and use digital stimulation and manual extraction of feces if not contraindicated by diagnosis of cardiac or neurological involvement.
Patient experiences increased comfort and relief from abdominal distention.	Effective bowel evacuation program is not established.	■ Ask dietitian for altered diet (including more fruits and vegetables). ■ Check if contraindication exists for increasing fluids to 3000 mL daily. ■ Obtain order from the healthcare provider to administer a different stool softener and bulk former or increase dosage. ■ Have patient increase physical activity, especially exercise of the abdominal muscles if not contraindicated by condition. ■ Ensure that patient begins bowel training program one half hour after a meal.
	Patient complains of severe and sudden abdominal pain, nausea, and distention.	■ Remove tubing, and notify healthcare provider immediately of possible perforation. (This is an uncommon complication.) ■ Assess vital signs. If you suspect cardiac dysrhythmias, remove bedpan and notify healthcare provider immediately. ■ Be prepared to administer emergency drugs, such as atropine. ■ If an IV is not in place, start an IV of 5% dextrose in water (D_5W) using a large-bore needle for emergency use.

EXPECTED OUTCOME	UNEXPECTED OUTCOME	POSSIBLE INTERVENTIONS
Enema is administered without difficulty.	Patient expels solution prematurely.	■ Calm and ease patient's distress by giving reassurance as you clean the equipment. ■ Place bedpan under patient. Place patient in semi-Fowler position with knees flexed. ■ Hold the rectal tube in patient's rectum between thighs. Slow the water flow, and continue with the enema.
Patient's skin remains free of erythema, excoriation, and infection.	Stoma becomes ulcerated or cut.	■ Examine pouching system to see if opening of pouch may be cutting into stoma. ■ Recut opening to exact size of stoma.
	Peristomal skin complications occur.	■ Evaluate cause of leakage. ■ Be sure pouch is cut to correct size. ■ Measure stoma at each pouch change for 4–6 weeks. Size will change as edema subsides. ■ Measure stoma at base. ■ May need to fill any creases around stoma with skin barrier paste. ■ Apply thin layer of ostomy powder over area and seal with an alcohol-free coating. ■ May need to use secondary skin barrier like Eakin seal. ■ May need to attach belt to minimize lateral leakage. ■ Change to a product like Durahesive that swells around stoma, preventing leakage. It holds up well to liquid output. ■ Be sure pouch is emptied before it is over one third full of stool or flatus, since an overfull pouch can break seal of pouch. ■ Pouches should not be changed more than once daily.
Dialysis Dialysis proceeds without complication (excess fluids and wastes removed from blood.)	Hypotension occurs during dialysis.	■ Administer normal saline, concentrated saline bolus, or albumin into extracorporeal circuit. ■ Place patient in shock position if tolerated. ■ Consider using smaller volume dialyzer, less ultrafiltration, or intermittent normal saline doses to maintain BP in future dialysis sessions. ■ Consider possible dialyzer reaction or myocardial infarction; notify healthcare provider for further assessment/diagnostic testing.
Vascular access site remains patent.	Patient states hand feels weak; neither thrill nor bruit can be assessed in fistula or graft.	■ Notify healthcare provider of potential clotting of fistula/graft (declotting should be attempted ASAP). ■ Prepare to possibly send patient to radiology for vascular procedure. ■ Review safety precautions to prevent constriction of blood flow in access extremity.
Patient demonstrates self-care after teaching.	Patient gains 3 kg (7 lb) between dialysis sessions; blood pressure is elevated.	■ Assess patient's understanding of fluid restriction (1500 mL/day); advise of hidden fluid in certain foods (ice cream, watermelon, etc.). ■ Encourage patient to control blood sugar (if diabetic) to help relieve thirst; decrease salt intake, but avoid salt substitute (many contain potassium salts). ■ Encourage patient to weigh daily.
Home Care Patient with an ostomy utilizes appropriate appliances and supplies to maintain bowel or bladder elimination.	Patient not coping with altered body image.	■ Refer to United Ostomy Associations of America, the Crohn's and Colitis Foundation of America, American Cancer Society, or the local enterostomal therapy nurse.

REVIEW Questions

1. The nurse notes that a *MALE MODE* bladder scan was completed for a female client during the previous shift. What data in the client's medical record was used to select this scan setting?
   1. Parent of two adult children
   2. Hysterectomy 10 years ago
   3. Lithotripsy for kidney stones 3 years ago
   4. Treated for urinary tract infection 6 months ago

2. The nurse prepares to collect a specimen for a urine culture from a client with an indwelling urinary catheter. Which action should the nurse complete first?
   1. Empty the urine collection bag.
   2. Swab the resealing port with alcohol.
   3. Insert the needle at a 45-degree angle.
   4. Clamp the drainage tubing below the port.

3. A client recovering from prostate surgery is receiving continuous bladder irrigation. What action should the nurse take when the drainage becomes bright red in color?
   1. Increase the rate of the irrigation fluid.
   2. Report the finding to the healthcare provider.
   3. Raise the height of the pole with the irrigation fluid.
   4. Disconnect the irrigation and hand-flush the bladder.

4. While changing a client's urostomy pouch, the nurse notes an area of skin excoriation around the stoma. What should the nurse do when applying the new pouch?
   1. Cut the skin barrier opening larger than the area of excoriation.
   2. Apply skin-prep liquid on the skin before applying the new pouch.
   3. Cut the skin barrier opening no more than 0.3 cm (⅛ in.) larger than the stoma.
   4. Cover the excoriated areas with a gauze bandage before applying the new pouch.

5. A client with a colostomy is instructed on self-irrigation to be performed at home after discharge. When observing a return demonstration of the procedure, which client action indicates that additional teaching is required?
   1. Instills the irrigation solution over 7 minutes
   2. Holds irrigation cone firmly against the stoma
   3. Hangs irrigation container on the shower curtain rod
   4. Fills irrigation container with 1000 mL of warm tap water

6. An older client is prescribed "enemas until clear" prior to a diagnostic test. Which part of the healthcare provider's order should the nurse question before administering the edema?
   1. Use a solution of tap water.
   2. Begin the enemas after the dinner meal.
   3. Wait at least 1 hour between each enema.
   4. Provide the enemas the evening before the test.

7. The nurse arrives at the home of a client who performs continuous ambulatory peritoneal dialysis (CAPD), at the time when the fluid is draining. Which observation should cause the nurse to be concerned?
   1. Drainage bag placed on a stool
   2. Draining continued for 10 minutes
   3. Thick white material in the drainage
   4. Tubing capped after draining completed

8. A client who receives hemodialysis treatments mentions that the hand with the arteriovenous fistula occasionally feels numb and cold. Which action should the nurse take first?
   1. Notify the healthcare provider.
   2. Transport the client to radiology.
   3. Assess the fistula for a thrill and bruit.
   4. Apply a tourniquet above the fistula site.

Note: For answers and rationales for the review questions, go to Appendix A or your Pearson MyLab Nursing and eText.

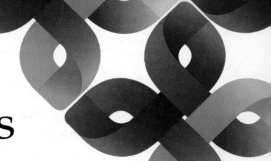

Chapter 5
Fluids and Electrolytes

Chapter at a Glance

❶ Nursing students may observe or assist with the following skills only with faculty permission and while under direct supervision of faculty or another RN.

» The Concept of Fluids and Electrolytes

Fluids and electrolytes help regulate body functions to maintain homeostasis. Fluids are found in two main compartments in the body: the extracellular compartment, which includes blood plasma, interstitial, and transcellular; and the intracellular compartment. Water is lost along with waste products when fluid leaves the body. To maintain a fluid balance, every day the body must take in water to replace the amount lost. Fluid excess and fluid deficit conditions can cause many problems that can become life threatening. Electrolytes are electrically charged ions that can conduct impulses. Extracellular fluid has a high concentration of sodium and chloride and a low concentration of potassium, calcium, magnesium, and phosphate. Intracellular fluid has a high concentration of potassium, magnesium, and phosphate, and a low concentration of sodium, chloride, and calcium. Electrolyte imbalances can result in serious, even life-threatening physical problems.

To correct a serious fluid deficiency, intravenous fluids can be ordered by the healthcare provider to give the patient enough fluids to balance the fluids lost. If there is an electrolyte imbalance also, electrolytes can be added to the intravenous fluids infusing into the patient. The nurse will initiate the intravenous infusion for fluid and electrolyte replacement, monitor the patient, and evaluate the effectiveness of this intervention.

Learning Outcomes

5.1 Show how to collect and measure fluids when monitoring a patient's intake and output.

5.2 Summarize five priority safety considerations when initiating an intravenous insertion site.

5.3 Differentiate between using an intravenous infusion pump and manually setting the flow rate to regulate infusion flow rate.

5.4 Summarize the sequence of steps in changing a central line dressing.

5.5 Explain assessment data to collect when evaluating an intravenous insertion site.

5.6 Give examples of six nursing interventions to encourage a patient to drink more fluids.

5.7 Give three examples of nursing measures that can be used with small children to discourage them from pulling at their intravenous insertion site.

5.8 Support the rationale for using sterile technique when flushing the lumens of a central line catheter.

The following feature links some, but not all, of the concepts related to assessment. They are presented in alphabetical order.

Concepts Related to
Fluids and Electrolytes

CONCEPT	RELATIONSHIP TO FLUIDS AND ELECTROLYTES	NURSING IMPLICATIONS
Cognition	Levels of electrolytes too high or too low can result in confusion and changes in cognitive processing.	■ Monitor electrolyte lab levels ■ Reorient patient to time and place as needed ■ Provide safety precautions to prevent injuries and accidents
Elimination	Fluid and electrolyte imbalances can be due to inadequate fluid intake.	■ Monitor intake and output for fluid balance ■ Monitor electrolyte lab levels ■ Encourage fluid intake as appropriate
Perfusion	Decreased fluid level in the vascular system means decreased perfusion.	■ Monitor patient's vital signs ■ Assess pulses, nail capillary refill, and color ■ Implement oxygen as ordered
Safety	Overhydration and dehydration can lead to cognitive changes that increase risk for unsafe behaviors and mobility.	■ Monitor patient's activities to prevent accidents ■ Assist patient getting out of and into bed ■ Assign someone to stay with patient as appropriate
Thermoregulation	Increased temperatures outside the body or inside the body can cause an increase in fluid loss.	■ Monitor patient's body temperature ■ Replace fluid loss by encouraging oral fluids or intravenous fluids as ordered ■ Adjust thermostat to cooler temperature

» Fluid Balance Measurement

Expected Outcomes

1. Patient's intake and output are calculated and reflect expected age-appropriate fluid amounts.
2. Intake and output measurements are accurately calculated and recorded during the shift.
3. Intake and output measurements for all shifts are totaled and documented for each 24-hour time period.

Fluid intake by parenteral or enteral tube or by oral routes is measured in milliliters and added together for the daily total intake. *Output* is a measurement of fluids that are expelled, drained, secreted, or suctioned from the body. *Sensible fluid loss,* or output that can be measured, includes urine, stool, vomitus, drainage from wounds, and nasogastric suction. *Insensible fluid loss,* or output that cannot be directly measured, includes sweat, sputum, mucus, tears, spit, and water loss through the skin by evaporation and water vapor with ventilation. Output for newborns and infants can be measured by weighing the diaper. Output for older children can be measured as for adults with a graduated cylinder and recorded in milliliters. **Table 5–1** » shows an example of the daily fluid intake and output for a healthy, average-size adult.

TABLE 5–1 Example of the Daily Fluid Intake and Output for an Average Adult

Source	Amount
Average Daily Intake (ml)	
Oral fluids	1200–1500
Water in foods	1000
Water as by-product of food metabolism	200
Total	2400–2700
Average Daily Output (ml)	
Urine	1400–1500
Lungs, skin, sweat	900–1000
Feces	100–200
Total	2400–2700

SKILL 5.1 Intake and Output: Measuring

Measurement and recording of all fluid intake and output (I&O) during a 24-hour period provide important data about the patient's fluid and electrolyte balance. Accurate measurement of I&O is documented for many adults and children, such as those receiving IV fluids or certain medications, after major surgery, and those with serious infections, renal disease or kidney damage, congestive heart failure, diabetes mellitus, dehydration or hypovolemia, or severe thermal burns.

Delegation or Assignment

Measurement and recording of normal oral fluid intake or urinary and gastrointestinal output may be delegated or assigned to the UAP. Measuring fluid intake and output from parenteral and enteral tubes and from wounds generally is not delegated or assigned to a UAP. The nurse remains responsible for the assessment, interpretation of abnormal findings, and determination of appropriate actions. Note that state laws for UAPs vary, so this task might be assigned to the UAP rather than delegated.

Equipment

- Graduated measuring container
- I&O tally sheet
- Sign to post in room indicating that the patient requires I&O recording

Preparation

- Three clinical measurements of fluid balance that the nurse can initiate independently are daily weights, vital signs, and fluid I&O.
- Assessing fluid I&O is an ongoing process that requires the nurse to have measuring devices and methods of recording easily accessible. Most agencies have a form for recording incremental I&O, usually a bedside record on which the nurse lists all items measured and the quantities per shift. These values will then be transferred onto the permanent chart record in the appropriate place (often on the vital signs record).

CAUTION! Hourly urine output of less than 0.5–1 mL/kg/hr or 24-hour urine output of less than 500 mL can indicate dehydration for an average-size healthy adult.

- Use the patient's own graduated receptacle when measuring output. Change gloves and perform hand hygiene between patients.

Procedure

1. Introduce self and verify the patient's identity using two identifiers. Explain to the patient what you are going to do, the reason for the examination, and how the patient can participate. Discuss how the findings will be used in planning further care or treatments.
2. Perform hand hygiene and observe other appropriate infection control procedures.

3. If necessary, record on the nursing care plan that the patient's I&O is to be measured, including when it should be totaled. In many cases, fluid balance is summed every shift and then totaled for the entire previous 24 hours. In extremely acute situations, the patient's I&O may be evaluated hourly so that changes in treatment can be implemented immediately.
4. *Recording intake:* Patients who wish to be involved in recording fluid intake measurements need to be taught how to compute the values and what to measure. Record each fluid item taken in, specifying the time and type of fluid. All of the following fluids need to be recorded:
   - *Oral fluids:* Includes water, milk, juice, soft drinks, coffee, tea, cream, soup, and any other beverages (**Table 5–2 》**). Include water taken with medications. To assess the amount of water taken from a water pitcher, measure what remains and subtract this amount from the volume of the full pitcher. Then refill the pitcher.
   - *Ice chips:* Record the fluid as approximately one half the volume of the ice chips consumed by the patient by chewing or letting them melt in the mouth. For example, if the ice chips fill a cup holding 200 mL and the patient consumed all of the ice chips, the volume consumed would be recorded as 100 mL.
   - *Foods that are or tend to become liquid at room temperature:* These include ice cream, sherbet, custard, and gelatin. Do not measure foods that are pureed, because purees are simply solid foods prepared in a different form.
   - *Tube feedings:* Remember to include the amount of water flush following medication administration, at the end of intermittent feedings, or during continuous feedings and the amount of water (if any) in the medication.
   - *Parenteral fluids:* The exact amount of intravenous fluid administered is to be recorded. Blood transfusions and fluids used to flush medications are included.

TABLE 5–2 Common Mealtime Fluid Portions

Container	Measurement	Container	Measurement
Coffee cup	240 mL (8 oz)	Sherbet/ice cream	120 mL (4 oz)
Commercial Styrofoam cup	240 mL (8 oz)	Popsicle	90 mL (3 oz)
Paper cup	180 mL (6 oz)	Soda	600 mL (20 oz)
Water pitcher	1000 mL (34 oz)	Soda	240 mL (8 oz)
Pint milk carton	240 mL (8 oz)	Gelatin/pudding	100 mL (3.4 oz)
Iced tea glass	300 mL (10 oz)	Nutritional supplement	240 mL (8 oz)
Soup bowl	180 mL (6 oz)	Juice	120 mL (4 oz)

*Remember: 30 mL = 1 oz

(continued on next page)

SKILL 5.1 Intake and Output: Measuring (*continued*)

- *Intravenous medications:* Intravenous medications that are prepared with solutions such as normal saline (NS) and are administered as an intermittent or continuous infusion must also be included (e.g., ceftazidime 1 g in 50 mL of sterile water). Most intravenous medications are mixed in 50–100 mL of solution.
- *Catheter or tube irrigant:* If the fluid used to irrigate urinary catheters, nasogastric (NG) tubes, and intestinal tubes or remaining after peritoneal dialysis is not aspirated after instillation, the remaining fluid volume must be measured and recorded.

5. *Recording output:* Inform patients, family members, and all caregivers that accurate measurements of the patient's fluid intake and output are required, explaining why and emphasizing the need to use a bedpan, urinal, commode, or in-toilet collection device (unless a urinary drainage system is in place). Instruct the patient not to put toilet tissue into the container with urine. Patients who wish to be involved in recording their own fluid output measurements need to be taught how to handle the fluids and to compute the values. To measure fluid output, measure the following fluids (remember to observe appropriate infection control precautions):

- *Urinary output:* Following each voiding, pour the urine into a measuring container, observe the amount, and record it and the time of voiding on the I&O form ❶. For patients with retention catheters, empty the drainage bag into a measuring container at the end of the shift (or at prescribed times if output is to be measured more often). Sometimes, urine output is measured hourly. If

the patient is incontinent of urine, estimate and record these outputs. For example, for a patient who is incontinent, the nurse might record "Incontinent × 3" or "Drawsheet soaked in 12-in. diameter." A more accurate estimate of the urine output of patients who are incontinent may be obtained by first weighing diapers or incontinent pads that are dry, and then subtracting this weight from the weight of the soiled items. Each gram of weight left after subtracting is equal to 1 mL of urine. If urine is frequently soiled with feces, the number of times the patient voided may be recorded rather than the volume of urine.

- *Vomitus and liquid feces:* The amount, appearance, and type of fluid and the time need to be specified.
- *Tube drainage, such as gastric or intestinal drainage:* The amount, appearance, and type of fluid and the time need to be specified.
- *Wound drainage and draining fistulas:* Wound drainage may be recorded by documenting the type and number of dressings or linen saturated with drainage or by measuring the exact amount of drainage collected in a vacuum drainage system (e.g., Hemovac) or gravity drainage system.

6. Document in the patient record using forms or checklists supplemented by narrative notes when appropriate. Fluid intake and output measurements are totaled at the end of the shift (every 8–12 hr), and the totals are recorded in the patient's permanent record ❷. Usually the staff on night shift totals the amounts of I&O recorded for each shift and records the 24-hour total. Check facility policy.

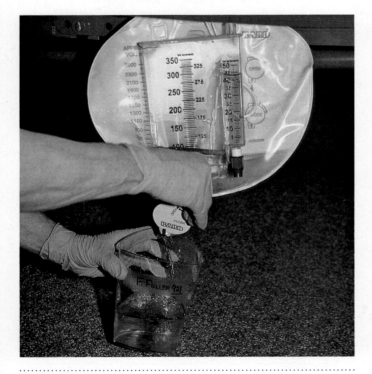

ROOM: 1243	NAME: Charlie Callaway MEDICAL RECORD NUMBER: 2872133				DATE: _____
Time	Oral Fluids	Parenteral Fluids	Urinary Output	Drainage	Other
0700	120 mL	0		0	0
0800	410 mL				
0900					
1000	90 mL				
1100			Foley		
1200	540 mL		catheter		
1300			draining		
1400					
1500	90 mL				
1600					
1700	640 mL		▼		
1800					
1900	90 mL				
Total for 12 hrs.	1,980 mL		985 mL		
2000					
2100					
2200	120 mL				
2300					
2400			Foley		
0100			catheter		
0200			draining		
0300					
0400					
0500					
0600					
0700	90 mL		▼ 780 mL		
Total for 24 hrs.	2,190 mL		1,765 mL		

❶ Empty urinal, bedpan, or Foley drainage bag into patient's individual (labeled) graduate cylinder and record amount of urine.

❷ Example of daily fluid I&O record.

SKILL 5.1 Intake and Output: Measuring (*continued*)

[date] 0830 Drank half a carton of milk, 1 cup of coffee, half a cup of water, and orange juice at breakfast for total intake 600 mL. Stated everything was good. Tolerated liquids without incident. *T. House*

CAUTION! Check all drainage receptacles such as Foley bag and NG canister at the beginning of each shift to ensure they were emptied from the previous shift and that there has not been excessive drainage.

Patient Teaching

- Consume six to eight (6-oz/180-mL) glasses of water daily unless contraindicated.
- Avoid excess amount of fluids high in salt.
- Limit caffeine and alcohol intake because they have a diuretic effect.
- Increase fluid intake before, during, and after strenuous exercise, particularly when the environmental temperature is high, and replace lost electrolytes from excessive perspiration as needed with commercial electrolyte solutions.
- Learn about and monitor side effects of medications that affect fluid balance (e.g., diuretics) and ways to handle side effects.
- Recognize possible risk factors for fluid imbalance such as prolonged or repeated vomiting, frequent watery stools, or inability to consume fluids because of illness.
- Seek prompt professional healthcare for notable signs of fluid imbalance such as sudden weight gain or loss, decreased urine volume, swollen ankles, shortness of breath, dizziness, or confusion.

Monitoring Fluid Intake and Output

- Teach and provide the rationale for monitoring fluid intake and output to the patient and family as appropriate. Include how to use a commode or collection device ("hat") in the toilet, how to empty and measure urinary catheter drainage, and how to count or weigh diapers.
- Instruct and provide the rationale for regular weight monitoring to the patient and family. Weigh at the same time of day, using the same scale and with the patient wearing the same amount of clothing.
- Educate and provide the rationale to the patient and family on when to contact a healthcare professional, such as in the case of a significant change in urine output; if weight goes up by more than 0.9–1.3 kg (2–3 lb) in a day or 2.2 kg (5 lb) in a week; if the patient loses a lot of weight or has prolonged episodes of vomiting, diarrhea, or inability to eat or drink; dry, sticky mucous membranes; extreme thirst; swollen fingers, feet, ankles, or legs; difficulty breathing, shortness of breath, or rapid heartbeat; and changes in behavior or mental status (U.S. National Library of Medicine, 2014).

Maintaining Fluid Intake

- Establish a 24-hour plan for ingesting the fluids. Generally, half of the desired total volume is given during the day, and the other half is divided between the evening and night, with most of that ingested during the evening. For example, if 2500 mL is to be ingested in 24 hours, the plan may specify 7 a.m.–3 p.m.: 1500 mL; 3 p.m.–11 a.m.: 700 mL; and 11 p.m.–7 a.m.: 300 mL.
- Set short-term outcomes that the patient can realistically meet. Examples include ingesting a glass of fluid every hour while awake, or a pitcher of water by noon.
- Explain to the patient the reason for the required intake and the specific amount needed.

- Identify fluids the patient likes and make available a variety of those items, including fruit juices, soft drinks, and milk (if allowed). Remember that beverages such as coffee and tea have a diuretic effect, so their consumption should be limited.
- Help patients select foods that tend to become liquid at room temperature (e.g., gelatin, ice cream, sherbet, custard), if these are allowed.
- Encourage patients when possible to participate in maintaining the fluid intake record. This assists them in the evaluation of the achievement of desired outcomes.
- Be aware of foods and beverages patients may prefer to eat or not according to their customs or cultures. For example, certain foods may be restricted from the diet, and other foods may be thought to have healing properties.

Helping Patients Increase Fluid Intake

- Teach family members the rationale for the importance of offering fluids regularly to patients who are unable to meet their own needs because of age, impaired mobility, cognition, or other conditions such as impaired swallowing due to a stroke.
- For patients who are confined to bed, supply appropriate cups, glasses, and straws to facilitate appropriate fluid intake and keep the fluids within easy reach.
- Make sure fluids are served at the appropriate temperature: hot fluids heated and cold fluids chilled.

Helping Patients Restrict Fluid Intake

- Explain the reason for the restricted intake and how much and what types of fluids are permitted orally.
- Help the patient decide the amount of fluid to be taken with each meal, between meals, before bedtime, and with medications.
- Identify fluids or fluid-like substances the patient likes and make sure that these are provided, unless contraindicated. A patient who is allowed only 200 mL of fluid for breakfast, for example, should receive the type of fluid the patient favors.
- Set short-term goals that make the fluid restriction more tolerable. For example, schedule a specified amount of fluid at 1- or 2-hour intervals between meals.
- Place allowed fluids in small containers such as a 120-mL (4-oz) juice glass to allow the perception of a full container.
- Periodically offer the patient ice chips as an alternative to water, because ice chips when melted are approximately half of the frozen volume.
- Provide frequent mouth care and rinses to reduce the thirst sensation.
- Instruct the patient to avoid ingesting or chewing salty or sweet foods (hard candy or gum), because these foods tend to produce thirst. Sugarless gum may be an alternative for some patients.

(*continued on next page*)

SKILL 5.1 Intake and Output: Measuring *(continued)*

Lifespan Considerations

NEWBORNS, INFANTS, AND CHILDREN

Newborns and infants are at high risk for fluid and electrolyte imbalance because:

- Their immature kidneys cannot concentrate urine.

- They have a rapid respiratory rate and proportionately larger body surface area than adults, leading to greater insensible losses through the skin and respirations.

- They cannot express thirst or actively seek fluids.

Vomiting and/or diarrhea in newborns, infants, and young children can lead quickly to electrolyte imbalance. Oral rehydration therapy (ORT) with electrolyte solutions such as Pedialyte can prevent the need for IV therapy and hospitalization.

OLDER ADULTS

Older adults are at high risk for fluid and electrolyte imbalance because of decreases in:

- Thirst sensation
- Ability of the kidneys to concentrate urine
- Intracellular fluid and total body water
- Response to body hormones that help regulate fluid and electrolytes

Other factors that may influence fluid and electrolyte balance in older adults are:

- Use of diuretics for hypertension and heart disease
- Decreased intake of food and water, especially in older adults with dementia or who are dependent on others to feed them and offer them fluids
- Impaired renal function; for example, in older adults with diabetes
- A change in mental status may be the first symptom of impairment and must be further evaluated to determine the cause

>> Intravenous Therapy

Expected Outcomes

1. The patient's fluid and electrolyte needs are met.
2. Intravenous (IV) catheter is inserted safely and without complications.
3. IV fluids infuse at the prescribed rate without complications.
4. IV catheter type/size/length is appropriate for the patient.
5. IV site remains clean without signs of infection or infiltration.
6. Central vascular line is properly placed without complication.

7. Central vascular line lumens remain patent and free of infection.
8. Central vascular catheter dressing is changed safely and without complications.
9. Blood samples are obtained safely and without complications.
10. Infusions of medications or fluids are accomplished safely and without complications.

SKILL 5.2 Central Line Dressing: Changing

Safety Note! *During scheduled clinical time, nursing students may have a learning opportunity to observe or assist with this skill only with faculty permission and with direct supervision from faculty or another RN.*

Sterile technique and supplies are used as precautions in preventing central line–associated bloodstream infections (CLABSIs) when following evidence-based guidelines for doing a central line dressing change. Changing dressings over the site are scheduled every 2 days for gauze dressings or every 7 days for a transparent semipermeable membrane (TSM) dressings, or follow facility policy. A dressing should also be changed when damp, loose, or visibly soiled (TJC, 2016).

Delegation or Assignment

Due to the need for sterile technique and technical complexity, changing a central line dressing is not delegated or assigned

to the UAP. The UAP may care for patients with central lines, and the nurse must ensure that the UAP knows what complications or adverse signs should be reported. The nurse remains responsible for the assessment, interpretation of abnormal findings, and determination of appropriate actions.

Equipment

- Central line dressing packaged kit

or

- Two face masks (one for the nurse and one for the patient)
- 2% chlorhexidine gluconate (CHG) wipes
- Clean gloves
- Sterile gloves
- Catheter securement device (according to facility policy)
- Disinfecting port protector caps (according to facility policy)
- TSM dressing (e.g., Op-Site, Tegaderm)
- Hypoallergenic 2.5-cm (1-in.) tape

SKILL 5.2 Central Line Dressing: Changing (*continued*)

- Dressing label
- Sterile drape

Preparation

- Review healthcare provider's orders and patient's plan of care.
- Review record for patient's allergies and date/time of last dressing change.
- Gather supplies.

Procedure

1. Introduce self and verify the patient's identity using two identifiers. Explain to the patient what you are going to do, why it is necessary, and how the patient can participate.
2. Perform hand hygiene and observe other appropriate infection control procedures.
3. Provide for patient privacy and assist the patient to a comfortable position, either sitting or lying. The patient should be supine if the tubing or injection cap is also being changed. **Rationale:** *An upright position during these techniques increases the chances of an air embolism forming.* Expose the central line site but provide for patient privacy.
4. Prepare the patient ❶.
   - Don a mask, and have the patient don a mask (if tolerated or as facility protocol indicates) and/or ask the patient to turn the head away from the insertion site. **Rationale:** *This helps protect the insertion site from the nurse's and patient's nasal and oral microorganisms. Turning the patient's head also makes the site more accessible.*

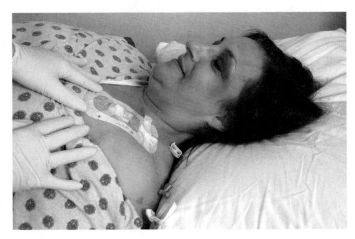

Source: Rick Brady/Pearson Education, Inc.

❶ Positioning patient flat on back for dressing change. Nurse will apply mask to patient, and have patient turn away from site. Gauze dressings are used only if the site is oozing. Gauze dressing must be changed every 48 hr or if soiled.

5. Prepare the equipment.
   - Establish a sterile field and place the sterile supplies.

6. Remove the old dressing.
   - Don clean gloves.
   - For a TSM dressing, pull both sides away from the insertion site, stretching it to lift it off the skin. For taped gauze dressings, hold the catheter with one hand and gently pull the tape in the direction of the catheter. **Rationale:** *This prevents catheter displacement and skin irritation.*
   - Inspect the skin for signs of irritation or infection. Inspect the catheter for signs of drainage. If infection is suspected, take a swab of the drainage for culture, label it, send it to the laboratory, and notify the healthcare provider. Measure the length of the external portion of the catheter extending from the skin exit site to the injection cap or infusion tubing. **Rationale:** *This measurement allows comparison with previous measurements to determine if the catheter is migrating in or out.*
7. Remove and discard gloves. Perform hand hygiene.
8. Cleanse the site.
   - Don sterile gloves.
   - Clean the catheter insertion site with CHG-based skin prep in a back-and-forth scrub motion, with plenty of friction for a minimum of 30 seconds. Let the skin air dry.
   - If possible, use one hand to lift the catheter so you can clean under it.
   - For additional protection against catheter-related bloodstream infections (CRBSIs), some facilities use CHG-impregnated sponges at the catheter exit site.
9. Apply the new dressing.
   - Apply the securement device.
   - Apply a new TSM dressing over the exposed catheter, including the hub. **Rationale:** *This type of dressing allows gas exchange but is impermeable to liquids and microorganisms. It also allows visualization of the site.*
10. Remove and discard gloves. Perform hand hygiene.
11. Label the dressing with catheter information, date and time of the dressing change, and your initials.
12. When the procedure is complete, perform hand hygiene and leave the patient safe and comfortable.
13. Complete documentation using forms, checklists, or electronic dropdown lists supplemented by nurse's notes or additional comments as appropriate.
    - Record the appearance of the catheter insertion site: presence of drainage, the type of dressing applied, patient complaints or concerns, and patency of tubing (if evaluated).

SAMPLE DOCUMENTATION

[date] 2030 Dressing changed on Broviac catheter. External portion 12.7 cm unchanged from previous. Skin without redness, drainage, or swelling. IV infusing freely. Transparent dressing applied using sterile technique. Tolerated without c/o discomfort. *J. Valenzuela*

SKILL 5.3 Central Line: Infusing Intravenous Fluids

Safety Note! *During scheduled clinical time, nursing students may have a learning opportunity to observe or assist with this skill only with faculty permission and with direct supervision from faculty or another RN.*

Fluids infuse through a central line catheter lumen. The types of fluids may include continuous infusions of specific fluids containing medications, nutritional fluids, or intermittent infusions such as IV antibiotics or other medications, flushes, or blood transfusion.

Delegation or Assignment

Due to the need for sterile technique and technical complexity, this skill is not delegated or assigned to the UAP. A UAP may care for patients with central lines, and the nurse must ensure that the UAP knows what complications or adverse signs should be reported to the nurse. The nurse remains responsible for the assessment, interpretation of abnormal findings, and determination of appropriate actions.

Equipment

- IV tubing administration set with needleless Luer-Lok connector if using needleless tubing
- Infusion pump
- Correct type of prescribed IV fluids
- Antimicrobial swabs
- 10-mL needleless syringe, if using needleless tubing, with 5 mL of preservative-free sterile 0.9% normal saline solution
- CLC2000 positive-pressure cap (or another brand) ❶
- Clean gloves and surgical mask

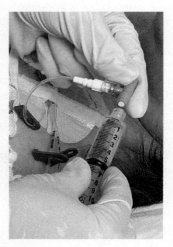

Source: Donna J. Duell

❶ Positive fluid displacement and positive end pressure prevent blood reflux into a catheter lumen. The device provides the saline flush to prevent clotting of the catheter.

Preparation

- Check healthcare provider's orders and patient's medication administration record for IV order.

- Check IV order with IV solution container.
- Take equipment to patient's room.

Procedure

1. Introduce self to patient and verify the patient's identity using two identifiers. Explain to the patient what you are going to do, why it is necessary, and how the patient can participate. Discuss how the results will be used in planning further care or treatments.
2. Perform hand hygiene and observe appropriate infection control procedures.
3. Provide for patient privacy and don gloves.
4. Hang prescribed IV solution on IV stand ❷ ❸.

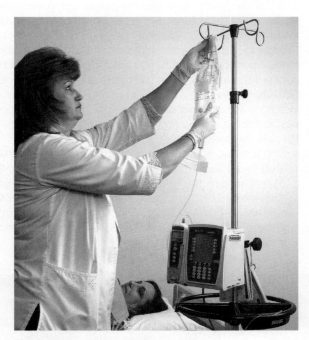

Source: Ronald May/Pearson Education, Inc.

❷ Hang IV solution on IV stand.

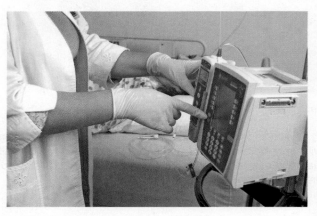

Source: Ronald May/Pearson Education, Inc.

❸ Attach point-of-care module and program.

SKILL 5.3 Central Line: Infusing Intravenous Fluids (*continued*)

5. Wipe access port with antimicrobial swab for 30 seconds and allow to air dry ④.

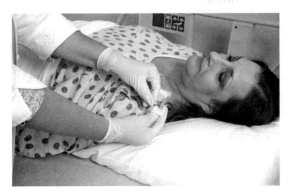

Source: Ronald May/Pearson Education, Inc.

④ Wipe access cap or positive-pressure clamp with antimicrobial swab and allow to air dry.

6. Unclamp lumen before attaching a 10-mL needleless syringe with saline flush to the lumen. (Clamp is not found on peripherally inserted central catheter [PICC] lines or Groshong valve catheter.) ⑤ ⑥.

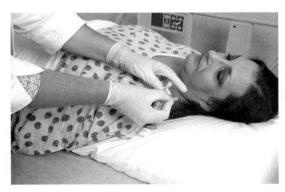

Source: Ronald May/Pearson Education, Inc.

⑤ Ensure clamp is open before attaching syringe.

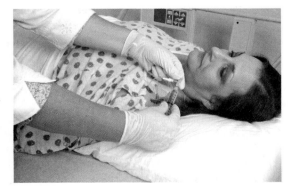

Source: Ronald May/Pearson Education, Inc.

⑥ Attach 10-mL needleless syringe with saline to pressure valve.

7. Aspirate for blood return, using very little force, to check for lumen patency and placement ⑦.

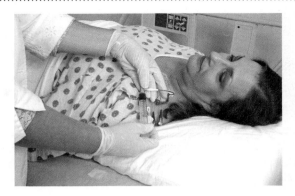

Source: Ronald May/Pearson Education, Inc.

⑦ Aspirate and check for blood return before infusing saline solution.

CAUTION! To minimize pressure on the catheter during injection, NEVER use less than a 10-mL syringe for central lines. Smaller syringes increase pressure within the catheter.

---

8. Instill saline solution using a push-pause-push motion. The central venous catheter (CVC) and tubing has a volume of 1–3 mL; therefore, about 5 mL of solution in a 10-mL syringe should be used to flush the catheter thoroughly. **Rationale:** *This clears the lumen of in-line dilute heparin.*

9. Maintain positive pressure when withdrawing syringe by clamping catheter before removing syringe or by maintaining pressure on syringe plunger before you clamp or use the CLC2000 positive-pressure cap. **Rationale:** *This prevents aspiration of blood into the lumen and decreases risk of catheter occlusion.*

10. Swab access port again with antimicrobial swabs for 30 seconds.

11. Insert IV tubing with Luer-Lok connector into access port. Unclamp lumen.

12. Set IV infusion pump to prescribed rate and begin infusing IV fluids ⑧.

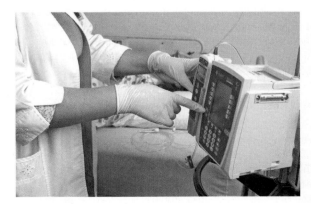

Source: Ronald May/Pearson Education, Inc.

⑧ After connecting IV tubing to catheter, turn on electric device to prescribed setting.

(*continued on next page*)

SKILL 5.3 Central Line: Infusing Intravenous Fluids (*continued*)

13. Ensure central line dressing is clean and intact.
14. When the procedure is complete, remove and discard gloves, perform hand hygiene, and leave the patient safe and comfortable.
15. Complete documentation using forms, checklists, or electronic dropdown lists supplemented by nurse's notes or additional comments as appropriate.

CAUTION! Nontunneled central vascular access devices (CVADs) have the highest infection rate of all types of CVADs; therefore, it is crucial that aseptic techniques be used in all aspects of catheter care.

SAMPLE DOCUMENTATION

[date] 0920 Labeled lumen for infusing fluids of nontunneled CVAD checked for patency. Blood flashback obtained then flushed with 5 mL NS using a 10-mL syringe in push-pause-push motion without difficulty. 1000 mL D_5 ½ NS bag of fluids connected to access needleless connector device. Unclamped IV tubing, IV infusion pump set at 100 mL/hr as ordered. CVAD site remains with dressing dry and intact. Tolerated procedure without complaint. *R. Greens*

SKILL 5.4 Central Line: Managing

Safety Note! *During scheduled clinical time, nursing students may have a learning opportunity to observe or assist with this skill only with faculty permission and with direct supervision from faculty or another RN.*

Central venous catheters (CVCs) are available with one, two, three, or four lumens. The triple-lumen catheter is commonly used because it provides multiple venous access. Each lumen has a color-coded port and specific uses. Color coding and port size may vary according to the manufacturer. The distal port is often used for the administration of blood products and for general venous access. The middle port is used for medication administration and provides a general venous access. The proximal port can be used as a general venous access to obtain blood for diagnostic tests or can be dedicated for the administration of total parenteral nutrition.

Delegation or Assignment

Due to the need for sterile technique and technical complexity, the maintaining and monitoring of central venous lines are not delegated or assigned to the UAP. The UAP may care for patients with central lines, and the nurse must ensure that the UAP knows what complications or adverse signs should be reported to the nurse.

Equipment

- Soft-tipped clamp without teeth
- Alcohol, 2% chlorhexidine gluconate (CHG) wipes
- Disinfecting port protector caps (according to facility policy)
- Transparent semi-permeable membrane (TSM) dressing
- 10-mL needleless syringe, if using needleless tubing, with 5 mL of preservative-free sterile 0.9% normal saline solution
- Heparin flush solution (e.g., 100 units heparin /mL or follow facility policy)
- Clean gloves
- Surgical masks
- Sterile gloves as needed

Preparation

- Review healthcare provider's orders and patient's plan of care.
- Review record for patient's allergies.
- Gather needed equipment and supplies.

Procedure

1. Prior to performing the procedure, introduce self and verify the patient's identity using two identifiers. Explain to the patient what you are going to do, why it is necessary, and how the patient can participate.
2. Perform hand hygiene and observe other appropriate infection control procedures.
3. Assist the patient to a comfortable position, either sitting or lying. Expose the IV site but provide for patient privacy.
4. Label each lumen of a multiple-lumen catheter.
   - Mark each lumen or port of the tubing with a description of its purpose (e.g., the distal lumen for infusing blood, the middle lumen for parenteral nutrition, and the proximal lumen for other IV solutions or for blood samples).

   or

   - Use a color code established by the facility to label the proximal, middle, and distal lumens. **Rationale:** *Labeling prevents mixing of incompatible medications or infusions and reserves each lumen for specific therapies.*
5. Monitor tubing connections.
   - Ensure that all tubing connections, such as injection ports, disinfecting port protector caps, or needleless connectors, are secured according to facility protocol.
   - Check the connections every 2 hours.
   - Tape cap ends if facility protocol indicates.
6. IV tubing change times that are commonly used are: (a) Primary continuous infusions other than lipids, blood, or blood products are changed every 96 hours (follow facility policy); (b) secondary tubing is changed every 72 hours (follow facility policy); (c) parenteral nutrition tubing is changed every 24 hours; (d) blood or blood products

SKILL 5.4 Central Line: Managing *(continued)*

tubing is changed every 4 hours. Facilities will use manufacturer's recommendations for specific medications and solution products in their policies.

7. Change the catheter site dressing according to facility policy.
   - Use strict aseptic technique (including the use of sterile gloves and mask) when caring for central lines and long-term venous access devices.
   - The frequency of dressing changes is dependent on the dressing material. TSM dressings or tape and gauze are acceptable; however, gauze dressings do not allow for visualization of the insertion site and need to be changed every 48 hours. In contrast, TSM dressings allow for visualization and can be left in place for a maximum of 7 days if they remain clean, dry, and intact ❶. All dressings should be changed when loose or soiled.

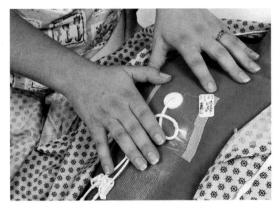

Source: Ronald May/Pearson Education, Inc.

❶ Applying a transparent dressing over insertion site.

   - Assess the site for any redness, swelling, tenderness, or drainage. Compare the length of the external portion of the catheter with its documented length to assess for possible displacement. Report and document any position changes or signs of infection.
   - Follow facility protocol for cleaning solutions and types of dressings. CHG is the preferred agent to clean the insertion site.
   - Clean the skin around the site with CHG solution, using a back-and-forth scrubbing motion for 30 seconds. Allow the site to air dry. A round dressing impregnated with CHG can also be applied to the insertion site to prevent catheter-related bloodstream infections (CRBSIs)
   - Apply a new stabilization device.
   - Apply a sterile dressing and secure it using tape.

8. Administer all infusions as ordered.
   - Use an IV pump for all fluids.
   - Maintain the fluid flow at the prescribed rate.
   - Whenever the line is interrupted for any reason, instruct the patient to perform the Valsalva maneuver. If the patient is unable to perform the Valsalva maneuver, place the patient in a supine position, and clamp the lumen of the catheter with a soft-tipped clamp. Place a strip of tape over the catheter (about 7.5 cm [3 in.] from

the end) before applying the clamp. **Rationale:** *The clamp is placed over the taped area to prevent damage to the tubing. A clamp without teeth prevents piercing.*

9. Cap lumens without continuous infusions, and flush them regularly.
   - Change the catheter cap as indicated by facility protocol. The catheter hub can be a source of infection ❷. Also available are commercial single-use Luer access valve disinfecting protection caps. This cap contains isopropyl alcohol, which cleans the needleless connector before access and also protects it from contamination between uses. The cap is twisted onto the needleless connector and left in place until the next access to the connector is needed. The nurse removes and discards the old cap, and the connector is ready for use without further wiping.

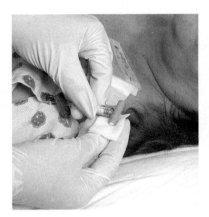

Source: Ronald May/Pearson Education, Inc.

❷ Wipe access cap with antimicrobial swab and allow to air dry.

   - The solution used and frequency of flushing are determined by facility protocol for the specific type of port being used. Heparin-induced thrombocytopenia (HIT) has been reported with the use of heparin flush solutions. If heparin is used as part of the flushing protocol, the concentration should not be in amounts that cause systemic anticoagulation but in the lowest possible concentration to maintain patency. Many facilities are switching to needleless IV connectors that can be flushed with normal saline solution only.
   - Wipe access port with antimicrobial swab for 30 seconds and allow to air dry.
   - Flush the catheter before and after each dose of medication ❸. **Rationale:** *The initial flush is to assess patency of the catheter, and the flush after administration of the medication is to ensure that the complete dose has entered the bloodstream.*
   - Use a 10-mL syringe to flush the catheter. **Rationale:** *Smaller syringes can exert too much pressure, which can damage the catheter.* Create turbulent flow with the flush by pushing, then pausing, and then pushing again, but do not use excessive force if you feel resistance. **Rationale:** *Turbulent flow may help keep the catheter free of residue,*

(continued on next page)

SKILL 5.4 Central Line: Managing (*continued*)

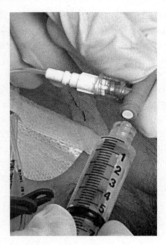

Source: Ronald May/Pearson Education, Inc.

❸ Flush a lumen regularly to prevent clotting of the catheter.

but forcing a blocked catheter can cause rupture of the catheter or push a clot free into the bloodstream.

- Blood reflux into the catheter lumen after flushing increases the risk of infection. This can be avoided by using a positive pressure flushing technique. The technique involves clamping the catheter while still instilling the last part of the flush, so that 0.5–1 mL of solution is left in the syringe, immediately after which the pressure is released on the syringe. Always follow manufacturer's recommendations for using injection caps.

CAUTION!
2016 National Patient Safety Goals (NPSGs)

GOAL 1: IDENTIFY PATIENTS CORRECTLY

Goal 01.01.01: Eliminate transfusion errors related to patient misidentification.

- Use at least two ways to identify patients. This is done to make sure the right patient gets the right medication or treatment.

Goal 01.03.01: Make sure that the correct patient gets the correct blood when receiving a blood transfusion.

- Match the blood or blood component to the order.
- Match the patient to the blood or blood component.

Source: Based on The Joint Commission (TJC). (2016). 2016 *Hospital national patient safety goals.* Retrieved from https://www.jointcommission.org/assets/1/6/2016_NPSG_HAP_ER.pdf.

---

10. Administer medications as ordered.
    - If a capped lumen used for medication has been flushed with heparin solution, flush the line with 5 mL of sterile normal saline in a push-pause-push motion according to facility protocol before giving the medication. **Rationale:** *Many medications are incompatible with heparin.*
    - After the medication is instilled through the lumen, flush with 5 mL sterile normal saline in push-pause-push

motion first, and then the heparin flush solution if indicated by facility protocol. **Rationale:** *The saline solution flushes the line of the medication. The heparin maintains the patency of the catheter by preventing blood clotting.*

11. Monitor the patient for complications.
    - Assess the patient's vital signs, skin color, mental alertness, appearance of the catheter site, and presence of adverse symptoms at least every 4 hours.
    - If an air embolism is suspected, give the patient 100% oxygen by mask, place the patient in a left Trendelenburg position, and notify the healthcare provider. **Rationale:** *Lowering the head increases intrathoracic pressure, decreasing the flow of air into the vein during inhalation. A left side-lying position helps prevent the air from moving to the pulmonary artery.*
    - If sepsis is suspected, replace a parenteral nutrition, blood, or other infusion with normal saline solution, change the IV tubing and dressing, save the remaining solution for lab analysis, record the lot number of the solution and any additives, and notify the healthcare provider immediately. When changing the dressing, take a culture of the catheter site as ordered by the healthcare provider or according to facility protocol.
    - If a lumen appears to be occluded, the cause could be thrombus, precipitate, or mechanical. An x-ray is prescribed to determine if the catheter is properly located. Fluoroscopy can demonstrate the presence of a thrombus by indicating the fluid path through the catheter. If drugs infused into the lumen might have created a precipitate, the pharmacist can assist in determining whether an acidic, alkaline, or lipid precipitate is likely and the appropriate solution to dissolve it. If the occlusion is mechanical, consult policy to determine if the nurse may reposition the catheter or if the healthcare provider must be notified.

12. When the procedure is complete, perform hand hygiene and leave the patient safe and comfortable.

13. Complete documentation using forms, checklists, or electronic dropdown lists supplemented by nurse's notes or additional comments as appropriate.
    - Record the date and time of any infusion started; type of solution, drip rate, and number of milliliters infusing per hour; dressing or tubing changes; appearance of insertion site; and all other nursing assessments.

SAMPLE DOCUMENTATION

[date] 1320 Sterile gloves and mask donned, patient given mask. Right subclavian central venous catheter (CVC) IV lumen port cleaned with CHG wipes and flushed with 5 mL saline with pulsating motion. Saline lock for catheter lumen administered. Catheter site without signs of infiltration or infection. TSM dressing remains dry and intact. Tolerated without discomfort. *C. Huffman*

SKILL 5.5 Implanted Vascular Access Devices: Managing

These central venous access devices allow frequent access to the veins without deep needlesticks. They remain in place for long periods of time (months or longer). Vascular access devices are commonly used to administer antibiotics, chemotherapy drugs, hyperalimentation, blood transfusions, or to provide multiple blood draws needed for diagnostic testing.

Delegation or Assignment

Due to the need for sterile technique and technical complexity, accessing an implanted vascular access device (IVAD) is not delegated or assigned to the UAP. The UAP may care for patients with such devices, and the nurse must ensure that the UAP knows what complications or adverse signs should be reported to the nurse. The nurse remains responsible for the assessment, interpretation of abnormal findings, and determination of appropriate actions.

Equipment

- IV solution container as ordered and IV tubing administration set

or

- Blood or blood product with transfusion set and priming saline

or

- Blood specimen tubes and syringe and needle
- Sterile gloves
- Clean gloves
- Masks
- 10-mL syringes with 5 mL of normal saline flush and 5-mL syringe of heparinized saline flush (100 units/mL of heparin) according to facility policy
- 2% lidocaine with subcutaneous syringe and needle (per facility policy)
- Chlorhexidine gluconate (CHG) swabs
- Straight or right-angled Huber needle with attached extension tubing and in-line clamp ❶
- Adhesive or hypoallergenic tape
- Dressing materials (e.g., 2 × 2 gauze, transparent semipermeable membrane [TSM] dressing)

Preparation

- Review healthcare provider's orders and patient's plan of care.
- Review patient's record for allergies.
- Gather necessary equipment and supplies.
- Attach the IV tubing to the infusion or transfusion container.
- Prime the infusion tubing with fluid.
- Prepare and label syringes of normal saline and heparinized saline. Connect the first of these to be used to the Huber needle. Saline followed by heparinized saline is used to flush the device before and after medications or periodically if not

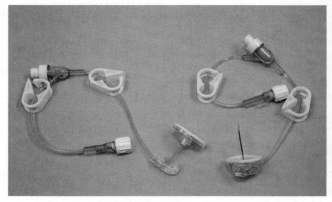

A

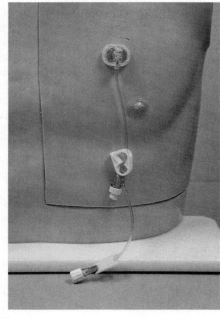

B

Sources: **A** *and* **B,** Ronald May/Pearson Education, Inc.

❶ **A,** An implantable venous access device and a right-angled Huber needle with extension set; **B,** A venous access device shown on a model.

in use (check facility policy). **Rationale:** *Heparinized saline may help prevent clotting. There is also some risk of heparin-induced thrombocytopenia, so heparin is not used without clear policy.*

Procedure

1. Prior to performing the procedure, introduce self and verify the patient's identity using two identifiers. Explain to the patient what you are going to do, why it is necessary, and how the patient can participate.
2. Provide for patient privacy and assist the patient to a comfortable position, either sitting or lying. Expose the IVAD site but provide for patient privacy.

(continued on next page)

SKILL 5.5 Implanted Vascular Access Devices: Managing (*continued*)

3. Perform hand hygiene. Apply face mask to patient and self.
4. Prepare the site.
   - Locate the IVAD device and its septum, that is, the disk at the center of the port where the needle will be inserted.
   - Prepare the skin by wiping it in a back-and-forth scrub motion using the CHG wipe (in accordance with facility policy) for 10 seconds and let the area air dry after applying solution.
   - Apply sterile gloves.
   - *Optional:* Inject 2% lidocaine subcutaneously over the needle insertion site. **Rationale:** *This anesthetizes the area for injection.* It may be ordered during the first few weeks after the implant surgery, when the area is tender and swollen and more pain from the needle puncture is felt. Other topical anesthetics may be used.
   - An ice pack may be placed over the site for several minutes to reduce discomfort from the needle puncture.
5. Insert the Huber needle.
   - Grasp the base of the IVAD device between two fingers of your nondominant hand to stabilize it. IVADs may have top entry or side entry ports, depending on the design.
   - Insert the needle at a 90-degree angle to the septum, and push it firmly through the skin and septum until it contacts the base of the IVAD chamber.
   - Avoid tilting or moving the needle when the septum is punctured. **Rationale:** *Needle movement can damage the septum and cause fluid leakage.*
   - When the needle contacts the base of the septum, aspirate for blood to determine correct placement. If no blood is obtained, remove the needle and repeat the procedure after having the patient move the arms and change position. **Rationale:** *Movement can free the catheter tip from the vessel wall, where it may be lodged.*
   - Infuse the 5 mL sterile normal saline flush using a push-and-pause motion. There should be no discomfort or sign of subcutaneous infiltration with infusion of the flush.
6. Prevent manipulation or dislodgement of the needle.
   - If the needle will remain in place for longer than needed to withdraw a blood sample or flush an unused port, secure the needle.
   - Support the Huber needle with 2 × 2 dressings and apply an occlusive transparent dressing to the needle site. Some manufacturer's devices include a safety lock to decrease accidental needlesticks and a patient comfort pad that sits between the needle hub and the skin.
   - Loop and tape the tubing. **Rationale:** *Looping prevents tension on the needle.*
7. Attach infusion tubing or an intermittent infusion access cap to the Huber needle.
   - A Huber needle can remain in place for 1 week before it needs to be changed.

- Wipe the infusion access port in a back-and-forth scrub motion using the CHG wipe (in accordance with facility policy) for 30 seconds and let the area air dry after applying solution. Infuse the 5 mL of sterile normal saline solution in a push-and-pause motion.
8. Perform a final flush with heparinized saline.
   - Clean the infusion access port again in a back-and-forth scrub motion using the CHG wipe (according to facility policy) for 30 seconds and let the area air dry. When flushing with the heparinized saline solution, maintain positive pressure, and clamp the tubing immediately before the flush is finished. **Rationale:** *These actions avoid reflux of the heparinized saline.*

OBTAINING A BLOOD SPECIMEN

To obtain a blood specimen:

- Clean the infusion access port in a back-and-forth scrub motion using the CHG wipe (according to facility policy) for 30 seconds and let the area air dry.
- Withdraw 10 mL of blood (or an amount according to facility policy) and discard it. **Rationale:** *This initial specimen may be diluted with saline and heparin from previous flushes.*
- Draw up the required amount of blood and transfer it to the appropriate containers.
- Clean the access port with CHG wipes in a back-and-forth scrub motion for 10 seconds. Flush with 5 mL of normal saline using a push-and-pause motion, according to facility policy. **Rationale:** *This thoroughly flushes the catheter of blood.*
- Clean the access port with CHG wipes in a back-and-forth motion for 10 seconds. Inject 5 mL of heparin flush solution to prevent clotting.

9. When the procedure is complete, remove and dispose of gloves, perform hand hygiene, and leave the patient safe and comfortable.
10. Complete documentation using forms, checklists, or electronic dropdown lists supplemented by nurse's notes or additional comments as appropriate.
    - Record the appearance of the IVAD site; any difficulty accessing the port and interventions used; presence of drainage; the type of dressing applied; infusions given; and patient complaints or concerns. Note any clinical signs indicating venous thrombosis (pain in the neck, arm, and/or shoulder on the side of the insertion site; neck and/or supraclavicular swelling); infection (redness and swelling at the site); and dislodgement of the needle or catheter (shortness of breath, chest pain, coolness in the chest).

SAMPLE DOCUMENTATION

[date] 0900 Implanted port right chest with skin intact and no swelling. Accessed with 20-gauge 2.5-cm (1-in.) Huber needle. Prompt blood return, flushed without difficulty. IV infusion begun. No c/o of discomfort. *G. Young*

SKILL 5.6 Infusion Device: Discontinuing

A peripheral intravenous catheter needs to be discontinued if the healthcare provider has written an order for it to be removed. Typical signs and symptoms of infiltration are erythema, inflammation, swelling, pain, or coolness noted at the catheter insertion site, a damp dressing, cessation of infusion, or absence of backflow of blood into the IV tubing when IV solution container is lowered.

Delegation or Assignment

In some states and agencies, removal of a peripheral IV catheter may be delegated or assigned to the UAP. In others, removal of IV infusions or devices is not delegated or assigned to the UAP. In any case, the nurse must ensure that the UAP knows what complications or adverse signs following removal should be reported to the nurse. In many states, a licensed practical nurse (LPN) or licensed vocational nurse (LVN) with special IV therapy training may discontinue IV infusions. Check the applicable state's nurse practice act. Note that state laws for UAPs vary, so this task might be assigned to the UAP rather than delegated.

Equipment

- Clean gloves
- Linen-saver pad
- Small sterile gauze pad and tape

Preparation

- Review healthcare provider's orders.
- Assess IV insertion site for signs and symptoms of infiltration.
- Gather needed supplies.

Procedure

1. Introduce self and verify the patient's identity using two identifiers. Explain to the patient what you are going to do, why it is necessary, and how the patient can participate. Explain the reason for discontinuing the IV and that the procedure should cause no discomfort other than that associated with removing the tape.
2. Perform hand hygiene and observe other appropriate infection control procedures.
3. Assist the patient to a comfortable position, either sitting or lying. Expose the IV site but provide for patient privacy. Place a linen-saver pad under the extremity that has the IV site.
4. Prepare the equipment.
   - Clamp the infusion tubing. **Rationale:** *Clamping the tubing prevents the fluid from flowing out of the IV catheter onto the patient or bed.*
   - Don clean gloves.
   - Remove the IV site dressing, ❶ stabilization device, and tape at the venipuncture site while holding the IV catheter firmly and applying countertraction to the skin. **Rationale:** *Movement of the IV catheter can injure the vein and cause discomfort to the patient. Countertraction prevents pulling the skin and causing discomfort.*
   - Assess the venipuncture site. **Rationale:** *Assess for signs of infection or phlebitis.*

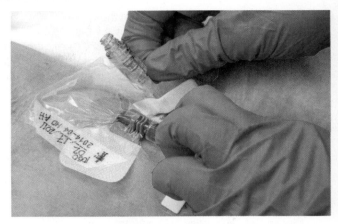

Source: Ronald May/Pearson Education, Inc.

❶ Remove the dressing and tape while holding the IV catheter firmly.

   - Apply the sterile gauze above the venipuncture site. Only touch the upper (top) portion of the gauze pad and maintain sterility of the lower (bottom) portion that is in contact with the venipuncture site.
5. Withdraw the catheter from the vein ❷.
   - Withdraw the catheter by pulling it out along the line of the vein. **Rationale:** *Pulling it out in line with the vein avoids pain and injury to the vein.* Do not press down on the sterile gauze pad while removing the catheter.
   - Immediately apply firm pressure to the site, using sterile gauze, for 2–3 min. **Rationale:** *Pressure helps stop the bleeding and prevents hematoma formation.*
   - Hold the patient's arm or leg above heart level if any bleeding persists. **Rationale:** *Raising the limb decreases blood flow to the area.*
   - Apply sterile gauze dressing. Instruct the patient to inform the nurse if the site begins to bleed at any time or the patient notes any other abnormalities in the area.

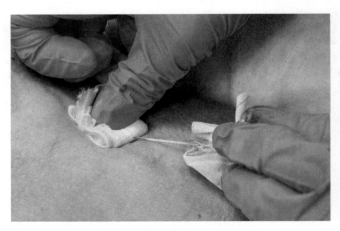

Source: Ronald May/Pearson Education, Inc.

❷ Withdraw the IV catheter from the vein. Do not apply pressure on the sterile gauze pad until the catheter is completely removed.

(continued on next page)

SKILL 5.6 Infusion Device: Discontinuing (*continued*)

6. Examine the catheter removed from the patient.
   - Check the catheter to make sure it is intact. **Rationale:** *If a piece of tubing remains in the patient's vein, it could move centrally (toward the heart or lungs).*
   - Report a broken catheter to the nurse in charge or healthcare provider immediately.
   - If the broken piece can be palpated, apply a tourniquet above the insertion site. **Rationale:** *Application of a tourniquet decreases the possibility of the piece moving until a healthcare provider is notified.*
7. Cover the venipuncture site.
   - Apply the new sterile dressing ❸. **Rationale:** *The dressing continues the pressure and covers the open area in the skin, preventing infection.*
   - Discard used supplies appropriately.

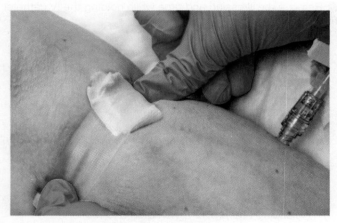

Source: Ronald May/Pearson Education, Inc.

❸ Apply new sterile dressing to the site with tape.

8. Remove and discard gloves.
9. Read the amount remaining in the IV solution container prior to discarding the IV solution.
10. When the procedure is complete, perform hand hygiene and leave the patient safe and comfortable.
11. Complete documentation using forms, checklists, or electronic dropdown lists supplemented by nurse's notes or additional comments as appropriate.
    - Record the amount of fluid infused on the I&O record and in the patient's chart, according to facility policy. Include the container number, type of solution used, time of discontinuing the infusion, and the patient's response.

SAMPLE DOCUMENTATION

[date] 2020 IV flow stopped and IV catheter removed per order of Dr. Jones. Local pressure applied to stop bleeding. IV site has no signs of infiltration or infection noted. Dressing applied when bleeding stopped. Received 750 mL of D_5 ½ NS IV fluids from IV bag. Tolerated procedure without complaint. *W. Hughes*

Lifespan Considerations
OLDER ADULTS

Older adult patients' veins may be fragile and roll easily, and the needle may easily puncture the wall of the vessel.

- Insert small-gauge, short catheter in distal vein first to preserve proximal vessel.
- Tourniquet (constricting band) may not be necessary for venipuncture. If used, it should be applied loosely.
- If used, release tourniquet as soon as venipuncture yields blood return to prevent excessive pressure in vein.
- Maintain close assessment of IV sites to promote long-term use of vessel.

Older adult patients may be prone to fluid and electrolyte disorders as a result of the normal aging process.

- Fluid replacement therapy requires close monitoring to prevent fluid overload, leading to pulmonary edema and electrolyte imbalance.
- Dehydration is a common reason for IV therapy.
- When infusing IV fluids, monitor closely for signs of fluid volume overload.
- Use an IV pump whenever infusing fluids into older adult patients. If dextrose solution is being infused, IV pumps *must* be used. Dextrose overload can lead to cerebral edema if infused too rapidly.

Stabilizing an IV catheter and dressing may be problematic due to older patients' fragile skin.

- Avoid excessive use of tape.
- Apply skin protector solution before dressing site.
- Use stretch mesh gauze to cover site and tubing to prevent catching on bed (avoid roll-type gauze).
- Observe the IV site carefully for signs of infiltration. Because of skin's loose folds and decreased tactile sensation, a large amount of fluid can sequester in subcutaneous tissue and go unnoticed before patient complains of pain.
- Check the IV site frequently when patient receives drugs that can cause irritation and even necrosis if they infiltrate.
- At first sign of phlebitis or infiltration, remove the IV and restart in a new site.

SKILL 5.7 Infusion Flow Rate Using Controller or IV Pump: Regulating

The purpose of intravenous fluid regulation is to control the amount of fluid a patient receives. Without careful control, the IV infusion could run at a rapid rate due to gravity and cause fluid or drug overload. Flow rate can be regulated manually, with a mechanical controller, or with a variety of infusion pumps to deliver IV fluids or medications accurately.

Delegation or Assignment

Due to the specific knowledge and skills in regulating infusion flow rate, this skill is not delegated or assigned to the UAP. The UAP may care for patients with IV pumps, and the nurse must ensure that the UAP knows what complications or adverse signs should be reported to the nurse. The nurse remains responsible for the assessment, interpretation of abnormal findings, and determination of appropriate actions. In many states, an LPN or LVN with special IV therapy training may manage intermittent infusion devices. Check the applicable state's nurse practice act.

Equipment

- Mechanical controller such as a Dial-A-Flo device
- IV tubing administration set
- Needleless connector (or needle connector)
- Prescribed IV fluid container, bag, or bottle
- Clean gloves
- Chlorhexidine gluconate (CHG) or alcohol swabs

For Infusion Pump Only

- Electronic infusion pump
- Infusion pump-compatible IV tubing administration set

Preparation

- Review healthcare provider's orders for type of IV fluids, medication additives, and flow rate (e.g., 1 L every 8 hr, or hourly flow rate such as 100 mL/hr).
- Check the patient's plan of care to support IV fluids therapy.
- Review the patient's record for allergies.
- Gather equipment and supplies.
- IV calorie calculation
  - 1000 mL D_5W provides 50 g of dextrose.
  - 50 g of dextrose provides 3.4 Cal/g; therefore, multiply 50 g × 3.4 Cal = 170 Cal.
  - 1000 mL D_5W provides 170 Cal.
  - Usual IV fluid maintenance is 2000–3000 mL/day (340–510 Cal/day).
- Conversion factors
  - 1 mL = 15 drops (gtts) = 60 micro drops (µgtts)
  - 1 drop (gtt) = 4 micro drops (µgtts)
  - 1 micro drop (µgtts)/min = 1 mL/hr
- IV tubing administration sets
  - Macro drip IV tubing (drop factor varies from 10, 15, and 20 gtt/mL)
    - Uses larger drops so has a quicker fluid flow infusion rate
    - Used to infuse a large volume of fluids to replace significant fluid loss
    - Used to provide a fluid challenge, or fluid bolus, for severe fluid deficit
    - May have complications from infusing too much fluid too quickly

- Micro drip IV tubing (drop factor 60 gtt/mL)
  - Uses smaller, micro drops, so effective for slow infusion
  - Used to titrate medications for better control
  - Used to deliver smaller fluid volume
  - Unable to provide high volume fluid rate
- Using a gravity controller device versus an infusion pump:
  - IV controllers use gravity to provide pressure, and infusion rates are calculated visually or mechanically by counting drops per minute. Some gravity control devices regulate the gravity flow of drops by constricting the IV tubing with roller clamps to allow a specified number of drops to be dispensed in the drip chamber every minute. Another type of manual controller has a dial that can be set to a fixed flow rate; for example, the Dial-A Flo device. Because the device cannot control the size of the drops dispensed, it is not as accurate as an IV pump.
  - Infusion, or volumetric, pumps control flow rate with a pumping action when the desired volume to be infused and time rate (mL/hr) is programmed. Volumetric pumps are used to deliver medium to large volumes of fluids. Set the volume control for approximately 50 mL less than the volume in the IV bag to prevent the tubing from being completely emptied prior to the container being changed. These pumps include several safety features; they (1) will stop if the IV line gets disconnected, (2) convert to a very slow maintenance rate or keep-vein-open (KVO) mode when the total volume to be infused has been infused, (3) have an alarm and will stop pumping when air is detected in the IV line, and (4) can switch to battery mode if main power fails.
- Factors that influence IV flow rates when using gravity for infusion follow:
  - Warm fluids drip faster than cold fluids.
  - The higher the bag is above the insertion site, the faster the infusion.
  - The larger the catheter diameter, the faster the flow rate.
  - The longer the catheter, the slower the flow rate because of resistance.
  - Manual control of IVs is not recommended because of the variables above, unless an IV pump is not available.
- If the alarm sounds when using an infusion pump, check the following:
  - Most devices have a message system that specifies the exact problem. You should be prepared to troubleshoot various components of the system.
  - *Infusion complete:* When the exact volume to be delivered is set and the volume limit has been reached, an alarm sounds and the machine goes to a KVO mode. Establish if the total volume of the container has been delivered; change the solution container if needed, and reset the volume to be infused.
  - *Occlusion:* All devices sound an alarm when they cannot maintain delivery in the face of increasing resistance. In this instance, check the insertion site for infiltration, and look for position problems, pinched tubing, closed clamp, turned stopcock, or clogged filter.
  - *Other problems:* Other messages may indicate "air in the line," "low battery," "cassette (improperly loaded)," or "free flow."

(continued on next page)

SKILL 5.7 Infusion Flow Rate Using Controller or IV Pump: Regulating (*continued*)

- *Nursing action:* Check trouble spots carefully, readjust, and restart the infusion.

Procedure

1. Introduce self and verify the patient's identity using two identifiers. Explain to the patient what you are going to do, why it is necessary, and how the patient can participate.
2. Perform hand hygiene and observe other appropriate infection control procedures.
3. Close regulating clamp on the IV set tubing before hanging IV container.
4. Spike IV solution container.

MECHANICAL CONTROLLER AND MANUAL SETTING

5. Fill drip chamber to minimum one third full. **Rationale:** *If the drip chamber is filled more than halfway, the drops may be miscounted.*
6. If the controller device is similar to a Dial-A-Flo (see ❸), connect it in-line with the primary IV tubing. If the controller device is electronic, attach it to the IV pole so that it will be below and in-line with the IV container, and then plug the machine into the electric outlet, unless battery power is used.
7. Prime the tubing by opening regulating clamp slowly and allowing tubing to fill with IV solution.
   Check manufacturer's drop-rate calibration on administration set package ❶.

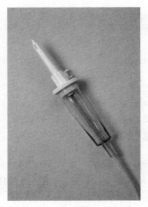 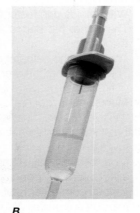

A   *B*

Source: *B,* George Draper/Pearson Education, Inc.

❶ Infusion set spikes and drip chambers: *A,* nonvented macrodrip; *B,* nonvented microdrip.

8. Use formulas to calculate flow rate.
   Flow rate
   $$\frac{\text{Total IV fluid mL}}{\text{Total hours to run}} = \text{mL/hr}$$
   Drops per minute (gtts/min)
   $$\frac{\text{mL/hr} \times \text{drop factor}}{60 \text{ min}} = \text{gtts/min}$$

9. Attach the IV drop sensor, and insert the IV tubing into the electronic controller.
   - Attach the IV drop sensor (electronic eye) to the drip chamber so that it is below the drip orifice and above the fluid level in the drip chamber ❷. **Rationale:** *This placement ensures an accurate drop count. If the sensor is placed too high, it can miss drops; if placed too low, it may mistake splashes for drops.*
   - Make sure the sensor is plugged into the controller.
   - Observe drip chamber; count the drops in 1 minute (or in 15 seconds and multiply by 4).

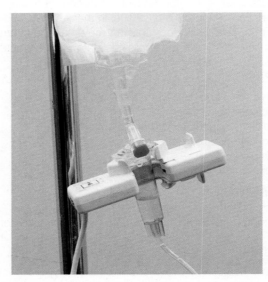

Source: George Draper/Pearson Education, Inc.

❷ The IV controller drop sensor.

10. Adjust the tubing clamp, for manually setting the flow rate, until the chamber drips the desired number of drops per minute (or 15-second increment). If using a Dial-A-Flo device ❸, dial in the rate of flow desired. If using an

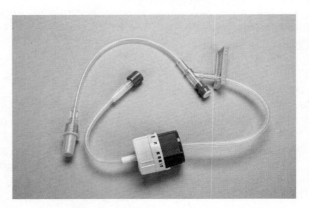

Source: Rick Brady/Pearson Education, Inc.

❸ The Dial-A-Flo mechanical gravity control device.

SKILL 5.7 Infusion Flow Rate Using Controller or IV Pump: Regulating (*continued*)

electronic controller, set volume control for the appropriate volume per hour; press the power button; close the door to the controller, and ensure that all tubing clamps are wide open. **Rationale:** *This enables the controller to regulate the fluid flow.*

- Count the drops for 15 seconds ❹, and multiply the result by 4. **Rationale:** *This verifies that the rate has been correctly set and the controller is operating accurately.* (*Note:* In some cases, the drops may fall at an uneven rate. If so, count the drops for 30–60 sec to verify that the per-minute rate is correct.)

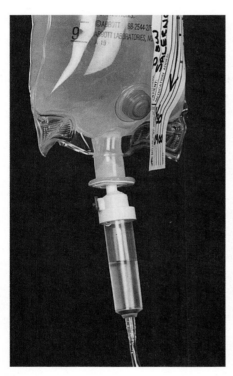

Source: Ronald May/Pearson Education, Inc.

❹ Count drops per minute to check accuracy of drip rate.

11. Monitor the flow rate frequently—adjustments to maintain desired delivery are often necessary.

CAUTION! Nurses need to check infusions at least every hour to ensure that the indicated milliliters per hour have infused and to assess the IV site. A strip of adhesive marking the exact time and/or amount to be infused should be taped to the solution container. Some agencies make premarked labels available.

---

12. An IV manual flow regulator controller, such as the Dial-A-Flo in-line device, can be used to regulate the flow of fluid instead of using the roller clamp.
13. Because this device is not an infusion pump, it is still necessary for the nurse to periodically count the drops to verify accuracy. Proceed to step 14 on page 310.

or

INFUSION PUMP ❺

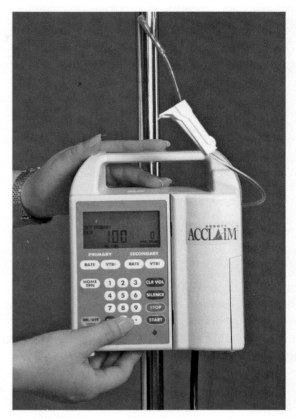

Source: Ronald May/Pearson Education, Inc.

❺ An infusion pump.

5. Fill the drip chamber to minimum one third full. **Rationale:** *This amount allows sufficient air space in drip chamber and creates a water seal to prevent air from entering tubing.*
6. Prime the tubing by opening regulating clamp slowly and allowing tubing to fill with IV solution. If using a cassette-type tubing, follow package instructions to correctly prime the cassette portion of the tubing that engages into the control device.
   Note: Check if tubing has an anti-free-flow device that must be opened prior to primary tubing.
7. Follow the manufacturer's instructions to load IV tubing into the pump, taking care to fit tubing and cassette into appropriate receptor sites. (One type of pump is a multiple-channel pump that can infuse three different IV solutions at one time.) Close device door and latch.
8. Check that the patient's venipuncture site is free from signs of vein irritation or infiltration.
9. Clean the insertion site with an antiseptic wipe and connect IV tubing to established infusion site.

(continued on next page)

SKILL 5.7 Infusion Flow Rate Using Controller or IV Pump: Regulating *(continued)*

10. Open the regulating clamp on administration set.
11. Turn the infusion pump ON.
12. Set the device parameters for operation, again following manufacturer's instructions or machine's setup prompts. Parameters may include:
    - Infusion (e.g., primary)
    - Volume to be infused
    - Rate (mL/hr)
    - Pressure (measure can vary; e.g., mmHg, cm H_2O, psi).
13. Start the device when parameters are set and observe that infusion is running properly.
14. Remove and discard gloves.
15. When the procedure is complete, perform hand hygiene and leave the patient safe and comfortable.
16. Check the patient's infusion site frequently.
17. Complete documentation using forms, checklists, or electronic dropdown lists supplemented by nurse's notes or additional comments as appropriate.

SAMPLE DOCUMENTATION

[date] 0630 Lactated Ringer's 1000 mL IV bag hung and connected to saline lock in left hand per order of Dr. Given. IV site shows no signs of infiltration or infection, dressing dry and intact. IV running at 75 mL/hr on IV pump. Tolerated without incident. *L. Maye*

Devices such as battery-operated controllers and infusion pumps with alarm systems facilitate a regulated flow. An infusion pump delivers fluids intravenously by exerting positive pressure on the tubing or on the fluid. In situations where the fluid flow is unrestricted, the pump pressure is comparable to that of gravity flow. However, if restrictions develop (increased venous resistance), the pump can maintain the flow by increasing the pressure applied to the fluid.

Newer systems are programmable and include drug libraries with dose rate calculators, automatic flushing between medications, dual or triple simultaneous line control, memory, multiple alarm settings (air in line, pressure/resistance, battery), schedule reminders, volume settings down to 0.1 mL, panel locks, and digital displays. Pumps can exert pressure on the tubing or on the fluid if restrictions develop (increased venous resistance) to maintain the fluid flow.

CAUTION! A *volume-control set,* ❻ or *Volutrol,* is used if the volume of fluid administered is to be carefully controlled. The set, which holds a maximum of 100 mL of solution, is attached below the solution container, and the drip chamber is placed below the set. Volume control sets are frequently used in pediatric settings, where the volume administered is critical.

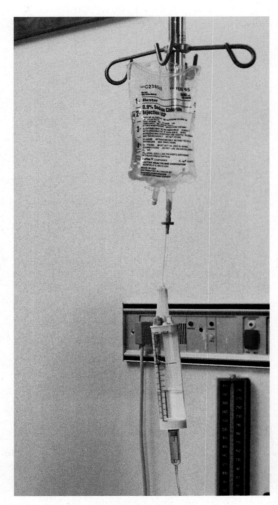

Source: Ronald May/Pearson Education, Inc.

❻ A Volutrol is used to control fluid volume.

SKILL 5.8 Infusion Intermittent Device: Maintaining

More commonly called a saline lock or heparin lock, this device maintains venous access that can be used when giving intermittent IV medications without continuous IV fluids running. The IV catheter is inserted into a peripheral vein, flushed with saline, capped off for later use, and then locked with a saline or heparin solution.

EVIDENCE-BASED PRACTICE

Saline versus Heparin Solution for Locking Catheters

Problem

Many times an IV infusion is converted to a saline or heparin lock, which means the IV catheter is flushed with saline and then capped

SKILL 5.8 Infusion Intermittent Device: Maintaining (*continued*)

off for later use to infuse fluids or administer medications. The catheter is said to be locked with saline or heparin solution so the inside of the catheter remains uncontaminated. The patency of the catheter is maintained by scheduled flushes of saline or heparin solution to keep the inside of the catheter clean and ready for use.

Flushing has been used to prevent catheter occlusion from blood, medication precipitates, or mechanical obstruction. Catheter locking is the injection of a small amount of solution following the flush. The solution, called catheter lock solution, stays in the catheter (and extension tubing set if used), when the catheter is not in use to prevent intraluminal obstruction. Using heparin as an anticoagulant and locking solution has been questioned for many years because of the high risks associated with it. Other catheter lock solutions have been tried such as urokinase, a thrombolytic agent.

Evidence

Using 10 mL of solution in a push-pause, pulsatile, or turbulent technique enhances the rinsing effect in the catheter. A flush amount of 20 mL is suggested after infusion of viscous products such as blood components, parenteral nutrition, and contrast media. The aim of a lock is to fill the catheter entirely. A survey among ICU nurses showed a 5–10 mL lock volume was being used for short-term central venous catheters. This means that if a heparin solution was used as the catheter lock solution, the heparin volume would be pushed into blood circulation with the next flush, and the patient would receive a dose of IV heparin. Research has shown such doses of heparin may lead to heparin-induced thrombocytopenia (HIT) and hypersensitivity to heparin. Adverse effects resulting from a variety of risks during the preparation of heparin solution flushes supports consideration of alternative locking solutions.

Evidence with peripheral catheters was found supporting the discontinued use of heparin locks in two meta-analyses using different concentrations of heparin. In another meta-analysis, evidence confirmed there was no significant difference in duration of patency or clotting between NS and a low-heparin solution, but there was a higher risk of clotting when locking with NS than with the higher concentration of heparin solution. Other studies report mixed results. The conclusion is the use of a low-dose heparin solution does not have an advantage over using a saline lock in peripheral catheters. Available evidence for other types of catheters is weak at this time because many of the studies lacked standardized variables, and so results are mixed.

Implications

The healthcare provider will determine whether a heparin solution or saline is used on saline locks and heparin locks and the amount of solution to use to flush the catheter. If the provider does not specify, follow facility policy for IV locks. Peripheral locks can be flushed with saline before and after each time they are used, between the administration of incompatible medications, during every shift, before and after a blood sample is taken, prn, and following recommendations of the manufacturer. To prevent complications, nurses need to use aseptic technique in preparing and administering flushes and solution when locking catheters. If using a heparin solution as a lock, monitor the patient for HIT such as symptoms of deep vein thrombosis, bleeding, stroke, myocardial infarction, pain or tenderness, discoloration, warm skin, sudden swelling, or symptoms of pulmonary embolism (shortness-of-breath, chest pain, anxiety, cough, and sweating).

Sources: Data from Wang, R., Zhang, M.G., Luo, O., He, L., Li, J.X., Tang, Y.J., ... Chen, X.Z. (2015). Heparin saline versus normal saline for flushing and locking peripheral venous catheters in decompensated liver cirrhosis patients: A randomized controlled trial. Retrieved from https://www.ncbi.nlm.nih.gov/pubmed/26252305; Molin, D. (2016). Normal saline versus heparin solution to lock totally implanted venous access devices: Results from a multicenter randomized trial. European Journal of Oncology Nursing 21, 272–273; Goossens, G. A. (2015). Flushing and locking of venous catheters: Available evidence and evidence deficit. Nursing Research and Practice. Retrieved from http://www.hindawi.com/journal

Delegation or Assignment

Due to the need for sterile technique and technical complexity, this procedure is not delegated or assigned to the UAP. The UAP may care for patients with such devices, and the nurse must ensure that the UAP knows what complications or adverse signs should be reported to the nurse.

In many states, a licensed practical nurse or licensed vocational nurse with special IV therapy training may manage intermittent infusion devices. Check the applicable state's nurse practice act.

Equipment

- Intermittent infusion cap or device ❶
- Clean gloves
- Transparent semipermeable membrane (TSM) dressing
- Sterile 2 × 2 or 4 × 4 gauze
- Sterile saline for injection (without preservative) in a prefilled syringe, a 3-mL syringe with a needleless infusion device, or heparin solution (follow healthcare provider's orders and facility policy)
- Alcohol wipes
- Tape
- Clean emesis basin

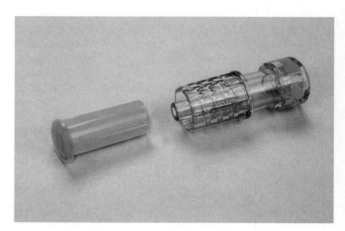

Source: Ronald May/Pearson Education, Inc.

❶ Intermittent infusion device with injection port.

Preparation

- Review healthcare provider's orders and the MAR.
- Check for the drug name, strength, and application instructions.
- Check patient allergy status.

Procedure

1. Prior to performing the procedure, introduce self and verify the patient's identity using two identifiers. Explain to the patient what you are going to do, why it is necessary, and how the patient can participate. Explain the reason for the

(*continued on next page*)

SKILL 5.8 Infusion Intermittent Device: Maintaining (*continued*)

intermittent device and that changing an IV to a saline lock should cause no discomfort other than that associated with removing tape from the IV tubing.

2. Perform hand hygiene and observe other appropriate infection control procedures.

3. Assist the patient to a comfortable position, either sitting or lying. Expose the IV site but provide for patient privacy. Don clean gloves.

4. Assess the IV site and determine the patency of the catheter. If the catheter is not fully patent or there is evidence of phlebitis or infiltration, discontinue the catheter and establish a new IV site.
   - Expose the IV catheter hub and loosen any tape that is holding the IV tubing in place or that will interfere with insertion of the intermittent infusion plug into the catheter.
   - Clamp the IV tubing to stop the flow of IV fluid.
   - Open the gauze pad and place it under the IV catheter hub. **Rationale:** *This absorbs any leakage that might occur when the tubing is disconnected.*
   - Open the alcohol wipe and intermittent infusion cap, leaving the plug in its sterile package.

5. Remove the IV tubing and insert the intermittent infusion plug into the IV catheter.
   - Stabilize the IV catheter with your nondominant hand and use the little finger to place slight pressure on the vein above the end of the catheter. Twist the IV tubing adapter to loosen it from the IV catheter and remove it, placing the end of the tubing into a clean emesis basin.
   - Pick up the intermittent infusion plug from its package and remove the protective sleeve from the male adapter, maintaining its sterility. Insert the plug into the IV catheter, twisting it to seat it firmly or engage the Luer-Lok.

6. Instill saline solution per facility policy (facility policy may state to instill a heparin solution instead of saline). **Rationale:** *Saline (or heparin solution) is used to maintain patency of the IV catheter when fluids are not infusing through the catheter.*

7. Cover the site with a TSM dressing ❷. **Rationale:** *The TSM dressing provides protection from infection, allows for ease of assessment of the venipuncture site, and also promotes comfort, preventing the plug from catching on clothing or bedding.*

8. Access the device to infuse fluids or medication.
   - Cleanse the cap with povidone-iodine or alcohol according to facility policy.
   - Use a threaded-lock needleless connector for infusions.

9. Flush the device with prescribed solution after each use or every 8–12 hr if not in use, according to facility policy ❸ ❹ ❺.

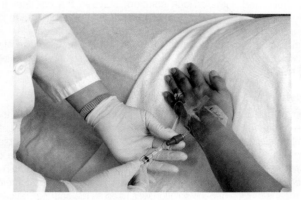

Source: Ronald May/Pearson Education, Inc.

❸ After swabbing injection port, attach syringe with normal saline (follow facility policy).

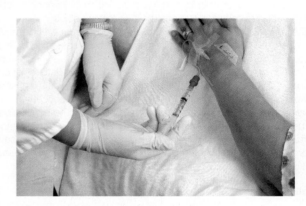

Source: Ronald May/Pearson Education, Inc.

❹ Gently flush the lock.

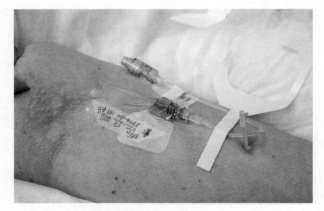

Source: Ronald May/Pearson Education, Inc.

❷ Intermittent infusion device in place.

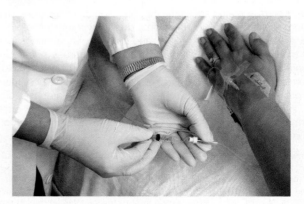

Source: Ronald May/Pearson Education, Inc.

❺ Remove the syringe and discard in sharps container.

SKILL 5.8 Infusion Intermittent Device: Maintaining (continued)

10. Remove and discard gloves. When the procedure is complete, perform hand hygiene and leave the patient safe and comfortable.
11. Instruct the patient to notify the nurse if the plug or catheter comes out; if the site becomes red, inflamed, or painful; or if any drainage or bleeding occurs at the site.
12. Complete documentation using forms, checklists, or electronic dropdown lists supplemented by nurse's notes or additional comments as appropriate. Record the date and time of converting the infusion device, the status of the IV insertion site, and any adverse responses of the patient.

SAMPLE DOCUMENTATION

[date] 1530 IV fluids stopped and converted IV catheter to saline lock per order of Dr. Clark. Received 700 mL D$_5$NS from IV bag. IV site has no signs irritation or infiltration. Needleless injection port attached to IV extension set tubing and flushed with 10 mL saline. Saline used to lock catheter without difficulty. Fresh TSM dressing applied over insertion site. Tolerated without complaint. *B. Marvin*

CAUTION! If the gauge of the catheter is small (i.e., 22 gauge or smaller), you may not get a blood return. This can be due to the collapse of the tip of the catheter as negative pressure is applied when attempting to aspirate blood. This does not always mean that the catheter is occluded. You may attempt to inject the saline gently while feeling for resistance. If any resistance is felt, it is possible that the catheter is occluded and needs to be removed and a new catheter inserted.

Patient Teaching

Teach the patient how to maintain a saline lock at home.

- Avoid manipulating the catheter or infusion plug and protect it from catching on clothing or bedding. A gauze bandage such as Kerlix or Kling may be wrapped over the plug to protect it when it is not in use.
- Cover the site with an occlusive dressing when showering; avoid immersing the site.
- Flush the catheter with saline solution as directed.
- Notify the healthcare provider if the plug or catheter comes out; or if the site becomes red, inflamed, or painful; or if any drainage or bleeding occurs at the site.

SKILL 5.9 Infusion: Initiating

Many patients require administration of fluids or medications directly through **intravenous** (into the vein) devices in healthcare facilities and in community settings. The intravenous route is the fastest way to deliver fluids and medications throughout the body. For information about blood administration, go to Chapter 12 in this book.

Delegation or Assignment

Due to the use of sterile technique, IV infusion therapy is not delegated or assigned to the UAP. The UAP may care for patients receiving IV therapy, and the nurse must ensure that the UAP knows how to perform routine tasks such as bathing and positioning without disturbing the IV. The UAP should also know what complications or adverse signs, such as leakage at the IV insertion site, should be reported to the nurse.

Equipment

- Clean gloves and mask
- IV tubing administration set
- Prescribed IV solution container (**Table 5–3 》》**)
- Labels for IV tubing and container
- IV pole
- Hypoallergenic tape
- IV infusion pump

Preparation

- Review healthcare provider's orders and patient's plan of care.

- Review patient's record for allergies.
- Make sure that the patient's clothing or gown can be removed over the IV apparatus if necessary. Many facilities provide special gowns that open over the shoulder and down the sleeve for easy removal.
- Gather needed equipment and supplies.

Procedure

PERIPHERAL LINE

1. Introduce self and verify the patient's identity using two identifiers. Explain to the patient what you are going to do, why it is necessary, and how the patient can participate. If possible, explain how long the infusion will need to remain in place.
2. Perform hand hygiene and observe other appropriate infection control procedures.
3. Apply a medication label to the IV fluids container if a medication was added ❶ ❷ ❸.
   - In many agencies, medications and labels are applied in the pharmacy; if they are not, insert the medication into the IV fluids container and apply the *Medication Added* label so it can be read easily when the container is hanging up and the type of IV fluid is still visible.
4. Apply a timing strip to the solution container if an IV pump is not available. A manual controller device or manual setting by counting drops in the drip chamber is used to set the flow rate to help maintain correct flow rate for

(continued on p. 315)

SKILL 5.9 Infusion: Initiating *(continued)*

TABLE 5–3 About Tonicity of Common IV Fluids

	IV Fluid	Description	Actions	Nursing Considerations
Hypertonic Solution	D_5LR	Dextrose 5% in Lactated Ringer's	■ Replaces fluid ■ Buffers pH ■ Provides calories	■ Irritating to veins ■ Monitor for fluid volume overload.
	$D_5 \frac{1}{2}$ NS	Dextrose 5% in 0.45% saline	■ Replaces electrolytes ■ Rehydrates	■ Irritating to veins ■ Common postoperative fluid
	D_5NS	Dextrose 5% in 0.9% saline	■ Replaces fluid, Na^+, Cl^-, calories	■ Irritating to veins ■ Monitor for fluid overload. ■ Monitor for hypernatremia. ■ Monitor for hyperchloremia.
Isotonic Solution	D_5W	■ Dextrose 5% in water	■ Raises total fluid volume ■ Rehydrates	■ Irritating to veins ■ Provides calories
	LR	■ Lactated Ringer's ■ Normal saline with electrolytes (K^+, Ca^{2+}) and buffer (lactate)	■ Replaces fluid ■ Buffers pH ■ Replaces electrolytes	■ May cause electrolyte imbalance ■ Commonly used during surgery
	NS	■ 0.9% NaCl in water	Increases plasma volume when RBCs are adequate	■ May increase fluid retention, edema ■ Helpful for Na^+ replacement but may cause hypernatremia ■ Monitor for hyperchloremia. ■ Dilutes hemoglobin ■ May worsen hypotension
Hypotonic Solution	½ NS	■ 0.45% NaCl in water	Increases total fluid volume	■ Supports renal function ■ Provides fluid replacement without extra glucose

Tonicity: ability of an extracellular fluid to alter the intercellular water amount in a cell; it influences osmosis by determining the direction that water flows.

Isotonic solution: having the same osmotic pressure within the cell as outside it, so water does not move into or out of the cell. Isotonic IV fluids do not promote osmosis, but increase extracellular fluid volume.

Hypotonic solution: having a lower concentration of NaCl outside the cell than within it (less than 0.9%), so water enters the cell. Hypotonic IV fluids promote osmosis of extracellular fluid into the cells.

Hypertonic solution: having a higher concentration of NaCl outside the cell than within it (more than 0.9%), so water leaves the cell. Hypertonic IV fluids promote osmosis of fluid out of the cells.

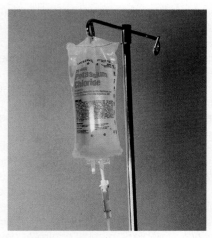

Source: Ronald May/Pearson Education, Inc.

❶ Most hospitals require a "Red Label" if potassium or other drugs are pre-added to the solution container.

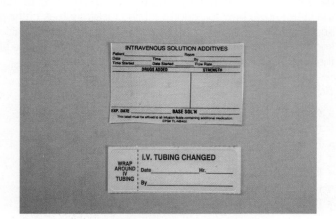

Source: Rick Brady/Pearson Education, Inc.

❷ *Top,* label indicating a medication added to an IV infusion; *Bottom,* label indicating when IV tubing changed.

SKILL 5.9 Infusion: Initiating *(continued)*

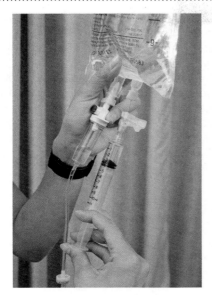

Source: Rick Brady/Pearson Education, Inc.

❸ Inserting a medication through the injection port of an infusing container.

the patient. Mark the strip to indicate the anticipated fluid level at hourly intervals, or follow facility policy.

5. Open and prepare the infusion set.
   • Remove tubing from the container and straighten it out.
   • Slide the tubing clamp along the tubing until it is just below the drip chamber to facilitate its access.
   • Close the clamp ❹.
   • Leave the ends of the tubing covered with the plastic caps until the infusion is started. **Rationale:** *This will maintain the sterility of the ends of the tubing.*
6. Spike the solution container ❺.
   • Using aseptic technique, expose the insertion site of the bag or bottle by carefully removing the protective cover so the insertion site remains sterile.

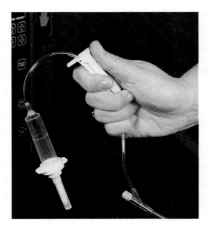

Source: Ronald May/Pearson Education, Inc.

❹ Clamp tubing before spiking IV fluid container.

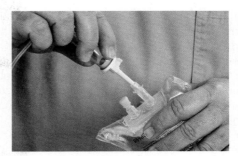

Source: Rick Brady/Pearson Education, Inc.

❺ Inserting the spike.

   • Remove the cap from the spike carefully so the spike remains sterile. Insert the spike into the insertion site of the bag or bottle without letting it touch any other part of the container.
7. Hang the solution container on the IV pole.
   • Adjust the IV pole so that the container is suspended about 1 m (3 ft) above the patient's head. **Rationale:** *This height is needed to enable gravity to overcome venous pressure and facilitate flow of the solution into the vein.*
8. Partially fill the drip chamber with solution.
   • Squeeze the chamber gently until it is half full of solution ❻. **Rationale:** *The drip chamber is partly filled with solution to form a water seal and prevent air from moving down the tubing.*
9. Prime the tubing as described below. The term *prime* means "to make ready," but in common use refers to flushing the tubing to remove air.

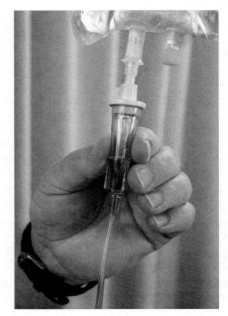

Source: Rick Brady/Pearson Education, Inc.

❻ Squeezing the drip chamber.

(continued on next page)

SKILL 5.9 Infusion: Initiating (*continued*)

• Remove the protective cap and hold the tubing over a container. Maintain the sterility of the end of the tubing and the cap.

• Release the clamp and let the fluid run through the tubing until all bubbles are removed. Tap the tubing with your fingers if necessary to help the bubbles move.

• Reclamp the tubing and replace the tubing cap, maintaining sterile technique.

• For caps with air vents, do not remove the cap when priming this tubing. **Rationale:** *The flow of solution through the tubing will cease when the cap is moist with one drop of solution.*

• If an infusion control pump or controller is being used, follow the manufacturer's directions for threading the tubing and setting the infusion rate.

10. Disconnect the used tubing or remove the cap on an intermittent device.

• Apply clean gloves.

• Place a sterile swab under the hub of the catheter. **Rationale:** *This absorbs any leakage that might occur when the tubing is disconnected.*

• Clamp the tubing. With the fourth or fifth finger of the non-dominant hand, apply pressure to the vein above the end of the catheter. **Rationale:** *This helps prevent blood from coming out of the IV catheter during the change of tubing.*

• Holding the hub of the catheter with the nondominant hand, remove the tubing or cap with the dominant hand using a twisting and pulling motion. **Rationale:** *Holding the catheter firmly but gently maintains its position in the vein.*

• Place the end of the used tubing or cap in a basin or other receptacle.

CENTRAL LINE

■ Apply clean gloves and mask. Give a mask to the patient to wear during this procedure as added protection against contamination. Position the patient with head turned away from catheter site during procedure for improved visualization and infection control.

■ Clean the junction of the catheter and tubing or cap with antiseptic, as required by facility protocol. **Rationale:** *This prevents the transfer of microorganisms from the patient's skin to the open catheter hub when it is detached; it also decreases the number of microorganisms at the catheter–tubing junction.*

■ Clamp the catheter and disconnect the tubing or cap using a twisting, pulling motion. If the catheter does not have a clamp, ask the patient to perform the Valsalva maneuver (that is, to take a deep breath and bear down). **Rationale:** *The Valsalva maneuver increases intrathoracic pressure, which reduces the risk of air entering the catheter.*

11. Connect the new tubing, and establish the infusion.

• Continue to hold the catheter and grasp the new tubing with the dominant hand.

• Remove the protective tubing cap and, maintaining sterility, insert the tubing end securely into the IV catheter hub.

• Open the clamp to start the solution flowing.

12. Ensure appropriate infusion flow.

• Remove and discard gloves and mask.

• Adjust the infusion rate of flow to the ordered flow rate.

13. Label the IV tubing.

• Label the tubing with the date and time of attachment and your initials **7**. This labeling may also be done when the container is set up. **Rationale:** *The tubing is labeled to ensure that it is changed at regular intervals (i.e., every 24–96 hr according to facility policy).*

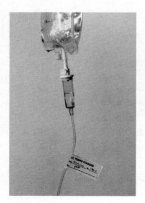

Source: Rick Brady/Pearson Education, Inc.

7 Tubing labeled with date, time, and nurse's initials.

CAUTION! The CDC has not established a recommendation for hang time (the amount of time an IV fluids container can hang before it needs to be changed, but common hang time is 24 hr). Follow facility policy and change fluids accordingly.

---

14. Loop the tubing and secure it with tape to the patient's skin. **Rationale:** *Looping and securing the tubing prevent the weight of the tubing or any movement from pulling on the IV catheter.*

15. When the procedure is complete, remove gloves. Perform hand hygiene and leave the patient safe and comfortable.

16. Complete documentation using forms, checklists, or electronic dropdown lists supplemented by nurse's notes or additional comments as appropriate. Record the infusion in the patient's chart. Some agencies provide a special form for this purpose **8**. Include the date and time of beginning the infusion; amount and type of solution used, including any additives (e.g., kind and amount of medications); container number; flow rate; and the patient's general response.

SAMPLE DOCUMENTATION

[date] 1010 D_5NS 1000 mL with 10 mEq potassium added hung using saline lock on left lower arm per order Dr. Drake. IV site flushed with 10 mL saline without difficulty and no signs of irritation or infiltration noted at site, TSM dressing remains intact. IV fluids going at 125 mL/hr via IV pump. Tolerated without complaint. *G. Vance*

SKILL 5.9 Infusion: Initiating (continued)

VENIPUNCTURE

DATE	TIME	SITE CODE	TYPE / GAUGE NEEDLE	INIT.	DC DATE	INIT.

CODES

SITE LOCATION:

RH	HAND	LH	HAND
RF	FOREARM	LF	FOREARM
RA	ANTECUBITAL	LA	ANTECUBITAL
RU	UPPER ARM	LU	UPPER ARM
RS	SUBCLAVIAN	LS	SUBCLAVIAN
RJ	JUGULAR	LJ	JUGULAR
RL	LEG	LL	LEG
VA	VASCULAR ACCESS		

SITE CONDITION:

A. PATENT WITHOUT REDNESS OR SWELLING OCCLUSIVE DRESSING INTACT
B. PATENT WITH MILD REDNESS AND/OR SWELLING OCCLUSIVE DRESSING INTACT
C. DRAINAGE (SEE NOTE)
D. DISLODGED / OCCLUDED
E. INFILTRATED
F. OCCLUSIVE DRESSING CHANGED

I.V. ORDERS

DATE ORDERED	INITIALS TRANS.	INITIALS CHECK	SOLUTION / ADDITIVE(S)	INFUSION RATE	DURATION

I.V.'s ADMINISTERED

DATE	TIME	INIT.	SITE LOC.	BOTTLE NUMBER	SOLUTION / ADDITIVE(S)	SHIFT	AMOUNT ABSORBED	AMOUNT REMAINING	TIME TUBING CHANGE	SITE COND.	TOTAL INFUSED
						0600					
						1400					
						2200					
						0600					
						1400					
						2200					
						0600					
						1400					
						2200					
						0600					
						1400					
						2200					
						0600					
						1400					
						2200					
						0600					
						1400					
						2200					

SIGN.

INIT.	SIGNATURE / TITLE	INIT.	SIGNATURE / TITLE	INIT.	SIGNATURE / TITLE

Intravenous Therapy Record

AFFIX PATIENT
I.D. LABEL HERE

MPN-105 86-6105-0

⑧ IV administration record.

SKILL 5.10 Infusion: Maintaining

Intravenous fluid therapy requires consistent monitoring and assessing for safety and effectiveness. Nurses monitor fluid status and IV management to avoid fluid imbalances due to flow rate problems (see step 7 below) and their assessment skills for early identification of infiltration complications including extravasation (see step 9 below). Nurses can instruct patients how to take care of their IV site and when to notify a nurse.

Delegation or Assignment

Due to the need for sterile technique and technical complexity, inspection of IV sites and regulation of IV rates are not delegated or assigned to the UAP. The UAP may care for patients with such devices, and the nurse must ensure that the UAP knows what complications or adverse signs should be reported to the nurse. In many states, an LPN or LVN with special IV therapy training may manage infusions. Check the applicable state's nurse practice act.

Equipment

- Clean gloves
- Saline flush
- Antiseptic swabs such as 2% chlorhexidine gluconate (CHG) with alcohol or 70% isopropyl alcohol
- Hypoallergenic tape

Preparation

- Review the healthcare provider's orders and patient's MAR.
- Review the patient's record for allergies.
- Gather equipment and supplies (anticipate you may need any of the above items listed under equipment when assessing IV fluids and saline locks on patients).

Procedure

1. Introduce self and verify the patient's identity using two identifiers. Explain to the patient what you are going to do, why it is necessary, and how the patient can participate.
2. Perform hand hygiene and observe other appropriate infection control procedures.
3. Position the patient appropriately.
   - Assist the patient to a comfortable position, either sitting or lying.
   - Expose the IV site but provide for patient privacy. Don clean gloves as appropriate.
4. Ensure that the prescribed solution is being infused.
   - Compare the label on the container (including added medications) to the healthcare provider's order. If the solution is incorrect, slow the rate of flow to a minimum to maintain the patency of the catheter. If the infusing solution is contraindicated for the patient, stop the infusion and saline-lock the catheter. **Rationale:** *Because IV tubing contains approximately 12–15 mL, it may be desirable to prevent even this much additional incorrect solution to infuse when the correct IV solution container is hung on the existing tubing. In this case, all tubing should be removed until new tubing, primed with the correct solution, can be started.*
   - Change the solution to the correct one, using new tubing if indicated.
5. Inform healthcare provider and charge nurse of the situation and complete an Incident Report Form following facility policy.
6. Complete documentation using forms, checklists, or electronic dropdown lists supplemented by nurse's notes or additional comments as appropriate.
7. Observe the rate of flow every hour.
   - Compare the rate of flow regularly, for example, every hour, against the infusion schedule. **Rationale:** *Infusions that are off schedule can be harmful to a patient.* To read the volume in an IV bag, pull the edges of the bag apart at the level of the fluid and read the volume remaining. **Rationale:** *Stretching the bag allows the fluid meniscus to fall to the proper level.*
   - Observe the position of the solution container. If it is less than 1 m (3 ft) above the IV site, readjust it to the correct height of the pole. **Rationale:** *If the container is too low, the solution may not flow into the vein because there is insufficient gravitational pressure to overcome the pressure of the blood within the vein.*
   - If too much fluid has infused in the time interval, check facility policy. The healthcare provider may need to be notified.
   - In some facilities, you will slow the infusion to less than the ordered rate so that it will be completed at the planned time. **Rationale:** *Solution administered too quickly may cause a significant increase in circulating blood volume (which is about 6 L in an adult). Hypervolemia may result in pulmonary edema and cardiac failure.* Assess the patient for manifestations of hypervolemia and its complications, including dyspnea; rapid, labored breathing; cough; crackles (rales); tachycardia; and bounding pulses.
   - In other facilities, if the order is for a specified amount of fluid per hour, the IV may be adjusted to the correct rate and the patient monitored for signs of fluid overload. In this case, make the appropriate revisions on the container time strip.
   - If the rate is too slow, check facility policy. Some facilities permit nursing personnel to adjust a rate of flow by a specified amount. Adjustments above this amount may require a healthcare provider's order. **Rationale:** *Solution that is administered too slowly can supply insufficient fluid, electrolytes, or medication for a patient's needs.*
   - If the prescribed rate of flow is 150 mL/hr or more, check the rate of flow more frequently, for example, every 15–30 min.
8. Inspect the patency of the IV tubing and catheter.
   - Observe the drip chamber. If it is less than half full, squeeze the chamber to allow the correct amount of fluid to flow in.
   - Inspect the tubing for pinches, kinks, or obstructions to flow. Arrange the tubing so that it is lightly coiled and

SKILL 5.10 Infusion: Maintaining (continued)

under no pressure. Sometimes the tubing becomes caught under the patient's body and the weight blocks the flow.

- Observe the position of the tubing. If it is dangling below the venipuncture site, coil it carefully on the surface of the bed. **Rationale:** *The solution may not flow upward into the vein against the force of gravity.*
- Determine IV catheter position. Some methods include:
  a. Aspirate the catheter for a blood return. Do this slowly and gently.
  b. Lower the solution container below the level of the infusion site and observe for a return flow of blood from the vein. **Rationale:** *A return flow of blood indicates that the IV catheter is patent and in the vein. Blood returns in this instance because venous pressure is greater than the fluid pressure in the IV tubing. Absence of blood return may indicate that the IV catheter is no longer in the vein or that the tip of the catheter is partially obstructed by a thrombus, the vein wall, or a valve in the vein. (Note:* With some catheters, no blood may appear even with patency because the soft catheter walls collapse during siphoning.)
- If there is leakage, locate the source. If the leak is at the catheter connection, tighten the tubing into the catheter. If the leak is elsewhere in the tubing, slow the infusion and replace the tubing. If leakage is substantial, estimate the amount of solution lost. If the IV insertion site is leaking, the catheter will have to be removed and IV access reestablished at a new site.

9. Inspect the insertion site for complications of IV fluid infiltration and extravasation.
   - In some situations, the IV catheter tip becomes displaced from inside the vein or the vein ruptures and causes IV fluids and medications to leak into tissue surrounding the vein. This is called infiltration, and if it occurs, stop the infusion and remove the catheter. Restart the infusion at another site.
   - Extravasation occurs when IV fluid or medication infiltrates and causes localized ischemia and necrosis of the tissue surrounding the vein where the IV catheter is located. Vesicants are medications or IV fluids, such as many chemotherapy drugs, promethazine, vancomycin, and dopamine, that can cause ischemia and necrosis.
   - For certain nonvesicant drugs, apply heat to the site; for isotonic or hypotonic fluid infiltration, choose heat or cold based on patient comfort and facility policy. **Rationale:** *Warmth promotes comfort and vasodilation, facilitating absorption of the fluid from interstitial tissues; cold restricts contact with additional tissue and limits the tissue affected by osmotic fluid shift.*
   - If the infiltration involves a vesicant IV solution or medication, the extravasation should be considered an emergency. Usually, vesicants are administered only through central venous infusions and by specially certified nurses.
   - Stop the infusion immediately.

- Disconnect the tubing from the catheter hub and attach a 3- or 5-mL syringe. Aspirate any fluid remaining in the hub and catheter.
- Photograph the site if that is facility policy.
- For a peripheral-short catheter, remove the dressing and withdraw the catheter. Use a dry gauze pad to control bleeding. Apply a new dry dressing. Do not apply excessive pressure to the area.
- For a central venous catheter, do not remove the catheter. Clamp and cap the catheter hub. Follow facility procedure for flushing when extravasation is suspected.
- Assess motion, sensation, and capillary refill distal to the injury. Measure the circumference of the extremity and compare it with the opposite extremity.
- Notify the healthcare provider and the charge nurse.
- The affected arm should be elevated and, depending on the drug, heat or cold therapy should be implemented.

CAUTION! Patients receiving hypertonic, acidic, or irritating agents, older patients with fragile veins, and pediatric patients who are active are at particular risk for IV site problems.

---

10. Inspect the insertion site for phlebitis (inflammation of a vein).
    - Inspect and palpate the site at least every 8 hours. Phlebitis can occur as a result of mechanical trauma or chemical irritation. Chemical injury to a vein can occur from IV electrolytes (especially potassium and magnesium) and medications. The clinical signs are redness, warmth, and swelling at the IV site and burning pain along the course of the vein.
    - If phlebitis is detected, discontinue the infusion, and apply warm or cold compresses to the venipuncture site. Do not use this injured vein for further infusions.
11. Inspect the IV site for bleeding.
    - Oozing or bleeding into the surrounding tissues can occur while the infusion is freely flowing but is more likely to occur after the catheter has been removed from the vein.
    - Observation of the venipuncture site is extremely important for patients who bleed readily, such as those receiving anticoagulants.
12. Instruct the patient to notify the nurse if:
    a. The solution stops dripping.
    b. The solution container is nearly empty.
    c. There is blood in the IV tubing.
    d. Discomfort or swelling is experienced at the IV site.
13. When the procedure is complete, perform hand hygiene and leave the patient safe and comfortable.
14. Complete documentation using forms, checklists, or electronic dropdown lists supplemented by nurse's notes or additional comments as appropriate.
    - Record the status of the IV insertion site and any adverse responses of the patient.

(continued on next page)

SKILL 5.10 Infusion: Maintaining (*continued*)

- Document the patient's IV fluid intake at least every 8 hours according to facility policy. Include the date and time; amount and type of solution used; container number; flow rate; and the patient's general response. In most agencies, the amount remaining in each IV container is also recorded at the end of the shift.

SAMPLE DOCUMENTATION

[date] 0512 C/o pain at IV site. Area tender to touch, small amount of swelling, no blood flashback noted. D_5NS IV fluids stopped, IV catheter removed and intact, dry sterile dressing applied to site. Heat moist washcloth in plastic bag applied to area. States it feels better from the warmth. Tolerated without incident. *G. Minor*

CAUTION! Some facilities use a single secondary tubing for all medications. The tubing is back-flushed with the primary solution prior to administering a new medication, providing the agents are compatible.

Regard IV systems as closed sterile systems and maintain as such. All entries into the tubing should be made through injection ports that are disinfected just before entry.

Patient Teaching

Teach the patient ways to help maintain the infusion system, for example:

- Avoid sudden twisting or turning movements of the arm with the catheter.
- Avoid stretching or placing tension on the tubing.
- Try to keep the tubing from dangling below the level of the IV catheter.
- Explain alarms if an electronic IV pump is used.
- Inform that the nurse will be checking the venipuncture site.

At Home

- Plant hangers, robe hooks, or over-the-door S hooks may be used to hang an IV container.
- Evaluate the patient's or caregiver's ability to operate the IV infusion pump at home.
- Emphasize the need for hand hygiene and clean technique when handling IV equipment. Set aside a clean area in the home to store the IV equipment.
- Discuss complications, such as infiltration, power failure, or equipment problems, and the measures to take when they arise.
- Make certain the patient knows how and where to obtain supplies.

SKILL 5.11 Infusion Pump and "Smart" Pump: Using

An infusion pump is a medical device that delivers fluids and medications into the vascular system in controlled amounts and rates. There are significant safety advantages over manual administration of fluids. There are many types of infusion pumps; some are stationary and others are portable. Nurses receive training on specific IV pumps utilized for patient care at the facility for which they work.

A smart infusion pump has additional software which can have a library of medications to be created with dosing guidelines, concentrations, and dose limits and thus can be used as a clinical resource. This pump can function as a normal infusion pump but then has additional computerized features including a dose log recording for record keeping, wireless connectivity to log all activity in real time, and the dose error reduction system to cross-check dosage orders against the drug being delivered. A soft alarm, for example, alerts you to a pump setting that doesn't match the facility's drug guidelines.

Delegation or Assignment

Due to the need for sterile technique and technical complexity, use of infusion devices is not delegated or assigned to the UAP. The UAP may care for patients with such devices, and the nurse must ensure that the UAP knows how to perform routine tasks such as positioning and changing gowns when a device is in place. The UAP should also know what complications or adverse signs, such as alarms, should be reported to the nurse.

Equipment

- Infusion pump or "smart" pump
- IV solution or medication as ordered
- IV pole
- IV tubing administration set
- Alcohol swabs and hypoallergenic tape
- Label for tubing
- Saline flush

Preparation

- Review healthcare provider's orders and patient's MAR.
- Review the use of the IV pump outside of the patient's room and be familiar with how to program it.
- Ensure that the tubing is the correct type for the device. Each manufacturer and model may require different tubing.
- Gather all equipment and supplies.

Procedure

1. Introduce self and verify the patient's identity using two identifiers. **Rationale:** *This ensures that the correct patient receives the infusion.* Explain to the patient what you are going to do, why it is necessary, and how the patient can participate. Explain what the IV pump sounds like during normal use, the various alarms, and to notify the nurse if an alarm sounds.

SKILL 5.11 Infusion Pump and "Smart" Pump: Using *(continued)*

2. Perform hand hygiene and observe other appropriate infection control procedures.
3. Provide for patient privacy as you prepare the patient.
   - Check the patient's identification band against the IV fluid container.
   - Assist the patient to a comfortable position, either sitting or lying. Expose the limb as needed but provide for patient privacy. Make sure that the clothing or gown can be removed over the IV apparatus if necessary. Some facilities provide special gowns that open over the shoulder and down the sleeve for easy removal.
4. Adjust the pump to be at eye level on the IV pole. **Rationale:** *Because the pump does not depend on gravity pressure, it can be placed at any level. Eye level is convenient for checking its functioning.*
   - Plug the machine into an electric outlet, unless battery power is used.
5. Set up the infusion.
   - Check the manufacturer's directions before using an IV filter or before infusing blood. **Rationale:** *Infusion pump pressures may damage filters or cause rate inaccuracies.*
   - Open the IV container, maintaining the sterility of the port, and spike the container with the administration set.
   - Place the IV container on the IV pole above the pump.
   - Fill the drip chamber.
   - Prime the tubing, and close the clamp. Some pumps have a cassette that must also be primed. Manufacturers give instructions for doing this. Often, the cassette must be tilted to be filled with fluid. Some pumps must have the power on and the tubing and cassette in place in order to perform priming.

Infusion Pump

6. Insert the IV tubing into the pump.
   - Press the power button to the "on" position.
   - Load the machine according to the manufacturer's instructions.
7. Initiate the infusion.
   - Perform venipuncture or verify saline lock is patent and without signs of infiltration with saline flush. Connect the tubing to the IV catheter.
8. Set the controls for the required drops per minute or milliliters per hour.
   - Press the start button.
   - Check the drip chamber to ensure that fluid is flowing from the container.
   Set the alarms. **Rationale:** *The alarms notify the nurse when a set volume of fluid has been infused or indicate malfunctioning of the equipment.* Proceed to step 10 below.

or

"Smart" Infusion Pump

6. Insert the IV tubing into the pump module and close the door to the pump ❶–❹. View-screen will ask which patient care area is being used. **Rationale:** *The pump automatically configures itself to provide the infusion parameters for that area.*

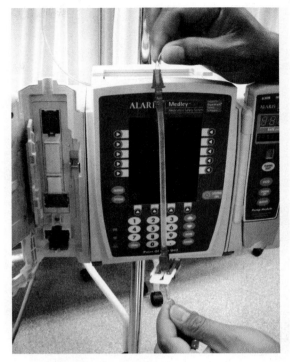

Source: Ronald May/Pearson Education, Inc.

❶ Hang IV bag on pole. Prime tubing and insert into pump module cassette.

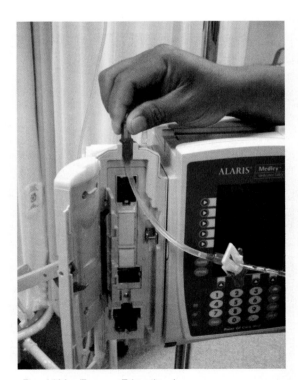

Source: Ronald May/Pearson Education, Inc.

❷ Place top of IV tubing into top of cassette; listen for click indicating it is seated.

(continued on next page)

SKILL 5.11 Infusion Pump and "Smart" Pump: Using (*continued*)

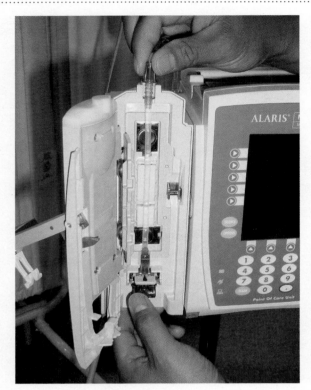

Source: Ronald May/Pearson Education, Inc.

❸ Insert white slide clamp into cassette; listen for click.

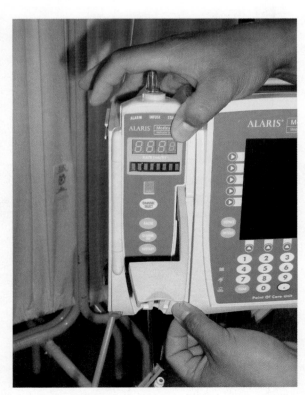

Source: Ronald May/Pearson Education, Inc.

❹ Close pump module door and lower locking lever.

7. Choose the intended drug and concentration from the list outlined on the screen ❺ ❻. Enter the ordered dose and infusion rate; the pump checks this information against the drug library. If what was programmed matches the pump's drug library, the pump allows the infusion to begin. Follow manufacturer's directions on how to program the pump. Each manufacturer's equipment is somewhat different.

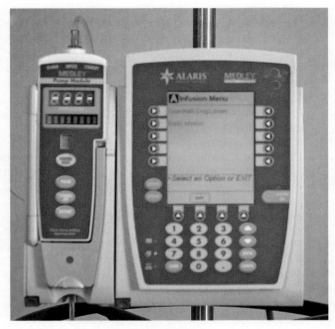

Source: Ronald May/Pearson Education, Inc.

❺ Select medication to be infused.

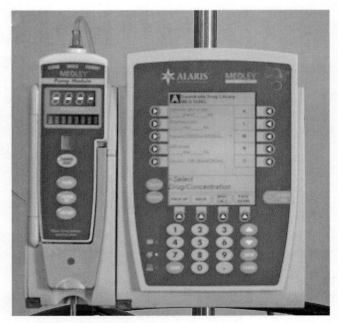

Source: Ronald May/Pearson Education, Inc.

❻ Check screen for drug name and infusion rate.

SKILL 5.11 Infusion Pump and "Smart" Pump: Using (continued)

8. If an audible and visual alert occurs, the programmed data are outside the specified limits. The alert informs you about which parameter is out of the recommended range. Depending on the medication or patient care area, the pump will sound a "soft" alarm or a "hard" alarm. Some facilities allow a soft alarm to be overridden. If you override the alarm, the infusion will begin. This alarm is considered a minor error ❼.

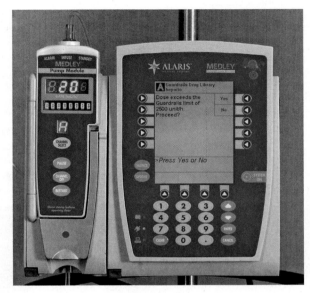

Source: Ronald May/Pearson Education, Inc.

❼ Check screen when "soft alert" sounds to determine problem.

CAUTION! Check the facility's policies and procedures to determine whether the pump can be run with the override or whether a verbal verification of the order with a healthcare provider or pharmacist must be obtained before proceeding.

9. When a hard alarm occurs, the pump shuts down. It cannot be overridden. Reprogram the pump with settings that are within your facility's specified limits to begin infusing when a hard alarm sounds.
   - The smart pump's software logs and tracks all alerts, recording the time, date, drug, concentration, and infusion rate, as well as any action taken, whether the pump is overridden or not.
10. Observe the screen to ensure medication is infusing at prescribed rate.
11. When the procedure is complete, perform hand hygiene and leave patient safe and comfortable.
12. Complete documentation using forms, checklists, or electronic dropdown lists supplemented by nurse's notes or additional comments as appropriate.
13. Monitor the infusion.
    - At least every hour, check the volume of fluid infused.
    - If the alarm sounds, begin at the patient level and check these points:
      a. IV site asymptomatic for infiltration or phlebitis.
      b. The tubing is not pinched, kinked, or disconnected.

c. The appropriate tubing clamps are fully open.
d. The sensors are correctly placed.
e. The rate/volume settings are accurate.
f. The drip chamber is correctly filled.
g. The container still has solution.
h. The time tape is accurate.
i. The IV container is correctly placed.

14. When the procedure is complete, perform hand hygiene and leave the patient safe and comfortable.
15. Complete documentation using forms, checklists, or electronic dropdown lists supplemented by nurse's notes or additional comments as appropriate. Record the date and time of starting the infusion, the type and amount of fluid being infused, the rate at which it is being infused, the infusion device used, the status of the IV insertion site, and any adverse responses of the patient.

SAMPLE DOCUMENTATION

[date] 1114 LR 1000 mL IV bag hung via IV pump to run at 125 mL/hr. Connected to saline lock IV site, right hand after patency checked—blood flashback occurred and saline 10 mL flushed without difficulty. Instructed to call nurse if alarm goes off. IV infusing at this time without incident. States she is ready to eat lunch now; procedure tolerated without complaint. *O. Chang*

CAUTION! Observe IV site frequently when pumps are used. IV pumps do not normally detect infiltration at the IV site. Infiltration does not produce enough pressure to trigger an alarm. Monitor for edema, cool skin, discomfort, and tenderness at the IV site.

Using a Bar-Code Medication Administration System

- If a facility uses a bar-code medication administration (BCMA) system, a computerized prescriber order entry (CPOE) system, automatic medication dispensing, and electronic medication records, smart pumps can provide a very high level of patient safety. The system will tell you which IV medications were ordered via a CPOE for your patient and when the medication is due.

- When the nurse enters the patient's room with the scanning device, she/he scans the bar-code labels on the medication, the patient's ID band, and the nurse's ID badge. The information from the bar-code label attached to the medication IV bag will be transmitted wirelessly to and programmed into the infusion pump. Two patient identifiers are still needed for safety.

- The pump will begin infusing only when scanning of all pieces of information is completed.

- The pump automatically communicates with a computer in the pharmacy, providing the status of the infusion.

(continued on next page)

SKILL 5.11 Infusion Pump and "Smart" Pump: Using (*continued*)

Lifespan Considerations

NEWBORNS, INFANTS, AND CHILDREN

- Emphasize to children that the IV controller or pump is not a toy and should not be touched. Children are naturally curious and will want to examine the equipment.
- Use a volume control infusion set (Volutrol, Buretrol, or Soluset) with a pump/controller for pediatric patients.
- Explain the procedure to young patients, encourage questions, and be alert for nonverbal cues. Children may not understand things that seem obvious to adults. For example, a child may think the IV therapy is a punishment.

OLDER ADULTS

- Check the IV flow rate frequently for older adults. Older adults are at increased risk to develop fluid overload if IV fluid is infused too rapidly.
- Check the IV site often for signs of infiltration. Veins become more fragile with aging.

SKILL 5.12 Infusion Syringe Pump: Using

Syringe pumps can provide continuous or intermittent low volume medications or fluids using a syringe. They usually have a maximum infusion rate, an alarm system, a keep-vein-open (KVO) rate, and a volume limit. Some of the syringe pumps have a lockout feature to limit access. A mini-infuser pump, which runs on batteries, provides controlled intermittent delivery of intravenous medication.

Delegation or Assignment

Due to the need for sterile technique and technical complexity, use of infusion devices is not delegated or assigned to the UAP. The UAP may care for patients with such devices, and the nurse must ensure that the UAP knows how to perform routine tasks such as positioning and changing gowns when a device is in place. The UAP should also know what complications or adverse signs, such as alarms, should be reported to the nurse.

Equipment

- Battery-operated or electronic syringe infusion pump
- Pharmacy-prepared and -labeled syringe with prescribed medication
- Microbore tubing with needleless access device
- Chlorhexidine gluconate (CHG) antiseptic wipes

Preparation

- Review healthcare provider's orders and the MAR.
- Check for the drug name, strength, and application instructions.
- Check patient allergy status.

Procedure

1. Check syringe label with healthcare provider's order for drug, dosage, and amount of drug to be delivered over specified time.
2. Ensure that medication is compatible with primary infusing solution.
3. Calculate amount of medication to be delivered per minute.
4. Attach microbore tubing to syringe, and holding syringe upright, expel air from medication syringe before priming tubing.

5. Holding syringe downward, carefully prime microbore tubing with medication (about 0.5 mL).
6. Insert syringe into cradle of pump, squeezing clamp around designated parts of syringe; attach pusher to plunger ❶.

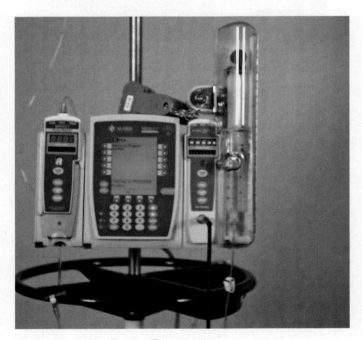

Source: Ronald May/Pearson Education, Inc.

❶ Smart pumps have syringe modules available for attachment to point-of-care computers. To attach such a module, follow manufacturer's directions.

7. Verify that IV site is free from infiltration and is patent.
8. Swab primary IV tubing port closest to patient.
9. Insert microbore cannula into port.
10. Set rate for drug delivery according to pharmacy specifications on syringe label, or as prescribed. Drug will be infused *independent* of the primary infusion rate.
11. Start syringe pump.
12. Check infusion indicator to verify pump is infusing.
13. Monitor for complications frequently.

SKILL 5.12 Infusion Syringe Pump: Using (*continued*)

14. For subsequent doses, the pharmacy dispenses a new syringe but microbore tubing may be reused for 72–96 hr (according to facility policy). A sterile cap is used each time a patient's primary tubing is accessed.
    Note: For other brands of syringe pumps, follow directions for setup and delivery of meds from manufacturer.
15. When the procedure is complete, perform hand hygiene and leave patient safe and comfortable.
16. Complete documentation using forms, checklists, or electronic dropdown lists supplemented by nurse's notes or additional comments as appropriate.

> **SAMPLE DOCUMENTATION**
>
> [date] 0800 Ampicillin 250 mg in 5 mL NS infused over 5 minutes with syringe infuser pump. IV site located left antecubital shows no signs infiltration or infection, dressing dry and intact. Tolerated with no immediate allergic reaction noted post 10 minutes. *W. Gnomes*

SKILL 5.13 Percutaneous Central Vascular Catheterization: Assisting

Safety Note! *During scheduled clinical time, nursing students may have a learning opportunity to observe or assist with this skill only with faculty permission and with direct supervision from faculty or another RN.*

The percutaneous central vascular catheter (PCVC) is usually inserted into the internal jugular or subclavian vein, with the catheter tip resting in the superior vena cava just above the right atrium. It is called a nontunneled catheter because it is inserted through the skin directly into a central vein in the chest or the neck (sometimes groin) for short-term therapy or in an emergent situation.

Delegation or Assignment

Due to the need for sterile technique and technical complexity of central lines, this skill is not delegated or assigned to the UAP. The UAP may care for patients with such devices, and the nurse must ensure that the UAP knows how to perform routine tasks such as positioning and changing gowns when a device is in place. The UAP should also know what complications or adverse signs, such as alarms, should be reported to the nurse.

Equipment

- Specific nontunneled catheter
- IV tubing administration set and solution container of ordered fluids
- Through-the-needle radiopaque central catheter
- Local anesthetic, syringes, and needles
- Sterile gloves, gown, masks, drapes, and sutures
- Antimicrobial swabs 2% chlorhexidine gluconate (CHG) swabs
- Intermittent infusion caps or positive-pressure device
- Prefilled syringes with preservative-free normal saline
- Transparent semipermeable membrane (TSM) dressing
- Securement device

Preparation

- Review healthcare provider's orders and the patient's MAR.
- Check patient's record for allergies.

- Verify informed signed consent for catheter placement in the patient's record.
- Gather needed equipment and supplies.

Procedure

1. Introduce self to patient and verify the patient's identity using two identifiers. Explain to the patient what you are going to do, why it is necessary, and how the patient can participate. Discuss how the results will be used in planning further care or treatments.
2. Perform hand hygiene and explain the procedure to the patient, including rationale for mask, positioning, and the Valsalva maneuver.
3. Provide for patient privacy and place patient in Trendelenburg position. **Rationale:** *This position prevents air embolism and helps distend subclavian and jugular veins.*
4. According to healthcare provider's preference, extend patient's neck and upper chest by placing a rolled pillow or blanket between shoulder blades. **Rationale:** *Usual insertion sites are either the subclavian or right jugular vein.*
5. Place mask on patient, and turn patient's head away from side of venipuncture. **Rationale:** *This facilitates filling the vessel with blood and prevents contamination.*
6. Maintain sterility while opening glove packet and sterile drape pack.
7. Open antimicrobial prep pads. Assist healthcare provider as needed.
8. The healthcare provider performs the central catheter insertion procedure.
   - It is recommended that the healthcare provider don a mask and hat (for head and facial hair cover), sterile gown, eye protection, and sterile gloves for this procedure.
   - The healthcare provider prepares the patient's skin, drapes area, and, using a sterile syringe and needle, draws up anesthetic to infiltrate the site.
   - As the healthcare provider inserts the catheter, instructions will be given to the patient to perform the Valsalva

(continued on next page)

SKILL 5.13 Percutaneous Central Vascular Catheterization: Assisting (*continued*)

maneuver to prevent air embolism. A 14-gauge needle is inserted into the subclavian vein, using the clavicle as a guide ❶ ❷.

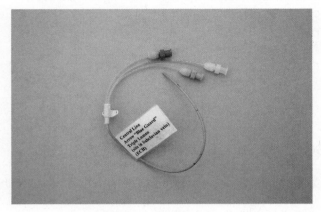

Source: Rick Brady/Pearson Education, Inc.

❶ Central line "Blue Guard." Triple-lumen catheter—subclavian vein.

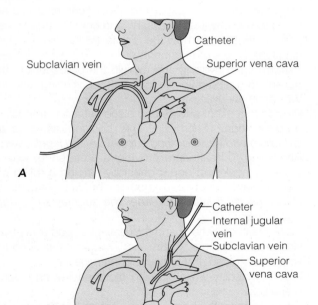

❷ Central venous catheters with *A,* subclavian insertion; *B,* left jugular vein insertion.

9. When catheterization is complete, the healthcare provider will insert injection cap, flush with 5 mL of normal saline, and (only according to facility policy) heparinize with 3 mL dilute heparin.
   - A securement device will be applied to the skin and catheter will be placed in the clamp.
   - The healthcare provider will cover securement device and catheter with sterile transparent dressing and label (according to facility policy).
10. The healthcare provider will prescribe an x-ray for validation of placement into superior vena cava before initiating infusion (unless emergency placement performed).
11. Monitor the patient's vital signs and breath sounds. *Rationale: Bleeding or pneumothorax may occur.*
12. When the procedure is complete, clean area, disposing of waste in appropriate container. Perform hand hygiene and leave the patient safe and comfortable.
13. Complete documentation using forms, checklists, or electronic dropdown lists supplemented by nurse's notes or additional comments as appropriate.

SAMPLE DOCUMENTATION

[date] 1330 Today is line day 3 for nontunneled PCVC. All three lumens capped at this time. Right subclavian insertion site is clean and dry without tenderness, redness, or signs of infection or infiltration. Able to move about bed and get up to chair with assistance. States is feeling better and looking forward to seeing her grandchildren. No complaints verbalized. *G. Rah*

CAUTION! All continuous IV infusions administered via a central line must have an electronic infusion pump in place.

Safety Considerations

Practice Guidelines to Prevent Central Line-Associated Bloodstream Infection (CLABSI)

HAND HYGIENE

- Use appropriate hand hygiene technique to decontaminate before donning gloves and after doffing gloves at each patient contact to reduce the patient's risk of CLABSI. Perform hand hygiene between patients.

BARRIER PRECAUTIONS

- Use full barrier personal protective equipment (PPE) precautions when inserting or assisting with insertion of central venous catheters, including peripherally inserted central catheter (PICC) lines. Include a cap that covers all hair, mask covering mouth and nose tightly, sterile gown, and sterile gloves. Full facial protection is worn if there is a risk of splashed blood or other body fluids.
- Cover the patient from head to toe with large sterile drape leaving small opening for insertion of catheter.

CHLORHEXIDINE SKIN ANTISEPSIS

- Prepare the site using 2% chlorhexidine gluconate (CHG) in 70% isopropyl alcohol.
- Pinch wings on chlorhexidine applicator to break open ampule. Hold applicator down to allow solution to saturate pad.

SKILL 5.13 Percutaneous Central Vascular Catheterization: Assisting *(continued)*

- Press sponge against skin and apply chlorhexidine using a back-and-forth friction rub for at least 30 seconds and then allow to air dry thoroughly, approximately 2 minutes. Do not wipe or blot area.
- If the patient is sensitive to this antiseptic, a single-patient povidone-iodine application may be used.
- Sterile technique is maintained throughout insertion of central venous catheters (CVCs).

CATHETER SITE SELECTION

- Use CVCs impregnated with antimicrobial agents, if they will be used for an extended period of time and risk of CLABSI is high.
- The catheter should have the minimum number of lumens necessary for the individual patient's care.
- Catheter should be inserted in the subclavian vein for nontunneled catheter.
- Selection of a central line placement site should take into consideration the patient's comfort, individual factors of the patient such as anatomic anomalies, risk of complications, potential for ambulation, and experience of the healthcare provider.

- It is recommended to use the subclavian or internal jugular veins unless a PICC line is used for adult patients. The internal jugular vein or femoral vein is most commonly used for children.

DRESSING

- A sterile dressing is applied (gauze, transparent dressing, or antimicrobial foam disc).

DAILY REVIEW OF LINE NECESSITY

- Risk for infection increases the longer a line stays in place.
- Include daily review of line necessity, with prompt removal of unnecessary CVC.
- Name the line day during rounds and in communications (e.g., "Today is line day 6.").

Source: Based on the Joint Commission (TJC). (2013). *CVC maintenance bundles.* Retrieved from https://www.jointcommission.org/assets/1/6/CLABSI_Toolkit_Tool_3-22_CVC_Maintenance_Bundles.pdf.

SKILL 5.14 PICC Line Dressing: Changing

Safety Note! *During scheduled clinical time, nursing students may have a learning opportunity to observe or assist with this skill only with faculty permission and with direct supervision from faculty or another RN.*

A peripherally inserted central catheter (PICC) is a long-term central intravenous line for delivering medications and fluids or withdrawing blood for frequent diagnostic tests. It can be inserted by a specially trained nurse or the healthcare provider.

Delegation or Assignment

Due to the need for sterile technique and technical complexity of central lines, this skill is not delegated or assigned to the UAP. The UAP may care for patients with such devices, and the nurse must ensure that the UAP knows how to perform routine tasks such as positioning and changing gowns when a device is in place. The UAP should also know what complications or adverse signs, such as alarms, should be reported to the nurse.

Equipment

- 2% chlorhexidine gluconate (CHG) antimicrobial swabs
- Securement device
- Transparent semipermeable membrane (TSM) dressing
- BioPatch disc (optional)
- Clean gloves
- Sterile gloves
- Surgical mask

Preparation

- Review healthcare provider's orders and patient's plan of care.

- Signed informed consent in patient's record for procedure (check facility policy for a nursing inserted PICC line).
- Review patient's record for allergies.
- Check patient's record for the last PICC line dressing change done.
- Gather equipment and supplies.

Procedure

1. Introduce self to patient and verify the patient's identity using two identifiers. Explain to the patient what you are going to do, why it is necessary, and how the patient can participate. Discuss how the results will be used in planning further care or treatments. Explain the procedure to the patient.
2. Perform hand hygiene and observe appropriate infection control procedures.
3. Provide for patient privacy. Perform hand hygiene and don mask and clean gloves.
4. Remove old transparent dressing by gently pulling in an upward direction ❶. **Rationale:** *This motion prevents dislodgement of the catheter.*
5. Check site for bleeding, infection, or signs of phlebitis. **Rationale:** *Bleeding may occur with arm use. Phlebitis is the most common complication.*
6. Discard old dressing and gloves. Perform hand hygiene.

CAUTION! Unless absolutely necessary, avoid blood pressure measurement in the arm with a PICC and avoid venipunctures on the extremity with a PICC line.

SKILL 5.14 PICC Line Dressing: Changing (*continued*)

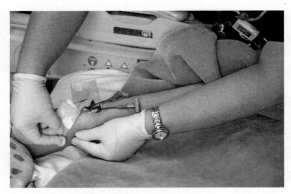

Source: Ronald May/Pearson Education, Inc.

❶ Remove dressing by gently pulling in an upward direction.

7. Prepare sterile supplies.
8. Don sterile gloves.
9. Clean exit site and catheter with antimicrobial swabs using back-and-forth scrub movement ❷.
   Note: The catheter is anchored by a securement device, which does not require suturing of PICC line. Approximately 2.5 cm (1 in.) of catheter extends from the insertion site.

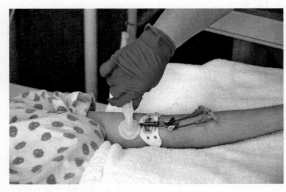

Source: Ronald May/Pearson Education, Inc.

❷ Cleanse site with CHG swab using back-and-forth motion.

10. Allow 30 seconds for antimicrobial solution to dry. Do not blow on arm or wave hand to hasten drying ❸. **Rationale:** *Waving hand or blowing may contaminate site—antibacterial action does not take effect until solution is dry.*
11. Replace and apply new securement device following manufacturer's instructions. The device should be changed at least every 7 days (follow facility policy) ❹.
12. Cover exit site with transparent semipermeable dressing. Avoid stretching the dressing. Press down on dressing to seal catheter site. No part of actual catheter should be outside transparent dressing.
    Note: Transparent dressings are not occlusive; they allow air to circulate through the semipermeable dressing and thus prevent perspiration from collecting under the dressing.
13. Remove gloves and mask.

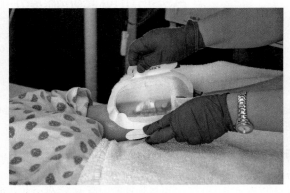

Source: Ronald May/Pearson Education, Inc.

❸ Allow site to dry before applying dressing. Place transparent dressing over site.

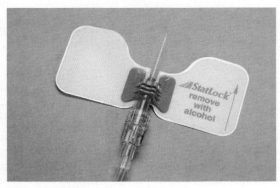

Source: Rick Brady/Pearson Education, Inc.

❹ StatLock device, the only evidence-based catheter stabilization device that meets national standards.

14. Initial and date dressing.
15. Change initial transparent dressing in 24 hours and then every 7 days or whenever it is soiled or loose. **Rationale:** *First dressing change is done to check insertion site.*
16. When the procedure is complete, perform hand hygiene and leave patient safe and comfortable.
17. Complete documentation using forms, checklists, or electronic dropdown lists supplemented by nurse's notes or additional comments as appropriate.

SAMPLE DOCUMENTATION

[date] 0750 Old TSM dressing removed from PICC line site right upper arm. Area clean and dry, no bleeding or discharge noted, denies tenderness, no phlebitis noted. Sterile technique used for cleaning of site with CHG wipes, allowed to dry. New securement device applied then covered with TSM dressing. Procedure tolerated without incident. *T. Barker*

SKILL 5.15 Venipuncture: Initiating

Safety Note! *During scheduled clinical time, nursing students may have a learning opportunity to observe or assist with this skill only with faculty permission and with direct supervision from faculty or another RN.*

Before preparing the infusion, first verify the healthcare provider's order indicating the type of solution, the amount to be administered, and the rate of flow or time over which the infusion is to be completed.

Prior to venipuncture, consider how long the patient is likely to have the IV, the kind of fluids to be infused, and medications the patient will be receiving or is likely to receive intravenously. These factors may affect choice of vein and catheter size. Review the patient record regarding previous venipuncture and patient allergies (e.g., to tape or povidone-iodine). Note any difficulties encountered and how they were resolved.

Delegation or Assignment

IV infusion therapy is not usually delegated or assigned to an unlicensed assistive personnel (UAP). The UAP may care for patients receiving IV therapy, and the nurse must ensure that the UAP knows how to perform routine tasks such as bathing and positioning without disturbing the IV. The UAP should also know what complications or adverse signs, such as leakage, should be reported to the nurse. In some states, the UAP may receive special IV therapy training to start IV infusions. Check the applicable state's nurse practice act.

Equipment

Substitute appropriate supplies if the patient has tape, antiseptic, or latex allergies.

- IV start kit if available, ❶ or collect separate items
- Hypoallergenic tape
- Clean gloves
- Tourniquet
- Antiseptic swabs such as 10% povidone-iodine or 2% chlorhexidine gluconate (CHG) with alcohol or 70% isopropyl alcohol

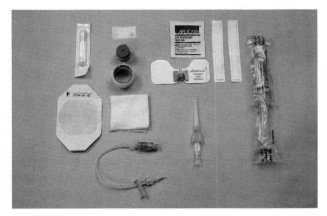

Source: Ronald May/Pearson Education, Inc.

❶ IV Start Kit contents.

- IV catheter (Choose an IV catheter of the appropriate type and size based on the size of the vein and the purpose of the IV. A 20- to 22-gauge catheter is indicated for most adults. Always have an extra catheter and ones of different sizes available.)
- Sterile gauze dressing or transparent semipermeable membrane (TSM) dressing
- Stabilization device
- Towel or disposable linen saver
- Local anesthetic (optional and per facility policy)

Preparation

- Review healthcare provider's orders and patient's MAR and plan of care.
- Review record for patient's allergies, especially latex products and betadine.
- If possible, select a time to perform the venipuncture that will minimize excessive movement of the affected limb. **Rationale:** *Moving the limb after insertion could dislodge the catheter.*
- Make sure the patient's clothing or gown can be removed over the IV apparatus if necessary. Some facilities provide special gowns that open over the shoulder and down the sleeve for easy removal.
- Review instructions for using the IV catheter because a variety of needle-safety devices are manufactured.
- Visitors or family members may be asked to leave the room if desired by the nurse or the patient.
- Gather needed equipment and supplies.

Procedure

1. Introduce self to patient and verify the patient's identity using two identifiers. Explain to the patient what you are going to do, why it is necessary, and how the patient can participate. Explain that venipuncture can cause discomfort for a few seconds, but there should be no ongoing pain after insertion. If possible, explain how long the IV will need to remain in place and how it will be used. Discuss how the results will be used in planning further care or treatments.
2. Perform hand hygiene and observe appropriate infection control procedures.
3. Assist the patient to a comfortable position, either sitting or lying. Expose the limb to be used but provide for patient privacy.
4. Select the venipuncture site ❷.
   - Use the patient's nondominant arm, unless contraindicated (e.g., mastectomy, fistula for dialysis). Identify possible venipuncture sites by looking for veins that are relatively straight. The vein should be palpable, but may not be visible, especially in patients with dark skin. Consider the catheter length; look for a site sufficiently distal to the wrist or elbow where the tip of the catheter will not be at a point of flexion. **Rationale:** *Sclerotic veins may make initiating and maintaining the IV difficult. Joint flexion increases the risk of irritation of vein walls by the catheter.*

(continued on next page)

SKILL 5.15 Venipuncture: Initiating (*continued*)

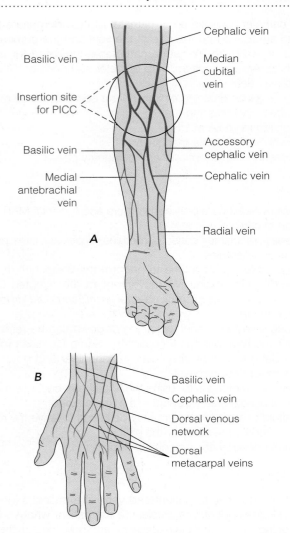

A

B

Cephalic vein
Basilic vein
Median cubital vein
Insertion site for PICC
Basilic vein
Accessory cephalic vein
Cephalic vein
Medial antebrachial vein
Radial vein

Basilic vein
Cephalic vein
Dorsal venous network
Dorsal metacarpal veins

❷ Commonly used venipuncture sites of the **A,** arm; **B,** hand. Part A also shows the site used for a peripherally inserted central catheter (PICC).

- If the site is very hairy, clip the hairs carefully with scissors. Shaving is not recommended. **Rationale:** *Shaving has the potential to cause microabrasions, which can increase the risk of infection.*
- Place a towel or linen saver under the extremity to protect linens (or furniture if in the home).

5. To help dilate the vein, place the extremity in a dependent position (lower than the patient's heart). **Rationale:** *Gravity slows venous return and distends the veins. Distending the veins makes it easier to insert the IV properly.*

6. Ask patient about allergy to latex. Apply a tourniquet ❸ firmly 15–20 cm (6–8 in.) above the venipuncture site if the blood pressure is within normal range. Explain that the tourniquet will feel tight. **Rationale:** *The tourniquet must be tight enough to obstruct venous flow but not so tight that it occludes arterial flow.*

- For older adults with fragile skin, instead of applying a tourniquet, place the arm in a dependent position to

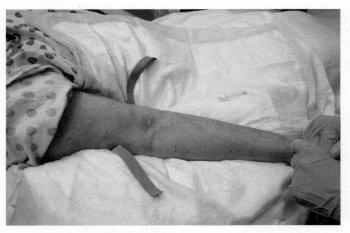

Source: Ronald May/Pearson Education, Inc.

❸ Apply tourniquet 15–20 cm (6–8 in.) above insertion site.

allow the veins to engorge. **Rationale:** *The tourniquet can cause tissue damage and may not be needed to allow the vein to dilate.*

7. If the vein is not sufficiently dilated:

- Massage or stroke the vein distal to the site and in the direction of venous flow toward the heart. **Rationale:** *This action helps fill the vein.*
- Encourage the patient to clench and unclench the fist. **Rationale:** *Contracting the muscles compresses the distal veins, forcing blood along the veins and distending them.*
- Lightly tap the vein with your fingertips. **Rationale:** *Light tapping may distend the vein.*
- If the preceding steps fail to distend the vein so that it is palpable, remove the tourniquet and wrap the extremity in a warm, moist towel for 10–15 min. **Rationale:** *Heat dilates superficial blood vessels, causing them to fill. Then repeat steps to dilate the vein.*

8. Minimize insertion pain as much as possible.

- Transdermal analgesic creams (e.g., EMLA, Synera) may be used, depending on policy and having healthcare provider's order.
- If permitted by facility policy and having healthcare provider's order, inject 0.03 mL of 1% lidocaine (without epinephrine) or normal saline intradermally over the site where you plan to insert the IV catheter.

9. Apply clean gloves and clean the venipuncture site ❹. **Rationale:** *Gloves protect the nurse from contamination by the patient's blood.*

- Clean the skin at the site of entry with a topical antiseptic swab (e.g., 2% CHG or alcohol). Some facilities may use an anti-infective solution such as povidone-iodine (check facility protocol). Check for allergies to iodine or shellfish before cleansing skin with Betadine or other iodine products.
- Use a back-and-forth motion for a minimum of 30 seconds to scrub the insertion site and surrounding area.
- Allow the site to air dry completely before insertion of the catheter.

SKILL 5.15 Venipuncture: Initiating *(continued)*

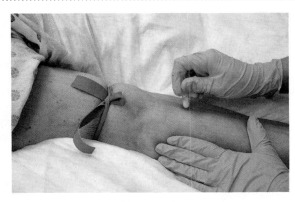

Source: Ronald May/Pearson Education, Inc.

④ **Use a back-and-forth-movement to cleanse the site with CHG or alcohol wipe.**

- Verify saline-filled syringe is attached to extension tubing and that the tubing has been primed (if facility policy) ⑤.

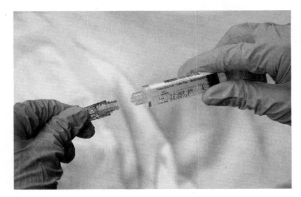

Source: Rick Brady/Pearson Education, Inc.

⑤ Attach saline-filled syringe to extension tubing.

10. Insert the catheter and initiate the infusion.
    - Remove the catheter assembly from its sterile packaging and inspect the needle tip ⑥. Remove the cover of the needle (stylet).

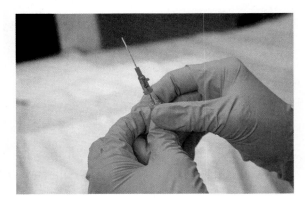

Source: Rick Brady/Pearson Education, Inc.

⑥ Inspect integrity of needle tip.

- Use the nondominant hand to pull the skin taut below the entry site. **Rationale:** *This stabilizes the vein and makes the skin taut for needle (stylet) entry. It can also make initial tissue penetration less painful.*
- Holding the over-the-needle catheter at a 15- to 30-degree angle with the needle (stylet) bevel up, insert the catheter through the skin and into the vein ⑦. A sudden lack of resistance is felt as the needle (stylet) enters the vein. Use a slow, steady insertion technique and avoid jabbing or stabbing motions.

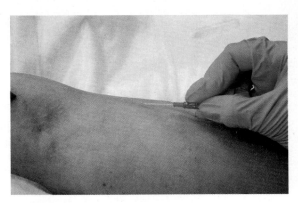

Source: Rick Brady/Pearson Education, Inc.

⑦ Insert needle, with bevel up, at 15- to 30-degree angle and slide needle into vein.

- Once blood appears in the lumen or clear "flashback" chamber, lower the angle of the catheter until it is almost parallel with the skin, and advance the needle (stylet) ⑧ ⑨ and catheter approximately 0.5–1 cm (about ¼ in.) farther. Holding the assembly steady, advance the catheter until the hub is at the venipuncture site. **Rationale:** *The catheter is advanced to ensure that it, and not just the needle (stylet), is in the vein.*

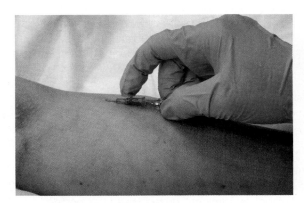

Source: Rick Brady/Pearson Education, Inc.

⑧ Advance catheter over needle until the hub is at the venipuncture site.

(continued on next page)

SKILL 5.15 Venipuncture: Initiating (*continued*)

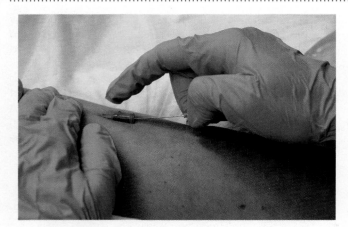

Source: Rick Brady/Pearson Education, Inc.

⑨ Separate, but do not completely remove, the stylet.

- If there is no blood return, try redirecting the catheter assembly again toward the vein. If the needle/stylet has been withdrawn from the catheter even a small distance, or the catheter tip has been pulled out of the skin, the catheter must be discarded and a new one used. **Rationale:** *Reinserting the needle (stylet) into the catheter can result in damage or slicing of the catheter. A catheter that has been removed from the skin is considered contaminated and cannot be reused.*

CAUTION! If no blood is observed and you did not feel the catheter enter the vein, pull back on entire catheter apparatus without exiting the skin. Reassess vein position, then reattempt venipuncture. If you are not successful, remove catheter and look for a different site. Remember the catheter is now contaminated and cannot be used again. Most facilities allow the nurse to attempt two venipunctures; if unsuccessful, the nurse must notify another professional to attempt venipuncture.

- If blood begins to flow out of the vein into the tissues as the catheter is inserted, creating a hematoma, the insertion has not been successful. This is sometimes referred to as a "blown vein." Immediately release the tourniquet and remove the catheter, applying pressure over the insertion site with dry gauze. Attempt the venipuncture in another site, in the opposite arm if possible. **Rationale:** *Placing the tourniquet back on the same arm above the unsuccessful site may cause it to bleed. Placing the IV below the unsuccessful site could result in infusing fluid into the already punctured vein, causing it to leak.*
- Release the tourniquet.
- Put pressure on the vein proximal to the catheter with a finger to eliminate or reduce blood oozing out of the catheter. Stabilize the hub with thumb and index finger of the nondominant hand.
- Remove the protective cap from the distal end of the tubing and hold it ready to attach to the catheter, maintaining the sterility of the end.

- Stabilize the catheter hub and apply pressure distal to the catheter with your finger. **Rationale:** *This prevents excessive blood flow through the catheter.*
- Carefully remove the needle (stylet), engage the needle-safety device (if it does not engage automatically), and attach the end of the infusion tubing **⑩** to the catheter hub. Place the needle (stylet) directly into a sharps container. If this is not within reach, place the needle (stylet) into its original package and dispose in a sharps container as soon as possible.

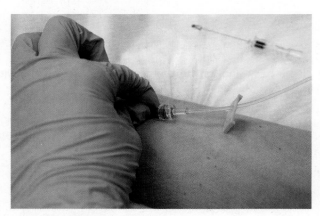

Source: Rick Brady/Pearson Education, Inc.

⑩ Attach extension tubing.

- Initiate the infusion or flush the catheter with sterile normal saline **⑪**. **Rationale:** *Blood must be removed from the catheter lumen and tubing immediately. Otherwise, the blood will clot inside the lumen.* Watch closely for any signs that the catheter has been infiltrated. Infiltration occurs when the tip of the IV is outside the vein and the fluid is entering the tissues instead. It is manifested by localized swelling, coolness, pallor, and discomfort at the IV site. **Rationale:** *Inflammation or infiltration necessitates removal of the IV catheter to avoid further trauma to the tissues.*

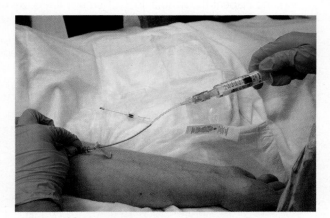

Source: Rick Brady/Pearson Education, Inc.

⑪ Backflush and instill 3 mL of saline. Observe for swelling at IV site.

SKILL 5.15 Venipuncture: Initiating (*continued*)

11. Stabilize the catheter and apply a dressing.
    - Secure the catheter according to the manufacturer's instructions and facility policy. Several methods are used to stabilize the catheter. If tape is used, it must be sterile tape or surgical strips and they should be applied only to the catheter adapter and not placed directly on the catheter–skin junction site. Use of a manufactured stabilization device is preferred.
    - Two methods are used for applying a dressing: a sterile gauze dressing secured with tape and a TSM dressing. Most common is the TSM, ⑫ because it allows for continuous assessment of the site; it is more comfortable than gauze and tape. Do not use ointment of any kind under a TSM dressing.

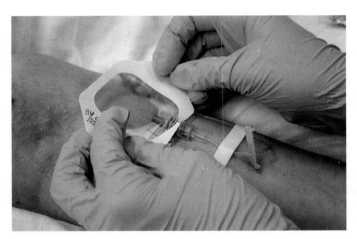

Source: Rick Brady/Pearson Education, Inc.

⑫ Place transparent dressing over the site.

- Label the dressing with the date and time of insertion; type, gauge, and length of catheter used; and your initials.
- Loop the tubing and secure it with tape. **Rationale:** *Looping and securing the tubing prevent the weight of the tubing or any movement from pulling on the IV catheter.*

12. Discard all used disposable supplies in appropriate receptacles. Cleanse any blood spills according to facility policy. Clean any reusable supplies.
13. Discard the tourniquet. Remove and discard gloves. Perform hand hygiene.
14. When the procedure is complete, perform hand hygiene and leave the patient safe and comfortable.
15. Complete documentation using forms, checklists, or electronic dropdown lists supplemented by nurse's notes or additional comments as appropriate. Record the date and time of the venipuncture; type, length, and gauge of the IV catheter; venipuncture site; how many attempts were made and the location of each attempt; and the type of dressing.

Lifespan Considerations

NEWBORNS, INFANTS, AND CHILDREN

- Because newborns and infants do not have large veins in the antecubital fossa, blood specimens for examination are usually taken with a heel stick, or if needed, from the external jugular and femoral veins (according to facility policy).
- Use a doll to demonstrate venipuncture for children and explain the procedure to the parents.
- Explain the procedure to the young patient, encourage questions, and be alert for nonverbal cues. Children may not understand things that seem obvious to adults. For example, a child may think the IV therapy is a punishment.
- Venipuncture can be extremely frightening for children. Many children will resist, cry, and even become combative. Parents, in turn, may become upset. Offering distractions and rewards may help. Helping the child to take deep, slow breaths can also trigger some degree of relaxation. Sometimes it is necessary to restrain the child. Most pediatric professionals believe that it is best if a person other than the child's parent holds the child, so the child doesn't associate the parent with the fear and pain. It is important for the parent to remain with the child, soothing the child with voice, closeness, and touch. Some parents are not able to do this, and they need support and understanding from nursing staff. A calm demeanor on the nurse's part (and relaxation breathing) will help ease this potentially upsetting situation for all concerned.
- A peripheral 22 or 24-gauge catheter in the shortest length can be used for an infant or child.
- Apply age-appropriate restraints, arm boards, gauze wrap, or other devices to protect the IV site.

OLDER ADULTS

- Skin may often be fragile and bruise easily. Select an IV site with adequate healthy tissue to support the IV catheter.
- To distend the vein, tap 2–3 times very lightly to prevent trauma.
- Consider not using a tourniquet. The older adult's superficial veins are often large enough to insert the needle (stylet) without further distention. Using a tourniquet can cause the vein to burst when the needle (stylet) enters.
- Minimize the use of alcohol and tape to avoid irritating sensitive skin.

(continued on next page)

SKILL 5.15 Venipuncture: Initiating (*continued*)

Practice Guidelines

VEIN SELECTION

- Use distal veins of the arm first; subsequent IV starts should be proximal to the previous site.

- Use the patient's nondominant arm whenever possible. **Rationale:** *This minimizes the patient's restricted mobility and function.*

- Select a vein that is:
  a. Easily palpated and feels soft and full
  b. Naturally splinted by bone
  c. Large enough to allow adequate circulation around the catheter.

- Avoid using veins that are:
  a. In areas of flexion (e.g., the antecubital fossa)
  b. Highly visible **Rationale:** *These veins tend to roll away from the needle (stylet).*
  c. Damaged by previous use, phlebitis, infiltration, or sclerosis
  d. Continually distended with blood, knotted, or tortuous
  e. In a surgically compromised or injured extremity (e.g., following a mastectomy) **Rationale:** *These sites may have impaired circulation and cause discomfort for the patient.*
  f. In the foot or legs unless arm veins are inaccessible, and with a healthcare provider's order. **Rationale:** *Lower extremity sites are more prone to thrombus formation and subsequent emboli.*

≫ Critical Thinking Options for Unexpected Outcomes

Not all unexpected outcomes require further nursing intervention; however, many times they do. When the patient demonstrates a change in signs/symptoms indicating an emerging problem, the nurse should immediately assess and troubleshoot what is happening. The assessment data must be processed quickly to formulate a hypothesis so the nurse can make a clinical judgment. The nurse then decides how best to resolve the problem and improve the patient's situation for a better outcome.

EXPECTED OUTCOME	UNEXPECTED OUTCOME	POSSIBLE INTERVENTIONS
Patient's intake and output are maintained within expected parameters of 200–300 mL of each other	Recorded I&O do not balance	■ Correlate I&O imbalance with weight changes. ■ Emphasize importance of accurate measurements to patient and family. ■ Check that entries into computer are accurate (i.e., entering 100 mL instead of 1000 mL). ■ Identify possible nonmeasurable sources of intake or output. ■ Report to charge nurse so she can ensure that all nurses are keeping accurate records. ■ Check if patient or family can help with keeping the I&O record. ■ Check the addition on the I&O record to see if an error was made.
	Fluid intake and output do not balance (intake greater than output).	■ Initiate daily weight measurements (weigh before breakfast, same scale, same clothing). ■ Compare losses or gains with patient's daily weight measurement. ■ Fluid intake and output generally are relatively equal (assuming numbers are accurate). Output should be about 500 mL less per 24 hours due to insensible fluid loss. ■ Determine whether treatment goal is to rehydrate or diurese the patient. ■ Use graduated container to accurately measure output in urine "hat." ■ Search for sources of unmeasured output (fever, wound drainage, diarrhea).
	Fluid output is greater than intake.	■ Analyze whether treatment goal (rehydration, diuresis) has been achieved. ■ Reposition patient cautiously, monitoring for possible orthostatic hypotension. ■ Identify when "dry weight" has been achieved (intake balances output after therapy received). ■ Search for sources of unrecorded intake (family offerings, flush solutions, ice chips, full-liquid foods).

EXPECTED OUTCOME	UNEXPECTED OUTCOME	POSSIBLE INTERVENTIONS
Fluid intake for adult is at least 2600 mL unless contraindicated by diagnosis.	Patient unable to maintain an intake of at least 2600 mL/day.	<ul><li>Ensure that fluid restriction is not ordered.</li><li>Offer fluids in small amounts more frequently.</li><li>Assess mouth for soreness.</li><li>Determine patient fluid preferences.</li><li>Determine patient preference for fluid to be hot, cold, or room temperature.</li><li>Consider "other" fluids such as gelatin, popsicles.</li><li>Assess patient's ability to use a straw (hemiplegic patient is often unable to suck through a straw).</li><li>Check if patient is able to drink fluids independently or if assistance is needed.</li><li>Ensure that adequate fluids are accessible at the bedside for the patient.</li><li>Do not administer fluids with a bulb syringe.</li><li>Address patient's toileting needs every 2 hr—some patients restrict their fluid intake for fear of incontinence.</li><li>Use a thickening additive in liquids to facilitate swallowing for the patient with aspiration precautions.</li></ul>
IV fluids infuse at prescribed rate without complications.	IV flow not maintained at appropriate rate.	<ul><li>Monitor IV fluid intake hourly.</li><li>Observe IV site for complications.</li><li>Restart IV immediately when infiltrated to ensure continuous IV fluid intake.</li><li>Document IV fluid intake every shift.</li><li>Account for interruption of primary infusion and the delivery of intermittent infusions of medications.</li><li>Check accuracy of IV administration equipment: electronic device, Dial-A-Flow, etc.</li><li>Inform healthcare provider of alterations in fluid received from what was ordered.</li></ul>
	IV solution does not flow properly.	<ul><li>Ensure that the control clamp is open.</li><li>Check that blood pressure readings are not taken on arm in which IV is running, because flow is impeded and a clot can form on the end of the needle.</li><li>Ensure that IV administration set is properly loaded. Check pump for flow problem indicator (e.g., cassette seating, air in line).</li><li>Check IV tubing from insertion site to IV solution for kinks/ obstructions.</li><li>Check for extremity causing positional obstruction to flow (e.g., elbow bent, arm rotated).</li></ul>
IV site remains clean, without signs of infection or infiltration.	Phlebitis is suspected at infusion site (tenderness, warmth, erythema, and pain).	<ul><li>Check infusion solution and medications being administered. (Potassium chloride and hypertonic solutions are particularly irritating to veins.)</li><li>Discontinue IV.</li><li>Apply warm compress per hospital policy.</li></ul>
	Infiltration occurs.	<ul><li>Place warm moist pack, using warm towel, enclose area from fingertips to elbow. Place extremity in plastic bag with open end at elbow. Leave in place no more than 10 minutes.</li><li>Elevate the affected extremity.</li></ul>
IV catheter inserted at an appropriate site without difficulty.	Venipuncture is unsuccessful for needle insertion.	<ul><li>Remove needle/catheter, apply pressure at insertion site until bleeding stops. (This prevents ecchymosis at site.) Apply bandage.</li><li>Apply small pressure dressing if patient on anticoagulant therapy.</li><li>Select another insertion site proximal to the infiltration area, or use another extremity.</li><li>Avoid the one-step entry method since this frequently results in a through-and-through vein puncture.</li><li>After two failed attempts, seek a more experienced person to perform venipuncture.</li><li>Place extremity in dependent position before placing tourniquet. Allows vein to fill.</li><li>Place warm compress on extremity to increase vasodilation, before placing tourniquet.</li></ul>

(continued on next page)

EXPECTED OUTCOME	UNEXPECTED OUTCOME	POSSIBLE INTERVENTIONS
Infusions of medications or fluids are accomplished without difficulty.	Secondary bag solution does not infuse adequately.	■ Check that primary IV bag is lower than secondary bag (if infusion device requires). ■ Check line for kinks and position. ■ Ensure that secondary needleless connector is properly attached in the primary injection port and second bag is sufficiently spiked. ■ Check that the roller clamp of the secondary tubing is open fully.
	Solution in primary IV tubing is incompatible with medication to be administered via secondary "piggyback."	■ Turn primary infusion off. ■ Before administering medication, flush primary tubing with solution compatible with medication (e.g., normal saline, 5% D/W). ■ Hang a separate solution compatible with medication and run through line to flush during drug administration.
	Central venous pressure (CVP) system does not infuse.	■ Check lines for kinks. Change patient's position. Check to make sure the manometer stopcock is in the IV→ patient position. ■ Obtain order for placing heparin in IV bag to maintain patency. ■ Notify healthcare provider and prepare for possible reinsertion.
Blood samples are obtained without difficulty.	Air enters central vein, producing air embolism from system being open at atmosphere.	■ Immediately clamp catheter and place patient in Trendelenburg position (turned to the left so right ventricle is uppermost). ■ Immediately inform healthcare provider and monitor until healthcare provider arrives. Assess vital signs and breath sounds. ■ Administer high-flow O_2 as necessary. ■ Prevent air embolism by having patient perform the Valsalva maneuver any time catheter is open to air, or use in-line catheter clamp. ■ Ensure patient has a patent peripheral IV line.
Central vascular line remains patent and free of infection.	Infection occurs at insertion site.	■ Prepare for catheter removal and possible reinsertion at another site. ■ If catheter is removed, cut off catheter tip with sterile scissors and place in sterile container. Send tip to laboratory for culture as ordered or facility policy. ■ Administer antibiotics as ordered. ■ Observe patient carefully for signs of systemic infection.
IV catheter maintains patency with use of CLC 2000 device.	Catheter appears to be or becomes occluded.	■ Reposition patient. ■ Ask patient to raise arms over head. ■ Follow facility policy and procedure. ■ Assess mechanical problem: tubing, pumps, catheter, clamps, insertion site, or securement device. ■ Assess nonthrombotic problem: medications infused, fluids or withdrawal of blood. Use of precipitate clearance agent is established by individual facility policies and procedures. ■ Assess thrombotic problem: use of thrombolytic clearance agents is established by individual facility policy and procedures. ■ Have patient perform the Valsalva maneuver. Turn head to one side. ■ Attempt to flush catheter with normal saline, using gentle pressure. ■ Notify healthcare provider for order to administer fibrinolytic agent or other agents.
	Central venous pressure (CVP) readings vary greatly.	■ Assess patency of setup. ■ Assess patient's level of pain; pain increases the CVP reading. ■ Assess if position of patient has been changed; raising the head of the bed alters the reading unless setup is adjusted. ■ Check that the marked area at midaxillary level is at the level of the patient's right atrium (fourth intercostal space [ICS]). ■ If patient has chronic obstructive pulmonary disease (COPD), heart failure, or hypovolemia, expect readings to differ from normal range. However, once baseline is established for individual patient, trends should be watched and evaluated against goals of therapy.

REVIEW Questions

1. The nurse reviews intake and output measurements collected by a UAP. Which measurement should the nurse investigate prior to reporting to the healthcare professional?
   1. Client weighing 121 lb with an 8-hour urine output of 110 mL
   2. Client weighing 132 lb with an 8-hour urine output of 480 mL
   3. Client weighing 143 lb with an 8-hour urine output of 650 mL
   4. Client weighing 154 lb with an 8-hour urine output of 980 mL

2. While changing the transparent semipermeable membrane (TSM) dressings on a client's central line, the nurse measures the catheter length as being 10.75 cm. This is a change from the previous measurement of 11.5 cm. What should the nurse do first?
   1. Pull back on the catheter.
   2. Complete the dressing change.
   3. Notify the healthcare provider.
   4. Document the discrepancy in length.

3. The nurse observes a new graduate nurse changing the intravenous fluid tubing for a client's central line infusion. For which action should the nurse intervene?
   1. Flushes the catheter with a 3-mL syringe
   2. Clamps catheter before removing the syringe
   3. Applies clean gloves after performing hand hygiene
   4. Cleanses access port with antimicrobial swab and allows to air dry

4. The nurse prepares to administer an intravenous medication through the middle port of a client's central venous catheter. Which action should the nurse take first before administering the medication?
   1. Lowering the head of the bed
   2. Changing the cap on the port
   3. Flushing the port with 3 mL heparin
   4. Flushing the port with 5 mL normal saline

5. The nurse inserts a Huber needle into a client's vascular access device in order to draw blood samples. Where should the nurse place the first 10 mL of blood withdrawn from the device?
   1. Trash can
   2. Sharps container
   3. Test tube for testing
   4. Biohazard waste container

6. An older client's intravenous infusion dressing is wet. What should the nurse do first?
   1. Remove the wet dressing.
   2. Clamp the infusion tubing.
   3. Lower the infusion container.
   4. Apply sterile gauze at the catheter site.

7. A client is prescribed to receive 3 L of dextrose 5% and 0.45% normal saline over 24 hours. The infusion set administers 20 gtts/mL. At how many drops per minute should the infusion set be calibrated in order to deliver this fluid? Calculate to the nearest whole number.

   ___gtt

8. A client is prescribed to receive 3 L of intravenous fluid over the next 12 hours. Which action should the nurse take to ensure that the correct amount is infused as prescribed?
   1. Chill the fluid prior to administering to the client.
   2. Use an intravenous catheter with a larger diameter.
   3. Insert a longer intravenous catheter prior to the infusion.
   4. Place the intravenous fluid at the level of the bed side rail.

9. A client's intravenous fluid infusion was changed to a keep-vein-open (KVO) rate at 1400 hours. When should the nurse change the client's fluid container and tubing?
   1. 0800 hours next day
   2. 1400 hours next day
   3. 2200 hours same day
   4. 2400 hours same day

10. A client receiving IV fluids reports burning pain along the vein being used for the infusion. What should the nurse do first?
    1. Apply a tourniquet.
    2. Clamp the infusion.
    3. Reposition the catheter.
    4. Lower the infusion bag.

11. The nurse turns off the smart pump and removes a client's intravenous catheter. What did the nurse most likely assess to make this clinical decision?
    1. Pump at eye level on the pole
    2. Erythema and swelling at the catheter site
    3. Catheter not flushed before starting the infusion
    4. Infusion tubing hanging below the level of the bed

12. The nurse assists in preparing a client for placement of a percutaneous central vascular catheter (PCVC) in the right subclavian vein. What should the nurse do before the procedure begins?
    1. Place the client into the left side-lying position.
    2. Turn the client's head toward the right shoulder.
    3. Place a rolled towel between the client's shoulder blades.
    4. Instruct to breathe deeply and cough when the puncture is made.

13. The nurse cleanses the site of a peripherally inserted central catheter (PICC) with antimicrobial-soaked swabs. What action should the nurse perform next?
    1. Wait 30 seconds for the solution to dry.
    2. Place a securement device over the catheter.
    3. Cover the insertion site with a transparent dressing.
    4. Assess the site for bleeding, infection, or signs of phlebitis.

Note: For answers and rationales for the review questions, go to Appendix A or your Pearson MyLab Nursing and eText.

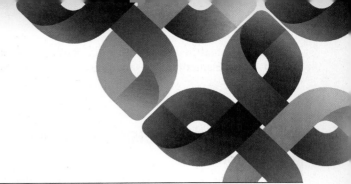

Chapter 6
Infection

Chapter at a Glance

» The Concept of Infection

Infection implies the invasion and colonization of microorganisms such as bacteria, viruses, or parasites that are not normally found within the body. An infection may remain localized, or it may spread throughout the body by way of the blood or lymphatic systems. There may or not be initial symptoms of an infection. An infectious disease, also called a *communicable* *disease,* can be spread directly or indirectly from one individual to another. If it is easily transmitted from one person to another, it is termed *contagious.* Preventing the transmission of pathogens and providing protection against them requires using appropriate safety precautions, personal protective equipment (PPE) and further infectious control protocols, and environmental controls.

Learning Outcomes

6.1 Summarize the reasoning for having more than one type of isolation precaution for infectious diseases and communicable infections.

6.2 Discuss priority safety considerations for removing specimens from an isolation room.

6.3 Differentiate the advantages and disadvantages of hand washing and using a waterless antiseptic for hand hygiene.

6.4 Contrast when to use a simple surgical mask and when to use a particulate filter respirator mask for isolation protocols.

6.5 Support the necessity of informing the hospital receiving department what type of isolation a patient needs and what precautions hospital personnel should follow when a patient who is in isolation is transported to another department for diagnostic tests.

6.6 Explain the rationale for doing frequent hand hygiene when providing nursing care to a group of patients.

6.7 Give examples of safety measures when transporting a patient outside an isolation room.

The following feature links some, but not all, of the concepts related to assessment. They are presented in alphabetical order

Concepts Related to
Infection

CONCEPT	RELATIONSHIP TO INFECTION	NURSING IMPLICATIONS
Assessment	Early recognition of signs and symptoms of infection means early treatment.	▪ Initial comprehensive assessment for risk factors for infection ▪ Continuous monitoring of trouble spots and preventive interventions
Immunity	Opportunistic pathogens can cause infection.	▪ Use standard precautions and other isolation protocols as appropriate ▪ Assist with hygiene measures
Oxygenation	Respiratory tract infections affect effective gas exchange.	▪ Encourage use of incentive spirometer ▪ Encourage effective coughing and deep breathing throughout day ▪ Implement oxygen therapy as ordered
Safety	Taking precautions helps to avoid hospital acquired illnesses.	▪ Protect patient and others with standard precautions and other isolation precautions as appropriate ▪ Perform procedures using aseptic techniques and clean techniques per facility protocols
Tissue Integrity	Treatment of tissue impairment can prevent infection. Surgical wound assessment and care to prevent infection.	▪ Assess tissue integrity to identify high risks for impairment ▪ Provide measures to maintain tissue integrity, positioning, movement, nutrition ▪ Assess surgical wound when dressing changed and keep site clean and dry

Planned nursing strategies to reduce the risk of transmission of organisms from one person to another include the use of meticulous asepsis. **Asepsis** is the freedom from infection or infectious material. There are two basic types of asepsis: medical and surgical. *Medical asepsis* includes all practices intended to confine a specific microorganism to a specific area, limiting the number, growth, and spread of microorganisms. *Surgical asepsis*, or *sterile technique*, refers to those practices that keep an area or object free of all microorganisms. It includes practices that destroy all microorganisms and spores (microscopic dormant structures formed by some pathogens that are very hardy and often survive common cleaning techniques).

≫ Medical Asepsis

Expected Outcomes

1. Care is delivered following hand hygiene to reduce potential pathogens on the hands.
2. The spread of microorganisms from healthcare workers or the environment to patients is prevented.
3. Patient-to-patient spread of endogenous and exogenous flora via healthcare worker is prevented.
4. Hospital personnel are protected from infection.

Medical asepsis prevents the transmission of infectious pathogens and controls infection by using clean technique practices to stop the microorganisms from growing and colonizing in a patient's environment. Some of these practices include bathing and helping patients with hygiene; keeping over-bed table clean and free from contaminating items such as used tissues; maintaining clean and dry linen on bed; keeping emesis basin, wash basin, and water pitcher clean and dry; and maintaining clean and dry dressings.

Standard precautions **(Figure 6–1 ≫)** (formerly known as *universal precautions*) are a type of isolation precaution to further extend medical asepsis practices. Standard precautions are basic preventive practices that are implemented with all patients and others to ensure disease transmission does not happen. They include:

▪ Performing frequent and effective hand hygiene, either hand washing with soap and water or doing a rub using a waterless alcohol-based product.

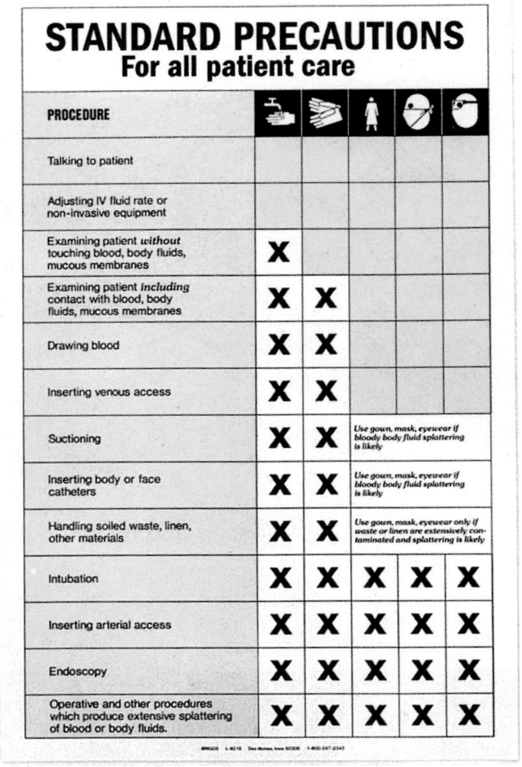

STANDARD PRECAUTIONS
For all patient care

PROCEDURE					
Talking to patient					
Adjusting IV fluid rate or non-invasive equipment					
Examining patient *without* touching blood, body fluids, mucous membranes	X				
Examining patient *including* contact with blood, body fluids, mucous membranes	X	X			
Drawing blood	X	X			
Inserting venous access	X	X			
Suctioning	X	X	*Use gown, mask, eyewear if bloody body fluid splattering is likely*		
Inserting body or face catheters	X	X	*Use gown, mask, eyewear if bloody body fluid splattering is likely*		
Handling soiled waste, linen, other materials	X	X	*Use gown, mask, eyewear only if waste or linen are extensively contaminated and splattering is likely*		
Intubation	X	X	X	X	X
Inserting arterial access	X	X	X	X	X
Endoscopy	X	X	X	X	X
Operative and other procedures which produce extensive splattering of blood or body fluids.	X	X	X	X	X

Source: Standard Precautions from *Clinical Nursing Skills: Basic to Advanced Skills*, 9e by Sandra F. Smith, Donna J. Duell, Barbara C. Martin, Michelle Aebersold and Laura Gonzalez. Copyright © 2017 by Pearson Education

Figure 6–1 》 Standard precautions.

- Using personal protective equipment (PPE) such as a gown, face mask, goggles, and frequently wearing clean gloves when there is anticipation of coming into contact with blood or other body fluids.
- Keeping clean items in contact only with other clean items, and if a clean item touches a contaminated item, considering the item now contaminated.
- Using space as a barrier when in contact with patients with respiratory symptoms, covering mouth and nose if coughing or sneezing, and performing hand hygiene if in contact with respiratory secretions.
- Disposing of syringes and needles appropriately in sharps container.
- Handling soiled or unclean items such as linen, emesis basin, urinal, or bed pan with gloved hands and away from clothing to avoid contamination.

SKILL 6.1 Hand Hygiene: Performing

Hand hygiene generally applies to routine hand washing using plain or antimicrobial soap; a hand rub using an alcohol-based antiseptic; or a surgical scrub using antimicrobial soap, which can be followed by an alcohol-based hand scrub product. Evidence supports appropriate and frequent hand washing as a primary measure for reducing the risk of transmitting pathogens.

Delegation or Assignment

Hand washing is not a delegated task; it is part of standard precautions and a responsibility of all healthcare personnel. The UAPs are expected to perform hand hygiene appropriately and as frequently as needed to help control the transmission of pathogens. The nurse can assess and evaluate the UAP effectively washing the hands and, if needed, additional instruction and practice may be given.

Equipment

- Soap and water for cleaning visible dirty hands and alcohol-based hand sanitizers for reducing the number of microorganisms on the hands (CDC, 2016)
- A nail-cleaning tool, such as a file or orangewood stick (a basic tool for manicures to clean fingernails and push back cuticles)
- Running warm water
- Paper towels
- Trash basket

Preparation

- For cleaning hands with soap and water, be at a sink with soap available and disposable towels.
- For cleaning hands with an alcohol-based hand sanitizer, use a portable dispenser.

Procedure

SOAP AND WATER

1. Stand in front of but away from sink. **Rationale:** *Uniform should not touch sink to avoid contamination.*
2. Ensure that paper towel is hanging down from dispenser.
3. Turn on water using foot pedal or faucet so that flow is adequate, but not splashing ❶.
4. Adjust temperature to warm. **Rationale:** *Cold water does not facilitate lathering and cleaning; hot is damaging to skin.*
5. Wet hands under running water, keeping hands below elbow level ❷. **Rationale:** *Wet hands facilitate distribution of soap over entire skin surface.*
6. Place 5–10 mL (1–2 teaspoons) of liquid soap on hands ❸. Thoroughly distribute over hands. Soap should come from a dispenser, not bar soap. **Rationale:** *This prevents spread of microorganisms.*

(continued on next page)

SKILL 6.1 Hand Hygiene: Performing *(continued)*

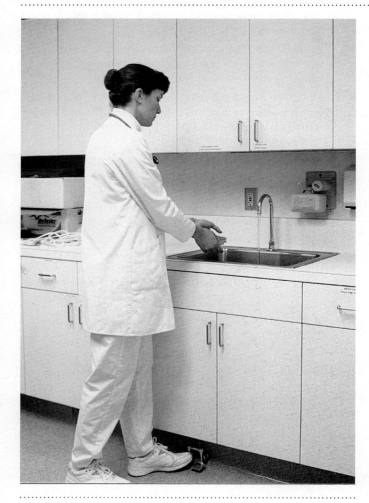

❶ Use foot pedals when available to prevent contamination of hands.

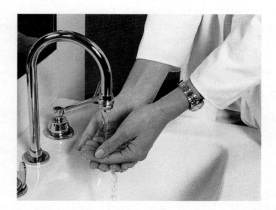

❷ To facilitate removal of pathogens, wet hands thoroughly before applying soap.

7. Rub vigorously, using a firm, circular motion, while keeping your fingers pointed down, lower than the wrists ❹. Start with each finger, then between fingers, then palm and back of hand. **Rationale:** *This creates friction on all surfaces.*

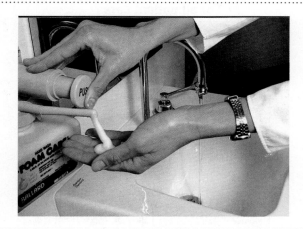

❸ Use a generous amount of soap and friction during hand washing procedure.

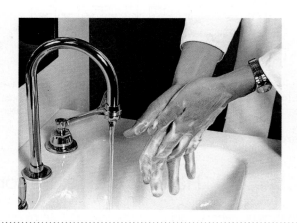

❹ Use a firm circular motion and keep fingers pointed down during hand washing to prevent contaminating arms.

8. Wash your hands for least 15 seconds before and after each direct contact with a patient or each use of patient care items to prevent spread of infection (CDC, 2013). **Rationale:** *Duration of washing is important to produce mechanical action and to allow antimicrobial products time to achieve desired effect.*

9. Clean under your fingernails with an orangewood stick. (This should be done at least at start of day and if hands are heavily contaminated.) Move rings up and down fingers to clean if rings are left on.

10. Rinse your hands under running water, keeping fingers pointed downward. **Rationale:** *This position prevents contamination of arms.*

11. Re-soap your hands, re-wash, and re-rinse if heavily contaminated.

12. Dry hands thoroughly with a paper towel, while keeping hands positioned with fingers pointing up. **Rationale:** *Moist hands tend to gather more microorganisms from the environment.*

SKILL 6.1 Hand Hygiene: Performing (*continued*)

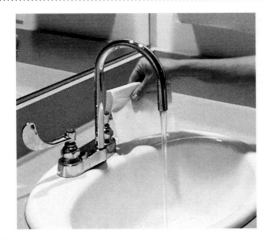

⑤ If foot pedal is not available, turn water faucet off using paper towel.

13. Turn off water faucet with dry paper towel, if not using foot pedal ⑤. **Rationale:** *This avoids recontaminating the hands.*
14. Restart procedure at step 5 if your hands touch the sink at any time between steps 5 and 13.

CAUTION! Antimicrobial soap or waterless agent should be used when identified resistant bacteria, colonization outbreaks, or hyperendemic infections are present with the exception of *Clostridium difficile* and *norovirus*, which are not killed by an alcohol-based gel.

---

or

ANTISEPTIC AGENTS (FOAMS OR GELS)

1. Check for soiled areas on hands and use waterless agent only if hands are clean. **Rationale:** *Hands soiled with dirt or organic matter require soap or detergents that contain antiseptic and water to effectively clean.*
2. Apply small amount of alcohol-based rub, foam, or gel (3–5 mL) on palm or hand ⑥.
3. Rub hands together vigorously, covering all surfaces, sides of hands and fingers. **Rationale:** *Failure to cover all surfaces can leave contaminated areas on the hands.*
4. Rub hands until dry—waterless agent will dry quickly and automatically without using a towel.
   Note: Disposable germicidal wipes are now available that are effective at killing 99.99% of harmful bacteria. These wipes are also effective at removing soil from hands because of natural friction when wiping. The wipes are made from cloth saturated with ethyl alcohol gel solution, free of fragrance and dye. These products are approved by the Environmental Protection Agency (EPA) for both hepatitis B and viruses.

For the technique of surgical hand antisepsis and scrub, see Skill 13.2 in Chapter 13.

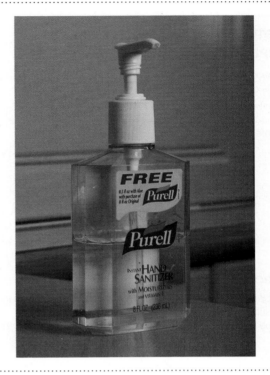

⑥ Waterless hand sanitizer kills 99.9% of the most common germs in 15 seconds.

EVIDENCE-BASED PRACTICE

Intervention Improves Hand Washing Practice

A 6-month program was run at Miami Children's Hospital to test the ability to improve hand washing compliance among healthcare providers. It involved an electronic monitoring system to confirm that providers engage in proper hand hygiene before patient contact. After healthcare providers apply soap or gel, they place their hands under wall-mounted sensors that verify that hand washing has taken place and send a signal to a specially designed badge worn by all staff and healthcare providers. When the clinician approaches the bedside, a bed monitor causes the badge to vibrate if appropriate hand hygiene has not taken place, thus reminding the healthcare provider to do hand washing before coming into contact with the patient. The system also generates customized reports to inform individualized provider education on hand hygiene as needed.

The program generated high levels of adherence to appropriate hand hygiene (94%). This led to significant reductions in the overall number of healthcare-associated infections (HAIs) (by 61%) and in non–*C. difficile* infections (91%). *C. difficile* HAIs were not meaningfully reduced, likely because these infections live on environmental surfaces for long periods of time; thus, they would have to be targeted by other types of infection prevention initiatives in addition to hand hygiene.

Source: Data from U.S. Department of Health & Human Services, Agency for Healthcare Research and Quality (2014).

(*continued on next page*)

SKILL 6.1 Hand Hygiene: Performing (*continued*)

Safety Considerations

COMPLIANCE STUDIES FOR HAND HYGIENE

- A study of 2800 opportunities for hand washing showed only a 48% compliance rate.

- Another study showed hands were washed for only 8.5–9.5 sec, although a minimum of 20 seconds is necessary to prevent spread of infection.

- Compliance with hand washing technique is higher among nurses than healthcare providers and other healthcare personnel; however, it is estimated to be only 30–50%.

Source: Data from Centers for Disease Control and Prevention (CDC) (2013).

>> Personal Protective Equipment (PPE) and Isolation Precautions

Expected Outcomes

1. Appropriate PPE and isolation measures are used for individual patients.
2. The transfer of microorganisms from healthcare workers or the environment to patients is prevented.
3. Cross-contamination among patients is prevented.
4. Hospital personnel and others are protected from contamination.

5. Appropriate equipment is provided and techniques for preventive measures are followed.
6. The incidence of healthcare-associated infections is reduced.
7. Immunosuppressed patients are prevented from acquiring healthcare-associated infections.

Isolation precautions help to prevent the transmission of infectious microorganisms by providing barriers between the microorganisms that can cause disease or illness and patients, healthcare personnel, visitors, and others in the healthcare environment. There are two major categories of isolation precautions: standard precautions and transmission-based precautions. Standard precautions are used whenever there is contact with any patients and all others. Performing hand hygiene frequently, wearing clean gloves when handling contaminated or unclean items, and wearing appropriate PPE are examples of basic prevention practices.

Transmission-based precautions are customized for specific pathogens in addition to standard precautions. One factor that determines which transmission-based precautions to use is based on how the pathogens are transmitted; direct or indirect contact, droplets, airborne, or vector-borne. For

example, *methicillin-resistant Staphylococcus aureus* (MRSA) and *C. difficile* are transmitted by contact, influenza and rubella are transmitted by droplets, and tuberculosis and varicella are airborne transmitted.

There are three transmission-based precautions: contact, airborne, and droplet precautions. For best practice in preventing infection transmission, each of these have specific guidelines about PPE, patient movement, air containment, and safety concerns. Consideration must be given to cleaning routines, placement of patients diagnosed with an infectious disease, transport of patients infected, individual point-of-care equipment, and availability and compliance using appropriate PPE. Visitors and others may need help in following isolation precautions generally posted outside the patient's room. Patients may need instructions concerning staying in their rooms as much as possible (**Table 6–1 >>**).

SKILL 6.2 Enteric Contact Precautions: Using

Enteric contact precautions are used for patients with active infection of pathogens such as *C. difficile*, rotavirus, or norovirus in the intestinal tract. The pathogens are transmitted in the patient's stool. Healthcare personnel must only perform soap and water hand washing instead of using an alcohol-based hand rub because the alcohol is not effective in removing the pathogens from the hands.

Delegation or Assignment

Donning (applying) ❶ and doffing (removing) ❷ PPE for enteric contact isolation is not a delegated task; it is following infection

control guidelines and appropriately using preventive precautions that are responsibilities of all healthcare personnel. The UAP is expected to apply and remove appropriate isolation attire each time entering or leaving an isolation room. The nurse can assess and evaluate the UAP's ability to complete this skill safely and, if needed, additional instruction and practice may be given.

Equipment

- Gown resistant to fluid penetration (as needed)
- Sterile or nonsterile gloves (usually nonsterile)

(*Text continues on p. 346.*)

TABLE 6–1 Types of Isolation Precautions

	Type of Precautions	When to Use These Types of Precautions	Recommended Precautions and PPE to Use
Tier One Standard Precautions	Standard precautions	■ Use with all patients. ■ Use when potential for contact with blood, excreted body fluids, mucous membranes, or open lesions	■ Hand hygiene ■ Gloves ■ Possibly gown, apron, mask, goggles, shoe covers
Tier Two Transmission-Based Precautions	Contact precautions	Pathogens transmitted by direct or indirect contact (touching), such as *methicillin-resistant Staphylococcus aureus* (MRSA) or vancomycin-resistant *Enterococcus* (VRE) in open wounds, diarrheal illnesses, RSV	■ Hand hygiene ■ Gloves, gown, and possibly goggles, apron
	Droplet precautions	Pathogens such as influenza, pertussis, respiratory syncytial virus infection (RSV), and bacterial meningitis transmitted by contact with tiny droplets of mucus or airway secretions from talking, coughing, and sneezing	■ Hand hygiene ■ Basic isolation mask and possibly gloves, gown, goggles
	Airborne precautions	Infectious disease pathogens such as tuberculosis (TB), chickenpox, measles transmitted through the air by droplet or dust particles	■ Hand hygiene ■ Fitted particulate respirator, such as an N95 respirator ■ Use a negative air pressure room. ■ Door is kept closed. ■ Possibly gloves, gown, goggles

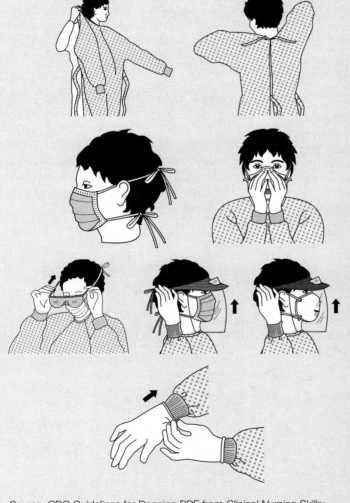

Source: CDC Guidelines for Donning PPE from *Clinical Nursing Skills: Basic to Advanced Skills*, 9e by Sandra F. Smith, Donna J. Duell, Barbara C. Martin, Michelle Aebersold and Laura Gonzalez. Copyright © 2017 by Pearson Education

❶ CDC guidelines for donning PPE.

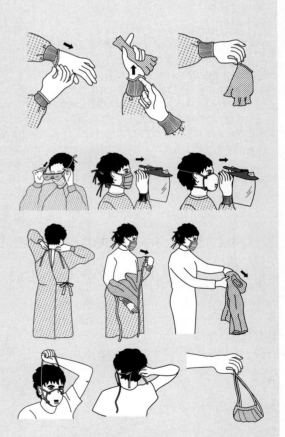

Source: CDC Guidelines for Safe Removal of PPE from *Clinical Nursing Skills: Basic to Advanced Skills*, 9e by Sandra F. Smith, Donna J. Duell, Barbara C. Martin, Michelle Aebersold and Laura Gonzalez. Copyright © 2017 by Pearson Education

❷ CDC guidelines for doffing PPE.

SKILL 6.2 Enteric Contact Precautions: Using *(continued)*

- Goggles or face shield (as needed)
- Isolation cart
- Appropriate isolation sign for patient's room door

Preparation

- Review healthcare provider's orders and the patient's MAR.
- Follow facility policies for isolation precautions.
- Determine PPE necessary when safely implementing interventions with the patient in isolation.
- Locate isolation cart with needed PPE next to the door of the patient's room.

CAUTION! If the nurse anticipates contact with a large volume of infective diarrhea or soiled sheets, a protective gown may be needed in addition to clean gloves.

Patient care items such as a stethoscope should not be used with a patient in Enteric Contact Precaution and then used with other patients unless properly cleaned and disinfected before reuse.

Procedure

1. Perform hand hygiene.
2. Don clean gloves and gown (if anticipate needing goggles or mask) at isolation cart.
3. Enter patient's room.
4. Introduce self to patient and parent. Verify the patient's identity using two identifiers. Explain to the patient and parent what you are going to do, why it is necessary, and how the patient can participate. Discuss how the results will be used in planning further care or treatments.
5. Use Contact Precautions for diapered or incontinent patients to control transmission of pathogens.
6. Provide for patient privacy.
7. Use assessment equipment located in the isolation room.
   - Use the thermometer, stethoscope, pulse oximeter, and sphygmomanometer with cuff in patient's room. Be sure to use an antiseptic wipe to clean ear tips of stethoscope before using it.
   - Call the results to a coworker to write down or write them on the dry erase board in the room so you can see results from doorway.
   - Replace equipment in appropriate area in room.
8. When procedure is complete, leave patient safe and comfortable.
9. Follow appropriate guidelines in doffing PPE items at the doorway and dispose of them in a red biohazard waste plastic bag after completing care.
10. Perform hand hygiene.
11. Complete documentation using forms, checklists, or electronic dropdown lists supplemented by nurse's notes or additional comments as appropriate.
12. Any child treated with isolation precautions should not be allowed in hospital playrooms to prevent transmission of pathogens. Any toys taken into an isolation room must be disinfected before being returned to the playroom.

SAMPLE DOCUMENTATION

[date] 0740 Remains in Enteric Contact Precautions. Moderate watery stool in diaper, light brown. Buttocks reddened, moisture barrier cream applied as ordered, new diaper applied. Mother has been in room throughout the night. Smiles when named called, no facial grimaces noted. *V. Jasper*

SKILL 6.3 Isolation, Attire: Donning and Doffing

Isolation precautions are used to prevent the transmission of pathogens. The three types of transmission-based precautions used are contact, droplet, and airborne. Isolation attire refers to the personal protective equipment (PPE) required for protection in each isolation type. PPE should be donned (or applied) and doffed (or removed) in specific sequences for best protection and prevention of contamination.

Delegation or Assignment

Donning and doffing isolation attire is not a delegated or assigned task; it is following infection control guidelines and appropriately using preventive precautions which are responsibilities of all healthcare personnel. The UAP is expected to apply and remove appropriate isolation attire each time entering or leaving an isolation room. The nurse can assess and evaluate the UAP's ability to complete this skill safely and, if needed, additional instruction and practice may be given.

Equipment

This list includes all major PPE options for isolation attire; specific attire depends on the type of exposure anticipated.

- Gown resistant to fluid penetration
- Sterile or nonsterile gloves (usually nonsterile)
- Goggles or face shield
- Basic isolation face mask or particulate respirator (N95)
- Head covering
- Shoe covers
- Isolation cart
- Appropriate isolation sign for door ❶

Preparation

- Review healthcare provider's orders and the patient's MAR.
- Follow facility policies for isolation precautions.
- Determine PPE necessary when safely implementing interventions with the patient in isolation.

SKILL 6.3 Isolation, Attire: Donning and Doffing (*continued*)

DROPLET PRECAUTIONS
(in addition to Standard Precautions)

Visitors, Report to Nurse's Station Before Entering Room

PRECAUCIONES de CONTAMINACIÓN por GOTAS

Visitantes – Por Favor de Reportarse a la Estación de Enfermeras Antes de Entrar al Cuarto

1. Wash hands when you enter and leave room.
2. Mask required when entering room.
3. Limit the movement/transport of patients from room to essential purposes only. During transport, minimize the spread of droplets by placing a surgical mask on the patients, if possible.

---

❶ Droplet isolation precautions.

CAUTION! Eye protection such as goggles, eye shield, or face shield should be worn for potential spray or splash of body fluids including blood and respiratory secretions. Personal eyeglasses and contact lenses should not be considered adequate eye protection.

- Locate isolation cart with needed PPE next to the door of the patient's room.
- Isolation precautions can increase an already stressful situation for a hospitalized child.

Younger children have limited cognitive abilities to understand the implications of isolation. The presence of people in gowns and masks is particularly frightening for them. To help decrease their fears, preparation is important. Letting the children see and play with the equipment lessens some of the anxiety. Healthcare workers should introduce themselves to the child before donning a mask. Frequent visits to the child can also lessen the fear and loneliness associated with isolation.

- Family members or others may want to visit the patient in isolation. Brochures and multi-language information sheets can help the patient understand what is happening and what the visitors can do to help be safe. Hand hygiene can be stressed to the patient, visitors, and also staff assigned to the patient in isolation. Visitors with children can be encouraged to check with the nurses' station first about safety of exposing the child to a contagious infectious disease like chickenpox or a wound that is infected with *S. aureus,* which the child can be instructed not to touch.

Procedure

DONNING ATTIRE ❷

Don necessary PPE outside the patient's room (use anteroom as available) ❸. Most facilities have portable isolation carts that are stocked with PPE and are available to locate outside the room of a patient on isolation precautions.

1. Complete hand hygiene.
2. If you need to wear a head covering and/or shoe covers, apply them at this step.
3. Take gown from isolation cart or cupboard. Put on a new gown each time you enter an isolation room.
4. Hold gown so that opening is in back when you are wearing the gown.
5. Put gown on by placing one arm at a time through sleeves. Pull gown up and over your shoulders.
6. Wrap gown around your back, tying strings at your neck.
7. Wrap gown around your waist, making sure your back is completely covered. Tie strings around your waist.
8. Don mask or respirator if indicated. **Rationale:** *Mask is required if there is a risk of splashing fluids.*
9. Don goggles, face shield, or mask, if indicated.
10. Don clean gloves and pull gloves over gown wristlets. **Rationale:** *This prevents contamination of exposed skin.*

DOFFING ATTIRE ❹

Doff PPE, except for a respirator when worn, at the doorway of the patient's room when leaving the room or in the anteroom. Discard disposable items in waste container and place other items in designated reprocessing container. After leaving the patient's room and closing the door, remove the respirator and discard in waste container.

1. Untie gown waist strings.
2. Remove gloves and dispose of them in garbage bag.
3. Next, untie neck strings, bringing them around your shoulders so that gown is partially off your shoulders.
4. Using your dominant hand and grasping the clean part of the wristlet, pull sleeve wristlet over your nondominant hand. Use your nondominant hand to pull sleeve wristlet over your dominant hand.
5. Grasp outside of gown through the sleeves at shoulders. Pull gown down over your arms.
6. Hold both gown shoulders in one hand. Carefully draw your other hand out of gown, turning arm of gown inside out. Repeat this procedure with your other arm.
7. Hold gown away from your body. Fold gown up, inside out.
8. Discard gown in appropriate place.
9. Remove goggles and/or mask and place in receptacle.
10. Remove head covering and/or shoe covers if applicable.
11. Complete hand hygiene. **Rationale:** *This prevents cross-infection to other patients.*

CAUTION! Some isolation gowns do not tie at the neck; they slip over the head. When removing these gowns, pull shoulders forward to loosen the Velcro at the neck area. Remove gown in the same manner as you would if tied at the neck.

(*continued on next page*)

SKILL 6.3 Isolation, Attire: Donning and Doffing (continued)

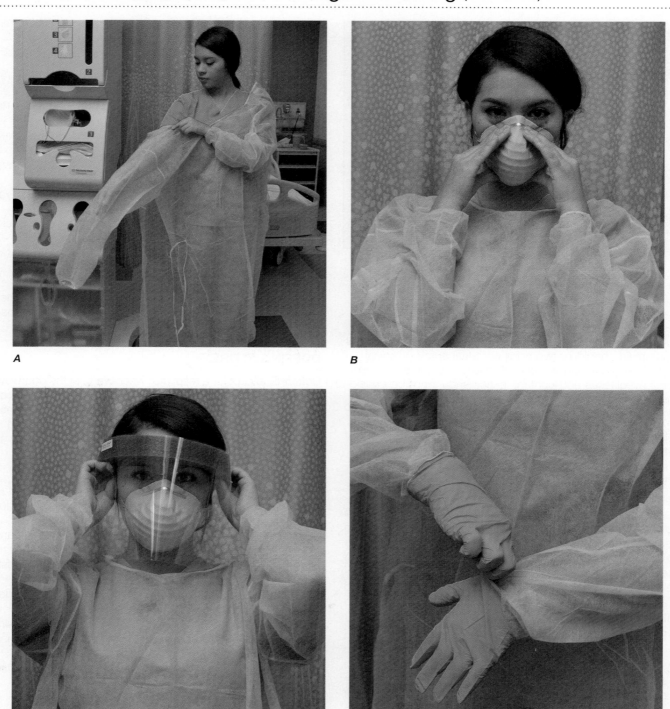

A

B

C

D

*Sources: **A–D,** Ronald May/Pearson Education, Inc.*

❷ ***A,*** Put on the gown; ***B,*** Don the mask; ***C,*** Put on the face shield; ***D,*** Put on gloves.

SKILL 6.3 Isolation, Attire: Donning and Doffing (*continued*)

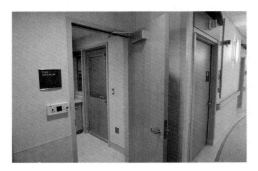

Source: Rick Brady/Pearson Education, Inc.

③ View from anteroom to patient's isolation room with directional airflow negative pressure ventilation system.

Patient Teaching

- All aspects of standard precautions and PPE apply equally in the clinic, home, or long-term care setting.
- Ensure that the supply of gloves, gowns, masks, and eyewear is adequate.
- Ensure that procedures are in place for removal and disposal of used materials.
- Teach the patient and family appropriate aspects of standard precautions.

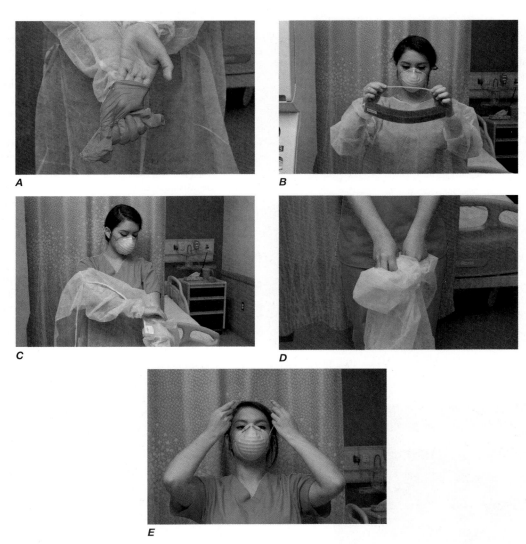

Sources: ***A–D,*** Ronald May/Pearson Education, Inc., ***E,*** Rick Brady/Pearson Education, Inc.

④ ***A,*** Remove gloves. Remove first glove by pulling it off so glove turns inside out. Place rolled-up glove in palm of second hand and remove second glove; ***B,*** Remove shield, taking care to hold it by the ties and not to touch the bottom of the shield; ***C,*** Remove gown by first untying string at waist or neck, and take it off by pulling down from the shoulders; ***D,*** Turn the gown inside out and pull arms out as you pull the gown off; ***E,*** Take off mask, holding it by the ties; be careful not to touch the bottom of the mask.

SKILL 6.4 Isolation, Patient and Others: Caring for

Isolation provides a controlled environment with specific precautions used to prevent infectious patients from infecting others. Isolation precautions provide protection for patients, healthcare workers, family members, and visitors.

Delegation or Assignment

Care for patients in isolation can be delegated or assigned to the UAP within the UAP job description. The UAP is expected to apply and remove appropriate isolation attire each time entering or leaving an isolation room. The nurse gives the UAP any instructions specific to the patient or procedure. The nurse remains responsible for the assessment, interpretation of abnormal findings, and determination of appropriate responses. Note that state laws for UAPs vary, so this task might be assigned to the UAP rather than delegated.

Equipment

This list includes all major personal protective equipment (PPE) options for isolation attire; specific attire depends on the type of exposure anticipated.

- Liquid soap
- Antibacterial gel for hand hygiene
- Disposable clean gloves
- Disposable apron or gown resistant to fluid penetration
- Goggles or face shield
- Clean, basic isolation mask or particulate respirator as appropriate
- Shoe covers or head covering as appropriate
- Thermometer capable of oral and rectal routes with sheaths to stay in isolation room as available or disposable thermometer
- Water-soluble lubricant
- Antimicrobial wipes
- Hypoallergenic tape (remains in isolation room)
- Sphygmomanometer with cuff to stay in isolation room
- Stethoscope to stay in isolation room
- Pulse oximeter
- Paper cups
- Isolation cart ❶ with PPE and supply of red isolation bags with the words "BIOHAZARDOUS WASTE" on them.
- Appropriate isolation sign for door

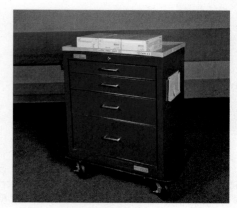

Source: Ronald May/Pearson Education, Inc.

❶ Place isolation cart outside patient's door when cart is required.

Preparation

- Review healthcare provider's orders and the patient's MAR.
- Follow facility policies for isolation precautions.
- Determine PPE necessary to safely implement interventions with the patient in isolation.
- Locate the isolation cart with PPE next to the door of the patient's room.
- Gather necessary equipment and supplies.

Procedure

1. Perform hand hygiene.
2. Don specific PPE at isolation cart for type of isolation precautions needed; enter patient's room.
3. Introduce self to patient and verify the patient's identity using two identifiers. Explain to the patient what you are going to do, why it is necessary, and how the patient can participate. Discuss how the results will be used in planning further care or treatments.
4. Observe appropriate infection control, including PPE, for the specific type of isolation precautions.
   - Perform hand hygiene before and after patient care and after disposing of soiled materials.
   - Don disposable gloves for any procedure and double gloves if tearing is likely during the procedure.
   - Don disposable gown or apron to protect clothing from becoming soiled.
   - Put on mask and protective eyewear if splattering is anticipated during the procedure (e.g., suctioning, wound irrigations).

CAUTION! If staff member has any type of open wound or weeping dermatitis, he or she should follow facility policy about providing care to patients in isolation precautions until condition is resolved.

---

5. Provide for patient privacy.
6. Use extraordinary care to avoid puncture wounds with needles and other sharp objects.
   - If puncture occurs, bleed wound and wash with soap and water.
   - Notify supervisor immediately and fill out unusual occurrence report.
7. Use disposable meal tray and food containers as available.
8. Have housekeeper clean spills of blood and body fluids with disinfectant soap per facility policy. Replace isolation bags in waste containers to keep them from overflowing.
9. Don't touch environmental surfaces except as necessary. Be mindful not to touch your face or adjust PPE with contaminated gloves.
10. Use assessment equipment located in the isolation room.
    - Use the thermometer, stethoscope, pulse oximeter, and sphygmomanometer with cuff in patient's room. Be sure to use an antiseptic wipe to clean ear tips of stethoscope before using it.

SKILL 6.4 Isolation, Patient and Others: Caring for (continued)

- Call the results to a coworker to write down or write them on the dry erase board in the room so you can see results from doorway.
  - Replace equipment in appropriate area in room.
11. When procedure is completed, leave the patient safe and comfortable.
12. Follow appropriate guidelines in doffing PPE items at the doorway and dispose of them in a red biohazard waste plastic bag after completing care.
13. Perform hand hygiene.
14. Complete documentation using forms, checklists, or electronic dropdown lists supplemented by nurse's notes or additional comments as appropriate.

Patient Teaching

Infection Precautions in the Home

- Wear disposable gloves when handling body fluids, linens, or other objects contaminated with body fluids.
- Use disposable gowns or aprons to protect clothing from becoming soiled.
- Use disposable mask for protection as appropriate.
- Follow appropriate care for linens and laundry:
  - Clothing or linen that is soiled with blood or body fluids should be stored in a plastic bag and washed separately with very hot water, detergent, and bleach.
  - Wear disposable gloves when touching soiled clothes or linen.
- Control the environmental temperature and airflow in the home (especially if patient has an airborne pathogen).
- Determine the advisability of visitors and family members in proximity to an infected patient in the home, especially if the visitors or family members are ill or have a depressed immune function.
- Perform proper hand hygiene (e.g., before eating, after toileting, before and after any home care treatment, after touching any body substances such as wound drainage) and related hygienic measures to all family members.
- Perform measures for disposing of trash.
  - Flush body wastes down the toilet.
  - Discard dressings, diapers, linen savers, or any materials soiled with secretions in a plastic bag. Discard into the regular trash.
- Use antimicrobial soaps and effective disinfectants.
- Reusable equipment and supplies should be washed using soap and water, and disinfected with a chlorine bleach solution.
- Discuss the signs and symptoms of infection and when to contact a healthcare provider.
- Keep medical supplies in a clean, dry location. If refrigeration is required, place medications in sealed plastic storage bag.
- Remind person with infection to avoid coughing, sneezing, or breathing directly on others. Cover the mouth and nose to prevent the transmission of airborne microorganisms.
- Have current proper immunizations of all family members.

Lifespan Considerations

NEWBORN, INFANT, AND CHILD

The majority of childhood infections are caused by viruses. In some cases, severe and even life-threatening infections occur. Considerations related to children include the following:

- Newborns and infants may not be able to respond to infections due to an underdeveloped immune system. As a result, in the first few months of life, infections may not be associated with typical signs and symptoms (e.g., a newborn or an infant with an infection may not have a fever).
- Newborns are born with some naturally acquired immunity transferred from the mother across the placenta.
- Breastfed newborns and infants enjoy higher levels of immunity against infections than formula-fed newborns and infants.
- Children who are immunocompromised (e.g., leukemia, HIV) or have a chronic health condition (e.g., cystic fibrosis, sickle cell disease, congenital heart disease) need extra precautions to prevent exposure to infectious agents.

OLDER ADULTS

Normal aging may predispose older adults to increased risk of infection and delayed healing. Anatomical and physiological agents that are protective when an individual is younger often change in structure and function with increasing age and then provide a decrease in their protective ability. Changes take place in the skin, respiratory tract, gastrointestinal system, kidneys, and immune system. Special considerations for older adults include the following:

- Nutrition may be poor in older adults. Certain components, especially adequate protein, are necessary to build up and maintain the immune system.
- Diabetes mellitus, which occurs more frequently in older adults, increases the risk of infection and delayed healing.
- The normal inflammatory response is delayed. Instead of displaying the redness, swelling, and fever usually associated with infections, atypical symptoms such as confusion and disorientation, agitation, incontinence, falls, lethargy, and general fatigue are often seen first.

Nursing interventions to promote prevention include the following:

- Provide and teach ways to improve nutritional status.
- Use strict aseptic technique (especially in healthcare facilities).
- Encourage older adults to have regular immunizations for flu and pneumonia.
- Be alert to subtle atypical signs of infection and act quickly to diagnose and treat.

SKILL 6.5 Isolation, Double-Bagging: Using

There are many types of large plastic bags that can be used to safely transport equipment, garbage, and contaminated items from an isolation environment to be disposed of properly or cleaned and disinfected adequately to be reusable. Some healthcare facilities use double-bagging, or putting one bag into another bag, for security and safety of containing contents while moving them. Other healthcare facilities use single, large, sturdy, red bags that are impervious to moisture and have the words "BIO-HAZARDOUS WASTE" on them. All facilities will double bag any bag that has a tear or is contaminated on the outside of the bag.

Delegation or Assignment

Double-bagging isolation waste or equipment may be delegated or assigned to the UAP. The UAP is expected to apply and remove appropriate isolation attire each time entering or leaving an isolation room. The nurse gives the UAP any instructions specific to the patient or procedure. The nurse remains responsible for the assessment, interpretation of abnormal findings, and determination of appropriate responses. Note that state laws for UAPs vary, so this task might be assigned to the UAP rather than delegated.

Equipment

- Disposable gloves
- Waste receptacle, rigid and puncture-proof
- Germicide
- Isolation cart
- Appropriate isolation sign for patient's room door

Preparation

- Review healthcare provider's orders and the patient's MAR.
- Follow facility policies for isolation precautions.
- Determine PPE necessary when safely implementing interventions with the patient in isolation.
- Locate isolation cart with needed PPE and supply of special, large, sturdy, isolation red bags next to the door of the patient's room.

Procedure

1. Perform hand hygiene and don clean gloves. Some nurses double glove to provide one more barrier layer.
2. Dispose of wastes contaminated with blood or body fluids.
   - Place waste products in impenetrable, heavy-duty plastic bag inside waste receptacle. Double bag if integrity of bag is compromised.
   - Remove gloves by rolling inside out (so contaminated side is on inside) and drop into plastic bag.
   - Seal plastic bag with tie.
   - Discard in patient's trash.
   - Perform hand hygiene with soap and water or germicide.
3. Dispose of body wastes, such as urine, feces, respiratory secretions, vomitus, and blood, by flushing them down the toilet. (This is true whether the toilet empties into a septic tank or a sewage system.)
4. Dispose of needles and sharp objects.
   - Do *not* remove needle from syringe or bend, break, clip, or recap after use.
   - Drop entire disposable safety syringe intact into rigid, puncture-proof receptacle provided by facility.
   - Complete hand hygiene.
5. Discard other trash.
   - Place in plastic bag.
   - Discard in patient's trash.

Note: Clothes and bedding do not need to be destroyed. They are laundered separately in hot water with a 10% bleach solution added to the detergent in the washer.

CAUTION! All items contaminated with blood, exudates, or other body fluids should be considered a possible risk of transmission of infectious diseases such as HIV or hepatitis B. These items should be disposed of by incineration, if possible. Use mechanisms for disposal of waste into normal trash only when incineration is not available.

SKILL 6.6 Isolation, Equipment, Specimens: Removing

Healthcare personnel use PPE as a barrier against infectious disease transmission. Standard precautions such as hand washing helps limit transmission of pathogens from patient to patient or patient to nurse. When it is moved from one patient to another, equipment also needs to be washed and decontaminated to prevent organisms such as *E. coli, S. aureus,* and *C. difficile* from being transmitted from patient to patient. These organisms can live on dry inanimate surfaces for many days and even months. Infection control must include equipment in the environment of patient care areas.

Delegation or Assignment

Removing equipment and specimens from isolation room can be delegated or assigned to the UAP. The UAP is expected to apply and remove appropriate isolation attire each time entering or leaving an isolation room. The nurse can request the UAP to report patient observations to the nurse for follow-up. Assessment and evaluation remain the responsibility of the nurse. Note that state laws for UAPs vary, so this task might be assigned to the UAP rather than delegated.

Equipment

- Antimicrobial agent and articles needed to wash equipment
- Red isolation bags with the words "BIOHAZARDOUS WASTE" on them
- Laundry bag
- Isolation cart
- Appropriate isolation sign for patient's room door

For Removing Specimen Only

- Appropriate specimen container for type of specimen being collected

SKILL 6.6 Isolation, Equipment, Specimens: Removing *(continued)*

Preparation

- Review healthcare provider's orders and the patient's medical record.
- Follow facility policies for isolation precautions.
- Determine PPE necessary when safely implementing interventions with the patient in isolation.
- Locate isolation cart with needed PPE and supply of special, large, sturdy, labeled BIOHAZARDOUS WASTE red bags next to the door of the patient's room.
- Gather antimicrobial agent and articles needed to wash equipment before bagging it to remove from isolation room if appropriate.

Procedure

1. Perform hand hygiene and don gloves.
2. At isolation cart, don PPE specific for type of isolation precautions needed; enter patient's room.
3. Introduce self to patient and verify the patient's identity using two identifiers. Explain to the patient what you are going to do, why it is necessary, and how the patient can participate. Discuss how the results will be used in planning further care or treatments.
4. Observe appropriate infection control, including PPE, for the specific type of isolation precautions.
   - Perform hand hygiene before and after patient care and after disposing of soiled materials.
   - Don disposable gloves for any procedure and double gloves if tearing is likely during the procedure or collecting the equipment and waste.
   - Don disposable gown or apron as appropriate to protect clothing from becoming soiled.
   - Put on mask and protective eyewear if splattering is anticipated during the procedure (e.g., suctioning, wound irrigations).
5. Provide for patient privacy.
6. Use extraordinary care to avoid puncture wounds with needles and other sharp objects.
   - If puncture occurs, bleed wound and wash with soap and water.
   - Notify supervisor immediately and fill out unusual occurrence report.

REMOVING CONTAMINATED EQUIPMENT AND WASTE

7. Perform hand hygiene and don gloves. Wash equipment with an antimicrobial agent ❶. **Rationale:** *Washing is preferred to spraying in order to ensure all surfaces are cleaned.*
8. Place equipment and trash in red isolation bags ❷ ❸, or follow facility policy. Double bag all bags when contamination on the outside of them or tears are noted.
   - Disposable glass: Place in isolation bag separate from burnable trash for disposal.
   - Garbage: Place in isolation bag for disposal as burnable trash.
   - Reusable equipment such as procedure trays: Bag separately and return to central supply room (CSR).

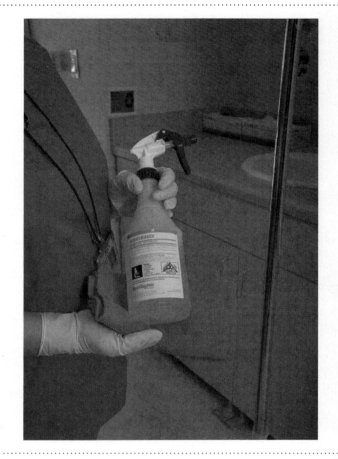

❶ Wash isolation equipment with antimicrobial agent.

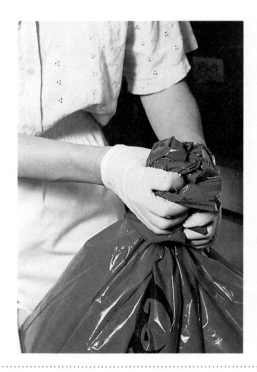

❷ Close bag securely and label contents, if necessary.

(continued on next page)

SKILL 6.6 Isolation, Equipment, Specimens: Removing *(continued)*

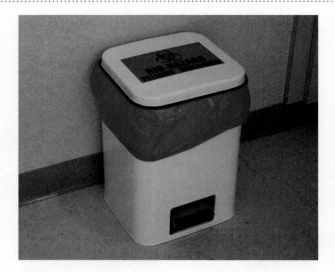

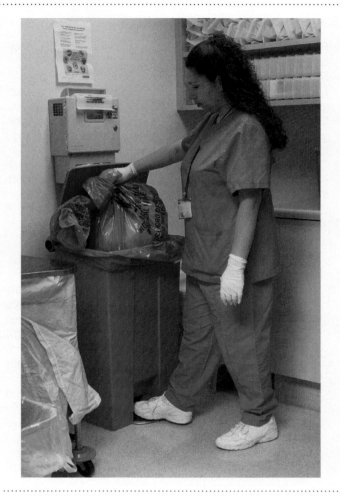

③ Place red biohazard bag in specified area for disposal.

> **Rationale:** *Appropriate separation of equipment from isolation room alerts central supply staff that it is contaminated and special handling needs to be carried out.*

- Rubber and plastic items: Bag items separately and return to CSR for gas sterilization.
- Dishes: Require no special precautions unless contaminated with infected material; then bag, label, and return to kitchen.
- Plastic or paper dishes: Dispose of these items in burnable trash bins.
- Soiled linens: Place in laundry bag, and send to separate area of laundry room for special care.
- Food and liquids: Dispose of these items by putting them in the toilet—flush thoroughly.
- Needles and syringes: Do not recap needles; place in puncture-resistant container.
- Sphygmomanometer and stethoscope: Disinfect using the appropriate cleaning protocol based on the infective agent.
- Thermometers: Dispose of electronic probe covers with burnable trash. If probe or machine is contaminated, clean with appropriate disinfectant for infective agent. If reusable thermometers are used, disinfect with appropriate solution.

9. Replace all bags ④, such as linen bag and waste bag, in appropriate container in room. Proceed to step 10 below.

or

REMOVING A SPECIMEN

7. Mark a specimen container with the patient's name, type of specimen, and the word "isolation" before entering the isolation room.
8. Perform hand hygiene, don appropriate PPE, including gloves. Collect specimen.
9. Place specimen container in a clean plastic biohazard bag ⑤ outside the room. **Rationale:** *Use clear bags so that laboratory personnel can see the specimen easily.*
10. When procedure is completed, leave patient safe and comfortable.

④ Set up new biohazard bag for continued use in patient's room.

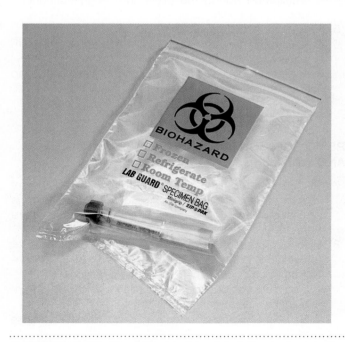

⑤ Biohazard bag for transportation of specimens from isolation room.

SKILL 6.6 Isolation, Equipment, Specimens: Removing (*continued*)

11. Follow appropriate guidelines in doffing PPE items at the doorway and dispose of them in a red biohazard waste plastic bag after completing care or preparing equipment to be removed.
12. Perform hand hygiene.
13. Send specimen to laboratory with appropriate laboratory request form, or take equipment and waste to the decontamination area of central supply room.
14. Complete necessary documentation using forms, checklists, or electronic dropdown lists supplemented by nurse's notes or additional comments as appropriate.

> **SAMPLE DOCUMENTATION**
>
> [date] 1625 Remains in contact isolation. Able to void for needed specimen. Urine in labeled container, deep amber with sedimentation noted, 35 mL. Specimen container placed in biohazard bag and sent to lab. Tolerated without incident. *H. Yarr*

SKILL 6.7 Isolation, Transporting Patient Outside Room

Sometimes patients in isolation need to be transported to other departments for diagnostic tests or medical therapies. PPE appropriate for the type of isolation precautions used with the patient will help limit exposure during transportation. For example, a basic isolation face mask will be worn by the patient with airborne isolation precautions and gloves will be worn by the transporters when moving a patient with contact isolation precautions.

Delegation or Assignment

Assisting the patient being transported from an isolation room to another department in the hospital may be delegated or assigned to the UAP. The nurse gives the UAP instructions specific to the type of PPE needed for protection during transport. The nurse can assess and evaluate the UAP's ability to complete this skill safely and, if needed, additional instruction may be given. Note that state laws for UAPs vary, so this task might be assigned to the UAP rather than delegated.

Equipment

- Transport vehicle (wheelchair or stretcher)
- Two bath blankets
- Basic isolation face mask for patient if needed
- Clean gloves
- Gown resistant to fluid penetration if needed
- Isolation cart

Preparation

- Review healthcare provider's orders and the patient's medical record.
- Follow facility policies for isolation precautions.
- Determine PPE necessary for specific isolation precautions.
- Locate isolation cart with needed PPE and supply of special large, sturdy red bags that are impervious to moisture with the words "BIOHAZARDOUS WASTE" on them next to the door of the patient's room.
- Appropriate isolation sign for patient's room door

Procedure

1. Perform hand hygiene.
2. Don recommended PPE for isolation precautions with patient.

3. Enter patient's room, introduce self and verify the patient's identity using two identifiers. Explain to the patient what you are going to do, why it is necessary, and how the patient will be transported to the other department. Discuss how the results will be used in planning further care or treatments.
4. If patient is being transported from a respiratory isolation room, instructions are given to wear a mask for the entire time out of isolation ❶. **Rationale:** *This prevents the spread of airborne microbes.*

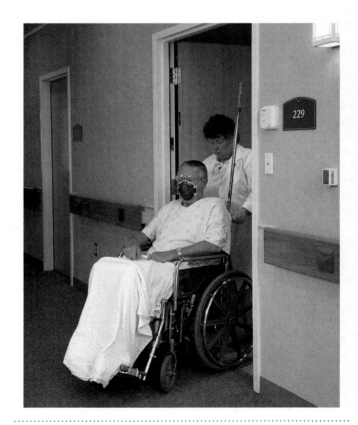

❶ Place surgical mask on patient if there is a need to transport the patient outside room.

(*continued on next page*)

SKILL 6.7 Isolation, Transporting Patient Outside Room (*continued*)

5. Cover the transport vehicle with a bath blanket if there is a chance of soiling when transporting a patient who has a draining wound or diarrhea.
6. Assist patient into transport vehicle. Cover patient with a bath blanket.
7. Tell receiving department what type of isolation patient needs and what precautions hospital personnel should follow.
8. When the patient returns to room, perform hand hygiene and don appropriate PPE.
9. Assist patient to bed or chair as patient desires.
10. Remove bath blanket and handle as contaminated linen.
11. Instruct others who helped transport patient to remove PPE and complete hand hygiene before they leave the area.
12. Wipe down transportation vehicle with an antimicrobial solution after every use.

13. Remove PPE and perform hand hygiene. Apply fresh PPE.
14. Move cleaned transportation vehicle out of room.
15. Leave patient safe and comfortable.
16. Remove PPE and discard in receptacle. Perform hand hygiene.

SAMPLE DOCUMENTATION

[date] 0730 Transported via blanket-covered wheelchair and basic isolation mask to x-ray department. X-ray dept. notified of need for using droplet precautions. Tolerated transporting to x-ray dept. without incident. *H. Grean*

SKILL 6.8 PPE, Clean Gloves: Donning and Doffing

Wearing clean gloves is effective in preventing contamination of healthcare workers' hands and in reducing transmission of pathogens in healthcare environments, but they do not provide complete protection against hand contamination such as with a needle stick. Be aware that glove use *does not* modify hand hygiene indications or replace hand hygiene actions (rubbing hands with alcohol-based product or washing hands with soap and water).

Delegation or Assignment

Wearing clean gloves as PPE is not a delegated task; it is part of preventive infection control behaviors and a responsibility of all healthcare personnel. The UAP is expected to apply and remove gloves each time there is an anticipation of coming in contact with blood-borne pathogens, body fluids, nonintact skin, and potentially infectious material. The nurse gives the UAP any instructions specific to the patient or procedure. The nurse remains responsible for the assessment, interpretation of abnormal findings, and determination of appropriate responses.

Equipment

- Clean gloves
- Trash receptacle

Preparation

- Review healthcare provider's orders and the patient's medical record.
- Many healthcare personnel carry an extra pair of clean gloves in their pocket, so they are readily available when needed.
  - Don a new pair of gloves:
    - After hand hygiene and for each patient
    - When anticipating contact with blood or another body fluid, regardless of the existence of sterile conditions
    - During contact precautions

- Doff gloves being worn:
  - As soon as gloves are damaged or damage is suspected
  - When contact with body fluid, nonintact skin, and mucous membrane has ended
  - When contact with a single patient and the surroundings or a contaminated body site on a patient has ended.

- Use guidelines to help decide the correct size of clean gloves to wear. Clean gloves come in sizes XS (extra small), S (small), M (medium), L (large), XL (extra-large), and XXL (extra extra-large) and vary slightly between manufacturers. Size is important because if the glove size is too small, it will constrict the fingers; if the size is too large, the extra glove material may get in the way of dexterity. There are size charts available from manufacturers to help in deciding which size glove to use. Measure the hand at the base of the fingers (over the knuckles), around the palm.

Procedure

DONNING GLOVES

1. Complete hand hygiene ❶. **Rationale:** *Donning gloves with unclean hands can transfer microorganisms outside gloves.*
2. Remove glove from glove receptacle ❷.
3. Hold glove at wrist edge and slip fingers into openings. Pull glove up to wrist.
4. Place gloved hand under wrist edge of second glove and slip fingers into opening.

DOFFING GLOVES

5. Remove glove by pulling off, touching only outside of glove at cuff, so that glove turns inside out.
6. Place rolled-up glove in palm of second hand.
7. Remove second glove by slipping one finger under glove edge and pulling down and off so that glove turns inside out. Both gloves are removed as a unit.

SKILL 6.8 PPE, Clean Gloves: Donning and Doffing *(continued)*

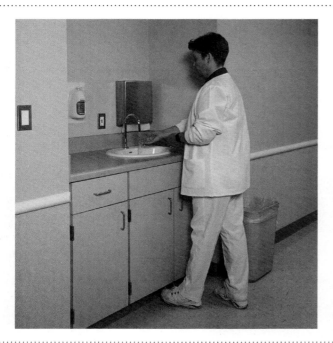

❶ Wash your hands or complete hand hygiene before donning gloves.

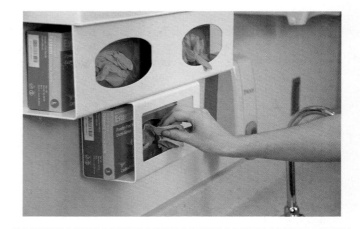

❷ Remove glove from dispenser.

8. Dispose of gloves in proper container, not at bedside ❸.
9. Complete hand hygiene.

CAUTION! Ungloved hands should not touch anything that is moist coming from a body surface. The moisture coming from a body surface should be considered potentially contaminated.

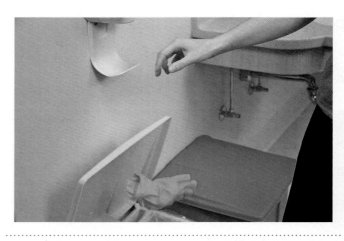

❸ Dispose of gloves in proper container, not at bedside. Complete hand hygiene.

SKILL 6.9 PPE, Face Masks: Donning and Doffing

There are two types of face masks worn for protection from liquid and airborne particles contaminating the face. One type is the basic isolation mask that is loose-fitting, covers the nose and mouth, and is secured with ear loops, elastic bands, or ties at the back of the head. This face mask creates a physical barrier between the mouth and nose and potential contaminants in the environmental air or splashes and large-particle droplets. The other type of face mask is actually a respirator which provides respiratory protection against airborne pathogens. To provide efficient filtration of airborne particles, every healthcare worker has to be fitted for the respirator to have the proper size needed in order to provide a tight seal over the nose and mouth. A commonly used respirator for airborne isolation is the N95 respirator, which means it will block at least 95% of very small particles.

Delegation or Assignment

Donning and doffing face masks is not a delegated task; it is part of infection control behaviors and a responsibility of all healthcare personnel. The UAP is expected to apply and remove a face mask for airborne isolation precautions. The nurse can assess and evaluate the UAP's ability to complete this skill safely and, if needed, additional instruction and practice may be given.

Equipment

- Clean, basic isolation face mask, particulate filter respirator mask (N95 mask), or contained air purifying respirators (CAPR), depending on precautions necessary
- Isolation cart
- Isolation precautions sign for patient's room door

Preparation

- Review healthcare provider's orders and the patient's medical record.

(continued on next page)

SKILL 6.9 PPE, Face Masks: Donning and Doffing (*continued*)

- Follow facility policies for isolation precautions.
- Ensure room designated airborne infection isolation room (AIIR) provides negative pressure in the room and has direct exhaust of air from the room to outside the building or recirculation of air using a HEPA filter for air to flow through before returning to air circulation.
- Determine PPE necessary when safely implementing interventions with the patient in isolation.
- Have an isolation cart with needed PPE and supply of special large, sturdy isolation red bags placed next to the door of the patient's room.
- A N95 or HEPA (high-efficiency particulate air) respirator mask is recommended for airborne infectious diseases, for example, influenza or suspected or confirmed multidrug-resistant tuberculosis.

Procedure

DONNING A FACE MASK OR RESPIRATOR

1. Perform hand hygiene.
2. Obtain face mask or respirator from box.

Face Mask ❶

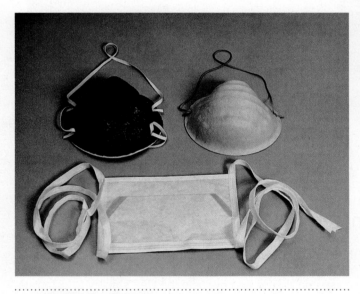

❶ Sample masks used for isolation protocol.

3. Determine which side of the mask is the top (the side that has a stiff bendable edge and molds to the shape of the nose) and which side is the front (the colored side of the mask is usually the front and should face away from you).
4. Position mask to cover your nose and mouth. Bend nose bar so that it conforms over bridge of your nose.
5. If you are using a mask with string ties, tie top strings on top of your head to prevent slipping. If you are using a cone-shaped mask, tie top strings over your ears. If you are using a mask with elastic bands, hold the mask to nose level and pull the top band over your head so it rests over the crown of your head. Pull the bottom band over your head so that it rests at the nape of your neck.

6. Tie bottom strings around your neck to secure mask over your mouth. There should be no gaps between the mask and your face.
7. *Important*: Change mask every 30 minutes or sooner if it becomes damp. **Rationale:** *Effectiveness is greatly reduced after 30 minutes or if mask is moist. Go to step 8 below.*

or

Respirator ❷

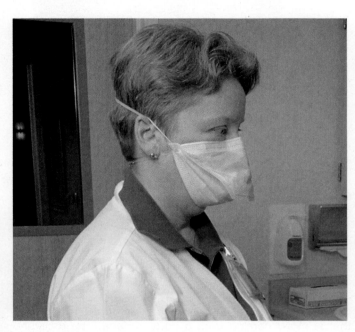

❷ Particulate filter respirator mask must be airtight.

3. Hold the respirator in your hands with the nosepiece toward your fingertips.
4. Position the respirator over your mouth and nose.
5. Pull the strap over your head.
6. Pull the shorter bottom strap over your head, below your ears.
7. Respirators should be replaced whenever they are damaged, soiled, or causing noticeably increased breathing resistance.

DOFFING A FACE MASK OR RESPIRATOR

8. Complete hand hygiene before removing mask or respirator.
9. If protective eyewear such as goggles or face shield are worn when there is a risk of splashes or sprays from blood, secretions, excretions, or body fluids, eyewear is removed before taking off mask or respirator.
10. Avoid touching the front of the mask or respirator.
11. To remove mask or respirator untie lower strings first, or slip bottom elastic band off and then the top band without touching mask or respirator. **Rationale:** *Only ties, bands, or loops are considered clean.*
12. Discard mask or respirator in a trash container.
13. Complete hand hygiene.

SKILL 6.9 PPE, Face Masks: Donning and Doffing (continued)

Safety Considerations

NEUTROPENIC PRECAUTIONS OR PROTECTIVE ISOLATION

In the past, healthcare facilities would implement a type of isolation called *reverse isolation*. This type of isolation was used to reduce the risk of contracting an infection from being exposed to potential environmental pathogens. Reverse isolation was used for immunosuppressed patients with cancer, after an organ transplant, or other neutropenic conditions. This category of isolation was deleted by the Centers for Disease Control and Prevention in the early 1980s because its effectiveness was not established through empirical data. There is no current evidence to support that reverse isolation reduces infection rates. Many healthcare facilities still provide immunosuppressed patients a preventative environment called *neutropenic precautions* or *protective isolation* ❸. Here are typical guidelines for neutropenic precautions or protective isolation:

- No PPE is recommended during routine care of neutropenic patients.
- Routine standard precautions are recommended for all patients when there is anticipation of contact with body fluids.
- Hand hygiene should be performed by staff and family or visitors entering the room.
- A visitor or family member with a respiratory or other infection should not visit the patient.
- No live plants or flowers are allowed in the room.
- No nonperishable fresh fruits or vegetables are allowed in the room.

> ### NEUTROPENIC PRECAUTIONS
> #### IMMEDIATE FAMILY ONLY
> #### TO HELP US PROTECT OUR PATIENTS
>
> 1. **KEEP DOOR CLOSED AT ALL TIMES.**
> 2. **WASH HANDS GOING IN AND OUT OF THE ROOM.**
> 3. **NO FLOWERS OR PLANTS ARE ALLOWED.**
> 4. **NO FRESH FRUITS OR VEGETABLES ARE ALLOWED.**
> 5. **NO PERSONS ALLOWED WITH INFECTIONS OR COLDS.**
>
> If you have any questions, please go the nurse's station, and we will be happy to answer them. Thank you.

❸ Neutropenic isolation precautions sign.

- The patient should be assigned to a private room but selective semiprivate room is acceptable.
- The door of the patient's room is to be kept closed.
- If available, the patient should have vital signs equipment used for the patient kept in the patient's room.
- The patient should wear a basic isolation mask when out of the room.
- Dietary foods should not include raw meats or seafood, deli foods, or partially cooked eggs.

❯❯ Critical Thinking Options for Unexpected Outcomes

Not all unexpected outcomes require further nursing intervention; however, many times they do. When the patient demonstrates a change in signs/symptoms indicating an emerging problem, the nurse should immediately assess and troubleshoot what is happening. The assessment data must be processed quickly to formulate a hypothesis so the nurse can make a clinical judgment. The nurse then decides how best to resolve the problem and improve the patient's situation for a better outcome.

EXPECTED OUTCOME	UNEXPECTED OUTCOME	POSSIBLE INTERVENTIONS
PPE and Isolation Precautions The transfer of microorganisms from healthcare workers or environment to patients is prevented.	Infection occurs in patient.	- Assess mode of transmission of microorganism. - Administer antibiotics specific to microorganism as ordered. - Review hand washing technique. - Attend in-service program on infection control procedures.
Hospital personnel and others are protected against contamination from blood or body fluids.	Contaminated blood or body fluids come in contact with skin or mucous membranes.	- Report incident, and complete unusual occurrence report (very important for follow-up legal and medical implications). - Follow hospital guidelines for postexposure prophylaxis (PEP). - HIV exposure should be immediately reported, because most hospitals offer azidothymidine (AZT) preventive therapy. This therapy should be administered within 1 hr and not more than 24 hr after exposure. - Obtain AIDS antibody test in ensuing months. - Continue to monitor own health status and carry out specific activities to build immune system. Maintain wellness activities to build immune system.

(continued on next page)

EXPECTED OUTCOME	UNEXPECTED OUTCOME	POSSIBLE INTERVENTIONS
Hospital personnel are protected from infection.	Hospital personnel become infected.	■ Request consultation therapy to handle feelings and learn new methods of coping with stress. ■ Change other aspects of your life to reduce stress. ■ Take measures to enhance immune system.
The incidence of healthcare-associated infections is reduced.	Healthcare-associated infection occurs in isolation environment.	■ Identify source of infection and contact the infection control practitioner for consultation. ■ Examine isolation precautions and hand washing practices among staff. ■ Provide educational activity on isolation precautions and hand washing to refresh awareness of appropriate guidelines.
PPE in the Home Setting Infections are treated appropriately and not transmitted to others living in the home or the nurse because effective preventive measures are utilized.	The home environment has potential infection sources.	■ Explain the necessity of keeping the environment free of potential organisms and of keeping it clean and uncluttered. ■ Instruct the patient and family members on proper hand hygiene technique. ■ Explain and develop a plan for family members to discard soiled dressings, diapers, etc., to prevent potentially infecting other household members.

REVIEW Questions

1. The nurse completes cleaning the perineum of a client who just had a bowel movement. Afterward, which approach should the nurse use to cleanse the hands?
   1. Rinse the gloves with warm water before removing them.
   2. Remove the gloves and wash the hands with antiseptic gel.
   3. Remove the gloves and wash the hands with soap and water.
   4. Wash the hands with soap and water followed by a waterless agent.

2. The nurse observes an unlicensed assistive personnel (UAP) provide care to a client in enteric contact precautions. For which UAP action should the nurse intervene?
   1. Washes hands with soap and water after removing gloves
   2. Leaves the room with the stethoscope draped around the neck
   3. Applies a gown before entering the room to place the client on a bedpan
   4. Places used gown in the biohazard receptacle before leaving the client's room

3. The nurse cares for a client with bacterial meningitis. When should the nurse remove the face mask when doffing PPE?
   1. After removing the gown
   2. After removing the gloves
   3. Before removing the gown
   4. Before removing the gloves

4. During a home visit, the nurse notes that a client's infected leg wound is draining purulent and serosanguineous fluid onto the bed sheets. What should the nurse instruct the spouse about the care of the client's bed linens?
   1. Wash in cool water.
   2. Wash separately with very hot water, detergent, and bleach.
   3. Soak in a solution of half-strength hydrogen peroxide before washing.
   4. Place into washer first while water is filling before adding other clothes.

5. The nurse irrigates and changes a client's abdominal wound dressing. Which item should the nurse flush down the commode?
   1. Used gloves
   2. Soiled dressing
   3. Wound drainage
   4. Irrigation syringe

6. A sputum sample is collected from a client in airborne precautions. What should the nurse do before sending this specimen to the laboratory?
   1. Place specimen container in plastic biohazard bag outside the room.
   2. Cleanse the outside of the specimen container with an antiseptic solution.
   3. Label the container with the client's name and personal identification information.
   4. Attach the sticker "isolation" to the outside of the container after the specimen is collected.

7. While transferring a client with a norovirus from the transportation cart to the bed, the nurse notes stool has seeped through the blankets that were covering the mattress. What action should be taken to disinfect the mattress on the cart appropriately?
   1. Apply antimicrobial gel to the mattress.
   2. Place soiled blankets with linen outside of the room.
   3. Wipe down the mattress with an antimicrobial solution.
   4. Cleanse the mattress with soap and water and allow to air dry.

8. The nurse enters the room of a client with seeping skin wounds. When should the nurse don gloves?
   1. After washing the hands
   2. Before washing the hands
   3. When touching the wounds
   4. When providing oral pain medication

Note: For answers and rationales for the review questions, go to Appendix A or your Pearson MyLab Nursing and eText.

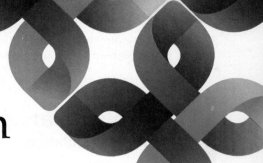

Chapter 7
Intracranial Regulation

Chapter at a Glance

❶ Nursing students may observe or assist with the following skills only with faculty permission and while under direct supervision of faculty or another RN.

≫ The Concept of Intracranial Regulation

Intracranial regulation is the ability of the cranial contents, such as the brain, blood, and cerebral spinal fluid, to maintain adequate intracranial pressure. All body systems and functions are interconnected with neurologic function, which means a change in intracranial regulation will alter the function of the central nervous system. Regulation includes a cranium that supports optimal brain function. An increase in pressure can be caused by a brain injury or other medical condition and can become life-threatening. A decrease in pressure or intracranial hypotension can be the result of an occult leak of cerebrospinal fluid or a lumbar puncture.

Learning Outcomes

7.1 Differentiate assessment data in the three categories included in the Glasgow Coma Scale: eye opening, verbal response, and motor response.

7.2 Support the reasoning for having a child in a side-lying and flexed position when having a lumbar puncture done.

7.3 Give examples of four early signs to assess for that indicate an increase in intracranial pressure in an older adult with a closed head injury.

7.4 Summarize the steps in determining a Glasgow Coma Score for the patient with an injury to the head.

7.5 Support why cerebrospinal fluid pressure readings using a manometer are monitored during a lumbar puncture when samples of cerebrospinal fluid are collected.

7.6 Explain why intracranial pressure monitoring would be implemented on a patient who fell off a ladder, hit the back of the head, and lost consciousness.

7.7 Give examples of two reasons a patient could not be assessed using the Glasgow Coma Scale.

7.8 Explain three actions the nurse can implement to support a patient during a lumbar puncture.

The following feature links some, but not all, of the concepts related to assessment. They are presented in alphabetical order.

Concepts Related to
Intracranial Regulation

CONCEPT	RELATIONSHIP TO INTRACRANIAL REGULATION	NURSING IMPLICATIONS
Cognition	Sensorium and state of consciousness may decrease when intracranial pressure (ICP) increases.	■ Frequent assessment of sensorium will assist nurse in identifying changes in cognition that may indicate changes in ICP. ■ Scoring patient using Glasgow Coma Scale provides assessment data for trending patient's neurologic status.
Communication	Changes in patient's condition happen quickly, and healthcare orders may need to be altered frequently.	■ Healthcare provider needs to be notified of changes in ICP measurements and monitoring of neurologic status by nurse efficiently. ■ Trends in ICP measurements need to be part of change-of-shift reporting.
Inflammation	Post severe head trauma, swelling of the brain can cause increased ICP.	■ Measuring and monitoring ICP provides data that may indicate inflammation of the brain tissue. ■ May become life-threatening.
Oxygenation	Adequate oxygen to all areas of the brain with increased ICP to avoid tissue damage.	■ Implement oxygen therapy as ordered. ■ If patient is unconscious, protect the airway.
Perfusion	Brain bleed may result from change in ICP.	■ Complications from bleeding due to increased ICP need to be addressed to avoid ischemic tissue damage. ■ Frequent assessment of ICP, neurologic status, vital signs, and sensorium need to be monitored.

Intracranial regulation focuses on the processes that affect intracranial compensation and adaptive neurologic function. All body functions, muscle movements, senses, mental processing, and emotions are regulated by the neurologic system. It takes in intrinsic and extrinsic information, processes it, interprets it, and causes motor or sensory responses.

Expected Outcomes

1. Lumbar puncture is performed with minimal discomfort and no untoward effects.
2. Appropriate tools are used to evaluate a neurologic patient's level of consciousness.
3. Ongoing assessment of a patient's brainstem reflexes and vital signs are used to determine compensating versus decompensating neurologic status.
4. Signs and symptoms of increased intracranial pressure are recognized.
5. Factors that increase intracranial hypertension are identified.
6. Measures to prevent/manage intracranial hypertension are initiated.
7. Patient responses to pain management and sedation are evaluated.

SKILL 7.1 Glasgow Coma Scale: Using

The Glasgow Coma Scale (GCS) has been used for several decades to evaluate level of consciousness (LOC) by requiring the patient to hear the examiner and respond with (1) eye opening, (2) oral responses, and (3) motor responses. Patients with a score of 8 or less are considered to be comatose and are typically intubated to protect the airway and facilitate mechanical ventilation if required. A "T" is added to their GCS score to indicate this functional limitation. Using this scale, a patient with a spinal cord injury and who is paralyzed may receive a coma score of 8, be intubated, but not be comatose. It follows that the GCS cannot be used to assess neurologic signs in patients who are unable to respond orally (e.g., patients who are intubated, sedated, aphasic, have impaired hearing, or altered level of consciousness).

Delegation or Assignment

Assessment of neurologic sensory and motor functions is not delegated or assigned to the UAP. However, signs and symptoms of problems may be observed during usual care and may be recorded by individuals other than the nurse. Abnormal findings must be validated and interpreted by the nurse.

SKILL 7.1 Glasgow Coma Scale: Using (*continued*)

Equipment

No equipment is needed for this skill.

Preparation

- Review healthcare provider's orders and the patient's medical record.
- Remember, the lowest score on the GCS is 3 and indicates a fully unresponsive patient. The highest score is 15 and indicates a completely awake and oriented patient.
- Use the pediatric GSC for newborns and infants.

Procedure

1. Introduce self to patient and verify the patient's identity using two identifiers. Explain to the patient what you are going to do, why it is necessary, and how the patient can participate. Discuss how the results will be used in planning further care or treatments.
2. Perform hand hygiene and observe appropriate infection control procedures.
3. Provide for patient privacy.
4. When the patient has an injury to the head or altered consciousness, assess each of the three categories of the Glasgow Coma Scale. In some cases the patient will need stimulation to obtain a response that can be scored. Initially, observe the patient to see if all categories can be assessed (e.g., the patient who is intubated cannot be assessed for verbal response).

STIMULANT CATEGORY	PHYSICAL OR AUDITORY RESPONSE MADE	COMMANDS GIVEN TO STIMULATE A RESPONSE	ACTIONS DONE TO STIMULATE A RESPONSE	RESPONSES OBSERVED
Eye opening	Opens eyes without being asked; looking around; opens eyes on command, trying to focus eyes	"Open your eyes." "Blink your eyes." "Look at me." "Follow my hand."	Touch patient's arm. Shake patient's arm.	Remains with eyes closed
Verbal response	Talking; making verbal sounds; responds to questions; is oriented, confused, or inappropriate	"Tell me your name." "Do you know where you are?" "What day is it?"	Speak louder and slower commands. Clap hands loudly.	Remains without speaking or making verbal sounds
Motor response	Making purposeful movements; trying to move; moves on command	"Move your legs." "Squeeze my hand." "Touch your head."	Give painful stimuli (i.e., sternal rub).	Remains without movement or having withdrawing or abnormal flexion or extension movements

5. Note the score for each category (**Table 7–1 ≫**). Document the total score and time performed. Total the scores for all three categories to get the Glasgow Coma Score.
6. Repeat the test at regular intervals to monitor if patient's condition is improving or becoming worse. **Rationale:** *Because the test provides a numeric score for altered consciousness, regular measurements help detect subtle changes in the patient's condition.*

TABLE 7–1 Glasgow Coma Scale for Assessment of Coma in Infants, Children, and Adults

Category	Score	Infant and Young Child Criteria	Older Child and Adult Criteria
Eye opening	4	Spontaneous opening	Spontaneous
	3	To loud noise	To verbal stimuli
	2	To pain	To pain
	1	No response	No response
Verbal response	5	Smiles, coos, cries to appropriate stimuli	Oriented to time, place, and person; uses appropriate words and phrases
	4	Irritable; cries	Confused
	3	Inappropriate crying	Inappropriate words or verbal response
	2	Grunts, moans	Incomprehensible words
	1	No response	No response
Motor response	6	Spontaneous movement	Obeys commands
	5	Withdraws to touch	Localizes pain
	4	Withdraws to pain	Withdraws to pain
	3	Abnormal flexion (decorticate)	Flexion to pain (decorticate)
	2	Abnormal extension (decerebrate)	Extension to pain (decerebrate)
	1	No response	No response

Sources: Based on Christensen, B. (2014). *Pediatric Glasgow Coma Scale.* Retrieved from http://emedicine.medscape.com/article/2058902-overview; Glasgow Coma Scale. (2014). *What is the Glasgow Coma Scale?* Retrieved from http://glasgowcomascale.org/what-is-gcs/; Jevon, P. (n.d.). *Annex 3.* Retrieved from http://www.sign.ac.uk/pdf/sign110_annex3.pdf

Add the score from each category to calculate the total score. The maximum score is 15, indicating the best possible level of neurologic functioning. The minimum score is 3, indicating total neurologic unresponsiveness.

(*continued on next page*)

SKILL 7.1 Glasgow Coma Scale: Using (*continued*)

Note: Because the Glasgow Coma Scale has limitations, the Full Outline of Un-Responsiveness (FOUR Score) Coma Scale ❶ is sometimes used for assessing the comatose patient, especially one with an acute metabolic or other nonstructural brain injury/disorder. FOUR Score detects early changes in consciousness, such as the inability to follow the examiner's commands, altered brainstem reflexes, and Cheyne–Stokes breathing. It is also used to differentiate vegetative from minimally conscious states, locked-in syndrome, uncal herniation, and brain death.

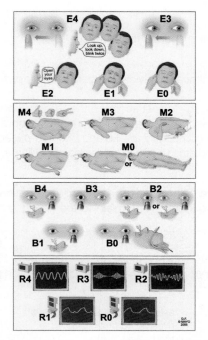

Source: Courtesy of and by permission of Mayo Foundation for Medical Education and Research. All rights reserved.

❶ Assessing coma in the neurologic patient using the Full Outline of Un-Responsiveness (FOUR) Score Coma Scale.

> ### SAMPLE DOCUMENTATION
>
> [date] 1820 Arouses easily, eye response 4, speech response 4, motor response 6, total GCS 14. Confused about what's going on at this time. Pupils slow but equal and reactant to light. V/S: T 37.11°C (98.8°F) (O), P 72, R 16, BP 112/76, 95% O_2 saturation. Daughter and other family present. Dressing on right forehead remains dry and intact. Resting quietly. *C. Napper*

SKILL 7.2 Intracranial Pressure: Monitoring and Caring for

Safety Note! *During scheduled clinical time, nursing students may have a learning opportunity to observe or assist with this skill only with faculty permission and with direct supervision from faculty or another RN.*

Intracranial pressure (ICP) is a measure that reflects equilibrium volumes of circulating blood, cerebrospinal fluid (CSF), and brain tissue within the skull. Increased ICP can be caused by an increase in volume of CSF or blood, or by the swelling of brain tissue from a severe head injury or illness such as encephalitis, hydrocephalus, brain tumor, or stroke. An increase in the pressure can damage the brain or spinal cord by restricting blood flow into the brain. Measuring and monitoring ICP pressure is done by inserting a sensor catheter device inside the head.

Delegation or Assignment

Due to specific knowledge and skills in regulating and monitoring ICP, this skill is not delegated or assigned to the UAP. The UAP may care for patients with an ICP transducer system and monitor, and the nurse must ensure that the UAP knows what complications or adverse signs should be reported to the nurse. The nurse remains responsible for the assessment, interpretation of abnormal finds, and determination of appropriate actions.

Equipment

- ICP transducer system and monitor
- Sterile gloves, mask, and gown

Preparation

- Review the patient's chart related to indications for intracranial pressure monitoring.
- Review the healthcare provider's orders for monitoring and drainage parameters.
- Verify the identity of the patient by checking the patient's identity band and asking patient to state name and birth date.
- Provide explanations to the patient and family or significant other about the need for ICP monitoring.
- Perform hand hygiene.

Procedure

1. Introduce self to patient and verify the patient's identity using two identifiers. Explain to the patient what you are going to do, why it is necessary, and how the patient can participate. Discuss how the results will be used in planning further care or treatments.
2. Perform hand hygiene and observe appropriate infection control procedures.
3. Provide for patient privacy.
4. Ensure that the fluid-filled transducer system ❶ ❷ ❸ is placed and maintained at the level of the foramen of Monro, the line between the top of the ear and the outer canthus of the eye. Balance the ICP transducer to zero for calibration according to hospital guidelines and when the patient's posi-

SKILL 7.2 Intracranial Pressure: Monitoring and Caring for (*continued*)

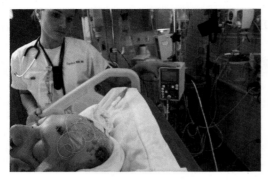

Source: Celina Burkhart/Pearson Education, Inc.

1 ICP microsensor (fiber optic catheter) senses changes in ICP. The system may be used to measure intraventricular parenchymal, subdural, or epidural pressure.

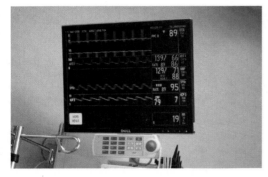

Source: Celina Burkhart/Pearson Education, Inc.

2 Monitor displays digital readouts and pressure waveforms of the ECG, arterial BP, SPO₂, and calculated CPP (MAP – ICP = CCP).

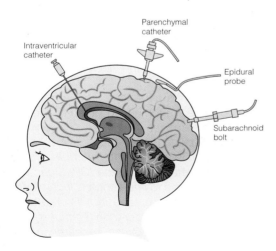

Source: Clinical Nursing Skills: Basic to Advanced Skills, 9e by Sandra F. Smith, Donna J. Duell, Barbara C. Martin, Michelle Aebersold and Laura Gonzalez. Copyright © 2017 by Pearson Education

3 Sites for ICP monitoring.

tion changes. **Rationale:** *This ensures the accuracy of pressure readings and waveforms by the transducer system.*

5. ICP monitoring is usually continuous **4** **5**. When an external ventricular drain is present, document ICP and

	UNCAL HERNIATION				
	Normal	Early	Late Third	Midbrain & Pons	Pons & Medulla	Terminal
RESPONSE	A&O MAE	Alert to Stuporous	Stuporous or Comatose	Stuporous or Comatose	Comatose →	
PUPILS	Perl	L>R / L=Sluggish	L>R / L=Unresponsive	Doll's eyes / Fixed	absent → / fixed	
MOTOR	MAE –	norm for patient	hemiplegia may be decorticate	decorticate or decerebrate	flaccid →	
RESPIRATIONS	eupnea	Cheyne Stokes or Hyperventilation	sustained hyperventilation		apneustic shallow / Cluster or Ataxic	
BP and PULSE	pulse	↕ pulse pressure				

Source: Clinical Nursing Skills: Basic to Advanced Skills, 9e by Sandra F. Smith, Donna J. Duell, Barbara C. Martin, Michelle Aebersold and Laura Gonzalez. Copyright © 2017 by Pearson Education.

4 Deterioration of level of consciousness precedes contralateral hemiparesis.

cerebral perfusion pressure (CPP) at the frequency ordered by the healthcare provider or by hospital protocol. Monitor and print ICP waveforms. See **Table 7–2 »**.

6. Assess the patient's responsiveness, vital signs, and neurologic status. Assess for signs of increased ICP. See **Table 7–3 »**. **Rationale:** *Patients with brain injuries are at risk for seizures and cerebral edema, which further compromise CPP.*

CAUTION! Cerebral perfusion pressure (CPP) is calculated by subtracting the ICP from the mean arterial pressure (MAP). (MAP is calculated by [(2 × diastolic) + systolic]/3.) Normal CPP is 60 to 150 mmHg. Normal ICP is 5 to 15 mmHg.

TABLE 7–2 ICP Waveforms and Implications

Waveform	Pressure (mmHg)	Implications
A	50–100	Symptoms related to cerebral dysfunction; changes in vital signs, respiratory pattern, and motor function; headache; and emesis
B	20–50	Decreasing level of consciousness, agitation, varying respiratory pattern
C	4–20	No clinical significance
Normal	4–15	Normal

(*continued on next page*)

SKILL 7.2 Intracranial Pressure: Monitoring and Caring for (continued)

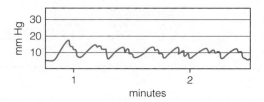

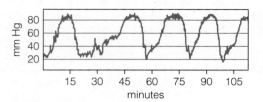

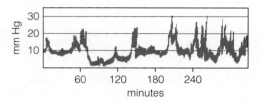

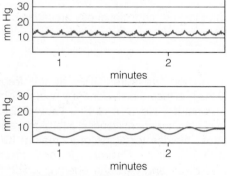

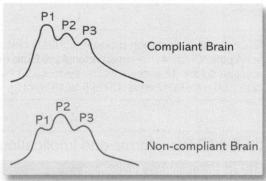

Source: Intracranial Pressure Waveforms from *Clinical Nursing Skills: Basic to Advanced Skills*, 9e by Sandra F. Smith, Donna J. Duell, Barbara C. Martin, Michelle Aebersold and Laura Gonzalez. Copyright © 2017 by Pearson Education

⑤ Intracranial pressure waveforms.

TABLE 7–3 Signs of Increased Intracranial Pressure

Timing of Signs	Signs
Early signs	Headache
	Visual disturbances, diplopia
	Vomiting without nausea
	Dizziness or vertigo
	Slight change in vital signs
	Pupils not as reactive or equal
	"Sunsetting" eyes
	Seizures
	Slight change in level of consciousness
Additional signs in newborns and infants	Bulging fontanelle
	Wide sutures, increased head circumference
	Dilated scalp veins
	High-pitched, catlike cry
Late signs	Significant decrease in level of consciousness
	Cushing triad:
	■ Increased systolic blood pressure and widened pulse pressure
	■ Bradycardia
	■ Irregular respirations
	Fixed and dilated pupils

7. Assess pain and comfort level. Administer sedation and pain medication as prescribed. **Rationale:** *Patients may experience pain at the catheter insertion site and pain from increased ICP. Medications promote the patient's comfort and help reduce elevations in ICP.*

8. Maintain the patient's position with the head at midline with the remainder of the body and the head of the bed elevated 15–30 degrees or according to healthcare provider's order. **Rationale:** *This position prevents compression of blood vessels in the neck and obstruction of venous blood flows.*

9. Monitor the patient's neurologic status during nursing care and continue or stop nursing interventions depending on patient's response. **Rationale:** *Anxiety, agitation, pain, hypoxia, hypertension, head position out of neutral alignment, some environmental stimuli, and nursing care procedures may elevate the ICP. Signs indicating poor patient response to interventions include deterioration in clinical signs, increase in ICP greater than 10 mmHg above baseline longer than 3 minutes, and wide-amplitude waveform and/or the appearance of plateau waves.*

10. When procedure is complete, perform hand hygiene and leave the patient safe and comfortable.

11. Complete documentation using forms, checklists, or electronic dropdown lists supplemented by nurse's notes or additional comments as appropriate.

12. Document the ICP reading, CPP, waveforms, and the patient's neurologic status at intervals specified by hospital guidelines or healthcare provider's order.

SKILL 7.2 Intracranial Pressure: Monitoring and Caring for *(continued)*

[date] 0430 V/S BP 134/72, P - 90, R - 26, T - 37.3°C (99.2°F), O$_2$ saturation 95% on 2 LPM via nasal cannula. Left pupil 2 mm, right pupil 3 mm. Arouses with verbal stimuli. Glasgow shows eye score-3, verbal score-4, and motor score-5.

Anxious about where she is. Reoriented to place, encouraged to remain calm and still. Mother at bedside. P1, P2, and P3 waveforms present on monitor in downward slope. ICP 11 mmHg. Insertion site of intraventricular catheter remains secured, dressing dry. *R. Hosea*

SKILL 7.3 Lumbar Puncture: Assisting

Safety Note! *During scheduled clinical time, nursing students may have a learning opportunity to observe or assist with this skill only with faculty permission and with direct supervision from faculty or another RN.*

In a lumbar puncture (LP, or spinal tap), cerebrospinal fluid (CSF) is withdrawn through a needle inserted into the subarachnoid space of the spinal canal between the third and fourth lumbar vertebrae or between the fourth and fifth lumbar vertebrae. At this level, the needle avoids damaging the spinal cord and major nerve roots. A lumbar puncture may be done to collect CSF for diagnostic tests, measure intracranial pressure or the pressure in the CSF, inject medications such as anesthetics, or inject radioactive dye for diagnostic imagery tests.

Delegation or Assignment

The nurse first determines that the UAP knows the correct way to assist and help hold the patient in the correct position for the lumbar puncture, while the nurse assists the healthcare provider to perform the lumbar puncture procedure. The nurse remains responsible for the assessment, interpretation of abnormal findings, and determination of appropriate responses. Note that state laws for UAPs vary, so this task might be assigned to the UAP rather than delegated.

Equipment

- Gather supplies for the procedure to be performed separately or use a disposable preassembled lumbar puncture set ❶.
  - Sterile sheet for sterile instrument tray and sterile sheet for puncture site

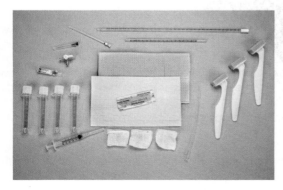

❶ A preassembled lumbar puncture set. Note the manometer at the top of the set.

- Sterile sponge sticks or cotton-tipped applicators to apply local povidone iodine or 2% chlorhexidine gluconate (CHG)
- 4 × 4 sterile gauze
- Four sterile test tubes
- Large sterile adhesive dressing
- Sterile manometer
- Sterile stopcock
- 1% lidocaine for local anesthetic
- Sterile 20-gauge needle and 18-gauge needle
- Sterile syringe and 25-gauge needle
- Sterile 20-gauge spinal needle
- Sterile gloves
- Personal protective equipment (PPE) if needed, gloves, gown, and mask

Preparation

- Review healthcare provider's orders and the patient's record.
- Check for patient allergies.
- Verify signed informed consent in front of the patient's record.
- Determine if the parent wants to be present during an uncomfortable procedure or to be available after the procedure to comfort the child. When the parent wishes to be present, discuss the parent's role (e.g., providing distraction or comfort during the procedure).
- Gather needed equipment and supplies.

Procedure

1. Introduce self to the patient (and parent if appropriate) and verify the patient's identity using two identifiers. Explain to the patient (and parent) what you are going to do, why it is necessary, and how the patient can participate. Explain the importance of remaining still during procedure. Discuss how the results will be used in planning further care or treatments.
2. Perform hand hygiene and observe appropriate infection control procedures.
3. Provide for patient privacy.
4. Assist the patient to the appropriate position.
   - The newborn or infant can be held in the desired position by holding the neck and thighs in your hands ❷.
   - Place the child in the side-lying or sitting position that is preferred by the practitioner. The assistant can hold the child in position by wrapping one arm behind the knees and the other behind the neck, keeping the back

(continued on next page)

SKILL 7.3 Lumbar Puncture: Assisting (*continued*)

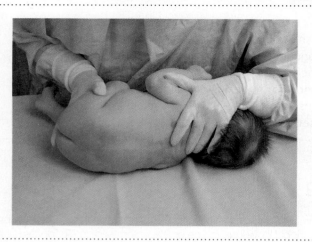

② Infant in side-lying and flexed position for a lumbar puncture.

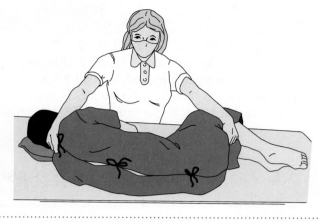

④ Supporting the adult for a lumbar puncture.

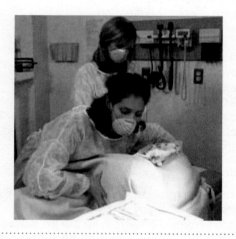

③ Child in side-lying and flexed position for a lumbar puncture.

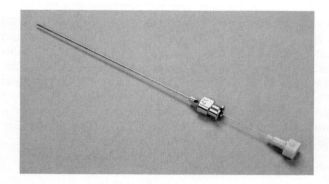

⑤ A spinal needle with the stylet protruding from the hub.

curved. **Rationale:** *This position ensures the best possible access to spinal processes and disc spaces.*

- The older child can be quite strong, and someone with enough strength will be needed to hold the child in the side-lying position. Lean over the child with your entire body, using your forearms against the thighs and around the shoulders and head ③. Alternatively, the older child may be in a seated position, bending forward and supported by the assistant.
- Be certain that the child has free air exchange. Another assistant may be assigned to monitor respirations and perform other assessments during the procedure.
- Instruct the adult to curl into a fetal position ④, a lateral position with the head bent toward the chest, the knees flexed onto the abdomen, and the back at the edge of the bed or examining table. Make sure the individual positioning and assisting the adult clearly understands what body parts must be held still and how to do this safely. **Rationale:** *In this position the back is arched, increasing the spaces between the vertebrae so that the spinal needle can be inserted readily.*

5. The UAP helps the patient maintain the lumbar puncture position, and the nurse monitors the patient, assists the

healthcare provider as necessary, and provides encouragement as needed. **Rationale:** *Holding the position helps prevent accidental needle displacement. Monitoring and reassuring the patient helps to maintain safety.*

6. Ask the patient to report headache or persistent pain at insertion site. **Rationale:** *This provides information about potential complications.*

7. During a lumbar puncture ⑤ ⑥, the healthcare provider frequently takes CSF pressure readings using a *manometer*, a glass or plastic tube calibrated in millimeters. The healthcare provider collects samples of CSF.

CAUTION! Normal spinal fluid is clear, colorless, and watery in appearance. Cloudy spinal fluid can indicate an infection or a buildup of white cells. If the fluid looks red, pink, or bloody, it can indicate bleeding or an obstruction in the spinal cord. Brown or yellow fluid may indicate an increase in protein or old bleeding.

---

8. After the procedure, apply a small sterile dressing over the puncture site. **Rationale:** *This protects the site from infection.*

9. Assist the patient to a dorsal recumbent position with one pillow or supine position. Monitor often.

10. When procedure is complete, discard waste in receptacle, perform hand hygiene, and leave patient safe and comfortable.

SKILL 7.3 Lumbar Puncture: Assisting (*continued*)

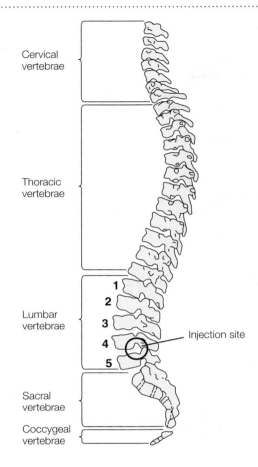

- Cervical vertebrae
- Thoracic vertebrae
- Lumbar vertebrae
  - 1
  - 2
  - 3
  - 4
  - 5
- Injection site
- Sacral vertebrae
- Coccygeal vertebrae

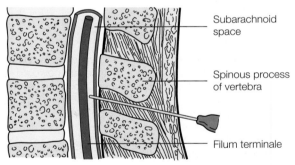

- Subarachnoid space
- Spinous process of vertebra
- Filum terminale

⑥ A diagram of the vertebral column, indicating a site for insertion of the lumbar puncture needle into the subarachnoid space of the spinal canal.

11. Label test tubes with patient information and date and time of collection. Send labeled specimens with lab slip to laboratory.
12. Complete documentation using forms, checklists, or electronic dropdown lists supplemented by nurse's notes or additional comments as appropriate.

SAMPLE DOCUMENTATION

[date] 1700 Instructed to curl into a fetal position, with the head bent toward the chest, the knees flexed onto the abdomen, and the back at the edge of the bed. Lumbar puncture procedure done by Dr. Westcott. Four test tubes with CSF collected, labeled, and sent to lab. Post procedure, repositioned to dorsal recumbent position. V/S 114/80, 88, 18. Resting quietly. Tolerated procedure without incident. *M. Downs*

CAUTION! Lumbar puncture requires that the child be held still to prevent injury and to ensure success in obtaining fluid. It is advisable to have an experienced staff member hold the child in position for the procedure.

Lifespan Considerations

CHILDREN

- Briefly demonstrate the procedure on a doll or stuffed animal. Allow time to answer questions.
- One member of the child healthcare team should stay in close physical contact with the child, maintain eye contact, and talk to and reassure the child during the procedure.

OLDER ADULTS

- Some patients need help maintaining the flexed position due to arthritis, weakness, or tremors.
- Provide an extra blanket to keep the patient warm during the procedure. Older adults tend to have a decreased metabolism and less subcutaneous fat.
- If the patient has a hearing loss, speak slowly, distinctly, and loudly enough, especially when unable to make eye contact.

≫ Critical Thinking Options for Unexpected Outcomes

Not all unexpected outcomes require further nursing intervention; however, many times they do. When the patient demonstrates a change in signs/symptoms indicating an emerging problem, the nurse should immediately assess and troubleshoot what is happening. The assessment data must be processed quickly to formulate a hypothesis so the nurse can make a clinical judgment. The nurse then decides how best to resolve the problem and improve the patient's situation for a better outcome.

EXPECTED OUTCOME	UNEXPECTED OUTCOME	POSSIBLE INTERVENTIONS
Lumbar puncture is performed with minimal discomfort and no untoward effects.	Patient has spinal fluid leak after lumbar puncture.	■ Keep patient in supine position. ■ Notify healthcare provider. ■ Keep sterile dressing over puncture site. Do not allow dressing to become wet. ■ If leak persists, healthcare provider may place patient in the Trendelenburg position to prevent headache. This position is contraindicated in patients with increased intracranial pressure or after a craniotomy.
Appropriate tools are used to evaluate a neurologic patient's level of consciousness.	Neurologic patient's comatose state cannot be determined using Glasgow Coma Scale due to inability to respond verbally.	■ Recognize that a nonverbal patient cannot respond to parameters assessed using the Glasgow Coma Scale. ■ Utilize the FOUR Score Coma Scale to assess separate components of eye response, motor response, brainstem reflexes, and respiration for the nonverbal patient.
Ongoing assessment of a patient's brainstem reflects, and vital signs are used, to determine compensating versus decompensating neurologic status.	Patient shows signs of decreasing level of consciousness.	■ Reassess to validate findings. ■ Notify healthcare provider of findings immediately.
Patient responses to pain management and sedation are evaluated.	Patient is very agitated with frequent nonpurposeful movements, despite increased frequency of sedative administration.	■ Try to find a cause for the patient's change in behavior. ■ Attempt an analgesic trial to determine whether the patient's pain is managed. This trial may be therapeutic as well as diagnostic.

REVIEW Questions

1. After morning care, the UAP reports that halfway through the bed bath, a client with a head injury stopped opening her eyes. What should the nurse do first?
   1. Reassess the client.
   2. Document the finding.
   3. Notify the healthcare provider.
   4. Explain that the client is sleeping.

2. The nurse decides to skip the Glasgow Coma Scale assessment for a client who was just transported from the emergency department. The nurse most likely makes this clinical decision because the client:
   1. Asked for something to eat
   2. Received multiple doses of diazepam for status epilepticus
   3. Reported severe pain when transferred from the stretcher to the bed
   4. Requested time alone to notify family of being admitted to the hospital

3. The nurse repositions a client with an external ventricular drain for continuous ICP monitoring. What should the nurse do before noting the current pressure reading?
   1. Lower the head of the bed.
   2. Measure current blood pressure.
   3. Balance the ICP transducer to zero.
   4. Ensure the transducer is at the midaxillary line.

4. A client with an external ventricular drain for continuous ICP monitoring has an ICP of 25 mmHg and a blood pressure of 178/90 mmHg. What should the nurse calculate this client's cerebral perfusion pressure to be, rounded to the nearest whole number?
   1. 63
   2. 65
   3. 94
   4. 153

5. A client with an external ventricular drain for continuous ICP monitoring had an ICP measurement of 15 mmHg at 0700 hours. At 0800 hours, the UAP reports that the client is "breathing funny." What ICP measurement should the nurse expect to assess in this client?
   1. 5 mmHg
   2. 10 mmHg
   3. 19 mmHg
   4. 32 mmHg

6. While triaging clients in the emergency department waiting room, the nurse immediately escorts a mother and newborn into an examination area. What assessment did the nurse use to make this clinical decision?
   1. Sucking on thumb
   2. Rapid respiratory rate
   3. High-pitching mewing cry
   4. Eyes open looking at mother

7. The nurse assesses a saturated dressing over the site of a lumbar puncture completed an hour ago on an adult client. What should the nurse anticipate being prescribed for this client?
   1. Pressure dressing
   2. Trendelenburg position
   3. Semi-Fowler position
   4. Intravenous fluid replacement

8. A client being prepared for a lumbar puncture asks why the fetal position is used. What should the nurse respond to this client?
   1. "It reduces the pain of the procedure."
   2. "It helps the procedure to be done faster."
   3. "It ensures the results of the procedure are positive for you."
   4. "It helps spread the vertebrae apart so that the needle can be inserted more easily."

Note: For answers and rationales for the review questions, go to Appendix A or your Pearson MyLab Nursing and eText.

Chapter 8
Metabolism

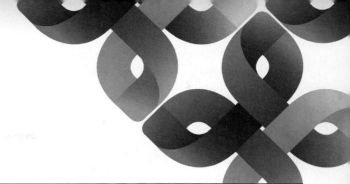

Chapter at a Glance

General Metabolism

Diabetes Care

❶ Nursing students may observe or assist with the following skills only with faculty permission and while under direct supervision of faculty or another RN.

» The Concept of Metabolism

Metabolism refers to the biochemical processes at the cellular level that happen to maintain body functions. They allow us to grow, repair damage, reproduce, and interact with our environment. The two components involved are *anabolism* (chemical reactions that require energy to build complex molecules) and *catabolism* (chemical reactions that break down complex molecules into smaller ones and releases energy). The digestive system breaks protein down to amino acids, fats into fatty acids, and carbohydrates into simple sugars. The body absorbs them and transports them to cells where metabolic chemical reactions occur to create energy from these compounds to be used or stored. Many hormones of the endocrine system, such as insulin and thyroxine, control the rate and type of metabolism.

Learning Outcomes

8.1 Give examples of four specific questions to ask a patient when obtaining subjective data to rule-out an endocrine dysfunction.

8.2 Discuss five hormones secreted by endocrine glands and the body functions they regulate.

8.3 Differentiate assessment characteristics of an abdomen without ascites and an abdomen with ascites.

8.4 Explain the importance of a patient voiding to empty the bladder just before having an abdominal paracentesis done.

8.5 Summarize three potential complications associated with diabetes mellitus.

8.6 Show the sequential steps in getting a blood sample and measuring blood glucose with a glucometer.

8.7 Give examples of interventions to implement when a patient with diabetes has hyperglycemia and hypoglycemia.

8.8 Explain six teaching points for a patient with diabetes to avoid complications.

The following feature links some, but not all, of the concepts related to assessment. They are presented in alphabetical order.

Concepts Related to
Metabolism

CONCEPT	RELATIONSHIP TO METABOLISM	NURSING IMPLICATIONS
Acid–Base Balance	Diabetic ketoacidosis causes metabolic acidosis.	▪ Uncontrolled diabetes causes unstable blood glucose, which affects acid–base balance. ▪ Measure and monitor blood glucose and treat with insulin using sliding scale as ordered.
Advocacy	Endocrine disorders are chronic conditions that can become progressively debilitating.	▪ Teach patient with chronic endocrine disorder how to self-manage and participate in decisions made concerning diet, medication, exercise, and complementary health approaches to maintain level of wellness and prevent complications and progression of disorder.
Mood and Affect	Chronic diseases can lead to chronic depression.	▪ Encourage and support patient's compliance with ordered treatment regimen. ▪ Assist patient in developing a support system. ▪ Provide patient community resources for counseling as needed.
Oxygenation	Collection of peritoneal fluid in the abdominal cavity causes displacement upward and limits lung expansion.	▪ Teach patient to take rest breaks when doing activities. ▪ Keep head of bed (HOB) elevated. ▪ Instruct patient to ask for assistance when up walking as needed. ▪ Provide oxygen therapy as ordered.
Safety	Treating blood glucose with insulin as needed 3–4 times a day requires safe and accurate measuring and monitoring of blood glucose.	▪ Ensure patient can accurately check blood glucose and safely self-administer insulin as ordered. ▪ Verify patient can recognize hyperglycemia and hypoglycemia symptoms to safely get help to correct the situation.

The primary function of the endocrine system is to regulate the body's internal environment. Hormones secreted by endocrine glands regulate growth, reproduction and sex differentiation, metabolism, and fluid and electrolyte balance. The endocrine system helps the body adapt to constant changes in the internal and external environment.

Hormones are chemical messengers of the body. They act on specific target cells, causing either an increase or decrease in body function. Hormone levels are regulated by a process called *negative feedback*. Negative feedback acts similar to the way the thermostat in a house regulates temperature. When too much hormone is released, the target cell sends back a message to reduce its hormone release. If too little hormone is released, the target cell sends back a message to increase the hormone to the normal level. **Figures 8–1** ⟫ and **8–2** ⟫ show selected endocrine glands and effects of their hormones on the body.

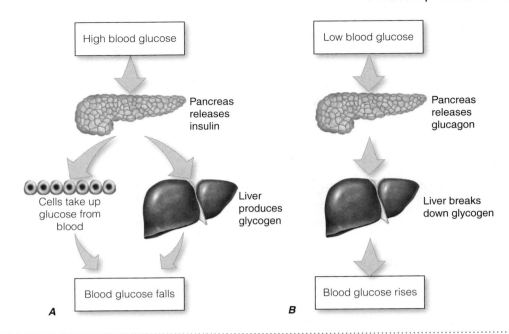

Figure 8–1 〉〉 Action of insulin and glucagon on blood glucose levels. **A,** High blood glucose is lowered by insulin release; **B,** Low blood glucose is raised by glucagon release.

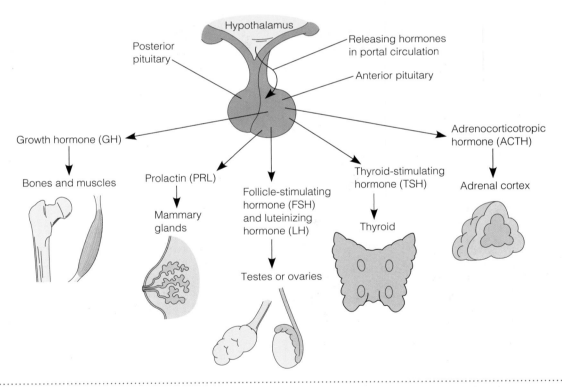

Figure 8–2 〉〉 Actions of the major hormones of the anterior pituitary.

» General Metabolism

Expected Outcomes

1. Assessment data supports differential endocrine disorder diagnoses.
2. Lifestyle changes assist in management of patient's altered health status.
3. Patient demonstrates understanding (verbalized knowledge) of behavioral modification strategies provided.
4. Paracentesis is completed without complications.

SKILL 8.1 Endocrine Disorders: Assessing

Because hormones affect all body systems, manifestations of endocrine dysfunction are often nonspecific. This makes assessment of endocrine function more difficult. However, subjective and objective data that support assessment of endocrine disorders can be collected.

Delegation or Assignment

Assessment of endocrine disorders is not delegated or assigned to the UAP. However, signs and symptoms of problems may be observed during usual care and may be recorded by individuals other than the nurse. Abnormal findings must be validated and interpreted by the nurse.

Equipment

- Platform scale with stature-measuring device (unless height and weight previously recorded in patient's record)
- Vital signs equipment, thermometer, blood pressure cuff, and pulse oximeter
- Stethoscope
- Clean gloves as needed

Preparation

- Review healthcare provider's orders and patient's nursing plan of care.
- Review patient's record for allergies, especially seafood and iodine (contrast dye).
- Gather equipment and supplies.

Procedure

1. Introduce self to patient and verify the patient's identity using two identifiers. Explain to the patient what you are going to do, why it is necessary, and how the patient can participate. Discuss how the results will be used in planning further care or treatments.
2. Perform hand hygiene and observe appropriate infection control procedures.
3. Provide for patient privacy.
4. Provide comfort and safety for patient and yourself, including raising bed to appropriate height for procedure.
5. Ask specific questions to obtain subjective data from the patient:
   - Changes in energy level and fatigue and how activities of daily living (ADLs) are affected
   - Increased sensitivity to heat or cold, weight loss or gain, diarrhea or constipation
   - Increased appetite, urination, or thirst; salt cravings
   - History of hypertension, abnormally fast or slow heart rate, palpitations, or shortness of breath
   - Changes in vision, excessive tearing, or swelling around the eyes
   - History of numbness or tingling in lips or extremities, nervousness, hand tremors, change in memory, mood, or sleep patterns
   - Thinning or loss of hair, dry or moist skin, brittle nails, easy bruising, or slow wound healing
   - History of taking any hormone replacements such as thyroid, steroids, or insulin
   - History of previous surgery, chemotherapy, or radiation, especially of the neck area, as well as brain surgery or a head injury
   - Any family history of diabetes mellitus, diabetes insipidus, goiter, obesity, Addison disease, or infertility
   - Changes in sexual function or secondary sex characteristics. Ask women about changes in menstruation or menopause.
6. Focus assessment to obtain objective data about the patient:
   - General appearance, vital signs, height, and weight. Note extremely short height.
   - Skin color, temperature, texture, and moisture. Observe for rough, dry or smooth, flushed skin. Note bronze color over knuckles, purple striae over the abdomen, and bruising.
   - Inspect the lower extremities for lesions and any signs of healing.
   - Assess the texture and condition of hair and nails. Observe for thinning and loss of hair, as well as thick or thin brittle nails. Look for excessive hair growth on face, chest, or abdomen.
   - Inspect the face for shape and symmetry. Inspect the eyes for the presence of exophthalmos (forward protrusion of the eyeballs). Determine visual acuity.
   - Inspect the neck for visible signs of masses. Gently palpate the thyroid gland from behind the patient ❶. Palpate only one side of the neck at a time.

CAUTION! Palpating the thyroid takes practice to do correctly without causing the patient to gag. Be especially gentle, and carefully use the fingertip pads when palpating the thyroid because of its location in front of the trachea and below the thyroid cartilage and cricoid cartilage. Some patients will be uneasy for you to reach around their neck from behind; it is acceptable to stand in front of the patient for this exam also.

SKILL 8.1 Endocrine Disorders: Assessing (continued)

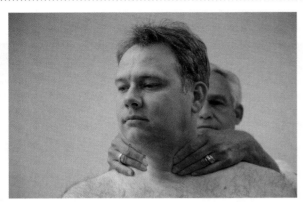

Source: Patrick Watson/Pearson Education, Inc.

....

1 Palpating the thyroid gland from behind the patient.

- Assess for increased size of hands and feet, trunk obesity, and thin extremities.
- Inspect men for gynecomastia (enlargement of the breasts).
- Evaluate muscle strength and deep tendon reflexes. Assess for the Chvostek sign (facial grimacing in response to tapping your finger at jaw) and Trousseau sign (carpal spasm when blood pressure cuff inflated higher than systolic pressure for 2–4 min).
- Assess ability to sense touch, hot/cold, and vibration in the extremities.
- Auscultate lungs for adventitious sounds and heart for extra heart sounds.
- Palpate hands and feet for edema.
- Perform hand hygiene and return bed to lowest height.

7. Review results of diagnostic tests.
   - To diagnose an endocrine disorder, several laboratory tests are used. **Table 8–1 》** lists these tests, their normal values, what the test measures and its significance, and any nursing implications for the test.
   - Other nonspecific laboratory tests are done to give clues about endocrine disorders. A chemistry panel, which includes serum electrolytes such as sodium, potassium, calcium, and phosphate, and blood glucose levels are used to monitor disease progression. For instance, serum sodium and blood glucose levels increase in Cushing syndrome but decrease in Addison disease. In people with diabetes, serum cholesterol and triglyceride levels help to evaluate the risk of developing atherosclerosis.

8. Review results of imaging studies. Imaging techniques used to diagnose endocrine disorders are noninvasive.

TABLE 8–1 Common Laboratory Tests for Endocrine Disorders

Test	Normal Adult Values	Explanation	Nursing Implications
Pituitary			
Growth hormone (GH)	Less than 5 ng/mL for men Less than 10 ng/mL for women	Used to evaluate growth hormone excess or deficiency. Increased values indicate acromegaly.	The patient must be fasting, well rested, and not physically or emotionally stressed.
Water deprivation test	1–5 pg/mL	Increased level indicates syndrome of inappropriate antidiuretic hormone (SIADH); decreased level means diabetes insipidus.	Tell patient to fast for 12 hours and to withhold fluids and smoking at midnight.
Thyroid			
Thyroid-stimulating hormone (TSH)	0.35–5.5 mcg/mL	This is the most sensitive test to evaluate thyroid function by measuring pituitary TSH secretion.	No fluid restriction is required. Avoid shellfish several days before test.
T_3 T_4	80–200 ng/dL 4.5–11.5 mcg/dL	Measures triiodothyronine (T_3) and thyroxine (T_4) to evaluate thyroid function. Increased level indicates hyperthyroidism; decreased reflects hypothyroidism.	No fluid restriction is required. Avoid shellfish several days before test.
Parathyroid			
Serum calcium	9–11 mg/dL	This test evaluates parathyroid function and calcium metabolism.	Fasting not required; however, it is part of a chemistry panel in which fasting is required.
Serum phosphate	2.5–4.5 mg/dL	It measures serum phosphate. Increased levels in both tests indicate hyperparathyroidism; decreased levels indicate hypoparathyroidism.	Fasting not required; however, it is part of a chemistry panel in which fasting is required.
Adrenal			
Cortisol	Between 8–10 a.m.: 5–23 mcg/dL Between 4–6 p.m.: 3–13 mcg/dL	This test measures total serum cortisol, which evaluates adrenal cortex function. Levels are increased in Cushing syndrome; decreased in Addison disease.	Advise patient to rest in bed 2 hours before blood is drawn. Explain that two blood samples are drawn—one between 8–10 a.m., the other between 4–6 p.m.
Aldosterone	4–30 ng/dL sitting position Less than 16 ng/dL supine position	Levels are drawn to diagnose hyperaldosteronism.	Ask patient to be in supine position for 1 hour before test is drawn.
Urinary 17-keto-steroids (17-KS)	5–15 mg/24 hr men 5–25 mg/24 hr women	17-KS are metabolites of testosterone, which are released from the adrenal cortex. Levels increase with Cushing syndrome and decrease in Addison disease.	Teach patient about 24-hour urine collection, which must be iced or refrigerated during collection.

(continued on next page)

SKILL 8.1 Endocrine Disorders: Assessing (continued)

TABLE 8–1 Common Laboratory Tests for Endocrine Disorders (continued)

Test	Normal Adult Values	Explanation	Nursing Implications
Pancreas			
Fasting blood glucose	70–100 mg/dL	This test measures circulating blood glucose level. Increases are seen in diabetes mellitus, acute pancreatitis; decreased level is seen in Addison disease.	This test is done fasting.
Glycosylated hemoglobin (HbA1c)	5.5–7%	Test used to measure glucose control during the previous 3 months. Levels are increased in newly diagnosed or poorly controlled diabetic. It is not used to diagnose diabetes mellitus.	No fasting is required.
Two-hour oral glucose tolerance test (OGTT)	Less than 125 mg/dL	Determines the level of glucose 2 hours after drinking 75 g of glucose. Glucose level should return to premeal levels, but in diabetics, the level is higher than 200 mg/dL.	Patient is NPO for 12 hours before test. Then patient must drink the entire 75 g of glucose and not eat anything else until blood is drawn.
Urine glucose	Negative	Estimates the amount of glucose in urine, which should be negative.	Collect a fresh urine sample; stagnant urine may alter test results.
Urine ketones	Negative	Measures ketones excreted in urine from incomplete fat metabolism. Positive result means lack of insulin or diabetic ketoacidosis.	Some drugs may interfere with both test results.
Urine test for microalbumin	0.2–1.9 mg/dL	Microalbumin is the earliest indicator for development of diabetic nephropathy. Elevated microalbumin levels increase the risk for end-stage renal disease.	Collect a fresh urine sample and send to laboratory for analysis.

MAGNETIC RESONANCE IMAGING (MRI)

- Used to identify tumors of the pituitary gland and hypothalamus.
- Patients with metallic implants cannot have an MRI due to its magnetic field.

COMPUTED TOMOGRAPHY (CT) SCAN

- In a thyroid scan, iodine-125 is injected IV.
  - Ask about allergies to iodine and seafood.
  - Abdominal CT is used to detect tumors of the adrenal gland and pancreas. "Cold spots," which do not take up the I-125, indicate malignancy.
- For the radioactive iodine (RAI) uptake test, iodine-131 or I-125 (capsule or liquid form) is given.
  - Increased uptake indicates Graves disease; decreased uptake means hypothyroidism.
  - Ask about allergies to iodine and seafood. Thyroid drugs or medications containing iodine are withheld for weeks before the study.

9. When the procedure is complete, perform hand hygiene and leave the patient safe and comfortable.
10. Complete documentation using forms, checklists, or electronic dropdown lists supplemented by nurse's notes or additional comments as appropriate.

SAMPLE DOCUMENTATION

[date] 1400 Back to room post CT Scan of neck. No complaints of itching, no redness, hives, or respiratory distress noted. VS T- 37.11°C (98.8°F) (oral), P-82, R-18, B/P-130/84, O$_2$Sat. 98% room air. States he's hungry, meal tray brought to bedside. Tolerated procedure without incident. *T. Moore*

SKILL 8.2 Endocrine Disorders: Complementary Health Approaches

Complementary health approaches are healthcare options that patients use along with conventional medical treatments and therapies. They include natural dietary supplements such as fish oil and herbs, relaxation exercises such as yoga and tai chi, meditation techniques, progressive relaxation, and guided imagery. Sometimes complementary health approaches are done by a trained specialist, such as massage therapist or acupuncturist. For safe coordination of their healthcare, patients need to discuss complementary health approaches they use with their healthcare providers. The National Center for Complementary and Integrative Health (NCCIH) is the federal agency doing scientific research and investigation for evidence about the use and value of complementary health approaches in improving health and healthcare.

Delegation or Assignment

The nurse must discuss the complementary health activity with the patient and then the patient's healthcare provider to determine if it can be done during the patient's stay in the healthcare facility. If the patient wants to learn relaxation

SKILL 8.2 Endocrine Disorders: Complementary Health Approaches (continued)

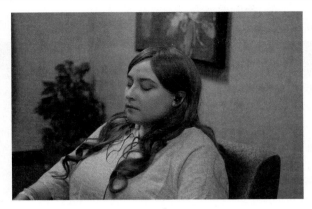

Source: Rick Brady/Pearson Education, Inc.

❶ Reduce environmental stimuli in the patient's room when teaching relaxation processes.

techniques during the hospital stay ❶, the nurse can teach the patient about controlled breathing exercises, progressive muscle relaxation, and guided imagery. These noninvasive pain management relaxation techniques can then be delegated or assigned to a UAP who is experienced with using the techniques and is comfortable helping the patient practice them. The nurse instructs the UAP to report patient observations to the nurse for follow-up. Assessment and evaluation of the effectiveness of the exercise remain the responsibility of the nurse (see Skill 3.3 for more information about these relaxation techniques).

Equipment

- No equipment is required for relaxation techniques.

Preparation

- Review healthcare provider's orders and patient's nursing plan of care.
- Review patient's record for allergies.

Procedure

1. Introduce self to patient and verify the patient's identity using two identifiers. Explain to the patient what you are going to do, why it is necessary, and how the patient can participate. Provide the patient information about how complementary health approaches work with a therapeutic regimen. Ask the patient about concerns with adjusting to an endocrine disorder. Discuss how the results will be used in planning further care or treatments.
2. Perform hand hygiene and observe appropriate infection control procedures.
3. Provide for patient privacy. Provide comfort and safety for the patient and yourself.
4. Focus on teaching patients how to meet physical and emotional needs for themselves and their families.
5. Depending on the endocrine disorder, discuss necessary lifestyle and behavioral modifications. **Table 8–2 »** lists selected strategies that apply.
6. When teaching is complete, perform hand hygiene and leave the patient safe and comfortable.
7. Complete documentation using forms, checklists, or electronic dropdown lists supplemented by nurse's notes or additional comments as appropriate.

SAMPLE DOCUMENTATION

[date] 1028 Asking about controlled breathing exercises to help relax. States, "I get so nervous around people." Discussion done about benefits of controlled breathing. Techniques demonstrated and practice from patient observed. States he wants to try this exercise next time he feels anxious around people looking at him. Encouragement and support provided. Continues to practice relaxation exercise quietly without incident. *W. Goodness*

TABLE 8–2 Select Endocrine Disorders and Common Strategies

Endocrine Disorders	Lifestyle/Behavioral Modification Strategy
Anterior Pituitary Gland	
Gigantism Dwarfism	■ Learn to cope with body image changes ■ Ask healthcare provider about massage therapy and meditation for anxiety about size ■ Learn to cope with possible surgery ■ Adapt environment to meet size needs ■ Need for lifetime hormone replacement therapy
Posterior Pituitary Gland	
Diabetes insipidus	■ Recognize excess fluid and electrolyte imbalance problems ■ Monitor weight daily ■ Maintain low-sodium diet ■ Need for periodic healthcare visits ■ Need for lifetime medication therapy ■ Ask healthcare provider about dietary supplements and their effects on blood glucose levels

(continued on next page)

SKILL 8.2 Endocrine Disorders: Complementary Health Approaches (*continued*)

TABLE 8-2 Select Endocrine Disorders and Common Strategies (*continued*)

Endocrine Disorders	Lifestyle/Behavioral Modification Strategy
Hyperthyroidism	
Graves disease	■ Learn to cope with body image changes of goiter and exophthalmos ■ Schedule rest times for fatigue ■ Maintain balanced diet and weight ■ Maintain cool environment ■ Wear tinted eyeglasses or eye shields to protect the cornea ■ Apply artificial tears as needed ■ Ask healthcare provider about special dietary foods that contain iodine or dietary supplements ■ Learn to cope with possible surgery ■ Learn coping strategies for emotional control ■ Need for lifetime medications ■ Need for periodic healthcare visits
Hypothyroidism	
Hashimoto thyroiditis	■ Learn to cope with body image of goiter ■ Slow movements, need for rest periods ■ Maintain warm environment ■ Maintain appropriate diet and weight ■ Monitor weight weekly ■ Ask the healthcare provider about using herbal supplements ■ Periodic healthcare visits ■ Utilize preventive infection practices ■ Use stool softeners or laxatives as prescribed ■ Need for lifetime medications
Myxedema coma	■ Have a plan to get immediate medical help with seizures or extreme lethargy ■ Need for lifetime medications ■ Ask the healthcare provider about diet and supplemental minerals to synthesize thyroid hormones
Adrenal Gland	
Cushing syndrome	■ Learn to cope with body image of buffalo hump over upper back, moon face, thinning of scalp hair, and increased body hair ■ Safety measures to prevent injuries, especially bone injuries and bruising ■ Utilize preventive infection practices ■ Ask the healthcare provider about ginseng and other herbs to enhance the body's ability to cope with mental stress ■ Maintain appropriate weight through fluid intake and meals ■ Need for lifetime medications ■ Learn to cope with possible surgery ■ Periodic healthcare visits ■ Seek counseling for depression
Addison disease	■ Monitor for hypotension, rapid pulse ■ Monitor serum electrolytes, mainly potassium ■ Ask healthcare provider about herbal therapy, yoga, and tai chi ■ Monitor daily fluid intake and output ■ Need to carry emergency kit containing parenteral cortisone and a syringe ■ Assess for signs of dehydration ■ Need for lifetime medications ■ Periodic healthcare visits

SKILL 8.3 Paracentesis: Assisting

Safety Note! *During scheduled clinical time, nursing students may have a learning opportunity to observe or assist with this skill only with faculty permission and with direct supervision from faculty or another RN.*

Normally the body creates just enough peritoneal fluid for lubrication. The fluid is continuously formed and absorbed into the lymphatic system. However, in some disease processes, a large amount of fluid accumulates in the abdominal cavity; this condition is called **ascites**. Normal ascitic fluid is serous, clear, and light yellow in color. An abdominal paracentesis is carried out to obtain a fluid specimen for laboratory study and to relieve pressure on the abdominal organs due to the presence of excess fluid. For more information about metabolism and ascites, see the Liver Disease exemplar in the Metabolism Module of Volume 1.

Delegation or Assignment

Assisting with a paracentesis is not delegated or assigned to the UAP. The nurse assists with the procedure and provides care to the patient while monitoring the patient during the procedure. The nurse can ask the UAP to report patient observations to the nurse for follow-up. Assessment and evaluation remain the responsibility of the nurse.

Equipment

- A prepackaged disposable paracentesis kit
- 4 one-liter vacuum bottles if anticipating many liters of fluid to be removed
- Clean gloves, sterile gloves, nonsterile gown

Preparation

- Verify signed informed consent for procedure is in front of patient's record.
- Review healthcare provider's orders and patient's nursing plan of care.
- Review patient's record for allergies.
- Gather equipment and supplies.

Procedure

1. Introduce self to patient and verify the patient's identity using two identifiers. Explain to the patient what happens during the procedure, that you will be present during the procedure, why it is necessary, and how the patient can participate. Discuss how the results will be used in planning further care or treatments.
2. Perform hand hygiene and observe appropriate infection control procedures.
3. Provide for patient privacy.
4. Have patient void just before the procedure. **Rationale:** *This reduces bladder size to minimize risk of puncturing the bladder.*
5. Help patient lie supine and assume a slightly recumbent position for procedure. If the patient is able, provide assistance to a Fowler position or sitting position on the side of the bed or in a chair with the legs spread apart. Explain the importance of remaining still during the procedure 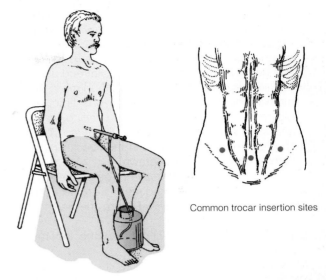.

Common trocar insertion sites

Source: Position Client in Chair to Facilitate Trocar Insertion and Drainage for Paracentesis from *Clinical Nursing Skills: Basic to Advanced Skills*, 9e by Sandra F. Smith, Donna J. Duell, Barbara C. Martin, Michelle Aebersold and Laura Gonzalez. Copyright © 2017 by Pearson Education.

❶ Position patient in chair to facilitate trocar insertion and drainage for paracentesis.

6. Provide verbal support; monitor for signs of distress during the procedure.
    - Using strict sterile technique, the healthcare provider makes a small incision midway between the umbilicus and the symphysis pubis on the midline. A trocar (a sharp, pointed instrument) and cannula (tube) are inserted. The trocar, which is inside the cannula, is then withdrawn ❷.

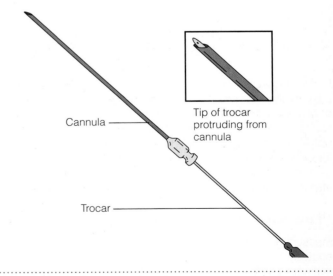

Cannula

Tip of trocar protruding from cannula

Trocar

❷ A trocar and cannula may be used for an abdominal paracentesis.

(continued on next page)

SKILL 8.3 Paracentesis: Assisting (continued)

- Tubing is attached to the cannula and the fluid flows through the tubing into a receptacle. If the purpose of the paracentesis is to obtain a specimen, the healthcare provider may use a long aspirating needle attached to a syringe rather than making an incision and using a trocar and cannula. Normally about 1500 mL is the maximum amount of fluid drained at one time, and it is drained very slowly. **Rationale:** *Limiting the amount and speed of fluid withdrawal prevents hypovolemic shock.* Some fluid is placed in the specimen container before the cannula is withdrawn.

7. The small incision may or may not be sutured; it is covered with a small sterile bandage. **Rationale:** *This helps prevent infection at the site.* Return the bed to lowest position.
8. Label and transport specimens to the laboratory as ordered.
9. Monitor the patient after the procedure.
10. When the procedure is complete, perform hand hygiene and leave the patient safe and comfortable.
11. Complete documentation using forms, checklists, or electronic dropdown lists supplemented by nurse's notes or additional comments as appropriate.

SAMPLE DOCUMENTATION

[date] 1340 Paracentesis per Dr. Grey. 16-gauge angiocath inserted RLQ with patient in supine slightly recumbent position. Fluid specimens collected before connected to vacuum bottle. 1250 mL of light yellow fluid removed. Band-aid applied to insertion site, remained dry with no fluid noted. Returned to semi Fowler position. P-92, R-20, B/P-146/90. Specimen containers labeled and sent to lab. Tolerated procedure without incident. *T. Mays*

Lifespan Considerations
OLDER ADULTS

- Provide pillows and blankets to help older adults remain comfortable during the procedure.
- Older adults may need to void more frequently and in smaller amounts.
- Monitor the patient for signs of hypovolemia after ascitic fluid removed. Older adults have less tolerance for fluid loss and may develop hypovolemia if a large volume of fluid is drained rapidly.

» Diabetes Care

Expected Outcomes

1. Accurate blood glucose level is obtained.
2. Patient actively participates in decisions about patient's care.
3. Medication therapeutic effect is achieved.
4. Patient's diabetic teaching is completed before discharge.

SKILL 8.4 Capillary Blood Specimen for Glucose: Measuring

Performing a capillary blood glucose test provides a quick and easy method of measuring blood glucose. In this test, a drop of blood is obtained via fingerstick of a child or adult or heelstick of a newborn or infant (the earlobe can also be used to obtain a blood sample if needed). It can be done as a self-test for people with diabetes or as a point-of-care test in a healthcare facility using a portable glucometer. Insulin administration after glucose measurement is described in Chapter 2.

Delegation or Assignment

Measuring a capillary blood specimen for glucose can be delegated or assigned to the UAP. The nurse can assess and evaluate the UAP's ability to complete this skill safely and accurately. The nurse remains responsible for the assessment, interpretation of abnormal findings, and determination of appropriate responses.

Equipment

- Portable glucometer
- Blood glucose reagent strip compatible with the glucometer
- 2 × 2 gauze
- Antiseptic swab
- Clean cotton ball or 2 × 2 gauze pad
- Clean gloves
- Sterile lancet (a sharp device to puncture the skin)
- Lancet injector (a spring-loaded mechanism that holds the lancet)
- Warm cloth or other warming device (optional)
- Band-aid if needed

Preparation

- Review healthcare provider's orders and patient's nursing plan of care.

SKILL 8.4 Capillary Blood Specimen for Glucose: Measuring *(continued)*

■ Review the type of glucometer and the manufacturer's instructions.
■ Gather equipment and supplies.

Procedure

1. Prior to performing the procedure, introduce self and verify the patient's identity using two identifiers. Explain to the patient that you are going to obtain a blood sample from a fingerstick to test for blood glucose, why it is necessary, and how the patient can participate. Discuss how the results will be used in planning further care or treatments.
2. Perform hand hygiene and observe other appropriate infection control procedures (e.g., gloves).
3. Provide for patient privacy.
4. Prepare the equipment.
   - Some glucometers turn on by inserting the test strip into the glucometer.
   - Calibrate the glucometer and run a control sample according to the manufacturer's instructions and/or confirm the code number.
5. Select and prepare the vascular puncture site.
   - Choose a vascular puncture site (e.g., the side of an adult's finger). Avoid sites beside bone. Wrap the finger first in a warm cloth, or hold a finger in a dependent (below heart level) position. If the earlobe is used, rub it gently with a small piece of gauze. **Rationale:** *These actions increase the blood flow to the area, ensure an adequate specimen, and reduce the need for a repeat puncture.*
   - Clean the site with an antiseptic swab or soap and water and allow it to air dry completely ❶. This will remove any residue from eating fruit or other contaminants on the skin that could impact the test result. The skin needs to be dried thoroughly to prevent dilution of the blood sample.
   - Some devices need a test strip inserted into the monitor at this point, following manufacturer's instructions ❷.

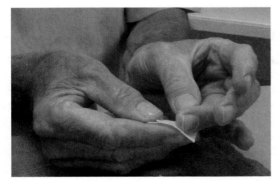

Source: Donna J. Duell

❶ Use soap and water or swab to cleanse finger before puncture.

6. Obtain the blood specimen.
   - Apply clean gloves.
   - Place the injector, if used, against the site, and release the needle ❸, thus permitting it to pierce the skin. Make sure the lancet is perpendicular to the site. **Rationale:** *The lan-*

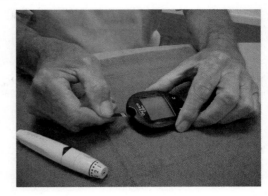

Source: Donna J. Duell

❷ Insert test strip into monitor (you have 30 sec to obtain a reading).

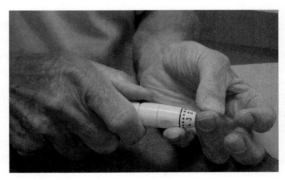

Source: Donna J. Duell

❸ Adjust Autolet depth, place on side of finger, and release.

cet is designed to pierce the skin at a specific depth when it is in a perpendicular position relative to the skin.
or
   - Prick the site with a lancet or needle, using a darting motion.
   - Gently squeeze (but do not touch) slightly proximal to the puncture site until a large drop of blood forms. The size of the drop of blood can vary depending on the meter. Some meters require as little as 0.3 mL of blood to test blood sugar accurately. A common practice to ensure accurate test results is to wipe the first drop of blood away, and use the second drop for testing.

CAUTION! Avoid "milking" or applying pressure to the fingertip to encourage blood flow. This can cause damage to the membrane of red blood cells that result in hemoglobin leaking into surrounding tissue fluid (hemolysis). Glucose results may be incorrectly lower than actual results. Free flowing blood is needed for best test results.

   - Hold the reagent strip under the puncture site until adequate blood covers the indicator square ❹. The pad will absorb the blood and a chemical reaction will occur. Do not smear the blood. **Rationale:** *Smearing the blood*

(continued on next page)

SKILL 8.4 Capillary Blood Specimen for Glucose: Measuring *(continued)*

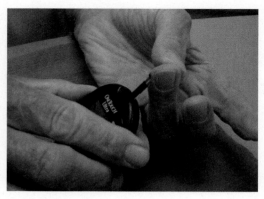

Source: Donna J. Duell

④ After gently massaging finger, place large drop of blood on test strip.

will cause an inaccurate reading. Some meters wick the blood by just touching the puncture site with the strip.
- Ask the patient to apply pressure to the skin puncture site with a 2 × 2 gauze. **Rationale:** *Pressure will assist hemostasis.*

7. Expose the blood to the test strip for the period and the manner specified by the manufacturer. As soon as the blood is placed on the test strip:
   - Follow the manufacturer's recommendations on the glucometer for the amount of time indicated by the manufacturer **⑤**. **Rationale:** *The blood must remain in contact with the test pad for a prescribed time to obtain accurate results.*
   - Some glucometers have the test strip placed in the machine before the specimen is obtained.

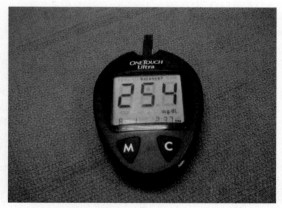

Source: Donna J. Duell

⑤ Wait 30 sec and note reading on monitor.

8. Measure the blood glucose.
   - Place the strip into the meter according to the manufacturer's instructions. Refer to the specific manufacturer's recommendations for the specific procedure.

- After the designated time, most glucometers will display the glucose reading automatically. Correct timing ensures accurate results.
- Turn off the glucometer and discard the test strip and 2 × 2 gauze in a biohazard container. Discard the lancet into a sharps container.

9. Remove and discard gloves. Perform hand hygiene.
10. Document the method of testing and results on appropriate documents in the patient's record. If appropriate, record the patient's understanding and ability to demonstrate the skill. The patient's record may also include an electronic dropdown list or flow sheet on which are recorded capillary blood glucose results and the amount, type, route, and time of insulin administration. Always check if a diabetic flow sheet is being used for the patient.
11. Check healthcare provider orders for sliding-scale insulin based on capillary blood glucose results. Administer insulin as prescribed (see Skill 2.35).

SAMPLE DOCUMENTATION

[date] 0720 Awake and alert. Fingerstick blood sample obtained from side of right middle fingertip for blood glucose test. Blood glucose level 102 per glucometer. No insulin required at this time per insulin sliding scale ordered. Tolerated without complaint. *P. Mann*

Lifespan Considerations
NEWBORNS AND INFANTS

The outer aspect of the heel is the most common site on newborns and infants for obtaining a capillary blood specimen. Placing a warm cloth on the newborn's or infant's heel often increases the blood flow to the area.

CHILDREN

- Use the side of a fingertip for a young patient older than age 2, unless contraindicated.
- When possible, allow the child to choose the puncture site.
- Praise the young patient for cooperating and assure the child that the procedure is not a punishment.

OLDER ADULTS

- Older adults may have arthritic joint changes, poor vision, or hand tremors and may need assistance using the glucose meter or obtaining a meter that accommodates these limitations.
- Older adults may have difficulty obtaining diabetic supplies due to financial concerns or homebound status.
- Older adults may have poor circulation. Warming the hands by wrapping with a warm washcloth for 3–5 min or placing the hand dependent for a few moments may help in obtaining a blood sample.

SKILL 8.4 Capillary Blood Specimen for Glucose: Measuring (*continued*)

Patient Teaching

Measuring Blood Glucose at Home

- Assess the patient's or caregiver's ability and willingness to perform blood glucose monitoring at home. There are many glucometers on the market with a variety of features and costs. The patient needs to learn the basics of performing blood glucose monitoring and then practice with the glucometer to be used at home, following the guidelines of the manufacturer.

- Demonstrate the proper use of the lancet and glucose meter, and provide written guidelines and pictures. Allow time for a return demonstration. The patient may need several visits to completely learn the procedure.

- Ensure the patient's ability to obtain supplies and purchase reagent strips. The strips are relatively expensive and may not be covered by the patient's insurance.

- Stress the importance of record keeping. Instruct the patient on when to do glucose monitoring, how to record the blood glucose levels, and when to notify the healthcare provider.

- Ensure children with diabetes who need to perform fingersticks know safe practices for cleaning blood from surfaces (household bleach is best) and about safe storage of equipment to prevent young children from having access to it.

- Assist child to identify a place in the school where the child can store glucose-monitoring equipment and perform the procedure in private.

EVIDENCE-BASED PRACTICE

Nasal Inhalation of Insulin for Diabetes Mellitus

The child and adult patient with diabetes must interrupt the daily schedule to check blood glucose and administer insulin injections as needed 3–4 times each day. These patients may resist having to do this and may become noncompliant with the therapeutic regimen of diet, exercise, medication treatment, and the schedule for measuring and monitoring blood glucose.

Research is actively being conducted by many pharmaceutical companies to find a less invasive option than injections to deliver insulin into the bloodstream; one such option is insulin via nasal inhalation. Although variables in types of insulin and data results are difficult to analyze, one insulin product has already been approved by the FDA and is called Afrezza (MannKind Corp). According to the manufacturing company, Afrezza, which is administered using a small inhaler, works best for patients with type 2 diabetes mellitus (T2DM). Many patients with diabetes would benefit from development of a noninvasive route for administering insulin to manage their diabetes. Such a product could positively impact compliance with therapeutic treatment among children and adults with diabetes.

Sources: Data from Modern Medicine Network. (2014). *Afrezza, fast-acting, inhaled insulin, is approved.* Retrieved from http://drugtopics.modernmedicine.com/drug-topics/content/tags/afrezza/afrezza-fast-acting-inhaled-insulin-approved?page=full; Pittas, A. (2015). *Inhaled insulin therapy in diabetes mellitus.* Retrieved from http://www.uptodate.com/contents/inhaled-insulin-therapy-in-diabetes-mellitus; Thompson, D. (2015). *Nasal spray may treat diabetics' low blood sugar. Trial found it easier to use than current remedy, an injection.* Retrieved from http://www.webmd.com/diabetes/news/20151218/nasal-spray-may-give-diabetics-faster-treatment-for-low-blood-sugar#1

SKILL 8.5 Diabetes: Managing

Metabolic disorders characterized by hyperglycemia (too much glucose in the blood) include prediabetes, undiagnosed diabetes, and diabetes mellitus. These conditions are due to an insufficient supply of insulin, ineffective insulin action, or both. Diabetes mellitus includes type 1 diabetes mellitus (T1DM), in which patients are insulin-dependent, and type 2 diabetes mellitus (T2DM), in which patients' therapy includes diet and exercise, oral medications, and/or insulin. A third type is gestational diabetes, usually a temporary condition occurring during pregnancy, in which therapy consists of diet and exercise and/or insulin. Blood glucose control is essential to reduce complications that most often affect the cardiovascular system, kidneys, eyes, and nerves. Go to Skill 2.35 for information about insulin administration for the patient with diabetes.

Safety Considerations

It is important for nurses to be able to recognize the signs and symptoms of hyperglycemia (blood glucose too high) and hypoglycemia (blood glucose too low) in patients with diabetes ❶. When a patient is recognized to have hypoglycemia, the blood glucose is usually checked twice to verify the glucose level. Most healthcare facilities have protocols to follow to begin treatment to raise the level of blood glucose. For example, for a patient with a blood glucose of 56 mg/dL that is awake and able to swallow, protocol may be to give the patient juice with sugar added, or soda, or 5 glucose tablets, or 2 tubes dextrose gel. Then the patient would receive 15 g of carbohydrate such as graham crackers, saltine crackers with peanut butter, or skim milk. Patient would be monitored and blood glucose would be rechecked after 15–20 min.

The nurse monitors for complications and teaches patients to be aware of potential complications associated with diabetes (**Table 8–3** ≫). The longer the patient has been diagnosed with diabetes, the greater the risk for complications. Frequent blood glucose monitoring with insulin injections, exercise, and a healthy diet can help reduce these risks.

(*continued on next page*)

SKILL 8.5 Diabetes: Managing *(continued)*

Hyperglycemia (high blood glucose)		Management
Fruity breath	Confusion	Check blood glucose
Nausea	Flushed skin	Have someone stay with patient
Drowsiness	Skin warm, dry	If insulin pump in use, check connectivity
Dry mouth	Blurred vision	Check blood or urine for ketones
Thirst	Increased respirations	Monitor patient
		Call healthcare provider

Hypoglycemia (low blood glucose)		Management
Weakness	Irritability	Check blood glucose (follow agency protocols for level of blood glucose)
Skin cool	Confusion	Stay with patient
Sweating	Anxiety	If patient is alert, give 15 grams simple fast-acting carbohydrate (orange juice, table sugar, glucose tablets, glucose gel)
Shaking	Increased pulse	Give Dextrose 50% IV per protocol if needed
Pallor	Headache	Monitor patient
		Recheck blood glucose after 15 minutes
		Call healthcare provider

❶ Symptoms and management of hyperglycemia and hypoglycemia.

TABLE 8–3 Potential Complications Associated with Diabetes Mellitus

Body Focus	Initial Complication	Further Complication	Late Development
Cardiovascular system	■ Atherosclerosis ■ Hypertension ■ Impaired peripheral circulation	■ Coronary artery disease ■ Stroke ■ Peripheral vascular disease	■ Myocardial infarction with heart failure ■ Lower leg ulcers ■ Gangrenous tissue and amputations of lower leg
Eyes	Diabetic retinopathy	■ Progressive blindness ■ Cataracts	■ Blurry vision ■ Loss of vision
Kidneys	Diabetic nephropathy	■ Albumin in urine ■ Hypertension, edema ■ Progressive renal insufficiency	■ End-stage renal disease ■ Renal failure
Nerves	Diabetic autonomic neuropathy	■ Sensory and motor impairment ■ Postural hypotension ■ Delayed gastric emptying, diarrhea ■ Impaired genitourinary function	■ Peripheral neuropathies begin in toes and progress upward; distal paresthesia, pain, cold sensation ■ Urinary retention ■ Frequent urinary tract infections ■ Sexual dysfunction ■ Increased risk for infection

Patient Teaching

Management of Potential Complications

- Maintain balance of nutrition, activity, and blood glucose levels.
- Monitor blood glucose levels regularly and give insulin and/or oral antidiabetic agents as prescribed.
- Rotate insulin injection sites.
- Eat appropriate meals and snacks at given times.
- Maintain skin integrity, especially feet.
- Have an adequate fluid intake appropriate for chronic conditions.
- Do not smoke.
- Assess for signs/symptoms of infection: fever, chills; cloudy, foul-smelling urine; tachycardia; red, swelling, or pain at skin breakdown site.

- Maintain good oral hygiene with a soft toothbrush.
- Be aware of environmental hazards to avoid injury.
- Develop an adequate support system with family and friends, or join a support group.
- Utilize community resources as needed.
- Have periodic medical assessment of general condition and any potential risk factors and a hemoglobin A1C lab test.
- Take all medications as prescribed.
- Report any change in chronic conditions to healthcare provider.
- Maintain self-care as able and secure assistance as needed.

SKILL 8.5 Diabetes: Managing (*continued*)

Safety Considerations

THE DIABETIC FOOT

People with diabetes mellitus have a high incidence of problems with their feet and subsequent amputations. Guidelines for management of the patient with diabetes foot care include:

- Inspect daily for injury, cuts, bruises, red areas, or burns from foot trauma occurring without knowing it happened.
- Inspect for cracks and fissures caused by dry skin, infections such as athlete's foot, and blisters.
- Avoid use of heating pads or ice packs on feet.
- Teach the patient to:
  - Practice meticulous care of toenails to avoid injury and ingrown toenails.
  - Avoid use of garters, knee stockings, or pantyhose.
  - Wear appropriate-fitting socks and shoes.
  - Never go barefoot.
  - Do not sit with legs crossed at the knees or ankles.
  - Seek early treatment of a superficial injury to avoid deeper progression.
  - Get bed rest, take antibiotics, and provide debridement wound care.

SICK-DAY MANAGEMENT

When an individual with diabetes is sick, blood glucose levels increase, even though food intake decreases. The individual may mistakenly alter or omit the insulin dose or oral antidiabetic agent, causing further problems. Dietary guidelines during illness focus on preventing dehydration and providing nutrition for promoting recovery. The nurse teaches the following sick-day management:

- Monitor blood glucose at least 4 times a day throughout the illness.
- Test urine for ketones if the blood glucose level is greater than 250 mg/dL.
- Continue to take the usual insulin dose or oral antidiabetic agent.
- Drink 240–360 mL (8–12 oz) of fluid each waking hour.
- Eat a small amount of carbohydrate every 1–2 hr, such as gelatin, fruit juice, or a popsicle.
- Call the healthcare provider if unable to eat for more than 24 hours or if vomiting and diarrhea last for more than 6 hours.

≫ Critical Thinking Options for Unexpected Outcomes

Not all unexpected outcomes require further nursing intervention; however, many times they do. When the patient demonstrates a change in signs/symptoms indicating an emerging problem, the nurse should immediately assess and troubleshoot what is happening. The assessment data must be processed quickly to formulate a hypothesis so the nurse can make a clinical judgment. The nurse then decides how best to resolve the problem and improve the patient's situation for a better outcome.

EXPECTED OUTCOME	UNEXPECTED OUTCOME	POSSIBLE INTERVENTIONS
General Metabolism Lifestyle changes assist in management of patient's altered health status.	Patient does not adhere to diet.	■ Elicit patient's feelings to determine reason for nonadherence. ■ Check method of diet preparation and administration to see if it is attractive and appealing. ■ Ensure that the environment is conducive to eating. ■ Collaborate with dietitian to discuss appropriate dietary choices with patient.
Paracentesis is completed without complications.	Urine output is blood tinged after paracentesis.	■ Notify healthcare provider at once; bladder may have been punctured during procedure. ■ Monitor vital signs for shock. ■ Maintain patient on bed rest. ■ Observe for urine output.
Diabetes Medication management of insulin injections is performed without complications.	Medication is administered using wrong parenteral route.	■ Notify healthcare provider after assessing patient; medications may need to be administered to reverse the action of the medication. ■ Monitor patient's response closely and report adverse findings immediately. ■ Medication administered by IM or IV rather than subcutaneously leads to faster absorption rates; therefore, ongoing assessment must be done to determine effects. (IV administration has immediate action.) ■ Complete unusual occurrence report according to facility policy.

(*continued on next page*)

EXPECTED OUTCOME	UNEXPECTED OUTCOME	POSSIBLE INTERVENTIONS
Basic diabetic teaching is done, including self-administration of insulin if required, before discharge.	Insufficient time to complete basic diabetic teaching, including self-administration of insulin if required, before discharge.	■ Collaborate with facility's diabetic nurse educator. ■ Continue to complete discharge teaching, and send to referral facility. ■ Notify healthcare provider of the situation (may need to schedule office visits to complete teaching). ■ Verbally communicate to referral facility and discuss discharge needs of patient (i.e., this may include home care nurse visits to ensure a patient with diabetes does appropriate diabetic checks and insulin is administered as needed).

REVIEW Questions

1. After assessing a client, the nurse reschedules serum thyroid tests for the following week. What information caused the nurse to make this clinical decision?
   1. Client smoked a cigarette 2 hours ago.
   2. Client was not supine for 1 hour before the test.
   3. Client ate crab cakes for dinner the previous day.
   4. Client did not abstain from food or fluids after midnight.

2. The nurse provides a schedule of beginning yoga classes for a client. Which health problem is this client most likely attempting to manage?
   1. Addison disease
   2. Myxedema coma
   3. Cushing syndrome
   4. Hashimoto thyroiditis

3. During a paracentesis, 1500 mL of fluid was removed from a client's abdomen over 10 minutes. Which assessment finding indicates the client is experiencing an adverse effect from this procedure?
   1. Warm, dry skin
   2. Heart rate 94 bpm
   3. Blood pressure 88/58 mmHg
   4. Respiratory rate 18/min and unlabored

4. The laboratory report from a paracentesis sample indicates the presence of urate crystals. What should this information indicate to the nurse?
   1. The client has unusual fluid in the peritoneum.
   2. The bladder was punctured during the procedure.
   3. The client has an undiagnosed electrolyte imbalance.
   4. There was not enough fluid removed during the procedure.

5. The UAP reports that a client's capillary blood glucose level could not be measured at 1600 hours because of "insufficient sample size." What should the nurse do?
   1. Ask another UAP to repeat the test.
   2. Observe the UAP perform the skill to determine competency.
   3. Document that the measurement was not able to be obtained.
   4. Notify the healthcare provider for changes in afternoon insulin dose.

6. The nurse reviews the process of measuring capillary blood glucose with a client newly diagnosed with type 2 diabetes mellitus. Which client statement indicates additional teaching is required?
   1. "I should let the alcohol dry before piercing my skin."
   2. "I should use a darting motion to puncture the skin for a sample."
   3. "I should warm my hands before attempting to get a blood sample."
   4. "I should press on the puncture site to make the blood flow better."

7. During a home visit, the nurse determines that a client with type 2 diabetes mellitus would benefit from additional teaching. What did the nurse observe to make this clinical decision?
   1. Client walking barefoot in the home
   2. Ashtray holding spare change and house keys
   3. Log of daily capillary glucose levels next to the monitor
   4. Glass of water placed on the table next to where the client sits

8. A client with type 2 diabetes mellitus is admitted for treatment caused by severe influenza. What should the nurse include in this client's plan of care?
   1. Monitor capillary glucose level twice a day.
   2. Restrict carbohydrate intake to 45 g/day.
   3. Encourage oral fluid intake to be 240 mL/hr.
   4. Hold prescribed medication if oral intake is 50% less than prescribed.

Note: For answers and rationales for the review questions, go to Appendix A or your Pearson MyLab Nursing and eText.

Chapter 9
Mobility

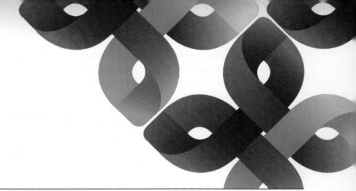

Chapter at a Glance

>> The Concept of Mobility

Mobility is independent, purposeful, and functional movement of the body or extremities by the musculoskeletal system, the brain and neuromuscular system, and energy. Joint mobility allows certain movement or range of motion movement around the joint. Stability of the joint results from support by ligaments, bones, and other connective tissue around the joint. Body movements include abduction, adduction, extension, flexion, rotation, and circumduction.

Impairment of mobility refers to a person's inability to use one extremity or more due to amputation, orthopedic or neuromuscular impairments, disease, accident, congenital disorder, or lack of manual dexterity or strength to walk, grasp, or lift objects. The use of assistive devices and equipment such as a wheelchair, walker, or crutches may be utilized to aid mobility. Nurses collaborate with physical therapists in providing patient education, assistance in positioning and movement, and training in adapting to changes from impaired mobility. Safety considerations are a priority to prevent injuries and accidents.

Learning Outcomes

9.1 Give examples of five safety guidelines of body mechanics to avoid complications from lifting and turning patients.

9.2 Support the advantages for older adults to perform range-of-motion exercises daily.

9.3 Explain various bed positions and give an example of how each one is used for patient care.

9.4 Give examples of assistive devices that can be used to help move a patient safely in bed or transfer a patient to a chair.

9.5 Summarize the steps in using a hydraulic lift to safely move a patient from the bed to a chair.

9.6 Differentiate safety measures when transporting a child patient and an adult patient to another department for a diagnostic test.

9.7 Differentiate between the various techniques of using crutches when walking.

9.8 Explain priority safety assessment observations for the patient in skin traction.

The following feature links some, but not all, of the concepts related to assessment. They are presented in alphabetical order.

Concepts Related to
Mobility

CONCEPT	RELATIONSHIP TO MOBILITY	NURSING IMPLICATIONS
Comfort	Acute and chronic pain can lead to decreased activity, causing changes in muscle and bone density.	■ Maintain pain management as ordered to encourage patient physical activity. ■ Integrate complementary health therapies for low-impact muscle exercises.
Health, Wellness, Illness	Physical activity maintains and increases joint movement, body strength, and feeling of well-being throughout the lifespan.	■ Physical activity at all ages and patient capabilities should be encouraged and supported to maintain well-being. ■ Range of motion exercises can be scheduled daily; passive, assisted, or active.
Perfusion	Poor circulation from staying in one position for long lengths of time can lead to complications.	■ Turning schedules can be used to reposition patients unable to move themselves as needed. ■ Assistance and support to be mobile in the bed or out of the bed can protect against circulation problems.
Safety	Manual lifting, moving, and patient positioning are high-risk interventions for back injuries and other musculoskeletal disorders.	■ Healthcare staff need to use assistive equipment and devices when moving, lifting, and positioning patients. ■ Two to three staff need to work together when moving, lifting, and transferring patients.
Skin Integrity	Patients who are less mobile are at high risk for skin breakdown.	■ Assess skin integrity when bathing or repositioning patients. ■ Keep patients clean and dry to prevent skin breakdown. ■ Turn and reposition patients every two hours to support adequate circulation and oxygenation.

In this chapter, readers will be given essential safe and efficient strategies for assisting patients to move and change positions. The use of assistive equipment, adequate numbers of staff, and proper body alignment of nurse and patient are discussed. Skills for assisting patients into various positions, turning patients in bed, and transferring patients from a bed to a chair or stretcher are included.

During all positional changes, the comfort and dignity of patients must be protected. Ensure modesty by preventing improper exposure throughout all positional changes. Protect dignity by giving careful and complete instructions, by not rushing, by encouraging patients to help themselves as much as possible, and by using a caring tone of voice and good eye contact.

>> Balance and Strength

Expected Outcomes

1. Correct body mechanics are utilized by caregiver.
2. Injuries are prevented to both the nurse and the patient.
3. Proper body mechanics facilitate patient care.
4. Patient maintains range of motion and muscle tone with range-of-motion exercises.
5. Patient is able to progress through range of motion with minimal to no pain.

SKILL 9.1 Body Mechanics: Using

Body mechanics relates to the movements and posture of the body. Using proper body mechanics (thus preventing strain and back injuries) helps to coordinate movements of healthcare facility personnel during lifting and moving patients.

Delegation or Assignment

Using proper body mechanics is not a delegated or assigned task; it is a safety prevention and a responsibility of all healthcare personnel. UAPs are expected to use safe and

SKILL 9.1 Body Mechanics: Using (*continued*)

efficient body mechanics. The nurse can assess and evaluate the UAP, and if needed, additional instruction and practice may be given.

Equipment

No equipment is required when using proper body mechanics. However, assistive moving equipment should be utilized by nurses and other healthcare personnel for enhanced safety for staff and patients.

Preparation

- Determine need for assistance in moving or turning a patient following OSHA lifting guidelines.
- All assistive equipment and devices need to be ready for use and easily accessible. Mechanical equipment needs to be maintained with slings and transfer sheets kept clean and stocked. Equipment should be charged. If any part is broken or malfunctioning, it should be taken to the maintenance department for repair or have an exchange agreement with a vendor for a loaner if the equipment needs to be sent to the manufacturer.
- Gather any assistive moving devices such as a gait belt and/or additional staff ❶.

Procedure

1. Introduce self to patient and verify the patient's identity using two identifiers. Explain to the patient what you are going to do, why it is necessary, and how the patient can participate.
2. Perform hand hygiene and observe appropriate infection control procedures.
3. Provide for patient privacy.
4. Provide comfort and safety for patient and self, including raising bed to appropriate height to support moving or lifting the patient. Don clean gloves as needed.
5. Utilize proper body mechanics for moving, turning, and lifting found in **Table 9–1** ❭❭.

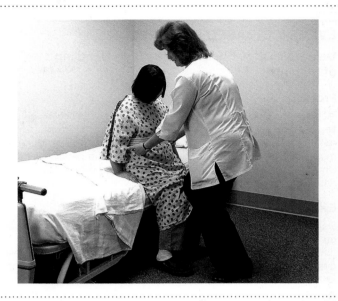

❶ Gait belts are routinely used to assist in manual transfer in most facilities.

6. When the procedure is complete, lower the bed if it was raised, perform hand hygiene, and leave patient safe and comfortable.
7. Complete documentation using forms, checklists, or electronic dropdown lists supplemented by nurse's notes or additional comments as appropriate.

SAMPLE DOCUMENTATION

[date] 2145 Returned to bed from chair via hydraulic lift. Tolerated without incident. States "I'm tired and ready to go to sleep now." *C. Holmes*

TABLE 9–1 Proper Body Mechanics for Moving, Turning, and Lifting

Action	Do	Don't
Balance (posture)	Align the body, keep back straight, hold abdomen firm and tuck buttocks in, have shoulders toward back slightly, have feet apart, head erect and facing forward.	Slouch, slump, hunch shoulders forward, or strain forward from waist or neck.
Balance (base)	Stand with feet apart and flat, with one foot slightly more forward.	Keep feet together when standing, moving, or lifting.
Lifting	Bend from the knees and hips and use the large leg muscles (squat).	Bend forward from the waist to reach or lift something.
Lifting	Push to move using legs.	Pull an object to move it.
Lifting	Stand close to object and lift it straight up.	Reach out arms or reach over something to lift up object.
Stabilizing	Pivot with the feet.	Twist your motion, especially when bending forward or carrying a load.
Stabilizing	Distribute weight evenly between both feet.	Have weight mainly on one foot.
Stabilizing	Keep load being carried close to the body.	Move a heavy load held away from the body.
Self-care	Vary exercise to include flexibility and strength of all muscle groups.	Always exercise the same group of muscles.
	Use assistive moving devices or ask for assistance when needed.	Carry too much weight or carry it too far alone.
	Assess weight and know own limitations.	Try to move weight and realize it's just too heavy.

(*continued on next page*)

SKILL 9.1 Body Mechanics: Using (*continued*)

EVIDENCE-BASED PRACTICE

Using Assistive Equipment for Safe Handling of Patients

Problem

Manual lifting, moving, and handling of patients in all healthcare settings such as acute, long-term, community-based, and home, is currently recognized as the greatest risk factor for work-related musculoskeletal overexertion injuries for healthcare personnel. In the United States, rates of these healthcare overexertion injuries are among the highest of all industries.

Evidence

Data from the Bureau of Labor Statistics show that the single greatest risk factor for overexertion injuries in healthcare workers is manual patient handling (lifting, moving, and repositioning of residents or patients without adequate assistive devices). Rising obesity rates in the United States have increased the physical demands on caregivers. Healthcare staff may feel an ethical duty to do all they can to assist patients and may put their own personal health and safety at risk.

Implications

Use of assistive moving devices and equipment provides safety for healthcare personnel and patients. Evidence-based research has shown that safe patient handling interventions can prevent overexertion injuries by replacing manual patient handling with safer methods. Professional organizations such as NIOSH and the CDC recommend manual lifting be eliminated whenever possible.

Source: Based on The National Institute for Occupational Safety and Health (NIOSH). Centers for Disease Control and Prevention (CDC). (2016). *Safe patient handling and movement (SPHM).* Retrieved from https://www.cdc.gov/niosh/topics/safepatient/; Occupational Safety and Health Administration (OSHA). U.S. Department of Labor. (2013). *Facts about hospital worker safety.* Retrieved from https://www.osha.gov/dsg/hospitals/documents/1.2_Factbook_508.pdf; Occupational Safety and Health Administration (OSHA). (2014). *Safe patient handling.* Retrieved from U.S. Department of Labor website https://www.osha.gov/SLTC/healthcarefacilities/safepatienthandling.html

SKILL 9.2 Range-of-Motion Exercises: Assisting

Range-of-motion (ROM) exercises focus on the movement of body joints to maintain flexibility and ability of joint motion as the patient is capable. If the patient is unable to exercise, assistance is needed to prevent stiffness of the joint from happening.

Delegation or Assignment

Assisting patients to do ROM exercises can be delegated or assigned to the UAP. It is important for the nurse to review the general guidelines for assisting a patient with ROM exercises to avoid injury to the UAP or patient. Emphasize the importance of reporting anything unusual to the nurse. If a patient has a recent spinal cord injury or some form of orthopedic trauma, the nurse or a physical therapist should assist the patient. Note that state laws for UAPs vary, so this task might be assigned to the UAP rather than delegated.

Equipment

No special equipment is needed other than a bed.

Preparation

- Review healthcare provider's orders and patient's nursing plan of care.
- Prior to initiating the exercises, review any possible restrictions with the healthcare provider or physical therapist. Also refer to the facility's protocol.

Procedure

1. Prior to performing the skill, introduce self and verify the patient's identity using two identifiers. Explain to the patient what you are going to do, why it is necessary, and how the patient can participate. Listen to any suggestions made by the patient or support people. Discuss the importance of ROM exercises in the plan of care.

2. Perform hand hygiene and observe other appropriate infection control procedures.
3. Provide for patient privacy. Provide comfort and safety for the patient and self.
   - Encourage patient to perform ROM exercises at least twice daily to maintain or improve mobility of joints. Assist the patient as needed or provide verbal cues.
   - Use a head to toe approach, repeating each motion three to four times.
   - When assisting the patient with movement, cradle the limb above and below the joint being exercised. **Rationale:** *This facilitates support and comfort. It also allows the nurse to detect ease/resistance to movement.*
   - Assess the patient for changes in cardiopulmonary status (e.g., dyspnea, fatigue, change in vital signs).
   - Discontinue exercises if patient complains of pain or discomfort.

CAUTION! Never force joint movements as patient may have stiffness, joint immobility, or rigidity of the bones of a joint due to injury, disease, or inactivity of the joint.

4. All body sites should be included in the patient's exercise session if possible. Follow the sequence in **Table 9–2 ≫**.
5. When exercising is complete, perform hand hygiene and leave patient safe and comfortable.
6. Complete documentation using forms, checklists, or electronic dropdown lists supplemented by nurse's notes or additional comments as appropriate. Document the following:
   - Type of ROM exercise (e.g., active, passive, active–assistive)
   - Joints exercised and their degree of joint motion
   - Length of exercise
   - Patient's tolerance level to the activity
   - Any abnormalities

(*Text continues on p. 393.*)

SKILL 9.2 Range-of-Motion Exercises: Assisting (*continued*)

TABLE 9–2 Range of Motion

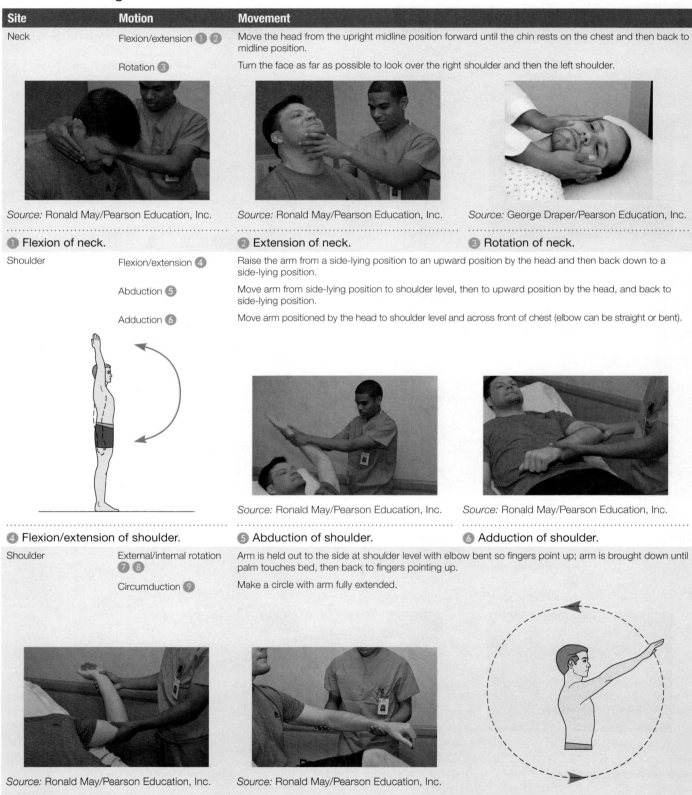

Site	Motion	Movement
Neck	Flexion/extension ① ②	Move the head from the upright midline position forward until the chin rests on the chest and then back to midline position.
	Rotation ③	Turn the face as far as possible to look over the right shoulder and then the left shoulder.

Source: Ronald May/Pearson Education, Inc. *Source:* Ronald May/Pearson Education, Inc. *Source:* George Draper/Pearson Education, Inc.

① Flexion of neck.   ② Extension of neck.   ③ Rotation of neck.

Site	Motion	Movement
Shoulder	Flexion/extension ④	Raise the arm from a side-lying position to an upward position by the head and then back down to a side-lying position.
	Abduction ⑤	Move arm from side-lying position to shoulder level, then to upward position by the head, and back to side-lying position.
	Adduction ⑥	Move arm positioned by the head to shoulder level and across front of chest (elbow can be straight or bent).

Source: Ronald May/Pearson Education, Inc. *Source:* Ronald May/Pearson Education, Inc.

④ Flexion/extension of shoulder.   ⑤ Abduction of shoulder.   ⑥ Adduction of shoulder.

Site	Motion	Movement
Shoulder	External/internal rotation ⑦ ⑧	Arm is held out to the side at shoulder level with elbow bent so fingers point up; arm is brought down until palm touches bed, then back to fingers pointing up.
	Circumduction ⑨	Make a circle with arm fully extended.

Source: Ronald May/Pearson Education, Inc. *Source:* Ronald May/Pearson Education, Inc.

⑦ External rotation of shoulder.   ⑧ Internal rotation of shoulder.   ⑨ Circumduction of shoulder.

(*continued on next page*)

SKILL 9.2 Range-of-Motion Exercises: Assisting (*continued*)

TABLE 9–2 Range of Motion (*continued*)

Site	Motion	Movement
Elbows	Flexion/extension ⑩	Move lower arm upward from side-lying position to shoulder level and then back down to side-lying position.
	Supination/pronation rotation ⑪	Lower arm is held straight in front of body, then turn the palm downward and back upward (just the forearm moves).
Wrists	Flexion/extension ⑫	Arm is held out to the side at shoulder level with elbow bent so fingers point up; move fingers of the hand downward and then back upward.

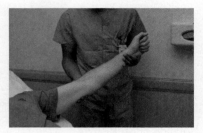

Source: Ronald May/Pearson Education, Inc.

⑩ Extension of elbow.

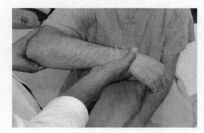

Source: Patrick Watson/Pearson Education, Inc.

⑪ Pronation rotation of elbow.

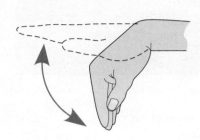

⑫ Flexion/extension of wrist.

Site	Motion	Movement
Fingers	Flexion/extension ⑬	Make a fist and then straighten the fingers.
	Abduction/adduction ⑭	Spread the fingers of the hand apart and then bring them back together.
Thumbs	Flexion/extension ⑮	Move the thumb across the palm toward the fifth finger and then move it away from the hand.

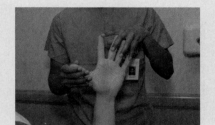

Source: Ronald May/Pearson Education, Inc.

⑬ Extension of fingers.

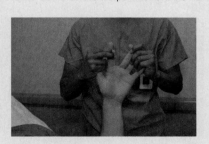

Source: Ronald May/Pearson Education, Inc.

⑭ Abduction/adduction fingers.

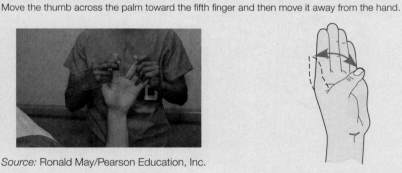

⑮ Flexion/extension of thumb.

Site	Motion	Movement
Hips	Flexion/extension ⑯	Lift leg and bend the knee; move the knee upward toward the chest and then back down; straighten the knee, and lower the leg to the bed.
	Internal/external rotation ⑰	Roll the foot and leg inward and then outward.
	Circumduction ⑱	Move the entire leg in a circle.

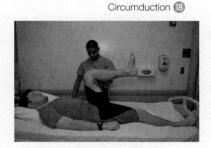

Source: Ronald May/Pearson Education, Inc.

⑯ Flexion of hip and knee.

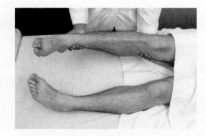

Source: George Draper/Pearson Education, Inc.

⑰ Internal rotation of hip.

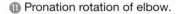

⑱ Circumduction of hip.

SKILL 9.2 Range-of-Motion Exercises: Assisting (*continued*)

TABLE 9–2 Range of Motion (*continued*)

Site	Motion	Movement
Legs	Abduction/adduction ⑲ ⑳	Move leg to the side away from the body and then back across and in front of the other leg.
Knees	Flexion/extension ㉑	Bend the knee and bring the heel toward the back of the thigh and then straighten the leg, returning the foot to the bed.

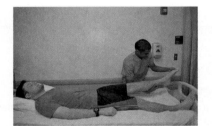

Source: Ronald May/Pearson Education, Inc.

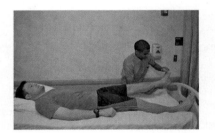

Source: Ronald May/Pearson Education, Inc.

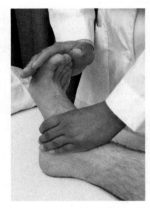

⑲ Abduction of leg.

⑳ Adduction of leg.

㉑ Flexion/extension of knee.

Site	Motion	Movement
Ankles	Flexion/extension ㉒ ㉓	Move the foot down and away from the leg; then move the foot back up toward the leg.
Toes	Flexion/extension ㉔	Curl the toes downward and then bend then upward.

Source: Ronald May/Pearson Education, Inc.

Source: Ronald May/Pearson Education, Inc.

Source: George Draper/Pearson Education, Inc.

㉒ Flexion of ankle.

㉓ Extension of ankle.

㉔ Extension of toes.

SAMPLE DOCUMENTATION

[date] 1000 Assisted ROM performed with bath. All joints ranged fully with 4 reps each. Resistance in shoulders resolved when pace slowed. Tolerated well, no c/o pain. *M. Foti*

Lifespan Considerations

CHILDREN

- Avoid hyperextension of joints. **Rationale:** *Some children may have lax ligaments, and overstretching can cause injury and pain.*

- In some children with impaired mobility, splinting of the wrist, knees, or ankles may be necessary.

- Children have developmental needs including the need to play. Performing ROM can be an opportunity for fun and for enhancing the child–caregiver relationship.

OLDER ADULTS

Changes in the Musculoskeletal System that Affect Nursing Care

- A small roll can be made of soft cloth to place in the palms to help prevent contractures of the fingers. *Ensure that the thumb is adducted with finger opposition.* **Rationale:** *Contractures occur when muscles atrophy and degenerate slowly and when tendons shrink and sclerose.*

- Range of motion of joints decreases from lack of adequate joint motion—that is, ankylosis.

(*continued on next page*)

SKILL 9.2 Range-of-Motion Exercises: Assisting (*continued*)

- Avoid hyperextending the joints of older adults. **Rationale:** *Such movements can cause pain or nerve damage because joints become less flexible with age.*
- Arthritis changes can cause contractures and enlarged, painful joints.
- Mobility level may be limited—muscle strength lessens and gait may be unsteady.
- Kyphosis may occur—cervical vertebrae may be flexed; intervertebral discs narrow.
- Osteoporosis may occur as a result of calcium loss from the bone and insufficient replacement.
- Osteoarthritis increases with age.

Safety Considerations

- Loss of muscle mass interferes with activities that require strength, such as bending down, dressing, and reaching for objects.
- Dexterity decreases, leading to a change in performing manipulative skills.
- Impaired mobility can lead to many subsequent problems, including depression, negative self-image, dependent behavior, and loss of independence.
- Effects of disability can influence the individual's body image, physical appearance, and bodily sensations.
- Vision problems may cause the patient to stumble or fall.

Patient Teaching

Teach the patient's family to do the following at home:

- Encourage patient to be mobile, and allow patient to be as mobile as possible.
- Assist the patient to perform ROM exercises at a slow pace 2–3 times daily.
- Use correct body mechanics to prevent muscle strain while assisting with the exercises.

- Assess ability to be mobile—gait, balance, posture, and whether the patient shuffles or is able to walk. Poor or unsteady mobility is often a direct cause of falling.
- Assess for certain medications the patient is taking that can cause vertigo, poor balance, blurred vision, weakness, or even drowsiness.
- Chronic diseases such as Parkinson disease, Alzheimer disease, and diabetes with peripheral neuropathy can all contribute to falls.
- Many older adult patients are fearful of falls and injuries when they are moving or walking.

≫ Moving and Transferring a Patient

Expected Outcomes

1. Patient's comfort is increased.
2. Skin remains intact without evidence of breakdown as a result of moving and turning.
3. Body alignment is maintained.
4. Assistive equipment and devices are used in patient transfers and repositioning as needed.
5. Caregiver is able to manage turning, repositioning, and assistive devices.

SKILL 9.3 Ambulating Patient: Assisting

Patients are encouraged to keep moving as able in healthcare facilities to help them maintain their usual level of functionality and to avoid complications of immobility such as pneumonia and deep vein thrombosis. Evidence supports ambulation of patients while in healthcare facilities, especially older adults, to maintain health and well-being.

Delegation or Assignment

Ambulation of patients is frequently delegated or assigned to the UAP. However, the nurse should conduct an initial assessment of the patient's abilities in order to direct the UAP in providing appropriate assistance. Any unusual events that arise from assisting the patient in ambulation must be validated and interpreted by the nurse. Note that state laws for UAPs vary, so this task might be assigned to the UAP rather than delegated.

Equipment

- Gait/transfer belt, whether or not the patient is known to be unsteady
- Wheelchair for following patient, or chairs along the route if the patient needs to rest
- Portable oxygen tank, if needed

Preparation

- Review healthcare provider's orders and patient's nursing plan of care.
- Be certain that others are available to assist you if needed. Also, plan the route of ambulation that has the fewest hazards and a clear path for ambulation.
- All assistive equipment and devices need to be ready for use and easily accessible. Mechanical equipment needs to be maintained, with slings and transfer sheets kept clean and

SKILL 9.3 Ambulating Patient: Assisting (*continued*)

stocked. Equipment should be charged. If any part is broken or malfunctioning, it should be taken to the maintenance department for repair or have an exchange agreement with a vendor for a loan if the equipment needs to be sent to the manufacturer.

Procedure

1. Prior to performing the procedure, introduce self and verify the patient's identity using two identifiers. Explain to the patient what you are going to do, why ambulation is necessary, and how the patient can participate. Discuss how this activity relates to the overall plan of care.
2. Perform hand hygiene and observe other appropriate infection control procedures.
3. Ensure that the patient is appropriately dressed to walk and has shoes or slippers with nonskid soles.
4. Prepare the patient for ambulation.
   - Have patient sit up in bed for at least 1 minute prior to preparing to dangle legs.
   - Assist the patient to sit on the edge of the bed and allow dangling for at least 1 minute (see Skill 9.8).
   - Assess the patient carefully for signs and symptoms of orthostatic hypotension (dizziness, lightheadedness, or a sudden increase in heart rate) prior to leaving the bedside. **Rationale:** *Allowing for gradual adjustment can minimize drops in blood pressure (and fainting) that occur with shifts in position from lying to sitting, and sitting to standing.*
   - Assist the patient to stand by the side of the bed for at least 1 minute until the patient feels secure.
   - Carefully attend to any IV tubing, catheters, or drainage bags. Keep urinary drainage bags below level of the patient's bladder.
   - Use a gait/transfer (walking) belt if the patient is slightly weak and unstable. Make sure the belt is pulled snugly around the patient's waist and fastened securely. Grasp the belt at the patient's back, and walk behind and slightly to one side of the patient ❶.

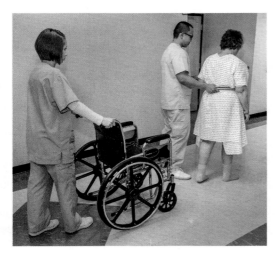

Source: Rick Brady/Pearson Education, Inc.

❶ Using a gait/transfer (walking) belt to support the patient.

5. Ensure patient safety while assisting the patient to ambulate.
   - Encourage the patient to ambulate independently if able, but walk beside the patient's weak side, if appropriate. If the patient has a lightweight IV pole because of infusing fluids, the patient may find that holding on to the pole while ambulating helps with balance.
   - Remain physically close to the patient in case assistance is needed at any point.
   - If it is the patient's first time out of bed following surgery, injury, or an extended period of immobility, or if the patient is quite weak or unstable, have an assistant follow you and the patient with a wheelchair in the event that it is needed quickly.
   - If the patient is moderately weak and unstable, walk on the patient's weaker side and interlock your forearm with the patient's closest forearm. Encourage the patient to press the forearm against your hip or waist for stability if desired. This patient should wear a gait/transfer belt, and the nurse should maintain a secure grasp of the belt.
   - If the patient is very weak and unstable, place your near arm around the patient's waist, and with your other arm support the patient's near arm at the elbow. Walk on the patient's stronger side. Again, the patient should wear a gait/transfer belt in case of an emergency.
   - If available, a nurse and a UAP can both support the patient, using a gait belt, during ambulation. Apply a gait belt before the patient gets out of bed. Each nurse should have one hand on the gait belt, at the back of the patient, and support the patient by holding on to the patient's forearm or the lower upper arm with the other hand. **Rationale:** *This provides a secure grip for each nurse.*
   - Walk in unison with the patient, using a smooth, even gait, at the same speed and with steps the same size as the patient's.
   - Ask the patient to straighten the back and raise the head so that the eyes are looking forward in a normal horizontal plane. **Rationale:** *Patients who are unsure of their ability to ambulate tend to look down at their feet, which makes them more likely to fall.*
6. Protect the patient who begins to fall while ambulating.
   - If a patient begins to experience the signs and symptoms of orthostatic hypotension or extreme weakness, quickly assist the patient into a nearby wheelchair or other chair, and help the patient to lower the head between the knees.
   - Stay with the patient.
   - If a chair is not close by, assist the patient to a horizontal position on the floor before fainting occurs.
     a. Assume a broad stance with one foot in front of the other. **Rationale:** *A broad stance widens your base of support. Placing one foot behind the other allows you to rock backward and use the femoral muscles when supporting the patient's weight and lowering the center of gravity (see the next step), thus preventing back strain.*
     b. Bring the patient backward so that your body supports the person. **Rationale:** *Patients who faint or start to fall usually pitch slightly forward because of*

(*continued on next page*)

SKILL 9.3 Ambulating Patient: Assisting *(continued)*

the momentum of ambulating. Bringing the patient's weight backward against your body allows gradual movement to the floor without injury to the patient.

   c. Allow the patient to slide down your leg, and lower the person gently to the floor, making sure the patient's head does not hit any objects.

   d. When the nurse and UAP are assisting the patient to walk, each one should place one hand under the patient's nearer axilla and continue to grasp the gait/transfer belt and lower the person gently to the floor or to a nearby chair. **Rationale:** *Placing the arms under the patient's axillae balances the patient's weight between the two people, preventing injury to the nurse, the UAP, and the patient. Keeping hold of the gait belt allows for more control and direction of the patient who can no longer effectively protect himself or herself.*

    • When the weakness subsides, assist the patient back to bed.

7. When walking is complete, perform hand hygiene and leave patient safe and comfortable.

8. Complete documentation using forms, checklists, or electronic dropdown lists supplemented by nurse's notes or additional comments as appropriate, including distance and duration of ambulation, description of the patient's gait (including body alignment) when walking, pace, activity tolerance when walking (e.g., pulse rate, facial color, any shortness of breath, feelings of dizziness or weakness), degree of support required, and respiratory rate and blood pressure after initial ambulation to compare with baseline data.

SAMPLE DOCUMENTATION

[date] 1030 Ambulated length of hall (36.3 m / 120 ft) and returned with minimal assistance of 2 staff. Denies feeling dizzy or weak. Steady gait, tolerated well. VS remain at baseline after walking. *B. Snyder*

Lifespan Considerations

CHILDREN

■ Children and adolescents who have suffered a sports injury (e.g., sprained ankle) may want to be more active than they should be. A cast, splint, or boot may be put in place to limit activity and assist in healing. Teach children the importance of appropriate activity and the use of assistive devices (e.g., crutches) if necessary. Help them focus on what they can do rather than what they cannot do (e.g., "You can stand at the free-throw line and shoot baskets").

OLDER ADULTS

■ Inquire how the patient has ambulated previously and/or check patient's history regarding the patient's abilities, and modify assistance accordingly.

■ Be cautious when using a transfer belt with a patient with osteoporosis. Too much pressure from the belt can increase the risk of vertebral compression fractures. If a patient has had abdominal surgery, it may be necessary to use a gait vest instead of a gait belt.

■ If assistive devices such as a walker or cane are used, make sure patients are supervised initially to learn the proper method of using them. Crutches may be much more difficult for older adults due to decreased upper body strength. In general, older individuals do much better with walkers than with crutches.

■ Break up the total desired patient mobility goal into shorter patient goals to build endurance, strength, and flexibility.

■ Be aware of any fall risks the older adult may have, such as:
   • Sensory changes such as decreased vision and hearing
   • Effects of medications
   • Neurologic disorders
   • Orthopedic problems
   • Presence of equipment that must accompany the patient when ambulating
   • Environmental hazards
   • Orthostatic hypotension

SKILL 9.4 Hydraulic Lift: Using

Manual or battery-powered lifts work to hoist patient for patient transfer. The patient sits in a sling while the hydraulic lift does the work of raising and lowering the patient when transferring the patient. Some lifts can safely move patients up to 204 kg (450 lb).

Delegation or Assignment

The skill of using a hydraulic lift can be delegated or assigned to UAPs who have demonstrated competent use of the equipment for the involved patient. The nurse remains responsible for the assessment, interpretation of abnormal findings, and determination of appropriate responses. Note that state laws for UAPs vary, so this task might be assigned to the UAP rather than delegated.

Equipment

■ Hydraulic lift (such as a mobile floor or ceiling-mounted lift) with any necessary accessories (such as the sling)

Preparation

■ Review healthcare provider's orders and patient's nursing plan of care.

■ All assistive equipment and devices need to be ready for use and easily accessible. Mechanical equipment needs to be maintained with slings and transfer sheets kept clean and stocked. Equipment should be charged. If any part is broken or malfunctioning, it should be taken to the maintenance department for repair or have an exchange

SKILL 9.4 Hydraulic Lift: Using *(continued)*

agreement with a vendor if the equipment needs to be sent to the manufacturer.

■ Obtain the lift and put in the patient's room. Arrange for assistance from others at a designated time.

Procedure

1. Prior to performing the procedure, introduce self and verify the patient's identity using two identifiers. Explain to the patient what you are going to do, why it is necessary, and how the patient can participate. Explain the procedure and demonstrate the lift. **Rationale:** *Some patients are afraid of being lifted and will be reassured by a demonstration.*
2. Wash hands and observe other appropriate infection control procedures.
3. Provide for patient privacy.
4. Prepare the equipment.
   - Lock the wheels of the patient's bed and raise the bed to the high position.
   - Put up the side rail on the opposite side of the bed and lower the side rail near you.
   - Position the lift so that it is close to the patient.
   - Place the chair that is to receive the patient beside the bed with wheels locked. Allow adequate space to maneuver the lift.
5. Position the patient on the sling ❶.

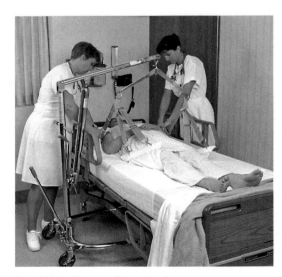

Source: Ronald May/Pearson Education, Inc.

❶ Place canvas piece under patient from knees to shoulders.

CAUTION! The remaining steps of this procedure need to be performed by at least two healthcare staff working together with the patient.

   - Roll the patient away from you.
   - Place the canvas seat or sling under the patient with the wide lower edge under the patient's thighs to the knees and the narrower upper edge up under the patient's shoulders. **Rationale:** *This places the sling under the*

patient's center of gravity and greatest part of body weight. Correct placement permits the patient to be lifted evenly, with minimal shifting.
   - Roll the patient toward you and pull the canvas sling through.
   - Roll the patient to the supine position and center the patient on top of the canvas sling.
6. Attach the sling to the swivel bar.
   - Wheel the lift into position, with the footbars under the bed on the side where the chair is positioned. Set the adjustable base at the widest position to ensure stability. Lock the wheels of the lifter.
   - Lower the side rail.
   - Move the lift arms directly over the patient and lower the horizontal bar by releasing the hydraulic valve. Lock the valve.
   - Attach the lifter straps or hooks to the corresponding openings in the canvas seat. Check that the hooks are correctly placed and that matching straps or chains are of equal length. Face the hooks away from the patient. **Rationale:** *This prevents the hooks from injuring the patient.*
7. Lift the patient gradually ❷.
   - Elevate the head of the bed to place the patient in a sitting position.
   - Ask the patient to remove eyeglasses and put them in a safe place. **Rationale:** *The swivel bar may come close to the face and cause breakage of eyeglasses.*
   - *Nurse 1:* Close the pressure valve and gradually pump the jack handle until the patient is above the bed surface. **Rationale:** *Gradual elevation of the lift is less frightening to the patient than a rapid rise.*
   - *Nurse 2:* Assume a broad stance and guide the patient with your hands as the patient is lifted. **Rationale:** *This*

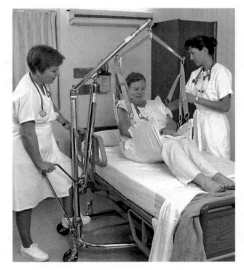

Source: Ronald May/Pearson Education, Inc.

❷ Raise patient off bed by turning release knob clockwise.

(continued on next page)

SKILL 9.4 Hydraulic Lift: Using *(continued)*

prepares the nurse to hold the patient and provide control during the movement.

- Check the placement of the sling before moving the patient away from the bed.

8. Move the patient over the chair.
   - *Nurse 1:* With the pressure valve securely closed, slowly roll the lift until the patient is over the chair. Use the steering handle to maneuver the lift.
   - *Nurse 2:* Guide movement by hand until the patient is directly over the chair. **Rationale:** *Slow movement decreases swaying and is less frightening. Guidance also decreases swaying and gives a sense of security.*

9. Lower the patient into the chair ❸.
   - *Nurse 1:* Release the pressure valve very gradually. **Rationale:** *Gradual release is less frightening than a quick descent.*
   - *Nurse 2:* Guide the patient into the chair.

10. Ensure patient comfort and safety.
    - Remove the hooks from the canvas seat. Leave the seat in place. **Rationale:** *The seat is left in place in preparation for the lift back to bed.*
    - Align the patient appropriately in a sitting position and return the patient's eyeglasses, if appropriate.
    - Apply a seat belt as needed.
    - Place the call bell within reach.

11. When the procedure is complete, perform hand hygiene and leave the patient safe and comfortable.

12. Complete documentation using forms, checklists, or electronic dropdown lists supplemented by nurse's notes or additional comments as appropriate, including the type of equipment, number of assistants needed, safety precautions taken, and the patient's physiological and psychological response.

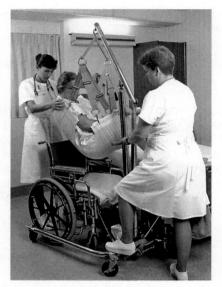

Source: Ronald May/Pearson Education, Inc.

❸ Use one nurse to stabilize patient as second nurse guides patient into chair.

SAMPLE DOCUMENTATION

[date] 0750 States "I'm ready to get up to the chair now." Hydraulic lift brought to room, UAP and I assisted patient into sling and transferred him to chair. Lift removed from room. Tolerated move without complaint. Call bell placed within reach, bedside table positioned in front of chair. *O. Hayward*

SKILL 9.5 Logrolling Patient in Bed

Logrolling is a technique used to turn a patient whose body must at all times be kept in straight alignment (like a log). An example is the patient with a spinal injury. Considerable care must be taken to prevent additional injury. This technique requires a minimum of two nurses, with preference of four to five staff, depending on facility policy. For the patient who has a cervical injury, one nurse must maintain the patient's head and neck alignment.

Delegation or Assignment

This skill can be delegated or assigned to the UAP after the nurse first determines that the UAP knows the correct logrolling technique. The nurse can assess and evaluate the UAP's ability to complete this skill safely and accurately. The nurse remains responsible for the assessment, interpretation of abnormal findings, and determination of appropriate responses. Note that state laws for UAPs vary, so this task might be assigned to the UAP rather than delegated.

Preparation

- Review healthcare provider's orders and patient's nursing plan of care.
- Determine if assistive devices will be required.
- All assistive equipment and devices need to be ready for use and easily accessible. Mechanical equipment needs to be maintained with slings and transfer sheets kept clean and stocked. Equipment should be charged. If any part is broken or malfunctioning, it should be taken to the maintenance department for repair or have an exchange agreement with a vendor for a loaner if the equipment needs to be sent to the manufacturer.
- Determine if any encumbrances to movement, such as an IV or an indwelling catheter, are present.
- Be aware of medications the patient is receiving, because certain medications may hamper movement or alertness of the patient.

SKILL 9.5 Logrolling Patient in Bed (*continued*)

■ Obtain assistance from other healthcare personnel. At least two or three additional people are needed to perform this skill safely.

Procedure

1. Prior to performing the procedure, introduce self and verify the patient's identity using two identifiers. Explain to the patient what you are going to do, why it is necessary, and how the patient can participate.
2. Perform hand hygiene and observe other appropriate infection control procedures.
3. Provide for patient privacy.
4. Position yourselves and the patient appropriately before the move.
   - Place the patient's arms across the chest. **Rationale:** *Doing so ensures that the arms will not be injured or become trapped under the body when the patient is turned.*
5. Pull the patient to the side of the bed.
   - Use a turn sheet or friction-reducing device to facilitate logrolling. First, stand with another nurse on the same side of the bed. Assume a broad stance with one foot forward, and grasp half of the fanfolded or rolled edge of the turn sheet or friction-reducing device. On a signal, pull the patient toward both of you ❶.
   - One nurse counts: "One, two, three, go." Then, at the same time, all staff members pull the patient to the side of the bed by shifting their weight to the back foot. **Rationale:** *Moving the patient in unison maintains the patient's body alignment.*

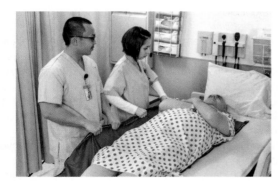

Source: Rick Brady/Pearson Education, Inc.

❶ Using a friction-reducing slide sheet, the nurses pull the sheet with the patient on it to the edge of the bed.

6. One person moves to the other side of the bed, and places supportive devices for the patient when turned.
   - Place a pillow where it will support the patient's head after the turn. **Rationale:** *The pillow prevents lateral flexion of the neck and ensures alignment of the cervical spine.*
   - Place one or two pillows between the patient's legs to support the upper leg when the patient is turned. **Rationale:** *This pillow prevents adduction of the upper leg and keeps the legs parallel and aligned.*

7. Roll and position the patient in proper alignment.
   - The person farthest from the patient assumes a stable stance.
   - This person reaches over the patient and grasps the far edges of the turn sheet or friction-reducing device ❷.
   - One nurse counts: "One, two, three, go." Then, at the same time, all nurses roll the patient to a lateral position.
   - The nurse behind the patient helps turn the patient and provides pillow supports to ensure good alignment in the lateral position.
   - Support the patient's head, back, and upper and lower extremities with pillows.
   - Raise the side rails and place the call bell within the patient's reach.

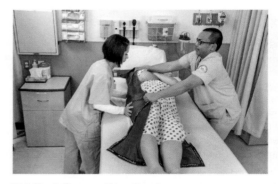

Source: Rick Brady/Pearson Education, Inc.

❷ The nurse on the right uses the far edge of the friction-reducing slide sheet to roll the patient toward him; the nurse on the left remains behind the patient and assists with turning.

8. When the procedure is complete, perform hand hygiene and leave patient safe and comfortable.
9. Complete documentation using forms, checklists, or electronic dropdown lists supplemented by nurse's notes or additional comments as appropriate, including:
   - Time and change of position moved from and position moved to
   - Any signs of pressure areas
   - Use of support devices
   - Ability of patient to assist in moving and turning
   - Response of patient to moving and turning (e.g., anxiety, discomfort, dizziness)

SAMPLE DOCUMENTATION

[date] 1512 Repositioned from back to left side using logrolling technique with 4 staff. Supported with pillows for comfort. Back skin shows no redness or dryness. Tolerated without complaint, able to hold arms on chest. G. Moore

SKILL 9.6 Moving Patient Up in Bed

Patients need to periodically be repositioned higher in the bed because throughout the day, they can slowly slide down toward the bottom of the bed. Positioning high at the top of the bed supports full lung expansion, is more comfortable, and makes the patient easily accessible for assessment or intervention.

Delegation or Assignment

The skills of moving and turning patients in bed can be delegated or assigned to the UAP. The nurse should make sure that any needed equipment and additional personnel are available to reduce risk of injury to the healthcare personnel. Emphasize the need for the UAP to report changes in the patient's condition that require assessment and intervention by the nurse. Note that state laws for UAPs vary, so this task might be assigned to the UAP rather than delegated.

Equipment

- Assistive moving devices such as pull and/or turn sheet, friction-reducing device, or a mechanical lift

Preparation

- Review healthcare provider's orders and patient's nursing plan of care.
- Determine if assistive devices will be required.
- All assistive equipment and devices need to be ready for use and easily accessible. Mechanical equipment needs to be maintained with slings and transfer sheets kept clean and stocked. Equipment should be charged. If any part is broken or malfunctioning, it should be taken to the maintenance department for repair or have an exchange agreement with a vendor for a loaner if the equipment needs to be sent to the manufacturer.
- Determine if any encumbrances to movement, such as an IV or an indwelling urinary catheter, are present.
- Be aware of medications the patient is receiving, because certain medications may hamper movement or alertness of the patient.
- Decide if assistance will be required from other healthcare personnel.
- Different cultures may have cultural variances regarding distance and space. It is important to explain the transfer process to patients, particularly if patients seem uncomfortable with having the nurse be close. Their culture may consider physical touch and closeness an invasion of personal space and privacy.

Procedure

1. Prior to performing the procedure, introduce self and verify the patient's identity using two identifiers. Explain to the patient what you are going to do, why it is necessary, and how the patient can participate. Listen to any suggestions made by the patient or support people.
2. Perform hand hygiene and observe other appropriate infection control procedures.
3. Provide for patient privacy.
4. Adjust the bed height and the patient's position.
   - Adjust the head of the bed to a flat position or as low as the patient can tolerate. **Rationale:** *Moving the patient upward against gravity requires more force and can cause back strain.*

- Raise the height of the bed as appropriate to enhance personnel safety (at the elbows).
- Verify bed wheels are locked and raise the rail on the side of the bed opposite you.
- Remove all pillows, then place one against the head of the bed. **Rationale:** *This pillow protects the patient's head from inadvertent injury against the top of the bed during the upward move.*
5. For the patient who is able to reposition without assistance:
   - Place the bed in flat or reverse Trendelenburg position (as tolerated by the patient). Stand by and instruct the patient to move self. Encourage the patient to reach up and grasp the upper side rails with both hands, bend knees, and push off with the feet and pull up with the arms simultaneously. Assess if the patient is able to move without causing friction to skin.
   - Ask if a positioning device is needed (e.g., pillow).
6. For the patient who is partially able to assist or who weighs more than 68 kg (150 lb):
   - Use a friction-reducing device such as a turn sheet and two to three assistants. **Rationale:** *Moving a patient up in bed is not a one-person task. During any patient handling, if the caregiver is required to lift more than 16 kg (35 lb) of a patient's weight, then it is recommended that assistive devices or equipment should be used (NIOSH, 2016).*
   - Place a drawsheet or a full sheet folded in half under the patient, extending from the shoulders to the thighs. Each person rolls up or fanfolds the turn sheet close to the patient's body on either side.
   - Both individuals grasp the sheet close to the shoulders and buttocks of the patient. **Rationale:** *This draws the weight closer to the nurse's center of gravity for balance and stability.*
   - Assist the patient to flex the hips and knees. Place the patient's arms across the chest. **Rationale:** *Ask the patient to flex the neck during the move and keep the head off the bed surface.*
   - Use a friction-reducing device and assistants to move the patient up in bed. Ask the patient to push on the count of three.
7. Position yourself and others appropriately, and move the patient ❶.
   - Face the direction of the movement, and then assume a broad stance with the foot nearest the bed behind

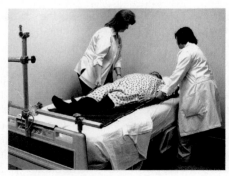

Source: Ronald May/Pearson Education, Inc.

❶ Use friction-reducing sheet and shift weight from back to front leg when moving patient up.

SKILL 9.6 Moving Patient Up in Bed (*continued*)

the forward foot and weight on the forward foot. Lean your trunk forward from the hips. Flex hips, knees, and ankles.

- Tighten your gluteal, abdominal, leg, and arm muscles and rock from the back leg to the front leg and back again. Then, shift your weight to the front leg as the patient pushes with the heels and pulls with the arms so that the patient moves toward the head of the bed.

8. For the patient who is unable to assist:
   - Use a hydraulic or battery-powered lift with supine sling or floor-based lift and two or more caregivers. Follow the manufacturer's guidelines for using the lift.
9. Elevate the head of the bed and provide appropriate support devices for the patient's new position (see Skill 9.7 for positioning patient).
10. When the procedure is complete, perform hand hygiene and leave patient safe and comfortable.

11. Complete documentation using forms, checklists, or electronic dropdown lists supplemented by nurse's notes or additional comments as appropriate, including:
    - Time and change of position moved from and position moved to.
    - Any signs of pressure areas.
    - Use of support devices.
    - Ability of patient to assist in moving and turning.
    - Response of patient to moving and turning (e.g., anxiety, discomfort, dizziness).

SAMPLE DOCUMENTATION

[date] 1210 Preparing to eat lunch. Assisted to move up in bed, HOB up, bedside table placed over bed. Able to push up with legs and arms on side rails. Tolerated without complaint. *W. Rogers*

SKILL 9.7 Positioning Patient in Bed

Positioning patients is a way to assist them to have body alignment, posture supporting physiologic well-being, and prevent complications of bedrest.

Delegation or Assignment

Positioning patients in bed can be delegated or assigned to the UAP. The nurse must give specific directions to the UAP about the appropriate positions for the patient and the reporting of any changes in skin integrity. The UAP should be encouraged to have the patient participate as much as possible in the position change. The nurse is responsible for evaluating the patient's comfort and alignment after the repositioning and for assessing skin integrity, particularly at pressure points. Note that state laws for UAPs vary, so this task might be assigned to the UAP rather than delegated.

Equipment

The following equipment can be used when positioning patients:

- Pillows—one to six, depending on patient need
- Trochanter rolls
- Footboard or suspension boots
- Hand rolls or wrist splints, if needed
- Folded towel
- Sandbag or rolled towel

Preparation

- Review healthcare provider's orders and patient's nursing plan of care.
- Check the position-change schedule for the next time and type of position change.
- Administer an analgesic, if appropriate, before changing the patient's position.

- Determine if any assistive devices will be required (e.g., friction-reducing device, mechanical lift).
- All assistive equipment and devices need to be ready for use and easily accessible. Mechanical equipment needs to be maintained with slings and transfer sheets kept clean and stocked. Equipment should be charged. If any part is broken or malfunctioning, it should be taken to the maintenance department for repair or have an exchange agreement with a vendor for a loaner if the equipment needs to be sent to the manufacturer.
- Determine if any encumbrances to movement, such as an IV or an indwelling urinary catheter, are present.
- Be aware of medications the patient is receiving, because certain medications may hamper movement or alertness of the patient.
- Obtain required assistance, as needed.

Procedure

1. Prior to performing the procedure, introduce self and verify the patient's identity using two identifiers. Explain to the patient what you are going to do, why it is necessary, and how the patient can participate.
2. Perform hand hygiene and observe other appropriate infection control procedures.
3. Provide for patient privacy.
4. Raise the height of the bed to bring the patient close to your center of gravity to avoid back strain.

FOWLER POSITION

- Position the patient.
  - Have the patient flex the knees slightly before raising the head of the bed. **Rationale:** *Slight knee flexion prevents*

(*continued on next page*)

SKILL 9.7 Positioning Patient in Bed (*continued*)

the patient from sliding toward the foot of the bed as the bed is raised. Be certain the patient's hips are positioned directly over the point where the bed will bend when the head is raised. If needed, assist the patient to move up toward the top of the bed before raising the head of the bed.

- Raise the head of the bed (HOB) to 45 degrees or the angle required and ordered for the patient. See **Table 9–3 ≫** for commonly used patient position bed settings.

- Provide supportive devices to align the patient appropriately.
  - Place a small pillow or roll under the lumbar region of the back if you feel a space in the lumbar curvature. **Rationale:** *The pillow supports the natural lumbar curvature and prevents flexion of the lumbar spine.*
  - Place a small pillow under the patient's head or have the patient rest the head against the mattress. **Rationale:** *Too many pillows beneath the head can cause neck hyperflexion.*

(*Text continues on p. 404.*)

TABLE 9–3 Bed Positions for Patient Care

Positions	Placement	Use
Low-Fowler ❶ 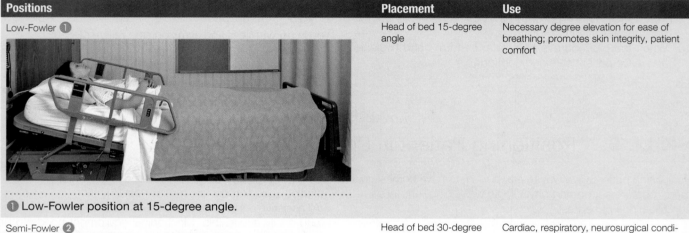 ❶ Low-Fowler position at 15-degree angle.	Head of bed 15-degree angle	Necessary degree elevation for ease of breathing; promotes skin integrity, patient comfort
Semi-Fowler ❷ 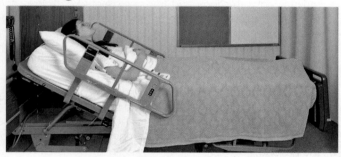 ❷ Semi-Fowler position at 30-degree angle.	Head of bed 30-degree angle	Cardiac, respiratory, neurosurgical conditions
Fowler ❸ 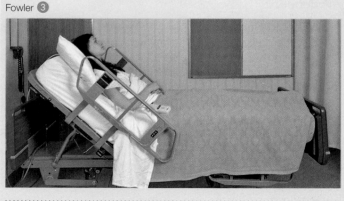 ❸ Fowler position at 45-60-degree angle.	Head of bed 45- to 60-degree angle; hips may or may not be flexed	Postoperative, gastrointestinal conditions; promotes lung expansion

SKILL 9.7 Positioning Patient in Bed (continued)

TABLE 9–3 Bed Positions for Patient Care (continued)

Positions	Placement	Use
High-Fowler ④ 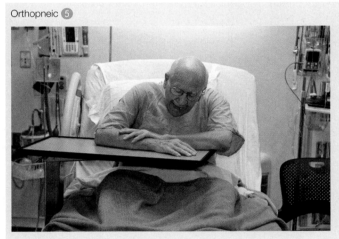	Head of bed 60-90-degree angle	Thoracic surgery, severe respiratory conditions

④ High-Fowler position at 60-90-degree angle.

Positions	Placement	Use
Orthopneic ⑤	Head of bed at 90 degrees or patient on side of bed leaning over bed table	Difficulty breathing, especially difficulty exhaling (COPD); can press the lower part of the chest against the table to aid exhalation

Source: Patrick Watson/Pearson Education, Inc.

⑤ Orthopneic position.

Positions	Placement	Use
Knee-gatch ⑥ 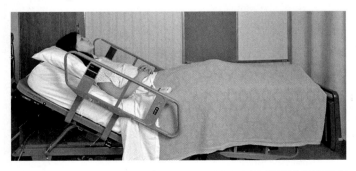	Lower section of bed (under knees) slightly bent	For patient comfort; contraindicated for vascular disorders

⑥ Elevated knee-gatch position.

(continued on next page)

SKILL 9.7 Positioning Patient in Bed *(continued)*

TABLE 9–3 Bed Positions for Patient Care *(continued)*

Positions	Placement	Use
Trendelenburg ⑦ 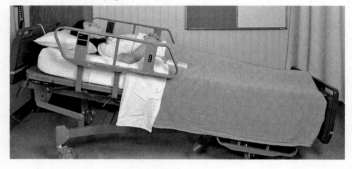 ⑦ Trendelenburg position.	Head of bed lowered and foot raised	Percussion, vibration, and drainage (PVD) procedure; promotes venous return
Reverse Trendelenburg ⑧ ⑧ Reverse Trendelenburg position.	Bed frame is tilted up with foot of bed down	Gastric conditions; prevents esophageal reflux

- Can place one or two pillows under the lower legs from below the knees to the ankles. Make sure that no pressure is exerted on the popliteal space and that the knees are flexed. **Rationale:** *Pressure against the popliteal space can damage nerves and vein walls, predisposing the patient to thrombus formation.*
- Avoid using the knee-gatch of a hospital bed to flex the patient's knees.
- Put a trochanter roll lateral to each femur (optional). **Rationale:** *This prevents external rotation of the hips.*
- Support the patient's feet with heel boots or a footboard. **Rationale:** *This prevents plantar flexion (foot drop).* The footboard should protrude several inches above the toes and be placed 1 inch away from the heels. **Rationale:** *This prevents undue pull on the Achilles tendon and discomfort.*
- Place pillows to support both arms and hands if the patient does not have normal use of them. **Rationale:** *These pillows prevent shoulder and muscle strain from the effects of downward gravitational pull, edema of the hands and arms, and flexion contracture of the wrist.* Arrange the pillows to support only the forearms and hands, up to the elbow. Proceed to step 5 below.

SUPINE POSITION

- Assist the patient to the supine position ⑨.

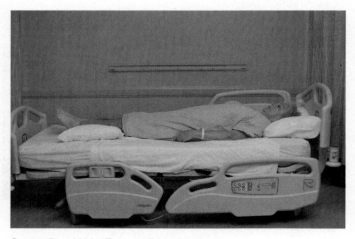

Source: Ronald May/Pearson Education, Inc.

⑨ Supine position.

SKILL 9.7 Positioning Patient in Bed (*continued*)

■ Provide supportive devices to align the patient appropriately.

- Place a pillow of suitable thickness under the patient's head and shoulders as needed. **Rationale:** *This prevents hyperextension of the neck.*
- Place a small pillow under the lower legs from below the knees to the ankles.
- *Optional:* Place trochanter rolls or sandbag laterally against the femurs. **Rationale:** *These prevent external rotation of the hips and legs.*
- Place a rolled towel or small pillow under the lumbar curvature if you feel a space between the lumbar area and the bed.
- Place a small pillow under thigh to flex knee slightly. **Rationale:** *This prevents hyperextension of knees.*
- Use heel boots or a footboard on the bed to support the feet. **Rationale:** *This prevents plantar flexion (footdrop).*
- If the patient is unconscious or has paralysis of the upper extremities, elevate the forearms and hands (*not* the upper arm) on pillows. **Rationale:** *This position promotes comfort and prevents edema.*
- If the patient has actual or potential finger and wrist flexion deformities, use hand rolls or wrist/hand splints ⑩. **Rationale:** *This prevents flexion contractures of the fingers.* Proceed to step 5 below.

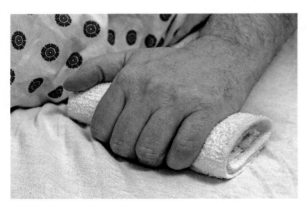

Source: Rick Brady/Pearson Education, Inc.

⑩ A hand roll may be made from a folded and rolled washcloth. It is used to maintain functional position of the wrist and fingers and to prevent contractures.

PRONE POSITION

■ Assist the patient to a prone position ⑪.
■ Provide supportive devices to position the patient appropriately.

- Turn the patient's head to one side, and either omit the pillow entirely if drainage from the mouth is being encouraged, or place a small pillow under the head to align the head with the trunk. **Rationale:** *This prevents flexion of the neck laterally.* Avoid placing the pillow under the shoulders. Verify patient's airway is open and not obstructed with a pillow.
- Place a small pillow or roll under the abdomen in the space between the diaphragm (or the breasts of a woman)

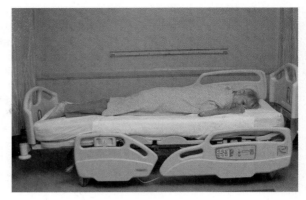

Source: Ronald May/Pearson Education, Inc.

⑪ Prone position.

and the iliac crests. **Rationale:** *The pillow prevents hyperextension of the lumbar curvature, difficulty breathing, and, for some women, pressure on the breasts.*

- Place a pillow under the lower legs from below the knees to just above the ankles. **Rationale:** *This raises the toes off the bed surface and reduces plantar flexion.* Proceed to step 5 on next page.

LATERAL POSITION

■ Assist the patient to a lateral position ⑫.
■ Provide supportive devices to align the patient appropriately.

- Place a pillow under the patient's head so that the head and neck are aligned with the trunk. **Rationale:** *The pillow prevents lateral flexion and discomfort of the major neck muscles.*
- Have the patient flex the lower shoulder and position it forward so that the body does not rest on it, in position of comfort.
- Place a pillow under the upper arm. **Rationale:** *This prevents internal rotation and adduction of the shoulder and downward pressure on the chest that could interfere with chest expansion during respiration.*

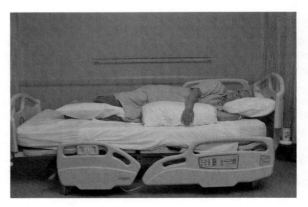

Source: Ronald May/Pearson Education, Inc.

⑫ Lateral (side-lying) position.

(*continued on next page*)

SKILL 9.7 Positioning Patient in Bed (*continued*)

- Place two or more pillows under the upper leg and thigh so that the extremity lies in a plane parallel to the surface of the bed. **Rationale:** *A position parallel to the bed prevents internal rotation of the thigh and adduction of the leg.*
- Ensure that the two shoulders are aligned in the same plane as the two hips. If they are not, pull one shoulder or hip forward or backward until all four joints are aligned in the same plane. **Rationale:** *Proper alignment prevents twisting of the spine.*
- Place a rolled pillow (fold pillow lengthwise) alongside the patient's back to stabilize the position. This pillow may not be needed when the patient's upper hip and knee are appropriately flexed.

5. When the procedure is complete, verify bed is in lowest position, perform hand hygiene and leave patient safe and comfortable.
6. Complete documentation using forms, checklists, or electronic dropdown lists supplemented by nurse's notes or additional comments as appropriate, including
   - Ways patient is able to assist with positioning.
   - Any signs of pressure areas or contractures.
   - Use of support/assistive devices and any special requirements.

SAMPLE DOCUMENTATION

[date] 1030 Turned to (L) side by 2 staff. Pillows under head, upper arm, & upper leg. Skin intact without redness noted. Tolerated without incident. *M. Lawrence*

Lifespan Considerations

NEWBORNS AND INFANTS

- Position newborns and infants on their back for sleep, even after feeding. This creates less risk of regurgitation and choking, and the rate of sudden infant death syndrome (SIDS) is significantly lower in newborns and infants who sleep on their backs.
- The skin of newborns can be fragile and may be torn (sheared) if the newborn or infant is pulled across a bed.

CHILDREN

- Carefully inspect the back of the head and dependent skin surfaces of all newborns, infants, and children confined to bed at least three times in each 24-hour period.

OLDER ADULTS

- In patients who have had cerebrovascular accidents (strokes), there is a risk of shoulder displacement on the paralyzed side from improper moving or repositioning techniques. Use care when moving, positioning in bed, and transferring. Pillows or foam devices are helpful to support the affected arm and shoulder and to prevent injury.
- Decreased subcutaneous fat and thinning of the skin may place older adults at risk for skin breakdown. Repositioning approximately every 2 hours (more or less, depending on the unique needs of the individual patient) helps reduce pressure on bony prominences and avoid tissue trauma.

SKILL 9.8 Sitting on Side of Bed (Dangling): Assisting

The patient assumes a sitting position on the edge of the bed to allow neurovascular equilibration before walking, moving to a chair or wheelchair, eating, or performing other activities.

Delegation or Assignment

Assisting the patient to sit on the side of the bed and dangle may be delegated or assigned to the UAP. The nurse instructs the UAP to report patient observations to the nurse for follow-up. Assessment and evaluation of effectiveness of the exercise remain the responsibility of the nurse. Note that state laws for UAPs vary, so this task might be assigned to the UAP rather than delegated.

Equipment

No equipment is needed for this skill.

Preparation

- Review healthcare provider's orders and patient's nursing plan of care.
- Determine if assistive devices will be required.

- Determine if any encumbrances to movement, such as an IV or an indwelling catheter, are present.
- Be aware of medications the patient is receiving, because certain medications may hamper movement or alertness of the patient.
- Decide if assistance will be required from other healthcare personnel.
- All assistive equipment and devices need to be ready for use and easily accessible. Mechanical equipment needs to be maintained with slings and transfer sheets kept clean and stocked. Equipment should be charged. If any part is broken or malfunctioning, it should be taken to the maintenance department for repair or have an exchange agreement with a vendor for a loaner if the equipment needs to be sent to the manufacturer.

Procedure

1. Prior to performing the procedure, introduce self and verify the patient's identity using two identifiers. Explain to the patient what you are going to do, why it is necessary, and how the patient can participate.

SKILL 9.8 Sitting on Side of Bed (Dangling): Assisting (*continued*)

2. Perform hand hygiene and observe other appropriate infection control procedures.
3. Provide for patient privacy.
4. Position yourself and the patient appropriately before performing the move.
   - Assist the patient to a lateral position facing you.
   - Raise the head of the bed slowly to its highest position.
   - Position the patient's feet and lower legs at the edge of the bed. **Rationale:** *This enables the patient's feet to move easily off the bed during the movement, and the patient is aided by gravity into a sitting position.*
   - Stand beside the patient's hips and face the far corner of the bottom of the bed (the angle in which movement will occur). Assume a broad stance, placing the foot nearest the patient forward. Lean your trunk forward from the hips.
5. Move the patient to a sitting position ❶.
   - Place one arm around the patient's shoulders and the other arm at the patient's thighs near the knees. **Rationale:** *Supporting the patient's shoulders prevents the patient from falling backward during the movement.*
   - Tighten your gluteal, abdominal, leg, and arm muscles.

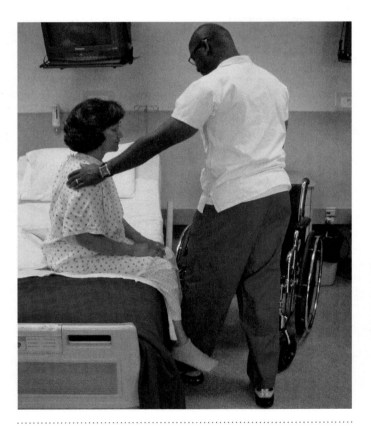

❶ Pivot patient to dangling position before placing feet on floor.

- Pivot on the balls of your feet in the desired direction facing the foot of the bed while guiding the patient's feet and legs off the bed. **Rationale:** *The weight of the patient's legs swinging downward increases downward movement of the lower body.*
- Keep supporting the patient until the patient is well balanced and comfortable. **Rationale:** *This movement may cause some patients to become lightheaded or dizzy.*
- Assess vital signs (i.e., pulse, respirations, and blood pressure) if indicated by the patient's health status.

CAUTION! If the patient becomes lightheaded, dizzy, or feeling "funny," assist the patient back to a lying position in bed and assess vital signs. Stay with the patient until patient feels better and vital signs are stable.

---

6. When assisting patient is complete, verify bed in lowest position, perform hand hygiene, and leave patient safe and comfortable.
7. Complete documentation using forms, checklists, or electronic dropdown lists supplemented by nurse's notes or additional comments as appropriate, including
   - Ability of patient to assist in moving and turning.
   - Response of patient to moving and turning (e.g., anxiety, discomfort, dizziness).

SAMPLE DOCUMENTATION

[date] 1310 Assisted to side of bed to dangle before getting up to chair. Denies dizziness or pain while sitting. No respiratory distress noted. Assisted to chair with help. Moving legs and arms for balance appropriately. Call bell placed in reach. Tolerated without incident. *C. Roy*

Patient Teaching

Positioning at Home

- Ensure height of the bed and the patient's leg length allows movements in and out of the bed.
- Ensure the mattress is not too soft. Bed boards are recommended for patients with back problems.
- Include application of body mechanics to prevent injury when turning and positioning patient and inquire about the possibility of using an assistive device in the home.
- Include basic principles of body alignment.
- Include checking the patient's skin for redness and integrity after repositioning the patient. Emphasize that reddened areas should not be massaged because it may lead to tissue trauma.

SKILL 9.9 Transferring Patient Between Bed and Chair

Sometimes patients desire to, and need to, get up out of bed and sit in a recliner chair, wheelchair, or portable commode chair, but are unable to do so without assistance. Nursing staff can assist patients to transfer from the bed to the chair in a variety of ways that are safe and efficient.

Delegation or Assignment

The skill of transferring a patient can be delegated or assigned to UAPs who have demonstrated safe transfer technique for the involved patient. It is important for the nurse to assess the patient's capabilities and communicate specific information about what the UAP should report back to the nurse. Note that state laws for UAPs vary, so this task might be assigned to the UAP rather than delegated.

Equipment

- Robe or appropriate clothing
- Slippers or shoes with nonskid soles
- Gait/transfer belt
- Chair, commode, wheelchair, or stretcher as appropriate to patient need
- Sliding board, if appropriate
- Mechanical lift, if appropriate

Preparation

- Review the healthcare provider's orders and the patient's nursing plan of care.
- Plan what to do and how to do it.
- Obtain essential equipment before starting (e.g., gait/transfer belt, wheelchair) and check that all equipment is functioning correctly.
- All assistive equipment and devices need to be ready for use and easily accessible. Mechanical equipment needs to be maintained with slings and transfer sheets kept clean and stocked. Equipment should be charged. If any part is broken or malfunctioning, it should be taken to the maintenance department for repair or have an exchange agreement with a vendor for a loaner if the equipment needs to be sent to the manufacturer.
- Remove obstacles from the area so patients do not trip, and make sure there are no spills or liquids on the floor on which patients could slip.

Procedure

1. Prior to performing the procedure, introduce self and verify the patient's identity using two identifiers. Explain the transfer process to the patient. During the transfer, explain step by step what the patient should do, for example, "Move your right foot forward."
2. Perform hand hygiene and observe other appropriate infection control procedures.
3. Provide for patient privacy.
4. Position the equipment appropriately.
   - Lower the bed to its lowest position so that the patient's feet will rest flat on the floor. Lock the wheels of the bed.
   - Place the wheelchair parallel to the bed as close to the bed as possible. Put the wheelchair on the side of the bed that allows the patient to move toward whichever side is stronger. Lock the wheels of the wheelchair and raise the footplate.

   or

   - For patients who have difficulty walking, place the wheelchair at a 45-degree angle to the bed. **Rationale:** *This enables the patient to pivot into the chair and lessens the amount of body rotation required.*

   or

   - For patients who cannot stand but are able to cooperate and possess sufficient upper body strength, use a sliding board to help them move without nursing assistance. **Rationale:** *This method not only promotes the patient's sense of independence but also preserves your energy.*
5. Prepare the patient.
   - Assist the patient to a sitting position on the side of the bed ❶.
   - Assess the patient for orthostatic hypotension before moving the patient from the bed.
   - Assist the patient in putting on a bathrobe and nonskid slippers or shoes.
   - Place a gait/transfer belt snugly around the patient's waist. Check to be certain that the belt is securely fastened.

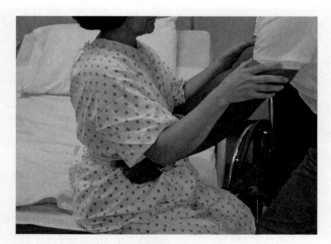

Source: Ronald May/Pearson Education, Inc.

❶ Move patient to side of bed using gait belt for support.

6. Give explicit instructions to the patient. Ask the patient to:
   - Move forward and sit on the edge of the bed with feet placed flat on the floor. **Rationale:** *This brings the patient's center of gravity closer to the nurse's.*
   - Lean forward slightly from the hips.
   - Place the foot of the stronger leg beneath the edge of the bed (or sitting surface) and put the other foot forward. **Rationale:** *A broader base of support makes the patient more stable during the transfer.*
   - Place the patient's hands on the bed surface (or available stable area) so that the patient can push down while standing. The patient can grasp your upper arms for support.

SKILL 9.9 Transferring Patient Between Bed and Chair (*continued*)

7. Position yourself correctly.
   - Stand directly in front of the patient. Lean the trunk forward from the hips. Hold the gait/transfer belt with the nearest hand; the other hand supports the back of the patient's shoulder. Flex the hips, knees, and ankles. Assume a broad stance, placing one foot forward and one back ❷.

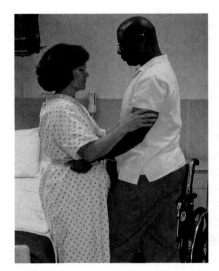

Source: Ronald May/Pearson Education, Inc.

❷ Stand with your foot between patient's feet; assist patient to standing position.

8. Assist the patient to stand, and then move together toward the wheelchair or sitting area to which you wish to transfer the patient. Count to three or give the verbal instructions of "Ready—Steady—Stand." On "three," or the word "stand," ask the patient to push down against the mattress/side of the bed while you transfer your weight from one foot to the other (while keeping your back straight) and stand upright, moving the patient forward (directly toward your center of gravity) into a standing position. (If the patient requires more than a very small degree of pulling, even with the assistance of two nurses, a mechanical device should be obtained and used.)
   - Support the patient in an upright standing position for a few moments. **Rationale:** *This allows the nurse an opportunity to ensure that the patient is stable before moving away from the bed.*
   - Together, pivot or take a few steps toward the wheelchair ❸, bed, chair, commode, or car seat.

CAUTION! When a patient has an injured lower extremity, movement should always occur toward the patient's unaffected (strong) side. For example, if the patient's right leg is injured and the patient is sitting on the edge of the bed preparing to transfer to a wheelchair, position the wheelchair on the patient's left side. **Rationale:** *In this way, the patient can use the unaffected leg most effectively and safely.*

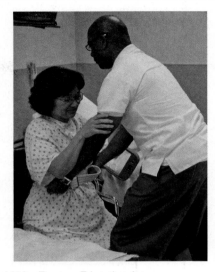

Source: Ronald May/Pearson Education, Inc.

❸ Grasping gait belt for safe transfer, use leg muscles to pivot patient into chair.

- Even if a patient is able to partially bear weight and is cooperative, it still may be safer to transfer a patient with the assistance of the nurse and UAP. If so, position yourselves on both sides of the patient, facing the same direction as the patient. Grasp the patient's transfer belt with the hand closest to the patient, and with the other hand support the patient's elbows. All three of you stand simultaneously, pivot, and move to the wheelchair. Reverse the process to lower the patient onto the wheelchair seat.
9. Assist the patient to sit.
   - Move the wheelchair forward or have the patient back up to the wheelchair (or desired seating area) and place the legs against the seat. **Rationale:** *Doing this minimizes the risk of the patient falling when sitting down.*
   - Make sure the wheelchair brakes are on.
   - Have the patient reach back and feel/hold the arms of the wheelchair.
   - Stand directly in front of the patient. Place one foot forward and one back.
   - Tighten your grasp on the transfer belt, and tighten your gluteal, abdominal, leg, and arm muscles.
   - Have the patient sit down while you bend your knees/hips and lower the patient onto the wheelchair seat ❹.
10. Ensure patient safety.
    - Ask the patient to push back into the wheelchair seat. **Rationale:** *Sitting well back on the seat provides a broader base of support and minimizes the risk of falling from the wheelchair.*
    - Remove the gait/transfer belt.
    - Lower the footplates and place the patient's feet on them, if applicable.

(continued on next page)

SKILL 9.9 Transferring Patient Between Bed and Chair (continued)

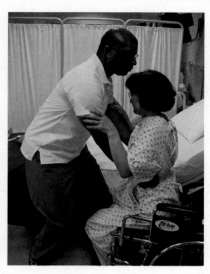

Source: Ronald May/Pearson Education, Inc.

④ Slowly lower patient into chair while holding gait belt securely.

11. When the patient is settled, perform hand hygiene and leave patient safe and comfortable.
12. Complete documentation using forms, checklists, or electronic dropdown lists supplemented by nurse's notes or additional comments as appropriate, including:
    - Patient's ability to bear weight and pivot
    - Number of staff needed for transfer and safety measures/precautions used
    - Length of time up in chair
    - Patient response to transfer and being up in chair or wheelchair

SAMPLE DOCUMENTATION

[date] 1630 Up to chair assisted by 2 staff. Able to walk slowly without incident. Denies dizziness or pain in legs. Waiting for family to visit. Tolerated ambulating without complaints. *H. Love*

SKILL 9.10 Transferring Patient Between Bed and Stretcher

Sometimes patients unable to stand and walk need to be transported to another department or healthcare facility for diagnostic tests, therapies, surgical procedures, or treatments. Nursing staff can assist patients to transfer from the bed to the stretcher for safe and efficient transport.

Delegation or Assignment

The skill of transferring a patient can be delegated or assigned to UAPs who have demonstrated safe transfer technique for the involved patient. It is important for the nurse to assess the number of staff needed, assistive devices needed, patient's ability to assist, and to communicate specific information about what the UAP should report to the nurse. Note that state laws for UAPs vary, so this task might be assigned to the UAP rather than delegated.

Equipment

- Stretcher
- Transfer assistive devices (e.g., rolling transfer board, friction-reducing device, lift) ① ②

Preparation

- Review healthcare provider's orders and patient's nursing plan of care.
- Obtain the necessary equipment and nursing personnel to assist in the transfer.
- All assistive equipment and devices need to be ready for use and easily accessible. Mechanical equipment needs to be maintained with slings and transfer sheets kept clean and stocked. Equipment should be charged. If any part is broken or malfunctioning, it should be taken to the maintenance

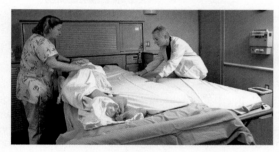

Source: Ronald May/Pearson Education, Inc.

① Positioning a rolling transfer board.

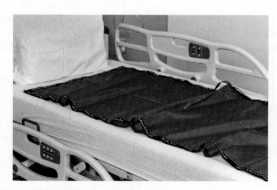

Source: Rick Brady/Pearson Education, Inc.

② Friction-reducing device with handles.

department for repair or have an exchange agreement with a vendor for a loaner if the equipment needs to be sent to the manufacturer.

SKILL 9.10 Transferring Patient Between Bed and Stretcher (*continued*)

Procedure

1. Prior to performing the procedure, introduce self and verify the patient's identity using two identifiers. Explain to the patient what you are going to do, why it is necessary, and how the patient can participate. Explain the transfer to the nursing personnel who are helping and specify who will give directions (one person needs to be in charge).
2. Perform hand hygiene and observe other appropriate infection control procedures.
3. Provide for patient privacy.
4. Adjust the patient's bed in preparation for the transfer.
   - Lower the head of the bed until it is flat or as low as the patient can tolerate.
   - Place the friction-reducing device under the patient and raise the bed so that it is slightly higher (i.e., about 1.3 cm [½ in.]) than the surface of the stretcher. **Rationale:** *It is easier for the patient to move down a slant.*
   - *Optional:* Use a transfer board ❸ or mechanical assistive devices and staff to assist. Turn the patient to a lateral position away from you, position the board close to the patient's back, and roll the patient onto the board. Pull the patient and board across the bed to the stretcher. Safety belts may be placed over the chest, abdomen, and legs.
   - Ensure that the wheels on the bed are locked.
   - Place the stretcher parallel to the bed next to the patient and lock the stretcher wheels.
   - *Optional:* Fill the gap that exists between the bed and the stretcher loosely with the bath blankets.
5. Transfer the patient securely to the stretcher.
   - If the patient can transfer independently, encourage the patient to do so and stand by for safety.
   - If the patient is partially able or not able to transfer:
     a. One caregiver needs to be at the side of the patient's bed, between the patient's shoulder and hip.
     b. The second and third caregivers should be at the side of the stretcher: one positioned between the patient's shoulder and hip, and the other between the patient's hip and lower legs.
     c. All caregivers should position feet in a walking stance.

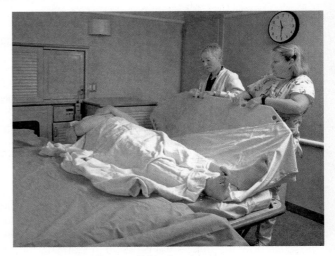

Source: Ronald May/Pearson Education, Inc.

❸ A smooth polyethylene transfer board for transferring patients.

   d. On a planned command, the caregivers at the stretcher's side pull and the caregiver at the bedside pushes the patient toward the stretcher.
6. Complete documentation using forms, checklists, or electronic dropdown lists supplemented by nurse's notes or additional comments as appropriate, including:
   - Equipment used
   - Number of people needed for transfer
   - Destination if reason for transfer is transport from one location to another

SAMPLE DOCUMENTATION

[date] 0930 Transferred to x-ray department stretcher with 3 staff members using a draw sheet. Tolerated move without complaint. Supine in good alignment on stretcher, sheet applied, then safety belt at waist. *L. Roger*

SKILL 9.11 Transporting: Newborn, Infant, Toddler

Safety of the newborn, infant, or toddler being transported from a secured pediatric unit to another department in the healthcare facility is a high priority. Parents are allowed to accompany their children, and specific IDs for parents and employees must be visual.

Delegation or Assignment

Assisting with routine noncritical transporting of newborns, infants, and toddlers can be delegated or assigned to UAPs that are working on the pediatric unit. They would have received specific training in keeping these patients safe during transporting to another department in the healthcare facility. They will

have specially coded ID badges designating they work on the pediatric unit. The nurse remains responsible for the assessment, interpretation of abnormal findings, and determination of appropriate responses. Note that state laws for UAPs vary, so this task might be assigned to the UAP rather than delegated.

Equipment

- Transporting vehicle (e.g., stretcher, crib, wheelchair)
- Wheeled poles for any necessary equipment
- Necessary supportive equipment such as oxygen tank or ventilation bags/masks
- Blankets

(*continued on next page*)

SKILL 9.11 Transporting: Newborn, Infant, Toddler (continued)

Preparation

- Review healthcare provider's orders and patient's nursing plan of care.
- Obtain necessary transporting equipment.
- Securely fasten intravenous lines, feeding lines, ECG leads, and other equipment. **Rationale:** *Lines that are securely fastened are less likely to be dislodged during transport.*
- Explain the transport to the family. **Rationale:** *Adequate explanation helps to decrease anxiety.*

Procedure

1. Introduce self to patient and parents, then verify the patient's identity using two identifiers. Explain to the patient and parents how the patient will be transported, why it is necessary, and how the patient can participate. Discuss how the results will be used in planning further care or treatments.
2. Perform hand hygiene and observe appropriate infection control procedures.
3. Provide for patient privacy.
4. Perform an assessment of the child. **Rationale:** *A baseline assessment provides comparison with later findings.*
5. The newborn or infant is placed in a bassinet or crib for transport. If the bassinet has a bottom shelf, it is used for carrying the IV pump or monitor.
6. The toddler is assisted to a high-top crib (may also be used for newborns and infants), with the side rails up and the protective top in place ❶. The child may be sitting or lying down. Alternatively, secure the child in a stroller or wheelchair of the proper size for the child's age ❷. Be sure to secure the child in the device with the seat safety strap. **Rationale:** *The child is secured to avoid falls and injury during transport.*

CAUTION! Stretchers should not be used because the mobile toddler may roll or fall off.

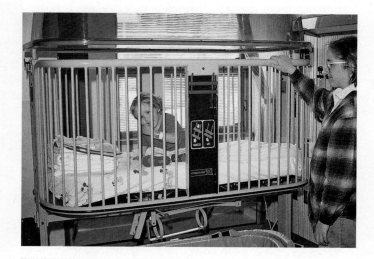

❶ High-top crib for newborn, infant, or toddler transport.

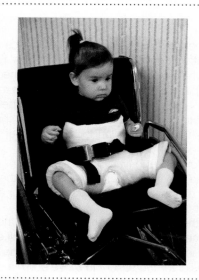

❷ Toddler in a wheelchair with a safety strap.

7. Attach intravenous poles and other equipment to the crib. When this is not possible, adequate personnel are needed to push all of the equipment. **Rationale:** *Lines can be more easily kept intact if they are on one transport vehicle.*
8. Keep the patient covered with blankets. **Rationale:** *Adequate covers help to prevent hypothermia resulting from a cool environment.*
9. Allow parents to accompany the child on the transport when possible. **Rationale:** *The parent's presence can provide a sense of security for the young child.*

CAUTION! Specialized wheelchairs and other equipment are available to carry enteral feeding solutions, motors necessary for equipment, and other supplies. These transporters are helpful for families when the child has a long-term disability, enabling them to take the child and equipment to school, stores, and other settings.

---

10. Complete documentation using forms, checklists, or electronic dropdown lists supplemented by nurse's notes or additional comments as appropriate, including the time the patient leaves the unit and where the patient is going, how the patient is traveling (i.e., via crib, wheelchair, or ambulation), who accompanies the patient, and how the patient responds.

SAMPLE DOCUMENTATION

[date] 0630 Placed in high-top crib, netting secured on top. Parents present and will accompany patient to surgical ready room. J. Bones, OR tech, and R. Willow, RN, transporting patient to OR. Crying softly but no distress noted. Off unit at 0646. *R. Willow*

SKILL 9.12 Turning Patient: Lateral or Prone Position in Bed

Assisting patients to turn while in bed can help prevent skin integrity problems for patients who cannot turn by themselves. Repositioning every 2 hours can prevent complications, support airway management, encourage lung expansion, and provide physiologic safety.

Delegation or Assignment

Turning patients in bed can be delegated or assigned to the UAP. The nurse must give specific directions to the UAP about the reporting of any changes in skin integrity. The UAP should be encouraged to have the patient participate as much as possible in turning. The nurse is responsible for evaluating the patient's comfort and alignment after the repositioning and for assessing skin integrity, particularly at pressure points. Note that state laws for UAPs vary, so this task might be assigned to the UAP rather than delegated.

Equipment

- Pillows
- Assistive devices as appropriate

Preparation

- Determine if any assistive devices will be required (e.g., friction-reducing device, mechanical lift).
- Determine if any encumbrances to movement, such as an IV or an indwelling urinary catheter, are present.
- Be aware of medications the patient is receiving, because certain medications may hamper movement or alertness of the patient.
- Use a Turn Schedule ❶ to keep staff rotating positions for patients who cannot turn by themselves to prevent complications of bed rest.
- Decide if assistance will be required from other healthcare personnel. **Rationale:** *Moving a patient is not a one-person task.*
- All assistive equipment and devices need to be ready for use and easily accessible. Mechanical equipment needs to be maintained with slings and transfer sheets kept clean and

stocked. Equipment should be charged. If any part is broken or malfunctioning, it should be taken to the maintenance department for repair or have an exchange agreement with a vendor for a loaner if the equipment needs to be sent to the manufacturer.

Procedure

1. Prior to performing the procedure, introduce self and verify the patient's identity using two identifiers. Explain to the patient that you are going to turn them in the bed, why it is necessary, and how the patient can participate.
2. Perform hand hygiene and observe other appropriate infection control procedures.
3. Provide for patient privacy.
4. Position yourself and the patient appropriately before performing the move. Other person(s) stand on the opposite side of the bed.
   - Adjust the head of the bed to a flat position or as low as the patient can tolerate. **Rationale:** *This provides a position of comfort for the patient.*
   - Raise the height of the bed appropriate to personnel safety (i.e., at the elbows).
   - Lock the wheels on the bed.
   - Move the patient closer to the side of the bed opposite the side the patient will face when turned. **Rationale:** *This ensures that the patient will be positioned safely in the center of the bed after turning.*
   - Use a friction-reducing device or mechanical lift (depending on level of patient assistance required) to pull the patient to the side of the bed. Adjust the patient's head and reposition the legs appropriately.

LATERAL POSITION

5. While standing on the side of the bed nearest the patient, place the patient's near arm across the chest. Abduct the patient's far shoulder slightly from the side of the body and externally rotate the shoulder ❷. **Rationale:** *Placing the arm away from the body and externally rotating the shoulder prevents that arm from being caught beneath the patient's body during the roll.*

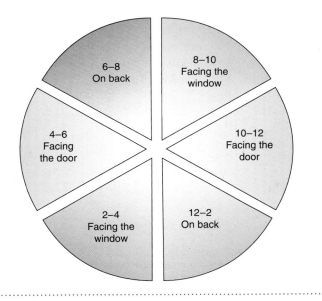

❶ Turn Schedule.

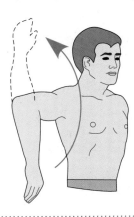

❷ External rotation of the shoulder prevents the arm from being caught beneath the patient's body when the patient is turned.

(continued on next page)

SKILL 9.12 Turning Patient: Lateral or Prone Position in Bed (continued)

- Place the patient's near ankle and foot across the far ankle and foot. **Rationale:** *This facilitates the turning motion.*
- The person on the side of the bed toward which the patient will turn should be positioned directly in line with the patient's waistline and as close to the bed as possible.

6. Roll the patient to the lateral position while maintaining proper alignment ❸. The second person standing on the opposite side of the bed helps roll the patient from the other side.
   - Place one hand on the patient's far hip and the other hand on the patient's far shoulder.
   - Position the patient in a side position with arms and legs positioned and supported properly. A pillow can be used to provide support under patient's back ❹. Proceed to step 7 below.

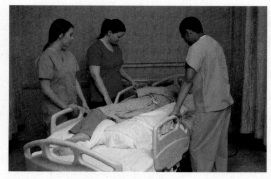

Source: Ronald May/Pearson Education, Inc.

❹ Maintain patient's position with pillow support under patient's back.

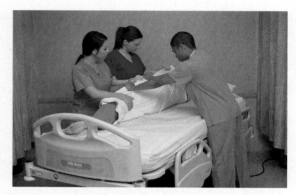

Source: Ronald May/Pearson Education, Inc.

❸ Maintain proper alignment while turning patient.

or

PRONE POSITION

5. While standing on the side of the bed nearest the patient, place the patient's near arm across the chest. Keep the patient's arm alongside the body for the patient to roll over.
   - Place the patient's near ankle and foot across the far ankle and foot.
   - The person on the side of the bed toward which the patient will turn should be positioned directly in line with the patient's waistline and as close to the bed as possible.

6. Roll the patient completely onto the abdomen for the prone position. **Rationale:** *It is essential to move the*

patient as close as possible to the edge of the bed before the turn so that the patient will be lying on the center of the bed after rolling. Never pull a patient across the bed while the patient is in the prone position. **Rationale:** *Doing so can injure a woman's breasts or a man's genitals.*

7. When the procedure is complete, verify bed is in lowest position, perform hand hygiene, and leave patient safe and comfortable.

8. Complete documentation using forms, checklists, or electronic dropdown lists supplemented by nurse's notes or additional comments as appropriate including:
   - Time and change of position moved from and position moved to
   - Any signs of pressure areas
   - Use of support devices
   - Ability of patient to assist in moving and turning
   - Response of patient to moving and turning (e.g., anxiety, discomfort, dizziness)

SAMPLE DOCUMENTATION

[date] 0400 Assisted to turn to right lateral side by UAP and me. No redness noted at lower back, denies discomfort, pillow placed at back for support. Positioned self for comfort. Tolerated without incident. *W. Mare*

≫ Patient Assistive Devices

Expected Outcomes

1. Feelings of physical and mental well-being increase.
2. Balance and muscle tone improve.
3. Patient progresses from being dependent to becoming independent in ambulation.
4. Complications of immobility are prevented with ambulation.

5. Patient correctly uses assistive devices without assistance.
6. Patient appropriately uses crutches to ambulate.
7. Crutches are measured correctly to prevent numbness or tingling in fingers.
8. Patient is able to resume routines of daily living.

SKILL 9.13 Cane: Assisting

When a patient has minor balance difficulties or a weak or injured leg, using a cane when walking or standing can provide the patient more balance and stability.

Delegation or Assignment

Due to the extent of knowledge required, teaching the patient to use assistive devices is not delegated or assigned to the UAP. The nurse or the physical therapist does the teaching. However, once the patient has demonstrated adequate skill, the UAP may assist the patient in ambulating with this equipment.

Equipment

- Appropriately sized cane with rubber tip(s)
- Gait/transfer belt, whether or not the patient is known to be unsteady
- Wheelchair for following patient, or chairs along the route if the patient needs to rest

Preparation

- Review healthcare provider's orders and patient's nursing plan of care.
- Ensure that the patient's path is free from clutter and hazards.

Procedure

1. Prior to performing the procedure, introduce self and verify the patient's identity using two identifiers. Explain to the patient what you are going to do, why it is necessary, and how the patient can participate. Discuss how this activity will be used in planning further care.
2. Perform hand hygiene and observe appropriate infection control procedures.
3. Ensure that patient is appropriately dressed for walking, especially in regards to stability of footwear.
4. Prepare the patient for walking.
   - Ask the patient to hold the cane on the stronger side of the body. **Rationale:** *This provides support and body alignment when walking.*
   - Position the tip of a standard cane (and the nearest tip of other canes) about 15 cm (6 in.) to the side and 15 cm (6 in.) in front of the near foot, so that the elbow is slightly flexed. **Rationale:** *In this position, the patient stands erect, with the center of gravity within the base of support.*
5. When maximum support is required, instruct the patient to move as follows:
   - Move the cane forward about 30 cm (1 ft), or a distance that is comfortable while the body weight is borne by both legs ❶.
   - Then, move the affected (weak) leg forward to the cane while the weight is borne by the cane and stronger leg.
   - Next, move the unaffected (stronger) leg forward ahead of the cane and weak leg while the weight is borne by the cane and weak leg.
6. If the patient requires minimal support from the cane, for instance just a little assist with balance, instruct the patient to follow these steps:
   - Move the cane and weak leg forward at the same time, while the weight is borne by the stronger leg ❷.

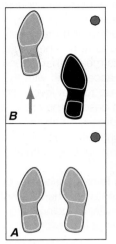
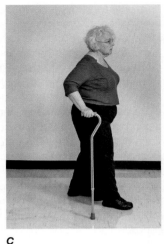

Source: **C,** Rick Brady/Pearson Education, Inc.

❶ Steps involved in using a cane to provide maximum support.

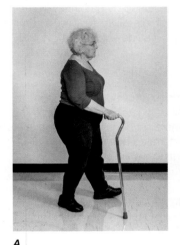
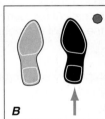

Source: **A,** Rick Brady/Pearson Education, Inc.

❷ Steps involved in using a cane when less than maximum support is required.

- Move the stronger leg forward while the weight is borne by the cane and the weak leg.
7. Ensure patient safety.
   - Walk beside the patient on the affected side. **Rationale:** *The patient is most likely to fall toward the affected side.*
   - Walk the patient for the time or distance indicated in the plan of care, being prepared to revise this plan if the patient's condition warrants it.
   - If the patient loses balance or strength and is unable to regain it, slide your hand up to the patient's axilla, and take a broad stance to provide a base of support. If there was any indication that this situation might occur, the patient should have had a gait belt placed before ambulation began. Have the patient rest against your

(continued on next page)

SKILL 9.13 Cane: Assisting (*continued*)

hip until assistance arrives, or gently lower yourself and the patient to the floor.

- For stair climbing, the phrase "up with the good, down with the bad" can help patients remember which pattern of movement to use. This means that when climbing stairs, the patient should ascend first with the good leg, bringing the weaker leg up to that level afterward. The pattern is reversed when descending stairs. This is also the pattern used with crutches on stairs.

8. When walking is complete, return patient to the room and assist to the bed or chair. Perform hand hygiene and leave patient safe and comfortable.

9. Complete documentation using forms, checklists, or electronic dropdown lists supplemented by nurse's notes or additional comments as appropriate, including the distance ambulated and any difficulties the patient experienced.

CAUTION! Instruct patients to use the cane opposite the side of pain or weakness to facilitate balance and decrease weight on painful extremities.

SAMPLE DOCUMENTATION

[date] 1307 Practiced with cane walking down hallway and back about 16 meters (52 ft). Able to correctly move cane when walking for best support. Denies lightheadedness or dizziness. No SOB noted. Back to chair in own room. Tolerated ambulation without incident, using cane correctly. *B. Korn*

SKILL 9.14 Crutches: Assisting

Crutches are assistive devices used by patients who have had surgery or have an injury or disability to one of their feet, ankles, knees, or legs. They provide support for mobility without using the affected leg.

Delegation or Assignment

Due to the extent of knowledge required, teaching the patient to use assistive devices is not delegated or assigned to the UAP. The nurse or the physical therapist does the teaching. However, once the patient has demonstrated adequate skill, the UAP may assist the patient in ambulating with this equipment

Equipment

- Appropriately sized crutches
- Gait/transfer belt, whether or not the patient is known to be unsteady
- Wheelchair for following patient, or chairs along the route if the patient needs to rest

Preparation

- Review healthcare provider's orders and patient's nursing plan of care.
- Ensure that the crutches are the proper length.

Procedure

1. Introduce self to patient and verify the patient's identity using two identifiers. Explain to the patient the need for crutches, why they are necessary, and how the patient can participate. Discuss how the results will be used in planning further care or treatments.

2. Perform hand hygiene and observe appropriate infection control procedures.

3. Provide for patient privacy.

4. Assist the patient to assume the tripod (triangle) position, the basic crutch stance used before crutch walking.
   - Ask the patient to stand and place the tips of the crutches 15 cm (6 in.) in front of the feet and out laterally

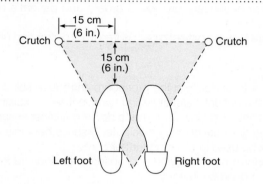

❶ The tripod position.

about 15 cm (6 in.). This is the starting position for all the different variations of ambulation with crutches ❶. **Rationale:** *The tripod position provides a wide base of support and enhances both stability and balance.*
   - Make sure the feet are slightly apart for a wide base.
   - Ensure that posture is erect; that is, the hips and knees should be extended, the back straight, and the head held straight and high. There should be no hunch to the shoulders and thus no weight borne by the axillae. The elbows should be extended sufficiently to allow weight bearing on the hands.
   - Stand slightly behind and on the patient's affected side. **Rationale:** *By standing behind the patient and toward the affected side, the nurse can provide support if the patient loses balance.*
   - If the patient is unsteady, place a walking belt around the patient's waist, and grasp the belt from above, not from below. **Rationale:** *A fall can be prevented more effectively if the belt is held from above.*

5. Teach the patient the appropriate crutch gait. Specific gaits are chosen based on patient capabilities and ability to bear weight. This varies from patient to patient.

SKILL 9.14 Crutches: Assisting (continued)

FOUR-POINT ALTERNATE GAIT

■ This is the most simple and safest gait, providing at least three points of support at all times, but it requires coordination. It is a slow gait because it requires the patient to move crutches and legs and shift weight constantly. To use this gait, the patient has to be able to bear some weight on both legs (❷, reading from bottom to top).

Step 4
Right foot advances

Step 3
Left crutch advances

Step 2
Left foot advances

Step 1
Right crutch advances

Tripod position

❷ The four-point alternate crutch gait.

■ Ask the patient to:
  ● Move the right crutch ahead a suitable distance (e.g., 10–15 cm [4–6 in.]).
  ● Move the left foot forward, preferably to the level of the crutch.
  ● Move the left crutch forward.
  ● Move the right foot forward.

THREE-POINT GAIT

■ To use this gait, the person must be able to bear entire body weight on the unaffected leg. It is a fast gait that requires strength in the three unaffected extremities. The two crutches and the unaffected leg bear weight alternately (❸, reading from bottom to top).
■ Ask the patient to:
  ● Move both crutches and the weaker leg forward.
  ● Move the stronger leg forward.

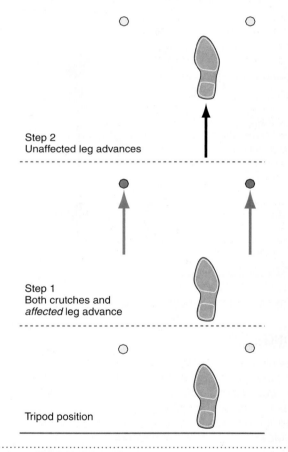

Step 2
Unaffected leg advances

Step 1
Both crutches and *affected* leg advance

Tripod position

❸ The three-point crutch gait.

TWO-POINT ALTERNATE GAIT

■ This gait is intermediate in pace and in required strength between the four-point gait and the three-point gait. It requires more balance than the four-point gait, because

(continued on next page)

SKILL 9.14 Crutches: Assisting *(continued)*

only two points support the body at one time; it also requires at least partial weight bearing on each foot. In this gait, arm movements with the crutches are similar to the arm movements during normal walking (❹, reading from bottom to top).

- Ask the patient to:
  - Move the left crutch and the right foot forward together.
  - Move the right crutch and the left foot ahead together.

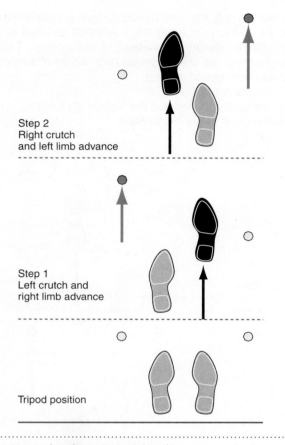

Step 2
Right crutch
and left limb advance

Step 1
Left crutch and
right limb advance

Tripod position

❹ The two-point alternate crutch gait.

SWING-TO GAIT

- People with paralysis of the legs and hips use the swing-to or swing-through gait. Prolonged use of these gaits results in atrophy of the unused muscles. The swing-to gait is the easier of these two gaits ❺.
- Ask the patient to:
  - Move both crutches ahead together.
  - Lift body weight by the arms and swing *to* the crutches.

SWING-THROUGH GAIT

- This gait requires considerable patient skill, strength, and coordination ❻.
- Ask the patient to:
  - Move both crutches forward together.
  - Lift body weight by the arms and swing through and beyond the crutches.

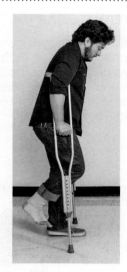

Source: Rick Brady/Pearson Education, Inc.

❺ The swing-to-crutch gait.

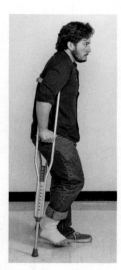

Source: Rick Brady/Pearson Education, Inc.

❻ The swing-through crutch gait.

6. Teach the patient to get into and out of a chair. Teach the patient to always leave the crutches within arms' reach when sitting or reclining, as they are needed for safe ambulation.

GETTING INTO A CHAIR

- Ensure that the chair has armrests and is secure or braced against a wall.
- Instruct the patient to:
  - Stand with the back of the unaffected leg centered against the chair.
  - Transfer the crutches to the hand on the affected side, hold the crutches by the hand bars, and then grasp the

SKILL 9.14 Crutches: Assisting *(continued)*

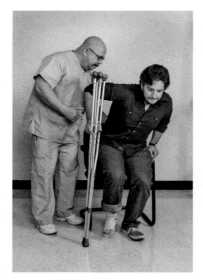

Source: Rick Brady/Pearson Education, Inc.

7 A patient using crutches getting into a chair.

arm of the chair with the hand on the unaffected side **7**. **Rationale:** *This allows the patient to support the body weight on the arms and the unaffected leg.*

- Lean forward, flex the knees and hips, and lower into the chair.

GETTING OUT OF A CHAIR

- Instruct the patient to:
  - Move forward to the edge of the chair and place the unaffected leg slightly under or at the edge of the chair. **Rationale:** *This position helps the patient stand up from the chair and achieve balance.*
  - Grasp the crutches by the hand bars in the hand on the affected side, and grasp the arm of the chair with the hand on the unaffected side. **Rationale:** *The body weight is placed on the crutches and the hand on the armrest to support the unaffected leg when the patient rises to stand.*
  - Push down on the crutches and the chair armrest while elevating the body out of the chair.
  - Assume the tripod position before moving.

7. Teach the patient to go up and down stairs.

GOING UP STAIRS

- Stand behind the patient and slightly to the affected side.
- Ask the patient to:
  - Assume the tripod position at the bottom of the stairs.
  - Transfer the body weight to the crutches and move the unaffected leg onto the step **8**.
  - Transfer the body weight to the unaffected leg on the step and move the crutches and affected leg up to the step.
  - Always have the crutches support the affected leg.
  - Repeat the steps above until the top of the stairs is reached.

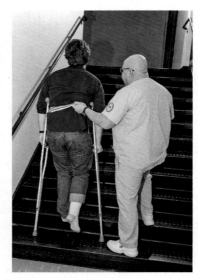

Source: Rick Brady/Pearson Education, Inc.

8 Climbing stairs: Place weight on the crutches while first moving the unaffected leg onto a step.

GOING DOWN STAIRS

- Stand one step below the person on the affected side.
- Ask the patient to:
  - Assume the tripod position at the top of the stairs.
  - Shift the body weight to the unaffected leg, and move the crutches and affected leg down onto the next step **9**.
  - Transfer the body weight to the crutches, and move the unaffected leg to that step. The crutches always support the affected leg.

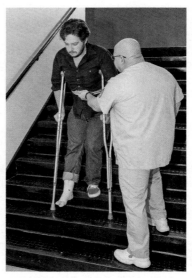

Source: Rick Brady/Pearson Education, Inc.

9 Descending stairs: Move the crutches and affected leg to the next step.

(continued on next page)

SKILL 9.14 Crutches: Assisting (*continued*)

■ Repeat the steps above until the bottom of the stairs is reached.

or

■ Ask the patient to:
  ● Hold both crutches in the outside hand and grasp the handrail with the other hand for support.
  ● Follow the steps for going up or down stairs.

8. Reinforce patient teaching.
9. When teaching is complete, perform hand hygiene and leave patient safe and comfortable.
10. Complete documentation using forms, checklists, or electronic dropdown lists supplemented by nurse's notes or additional comments as appropriate, including the patient's progress, distance ambulated, and any difficulties the patient experienced, including changes in vital signs as compared to baseline.

SAMPLE DOCUMENTATION

[date] 1500 Attempted crutch walking up steps. Unable to lift affected leg to next step, balance remained stable. Became dyspneic and upset. Vital signs (when seated) at baseline after activity. Reassured that this skill takes time. Encouraged to continue seated leg exercises and frequent ambulation. Will try again tomorrow. *B. Schneider*

Patient Teaching

Teach patient the following about crutches:

■ The weight of the body should be borne by the arms rather than the axillae (armpits). Continual pressure on the axillae can injure the radial nerve and may cause pain, numbness, and tingling.

■ Maintain an erect posture as much as possible to prevent strain on muscles and joints and to maintain balance.

■ Each step taken with crutches should be a comfortable distance. Start with a small rather than a large step.

■ Inspect the crutch tips regularly, and replace them if worn.

■ Keep the crutch tips dry and clean to maintain their surface friction. If the tips become wet, dry them well before use.

■ Wear a shoe with a low heel that grips the floor and has rubber soles. Adjust shoelaces so they cannot come untied or reach the floor where they might catch on the crutches. Consider shoes with alternative forms of closure (e.g., Velcro), especially if it is not easy to bend to tie laces.

Safety Considerations
MEASURING PATIENTS FOR CRUTCHES ⑩

When nurses measure patients for axillary crutches, it is most important to determine the correct length for the crutches and the correct placement of the hand piece.

Two methods are used to measure crutch length:

1. The patient lies in the supine position, and the nurse measures from the anterior fold of the axilla to a point 2.5 cm (1 in.) lateral from the heel of the foot.
2. The patient stands erect and positions the crutch tips 5 cm (2 in.) in front of and 15 cm (6 in.) to the side of the feet. The nurse makes sure the shoulder rest of the crutch is at least two finger-widths—that is, 2.5–5 cm (1–2 in.)—below the axilla.

To determine the correct placement of the hand bar:

1. The patient stands upright and supports the body weight by the hand grips of the crutches.
2. The nurse measures the angle of elbow flexion. It should be about 30 degrees. A *goniometer* (a handheld instrument used to measure joint angles) may be used to verify the correct angle.

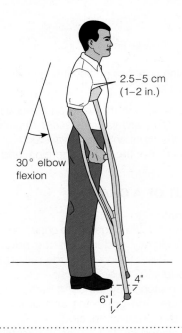

2.5–5 cm (1–2 in.)

30° elbow flexion

4"

6"

⑩ The standing position for measuring the correct length for crutches.

SETTING CRUTCH HEIGHT FOR CHILDREN

■ While the child is standing, the child's elbows should be slightly and comfortably flexed.

■ Place the tip of the crutches about 8–15 cm (3–6 in.) to the upper, outer border of the toes on each foot.

■ The upper pad on the crutches should now be lightly placed in the child's axilla. **Rationale:** *Crutches that are too high can put pressure on the brachial plexus, causing pain and injury. Crutches that are too low require that the child bend over to walk, and can cause injury to or discomfort of the back and neck.*

■ The child should be taught safe crutch walking, a procedure generally taught by a physical therapist or other specialist.

SKILL 9.15 Walker: Assisting

A walker is an assistive device for patients with leg weakness to improve their balance, or who need a wider base of support to improve their mobility.

Delegation or Assignment

Due to the extent of knowledge required, teaching the patient to use assistive devices is not delegated or assigned to the UAP. The nurse or the physical therapist does the teaching. However, once the patient has demonstrated adequate skill, the UAP may assist the patient in ambulating with this equipment.

Equipment

- Walker of appropriate size
- Gait/transfer belt, whether or not the patient is known to be unsteady
- Wheelchair for following patient, or chairs along the route if the patient needs to rest

Preparation

- Review the healthcare provider's orders and patient's nursing plan of care.
- Ensure patient has adequate arm strength to use walker.
- Ensure walker is at correct height. The walker should reach to the level of the patient's hip joint, and the elbows should be bent at about a 30-degree angle while using it.
- Ensure patient has a clear path free from obstacles.
- Use shoes that support the feet and are resistant to skidding and slipping.

Procedure

1. Introduce self to patient and verify the patient's identity using two identifiers. Explain to the patient that you are going to teach how to safely use a walker, why it is necessary, and how the patient can participate. Discuss how the results will be used in planning further care or treatments.
2. Perform hand hygiene and observe appropriate infection control procedures.
3. Provide for patient privacy.
4. Give the patient these instructions when maximum support is required:
   - Move the walker ahead about 15 cm (6 in.) while your body weight is borne by both legs.
   - Then move the right foot up to the walker while your body weight is borne by the left leg and both arms.
   - Next, move the left foot up to the right foot while your body weight is borne by the right leg and both arms.
5. Give the patient these instructions if one leg is weaker than the other:
   - Move the walker and the weak leg ahead together about 15 cm (6 in.) while your weight is borne by the stronger leg ❶.
   - Then move the stronger leg ahead while your weight is borne by the affected leg and both arms.
6. When teaching is complete, perform hand hygiene and leave patient safe and comfortable.
7. Complete documentation using forms, checklists, or electronic dropdown lists supplemented by nurse's notes or

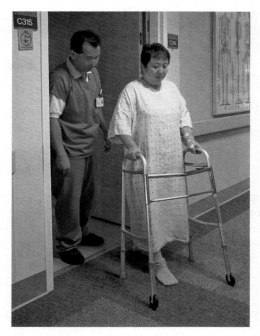

Source: Sandra Smith/Pearson Education, Inc.

❶ Instruct patient to move weaker side first.

additional comments as appropriate, including the distance ambulated, any difficulties the patient experienced, and changes in vital signs in relation to baseline.

SAMPLE DOCUMENTATION

[date] 1320 Walker sized by physical therapist. Instructions including a demo of using the walker done. Patient practiced using walker with physical therapist, short walk of 4.6 m (15 ft.), then returned to chair in room. States the walker helped her keep her balance more. No distress noted, tolerated practice without incident. *M. Boom*

Safety Considerations
CHILDREN

- Children learn and adapt quickly to the use of assistive devices.
- Care should be taken to check regularly that the child is using proper technique.
- Children may reach the point where they prematurely believe they no longer need them.

OLDER ADULTS

- Older adults' conditions can change rapidly. Check regularly to see that the current assistive device is the most appropriate one and that it fits the patient properly.

(continued on next page)

SKILL 9.15 Walker: Assisting *(continued)*

- Reinforce teaching regarding proper use of mechanical aids. Patients can easily fall into bad habits such as leaning the axillae on the crutches.

- Be aware that there may be a social stigma attached to the use of walkers in the minds of older adults. They may avoid using needed devices because of a need to perceive themselves as other than "old."

Patient Teaching

Using Assistive Devices at Home

- Ensure with patient and family that home lighting is adequate, nonskid rugs are used, clutter on floors is minimized, and non-slippery floor products are used for safety.
- Recommend nonskid strips be placed on outside steps and inside stairs that are not carpeted.
- Ensure that chairs are high enough to sit on and rise from comfortably, with sturdy arms from which to push up against when rising.

- Reinforce using proper gaits with canes, crutches, and walkers. Ask the patient to demonstrate how the appliance is normally used.
- Ensure that the equipment is properly maintained and stored out of the way when not in use.
- Suggest applying tennis balls with a cross cut in them over walker tips to make sliding easier.

≫ Traction and Cast Care

Expected Outcomes

1. Extremity is maintained in correct alignment.
2. Pin site remains free of infection.
3. Cast integrity is maintained to provide adequate site immobilization.

4. Patient experiences minimal swelling.
5. Neurovascular complications do not occur.

SKILL 9.16 Cast, Initial: Caring for

A cast is used to immobilize a fractured or injured bone and maintain it in good alignment while it heals. Underneath the hard plaster or fiberglass exterior is soft cotton padding applied to the extremity for comfort and protection for the skin. Cast splints can be used to support proper bone and joint development in children.

Delegation or Assignment

The nurse should perform baseline assessment of new casts (**Table 9–4 ≫**). Care of patients with stable casts may be delegated or assigned to the UAP. The status of the cast is

TABLE 9–4 Cast Materials

Type of Material	Description	Application	Setting Time and Weight-Bearing Restrictions
Plaster (or plaster of paris products)	Open-weave cotton rolls or strips saturated with powdered calcium sulfate crystals (gypsum)	Applied after being soaked in tepid water for a few seconds until bubbling stops	Dries in 48 hr, no weight bearing allowed until dry
Synthetics; polyester and cotton (e.g., Hygia Cast, Nemoa)	Open-weave polyester and cotton tape permeated with water-activated polyurethane resin	Applied after being soaked in cool water, 26°C (80°F); used within 2–3 min of soaking	Sets in 7 min, weight bearing allowed in 15 min
Fiberglass; water-activated (e.g., Scotchcast, Delta-Lite) or light-cured (e.g., Lightcast II); fiberglass-free/latex-free (e.g., Delta-Cast Elite, FlashCast Elite)	Open-weave fiberglass tape impregnated with water-activated polyurethane resin or photosensitive polyurethane resin	Applied after being immersed in tepid water for 10–15 sec or applied with gloves or silicone-type hand cream to keep it from sticking	Sets in 7–15 min, weight bearing allowed in 20–30 min; light-cured version sets after being exposed for 3 min to a special ultraviolet lamp (curing), weight bearing allowed immediately
Thermoplastic (e.g., Hexcelite)	Knitted thermoplastic polyester fabric in rigid rolls	Applied after being heated in water at 76°C–82°C (170°F–180°F) for 3–4 min to make the rolls soft and pliable	Remove excess water by squeezing between towels before applying. Cured when cool to touch, then weight bearing allowed

SKILL 9.16 Cast, Initial: Caring for (continued)

observed during usual care and may be recorded by individuals other than the nurse. However, assessment of complications from the cast requires the expertise of a nurse. Abnormal findings detected by the UAP must be validated and interpreted by the nurse. Note that state laws for UAPs vary, so this task might be assigned to the UAP rather than delegated.

Equipment

- Pillows to support the casted areas
- Ice packs
- Pen
- Absorbent pads and protectors
- Clean gloves

Preparation

- Review healthcare provider's orders and patient's nursing plan of care.
- Review the patient record to determine the reason for the cast and the initial status of the patient's extremity. Examine the record regarding pain assessment findings and interventions.

Procedure

1. Introduce self to patient (and parents) and verify the patient's identity using two identifiers. Explain to the patient (and parents) what you are going to do, why it is necessary, and how the patient can participate. Discuss how the results will be used in planning further care or treatments.
2. Perform hand hygiene and observe appropriate infection control procedures.
3. Provide for patient privacy. Don clean gloves if cast still wet.
4. Assess the neurovascular status of the affected limbs.
   - Assess the toes or fingers for nerve and circulatory impairments every 30 minutes for 4 hours following cast application, and then every 3 hours for the first 24–48 hr or until all signs and symptoms of impairment are negative. Increase the frequency of neurovascular assessments in accordance with the patient's condition (e.g., presence of circulatory impairment). **Rationale:** *Rapid swelling under a cast can cause neurovascular problems, so frequent neurovascular assessments by the nurse are a priority.*

CAUTION! When casting material inhibits palpation of peripheral pulses, assess capillary refill and for edema, comfort level, and other parameters of circulation-motor-sensory status (C-M-S check) as an indication of neurovascular status.

---

5. Support and handle the cast appropriately.
   - Immediately after the cast is applied, place it on pillows. Avoid using plastic or rubber pillows. **Rationale:** *The pillows provide even pressure and support the curves of the cast and promote venous blood return, thereby decreasing the possibility of swelling.*

- Until a cast has set or hardened, which is dependent on the type of casting material used, support the cast in the palms of your hands rather than with your fingertips, and extend your fingers so that your fingertips do not touch the plaster. **Rationale:** *Fingertip pressure can cause dents in unset plaster and subsequent skin pressure areas.*
- When the cast is set, continue to handle the cast with your palms only, but you may then wrap your fingers around the contour of the cast.

6. Implement measures to reduce swelling.
   - Control swelling by elevating arms or legs higher than the heart on pillows ❶. Generally, three pillows are needed to achieve high elevation of a leg. As circulation improves and healing progresses, the elevation can be gradually reduced to two pillows (moderate elevation) and then to one pillow (low elevation). **Rationale:** *Swelling can cause neurovascular impairment.*

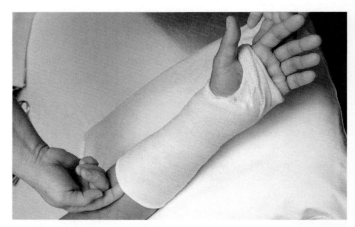

Source: Ronald May/Pearson Education, Inc.

❶ Position extremity above heart level to reduce edema formation. Check cast for tightness. The nurse should be able to insert one to two fingers between cast and skin.

- Apply ice packs to control perineal edema associated with a hip spica cast. Although ice packs are a less effective method of control than elevation, elevation of the area is obviously difficult.
- Report excessive swelling and indications of neurovascular impairment to the healthcare provider or nurse in charge. The healthcare provider may bivalve a cast if it appears to be too tight. Bivalving a cast is cutting the cast partially or completely and wrapping it with bandage material to hold it together. **Rationale:** *This relieves the pressure of the cast but still provides support.*

7. Use appropriate means to dry the plaster cast thoroughly.
   - Extremity plaster casts usually take 24–48 hr to dry completely; spica or body casts require 48–72 hr. Drying time depends on the temperature, humidity, size of the cast, and method used for drying. The cast is dry

(continued on next page)

SKILL 9.16 Cast, Initial: Caring for (continued)

when it no longer feels damp. A dry cast feels dry, looks white and shiny, and is odorless, hard, and resonant when tapped. Synthetic casts take only 10–15 min to harden completely.

- Expose the cast to the circulating air. Place sheets and blankets only over areas that do not have the cast.
- Check facility policy about the recommended turning frequency for patients with different kinds of casts. **Rationale:** *Frequent turning promotes even drying of the cast.*
- Every 2–4 hr, turn the patient with an extremity cast or body spica.

CAUTION! Do not use abductor bars (incorporated into cast) for moving the patient. Move the patient as a unit instead.

- Use regular pillows. **Rationale:** *Plastic or rubber pillows hinder drying and do not allow the heat of a drying cast to dissipate.*
- Do not facilitate drying by artificial means (i.e., by using a fan, hair dryer, infrared lamp, or electric heater). **Rationale:** *Artificial methods dry the outer surface of the cast while the inner portion remains soft and spongy. Such a cast cracks readily at points of strain.*

8. Monitor bleeding if an open reduction was done or if the injury was a compound fracture.
   - Monitor bloodstains or other drainage ❷ on the cast for 24–72 hr after surgery or injury, or longer if necessary.

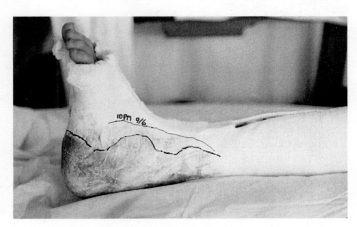

Source: Ronald May/Pearson Education, Inc.

❷ Observe casted extremity frequently to monitor and mark drainage or blood. Assess dependent area for both as well.

- Outline the stained area or any drainage noted with a pen at least every 8 hours if it is changing, and note the time and date, so that any further bleeding can be determined.

CAUTION! If the patient has had an open reduction, wound drainage will be absorbed and spread rapidly, or seep down the back of cast. The visible drainage does not necessarily indicate the amount of actual drainage.

Inspect all cast surfaces and mark drainage regularly if it is increasing. Bleeding should not persist after 24 hours.

9. Assess pain and pressure areas.
   - Never ignore complaints of pain, burning, swelling, or pressure. If a patient is unable to communicate, be alert to changes in temperament, restlessness, or fussiness that may indicate a problem. **Rationale:** *Compartment syndrome is a serious complication that can result when swelling and pressure within the closed fascial compartment build to dangerous levels, preventing nourishment from reaching nerve and muscle cells. Apply ice, put extremity in neutral position, and notify healthcare provider immediately. An absent or diminished distal pulse necessitates immediate surgical action to allow expansion and blood flow and prevent nerve damage.*
   - Determine particularly whether the pain is persistent and if it occurs over a bony prominence or joint.
   - Do not disregard a cessation of persistent pain or discomfort complaints from the patient. **Rationale:** *Cessation of complaints can indicate a skin slough. When a skin slough occurs, superficial skin sensation is lost and the patient no longer feels pain.*
   - When a pressure area under the cast is suspected, the healthcare provider may either bivalve the cast so that all of the skin beneath the cast can be inspected or cut a window in the cast over only the area of concern. When a cast is windowed:
     a. Retain the piece (cast and padding) that was cut out. Some healthcare providers order that it be taped back if no skin problem is present, but left out if a pressure area is present. **Rationale:** *Putting back the piece prevents window edema.*
     b. Inspect the skin under the window at scheduled time intervals.

Safety Considerations

Assess circulation and neurological status every 15 min after surgery or cast placement and then progress to every 30 min, 60 min, and 2 hr. Report abnormal findings or changes in condition. Include the following observations on the involved extremities:

- Distal pulses
- Color
- Warmth
- Sensation
- Capillary refill
- Edema
- Movement
- Pain, tingling

Rationale: *Circulation and nerves under the cast can be injured if it is too tight.*

Neurovascular impairment under a cast is an emergency. If assessments indicate impaired circulation or neurologic status, notify the healthcare provider immediately. Have a cast cutter at the bedside so the cast can be removed if needed and the pressure relieved.

SKILL 9.16 Cast, Initial: Caring for (continued)

10. When the procedure is complete, perform hand hygiene and leave patient safe and comfortable.

11. Complete documentation using forms, checklists, or electronic dropdown lists supplemented by nurse's notes or additional comments as appropriate, including whether or not there are problems.

SAMPLE DOCUMENTATION

[date] 1100 Cast still damp, elevated on one pillow. Fingers warm to touch, color pink, full ROM of fingers, no numbness or tingling. Arm pain at 2/10. Declined pain med. Tolerated assessment without complaint. *E. Mitchell*

Lifespan Considerations

CHILDREN

■ Teach parents of young children ways to prevent the child from placing small items inside the cast. Serious infections and damage to tissues can occur as a result of sticking anything inside the cast.

Parents also need to ensure that the top of a body cast is covered during meals so that food does not fall inside the cast.

■ If possible, allow the child to choose the color of the synthetic cast. Wearing a cast can cause disturbances in body image and self-concept. Education regarding cast care, how to adapt activities of daily living (ADLs), efficient ambulation, and what to expect as far as cast removal will help the child cope effectively.

■ Reassure the child that the saw used for windowing, bivalving, and removing the cast is not painful. It rapidly vibrates back and forth rather than rotates, so injury from the blade is unlikely. The saw is rather loud and can scare children, so have an adult present to support the child during these procedures. Let the child keep the cast pieces when removed if desired and they are no longer needed.

OLDER ADULTS

■ Older adults who are immobilized are at increased risk for skin breakdown and pressure ulcers.

■ Wound healing may be slower in older adults than in younger patients.

■ Older adults may be less able to manage the additional weight and imbalance caused by a cast.

■ Take appropriate steps in planning for use of crutches or other mobility devices to keep older adults moving safely.

Patient Teaching

■ For itching, suggest that the patient use a hair dryer on cool, a vacuum cleaner on reverse, or an ice bag over the outside of the itching area. Emphasize the importance of not putting anything inside the cast, because serious infections and tissue damage can occur.

■ Look a few times a day for indications of extreme coldness or blueness of toes or fingers; extreme continuous swelling of casted toes or fingers; numbness or tingling ("pins and needles" sensation) in casted toes or fingers; continuous or increasing pain; foul odor from within the cast; unexplained fever; inability to move the toes or fingers; or a weakened, cracked, loose, or tight cast. If any of these problems occur, call the healthcare provider immediately.

■ Keep the plaster cast dry.

■ Avoid strenuous activity and follow medical advice about exercise.

■ Elevate the arm or leg frequently to prevent dependent edema.

■ Move the toes or fingers frequently.

■ Look at the skin around the cast edges frequently, and keep it clean and dry.

■ Suggest modifications that may be necessary in clothing, toileting, sleeping, and other activities.

SKILL 9.17 Cast, Ongoing for Plaster and Synthetic: Caring for

Cast care is important to keep the integrity of the cast intact to maintain support, protection, and alignment while the bone and tissue heal and to avoid complications when the cast integrity is breeched.

Delegation or Assignment

Care of patients with stable casts may be delegated or assigned to the UAP. The status of the cast is observed during usual care and may be recorded by individuals other than the nurse. However, assessment of complications from the cast requires the expertise of a nurse. Abnormal findings detected by the UAP must be validated and interpreted by the nurse. Note that state laws for UAPs vary, so this task might be assigned to the UAP rather than delegated.

Equipment

Assemble any of the following equipment items necessary to complete patient care:

■ Pillows to support the casted areas
■ Damp cloth
■ Swab
■ Alcohol
■ Acetone or nail polish remover
■ Waterproof tape or adhesive strips
■ Bib or towels
■ Fracture bedpan
■ Plastic covering

(continued on next page)

SKILL 9.17 Cast, Ongoing for Plaster and Synthetic: Caring for (continued)

- Soap and water
- Handheld blow dryer
- Mineral, olive, or baby oil

Preparation

- Review healthcare provider's orders and patient's nursing plan of care.
- Review the patient record to determine previous status of the cast and the patient's extremities. Examine the record regarding pain assessment findings and interventions.

Procedure

1. Prior to performing the procedure, introduce self to the patient (and parents) and verify the patient's identity using two identifiers. Explain to the patient (and parents) what you are going to do, why it is necessary, and how the patient can participate. Discuss how the results will be used in planning further care or treatments.
2. Perform hand hygiene and observe other appropriate infection control procedures.
3. Provide for patient privacy as indicated.
4. Continue to assess the patient for problems.
   - Assess the neurovascular status of the affected limb at regular intervals in accordance with facility protocol.
   - Inspect the skin near and under the cast edges whenever neurovascular assessments are made and/or whenever the patient is turned.
   - Check the cast daily for a foul odor. **Rationale:** *This kind of odor may indicate skin excoriation from pressure or an infected area beneath the cast.*
5. Implement measures to prevent skin irritation at the edges of the cast.
   - Wash crumbs of plaster from the skin with a damp cloth and feel along the cast edges to check for rough edges or areas that press into the patient's skin. **Rationale:** *Small bits of plaster frequently break off from rough edges, and if they fall inside the cast, they can cause discomfort and irritation.*
   - Remove the resin of synthetic casting materials with a swab moistened with alcohol, acetone, or nail polish remover. Check the manufacturer's directions.
   - When it is dry, cover any rough edges and protect areas of the cast that may come in contact with urine. "Petal" the edges with small strips of waterproof tape or moleskin as follows:
     - a. Cut several strips of 2.5-cm (1-in.) adhesive, 5–7.5 cm (2–3 in.) long. Then curve all corners of each strip. **Rationale:** *Square or pointed ends tend to curl.*
     - b. Insert one end of each strip as far as possible inside the cast, and bring the other end out over the cast edge ❶.
     - c. Press the petals firmly against the plaster, overlapping successive petals slightly ❷.
6. Provide skin care to all areas vulnerable to pressure.
   - Assess all areas at least every 4 hr and provide periodic care.
     - a. Reach under the cast edges as far as possible and massage the area.

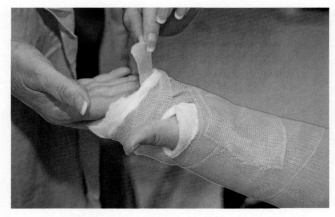

Source: Rick Brady/Pearson Education, Inc.

❶ Gently insert the strip under the cast and fold over the exposed edge.

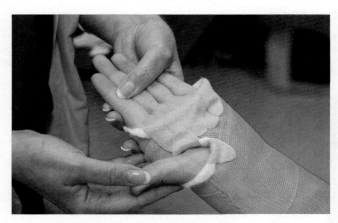

Source: Rick Brady/Pearson Education, Inc.

❷ Overlapping the strips ensures that there are no remaining exposed cast edges.

7. Keep the cast clean and dry. Cover it with a plastic bag during bathing or toileting.
8. Use pain-control measures as needed and reassess pain. Report immediately worsening pain or pain that is not controlled by prescribed medication.

PLASTER CAST

- Place a bib or towel over a body cast to catch spills. If a spill does wet the cast, allow the area to air-dry.
- Use a fracture bedpan for people with long leg, hip spica, or body casts. **Rationale:** *The flat end placed correctly under the patient's buttocks lessens the chance of spillage and minimizes the amount of lifting required by the patient and/or nurse.*
- Before placing the patient on the bedpan, tuck plastic or other waterproof material around the top of a long leg cast or around the perineal cutout. For a perineal cutout, funnel one end of the plastic into the bedpan.
- Remove the plastic when elimination is completed. **Rationale:** *If left in place, waterproof material makes the*

SKILL 9.17 Cast, Ongoing for Plaster and Synthetic: Caring for (continued)

cast edge airtight and prevents evaporation of perspiration, which is irritating to the skin.
- For people with long leg casts, keep the cast supported on pillows while the patient is on the bedpan. **Rationale:** *If the cast dangles, urine may run down the cast.*
- For patients with hip spica casts, support both extremities and the back on pillows so that they are as high as the buttocks. **Rationale:** *This prevents urine from running back into the cast.*
- When removing the bedpan, hold it securely while the patient is turning or lifting the buttocks. **Rationale:** *This prevents dripping and spilling.*
- After removing the bedpan, thoroughly clean and dry the perineal area.

SYNTHETIC CAST

- Wash the soiled area with warm water and a mild soap.
- Thoroughly rinse the soap from the cast.
- Dry thoroughly to prevent skin maceration and ulceration under the cast.
- If the cast is immersed in water, dry the cast and underlying padding and stockinette thoroughly. First, blot excess water from the cast with a towel. Then, use a handheld blow dryer on the cool or warm setting, directing the air stream in a sweeping motion over the exterior of the cast for about 1 hour or until the patient no longer feels a cold clammy sensation like that produced by a wet bathing suit. **Rationale:** *This drying procedure is essential to prevent skin maceration and ulceration.*

9. Turn and position the patient in correct alignment to prevent the formation of pressure areas.
   - Place pillows so that:
     a. Body parts press against the edges of the cast as little as possible.
     b. Toes, heels, elbows, and so on, are protected from pressure against the bed surface.
     c. Body alignment is maintained.
   - Plan and implement a turning schedule that will incorporate all of the possible positions (see Skill 9.12). Generally, patients can be placed in lateral, prone, and supine positions unless surgical procedures or any other factors contraindicate them. Attach a trapeze to the overhead frame to enable the patient to assist with moving. **Rationale:** *Repositioning prevents pressure areas.*
   - Turn people with large casts or those unable to turn themselves at least once every 4 hr. If the person is at risk for skin breakdown, turn every 1–3 hr as needed.
   - When turning the patient in a long leg cast to the unaffected side, place a pillow between the legs to support the cast.
   - Use at least three individuals to turn a person in a *damp* hip spica cast. When the cast is dry, the individual can usually turn with the assistance of one nurse. To turn a patient from the supine to prone position, follow these steps:
     a. Remove the support pillows only when an assistant is supporting the cast.
     b. Move the patient to one side of the bed.

c. Ask the patient to place the arms above the head or along the sides.
d. Have two assistants go to the other side of the bed while you remain to provide security for the person who is at the edge of the bed.
e. Place pillows along the bed surface to receive the cast when the patient turns.
f. Roll the patient toward the two assistants and onto the pillows.
g. Adjust the pillows as needed so that they provide proper support and comfort, and prevent pressure areas.

10. Encourage range-of-motion (ROM) and isometric exercises (see Skill 9.2).
    - Unless contraindicated, encourage active ROM exercises for all joints on the unaffected extremities, as well as on the joints proximal and distal to the cast. If active exercises are contraindicated, implement active–assistive or passive exercises, depending on the patient's abilities and disabilities. **Rationale:** *Exercise helps prevent joint stiffness, muscle atrophy, and venous stasis.*
    - Encourage the patient to move toes and/or fingers of the casted extremity as frequently as possible. **Rationale:** *Moving these extremities enhances peripheral circulation and decreases swelling and pain.*
    - Teach isometric (muscle-setting) exercises for extremities in a cast. **Rationale:** *Isometric exercise will minimize muscle atrophy in the affected limb.*
      a. Teach the isometric exercises on the patient's unaffected limb before the person applies it to the affected limb.
      b. Demonstrate muscle palpation while the patient is carrying out the exercise. **Rationale:** *Palpation enables the person to feel the changes that occur with muscle contraction and relaxation.*
    - Determine if the patient can be safely assisted out of bed. To protect both the nurse and the patient, ensure that sufficient caregivers and assistive equipment are available and properly used. Healthcare facilities should have a designated process for the use of "lift teams." Safe Patient Handling legislation in the United States has been introduced in many states. The most current bill at the federal level is the Nurse and Healthcare Worker Protection Act of 2015 (NIOSH, 2016). Some facilities have Safe Patient Handling programs, and others support the program but have not yet initiated it.

11. Provide patient teaching to promote self-care, comfort, and safety.
    - Teach people immobilized in bed with large body casts ways to turn and to move safely by using a trapeze, the side rails, and other such devices.
    - Instruct patients with leg casts about ways to walk effectively with crutches.
    - Instruct people with arm casts how to apply slings.
    - Teach patients how to safely resolve itching under the cast. Discourage the person from using long sharp objects to scratch under the cast. **Rationale:** *These*

(continued on next page)

SKILL 9.17 Cast, Ongoing for Plaster and Synthetic: Caring for (continued)

objects can break the skin and cause an infection, because bacteria flourish in the warm, dark, moist environment under the cast. Sticking objects under a cast can also cause folding or bunching of padding material and subsequent pressure and discomfort.

- When healing is complete and the cast is removed, the underlying skin is usually macerated, pale, flaky, and encrusted, since layers of dead skin have accumulated. Instruct patients to remove this debris gently and gradually:
  a. Apply oil (e.g., mineral, olive, or baby oil).
  b. Soak the skin in warm water and dry it.
  c. Caution the patient not to rub the area too vigorously. **Rationale:** *Vigorous rubbing can cause bleeding or excoriation of fragile skin.*

d. Repeat steps a and b for several days. **Rationale:** *Gradual removal of skin exudates reduces skin irritation.*

12. When the procedure is complete, perform hand hygiene and leave patient safe and comfortable.
13. Complete documentation using forms, checklists, or electronic dropdown lists supplemented by nurse's notes or additional comments as appropriate.

> **SAMPLE DOCUMENTATION**
>
> [date] 1000 Cast intact, leg elevated on 2 pillows. Toes warm to touch, pink, capillary refill 2 seconds. Moves toes readily and fully; states no numbness or tingling. Pain 0/10. *B. Snyder*

SKILL 9.18 Traction, Skin and Skeletal: Caring for

Skin traction uses ropes, pulleys, and weights to pull on a body part that has an injury with joint dislocation, bone fracture, chronic bone deformity, or muscle spasm to realign the area usually in preparation for surgical repair. Skeletal traction includes using pins, wires, or screws to stabilize and realign an injured or fractured bone during surgical repair.

Delegation or Assignment

Care of patients with stable traction may be delegated or assigned to the UAP. Assessment and pin site care with skeletal traction must be performed by the nurse. The status of the traction is observed during usual care and may be recorded by individuals other than the nurse. However, assessment of complications from the traction requires the expertise of a nurse. Abnormal findings detected by the UAP must be validated and interpreted by the nurse. Note that state laws for UAPs vary, so this task might be assigned to the UAP rather than delegated.

Equipment

- Over-the-bed trapeze bar if appropriate
- Pads

For Skin Traction Only
- Orthopedic traction apparatus, including traction straps, ropes, pulleys, and weights
- Elastic wrap

For Skeletal Traction Only
- Supplies for providing pin site care according to facility policy (e.g., normal saline, cotton-tipped swabs, gauze dressings, clean or sterile gloves)

Preparation

- Determine the following: bruises and abrasions in the area where the traction is to be applied, any history of circulatory

problems and skin allergies, mental and emotional status, and ability to understand activity restrictions.
- Check healthcare provider's order for type of traction, and inspect the traction apparatus regularly.
- Determine the degree of movement permitted and any special precautions (e.g., bed positions permitted).
- Gather equipment needed and review proper setup.
- Double check the weights to be certain they are the same as those ordered.

Procedure

1. Introduce self to patient (and parents) and verify the patient's identity using two identifiers. Explain to the patient (and parents) the type of traction and what it involves, why it is necessary, and how the patient can participate. Discuss how the results will be used in planning further care or treatments.
2. Perform hand hygiene and observe appropriate infection control procedures.
3. Provide for patient privacy.

SKIN TRACTION

4. Maintain the patient in the appropriate traction position.
   - Maintain the patient in the supine position unless there are other orders. **Rationale:** *Changing position can change the body alignment and the amount of force supplied by the traction.*
   - Maintain body alignment when turning the patient. In some cases, the person can turn to a lateral position if a pillow placed between the legs maintains body alignment. Refer to the patient's record for information about permitted movement.

(continued on next page)

SKILL 9.18 Traction, Skin and Skeletal: Caring for (continued)

- Provide a trapeze to assist the patient to move and lift the body for back care if the patient is unable to turn ❶.
- Provide a fracture bedpan as required to minimize the patient's movement during elimination.

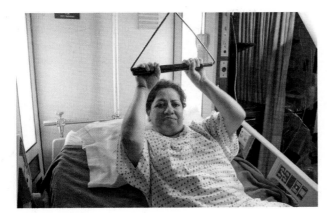

Source: Rick Brady/Pearson Education, Inc.

❶ A trapeze attached to an overhead frame facilitates patient mobility and nursing care. Patient uses both hands for repositioning to avoid twisting and back strain.

5. Assess the neurovascular status of the affected extremity every 30 min initially, and then every 1–2 hr for the first 24 hr. If the patient's status is stable, then assess every 4 hr during the traction. If the patient's status is not normal, continue assessments hourly. Include the following areas:
   - Proper position of traction
   - Proper body alignment ❷
   - Neurovascular status of the extremity
   - Skin condition under and around the traction application
   - Skin on prominences exposed to the surface of the bed
   - Vital signs
   - Pain and psychological status. **Rationale:** *Traction can lead to skin breakdown or neurovascular impairment. Infections can result, especially with internal traction. Children may be pulled out of correct alignment by traction and movement in bed and may require frequent repositioning.*

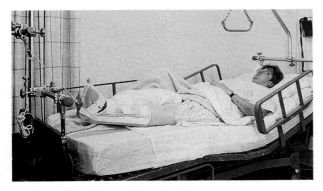

Source: Ronald May/Pearson Education, Inc.

❷ Ensure patient is positioned correctly in bed.

Patient Teaching

Preventing Problems Associated with Immobility

- Teach the patient deep-breathing and coughing exercises to prevent hypostatic pneumonia.
- Teach the patient appropriate exercises to maintain and develop muscle tone, prevent muscle contracture and atrophy, and promote blood circulation:
- Teach range-of-motion (ROM) exercises (discussed earlier in this chapter).
- Teach isometric exercises, like tightening the knees, to strengthen the quadriceps. Pushing the knees down without moving them also strengthens the hamstring muscles. Tensing the buttocks and the inner thighs promotes stabilization of the hips. Tensing the inner thighs also helps stabilize the knees.
- Circulation to the extremities can be promoted by encouraging the patient to flex and extend the feet and to perform the isometric exercises.
- Specific exercises to strengthen the biceps and triceps in preparation for using crutches can be taught as indicated. For example, raising the buttocks off the bed by pushing down with the arms develops the triceps, and pulling the body up with a trapeze develops the biceps.

6. Provide protective devices and measures to safeguard the skin.
   - Place heel protectors or sheepskins under the heels, sacrum, shoulders, and other pressure areas.
   - Change or clean the sheepskin lining at least weekly.
   - Massage the skin with rubbing alcohol or lotion every 4 hr, or if redness and signs of pressure appear, every 2 hr. **Rationale:** *Alcohol tends to toughen the skin and leave it less vulnerable to breakdown. Because alcohol is drying to the skin, however, lotion may be preferred for those who have dry skin (e.g., older adults).*
   - Make sure the spreader bar is wide enough to prevent the traction tape from rubbing on the patient's bony prominences.
7. Remove only intermittent nonadhesive skin traction in accordance with facility protocol or orders. To remove nonadhesive skin traction:
   - Remove the weights first.
   - Unwrap the bandage and provide skin care.
   - Rewrap the limb and slowly reattach the weights. Proceed to step 8 on page 431.

Safety Considerations

Perform a detailed follow-up examination based on findings that deviated from expected or normal for the patient. The patient should be able to demonstrate usual ROM in all unaffected body joints, move all fingers or toes of the affected extremity, feel normal sensation and have normal skin color and temperature in all fingers or toes of the affected extremity, and be free of pressure signs (pallor, redness, increased warmth or tenderness) over pressure areas. Relate findings to previous assessment data if available. Report significant deviations from normal to the healthcare provider.

(continued on next page)

SKILL 9.18 Traction, Skin and Skeletal: Caring for (continued)

CAUTION! Do not apply Buck traction over or under a calf compression device. Foot pumps (only around the foot) are acceptable for deep venous thrombosis prophylaxis.

or

SKELETAL TRACTION

4. Inspect the traction apparatus ❸:
   - Is the appropriate countertraction provided? For example, is the foot of the bed elevated 2.5 cm (1 in.) for every pound of traction, or is the knee of the bed flexed 20–30 degrees?
   - Are the correct weights applied? For example, Buck traction should have no more than 2.3 kg (5 lb).
   - Is there free play of the ropes on the pulleys; that is, does the groove of the pulley support the rope? Are the knots positioned no closer than 30 cm (12 in.) to the nearest pulley?
   - Do all weights hang freely and not rest against or on the bed or floor when the bed is in the lowest position?
   - Are the ropes intact—that is, not frayed, knotted, or kinked between their points of attachment?
   - Are the ropes securely attached with slipknots and the short ends of ropes attached with tape?
   - Is the line of the traction straight and in the same plane as the long axis of the bone?
   - Are bedclothes and other objects free from the traction?
   - Is the spreader bar wide enough to prevent the traction tape from rubbing on bony prominences?

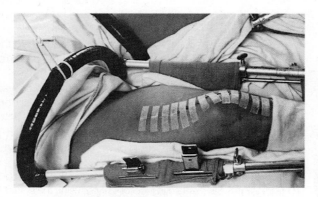

Source: Ronald May/Pearson Education, Inc.

❸ A Thomas splint is an example of skeletal traction of an extremity. It is used for balanced suspension with fracture of a femur.

5. Maintain the patient in the appropriate traction position. Check that the head, knee, and foot of the bed are properly elevated.
   - For patients with skull tongs or a halo ring, turn the patient as a unit. Do not allow the neck to twist. A special bed may be required.
   - If skull tongs or pins become dislodged, support the head, remove the weights, place sandbags or liter fluid bags on either side of the head to maintain alignment, and notify the healthcare provider immediately.

CAUTION! Skeletal traction is never released without a healthcare provider's order.

6. Assess the neurovascular status of the affected part ❹.
   - Conduct a neurovascular assessment every hour for the first 24 hr. If the patient's status is "normal," then assess every 4 hr during the traction. If the patient's status is not normal, continue assessments hourly.

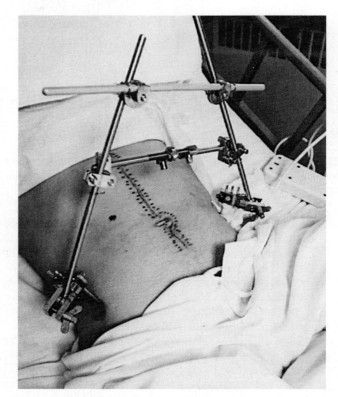

Source: Ronald May/Pearson Education, Inc.

❹ A Hoffman frame traction is an external fixator used for complex fractures, usually including extensive soft tissue, nerve, and vessel damage.

7. Provide pin site care daily ❺ if indicated by the healthcare provider's orders and facility protocol emphasizing reduction of the potential for infection.
   - Carefully inspect the site. Regular inspection of the pin site ensures early detection of minor infections, as manifested by signs of serosanguineous drainage, crusting, swelling, and erythema.
   - Use clean or sterile technique as facility protocol dictates. **Rationale:** *Sterile technique is most often used in the hospital setting, clean technique in the ambulatory setting.*
   - According to facility policy, remove crusts using normal saline or other agent such as diluted alcohol, povidone-iodine, or hydrogen peroxide recommended by the

SKILL 9.18 Traction, Skin and Skeletal: Caring for *(continued)*

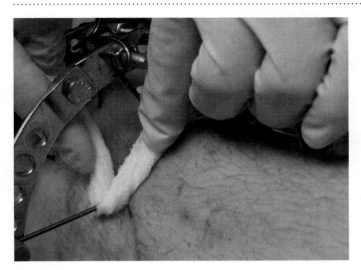

Source: Alex. Heinrich/doc-stock/Alamy Stock Photo

⑤ Pin site care for external fixation.

facility. Use a cotton-tipped swab with a gentle, rolling technique to reduce irritation to the tissue. **Rationale:** *Removing crusted secretions permits the pin site to drain freely. Initial crusts around pins do not create a problem and can serve as a barrier to infection, but accumulated crusts around external fixator pins may cause secondary infection.*

- If purulent (containing pus) drainage is present, notify the healthcare provider and obtain specimens for culture and sensitivity.
- Apply sterile ointment if ordered. Determine facility practices regarding pin site care; ointment could interfere with proper drainage.
- Loosely apply gauze dressing around pin site.
- Adjust frequency of care according to the amount of drainage. If no drainage is present, daily site care is adequate. If drainage is present, perform site care every 8 hr.
- Dispose of soiled equipment according to facility protocol.
- Remove and discard gloves. Perform hand hygiene.

8. When the procedure is complete, perform hand hygiene and leave patient safe and comfortable.
9. Provide teaching and evaluation of technique if the family will maintain traction at home.
10. Complete documentation using forms, checklists, or electronic dropdown lists supplemented by nurse's notes or additional comments as appropriate.

SAMPLE DOCUMENTATION

[date] 1230 Traction maintained at 9 kg (20 lb) with FOB ↑ 50 cm (20 in.). Skin intact and pink, sensation present, no pain. Pin sites clean and dry without sign of infection. No complaints at this time. *G. Merritt*

Lifespan Considerations
NEWBORNS, INFANTS, AND CHILDREN

- Bryant traction **⑥** is an adaptation of a bilateral Buck extension. It is used to stabilize fractured femurs or correct congenital hip dislocations in young children under 17.5 kg (35 lb). The skin traction is applied to both the affected and the unaffected leg to maintain the position of the affected leg. A spreader bar attached to the strips or positioning of the pulleys maintains leg alignment. Unless otherwise ordered, the hips are flexed at right angles (90 degrees) to the body with the knees extended, and the buttocks raised about 2.5 cm (1 in.). Pressure areas include skin over the tibia, malleoli, hamstring tendon, soles of feet, and upper back.

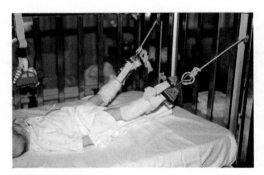

Source: Mediscan/Alamy Stock Photo

⑥ Bryant traction. Ensure that the sacrum is elevated sufficiently to allow the nurse to slip a hand between the child's buttocks and the bed.

OLDER ADULTS

- Adhesive skin traction should not be used due to the increased fragility of older adults' skin.
- Skin breakdown can occur more easily with any form of traction in older adults than in younger patients.

Patient Teaching

Traction at Home

- Patients who use electrical cervical traction or over-the-door mechanical systems need instructions about using the system several times a day for up to 30 min at a time. A physical therapist should establish the system and conduct initial patient and family teaching. The nurse can reinforce proper technique and assess effectiveness during home or clinic visits.
- Patients in halo-thoracic vest traction are ambulatory and need not be hospitalized. They, along with the family, need instructions regarding hygiene and care of the device, and when to contact the healthcare providers must be reinforced.
- Children are increasingly being treated with traction at home. The family needs instructions about how to set up and maintain the traction. They also need to be taught how to troubleshoot the traction and what to look for with the extremity involved. The nurse can evaluate the effectiveness of the traction during home or clinic visits.

Critical Thinking Options for Unexpected Outcomes

Not all unexpected outcomes require further nursing intervention; however, many times they do. When the patient demonstrates a change in signs/symptoms indicating an emerging problem, the nurse should immediately assess and troubleshoot what is happening. The assessment data must be processed quickly to formulate a hypothesis so the nurse can make a clinical judgment. The nurse then decides how best to resolve the problem and improve the patient's situation for a better outcome.

EXPECTED OUTCOME	UNEXPECTED OUTCOME	POSSIBLE INTERVENTIONS
Balance and Strength Correct body mechanics are utilized by caregiver.	Incorrect body mechanics are used while giving patient care.	▪ Identify areas of your body where you feel stress and strain. ▪ Evaluate the way you use body mechanics. ▪ Attend an in-service program on using body mechanics appropriately. ▪ Concentrate on how you are using your body when moving and turning patients. ▪ Position bed and equipment at a comfortable height and proximity to working area. ▪ Use your longest and strongest muscles to prevent injury.
Injuries are prevented to both the nurse and the patient.	Nurse injures self while giving patient care.	▪ Prevent future episodes of injury by increasing physical activity and exercises, changing ergonomics, and evaluating use of orthosis. ▪ Report any back strain immediately to supervisor. ▪ Complete unusual occurrence form. ▪ Go to health service or emergency department for evaluation and immediate care. ▪ Evaluate any activities that led to injury to determine incorrect use of body mechanics. ▪ Prevent additional injury by obtaining assistance when needed. ▪ Use devices such as turning sheets or assistive devices to assist in turning difficult patients.
Positioning a Patient Use of proper body mechanics facilitates patient care.	Nurse uses poor body mechanics and injures patient.	▪ Assess the extent of patient's injury. ▪ Notify patient's healthcare provider. ▪ Complete unusual occurrence form. ▪ Carry out healthcare provider's orders for follow-up treatment.
Moving and Transferring Mechanical equipment and devices are used in patient transfers and repositioning as needed.	Patient unable to assist with movement.	▪ Use a friction-reducing sheet to provide more support for patient. ▪ Obtain additional assistance to help with moving heavy weight.
	Patient afraid of using assistive device.	▪ Request healthcare provider's order for therapeutic mattress or dressings for pressure ulcer(s) care. ▪ Explain use of equipment (i.e., comfort and safety in transferring). ▪ Demonstrate equipment before using.
Patient is moved safely using appropriate device. Body alignment is maintained.	Patient unable to maintain any type of position without assistance.	▪ Use trochanter roll to prevent external rotation of patient's hip. ▪ Use foam bolsters to maintain side-lying positions. ▪ Use folded towels, blankets, or small pillows to position patient's hands and arms to prevent dependent edema.
Appropriate assistive devices are utilized to transfer patient.	Unable to transfer patient from bed to wheelchair due to excessive weight.	▪ Determine if wheelchair without arms or transfer board can aid in transfer. ▪ Contact supply services to obtain mechanical assist devices. ▪ Ask other staff if they can assist with transfer.
Injuries are prevented to both the nurse and the patient.	Injury occurs to patient when caregiver attempts transfer to wheelchair.	▪ Do not continue to reposition patient, place in bed. ▪ Complete sensory, motor, and pain assessment. ▪ Notify healthcare provider. ▪ Document findings.
Patient is able to progress through range-of-motion (ROM) exercises with minimal to no pain.	Patient experiences pain and discomfort during ROM exercises.	▪ Assess amount and type of pain and report findings to healthcare provider. ▪ Reevaluate your technique in assisting the patient performing the exercises. ▪ Start exercises with less stress on joints. Do exercises for a shorter period of time and gradually increase time and range of joint mobility.
Patient progresses from being dependent to becoming independent in ambulation.	Patient experiences vertigo or feels faint.	▪ If in the patient's room, help the patient return to the chair or bed. ▪ If in the hall, ease the patient down the wall to the floor. Do not attempt to hold the patient. ▪ Call for help.
Feelings of physical and mental well-being increase.	Patient is too weak to ambulate.	▪ Provide active and assistive ROM before attempting ambulation. ▪ Begin ambulation protocol as soon as possible using assistive device.

EXPECTED OUTCOME	UNEXPECTED OUTCOME	POSSIBLE INTERVENTIONS
Balance and muscle tone improve.	Patient is heavy or has poor balance.	■ Ask other nursing staff to help you ambulate the patient until able to walk independently. ■ If necessary, enlist the aid of a stronger assistant whose presence may give the patient additional psychological as well as physical support. ■ Gradually increase ambulation as muscle tone improves and balance improves. ■ Request assistance for ambulation from physical therapist. ■ Obtain walker to assist patient with ambulation. The walker will also provide reassurance to patient.
Assistive Devices Patient appropriately uses crutches to ambulate.	Patient fears falling while dependent on crutches.	■ Place safety or gait belt on patient until he/she feels confident. ■ Observe as the patient practices the procedures to make sure that the steps are being completed correctly for each gait. ■ Slow down crutch protocol until patient gains confidence at every level of mastery (e.g., four-point gait to two-point gait). ■ Remain with patient and give verbal reassurance and feedback for improvement.
	Patient not stable ambulating with crutches or cane.	■ Place safety belt on patient and ambulate with walker. ■ Increase both upper and lower muscle strength to increase ambulation with cane or crutches.
Patient uses assistive devices correctly without assistance.	Slipping occurs with crutch walking.	■ Check crutch tips to ensure they cover all metal or wood. ■ Observe the patient's stance or gait to determine if it is too broad. ■ Be sure that floor surface is dry and free of scatter rugs.
Crutches are measured correctly to prevent numbness or tingling in fingers.	Patient complains of numbness and tingling in fingers when crutch walking.	■ Remeasure distance between axilla and crutch bars to determine if two fingerbreadths can be inserted. ■ Observe patient's gait to determine if patient is leaning on crutch inappropriately.
Caregiver is able to manage turning, repositioning, and assistive devices.	Unable to lift patient up in bed with single healthcare worker.	■ If a second person is available, utilize him/her to assist in moving. ■ Use sliding board if two healthcare workers are available. ■ Use a hydraulic lift to assist with moving the patient up in bed or getting out of bed.
Assistive Devices Patient progresses from being dependent to becoming independent in ambulation.	Patient is not ambulating.	■ Discuss with caregiver and patient reasons why patient is not ambulating. ■ If patient is afraid of falling, ensure that a gait belt is worn and the patient uses a walker to start with and then moves to a cane, if possible. ■ Use two individuals to assist with walking, if available.
Traction and Cast Care Extremity is maintained in correct alignment.	Patient in skeletal traction keeps migrating to foot of bed.	■ Without releasing traction, use pull sheet and an assistant to reposition patient up in bed. Use a vest restraint if appropriate. ■ Elevate lower part of bed to provide countertraction. ■ Increase weight of countertraction at head of bed.
Neurovascular complications do not occur.	Patient experiences "tightness" in thigh after fracture of the femur.	■ Measure thigh circumference and compare with contralateral thigh. ■ Assess for presence of ecchymosis. ■ Monitor vital signs closely for hypovolemia (several units of blood may be sequestered in the thigh after fracture of the femur). ■ Notify healthcare provider for significant changes.
	Patient in Buck traction is unable to dorsiflex the foot.	■ Release proximal strap as it may be compressing peroneal nerve over head of fibula. ■ Assess sensation over dorsum of foot and between big and second toes. ■ Notify healthcare provider.
	Patient develops pain not relieved by analgesics, pain that worsens with extremity elevation and passive stretching of digits.	■ Maintain extremity in neutral position. ■ Notify orthopedic technician immediately; windowing or bivalving of cast may be indicated. ■ Suspect acute compartment syndrome and notify healthcare provider immediately to obtain measurement of compartment pressure. ■ Fasciotomy may be indicated if tissue swelling or external device compromises circulation within a muscle compartment.
Pin site remains free of infection.	Halo pin site appears to be infected.	■ Notify healthcare provider. ■ Obtain culture of drainage for antibiotic sensitivity studies. ■ Cleanse pin site as prescribed, using aseptic technique and separate applicator for each site. ■ Remove crusts to allow drainage. ■ Monitor for systemic signs of infection.

(continued on next page)

EXPECTED OUTCOME	UNEXPECTED OUTCOME	POSSIBLE INTERVENTIONS
Cast integrity is maintained to provide adequate site immobilization.	Cast cracks from improper drying or stress.	■ Notify healthcare provider immediately. ■ Reassure patient. ■ Do not reposition patient until healthcare provider assesses.
	Cast edges begin to crumble.	■ "Petal" edges of cast with 1- to 2-in. strips of tape. ■ Place half of tape inside cast, pull tape over cast, and anchor on outside of cast. ■ Continue to petal cast until all edges are covered.
Patient experiences minimal swelling.	Fingers swell after application of arm cast.	■ Assess that there is room for two fingers to be slipped under cast. ■ Apply ice alongside of cast and maintain elevation after cast application. ■ Maintain arm positioning with hand higher than elbow. ■ Encourage patient to exercise fingers to help reduce edema. ■ Monitor neurovascular status frequently.

REVIEW Questions

1. The nurse has instructed the spouse of a client recovering from Guillain-Barré on range of motion exercises to perform at home. Which observation indicates that additional teaching is required?
   1. Supported the knee to rotate the ankle
   2. Supported the arm above and below the elbow
   3. Started at the head by flexing the neck forward
   4. Rolled the foot and leg inward and then outward

2. A client becomes dizzy while ambulating with a nurse for the first time after surgery and starts to fall forward. Which action should the nurse take first?
   1. Widen his or her own stance
   2. Pull up on the client's arm
   3. Tighten the grip on the gait belt
   4. Have the client look down at the floor

3. The nurse observes the UAP logroll a client. For which action should the nurse intervene?
   1. Client's arms crossed over the chest
   2. Two pillows placed between the client's legs
   3. Pillow placed to support the client's head after the turn
   4. Client's upper body moved, followed by the lower body

4. A client needs to be moved up in bed. What should the nurse do once a draw sheet is placed under the client?
   1. Lower the head of the bed
   2. Raise the height of the bed
   3. Place a pillow against the head of the bed
   4. Grasp the draw sheet at the shoulders and hips

5. A client with a left lower leg wound needs to be transferred to a wheelchair. In which position should the nurse place this device?
   1. Facing the bed
   2. Parallel to the bed on client's right side
   3. On the left side of the client
   4. At a 45-degree angle to the bed

6. A client who was placed in the prone position is located near the left side rail. What should the nurse do to ensure proper positioning of this client?
   1. Reverse the turn and start over.
   2. Place pillows against the left raised side rail.
   3. Slide the client toward the center of the bed.
   4. Move the body in segments toward the center of the bed.

7. The nurse is ambulating a client who is using a newly prescribed cane. What should the nurse instruct the client to do after moving the cane forward?
   1. Move the weak leg ahead of the cane
   2. Move the strong leg ahead of the cane
   3. Move the weak leg to the level of the cane
   4. Move the strong leg to the level of the cane

8. The nurse observes a client use crutches to walk down a set of stairs. Which action indicates that the nurse needs to review the process for safety?
   1. Flexes elbows at a 30-degree angle
   2. Supports body weight by hands on the hand bars
   3. Assumes the tripod position at the top of the stairs
   4. Moves crutches and unaffected leg to the lower step

9. A client with right leg weakness is prescribed to use a walker. Which direction should the nurse provide when instructing on the use of this device?
   1. Move the walker ahead of the right foot
   2. Move the right foot and walker together
   3. Move the right foot up to the walker first
   4. Move the left foot and the walker together

10. Two hours after the application of a fiberglass cast, the client complains of severe pain. What should the nurse do first?
    1. Apply ice to the limb
    2. Provide pain medication
    3. Notify the healthcare provider
    4. Elevate the limb on two pillows

11. When a client's long leg cast is removed, the skin under it is macerated and crusted. Which action should the nurse take to cleanse this client's leg?
    1. Apply oil and soak the leg in warm water
    2. Scrub the leg with soap and a soft washcloth
    3. Brush off the crusted skin with a dry washcloth
    4. Apply antibiotic ointment to open areas and cover with gauze

12. Two pins on a client's external fixator device have purulent drainage. What action should the nurse take first?
    1. Cleanse with peroxide
    2. Apply sterile ointment
    3. Notify the healthcare provider
    4. Obtain a specimen for culture and sensitivity

Note: For answers and rationales for the review questions, go to Appendix A or your Pearson MyLab Nursing and eText.

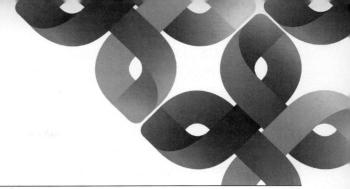

Chapter 10
Nutrition

Chapter at a Glance

Healthy Eating Habits

SKILL 10.1 **Body Mass Index (BMI):** Assessing
SKILL 10.2 **Diet, Therapeutic:** Managing
SKILL 10.3 **Eating Assistance:** Providing
SKILL 10.4 **Mealtime:** Complementary Health Approaches
SKILL 10.5 **Nutrition:** Assessing

Enteral Nutrition Using a Feeding Tube

SKILL 10.6 **Feeding, Continuous, Nasointestinal/ Jejunostomy with a Small-Bore Tube:** Administering ❶
SKILL 10.7 **Feeding, Gastrostomy or Jejunostomy Tube:** Administering ❶

SKILL 10.8 **Gastric Lavage:** Performing ❶
SKILL 10.9 **Nasogastric Tube:** Feeding
SKILL 10.10 **Nasogastric Tube:** Flushing and Maintaining
SKILL 10.11 **Nasogastric Tube:** Inserting ❶
SKILL 10.12 **Nasogastric Tube:** Removing

Parenteral Nutrition Using Intravenous Infusion

SKILL 10.13 **Lipids, IV Infusion:** Providing ❶
SKILL 10.14 **Total Parental Nutrition (TPN), IV Infusion:** Providing ❶

❶ Nursing students may observe or assist with the following skills only with faculty permission and while under direct supervision of faculty or another RN.

≫ The Concept of Nutrition

Nutrition is the process of taking in foods and beverages for nutrients. The body needs six types of nutrients: proteins, water, vitamins, minerals, carbohydrates, and lipids. These nutrients are broken down in the digestive system to molecules small enough for the body to absorb. Then they are transported to cells for further metabolic chemical reactions to make energy, regulate body functions, and build and maintain body cells. The body needs all of these nutrients to maintain a state of wellness. Too much or too little of any of the nutrients can affect body functions. Patients whose digestive tract can function but who cannot eat enough to meet nutritional needs and patients who are seriously ill or undernourished may need to receive enteral tube nutrition, or tube feeding. Patients who are not able to eat foods and drink water, have severe malabsorption disorders, or have a digestive tract that does not function may receive partial or complete parenteral nutrition, or intravenous feeding. Nursing care for patients receiving enteral tube feedings and parenteral nutrition includes management of the process and monitoring for complications and patient response.

Learning Outcomes

10.1 Differentiate nutritional requirements between the newborn, infant, child, adult, and older adult.

10.2 Give examples of four dietary data categories of eating patterns when taking a nutritional assessment.

10.3 Explain how eating habits developed as children can influence eating habits as adults.

10.4 Summarize five safety considerations when assisting a patient with dysphagia to eat.

10.5 Differentiate between the various methods used to determine appropriate nasogastric tube placement.

10.6 Differentiate between using an open system for administering tube feedings and using a closed system.

10.7 Support the reasoning of using sterile technique when administering total parenteral nutrition.

10.8 Give examples of safety considerations when infusing intravenous lipids.

The following feature links some, but not all, of the concepts related to assessment. They are presented in alphabetical order.

Concepts Related to
Nutrition

CONCEPT	RELATIONSHIP TO NUTRITION	NURSING IMPLICATIONS
Digestion	It functions to breakdown food into molecules for absorption to meet body needs.	■ Provide food consistency for individual patient to help absorption. ■ Ensure adequate fluid intake. ■ Provide adequate variety of nutrients in diet.
Elimination	Appropriate fluid intake and fiber helps prevent constipation.	■ Maintains fluid balance in body. ■ Fiber provides bulk in bowels which aids natural fecal evacuation.
Fluids and Electrolytes	Fluid intake and fluid output need to be balanced for homeostasis.	■ Adequate fluid intake from beverages and high water-content foods help to maintain fluid balance.
Infection	A healthy immune system helps prevent infections.	■ Encourage a variety of nutrients in diet for vitamins, minerals, amino acids, and essential fatty acids.
Tissue Integrity	A diet rich in protein is needed to support wound healing.	■ Encourage protein in patient's diet to aid in wound healing.

≫ Healthy Eating Habits

Expected Outcomes

1. Patient maintains body mass index appropriate for age, size, and activity.
2. Patient's nutritional needs are met with a balanced diet appropriate for developmental age.
3. Patient experiences no complications while eating.
4. Patient with dysphagia maintains appropriate body weight.
5. Patient demonstrates understanding (verbalized knowledge) of dietary information provided.

SKILL 10.1 Body Mass Index (BMI): Assessing

The body mass index (BMI) uses a formula of kilograms per square meter (kg/m^2) to assess nutritional status and total body weight relative to height. Beginning at age 2 years, the BMI can be easily determined after plotting the length/height and weight on the standardized growth curves. Tracking changes in BMI can provide clues to nutritional problems, including obesity, health promotion issues, or illness.

Delegation or Assignment

Due to specific knowledge and skill in determining a BMI, this skill is not delegated or assigned to the UAP. The nurse remains responsible for the assessment, interpretation of abnormal finds, and determination of appropriate actions.

Equipment

■ Weigh scale appropriate for age
■ Tape measure, measuring board, or height-measuring device appropriate for age

Preparation

■ Review healthcare provider's orders and patient's nursing plan of care.
■ Gather equipment and supplies.

Procedure

1. Introduce self to patient (and parents) and verify the patient's identity using two identifiers. Explain to the patient (and parents) that you are going to weigh the patient and measure the patient's height (or length) to determine the patient's BMI, and how the patient can participate. Discuss how the results will be used in planning further care or treatments.
2. Perform hand hygiene and observe appropriate infection control procedures.
3. Provide for patient privacy and safety.
4. Weigh the patient and measure patient's height, or length (also see Skill 1.2 and Skill 1.4). Use a BMI table to determine patient's BMI (**Table 10–1 ≫**).
5. Compare patient's BMI to standard growth chart appropriate for age and size of patient.
6. To calculate BMI manually, the formula is kg/m^2. Follow these steps:
   ● Weight is converted to kilograms. If the weight is in pounds, divide that number by 2.2 to get kilograms (2.2 pounds = 1 kilogram).
   For example, if the weight is 154 pounds, 154 ÷ 2.2 = 70 kilograms

SKILL 10.1 Body Mass Index (BMI): Assessing *(continued)*

TABLE 10–1 Body Mass Index (BMI) Table

	Normal						Overweight						Obese				
BMI	19	20	21	22	23	24	25	26	27	28	29	30	31	32	33	34	35
Height (in.)								Weight (in pounds)									
4′10″ (58″)	91	96	100	105	110	115	119	124	129	134	138	143	148	153	158	162	167
4′11″ (59″)	94	99	104	109	114	119	124	128	133	138	143	148	153	158	163	168	173
5′ (60″)	97	102	107	112	118	123	128	133	138	143	148	153	158	163	168	174	179
5′1″ (61″)	100	106	111	116	122	127	132	137	143	148	153	158	164	169	174	180	185
5′2″ (62″)	104	109	115	120	126	131	136	142	147	153	158	164	169	175	180	186	191
5′3″ (63″)	107	113	118	124	130	135	141	146	152	158	163	169	175	180	186	191	197
5′4″ (64″)	110	116	122	128	134	140	145	151	157	163	169	174	180	186	192	197	204
5′5″ (65″)	114	120	126	132	138	144	150	156	162	168	174	180	186	192	198	204	210
5′6″ (66″)	118	124	130	136	142	148	155	161	167	173	179	186	192	198	204	210	216
5′7″ (67″)	121	127	134	140	146	153	159	166	172	178	185	191	198	204	211	217	223
5′8″ (68″)	125	131	138	144	151	158	164	171	177	184	190	197	203	210	216	223	230
5′9″ (69″)	128	135	142	149	155	162	169	176	182	189	196	203	209	216	223	230	236
5′10″ (70″)	132	139	146	153	160	167	174	181	188	195	202	209	216	222	229	236	243
5′11″ (71″)	136	143	150	157	165	172	179	186	193	200	208	215	222	229	236	243	250
6′ (72″)	140	147	154	162	169	177	184	191	199	206	213	221	228	235	242	250	258
6′1″ (73″)	144	151	159	166	174	182	189	197	204	212	219	227	235	242	250	257	265
6′2″ (74″)	148	155	163	171	179	186	194	202	210	218	225	233	241	249	256	264	272
6′3″ (75″)	152	160	168	176	184	192	200	208	216	224	232	240	248	256	264	272	279

Source: Data from National Heart, Lung, and Blood Institute (NHLBI). (1998). *Clinical guidelines on the identification, evaluation, and treatment of overweight and obesity in adults: The evidence report.* Bethesda, MD: Author.

- Height needs to be in meters. If the height is in inches, multiply that number by 0.0254 to get meters (1 in. = 0.0254 m).
  For example, if the height is 56 inches (4 ft. 8 in.), 56 × 0.0254 = 1.4224 meters
- Square the number of meters. Multiply the number of meters by itself.
  For example, if the height measures 1.4224 meters, $1.4224 \times 1.4224 = 2.0232$ meters^2
- Calculate the BMI for kilograms. Divide kilograms of weight by height in meters squared.
  For example, if the weight is 70 kilograms and the patient is 1.4224 meters tall, the meters squared is 2.0232, so: 70 kg ÷ 2.0232 (meters^2) = 34.5986, rounded to a BMI of 35.

- Calculate the BMI for pounds. If the patient weighs 154 pounds and is 4 ft. 8 in. tall, using the math above:

  154 pounds = 70 kilograms, 4 ft. 8 in. = 56 inches, which = 1.4224 meters; meters^2 = 2.0232, so: 70 ÷ 2.0232 (meters^2) = 34.5986, rounded to a BMI of 35.

7. When the procedure is complete, perform hand hygiene and leave patient safe and comfortable.
8. Document the BMI using forms, checklists, or electronic dropdown lists supplemented by nurse's notes or additional comments as appropriate.

SKILL 10.2 Diet, Therapeutic: Managing

Alterations in a patient's diet are often needed to treat a disease process such as diabetes mellitus, to prepare for a special examination or surgery, to increase or decrease weight, to restore nutritional deficits, or to allow an organ to rest and promote healing. It is a skill to know how to live on a special diet. Diets can be modified in texture, kilocalories, specific nutrients, seasonings, or consistency.

(continued on next page)

SKILL 10.2 Diet, Therapeutic: Managing (*continued*)

TABLE 10–2 Lifestyle and Behavioral Modification Strategies to Help Maintain Common Therapeutic Diets

Therapeutic Diet	Modification Strategies
Bland diet	■ Have frequent, small feedings during active stress periods. ■ Avoid foods that are fatty, fried, spicy, raw, or difficult to chew. ■ Include cottage cheese, carrots, peas, ripe bananas, cream of wheat, lean meat, chicken, eggs, creamy peanut butter, and broth soup.
Blenderized liquid diet	■ Use blender to bring food and liquid to a liquid form (used in addition to standard enteral feeding formula at home by many patients). ■ Liquefy whole foods in blender with juice, broth, milk, or water.
Mechanical soft diet	■ Uses foods that have smooth consistency and can be easily digested (if trouble with chewing and swallowing). Allows variations in taste that are not allowed on a soft diet but are a pureed consistency. ■ Include all liquids, yogurt, eggs, soft cooked vegetables, mashed potatoes, bananas, applesauce, white rice, pasta, cake, and sauces.
Postoperative diet progression	■ *Clear liquid diet:* 1000–1500 mL/day of liquid foods such as water, tea, broth, gelatin, and pulp-free juices or clear carbonated beverages. ■ *Full liquid diet:* Includes any food that is liquid at room temperature—clear liquids, milk and milk products, custards, puddings, creamed soups, sherbet, ice cream, and any fruit juice. ■ *Soft diet:* Includes items in a full liquid diet plus pureed vegetables, eggs (not fried), milk, cheese, fish, fowl, tender beef, veal, potatoes, and cooked fruit. Include foods that are easy to chew and digest and low in fiber; do not include gas-forming foods. ■ *Regular diet:* Take into consideration food tolerances and preferences.
Providing consistent carbohydrate diet	■ Refined or simple sugars are limited. ■ Counting grams of carbohydrates and using the glycemic index (describes how much blood glucose level rises with a specific food when compared with an equivalent amount of glucose) are nutritional tools for managing diabetes. ■ Equal (consistent) amount of carbohydrate is provided at each meal to ease management of blood sugars. ■ Eat a mixture of protein, carbohydrates, and fat. ■ Restricted foods are simple carbohydrates; for example, juices, white sugar, and white flour. Teach patient to read food labels.
Pureed diet	■ Mash, mince, or grind foods. ■ Do not mix all pureed food together or feed out of one bowl or dish. Try to keep foods separate and eat alternately, with dessert last.
Restricting dietary fat	■ Restrict total fat to less than 30% of calories, restrict saturated fat to 7% of calories, and reduce cholesterol to 200 mg/day. ■ Higher percentage may be allowed if saturated and trans fats are replaced with monounsaturated fats found primarily in plant products (olive oil, canola oil, avocados, pecans, almonds); use low-fat or nonfat products; increase intake of fruits and vegetables, whole grains, legumes, and seeds. ■ Limit high-cholesterol foods found in animal products, such as egg yolk, red meat, shellfish, organ meats, bacon, and pork. ■ Avoid such foods as gravies, fatty meat and fish, cream, fried foods, rich pastries, whole-milk products, cream soups, salad and cooking oils, nuts, and chocolate.
Restricting dietary protein	■ Decrease protein allowance to 0.5–0.6 g/kg/day (predialysis). ■ Limit high-protein foods, such as eggs, meat, milk, and milk products.
Restricting mineral nutrients (sodium, potassium)	1. *Low sodium (LS) diet:* ■ Restrict salt in cooking and eliminate adding salt to food at the table. ■ Avoid salty foods like bacon, ham, pizza, bread with salted tops, crackers, canned meat, cold cuts, processed cheese, olives, pickled vegetables, vegetable juices, canned soup, soy sauce, and bottled salad dressings. ■ Choose low-sodium foods such as eggs, fresh beef or poultry, milk, rice, pasta, corn, noodles, fresh potatoes, mayonnaise, and dried fruit. ■ Be aware of sodium content of some medications (e.g., antacids). 2. *No added sodium (NAS) diet:* ■ Avoid processed foods, eat fresh fruits and vegetables, drink coffee and tea, check for added salt in proteins, eat salt-free nuts, check dairy products for sodium levels, and dried grains.
Providing nutrient-enhanced diets	1. *High-iron diet:* ■ Include foods high in iron content, such as meats (especially organ meats), egg yolks, seafood (especially shellfish), and plant-based sources such as whole-wheat products, leafy vegetables, nuts, dried fruit, and legumes. ■ Vitamin C enhances absorption of plant-based iron. 2. *High-calcium diet:* ■ Increase normal adult intake of 1 g/day to 1.5 g/day for postmenopausal female. ■ Use *fortified* low-fat and nonfat dairy products, fruit juices, and oatmeal. ■ If lactose intolerant, use leafy green vegetables and non-liquid dairy products (cheese, yogurt) or lactose-free dairy products, fish products, and almonds. ■ Vitamin D promotes calcium absorption.

SKILL 10.2 Diet, Therapeutic: Managing (*continued*)

Delegation or Assignment

Teaching a patient how to manage a therapeutic diet is not delegated or assigned to the UAP. The nurse instructs the UAP to report patient observations to the nurse for follow-up. Assessment and evaluation of effectiveness of the exercise remain the responsibility of the nurse.

Equipment

No equipment is required for this skill.

Preparation

- Review healthcare provider's orders and patient's nursing plan of care.
- Gather written information about the patient's therapeutic diet to give to the patient.

Procedure

1. Introduce self to patient and verify the patient's identity using two identifiers. Explain to the patient you are going to discuss eating modifications, why they are necessary, and how the patient can participate. Discuss how the results will be used in planning further care or treatments.
2. Perform hand hygiene and observe appropriate infection control procedures.
3. Provide for patient privacy. **Rationale:** *A quiet environment will allow greater focus.*
4. Assess what the patient knows about the healthcare provider's prescribed diet for the patient. Keep a low-key, professional tone when discussing the need for dietary changes. **Rationale:** *The thought of changing eating habits may be difficult for patients.*
5. Engage the patient in developing eating modifications related to the new diet regimen (**Table 10–2 》**). Help the patient identify lifestyle and behavioral changes that will be needed. **Rationale:** *Lifestyle and behavioral changes require full involvement on the patient's part. The nurse helps prepare the patient to take the initiative and assume responsibility for the patient's own health.*
6. Offer to have the dietician stop by to explain how to read food labels and further discuss the patient's therapeutic diet.
7. When the discussion is complete, perform hand hygiene and leave the patient safe and comfortable.
8. Complete documentation using forms, checklists, or electronic dropdown lists supplemented by nurse's notes or additional comments as appropriate, including type of diet, patient or family teaching provided, nutritional consult requested, tolerance of diet progression, and community facility referral offered.

SAMPLE DOCUMENTATION

[date] 1020 Discussion with patient about new therapeutic bland diet. Expressed interest in more information he could share with his family. Written guidelines given to patient and reviewed. Stated he would like me to ask the dietician to stop by and talk with him more about his new eating habits. Actively participated in discussion without incident. *R. Meadows*

Patient Teaching

Healthy Eating on a Therapeutic Diet

- Discuss importance of properly fitted dentures and dental care.
- Discuss safe food preparation and preservation techniques as appropriate.
- Discuss the purpose of the diet.
- Discuss allowed and excluded foods.
- Explain the importance of reading food labels when selecting packaged foods.
- Include family or significant others in the discussions.
- Reinforce information provided by the dietitian or nutritionist as appropriate.
- Discuss herbs and spices as alternatives to salt and substitutes for sugar.
- Discuss physiological, psychological, and lifestyle factors that predispose to weight changes.
- Discuss ways to adapt eating practices by using smaller plates, taking smaller servings, chewing each bite a specified number of times, and putting fork down between bites.
- Discuss ways to control the desire to eat by taking a walk, drinking a glass of water, or doing slow deep-breathing exercises.
- Discuss stress reduction techniques.
- Provide information about available community resources (e.g., weight-loss groups, Meals-on-Wheels, dietary counseling, exercise programs, self-help groups).
- Discuss factors contributing to inadequate nutrition and weight changes.
- Discuss ways to manage, minimize, or alter the factors contributing to malnourishment.

Teaching Parents Dietary Management

For Newborns and Infants

- Encourage parents to provide only breast milk or formula until the newborn or infant reaches the age of 6 months. **Rationale:** *Breast milk provides all of a newborn's or infant's needs and is associated with some benefits (reduced incidence of allergies, diarrhea) and some protection (transmission of mother's immunities).*

(*continued on next page*)

SKILL 10.2 Diet, Therapeutic: Managing (*continued*)

- Give feedings when the newborn or infant cries for food, not by the clock.
- Introduce one food at a time, starting with foods with low allergy potential, such as rice cereal.
- Do not lay the newborn or infant down to sleep with a bottle. **Rationale:** *Any liquid other than water can cause tooth decay, even in erupting teeth.*

For Toddlers

- Teach parents about potential for choking and about what foods to avoid.
- Offer a variety of finger foods from all food groups but do not be concerned about quantity. Provide small portions. **Rationale:** *Toddlers may have a very low intake due to slower growth during this period.*
- Make foods available at meal and snack times only. Do not force food intake. **Rationale:** *This helps to prevent tantrums related to eating times.*
- Encourage involvement in snack preparation. **Rationale:** *Even at an early age, children can begin to learn about good nutrition.*
- Do not use food as a bribe.

For School-Age Children

- Teach parents that habits formed in early years will affect their children for life. It is important to give them information about good food choices and to help them participate in healthy practices such as school breakfast and lunch programs.
- Provide nutritious foods following the federal government's MyPlate nutrition guide. Provide small portions.
- Recognize children's likes and dislikes. Do not force children to eat foods they dislike, but do not limit family intake to their limited choices.

For Teens

- Recognize the importance of peer pressure.
- Encourage teens planning a party or gathering to find healthful choices that will appeal to their age group.
- Engage teens in making decisions about meal planning.
- Help overweight teens think of rewards other than food and provide positive reinforcement that is not food (e.g., a movie, a manicure).
- Provide healthful foods and avoid criticism during mealtimes.

SKILL 10.3 Eating Assistance: Providing

Patients may need assistance in preparing and consuming foods and liquids on their meal trays. This is an opportunity to observe the patient's ability to self-feed and note any difficulties with chewing and swallowing.

Delegation or Assignment

Assisting or feeding a patient is often delegated or assigned to the UAP. It is, however, the responsibility of the nurse to assess the patient's ability to eat and to identify actual or potential risk factors that may affect the patient's nutritional status. The nurse must instruct the UAP about strategies that promote the patient's nutritional health as well as the importance of the UAP reporting any unusual or different patient behaviors to the nurse. Note that state laws for UAPs vary, so this task might be assigned to the UAP rather than delegated.

Equipment

- Meal tray with the correct food and fluids
- Extra napkin or small towel
- Straw, special drinking cup, weighted glass, or other adaptive feeding aid as required

Just for the Patient with Dysphagia

- Penlight to inspect oral cavity
- Oral suction catheter connected to suction source

Preparation

- Review healthcare provider's orders and patient's nursing plan of care.
- Assist the patient to the bathroom or onto a bedpan or commode if the patient needs to urinate.

- Offer the patient assistance in washing the hands prior to a meal. If the patient has problems with oral hygiene, brushing the teeth or using a mouthwash can improve the taste in the mouth and hence the appetite.
- Clear and clean the overbed table so that there is space for the tray.

Just for the Patient with Dysphagia

- Pay attention to specific instructions for feeding technique (diet and positioning) prescribed by speech or swallowing specialist; for example, use cornstarch, food starch, or rice cereal to modify consistency or thicken beverages and pureed foods, as prescribed. **Rationale:** *Patients with swallowing problems find it easier to swallow thickened liquids.*
- Check if patient is receiving both oral and enteral feeding; stop the enteral solution about 1 hour before oral feeding.
- Check that patient has not recently received sedating medication.
- Eliminate environmental distractors such as television, radio.
- Provide a 30-minute rest period before mealtime.
- Ensure that temperature of food is appropriate.

Procedure

1. Prior to feeding the patient, introduce self and verify the patient's identity using two identifiers. Explain to the patient what you are going to do, why it is necessary, and how the patient can participate.
2. Perform hand hygiene and observe other appropriate infection control procedures.
3. Provide for patient privacy if appropriate.

SKILL 10.3 Eating Assistance: Providing (*continued*)

ASSISTING EATING

4. Position the patient and yourself appropriately.
   - Assist the patient to a comfortable position for eating. Most people sit during a meal; if it is permitted, assist the patient to sit in bed ❶ or in a chair.
   - If the patient is unable to sit, assist the patient to a lateral position. **Rationale:** *It is easier to swallow in a lateral position than in a back-lying position.*
   - If the patient requires assistance with feeding, assume a sitting position, if possible, beside the patient.

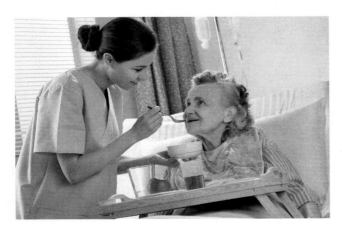

Source: Alexander Raths/Shutterstock

❶ A supported sitting position contributes to a patient's comfort while eating.

5. Assist the patient as required.
   - Check tray for the patient's name, the type of diet, and completeness. If the diet does not seem to be correct, check it against the patient's chart. Do *not* leave an incorrect diet for a patient to eat.
   - Encourage the patient to eat independently, assisting as needed.
   - Remove the food covers, butter the bread, pour the drink, and cut the meat, if needed.
   - For a patient with a visual impairment, identify the placement of the food as you would describe the time on a clock. For instance, say "The potatoes are at 8 o'clock, the chicken at 12 o'clock, and the green beans at 4 o'clock" ❷.
6. If the patient needs assistance with feeding:
   - Ask in which order the patient desires to eat the food.
   - Use normal utensils whenever possible.
   - If the patient has a visual impairment, tell which food you are giving.
   - Warn the patient if the food is hot or cold.
   - Allow ample time for the patient to chew and swallow the food before offering more.
   - Provide fluids as requested or, if the patient is unable to ask, offer fluids after every three or four mouthfuls of solid food.
   - Use a straw or special drinking cup for fluids that would spill from normal containers.

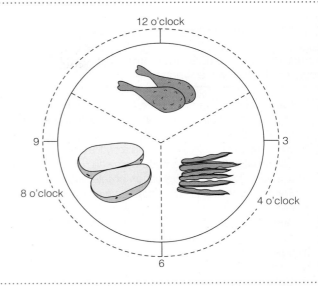

❷ For a patient with a visual impairment, the nurse can use the clock system to describe the location of food on the plate.

   - Make the time a pleasant one, choosing topics of conversation that are of interest to the patient, if the individual wants to talk. Proceed to step 7.

or

PATIENT WITH DYSPHAGIA

4. Maintain bed in LOW position.
5. Preparing for the patient to eat
   - Assist patient to sit upright (90 degrees) in a chair or in bed with hips flexed, shoulders and face slightly forward, and chin parallel to the floor or slightly tucked. **Rationale:** *Gravity assists proper bolus movement to the stomach.*
   - Be aware that prescribed position is different for specific forms of dysphagia. Some types of dysphagia require patient positioning to one side, with head rotated toward the stronger or weaker side, or even side-lying. Instructions should be placed in patient's record and care plan and posted at patient's head of bed.
   - Place towel over patient's chest.
   - Place tray on overbed table and towel under plate. **Rationale:** *This stabilizes plate while feeding.*
   - Suction oral secretions before feeding, if necessary.
   - Sit at patient's side.
6. When patient is eating,
   - Encourage self-feeding.
   - Instruct patient to take (or offer) small portions of food at first (0.5–1 tsp at a time), bites manageable in size but large enough to require chewing.
   - Instruct patient to eat food first, without accompanying liquid, reserving all liquid intake until after finishing food (although some authorities recommend alternating solids with liquids).
   - Instruct patient to perform an exaggerated sucking motion at the beginning of each swallow with chin tucked slightly.

(*continued on next page*)

SKILL 10.3 Eating Assistance: Providing (*continued*)

CAUTION! The use of a straw increases risk of aspiration because the patient with dysphagia has less control over the amount of fluid intake. Similarly, the patient with dysphagia should not be fed with a syringe.

- Patients with advanced dementia may not remember how to chew or swallow. Demonstrating chewing and gently stroking the area under the patient's chin with a downward motion during swallowing may be helpful cues.
- Allow patient to concentrate on swallowing without distractions such as conversation or television. **Rationale:** *For the patient with dysphagia, swallowing takes concentration; talking increases risk for aspiration.*
- Avoid rushed or forced feeding and make sure patient is swallowing every mouthful.
- Visually inspect oral cavity and under dentures for retained food.
- Observe patient closely for evidence of aspiration (e.g., cough, drooling, voice change such as hoarseness or a gurgling noise after swallowing), and suction oropharynx if indicated.
- Maintain patient in a sitting position for 30 minutes after eating.

7. After the meal, ensure patient is comfortable and safe.
   - Assist the patient to clean the mouth and hands.
   - Reposition the patient.
   - Remove the food tray from the bedside.

8. Complete documentation using forms, checklists, or electronic dropdown lists supplemented by nurse's notes or additional comments as appropriate, including the amount of fluid intake and the percent of the meal consumed, any pain, fatigue, or nausea experienced, or if the patient is not eating.

SAMPLE DOCUMENTATION

[date] 1235 Sitting in chair, ate 90% of lunch, PO intake 245 mL. No difficulty or distress noted. States he is ready to get back in bed to rest now. *G. Knowles*

Lifespan Considerations
OLDER ADULTS

- Offer fluids frequently to prevent dry mouth.
- Allow more time to eat.
- Observe for dysphagia and adapt the older patient's diet accordingly.
- Evaluate problems that can interfere with eating such as ill-fitting dentures, sore gums, constipation, diarrhea, or a special diet.
- Encourage the patient to remain independent when possible.

SKILL 10.4 Mealtime: Complementary Health Approaches

Complementary health approaches can be combined with conventional medicine to help patients maintain or improve their level of health and wellness through nutrition including food choices, herbal and dietary supplements, vitamins, and minerals.

Delegation or Assignment

Teaching a patient about complementary health approaches for mealtime is not delegated or assigned to the UAP. The nurse is responsible for assessing the patient's willingness to participate in complementary relaxation behaviors in addition to the medical treatments. The nurse teaches the patient about the techniques of relaxation at mealtime and complementary approaches that support nutrition. The nurse instructs the UAP to report patient observations to the nurse for follow-up. Assessment and evaluation of effectiveness of the exercise remain the responsibility of the nurse.

Equipment

- No equipment is required for this skill.

Preparation

- Allow 10–15 min of uninterrupted time for the discussion. Ensure that the environment is private, quiet, comfortable,

and at a temperature that suits the patient. The patient should have an empty bladder. **Rationale:** *Interruptions or distractions interfere with the patient's ability to achieve full relaxation.*

Procedure

1. Introduce self to patient (and parents) and verify the patient's identity using two identifiers. Explain to the patient (and parents) what you are going to do, why it is necessary, and how the patient can participate. Discuss how the results will be used in planning further care or treatments. Explain the rationale and benefits of complementary health approaches. Ask the patient about nutritional goals. This type of therapy can provide relaxation and feelings of empowerment, lead to creative problem solving, and facilitate healing. Carefully explain to the patient that when deciding to try natural and herbal supplements, it is important to remember that the supplements can have side effects and drug or food interactions. Emphasize the need for the healthcare provider to know what supplements are being taken.
2. Perform hand hygiene and observe appropriate infection control procedures.
3. Provide for patient privacy.

SKILL 10.4 Mealtime: Complementary Health Approaches (continued)

4. Assess usual mealtime patterns.
   - Ask the patient to describe what mealtime is like, noise level, eating in a hurry or while doing something else.
   - Encourage the patient to name specific elements of a relaxed eating experience.
   - Ask if the patient consumes a healthy diet that provides essential nutrients.
5. Provide patients with the following techniques for increasing relaxation at mealtime:
   - Brush your teeth before mealtime. This improves the ability to taste.
   - Sit for a moment before eating, closing your eyes and taking two or three relaxed breaths.
   - Focus on the process of eating.
   - Eat healthful, familiar food that you like.
   - Take small portions and eat them slowly, putting the fork down between bites.
   - Avoid unpleasant or uncomfortable activities immediately before or after a meal.
   - Eat in a clutter-free, clean environment that is free of unpleasant sights and odors.
   - Reduce psychological stress. Do not eat while discussing difficult topics or arguing.
   - Build awareness of stress signs, anger, anxiety, eating disorders, fatigue, and restlessness.
   - Avoid consuming stressors such as caffeine, alcohol, sugar, junk foods, and food products with preservatives. A diet of high-stress foods can result in hypertension,

high cholesterol, unstable blood sugar levels, and a rapid, bounding pulse rate.
6. Complementary health approaches
   - Herbal remedies
   - Aromatherapy
   - Acupuncture
   - Yoga or tai chi
   - Deep breathing, progressive muscle relaxation, or mediation (see Skill 3.3).
   - Eating small, well-balanced meals throughout the day keeps energy up and stabilizes mood.
7. When the session is complete, perform hand hygiene and leave the patient safe and comfortable.
8. Complete documentation using forms, checklists, or electronic dropdown lists supplemented by nurse's notes or additional comments as appropriate.

SAMPLE DOCUMENTATION

[date] 1845 States willingness to learn more about complementary health approaches to help her reduce stressful eating behaviors. Actively participated in discussion. Looking forward to trying the relaxation techniques at mealtime. Tolerated without incident. *B. Prime*

SKILL 10.5 Nutrition: Assessing

Doing a nutritional assessment includes objective and subjective data about the patient's nutrient and food consumption, acute and chronic medical history, medications, herbs and supplements history, and lifestyle. This data can assist in evaluating the patient's nutritional status.

Delegation or Assignment

Due to specific knowledge and skill in nutritional assessment, this skill is not delegated or assigned to the UAP. The nurse remains responsible for the assessment, interpretation of abnormal findings, and determination of appropriate actions.

Equipment

No equipment is required for this skill.

Preparation

- Review healthcare provider's orders and patient's nursing plan of care.
- Review patient's record for allergies.

EVIDENCE-BASED PRACTICE

Assessment of Older Adults for Malnutrition

The Mini-Nutritional Assessment (MNA) is an assessment tool that helps identify older adults who are malnourished or at risk for

malnutrition. This tool has been modified and shortened over the years but has not lost its validity or accuracy. Currently, the MNA consists of six questions to screen older adults so there is a faster response for intervention. These questions address eating patterns and changes in them such as decreased appetite, recent weight changes, activity level, cognitive memory or emotional concerns, and body mass index (BMI).

Source: Data from Nestlé Nutrition Institute. (2016). *MNA mini nutritional assessment.* Retrieved from http://www.mna-elderly.com/default.html

---

Procedure

1. Introduce self to patient (and parents) and verify the patient's identity using two identifiers. Explain to the patient (and parents) that you are going to do a nutritional assessment, why it is necessary, and how the patient can participate. Discuss how the results will be used in planning further care or treatments.
2. Perform hand hygiene and observe appropriate infection control procedures.
3. Provide for patient privacy.
4. Initial screening is performed on hospital admission and includes:
   - Changes in body weight of less than or equal to 4.5 kg (10 lb) in the last 6 months
   - Nausea, vomiting, diarrhea lasting more than 5 days

(continued on next page)

SKILL 10.5 Nutrition: Assessing (continued)

- Declining food intake, difficulty chewing/swallowing, and time/duration of recent hospitalizations. If results of this initial screening classify the patient at "nutrition risk," a dietitian consult is indicated.

5. Further nutritional data such as types of food eaten, how often specific foods are eaten, portion sizes, and number of servings of food categories consumed daily can be collected with a dietary questionnaire. Specific questions about food allergies, food intolerances, foods avoided, cultural food preferences, and information about constipation, gas, vomiting, or frequency of heartburn can be included.

6. Objective and subjective measurements of nutritional status can be obtained as listed in **Table 10–3 ≫**.
   - Weight in relation to height (body mass index)
   - Food log data of nutrient intake and calorie counts
   - Laboratory tests: serum albumin, transferrin, and prealbumin; tests of cellular immunity; and total lymphocyte count

TABLE 10–3 Nutritional Assessment Parameters

Clinical Assessment	Normal	Abnormal
Dietary Data		
Appetite	Remains unchanged	Increased or decreased recently
		Particular cravings
Nutritional intake	Adequate foods and fluids to supply body nutrients	Elimination of certain food categories that results in limited nutrients
	Nonallergic response to major food groups	Emphasis on some food groups (sugar) to the exclusion of others (vegetables)
		Allergic response to certain foods
Caloric intake	Average 28 kcal/kg/day	Constant use of fad diets to lose weight
		Use of drugs or chemicals that interfere with appetite or nutrient assimilation
Meal patterns	3–6 home-prepared meals/day	Fast-food or packaged foods
	Adequate time and calm atmosphere for meals	Missed meals, constant snacking, or overeating
		Eating "on the run" or hurried
General Appearance		
Global observations	Alert, responsive, healthy-appearing eyes and skin	Listless, dull, nonresponsive
		Skin and eyes appear unhealthy
Physical factors	Adequate chewing and swallowing capability	Teeth or gums in poor condition or ill-fitting dentures
	Mouth and gums healthy so food can be ingested	Swallowing impairs ingestion
	Physical exercise adequate for calorie intake	Inadequate physical exercise to burn calories
Presence of disease	No disease process that interferes with nutrient assimilation	Disease present that interferes with ingestion, digestion, assimilation, or excretion
	No congenital condition or postsurgery condition that interferes with nutrient assimilation	Congenital condition, rehabilitation phase, or postsurgery that interferes with food assimilation
Elimination schedule	Regular, adequate elimination of foods	Irregular or painful elimination
	Absence of constant flatus, discharge, or mucus	Presence of constant flatus
		Presence of discharge, blood, or mucus
Anthropometric Measurements		
Height (see Skill 1.2)	For bedridden patients, measure arm span—fully extend arms to a 90-degree angle to body and measure from tip of one middle finger to the tip of other middle finger for estimated height.	Loss of 5–8 cm (2–3 in.) in height may indicate osteoporosis.
Weight—compared to ideal and usual body weight (see Skill 1.4)	Ideal body weight	Changed—markedly increased or decreased recently: important indicator of changed nutritional status
	45 kg (100 lb) (female); 48 kg (106 lb) (male) for 1.524 m (5 feet) height + 2.2 kg (5 lb) for each 1 in. over 1.524 m (5 feet) (female) and 3 kg (6 lb) for each 0.0254 m (1 in) over 5 feet (male); small frame minus 10%; large frame plus 10%	Loss of more than 10% weight for prior 6 months should be clinically evaluated.
Body mass index ratio of weight in kilograms and height in meters (see Skill 10.1)	18.5–24.9	Less than 18.5—underweight
		25–29—overweight
		30–39—obese
Triceps skinfold thickness measurement (use skinfold calipers with mm)	Standard values—male to female 12.5–16.5	If values change over months, may indicate a chronic condition.
Circumference of upper arm (use tape measure with cm)	29.3–28.5	
Midarm muscle circumference (use tape measure with cm)	25.3–23.2	Hydration status may influence results.

SKILL 10.5 Nutrition: Assessing (*continued*)

TABLE 10–3 Nutritional Assessment Parameters (*continued*)

Clinical Assessment	Normal	Abnormal
Biochemical Assessments*		
Serum albumin	3.5–5.0 g/dL	Examples of possible disease conditions: Decrease signifies lowered nutritional status—protein deficient
Serum transferrin binds iron to plasma and transports to bone marrow.	200–430 mg/dL	Reduced levels may indicate chronic diseases and protein deficiency. Elevated levels—anemias, liver damage, lead toxicity
Hemoglobin	Male—13.5–17 g/dL Female—12–15 g/dL	Decreased related to iron deficiency (anemias and leukemia)
Prealbumin (PA) serum	20–50 mg/dL	Decreased—protein wasting diseases, malnutrition (10.7 indicates severe nutritional deficiency) Elevated—Hodgkin's disease
Blood urea nitrogen: creatinine ratio	10:1–20:1	Reflects nitrogen imbalance and inadequate renal functioning; increased ratio noted with congestive heart failure, decreased ratio with impaired renal perfusion
24-hr urinary nitrogen	Positive balance	Inadequate protein intake
Sociocultural Data		
Cultural–religious factors	Ability to afford adequate foods in all food categories Cultural beliefs that do not eliminate whole food groups Religious beliefs that do not eliminate whole food groups	Economic position that precludes purchase of adequate food Religious or cultural beliefs that interfere with receiving balanced diet (macrobiotic diets) Inadequate knowledge, experience, or intelligence to prepare healthy meals
Ethnicity	Traditional foods that do not eliminate whole food groups	Beliefs and ethnic preference that eliminate major nutrients from the diet
Lifestyle	Well-balanced meals that include all nutrients Food does not lose all nutrient value in preparation	Fast-paced stressful lifestyle that incorporates fast food or convenience foods deficient in nutrients or imbalanced (high-fat)

*Laboratory test parameters differ among laboratories. Check the reference range for the specific lab where the patient's blood or urine was tested.

- Evaluation of body composition by anthropometric measurements (triceps skinfold, midarm muscle circumference).
7. When assessment is complete, perform hand hygiene, and leave patient safe and comfortable.
8. Complete documentation using forms, checklists, or electronic dropdown lists supplemented by nurse's notes or additional comments as appropriate.

SAMPLE DOCUMENTATION

[date] 0740 Nutrition history obtained including current food likes and dislikes. Weight 57.3 kg (126 lb), height 5 ft 5 in, BMI 21. Denies change in body weight in past 6 months. Denies change in dietary habits past 6 months, food allergies, or foods she doesn't like to eat. States bowel and bladder habits routine without nausea, vomiting, or constipation. Friendly and talkative. Tolerated assessment without incident. *R. Beaker*

Patient Teaching

About Nutrition

Children

- Reinforce to parents that children learn lifelong good and bad eating habits from them.
- Reinforce to parents that eating can become a source of conflict if they try to tell the child what and how much to eat, or if the child tries to tell the parent what foods should be eaten.
- Children's access to "junk food" should be limited, but completely forbidding a food may also create conflict.

Older Adults

- Reinforce they should not change their diet significantly without consulting their healthcare provider because drug dosage may have been based on the older adult's previous dietary intake.

(*continued on next page*)

SKILL 10.5 Nutrition: Assessing (*continued*)

- Ensure they know some medications increase appetite, such as glucocorticoids, and some medications decrease appetite by their actions or by causing an unpleasant taste.
- Ensure they know certain tablets should not be crushed to be given by mouth or by gastric tubes, such as enteric-coated or slow-release medications.
- Use community resources to help buy food if economically necessary for the older adult, especially if a prescribed diet requires expensive supplements.
- Ensure caregivers know conditions such as neuromuscular disorders and dementia can make it difficult for older adults to eat or to be fed. Safety should always be a priority concern with

attention paid to prevent aspiration. All healthcare personnel and family caregivers should be taught proper techniques to reduce this risk. Effective techniques include:

- Use the chin-tuck method when feeding patients with dysphagia. Having patients flex the head toward the chest when swallowing will decrease the risk of aspiration into the lungs.
- Use foods of prescribed consistency. Many older adults can more easily swallow foods with thicker consistency than thin liquids.
- Try to provide food preferences. The family can help provide this information.

≫ Enteral Nutrition Using a Feeding Tube

Alternative feeding methods to ensure adequate nutrition include enteral (through the gastrointestinal system) methods. **Enteral nutrition** is provided when the patient is unable to ingest foods or the upper gastrointestinal tract is impaired but the remainder of the intestinal tract is functional. Enteral feedings are administered through nasogastric and small-bore feeding tubes or through gastrostomy or jejunostomy tubes.

Expected Outcomes

1. Patient's nutritional needs are met with nasogastric feeding.
2. Patient's nutritional needs are met with continuous enteral feeding.
3. Gastrostomy tube site is free of signs of irritation/inflammation.
4. Patient experiences no complications with nasogastric feeding.

SKILL 10.6 Feeding, Continuous, Nasointestinal/Jejunostomy with a Small-Bore Tube: Administering

Safety Note! *During scheduled clinical time, nursing students may have a learning opportunity to observe or assist with this skill only with faculty permission and with direct supervision from faculty or another RN.*

A nasointestinal tube is inserted into the naris, passing through the nasopharynx, esophagus, stomach, and enters the intestines. A feeding jejunostomy tube is inserted through the abdomen and into the jejunum, a section of the small bowel, for instilling nutritional solutions to provide the patient nutrition. Small bore tubes are more comfortable but become clogged more often than large bore tubes.

Delegation or Assignment

Due to the need for sterile technique and technical complexity, the maintaining and monitoring of nasointestinal or jejunostomy tubes or nutritional solutions are not delegated or assigned to the UAP. The UAP may care for patients with these feeding tubes. The nurse must ensure that the UAP knows what complications or adverse signs should be reported to the nurse.

Equipment

- Prescribed formula in closed container (ready-to-infuse system preferred; note expiration date)
- Antimicrobial swabs
- Formula reservoir or bag if necessary for open system (date and replace daily)
- Container of ready-to-use sterile formula (cover, label for patient, refrigerate unused portion, and discard in 48 hours) or closed system formula ❶
- Administration tubing compatible with pump (replace daily)
- Infusion pump (not to exceed 40 psi)
- Label or pen
- 60-mL sterile syringe
- Sterile normal saline solution or warm water
- Clean gloves

Preparation

- Review healthcare provider's orders for feeding formula type and rate of administration. Review patient's nursing plan of care.
- Check x-ray report for tube placement.

SKILL 10.6 Feeding, Continuous, Nasointestinal/Jejunostomy with a Small-Bore Tube: Administering (*continued*)

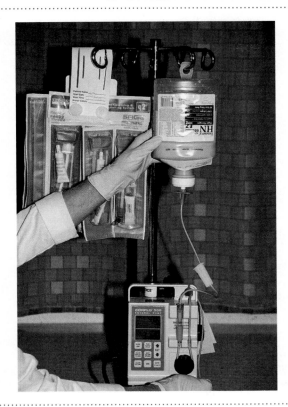

❶ Closed system formula can hang to 48 hr if sterile technique is used.

- Gather equipment.
- Don clean gloves if indicated.

Procedure

1. Introduce self to patient and verify the patient's identity using two identifiers. Explain to the patient what you are going to do, why it is necessary, and how the patient can participate. Discuss how the results will be used in planning further care or treatments.
2. Perform hand hygiene and observe appropriate infection control procedures.
3. Provide for patient privacy.
4. Check length of exposed tubing. **Rationale:** *An increase in length may indicate tube tip has dislocated upward, from duodenum to stomach, or from stomach into the esophagus.*
5. If using reservoir or bag for continuous intestinal feeding, rinse bag with sterile water, and fill with enough formula to limit hang time. Do not allow the feeding solution to hang longer than 4 to 8 hours. Check facility policy or manufacturer's recommendations regarding time limits.
   Note: Bring unused formula to room temperature before use. **Rationale:** *This reduces the risk of infection, because the advancement of the tube to intestine places it in a less protected (alkaline) environment.*

Safety Considerations

- If patient is receiving continuous feeding, maintain head of bed (HOB) elevation at 30–45 degrees at all times. Turn off feeding 1 hour before patient must be repositioned at less than 30-degree elevation for any procedure or transport.
- Transition from nutrition support to oral feeding requires careful monitoring. Enteral tubes or parenteral access should not be removed until the patient has tolerated oral nutrition for 2–3 days or as healthcare provider orders.
- Enteral nutrition via nasointestinal or orointestinal infusion should be withheld if the patient is hypotensive (mean arterial pressure [MAP] less than 60 mmHg), especially if receiving catecholamine agents to maintain hemodynamic stability. Signs of intolerance may indicate gut ischemia.

6. Disinfect ports with antiseptic swab before and after handling.
7. Connect administration tubing to formula reservoir (container or bag) and prime tubing per manufacturer's instructions.
8. Thread tubing through pump per manufacturer's instructions ❷.
9. Note mark on patient's feeding tube to determine if migration has occurred.

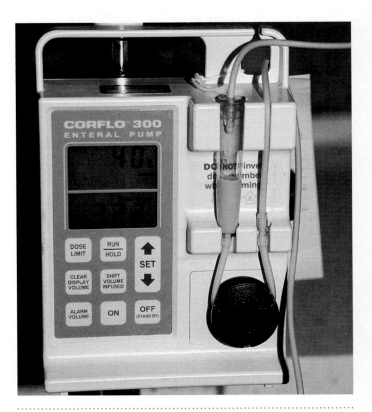

❷ Thread tubing through pump per manufacturer's instructions. Pump pressure must not exceed 40 psi.

(*continued on next page*)

SKILL 10.6 Feeding, Continuous, Nasointestinal/Jejunostomy with a Small-Bore Tube: Administering (*continued*)

10. Connect primed formula tubing to patient's small-bore feeding tube. Initiate feeding with isotonic (300 mOsm) or slightly hypotonic formula. **Rationale:** *This prevents dumping syndrome (cramping and diarrhea).*
Note: Alternate method is to connect formula tubing to patient's surgically established jejunostomy feeding tube ❸.

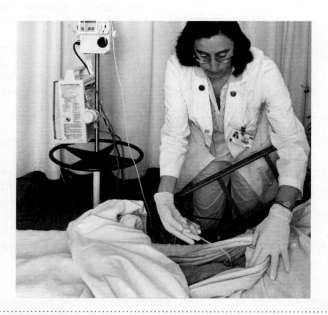

❸ Connect continuous feeding system to patient's surgically placed jejunostomy tube.

11. Start feeding at slow constant infusion rate (25–50 mL/hr). **Rationale:** *Slow increase in feeding volume is better tolerated. (Maximum rate is 100–150 mL/hr.)*
12. If patient tolerates feeding, increase rate in 8–24 hours (increase by 25–50 mL/hr to prescribed rate).
13. Keep patient's HOB elevated at 30–45 degrees, or maintain patient with obesity in reverse Trendelenburg position ❹. **Rationale:** *This lowers intra-abdominal pressure and reduces the risk of aspiration.*
14. Prep side port with antimicrobial swab and, using 60-mL syringe, flush small-bore continuous feeding tube every 4 hours; flush before and after medication administration with 15 mL sterile water or saline ❺. **Rationale:** *This prevents tube clogging.*
15. Check residual volume regularly. **Rationale:** *Small-bore feeding tube residuals are usually less than 10 mL. Residuals as much as 50 mL may indicate upward displacement from the bowel into the stomach.*
16. When the procedure is complete, perform hand hygiene and leave patient safe and comfortable.
17. Complete documentation using forms, checklists, or electronic dropdown lists supplemented by nurse's notes or additional comments as appropriate, including:
    * External length of exposed tubing
    * Methods of validating tube placement

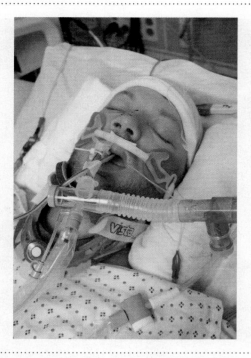

❹ Maintain head-of-bed (HOB) elevation at 30–45 degrees to reduce risk of aspiration in patients receiving continuous enteral feeding.

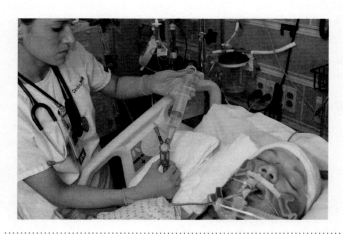

❺ Use 60-mL syringe to flush feeding tube with 15 mL sterile water or saline every 4 hr, and before and after medication administration. Do not use tap water.

* Quantity and character of aspirated residuals (color, pH, other tests)
* Amount and type of formula administered
* HOB elevation during and following feeding

Additional daily documentation includes:

* Frequency of tube irrigation and irrigant used
* Abdominal assessment findings (distention, nausea, vomiting, flatus, bowel movement)
* Bowel elimination pattern and characteristics

SKILL 10.6 Feeding, Continuous, Nasointestinal/Jejunostomy with a Small-Bore Tube: Administering (*continued*)

- Daily weight
- Intake and output
- Tube site assessment and dressing application
- Oral hygiene provided

SAMPLE DOCUMENTATION

[date] 0800 Awake and alert. Exposed tube marking remains same. 1 kcal/mL nutritional formula continues at 75 mL/hr via feeding pump. Jejunostomy tube insertion site remains without redness or tenderness. Dressing dry and intact. Remains in Fowler's position. Denies abdominal cramping or discomfort at this time. No complaints verbalized. *P. Mapps*

Safety Considerations

- Many devices, both enteral and parenteral are the color purple. However, while enteral connectors are now being made purple so the nurse will note that this is not an IV device color, two manufacturers use purple for peripherally inserted central (PIC) catheters. Thus, the risk for enteral misconnection may actually be increased.

- Patients who are obese cannot efficiently mobilize fat stores. Instead, they use protein as a primary source of energy, have marked loss of muscle and lean body mass, and become nutrient depleted when critically ill. In these and other protein-deficient patients, nutrient support can cause refeeding syndrome. This adverse response is characterized by volume overload, heart failure, pulmonary edema, glucose intolerance, excess carbon dioxide production (a by-product of glucose metabolism), increased respiratory work, and respiratory failure.

SKILL 10.7 Feeding, Gastrostomy or Jejunostomy Tube: Administering

Safety Note! *During scheduled clinical time, nursing students may have a learning opportunity to observe or assist with this skill only with faculty permission and with direct supervision from faculty or another RN.*

Enteral feedings can provide nutritional solutions directly into the stomach or jejunum. This is especially helpful for patients who are not able to orally consume enough nutrients daily for physical reasons, such as chronic neuromuscular disorders, mechanical dysphagia, stomach dysfunction, and chronic malnutrition.

Delegation or Assignment

Administering feedings through a gastrostomy or jejunostomy tube is not delegated or assigned to the UAP. Some agencies, however, may allow a trained UAP to administer a feeding. In this case, it is the responsibility of the nurse to assess tube placement and determine that the tube is patent. The nurse should reinforce major points, such as making sure the patient is sitting upright, and instruct the UAP to report any difficulty administering the feeding or any complaints voiced by the patient. Abnormal findings must be validated and interpreted by the nurse.

Equipment

- Correct amount of feeding solution
- Graduated container and tubing with clamp to hold the feeding
- 60-mL catheter-tip syringe

For a Tube that Remains in Place

- Mild soap and water
- Clean gloves
- Petrolatum, zinc oxide ointment, or other skin protectant
- Precut 4 × 4 gauze squares
- Uncut 4 × 4 gauze squares

For Tube Insertion

- Clean gloves
- Moisture-proof bag
- Water-soluble lubricant
- Feeding tube (if needed)

Preparation

- Before starting a gastrostomy or jejunostomy feeding, determine the type and amount of feeding to be instilled, frequency of feedings, and any pertinent information about previous feedings (e.g., the positioning in which the patient best tolerates the feeding).
- Review healthcare provider's orders for type and amount of feeding, review patient's nursing plan of care.
- Gather needed equipment and supplies.

Procedure

1. Introduce self and verify the patient's identity using two identifiers. Explain to the patient what you are going to do, why it is necessary, and how the patient can participate ❶. Inform the patient that the feeding should not cause any discomfort but may cause a feeling of fullness.

(continued on next page)

SKILL 10.7 Feeding, Gastrostomy or Jejunostomy Tube: Administering (*continued*)

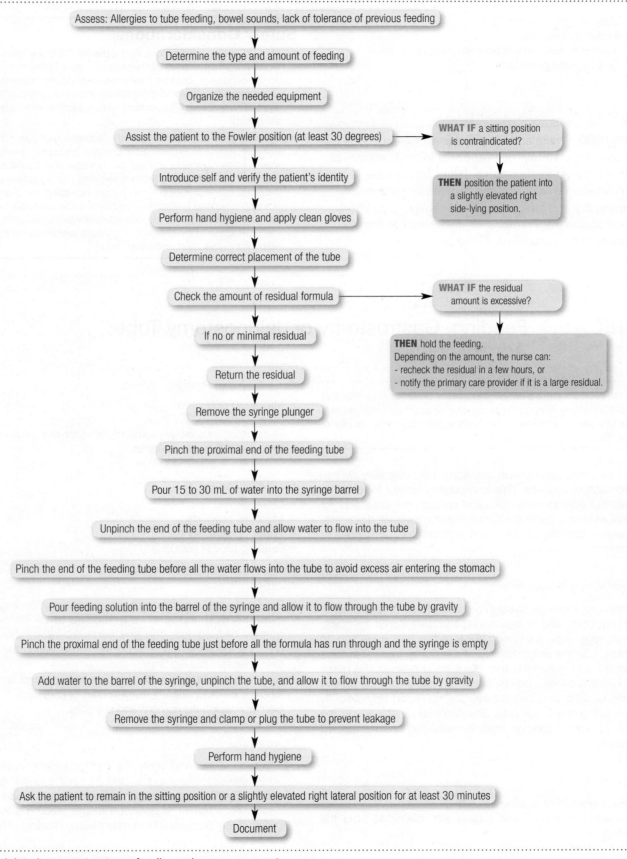

Assess: Allergies to tube feeding, bowel sounds, lack of tolerance of previous feeding

Determine the type and amount of feeding

Organize the needed equipment

Assist the patient to the Fowler position (at least 30 degrees)

WHAT IF a sitting position is contraindicated?

THEN position the patient into a slightly elevated right side-lying position.

Introduce self and verify the patient's identity

Perform hand hygiene and apply clean gloves

Determine correct placement of the tube

Check the amount of residual formula

WHAT IF the residual amount is excessive?

THEN hold the feeding.
Depending on the amount, the nurse can:
- recheck the residual in a few hours, or
- notify the primary care provider if it is a large residual.

If no or minimal residual

Return the residual

Remove the syringe plunger

Pinch the proximal end of the feeding tube

Pour 15 to 30 mL of water into the syringe barrel

Unpinch the end of the feeding tube and allow water to flow into the tube

Pinch the end of the feeding tube before all the water flows into the tube to avoid excess air entering the stomach

Pour feeding solution into the barrel of the syringe and allow it to flow through the tube by gravity

Pinch the proximal end of the feeding tube just before all the formula has run through and the syringe is empty

Add water to the barrel of the syringe, unpinch the tube, and allow it to flow through the tube by gravity

Remove the syringe and clamp or plug the tube to prevent leakage

Perform hand hygiene

Ask the patient to remain in the sitting position or a slightly elevated right lateral position for at least 30 minutes

Document

❶ Administering a gastrostomy feeding using an open system.

SKILL 10.7 Feeding, Gastrostomy or Jejunostomy Tube: Administering (*continued*)

2. Perform hand hygiene and observe other appropriate infection control procedures.
3. Provide for patient privacy. Don gloves. Raise bed to appropriate height for the procedure.
4. Assist the patient to a Fowler position (at least 30 degrees elevation) in bed or a sitting position in a chair, the normal position for eating. If a sitting position is contraindicated, a slightly elevated right-side-lying position is acceptable. **Rationale:** *These positions enhance the gravitational flow of the solution and prevent aspiration of fluid into the lungs.*
5. Insert a feeding tube, if one is not already in place.
   - Remove the dressing. Then discard the dressing and gloves in the moisture-proof bag. Perform hand hygiene.
   - Apply new clean gloves.
   - Lubricate the end of the tube, and insert it into the ostomy opening 10–15 cm (4–6 in.).
6. Check the location and patency of a tube that is already in place.
   - Determine correct placement of the tube by aspirating secretions and checking the pH of the return. Follow facility policy if the pH is 6 or higher.
   - If the tube is placed in the stomach, aspirate all contents and measure the amount before administering the feeding. **Rationale:** *This is done to evaluate absorption of the last feeding; that is, whether undigested formula from a previous feeding remains. If the tube is in the small intestine, residual contents cannot be aspirated.*
   - Follow facility policy for amount of residual formula. This may include withholding the feeding, rechecking in 3–4 hr, or notifying the healthcare provider if a large residual remains.
   - Reinstill the gastric contents into the stomach if this is the facility policy or healthcare provider's order. **Rationale:** *Removal of the contents could disturb the patient's electrolyte balance.*
   - For continuous feedings, check the residual every 4–6 hr and hold feedings according to facility policy.
   - Remove the syringe plunger. Pour 15–30 mL of water into the syringe, remove the tube clamp, and allow the water to flow into the tube. **Rationale:** *This determines the patency of the tube. If water flows freely, the tube is patent.*
   - If the water does not flow freely, notify the nurse in charge and/or healthcare provider.
7. Administer the feeding.
   - Check the expiration date of the feeding.
   - Warm the feeding to room temperature. **Rationale:** *An excessively cold feeding may cause abdominal cramps.*

- Hold the barrel of the syringe 7–15 cm (3–6 in.) above the ostomy opening.
- Slowly pour the solution into the syringe and allow it to flow through the tube by gravity.
- Just before all of the formula has run through and the syringe is empty, add 30 mL of water. **Rationale:** *Water flushes the tube and preserves its patency.*
- If the tube is to remain in place, hold it upright, remove the syringe, and then clamp or plug the tube to prevent leakage.

8. Ensure patient comfort and safety.
   - After the feeding, ask the patient to remain in the sitting position or a slightly elevated right lateral position for at least 30 minutes. **Rationale:** *This minimizes the risk of aspiration.*
   - Assess status of peristomal skin. **Rationale:** *Gastric or jejunal drainage contains digestive enzymes that can irritate the skin.* Document any redness and broken skin areas.
   - Check orders about cleaning the peristomal skin, applying a skin protectant, and applying appropriate dressings. Generally, the peristomal skin is washed with mild soap and water at least once daily. The tube may be rotated between thumb and forefinger to release any sticking and promote tract formation. Petrolatum, zinc oxide ointment, or other skin protectant may be applied around the stoma, and precut 4 × 4 gauze squares may be placed around the tube. The precut squares are then covered with regular 4 × 4 gauze squares, and the tube is coiled over them.
   - Observe for common complications of enteral feedings: aspiration, hyperglycemia, abdominal distention, diarrhea, and fecal impaction. Report findings to the healthcare provider. Often, a change in formula or rate of administration can correct problems.
   - When appropriate, teach the patient how to administer feedings and when to notify the healthcare provider concerning problems.
9. Remove and discard gloves. Perform hand hygiene. Reposition bed to lowest height.
10. Complete documentation using forms, checklists, or electronic dropdown lists supplemented by nurse's notes or additional comments as appropriate.

SAMPLE DOCUMENTATION

[date] 2045 No fluid aspirated from gastrostomy tube. Placed in Fowler position. 30 mL water flowed freely by gravity through tube. 250 mL room-temperature Ensure formula given over 20 minutes. No complaints of discomfort. *L. Traynor*

SKILL 10.8 Gastric Lavage: Performing

Safety Note! *During scheduled clinical time, nursing students may have a learning opportunity to observe or assist with this skill only with faculty permission and with direct supervision from faculty or another RN.*

Gastric lavage is a quick way to irrigate or wash out stomach contents with water or saline during an emergency such as an overdose of medications, accidental poisoning, or large amount of blood from a stomach hemorrhage. It is also used before and after certain surgical procedures to remove gastric contents.

Delegation or Assignment

Gastric lavage is not delegated or assigned to the UAP. However, signs and symptoms of problems may be observed during usual care and may be recorded by individuals other than the nurse. Abnormal findings must be validated and interpreted by the nurse.

Equipment

- Large-bore (37- to 40-Fr) soft Ewald or orogastric tube (*Note:* Patient must have cuffed endotracheal tube in place if comatose.)
- Large irrigating syringe with adapter
- Container for aspirate
- Lavage fluid, normal saline, or lukewarm water
- Activated charcoal for drug/toxin adsorption
- Container for specimen
- Water-soluble lubricant
- Standby suction available
- Towel
- Pen and tape
- Clean gloves

Preparation

- Review healthcare provider's orders for gastric lavage and solution to be used.
- Determine if patient is alert or comatose.
- Gather equipment and supplies.

Procedure

1. Introduce self to patient and verify the patient's identity using two identifiers. Explain to the patient what you are going to do, why it is necessary, and how the patient can participate. Discuss how the results will be used in planning further care or treatments.
2. Perform hand hygiene and observe appropriate infection control procedures.
3. Provide for patient privacy and don gloves.
4. Provide comfort and safety for patient and yourself, including raising bed to appropriate height for procedure.
5. Per facility protocol (healthcare provider may insert), measure for tube insertion the distance from bridge of nose to earlobe to xiphoid process and mark with tape or a pen.
6. Place patient in head-down, left side-lying position. **Rationale:** *This reduces the risk of aspiration if patient vomits.*
7. Lubricate tube with water-soluble lubricant.
8. Insert tube nasogastrically or orogastrically, about 50 cm (20 in.). Tape tube down to stabilize its position.
9. Aspirate gastric contents with syringe before instilling solution. Save specimen for analysis.
10. Repeatedly instill 50–100 mL normal saline or water and aspirate contents. **Rationale:** *Some authorities recommend water to lavage the stomach of blood since it breaks up clots more easily than saline solution, is less expensive, and is readily available.*

CAUTION! Gastric lavage used to remove unabsorbed poison or drug ingestion is generally ineffective if more than 60 minutes have passed. After that, the procedure may delay administration of activated charcoal or antidotes. It is not used for corrosive agents or petroleum distillates due to risk of aspiration.

---

11. Carefully monitor volume instilled and character and volume of aspirated contents. **Rationale:** *This will assist in determining net volume if there is blood loss.*
12. Continue repeating process until gastric return is clear, or as ordered.
13. Stomach will be left empty for decontamination. Activated charcoal may be instilled (as ordered) or a saline cathartic may be given. **Rationale:** *Activated charcoal adsorbs drugs in the stomach or intestine.*
14. Pinch tube for removal, wrap in towel, and dispose of equipment.
15. When the procedure is complete, remove and discard gloves. Perform hand hygiene. Return bed to lowest height.
16. Complete documentation using forms, checklists, or electronic dropdown lists supplemented by nurse's notes or additional comments as appropriate.

SAMPLE DOCUMENTATION

[date] 0300 Awake and alert. 37 Fr Ewald tube inserted left nares with small amount difficulty. Encouraged not to fight and to lie still. Two UAPs assisting to hold patient from pulling tube out. Tube tested for placement, aspirated 25 mL gastric contents with tablet fragments. Lavaged with sterile saline until returned clear, 1200 mL saline used. Returned 1350 gastric with saline contents. 100 g activated charcoal slurry instilled down Ewald tube as ordered. Ewald tube removed without incident. Quietly crying at this time, support given. *J. Keys*

SKILL 10.9 Nasogastric Tube: Feeding

A nasogastric (NG) tube is inserted in the naris and placed in the stomach to provide nutritional solutions and administer medications over a short period of time when patients are unable to or have difficulty with swallowing or eating. An NG tube may be inserted for patients who are comatose, have had recent surgery, or are premature newborns or infants.

Delegation or Assignment

Administering a tube feeding requires application of knowledge and problem solving, and it is not usually delegated or assigned to the UAP. Some agencies, however, may allow a trained UAP to administer a feeding. In this case, it is the responsibility of the nurse to assess tube placement and determine that the tube is patent. The nurse should reinforce major points, such as making sure the patient is sitting upright, and instruct the UAP to report any difficulty administering the feeding or any complaints voiced by the patient.

Equipment

- Correct type and amount of feeding solution
- 60-mL catheter-tip syringe
- Emesis basin
- Clean gloves
- pH test strip or meter
- Large syringe or calibrated plastic feeding bag with label and tubing that can be attached to the feeding tube or prefilled bottle with a drip chamber, tubing, and a flow-regulator clamp
- Measuring container from which to pour the feeding (if using open system)
- Water (60 mL unless otherwise specified) at room temperature
- Feeding pump as required

Preparation

- Review healthcare provider's orders for type of formula and rate of instilling it. Review patient's nursing plan of care.
- Gather equipment and supplies.

CAUTION! Do not add colored food dye to tube feedings. Previously, blue dye was often added to assist in recognition of aspiration. However, the United States Food and Drug Administration (USFDA) reports cases of many adverse reactions to the dye, including toxicity and death.

Procedure

1. Introduce self and verify the patient's identity using two identifiers. Explain to the patient what you are going to do, why it is necessary, and how the patient can participate. Inform the patient that the feeding should not cause any discomfort but may cause a feeling of fullness.
2. Perform hand hygiene and observe other appropriate infection control procedures.
3. Provide privacy for this procedure if the patient desires it. **Rationale:** *Tube feedings are embarrassing to some people.*

4. Assist the patient to a Fowler position (45–60 degrees elevation) in bed or a sitting position in a chair, the normal position for eating. If a sitting position is contraindicated, a slightly elevated right side-lying position is acceptable. **Rationale:** *These positions enhance the gravitational flow of the solution and prevent aspiration of fluid into the lungs.*
5. Assess tube placement prior to initiating a feeding or three times per day for continuous feedings.
   - Apply clean gloves.
   - Examine the placement mark on the tube to determine if it has advanced or slipped out.
   - Attach the syringe to the open end of the tube and aspirate. Check the pH.
   - Allow 1 hour to elapse before testing the pH if the patient has received a medication.
   - Use a pH meter rather than pH paper if the patient is receiving a continuous feeding. Follow facility policy if the pH is 6 or higher.
6. Assess residual feeding contents.
   - If the tube is placed in the stomach, aspirate all contents and measure the amount before administering the feeding. **Rationale:** *This is done to evaluate absorption of the last feeding; that is, whether undigested formula from a previous feeding remains.*
   - If 100 mL (or more than half of the last feeding) is withdrawn, check with the nurse in charge or refer to facility policy before proceeding. The precise amount of residual requiring intervention is usually determined by the healthcare provider's order or by facility policy. **Rationale:** *At some agencies, a feeding is delayed when the specified amount or more of formula remains in the stomach.*

   or

   - Reinstill the gastric contents into the stomach if this is the facility policy or healthcare provider's order. **Rationale:** *Removal of the contents could disturb the patient's electrolyte balance.*
   - If the patient is on a continuous feeding, check the gastric residual every 4–6 hr or according to facility protocol.
7. Administer the feeding.
   - Before administering feeding:
     a. Check the expiration date of the feeding.
     b. Warm the feeding to room temperature. **Rationale:** *An excessively cold feeding may cause abdominal cramps.*
     c. When an open system is used, clean the top of the feeding container with alcohol before opening it.

FEEDING BAG (OPEN SYSTEM)

- Hang the labeled bag from an infusion pole about 30 cm (12 in.) above the tube's point of insertion into the patient.
- Clamp the tubing and add the formula to the bag.
- Apply a label that indicates the date, time of starting the feeding, and nurse's initials on the feeding bag.

(continued on next page)

SKILL 10.9 Nasogastric Tube: Feeding (continued)

- Open the clamp, run the formula through the tubing to prime it, and reclamp the tube to prevent instilling air into the stomach.
- Attach the bag to the feeding tube ❶ and regulate the drip by adjusting the clamp to the drop factor on the bag (e.g., 20 drops/mL) if not placed on a pump. Proceed to step 8 below.

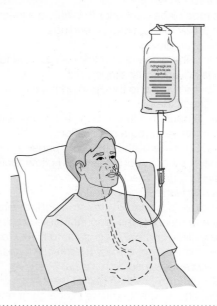

❶ Using a calibrated plastic bag to administer a tube feeding.

SYRINGE (OPEN SYSTEM)

- Remove the plunger from the syringe and connect the syringe to a pinched or clamped nasogastric tube to prevent instilling air into the stomach.
- Add the feeding to the syringe barrel ❷.
- Permit the feeding to flow in slowly at the prescribed rate. Raise or lower the syringe to adjust the flow as needed. Pinch or clamp the tubing to stop the flow for a minute if the

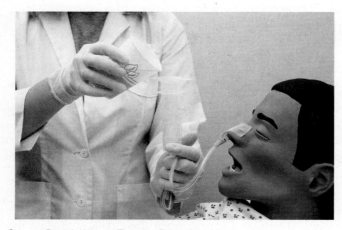

Source: Patrick Watson/Pearson Education, Inc.

❷ Using the barrel of a syringe to administer a tube feeding.

patient experiences discomfort from flatus, cramps, or vomiting. Proceed to step 8 below.

PREFILLED BOTTLE WITH DRIP CHAMBER (CLOSED SYSTEM)

- Remove the screw-on cap from the container and attach the administration set with the drip chamber and tubing.
- Close the clamp on the tubing.
- Hang the container on an intravenous pole about 30 cm (12 in.) above the tube's insertion point into the patient.
- Squeeze the drip chamber to fill it to one third to one half of its capacity.
- Open the tubing clamp, run the formula through the tubing to prime it, and reclamp the tube to prevent instilling air into the stomach.
- Attach the feeding set tubing to the feeding tube and regulate the drip rate to deliver the feeding over the desired length of time. Using a feeding pump is another option to manually setting the drip rate. Proceed to step 8 below.

CONTINUOUS-DRIP FEEDING

- Interrupt the feeding at least every 4–6 hr, or as indicated by facility protocol or the manufacturer, and aspirate and measure the gastric contents. **Rationale:** *This determines adequate absorption and verifies correct placement of the tube.*
- Determine facility protocol regarding withholding a feeding. Many agencies withhold the feeding if more than 75–100 mL of residual is aspirated. If the feeding is withheld, flush the tubing with water to prevent formula from clogging the tube.
- To prevent spoilage or bacterial contamination, do not allow the feeding solution to hang longer than 4–8 hr. Check facility policy or manufacturer's recommendations regarding time limits.
- Follow facility policy regarding how frequently to change the feeding bag and tubing. Changing the feeding bag and tubing every 24 hours reduces the risk of contamination.

8. Flush the feeding tube before all of the formula has run through the tubing.
   - Instill a flush of 50–100 mL of water through the feeding tube or medication port depending on facility policy.
   - Be sure to add the water before the feeding solution has drained from the neck of a syringe or from the tubing of an administration set to prevent instilling air into the stomach.
9. Clamp the feeding tube before all of the water is instilled to prevent air from entering the tube.
10. Ensure patient comfort and safety.
    - Secure the tubing to the patient's gown to minimize pulling of the tube with movement.
    - Ask the patient to remain sitting upright in Fowler position or in a slightly elevated right lateral position for at least 30 minutes to prevent the potential aspiration of the feeding into the lungs.
    - Check the facility's policy on the frequency of changing the NG tube and the use of smaller lumen tubes if a large-bore tube is in place. **Rationale:** *These measures*

SKILL 10.9 Nasogastric Tube: Feeding (*continued*)

prevent irritation and erosion of the pharyngeal and esophageal mucous membranes.

- Remove and discard gloves. Perform hand hygiene.

11. Dispose of equipment appropriately.
    - If the equipment is to be reused, wash it thoroughly with soap and water so that it is ready for reuse.
    - Change the equipment every 24 hours or according to facility policy.
12. Remove and discard gloves. Perform hand hygiene, and leave patient safe and comfortable.
13. Complete documentation using forms, checklists, or electronic dropdown lists supplemented by nurse's notes or additional comments as appropriate, including:
    - The amount and kind of feeding solution taken, duration of the feeding, and assessments of the patient.
    - The volume of the feeding and water administered on the patient's intake and output record.
14. Monitor the patient for possible problems.
    - Carefully assess patient receiving tube feedings for problems.
    - To prevent dehydration, give the patient supplemental water in addition to the prescribed tube feeding as ordered.

SAMPLE DOCUMENTATION

[date] 1330 Aspirated 20 mL pale yellow fluid from NG tube, pH 5. Returned residual. Placed in Fowler position. 1 liter room-temperature ordered formula begun @ 60 mL/hour on pump. No nausea reported. *L. Traynor*

Lifespan Considerations

NEWBORNS AND INFANTS

- Feeding tubes may be reinserted at each feeding to prevent irritation of the mucous membrane, nasal airway obstruction, and stomach perforation that may occur if the tube is left in place continuously. Check facility practice.

CHILDREN

- Position a small child, infant, or newborn in your lap, provide a pacifier, and hold and cuddle the child during feedings. This promotes comfort, supports the normal sucking instinct of the newborn or infant, and facilitates digestion.

OLDER ADULTS

- Physiological changes associated with aging may make the older adult more vulnerable to complications associated with enteral feedings such as:
  - Increased amount of time to empty stomach associated with medical conditions such as hiatal hernia and diabetes mellitus.
  - Diarrhea from administering the feeding too fast.
  - Dehydration if concentration is too high.
  - Hyperglycemia if the feeding has a high concentration of glucose.

Patient Teaching

Managing NG Tube Feedings

Teach the patient the following so that the patient can manage the NG tube feeding.

- Formula name, how to mix or prepare it, how much, and how often it is to be given; how to inspect containers of formula for expiration date, leaks, and cracks; how to use aseptic techniques such as swabbing the container's top with alcohol before opening it and changing the syringe administration set and reservoir every 24 hours.
- Importance of refrigerating diluted or reconstituted formula and formula that contains additives.
- How to assess for tube placement using pH measurement before administering the feeding, including what to do if pH is greater than 6 or higher.
- How to do hand hygiene properly; how to fill and hang the feeding bag; how to operate an infusion pump and set the rate, if indicated; and what position the patient should be in during and after the feeding.
- Importance of monitoring the patient's temperature, weight, and intake and output every day.
- Need to observe for indications of infection such as fever, increased respiratory rate, decrease in urine output, increased stool frequency, and altered level of consciousness.
- Need to know where to find emergency telephone numbers of home care facility, nursing clinician, and/or healthcare provider, or other 24-hour on-call emergency service.

SKILL 10.10 Nasogastric Tube: Flushing and Maintaining

Regular flushing of a nasogastric tube if feeding is not in progress can prevent it from becoming blocked. It is also important to flush the tube before and after administering medications through it.

Delegation or Assignment

Due to the need for knowledge and skills of technical complexity, the maintaining and monitoring of nasogastric tubes is not delegated or assigned to the UAP. The UAP may care for patients with nasogastric tubes. The nurse must ensure that the UAP knows what complications or adverse signs should be reported to the nurse.

Equipment

- Disposable irrigation set with 60-mL syringe with catheter tip
- Emesis basin
- Towel

(*continued on next page*)

SKILL 10.10 Nasogastric Tube: Flushing and Maintaining *(continued)*

- Normal saline irrigation solution
- Intake and output (I&O) record sheet
- Clean gloves

Preparation

- Check healthcare provider's orders and patient's nursing plan of care.
- Gather supplies.

Procedure

1. Introduce self to patient and verify the patient's identity using two identifiers. Explain to the patient what you are going to do, why it is necessary, and how the patient can participate. Discuss how the results will be used in planning further care or treatments.
2. Perform hand hygiene and observe appropriate infection control procedures.
3. Provide for patient privacy, and don clean gloves.
4. Place patient in semi-Fowler position. Position bed at an appropriate height.
5. Disconnect nasogastric (NG) tube from suction source if used.
6. Place towel under NG tube to protect sheets and place emesis basin nearby.
7. Check NG tube placement ❶. **Rationale:** *Solution could be instilled in lungs if NG tube is not in the stomach.*
8. Draw up 20–30 mL normal saline into irrigating syringe.

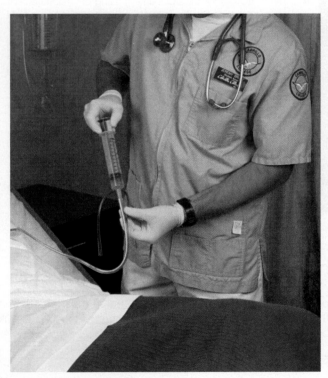

Source: Ronald May/Pearson Education, Inc.

❶ Aspirate secretions to check tube placement before instilling saline solution.

9. Gently instill normal saline (NS) into NG tube or remove syringe plunger, pour NS into syringe barrel, and allow solution to flow in by gravity ❷.

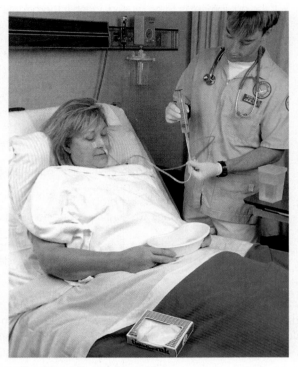

Source: Ronald May/Pearson Education, Inc.

❷ Gently instill normal saline into nasogastric (NG) tube by syringe, or allow solution to flow by gravity.

CAUTION! If secretions siphon into blue vent lumen of a Salem Sump tube, clear it by instilling 20 mL of normal saline followed by 20 mL of air. Air vent must be cleared of secretions to restore proper functioning.

---

10. Repeat procedure if necessary.
11. Reconnect NG tube to suction or plug tube. Place bed in lowest position.
12. When the procedure is complete, remove and discard gloves. Perform hand hygiene and leave patient safe and comfortable.
13. Complete documentation using forms, checklists, or electronic dropdown lists supplemented by nurse's notes or additional comments as appropriate.

SAMPLE DOCUMENTATION

[date] 1400 Tube placement checked, pH 4.85 from 15 mL aspirate, light brown gastric secretions. 20 mL saline instilled in tube via gravity to flush tube without incident. Tolerated without complaint. Resting in bed. *W. Howell*

SKILL 10.10 Nasogastric Tube: Flushing and Maintaining (*continued*)

Safety Considerations

- If water rather than normal saline is used to flush enteral decompression tubes, the production of gastric secretions will increase and increasing amounts of electrolytes will be washed out. Similarly, if the patient is NPO but ingests ice chips ad lib, electrolyte imbalance due to washout can occur, causing metabolic alkalosis.

- Limit the use of ice chips by substituting chips made from an electrolyte solution, and provide oral hygiene to keep the patient's mucous membranes moist for comfort.

- If the patient is receiving adequate parenteral hydration (IV fluids), excessive thirst should not be experienced.

SKILL 10.11 Nasogastric Tube: Inserting

Safety Note! *During scheduled clinical time, nursing students may have a learning opportunity to observe or assist with this skill only with faculty permission and with direct supervision from faculty or another RN.*

A nasogastric (NG) tube is inserted into a naris and advanced down to the stomach. The tube can be used for feeding patients formula and administering medications or it can be connected to a suction system to drain gastric secretions.

Delegation or Assignment

This skill is not delegated or assigned to the UAP. The UAP, however, can assist with the oral hygiene needs of a patient with a nasogastric tube. Insertion of an NG tube is an invasive procedure requiring application of knowledge (e.g., anatomy and physiology, risk factors) and problem solving. In some agencies, only healthcare providers with advanced training are permitted to insert NG tubes that require use of a stylet.

Equipment

- Large- or small-bore tube (nonlatex preferred)
- Nonallergenic adhesive tape, 2.5 cm (1 in.) wide
- Clean gloves
- Water-soluble lubricant
- Facial tissues
- Cup of ice with spoon or cup of water with drinking straw
- 20- to 60-mL syringe with an adapter
- Emesis or wash basin, depending on amount of gastric secretions anticipated
- pH test strip or meter
- Bilirubin dipstick
- Stethoscope
- Disposable pad or towel
- Clamp or plug (optional)
- Antireflux valve for air vent if Salem Sump tube is used
- Suction apparatus with tubes and canister connected
- Safety pin and elastic band
- CO_2 detector (optional)

Preparation

- Review healthcare provider's orders relative to inserting an NG tube. Review patient's nursing plan of care.
- Gather needed equipment and supplies.

CAUTION!

- Nurses do not insert or withdraw an NG tube for patients recovering from gastric surgery. The suture line could be interrupted, or hemorrhage could occur. The healthcare provider should be notified of dislodgement.
- Never insert an NG tube in a patient after nasal, craniofacial, or hypophysectomy surgery.

Procedure

1. Introduce self and verify the patient's identity using two identifiers. Explain to the patient that you are going to insert a nasogastric tube, why it is necessary, and how the patient can participate. The passage of a gastric tube is unpleasant because the gag reflex is activated during insertion. Establish a method for the patient to indicate distress and a desire for you to pause the insertion. Raising a finger or hand is often used for this.
2. Perform hand hygiene and observe other appropriate infection control procedures.
3. Provide for patient privacy. Raise bed to appropriate height.
   - Assist the patient to a high-Fowler position if the patient's health condition permits, and support the head on a pillow. **Rationale:** *It is often easier to swallow in this position, and gravity helps the passage of the tube.*
4. Assess the patient's nares.
   - Don clean gloves.
   - Ask the patient to hyperextend the head as able to and, using a flashlight, observe the mucosa of each naris for any irritations or lesions and the passageway for any obstructions or septum deformity.
   - Assess for patency by asking the patient to breathe through one naris while occluding the other.
   - Select the naris that has the greater airflow for inserting the NG tube.
5. If a large-bore tube (e.g., Salem Sump tube) is being used, place the tube in a basin of warm water while preparing the patient. **Rationale:** *This allows the tubing to become more pliable and flexible.*

(*continued on next page*)

SKILL 10.11 Nasogastric Tube: Inserting (*continued*)

6. Determine how far to insert the tube. (Measure the tube.)
   - Use the tube to mark off the distance from the tip of the patient's nose to the tip of the earlobe and then from the tip of the earlobe to the tip of the xiphoid ➊. **Rationale:** *This length approximates the distance from the naris to the stomach. This distance varies among individuals.*
   - Mark this length with adhesive tape if the tube does not have markings.

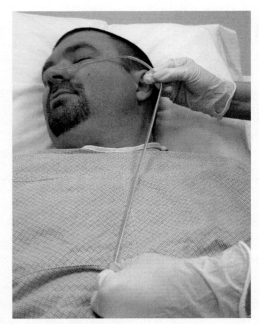

Source: Patrick Watson/Pearson Education, Inc.

➊ Measuring the appropriate length for a nasogastric (NG) tube.

7. Insert the tube.
   - Lubricate the tip of the tube well with water-soluble lubricant to ease insertion ➋. **Rationale:** *A water-soluble lubricant dissolves if the tube accidentally enters the lungs.*
   - Insert the tube, with its natural curve toward the patient, into the selected naris ➌. Ask the patient to hyperextend the neck, and gently advance the tube toward the nasopharynx ➍. **Rationale:** *Hyperextension of the neck reduces the curvature of the nasopharyngeal junction.*
   - Direct the tube along the floor of the nostril and toward the ear on that side. **Rationale:** *Directing the tube along the floor avoids the turbinates along the lateral wall.*
   - Slight pressure and a twisting motion are sometimes required to pass the tube into the nasopharynx, and patient's eyes may water at this point. **Rationale:** *Tears are a natural body response.* Provide the patient with tissues as needed.
   - If the tube meets resistance, withdraw it, relubricate it, and insert it in the other naris. **Rationale:** *The tube*

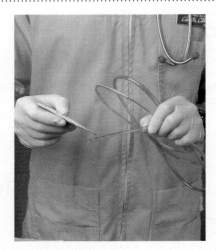

Source: Ronald May/Pearson Education, Inc.

➋ Lubricate first 10 cm (4 in.) of NG tube with water-soluble lubricant.

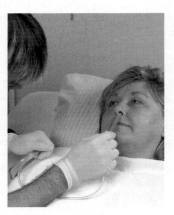

Source: Ronald May/Pearson Education, Inc.

➌ Insert NG tube through patient's more patent nostril.

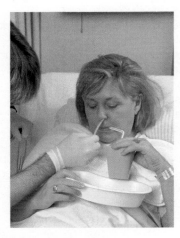

Source: Ronald May/Pearson Education, Inc.

➍ Instruct patient to flex head forward and take sips of water as tube is advanced.

SKILL 10.11 Nasogastric Tube: Inserting (*continued*)

should never be forced against resistance because of the danger of injury.

- Once the tube reaches the oropharynx (throat), the patient will feel the tube in the throat and may gag and retch. Ask the patient to tilt the head forward, and encourage the patient to drink (or eat ice chips) and swallow. **Rationale:** *Tilting the head forward facilitates passage of the tube into the posterior pharynx and esophagus rather than into the larynx; swallowing moves the epiglottis over the opening to the larynx.*
- If the patient gags, stop passing the tube momentarily. Have the patient rest, take a few breaths, and take sips of water (or ice chips) to calm the gag reflex.

CAUTION! Coughing and choking are normal responses for some patients; however, choking and coughing plus cyanosis or inability to speak indicate that the tube may be in the airway. If this occurs, immediately pull the NG tube out of the naris, wait a few minutes and reinsert the tube.

- In cooperation with the patient, pass the tube 5–10 cm (2–4 in.) with each swallow, until the indicated length is inserted ⑤.
- If the patient continues to gag and the tube does not advance with each swallow, withdraw it slightly, and inspect the throat by looking through the mouth. **Rationale:** *The tube may be coiled in the throat.* If so, withdraw it until it is straight, and try again to advance it to the stomach.
- If a CO_2 detector is used, after the tube has been advanced approximately 30 cm (12 in.), draw air through the detector. Any change in color of the detector indicates placement of the tube in the respiratory tract. Immediately withdraw the tube and reinsert ⑥.

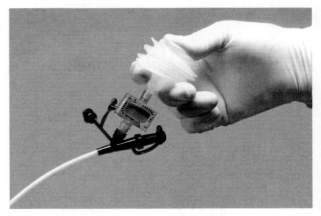

Source: Patrick Watson/Pearson Education, Inc.

⑥ After drawing air into the tube using a syringe or attached bellows, match the sensor color to the legend on the detector. This example shows purple—no CO_2 present.

EVIDENCE-BASED PRACTICE

Determining Proper NG Tube Placement

Problem

Nurses do blind insertions of nasoenteric and nasogastric tubes at the bedside. There is a risk for misplacement of the feeding tube in the tracheobronchial area, in the esophagus when not advanced far enough into the stomach, or not advanced far enough in the small intestines.

Evidence

Cases of patients having severe complications of feeding tube misplacement have been studied. One study was done using 9931 patients that had a narrow-bore nasoenteric tube inserted. Of this number, 187 patients had the tube misplaced in the tracheal-bronchus, of which 35 of these patients had to be treated for a pneumothorax, and 5 of them died as a result.

Implications

The most accurate and recommended verification of correct tube placement is with radiographic confirmation before tube feeding is initiated. There are several bedside methods to check for correct tube placement. The American Association of Critical-Care Nurses recommends using two of the following methods to verify tube placement of the tube: (1) observe for signs of respiratory distress when inserting the tube; (2) measure pH of aspirate from tube; (3) use colorimetric capnometry to detect carbon dioxide during tube placement; (4) assess aspirate from tube.

Sources: American Association of Critical-Care Nurses (AACN). (2016). AACN Practice Alert. *Initial and ongoing verification of feeding tube placement in adults.* Retrieved from https://www.aacn.org/clinical-resources/practice-alerts/initial-and-ongoing-verification-of-feeding-tube-placement-in-adults; Loo, Y. (2015). *Pneumothorax from nasogastric feeding tube in a patient with tracheostomy tube.* Retrieved from http://jaccr.com/pneumothorax-from-nasogastric-feeding-tube-in-a-patient-with-tracheostomy-tube/; Amirlak, B., Amirlak, I., Awad, Z. T., & Forse, R. (2014). *Pneumothorax following feeding tube placement: Precaution and treatment.* Retrieved from https://www.researchgate.net/publication/230573733

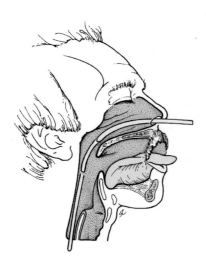

⑤ NG tube inserted through naris to stomach.

(*continued on next page*)

SKILL 10.11 Nasogastric Tube: Inserting (*continued*)

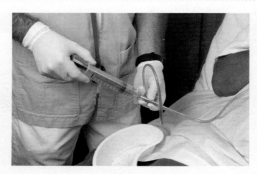

Source: Ronald May/Pearson Education, Inc.

❼ Aspirate gastric contents to check color and pH.

8. Aspirate stomach contents and check the pH, which should be acidic **❼** for tube placement. **Rationale:** *Testing pH is one way to determine location of a feeding tube. Gastric contents are commonly pH 1–5; pH of 6 or greater would indicate the contents are from lower in the intestinal tract or in the respiratory tract.*
   - Aspirate can also be tested for bilirubin. Bilirubin levels in the lungs should be almost zero, while levels in the stomach will be approximately 1.5 mg/dL and in the intestine over 10 mg/dL.
   - Almost all nasogastric tubes are radiopaque, and placement can be confirmed by x-ray. Check facility policy.
   - Place a stethoscope over the patient's epigastrium and inject 5–20 mL of air into the tube while listening for a whooshing sound. Although still one of the methods used, do not use this method as the *primary* method for determining placement of the feeding tube. **Rationale:** *This method does not guarantee tube position.*
   - If the signs indicate placement in the lungs, remove the tube and begin again.
   - If the signs do not indicate placement in the lungs or stomach, advance the tube 5 cm (2 in.), and repeat the tests.
9. Secure the tube by taping it to the bridge of the patient's nose **❽**.
   - If the patient has oily skin, wipe the nose first with alcohol to remove oil from the skin.
   - Cut 7.5 cm (3 in.) of tape, and split it lengthwise at one end, leaving a 2.5-cm (1-in.) tab at the end.
   - Place the tape over the bridge of the patient's nose, and bring the split ends either under and around the tubing, or

under the tubing and back up over the nose. Ensure that the tube is centrally located prior to securing with tape to maximize airflow and prevent irritation to the side of the nares. **Rationale:** *Taping in this manner prevents the tube from pressing against and irritating the edge of the nostril.*

10. Once the correct position has been determined, attach the tube to a suction source or feeding apparatus as ordered, or clamp the end of the tubing.
11. Secure the tube to the patient's gown by looping an elastic band around the end of the tubing, and attach the elastic band to the gown with a safety pin. Another method is to attach a piece of adhesive tape to the tube, and pin the tape to the gown. **Rationale:** *The tube is attached to prevent it from dangling and pulling.*
12. Remove and discard gloves. Perform hand hygiene. Return bed to lowest position and leave patient safe and comfortable.
13. Establish a plan for providing daily nasogastric tube care.
    - Inspect the nostril for discharge and irritation.
    - Clean the nostril and tube with moistened, cotton-tipped applicators.
    - Apply water-soluble lubricant to the nostril if it appears dry or encrusted.
    - Change the adhesive tape as required to secure the tube and prevent skin trauma from either tape or pressure of the tube against the naris.
    - Give frequent mouth care. Due to the presence of the tube, the patient may breathe through the mouth.
14. If suction is applied, ensure that the patency of both the nasogastric and suction tubes is maintained.
    - Irrigations of the tube may be required at regular intervals. In some agencies, irrigations must be ordered by the healthcare provider. Prior to irrigation, always recheck placement.
    - If a Salem Sump tube is used, follow facility policies for irrigating the vent lumen with air to maintain patency of the suctioning lumen. Often, a sucking sound can be heard from the vent port if it is patent.
    - Keep accurate records of the patient's fluid intake and output, and record the amount and characteristics of the drainage.
15. Complete documentation using forms, checklists, or electronic dropdown lists supplemented by nurse's notes or additional comments as appropriate, including the insertion of the tube, the type of tube, how correct placement was determined, type of suction if used, color and amount of gastric secretions, and patient responses (e.g., discomfort, abdominal distention).

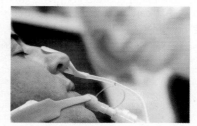

Source: Bodenham/LTH NHS Trust/Science Source

❽ A nasogastric tube taped to the bridge of the nose. Bodenham, LTH NHS Trust/Science Source

SAMPLE DOCUMENTATION

[date] 1030 Feeding tube (8 Fr) inserted without difficulty through (R) naris with stylet in place. To x-ray to check placement. Radiologist reports tube tip in stomach. Stylet removed. Aspirate pH 4. Tube secured to nose. Verbalizes understanding of need to not pull on tube. *L. Tray*

SKILL 10.11 Nasogastric Tube: Inserting (*continued*)

Safety Considerations

SALEM SUMP TUBE ❾

The Salem Sump tube is a double-lumen nasogastric tube. The blue lumen is used for decompression. It has a blue pigtail that provides an air vent to allow atmospheric pressure to enter the stomach to prevent tube adherence to gastric mucosa when the tube is attached to suction. It is NOT used for irrigation, obtaining a speci-

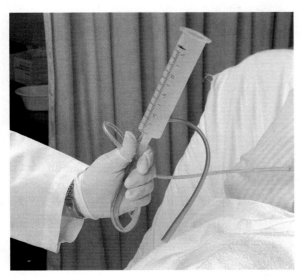

Source: Ronald May/Pearson Education, Inc.

❾ The nasogastric Salem Sump tube.

men, or connecting to the suction set-up. However, if the vent lumen is blocked and requires flushing, after the flush the pigtail should be cleared with an injection of 20 mL air. The pigtail should be kept above the level of the patient's stomach to prevent stomach contents from siphoning into the air vent lumen, making it dysfunctional.

Lifespan Considerations

NEWBORNS, INFANTS, AND YOUNG CHILDREN

- Restraints may be necessary during tube insertion and throughout therapy. **Rationale:** *Restraints will prevent accidental dislodging of the tube.*
- Place the newborn or infant in an infant seat or position the newborn or infant with a rolled towel or pillow under the head and shoulders.
- When assessing the nares, obstruct one of the newborn's or infant's nares and feel for air passage from the other. If the nasal passageway is very small or is obstructed, an orogastric tube may be more appropriate.
- Measure appropriate nasogastric tube length from the nose to the tip of the earlobe and then to the point midway between the umbilicus and the xiphoid process.
- If an orogastric tube is used, measure from the tip of the earlobe to the corner of the mouth to the xiphoid process.
- Do not hyperextend or hyperflex a newborn's or infant's neck because it could occlude the airway.
- Tape the tube to the area between the end of the nares and the upper lip as well as to the cheek.

SKILL 10.12 Nasogastric Tube: Removing

Delegation or Assignment

Due to the need for assessment and the technical complexity of removing a nasogastric tube, this skill is not delegated or assigned to the UAP. Abnormal findings must be validated and interpreted by the nurse.

Equipment

- Disposable pad or towel
- Tissues
- Clean gloves
- 60-mL syringe (optional)
- Plastic trash bag

Preparation

- Confirm the healthcare provider's order to remove the nasogastric tube.
- Provide tissues to the patient to wipe the nose and mouth after tube removal.

Procedure

1. Introduce self and verify the patient's identity using two identifiers. Explain to the patient that you are going to remove the nasogastric tube, why it is necessary, and how the patient can participate.
2. Perform hand hygiene and observe other appropriate infection control procedures (e.g., clean gloves).
3. Provide for patient privacy. Position bed at appropriate height for the procedure.
4. Assist the patient to a sitting position if health permits. Place the disposable pad or towel across the patient's chest to collect any spillage of secretions from the tube.
5. Detach the tube.
   - Don clean gloves.
   - Disconnect the nasogastric tube from the suction apparatus, if present.
   - Unpin the tube from the patient's gown.
   - Remove the adhesive tape securing the tube to the nose.

(continued on next page)

SKILL 10.12 Nasogastric Tube: Removing (*continued*)

6. Remove the nasogastric tube.
   - *Optional:* Instill 50 mL of air into the tube. **Rationale:** *This clears the tube of any contents, such as feeding or gastric drainage, and decreases the chances of dragging any drainage through the esophagus and nasopharynx.*
   - Ask the patient to take a deep breath and to hold it ❶. **Rationale:** *This closes the glottis, thereby preventing accidental aspiration of any gastric contents.*
   - Pinch the tube with the gloved hand. **Rationale:** *Pinching the tube prevents any contents inside the tube from draining into the patient's throat.*
   - Smoothly withdraw the tube ❷.
   - Place the tube in the plastic bag. **Rationale:** *Placing the tube immediately into the bag prevents the transference of microorganisms from the tube to other articles or people.*
   - Observe the intactness of the tube end.

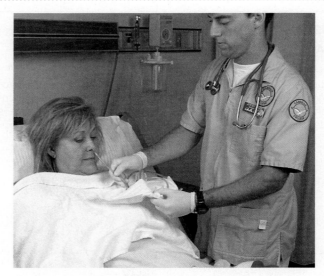

Source: Ronald May/Pearson Education, Inc.

❷ Have patient hold breath. Remove NG tube with continuous steady pull.

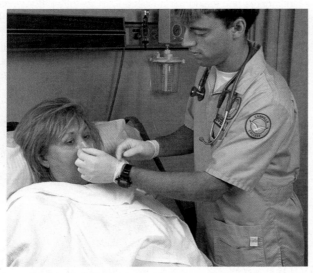

Source: Ronald May/Pearson Education, Inc.

❶ Clamp tube, unpin tube from gown, and loosen tape on nose securing nasogastric (NG) tube.

7. Ensure patient comfort.
   - Provide mouth care if desired.
   - Assist the patient as required to blow the nose. **Rationale:** *Excessive secretions may have accumulated in the nasal passages.*

8. Dispose of the equipment appropriately.
   - Place the pad, bag with tube, and gloves in the receptacle designated by the facility.
   - Place bed in lowest position. Remove and discard gloves. Perform hand hygiene.
9. When the procedure is complete, leave patient safe and comfortable.
10. Complete documentation using forms, checklists, or electronic dropdown lists supplemented by nurse's notes or additional comments as appropriate, including removal of the tube, the amount and appearance of any drainage if connected to suction, and any relevant assessments of the patient.

SAMPLE DOCUMENTATION

[date] 1500 NG tube removed intact without difficulty. Oral & nasal care given. No bleeding or excoriation noted. States is hungry & thirsty. 60 mL apple juice given. No c/o nausea. *L. Traynor*

≫ Parenteral Nutrition Using Intravenous Infusion

Expected Outcomes

1. Lipids infuse within time frame.
2. Adequate calories and essential fatty acids are provided to patients unable to ingest orally.
3. Total parenteral nutrients provided without complications or adverse effects.
4. Normal pancreatic function is maintained.

SKILL 10.13 Lipids, IV Infusion: Providing

Safety Note! *During scheduled clinical time, nursing students may have a learning opportunity to observe or assist with this skill only with faculty permission and with direct supervision from faculty or another RN.*

Lipid emulsions provide patients a source of essential fatty acids and a non-glucose high energy supply that can reduce the level of glucose taken in to meet the body's need for an energy source. They are given with total parenteral nutrition to supply essential fatty acids.

Delegation or Assignment

Due to the need for sterile technique and technical complexity, administration of lipids is not delegated or assigned to the UAP. The UAP may care for patients receiving lipids, and the nurse must ensure that the UAP knows what complications or adverse signs should be reported to the nurse.

Equipment

- IV lipid solution in container ①
- Nonphthalate vented IV tubing infusion set (to prevent pooling of fat in IV tubing)
- Needleless cannula
- 2% chlorhexidine gluconate swabs
- Infusion pump

Note: Many facilities do not infuse lipids alone but combine with total parenteral nutrition (TPN) infusion as an IV piggyback solution.

Preparation

- Review healthcare provider's orders and the MAR.
- Obtain lipid emulsion (refrigerated) from the pharmacy and warm the solution to room temperature (may take 1–2 hr).
- Examine solution for separation of emulsion into layers or fat globules or for accumulation of froth. Do not use if any of these appear.
- Label bottle with patient name, medical record number, room number, date, time, flow rate, bottle number, and start and stop times.
- Gather needed equipment and supplies.

Procedure

1. Introduce self to patient and verify the patient's identity using two identifiers. Explain to the patient that you are going to hang a lipid solution to infuse, why it is necessary, and how the patient can participate. Discuss how the results will be used in planning further care or treatments.
2. Perform hand hygiene and observe appropriate infection control procedures.
3. Provide for patient privacy.
4. Take vital signs for baseline assessment. **Rationale:** *Baseline information is needed because an immediate reaction can occur.*
5. Perform hand hygiene, and then swab stopper on IV bottle with antimicrobial swab and allow to dry.
6. Attach vented non–polyvinyl chloride (non-PVC) infusion set to bottle, twisting the spike to prevent particles from stopper falling into the emulsion, or spike bag with regular IV tubing ②.

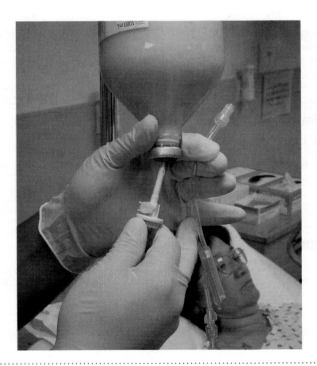

① Lipids are administered from glass container or non–polyvinyl chloride (non-PVC) infusion sets.

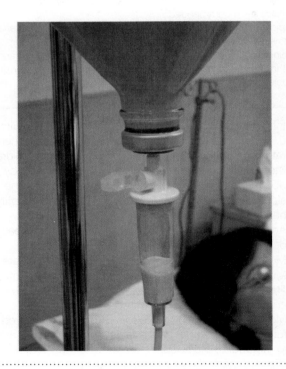

② Vented tubing is required for lipid infusion.

(continued on next page)

SKILL 10.13 Lipids, IV Infusion: Providing (continued)

7. Hang IV bottle at least 75 cm (30 in.) above IV site. **Rationale:** *Due to solution viscosity, lipid emulsion needs to be at this height to prevent it from backing up into infusion tubing.*

8. Fill drip chamber two thirds full, slightly open clamp on the tubing, and prime the tubing slowly. **Rationale:** *Priming more slowly reduces chance of air bubbles with this solution.*

9. Attach the tubing to the IV site.

10. If piggybacking lipids into hyperalimentation, use port closest to patient, below tubing filter ❸.

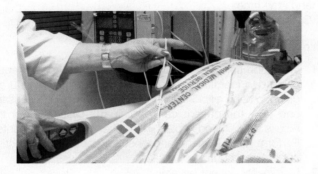

❸ Check facility policy regarding use of in-line filters for lipid administration. Filters are not recommended by the Centers for Disease Control and Prevention (CDC), but the Infusion Nurses Society favors them.

Safety Considerations

Administration sets that contain di-(2-ethylhexyl) phthalate (DEHP) plasticizers extract lipids from the infusion set. Therefore, use of a separate administration set, glass infusate container, or special non-PVC IV bag is recommended.

Lipid emulsions alone promote growth of specific bacteria and yeasts as soon as 6 hours after the infusion. However, when lipids are combined with a TPN solution (amino acids, lipid emulsion, and glucose) in the same bag, they do not appear to support any greater microbial growth than non–lipid-containing TPN fluids. Thus, lipids in TPN solution can hang safely for 24 hr.

11. Infuse lipid solutions initially at 1 mL/min for adults and 0.1 mL/min for children for first 15–30 min. Then increase rate to 2 mL/min for adults and 0.2 mL/min for children.

12. Monitor vital signs according to facility policy and observe for side effects during first 30 min of the infusion. If side effects occur, stop the infusion and notify the healthcare provider.

13. Adjust flow to prescribed IV rate if no adverse reactions occur.

14. Monitor and maintain the infusion at the ordered rate.

15. Monitor serum lipids 4 hr after discontinuing infusion. **Rationale:** *If you draw blood too soon after infusion is completed, incorrect blood values result.*

16. Monitor liver function tests for evidence of impaired liver function. **Rationale:** *These tests indicate the liver's ability to metabolize the lipids.*

17. Discard partially used bottles/bags. **Rationale:** *This action prevents contamination.*

Safety Considerations

Observe for IV lipid side effects after starting lipid infusion:

Chills	Headache	Vertigo
Chest and back pain	Diaphoresis	Cyanosis
Fever	Pressure over the	Sleepiness
Nausea and vomiting	eyes	Allergic reactions
Flushing	Dyspnea	Thrombophlebitis.

18. Discard administration set after each unit unless additional units are administered consecutively.

19. Continue to monitor vital signs, and observe patient for adverse reactions during the entire process of infusion.

20. When the procedure is complete, perform hand hygiene and leave patient safe and comfortable.

21. Complete documentation using forms, checklists, or electronic dropdown lists supplemented by nurse's notes or additional comments as appropriate.

SAMPLE DOCUMENTATION

[date] 0730 Lipids bag connected to piggyback IV tubing, line primed. Needleless connector port cleaned, air dried, and lipids bag connected to port below tubing filter. Rate set at 1 mL/min infused for 15 minutes without complication. Rate increased to 2 mL/min. Tolerating infusion without difficulty or complaint. *T. Jay*

CAUTION! In-line filters are not recommended by the Centers for Disease Control and Prevention (CDC) as a routine infection control measure; however, the Infusion Nurses Society favors the use of filters. Always check hospital policies and procedures to determine use of filters.

Safety Considerations

IV LIPID INFUSION

- IV lipid solutions are isotonic and provide 1.1 kcal/mL of solution in a 10% solution or 2.0 kcal/mL in a 20% solution.
- Do not put additives into IV lipid bottle.
- Do not use an IV filter because the particles are large and cannot pass through.

FOR ADULTS

- Lipid 10%: Up to 500 mL 4–6 hr on first day to maximum of 2.5 g/kg body weight per day. Do not exceed 60% of patient's total caloric intake per day.
- Liposyn 10%: No more than 500 mL/day in 4–6 hr.

FOR CHILDREN

- Lipid 10%: Up to 1 g/kg in 4 hr. Do not exceed 60% of total caloric intake.

SKILL 10.14 Total Parenteral Nutrition (TPN), IV Infusion: Providing

Safety Note! *During scheduled clinical time, nursing students may have a learning opportunity to observe or assist with this skill only with faculty permission and with direct supervision from faculty or another RN.*

Total parenteral nutrition (TPN) means all the nutrition a patient takes into the body is provided intravenously using a large central vein in the neck or chest. The patient is totally dependent on TPN and not getting nutrition from any other source, such as oral ingestion or enteral feedings. TPN is highly concentrated and usually hyperosmolar, so considered caustic and can only be given in a central large-diameter vein. TPN is different from partial parenteral nutrition (PPN). PPN has fewer nutrients in the mixture and can be administered through a peripheral IV line. The patient also receives nutrition from an additional source, such as tube feeding, when receiving PPN.

Delegation or Assignment

Due to the need for sterile technique and technical complexity, administration of TPN is not delegated or assigned to the UAP. The UAP may care for patients receiving TPN, and the nurse must ensure that the UAP knows what complications or adverse signs should be reported to the nurse.

Equipment

- TPN solution
- Timing tape
- Infusion pump
- Tubing with filter
- Clean gloves
- Surgical masks
- Antimicrobial swabs
- 10-mL needleless syringe, if using needleless tubing, with 5 mL of preservative-free 0.9% normal saline solution
- CLC2000 positive-pressure cap (or another brand)

Preparation

- Review the patient record regarding previous TPN. Note any complications and how they were managed.
- Check healthcare provider's orders for TPN solution and flow rate. Inspect and prepare solution.
- Remove the ordered TPN solution from the refrigerator 1 hr before use, and check each ingredient and the proposed rate against the order on the chart. **Rationale:** *Infusion of a cold solution can cause pain, hypothermia, and venous spasm and constriction.*
- Inspect the solution for cloudiness or presence of particles, and ensure that the container is free from cracks. For lipids, examine the bag for separation of emulsion, fat globules, or froth.
- Ensure that correct placement of the central line catheter has been confirmed by x-ray examination. If a multi-lumen

catheter is used to administer TPN, one port is designated exclusively for TPN and is so labeled.
- Before administering any TPN solution:
  a. Check its expiration date. Most solutions must be used within 24 hours of preparation, unless they are refrigerated.
  b. The nurse checks the TPN solution nutrients (calories, minerals, vitamins, nutrients, trace elements, electrolytes, and any added medications) listed on the bag against the order written by the healthcare provider. (Some agencies require that two nurses check the TPN solution, similar to checking blood products.) **Rationale:** *This is another check that ensures the solution was properly prepared by the pharmacist.*
  c. Apply a timing tape on the solution container.
- Gather all equipment and supplies.

Procedure

1. Introduce self and verify the patient's identity using two identifiers. Explain to the patient what you are going to do, why it is necessary, and how the patient can participate.
2. Provide for patient privacy and prepare the patient.
   - Assist the patient to a comfortable position, either sitting or lying. If necessary, expose the central line site but provide for patient privacy.
3. Perform hand hygiene and observe other appropriate infection control procedures.
4. Use strict aseptic technique, don gloves and mask (per facility policy).
5. Verify patency of TPN lumen.
   - Wipe access port with antimicrobial swab and allow to air dry.
   - Insert needleless cannula from saline flush syringe and unclamp lumen.
   - Aspirate for blood return, using very little force, to check lumen patency and placement.
   - Instill 5 mL of solution in a 10-mL syringe to flush the catheter thoroughly.
   - Maintain positive pressure when withdrawing syringe by clamping catheter before removing syringe or by maintaining pressure on syringe plunger before you clamp or use the CLC2000 positive-pressure cap.
   - Swab access port again with antimicrobial swabs.
6. Change the solution container to the TPN solution ordered.
   - Ensure that the tubing has an in-line filter connected at the end of the TPN tubing. For plain TPN, use a 0.22-micron filter. For TPN with lipids, the filter must be 1.2 microns ❶. Plain lipids are infused without a filter. **Rationale:** *The filter traps bacteria and particles that can form in the TPN solution.*
   - Attach and connect the tubing to an infusion pump. **Rationale:** *A pump eliminates the changes in flow rate that occur with alterations in the patient's activity and position.*

(continued on next page)

SKILL 10.14 Total Parenteral Nutrition (TPN), IV Infusion: Providing (*continued*)

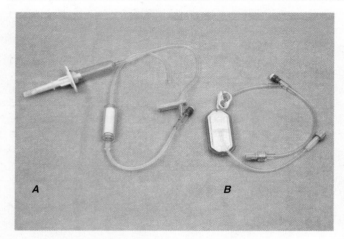

Source: Patrick Watson/Pearson Education, Inc.

❶ **A,** A 0.22-micron filter used for total parenteral nutrition (TPN); **B,** A 1.2-micron filter for use with TPN-containing lipids.

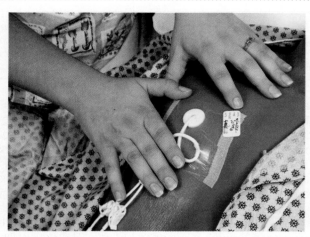

Source: Donna J. Duell

❸ Nontunneled catheter used to deliver parenteral nutrition.

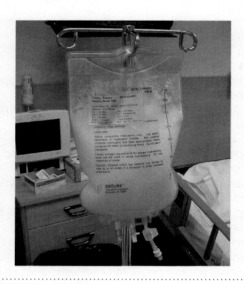

❷ Total parenteral nutrition.

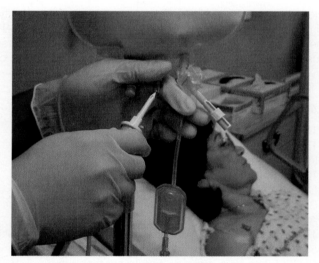

Source: Ronald May/Pearson Education, Inc.

❹ In-line filter used when administering TPN solution.

- Attach the TPN solution to the IV administration tubing ❷ ❸ ❹. If a multiple-lumen tube is in place, attach the infusion to the dedicated and TPN-labeled lumen.
- If lipids are being infused separately from the TPN, connect the lipid tubing to the injection port closest to the patient (below the TPN filter).
7. Regulate and monitor the flow rate.
   - Establish the prescribed rate of flow and monitor the infusion at least every 30 min.
   - Never accelerate an infusion that has fallen behind schedule. **Rationale:** *Wide fluctuations in blood glucose can occur if the rate of TPN infusion is irregular.*

- Never interrupt or discontinue the infusion abruptly. If TPN solution is temporarily unavailable, infuse a solution containing at least 5–10% dextrose. **Rationale:** *This prevents rebound hypoglycemia.*
- During the initial stage of a lipid infusion (i.e., the first hour), closely monitor vital signs and signs of any side effects (e.g., fever, flushing, diaphoresis, dyspnea, cyanosis, headache, nausea, or vomiting).
- Start lipid infusions very slowly according to the healthcare provider's orders, the manufacturer's directions, and facility policy. For a 10% emulsion, start at 1 mL/min for the first 5 minutes, then up to 4 mL/min for the

SKILL 10.14   Total Parenteral Nutrition (TPN), IV Infusion: Providing (*continued*)

next 25 minutes. If well tolerated, set ordered rate thereafter.

8. Monitor the patient for complications.
   - Change the administration set and filter every 24 hr.
   - Monitor the vital signs every 4 hr. If fever or abnormal vital signs occur, notify the healthcare provider. **Rationale:** *An elevated temperature is one of the earliest indications of catheter-related sepsis.*
   - Collect double-voided urine specimens in accordance with facility policy, and test the urine for specific gravity. If the specific gravity is abnormal, notify the healthcare provider, who may alter the constituents of the TPN solution.
   - Assess capillary (fingerstick) blood glucose levels every 6 hr according to facility protocol. **Rationale:** *Blood glucose is tested to make certain the infusion is not running too rapidly for the body to metabolize glucose or too slowly for caloric needs to be met.* Notify the healthcare provider of abnormal glucose levels. For hyperglycemia, supplementary insulin may be ordered subcutaneously or added directly to the TPN solution. For hypoglycemia, the infusion rate may need to be increased.
   - Measure the daily fluid intake and output and calorie intake. **Rationale:** *Precise replacement for fluid and electrolyte deficits can then be more readily determined.*
   - Monitor the results of laboratory tests (e.g., serum electrolytes and blood urea nitrogen) and report abnormal findings to the healthcare provider.

9. Assess weight and anthropometric measurements.
   - Weigh the patient daily, at the same time and in the same garments. A gain of more than 0.5 kg (1.1 lb) per day indicates fluid excess and should be reported.
   - Measure arm circumference and triceps skinfold thickness weekly or in accordance with facility protocol to assess the physical changes.

10. When the procedure is complete, perform hand hygiene and leave patient safe and comfortable.

11. Complete documentation using forms, checklists, or electronic dropdown lists supplemented by nurse's notes or additional comments as appropriate, including the type and amount of TPN infusion, rate of infusion, vital signs every 4 hr, fingerstick blood glucose levels as ordered, patient's weight daily, and anthropometric measurements.

SAMPLE DOCUMENTATION

[date] 2030 Awake and alert. Central line single lumen non-tunneled site right chest dressing dry and intact. TPN solution hung and connected to infusion pump. Lumen checked for patency, blood flashback obtained then flushed with 5 mL saline using a 10-mL syringe without complication. TPN IV line connected to access needleless connector, IV tubing unclamped, IV infusion pump set at 75 mL/hr as ordered. Tolerated procedure without incident. *K. Tuner*

Safety Considerations

- TPN and lipids are frequently infused together in the same bottle to prevent microorganism growth from lipid emulsion.
- Do not "catch up" a deficit in infused volume. Doing so could result in complications for the patient. To ensure constant flow rate, check rate every 2 hr.
- No medication or blood products are to be added or piggybacked into a TPN line.
- No blood specimen should be withdrawn from an IV line infusing TPN.
- TPN is never stopped abruptly. It should be tapered off.

≫ Critical Thinking Options for Unexpected Outcomes

Not all unexpected outcomes require further nursing intervention; however, many times they do. When the patient demonstrates a change in signs/symptoms indicating an emerging problem, the nurse should immediately assess and troubleshoot what is happening. The assessment data must be processed quickly to formulate a hypothesis so the nurse can make a clinical judgment. The nurse then decides how best to resolve the problem and improve the patient's situation for a better outcome.

EXPECTED OUTCOME	UNEXPECTED OUTCOME	POSSIBLE INTERVENTIONS
Healthy Eating Habits Patient's nutritional needs are met with a balanced diet appropriate for developmental age.	Patient is nauseated and vomits.	■ Withhold food if patient is nauseated or vomiting. ■ Provide antiemetic or patient's preferred comfort measures (cold cloth to throat, soda drink). ■ Identify potential source for nausea: specific foods or odors, experience of pain, side effects of medication (e.g., morphine sulfate), or positional changes.
	Older patient with visual impairment only eats food on one half of food tray.	■ Patient may have homonymous hemianopia due to cerebrovascular accident (CVA) and is unable to see the half of the tray on the paralyzed side. ■ Move food tray so that ignored side is within patient's restricted range of vision (move tray leftward if patient has had a left CVA and right side of tray has been ignored). ■ Encourage patient to turn head so that patient's visual field includes the half of tray with food that has not been seen or eaten.
Patient experiences no complications while consuming nutrients.	Patient has signs of aspirating food (coughing, hoarseness, noisy breathing).	■ Request speech pathologist consult for swallow evaluation. ■ Ensure that caregivers are following individualized feeding instructions/precautions (e.g., patient positioning, use of thickening agents, avoiding use of straws). ■ Remind patient not to talk while eating and to concentrate on swallowing.
Enteral Nutrition Using a Feeding Tube Patient's nutritional needs are met with nasogastric (NG) feeding.	NG tube feedings are delayed/skipped due to large residual volumes.	■ Assess for adequate GI function (no abdominal distention; no nausea or vomiting; presence of flatus, bowel movement). If residual is less than or equal to 500 mL, continue feeding, but closely monitor patient's response. ■ Change to continuous rather than intermittent feeding. ■ Continue measures to prevent aspiration. ■ Consider postpyloric feeding.
Patient experiences no complications with NG feeding.	Patient develops diarrhea with enteral feeding.	■ Use closed system if possible to prevent contamination. ■ Don clean gloves when setting up or opening system; use sterile technique if patient is immunocompromised or critically ill. ■ Flush bag before refilling with formula. ■ Use prepackaged, ready-to-use sterile feeding formulas. If using open system, cover, label, and refrigerate unused formula and discard in 24 hr. ■ Lower height of the feeding bag or syringe to slow down the rate of feeding. ■ Disinfect ports before and after any handling. ■ Consult dietitian about osmolarity of formula (hyperosmolar or high-fiber formula may cause diarrhea).
Patient's nutritional needs are met with continuous enteral feeding.	Small-bore feeding tube fails to advance into duodenum.	■ Determine if gastric feeding is acceptable (patient does not have gastroparesis, reflux esophagitis, high risk for aspiration, absence of gag or cough reflex). ■ Administer prokinetic agent before rather than after tube insertion. ■ Suggest tube be advanced under fluoroscopy.
Gastrostomy tube site is free of signs of irritation/inflammation.	Gastrostomy tube site becomes irritated.	■ Apply plain antacid (e.g., Mylanta) as ordered to area if condition is mild. ■ Use skin prep barrier followed by antifungal powder followed by skin prep barrier. ■ Request tube with external bar or disc be replaced with plain tube that is sutured into place (bars and discs may embed into skin).
Parenteral Nutrition Using Intravenous Infusion Parenteral nutrients provided without complications or adverse effects.	Patient develops dyspnea, cyanosis, or allergic reaction, such as nausea, vomiting, increased temperature, or headache.	■ Stop infusion immediately, and notify healthcare provider.
	Patient develops hyperlipidemia or hypercoagulability.	■ Monitor laboratory results, particularly liver function tests, and notify healthcare provider when any abnormality occurs.
Adequate calories and essential fatty acids are provided to patients unable to ingest orally.	Patient's serum triglyceride and liver function test results remain elevated.	■ Continue IV lipid infusion. ■ Begin the feeding with a weaker concentration of formula, and increase the concentration slowly as ordered. ■ Repeat lab values.
Lipids infuse within time frame.	Patient experiences side effects and cannot continue with lipid infusion.	■ Reassess patient's ability to tolerate fat solution. ■ Notify healthcare provider for order to discontinue fat solution, and administer hyperalimentation solution. ■ Monitor liver function test results.

REVIEW Questions

1. A client with chronic renal failure who weighs 165 lb is prescribed a diet that limits protein to 0.6 g/kg/day. How many grams of protein per day should the nurse instruct this client to consume?
   _____ grams/day

2. The nurse instructs a client with cardiovascular disease on a prescribed low-fat diet. Which food choice indicates that the client would benefit from additional teaching?
   1. Snack bag of almonds
   2. Cream of mushroom soup
   3. Whole wheat roll with margarine
   4. Salad with romaine lettuce and olive oil

3. The nurse observes the UAP helping a client with dysphagia to eat breakfast. At which action by the UAP should the nurse intervene?
   1. Asking the client to answer questions while eating
   2. Sitting the client upright in a chair
   3. Placing a towel under the tray
   4. Offering liquids without a straw

4. The nurse provides 240 mL of feeding through a client's gastrostomy tube. What should the nurse do to ensure that the tube remains patent?
   1. Clamp the feeding tube.
   2. Follow the feeding with 60 mL of sterile normal saline.
   3. Position the client upright for 30 minutes after the feeding.
   4. Follow the last amount of feeding with 30 mL of water.

5. The nurse aspirates 200 mL of formula through the nasogastric tube of an older client receiving a continuous feeding. Which health problem should the nurse consider might be affecting the absorption of this client's feeding?
   1. Heart failure
   2. Diverticulitis

3. Diabetes mellitus
4. Parkinson disease

6. After inserting a nasogastric tube, the client is not coughing despite the nurse not being able to auscultate sounds over the epigastric area. What action should the nurse take?
   1. Look inside the client's mouth.
   2. Advance the tube another 5 cm (2 in.).
   3. Place the end of the tube in a container of water.
   4. Remove the tube and insert it through the other naris.

7. While removing a nasogastric tube, the client begins to cough. Which nursing action could have prevented the client's response?
   1. Instilling 50 mL of air into the tube
   2. Flushing the tube before removing it
   3. Placing the client into a side-lying position
   4. Having the client take a deep breath and hold it

8. An adult client is prescribed 500 mL of intralipids to be infused at 1 mL/min for 15 min and then 2 mL/min for the remainder of the infusion. If the infusion is started at 1000 hours, when should the nurse expect to discontinue the infusion?
   1. 1200 hours
   2. 1400 hours
   3. 1600 hours
   4. 1800 hours

9. The nurse notices that a client's infusion of total parenteral nutrition (TPN) has less than 100 mL remaining even though the pump was programmed to infuse at a much slower rate. What should the nurse do first?
   1. Stop the infusion.
   2. Weigh the client.
   3. Measure capillary blood glucose.
   4. Place an infusion bag of normal saline at the bedside.

Note: For answers and rationales for the review questions, go to Appendix A or your Pearson MyLab Nursing and eText.

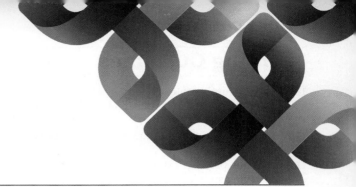

Chapter 11
Oxygenation

Chapter at a Glance

❶ Nursing students may observe or assist with the following skills only with faculty permission and while under direct supervision of faculty or another RN.

» The Concept of Oxygenation

Oxygenation refers to the process of supplying oxygen to the body. Oxygenation is assessed by using a pulse oximeter and arterial blood gases. *Ventilation* refers to the mechanics of moving air in and out of the body, inhaling oxygen and exhaling carbon dioxide. Ventilation is assessed by chest movement, auscultation of breath sounds, compliance of the lungs when expanding, and the respiratory rate. Both of these respiratory physiological processes are essential in providing oxygen necessary to perform cellular activities and remove carbon dioxide waste. The circulatory system transports oxygen to body cells and carbon dioxide away from them. Oxygen is transported dissolved in the blood and by chemical combination with hemoglobin in red blood cells. Supplemental oxygen is used when normal lung function is reduced and patients do not get enough oxygen naturally in acute and chronic conditions. Supplemental oxygen can be delivered by several methods and devices, depending on the percentage of oxygen needed. Other breathing treatments that provide assisted breathing are continuous positive airway pressure (CPAP) and bilevel positive airway pressure (Bi-PAP). Priority consideration for oxygenation is airway management. Artificial airways may be used to facilitate air passage to and from the lungs. Nurses collaborate with respiratory therapists in monitoring oxygen therapy delivery systems and patients receiving oxygen therapy.

Learning Outcomes

11.1 Give examples of teaching points to help a patient expectorate sputum when collecting a specimen in a sputum container.

11.2 Support advantages of having a patient use an incentive spirometer.

11.3 Explain priority safety considerations for the patient receiving supplemental oxygen.

11.4 Summarize five early signs/symptoms of hypoxia.

11.5 Show the sequential steps in opening and maintaining the airway of an unresponsive adult.

11.6 Summarize how to use a bulb syringe to suction a newborn's or infant's nose or mouth to remove secretions.

11.7 Give examples of priority safety measures when providing tracheostomy care.

11.8 Differentiate the significance of seeing continuous bubbling in the suction control chamber and seeing continuous bubbling in the water-seal chamber of a chest tube closed drainage system.

The following feature links some, but not all, of the concepts related to assessment. They are presented in alphabetical order.

Concepts Related to
Oxygenation

CONCEPT	RELATIONSHIP TO OXYGENATION	NURSING IMPLICATIONS
Acid–Base Balance	Respiratory acidosis and alkalosis imbalances	<ul><li>Monitor oxygen saturations with vital signs.</li><li>Support patient with hyperventilation or hypoventilation.</li><li>Maintain open airway.</li></ul>
Cognition	Acute hypoxia can result in decreased cognition and confusion.	<ul><li>Monitor oxygen saturations with vital signs.</li><li>Rule out physical reason for signs and symptoms (S/S).</li><li>Determine the cause of acute hypoxia.</li></ul>
Comfort	Respiratory rate increases with pain and could result in respiratory alkalosis.	<ul><li>Treat pain with ordered medications.</li><li>Encourage patient to slow breathing rate.</li><li>Monitor oxygen saturations and vital signs.</li></ul>
Fluids and Electrolytes	Fluid volume excess can cause lung congestion and impaired gas exchange in lungs.	<ul><li>Monitor intake and output.</li><li>Administer medications as ordered.</li><li>Implement oxygen therapy as ordered.</li><li>Keep HOB high Fowler position.</li></ul>
Safety	Acute hypoxia can cause acute confusion.	<ul><li>Assign someone to stay with patient as needed.</li><li>Encourage patient to call for help to get out of bed.</li><li>Monitor oxygen saturations and vital signs.</li></ul>

Living cells require a consistent supply of oxygen. There are three actions necessary to make this process happen: (1) Air needs to be transported to and from the lungs, so there needs to be a patent airway. (2) Oxygen (O_2) exchange and carbon dioxide (CO_2) exchange need to take place in the lungs. An adequate percentage of O_2 must be breathed in and available to diffuse into the blood, and CO_2 must be breathed out. (3) The O_2 needs to be transported and made available to all body cells by the cardiovascular system.

Most people in good health give little thought to their respiratory function. Changing position frequently, ambulating, and exercising usually maintain adequate ventilation and gas exchange. Many people tend to breathe in a shallow fashion and do not draw air into the lowest regions of the lungs, thus limiting potential gas exchange. This chapter includes interventions to support mechanics of respiration and ventilation.

›› Assessment

Expected Outcomes

1. Patient receives instructions about all specimen collection procedures before they are begun.

2. Specimens are collected following common guidelines and facility procedures.

SKILL 11.1 Nose and Throat Specimen: Collecting

When someone is having upper respiratory symptoms such as a runny nose or throat discomfort when swallowing, secretions are collected from the nose or nasopharyngeal area using a special culture tube and swab for a culture and sensitivity (C&S) lab test. The results usually take 48 hours and help the healthcare provider to decide the best treatment for the symptoms.

Delegation or Assignment

Obtaining nose and throat specimens is an invasive skill that requires the application of scientific knowledge and potential problem solving to ensure patient safety. Therefore, the nurse needs to perform this skill and does not delegate or assign it to the UAP.

Equipment

- Clean gloves
- Two sterile, cotton-tipped swabs in sterile culture tubes with transport medium
- Penlight
- Tongue blade (if swabbing the throat)
- Otoscope with a nasal speculum (optional, not usually used by the generalist nurse)
- Completed label for each specimen container
- Completed laboratory requisition

Preparation

- Review healthcare provider's orders and patient's nursing plan of care.
- Gather needed equipment and supplies.

Procedure

1. Introduce self and verify the patient's identity using two identifiers. Explain to the patient you are going to use a cotton swab to collect secretions from the nose or back of throat (depending on healthcare provider's order), why it is necessary, and how the patient can participate. Discuss how the results will be used in planning further care or treatments. Inform the patient that he may gag while swabbing the throat or feel like sneezing during the swabbing of the nose; however, the procedure will take less than one minute.
2. Perform hand hygiene and observe other appropriate infection control procedures.
3. Provide for patient privacy.
4. Prepare the patient and the equipment:
   - Assist the patient to a sitting position. **Rationale:** *This is the most comfortable position for many people and the one in which the pharynx is most readily visible.*
   - Don gloves if the patient's mucosa will be touched.
   - Open the culture tube and place it on the sterile wrapper. **Rationale:** *This prevents microorganisms from entering the tube.*
   - Remove one sterile applicator and hold it carefully by the stick end, keeping the remainder sterile. The swab end is kept from touching any objects that could contaminate it.

THROAT SPECIMEN

5. Ask the patient to tilt the head back, open the mouth, extend the tongue, and say "ah." **Rationale:** *When the tongue is extended, the pharynx is exposed. Saying "ah" relaxes the throat muscles and helps minimize contraction of the constriction muscle of the pharynx (the gag reflex).*
6. Use a penlight to illuminate the posterior pharynx while depressing the tongue with a tongue blade ❶. Depress the anterior third of the tongue firmly without touching the throat. **Rationale:** *Touching the throat stimulates the gag reflex. Check for inflamed areas.*

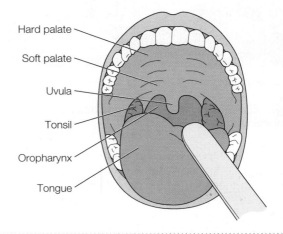

❶ Depressing the tongue to view the pharynx.

7. Insert a swab into the mouth without touching any part of the mouth or tongue.
8. Gently and quickly swab along the tonsils making sure to contact any areas on the pharynx that are particularly erythematous (reddened) or that contain exudates (purulent drainage). **Rationale:** *Rotating the swab where exudate is present may maximize the amount of specimen collected.*
9. Remove the swab without touching the mouth or lips ❷.

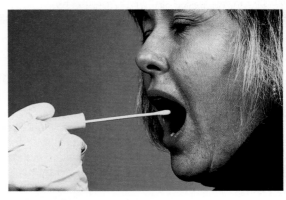

Source: Ronald May/Pearson Education, Inc.

❷ After swabbing throat, remove applicator stick, being careful not to touch any part of the mouth.

(continued on next page)

SKILL 11.1 Nose and Throat Specimen: Collecting (*continued*)

10. Insert the swab into the sterile tube without allowing it to touch the outside of the container ❸. Push the tip of the swab into the liquid medium. Make sure the swab is placed in the correctly labeled tube. **Rationale:** *Touching the outside of the tube could transmit microorganisms to it and then to others.*

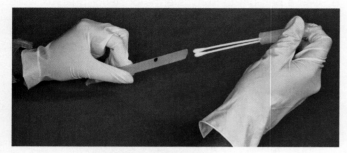

Source: Ronald May/Pearson Education, Inc.

❸ Push applicator stick into specimen tube, being careful not to contaminate stick.

11. Crush the ampule of culture medium at the bottom of the tube. Place the top securely on the tube, taking care not to touch the inside of the cap. **Rationale:** *Touching the inside of the cap could transmit additional microorganisms into the tube.*
12. Repeat the above steps with the second swab and discard the tongue blade in the waste container. Proceed to step 13.

NASAL SPECIMEN

5. Ask the patient to blow her nose to clear her nasal passages. Check nostrils with a penlight to check for patency.
6. Ask the patient to tilt the head back, use the penlight to illuminate the naris.
7. Insert the sterile swab carefully along the septum and the floor of the nose.
8. When the area of mucosa that is reddened or contains exudate is reached, rotate the swab quickly.
9. Remove the swab without touching the nasal passage.

10. Insert the swab into the culture tube.
11. Crush the ampule at the bottom of the tube and push the tip of the swab into the liquid medium.
12. Repeat the above steps for the other naris.
13. Remove and discard gloves. Perform hand hygiene and leave patient safe and comfortable.
14. Label and transport the specimens to the laboratory.
15. When the procedure is complete, perform hand hygiene and leave patient safe and comfortable.
16. Complete documentation using forms, checklists, or electronic dropdown lists supplemented by nurse's notes or additional comments as appropriate including the collection of the nose and/or throat specimens, assessments of the nasal mucosa and pharynx, and any discomfort the patient experienced.

SAMPLE DOCUMENTATION

[date] 1115 Awake and alert, sitting in chair. Swab of throat done. Tolerated without complaint. Mucosa reddened with white pus pockets noted on both swollen tonsils. Specimen to lab for C&S. *G. York*

Lifespan Considerations
NEWBORNS AND INFANTS

- When taking a throat swab on a newborn or infant, avoid occluding the nose because newborns and infants normally breathe only through the nose.

CHILDREN

- Have a parent stand the young child between the parent's legs with the child's back to the parent and the parent's arms gently but firmly around the child. As the parent tips the child's head back, ask the child to open wide and stick the tongue out. Assure the child that the procedure will be over quickly and may "tickle" but should not hurt.

SKILL 11.2 Peak Expiratory Flow Rate: Measuring

The peak expiratory flow rate (PEFR) is the maximum flow rate that occurs during a forced exhalation by an individual. A portable peak flow meter is used to measure the PEFR. Monitoring of PEFR can show trends for several chronic respiratory conditions such as asthma and emphysema, and is used by healthcare providers to make decisions about best treatments for patients.

Delegation or Assignment

PEFR measurement may be delegated or assigned to a trained UAP. The nurse should double check any values found to be abnormal or significantly different from previous results and must

interpret the findings. Modifications in the treatment regimen may not be initiated by the UAP. Note that state laws for UAPs vary, so this task might be assigned to the UAP rather than delegated.

Equipment

- Peak flow meter

Preparation

- Review healthcare provider's orders and patient's nursing plan of care.
- Gather equipment needed.

SKILL 11.2 Peak Expiratory Flow Rate: Measuring (*continued*)

Procedure

1. Introduce self and verify the patient's identity using two identifiers. Explain to the patient you are going to use a peak flow meter to check the patient's peak flow, why it is necessary, and how the patient can participate. Discuss how the results will be used in planning further care or treatments. Normal or expected PEFR is established based on age and size, and a reference chart is included with each peak flow meter. Patients may be taught to use their own individual peak flow meter to anticipate early changes in their condition as part of their self-care plan.
2. Perform hand hygiene and observe other appropriate infection control procedures.
3. Provide for patient privacy.
4. Position the patient. If possible, the patient should be sitting with the chest free from contact with the bed or chair. If not possible, place the patient in semi-Fowler or high-Fowler position.
5. Reset the marker on the flow meter to the zero position ❶.

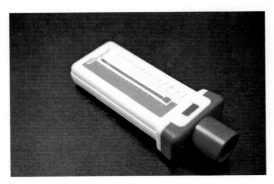

Source: Emmanuel Rogue/MediaforMedical SARL/Alamy Stock Photo

❶ Peak flow meter with marker in the zero position.

6. Assist the patient to use the flow meter.
   - Ask the patient to take a deep breath in ❷.

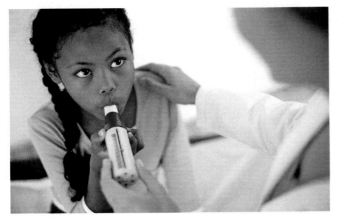

Source: Ian Hooton/Science Photo Library/Alamy Stock Photo

❷ PEFR measurement.

- Patient places the mouthpiece in the mouth with the teeth around the opening and the lips forming a tight seal.
- Have the patient exhale as quickly and forcefully as possible ❸. If you suspect the patient is exhaling a significant amount of air through the nose, apply a nose clip.

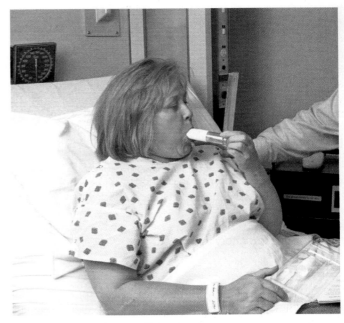

Source: Ronald May/Pearson Education, Inc.

❸ Have patient blow out through mouth as hard and fast as possible—indicator moves up scale to record peak expiratory flow (L/min).

7. Perform step 6 two more times, allowing the patient to rest for 5–10 seconds in between. Record the highest PEFR level achieved.
8. When the procedure is complete, perform hand hygiene and leave patient safe and comfortable.
9. Complete documentation using forms, checklists, or electronic dropdown lists supplemented by nurse's notes or additional comments as appropriate.

SAMPLE DOCUMENTATION

[date] 1412 Sitting in chair with parent beside him. Able to hold peak flow meter with me, asked to blow out the candle really hard as he could, completed the forced expiration without difficulty. PERF is 214 at this time. Tolerated without complaint, cooperative and smiling without respiratory distress noted. *E. Bell*

SKILL 11.3 Sputum Specimen: Collecting

Sputum specimens are obtained with deep coughing by the patient to collect tracheal-bronchial secretions (not just saliva) for a variety of lab diagnostic test such as a culture and sensitivity (C&S) lab analysis.

Delegation or Assignment

The UAP can obtain a sputum specimen that is expectorated by a patient. It is important to instruct the UAP about when to collect the specimen, how to position the patient, and how to correctly collect the specimen. A nurse, not a UAP, obtains a sputum specimen by use of pharyngeal suctioning because this is an invasive, sterile process that requires knowledge application and problem solving. Note that state laws for UAPs vary, so collection of expectorated specimens might be assigned to the UAP rather than delegated.

Equipment

- Sterile specimen container with a cover
- Clean gloves (if assisting the patient)
- Disinfectant and swabs, or liquid soap and water
- Paper towels
- Completed label
- Completed laboratory requisition
- Mouthwash

Preparation

- Review healthcare provider's orders and patient's nursing plan of care.
- Gather the appropriate supplies.

Procedure

1. Introduce self and verify the patient's identity using two identifiers. Explain to the patient what you are going to do, why it is necessary, and how the patient can participate. Discuss how the results will be used in planning further care or treatments. Give the patient the following information and instructions:
   - The purpose of the test, the difference between sputum and saliva, and how to provide the sputum specimen
   - Not to touch the inside of the sputum container or lid
   - To expectorate the sputum directly into the sputum container
   - To keep the outside of the container free of sputum, if possible
   - How to hold a pillow firmly against an abdominal incision if the patient finds it painful to cough
   - The amount of sputum required (usually 4–10 mL [1–2 tsp] of sputum is sufficient for analysis).
2. Perform hand hygiene and observe other appropriate infection control procedures.
3. Provide for patient privacy.
4. Provide necessary assistance to collect the specimen.
   - Assist the patient to a sitting position (e.g., high-Fowler or semi-Fowler position, or on the edge of a bed or in a chair). **Rationale:** *These positions allow maximum lung ventilation and expansion.*

- Ask the patient to hold the sputum cup on the outside, or, for a patient who is not able to do so, put on gloves and hold the cup for the patient.
- Ask the patient to breathe deeply and then cough up secretions ❶. **Rationale:** *A deep inhalation provides sufficient air to force secretions out of the airways and into the pharynx.*
- Hold the sputum cup so that the patient can expectorate into it, making sure that the sputum does not come in contact with the outside of the container.
- Assist the patient to repeat coughing until a sufficient amount of sputum has been collected.
- Cover the container with the lid immediately after the sputum is in the container ❷. **Rationale:** *Covering the container prevents the inadvertent spread of microorganisms to others.*

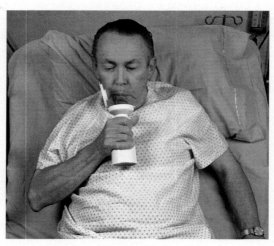

Source: Ronald May/Pearson Education, Inc.

❶ Instruct patient to lift hinged lid of sputum collection system and expectorate directly into sterile container.

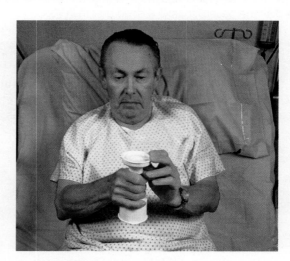

Source: Ronald May/Pearson Education, Inc.

❷ Instruct patient to obtain 1–2 tsp of sputum, close and seal lid of container.

SKILL 11.3 Sputum Specimen: Collecting *(continued)*

- If spillage occurs on the outside of the container, clean the outer surface with a disinfectant. Some agencies recommend washing the outside of all containers with liquid soap and water and then drying with a paper towel.
  - Remove and discard the gloves. Perform hand hygiene.
5. Ensure patient comfort and safety.
  - Assess the patient for respiratory difficulty and provide oxygen per the healthcare provider's orders.
  - Assist the patient in rinsing the mouth with a mouthwash as needed.
  - Assist the patient to a position of comfort that allows maximum lung expansion as required.
6. Label and transport the specimen to the laboratory.
  - Ensure that the specimen label and the laboratory requisition contain the correct information. Attach the label and requisition securely to the specimen.
  - Arrange for the specimen to be sent to the laboratory immediately. **Rationale:** *Bacterial cultures must be started immediately before any contaminating organisms can grow, multiply, and produce false results.*
7. Complete documentation using forms, checklists, or electronic dropdown lists supplemented by nurse's notes or additional comments as appropriate including the amount, color, consistency (e.g., thick, tenacious, watery), evidence of hemoptysis (blood in the sputum), odor of the sputum, any measures needed to obtain the specimen (e.g., postural drainage), any discomfort experienced by the patient, and any interventions implemented to ensure adequate air exchange postprocedure (such as O_2 saturation monitoring or administration of O_2).

SAMPLE DOCUMENTATION

[date] 1310 Sitting on side of bed. Instructed to deep cough and put secretions in container. Specimen in container without difficulty. Productive cough of deep yellow tenacious foul-smelling moderate amount of sputum. Tolerated procedure without SOB but felt fatigued, back to bed resting. Specimen to lab. *C. Jays*

≫ Interventions

Expected Outcomes

1. Promote gas exchange through the use of a sustained maximal inspiration device (incentive spirometer), controlled breathing to sustain maximal expiration (pursed-lip breathing), chest physiotherapy to mobilize secretions, and positioning to support respirations.
2. Encourage breathing exercises to minimize or reverse atelectasis in the lungs.
3. Prevent pulmonary complications for the immediate postoperative patient.
4. Maximize ability of patient with chronic obstructive pulmonary disease (COPD) to maintain airway patency, decrease shortness of breath, control breathing rate, and maximize breathing effectiveness.

When people become ill, their respiratory function may be inhibited because of pain and immobility. The result of inadequate chest expansion is pooling of respiratory secretions, which ultimately harbor microorganisms and promote infection. In addition, shallow respirations may potentiate alveolar collapse, which may cause decreased diffusion of gases and subsequent hypoxemia. This situation is often compounded when opioids are given for pain, because they further depress the rate and depth of respiration.

The semi-Fowler or high-Fowler position allows maximum chest expansion and encourages deeper breaths in patients. The nurse should encourage patients to turn from side to side frequently so that each side of the chest experiences maximum expansion. Sitting in a chair and ambulating also increase lung capacity and encourage deeper breaths.

Patients in respiratory distress must sit up to relieve their dyspnea or labored breathing. This is called the **orthopneic position**, which is an adaptation of the high-Fowler position. Patients will often then lean over their overbed tables (which are raised to a suitable height), sometimes with a pillow for support. A patient in this position can also press the lower part of the chest against the table to help with exhalation. Some patients also sit upright and lean on their arms or elbows. This is called the **tripod position**.

Breathing exercises are frequently indicated for patients with restricted chest expansion, such as people with **chronic obstructive pulmonary disease (COPD)** or patients recovering from thoracic or abdominal surgery. Instructing and encouraging the patient to take deep, sustained breaths is among the safest, most effective, and least expensive strategies for keeping the lungs expanded. **Abdominal (diaphragmatic) breathing** permits deep, full breaths with little effort (see Skill 13.1).

SKILL 11.4 Chest Physiotherapy: Preparing Patient

Chest physiotherapy (CPT) is implemented by physical therapists, respiratory therapists, or nurses to help loosen tracheal-bronchial secretions so they will be more mobile when the patient coughs to move them out of the respiratory tract to be expectorated. The different interventions that can be provided manually or by electronic devices include vibration, percussion, postural drainage, controlled breathing, and controlled coughing.

Delegation or Assignment

Teaching and performing CPT techniques are not delegated or assigned to the UAP. In most healthcare facilities, physical therapists are responsible for providing CPT to the patient. Assessment and evaluation of effectiveness of CPT is the responsibility of the nurse and respiratory therapist. The nurse instructs the UAP to report patient observations to the nurse for follow-up.

Equipment

- Hospital bed or other surface to place patient in head-down position
- Gown or towel (optional)
- Tissues
- Container for sputum
- Clean gloves
- Stethoscope
- Pulse oximeter (if indicated)
- Mouthwash/oral hygiene product

Preparation

- Review healthcare provider's orders for CPT and patient's nursing plan of care.
- Schedule CPT to be administered before or at least two hours after meals to prevent vomiting.
- Establish the location of lung segments if the entire lung field is to undergo CPT ❶. **Rationale:** *Usually, the lower areas are the most affected.*

Procedure

1. Introduce self and verify the patient's identity using two identifiers. Explain to the patient what chest physiotherapy is, why it is necessary, and how the patient can participate. Discuss how the results will be used in planning further care or treatments. Many times family members learn the techniques of CPT ❷ ❸ for when the patient is at home.
2. Perform hand hygiene and observe other appropriate infection control procedures.
3. Provide for patient privacy.
4. Auscultate chest for breath sounds and adventitious sounds prior to therapy.

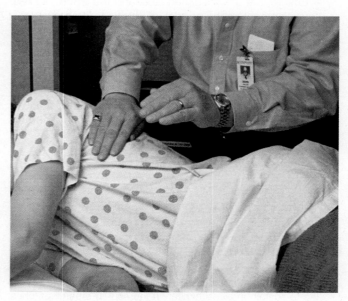

Source: Ronald May/Pearson Education, Inc.

❷ Perform percussion and vibration with each position change.

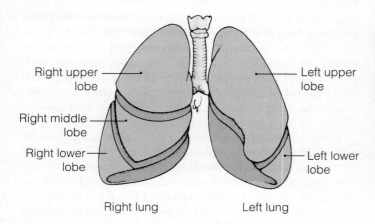

Source: Ronald May/Pearson Education, Inc.

❸ Place hands flat over area to be vibrated, keeping wrist soft.

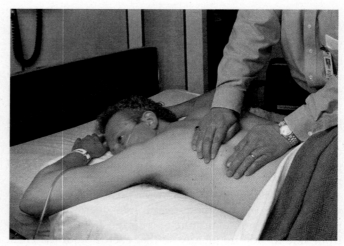

❶ Lobes of the lungs.

SKILL 11.4 Chest Physiotherapy: Preparing Patient (*continued*)

5. Obtain pulse oximetry (SPO$_2$) if indicated before therapy.
6. Collaborate with physical therapist to support best patient outcomes from therapy.
7. Auscultate lungs after therapy. Obtain pulse oximetry if indicated after therapy.
8. Reinforce teaching and techniques of CPT with patient and family.
9. When the procedure is complete, perform hand hygiene and leave patient safe and comfortable.
10. Complete documentation using forms, checklists, or electronic dropdown lists supplemented by nurse's notes or additional comments as appropriate.

SAMPLE DOCUMENTATION

[date] 0925 Sitting on side of bed. Lung sounds mix of gurgles and wheezing left lower side. O$_2$ Saturation 93% room air. Physical therapy here to do CPT maneuvers with patient. Wife in room observing. Productive cough for large amount yellow-green thick sputum. Rest period × 10 minutes then able to proceed. Lung sounds remain with mix of gurgles and wheezing left lower side, O$_2$ Saturation 94% room air. No complaints or SOB noted. *R. Roy*

SKILL 11.5 Incentive Spirometer: Using

The incentive spirometer is a device that helps patients take long, slow, deep breaths, much like with yawning or sighing. Deep breathing helps to expand the lungs fuller to prevent complications like pneumonia in patients that are not as active as usual due to illness or surgery.

Delegation or Assignment

The nurse is responsible for teaching patients how to use an incentive spirometer, assessing the patient's performance, and evaluating the outcomes of the therapy. The UAP, however, can reinforce and assist patients in using the incentive spirometer. The nurse should inform the UAP of the key points to using the incentive spirometer correctly. Note that state laws for UAPs vary, so this task might be assigned to the UAP rather than delegated.

Equipment

- Flow-oriented or volume-oriented incentive spirometer (sustained maximal inspiration [SMI] device)
- Mouthpiece or breathing tube
- Label for mouthpiece
- Progress chart
- Nose clip (optional)

Preparation

- Review healthcare provider's orders and patient's nursing plan of care.
- This skill should not be performed immediately after a meal or other physically stressful activity.

Procedure

1. Introduce self and verify the patient's identity using two identifiers. Explain to the patient what you are going to do, why it is necessary, and how the patient can participate. Discuss how the results will be used in planning further care or treatments.
2. Perform hand hygiene and observe other appropriate infection control procedures.
3. Provide for patient privacy.
4. Prepare the patient.
   - Assist the patient to an upright position in bed or on a chair. If the person is unable to assume a sitting position for a flow spirometer, have the person assume any position. **Rationale:** *A sitting position facilitates maximum ventilation of the lungs.*

FLOW-ORIENTED

Instruct the patient to use the spirometer as follows:

5. Hold the spirometer in the upright position. **Rationale:** *A tilted spirometer requires less effort to raise the balls or disks; a volume-oriented device will not function correctly unless upright.*
6. Exhale normally.
7. Seal the lips tightly around the mouthpiece, ❶ take in a slow deep breath to elevate the balls, and then hold the breath for 2 seconds initially, increasing to 6 seconds (optimum) to keep the balls elevated if possible.
8. Instruct the patient to *avoid* brisk low-volume breaths that snap the balls to the top of the chamber. The patient may use a nose clip if the person has difficulty breathing only through the mouth. **Rationale:** *A slow, deep breath ensures maximal ventilation. Greater lung expansion is achieved with a very slow inspiration than with a brisk shallow breath. Sustained elevation of the balls ensures adequate ventilation of the alveoli (lung air sacs).*
9. Have patient remove the mouthpiece and exhale normally.
10. Teach patient to cough productively, as needed, after using the spirometer. **Rationale:** *Deep ventilation may loosen secretions and stimulate coughing. Effective coughing can facilitate the removal of the loose secretions.*
11. Tell patient to relax and take several normal breaths before using the spirometer again.
12. Have patient repeat the procedure for a total of 10 breaths, encouraging the patient to take progressively deeper breaths up to the maximal goal.

(*continued on next page*)

SKILL 11.5 Incentive Spirometer: Using *(continued)*

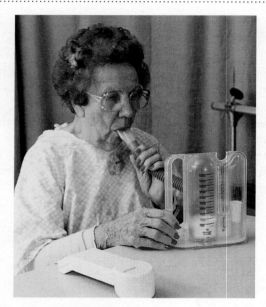

Source: Ronald May/Pearson Education, Inc.

❶ Patient places mouth tightly around mouthpiece and inhales slowly, while watching yellow flow rate indicator, to promote lung expansion.

13. Repeat series of breaths once each hour while awake. **Rationale:** *Practice increases inspiratory volume, maintains alveolar ventilation, and prevents atelectasis (collapse of the air sacs).* Proceed to step 14.

VOLUME-ORIENTED

5. Verify the spirometer is set to "target" volume. **Rationale:** *This provides an incentive and motivation for the patient. The nurse can start low and increase the "target" after patient success.*
6. Instruct the patient to exhale normally.
7. Have patient seal the lips tightly around the mouthpiece and take in a slow, deep breath until the piston is elevated to the predetermined level. The piston level may be visible to the patient to identify the volume obtained.
8. Instruct to hold the breath for 6 seconds to ensure maximal alveolar ventilation.
9. Have patient remove the mouthpiece and exhale normally.
10. Encourage patient to cough productively, as needed, after using the spirometer. **Rationale:** *Deep ventilation may loosen secretions and stimulate coughing. Effective coughing can facilitate the removal of the loose secretions.*
11. Have patient relax and take several normal breaths before using the spirometer again, then repeat the procedure for a total of 10 breaths. Encourage the patient to take progressively deeper breaths up to the maximal goal.
12. Have patient repeat series of breaths once each hour while awake. **Rationale:** *Practice increases inspiratory volume, maintains alveolar ventilation, and prevents atelectasis.*
13. Encourage the patient to record the top volume achieved at each hour while performing the technique. **Rationale:**

This facilitates cooperation of the patient and assists in evaluating outcomes of the skill.

14. Clean the mouthpiece with water and shake it dry. Label the mouthpiece and a disposable incentive spirometer with the patient's name and leave it at the bedside for the patient to use as prescribed.
15. When the procedure is complete, perform hand hygiene and leave patient safe and comfortable.
16. Complete documentation using forms, checklists, or electronic dropdown lists supplemented by nurse's notes or additional comments as appropriate including type of spirometer, number of breaths taken, volume or flow levels achieved, patient response, and results of auscultation. Also include, when appropriate, patient education and the ability of the patient to perform the procedure without prompting.

SAMPLE DOCUMENTATION

[date] 1030 Coarse rales in RLL. Instructed on use of incentive spirometer (IS). Able to use correctly and raise one ball for 3 seconds. Use of IS stimulated cough, resulting in production of small amount light-colored thick mucus. Encouraged to continue using IS each hour. *S. Lee*

Lifespan Considerations

CHILDREN

- Consider the developmental level of the child when choosing a method to promote breathing exercises. Examples include an incentive spirometer, pinwheels, or other blow toys.
- Use of the incentive spirometer can be presented as a game for young patients. Demonstrate the procedure beforehand and show the child how to take slow, deep breaths.
- Nasal clips may be needed if the younger patient does not understand how to refrain from breathing through the nose.

OLDER ADULTS

- Older adults may have trouble sealing their lips around the mouthpiece of a spirometer because of dentures or a dry mouth.

Patient Teaching

- Ensure the patient knows how to use and clean the incentive spirometer.
- Make certain the patient understands how often to use the incentive spirometer.
- Have the patient demonstrate the use of the incentive spirometer.
- Evaluate the patient's ability to use the incentive spirometer.
- Offer written material to reinforce verbal instructions.

SKILL 11.6 Pursed-Lip Breathing

Pursed-lip breathing helps the patient develop control over breathing. The pursed lips create a resistance to the air flowing out of the lungs, thereby prolonging exhalation and preventing airway collapse by maintaining positive airway pressure. The patient purses the lips as if about to whistle and breathes out slowly and gently, tightening the abdominal muscles to exhale more effectively.

Delegation or Assignment

The UAP can reinforce and assist patients in performing breathing exercises. However, the nurse is responsible for teaching the patient the breathing exercises, evaluating the effectiveness of the teaching, and assessing the outcomes of the breathing exercises (e.g., ease of breathing, effectiveness of cough, breath sounds). Note that state laws for UAPs vary, so this task might be assigned to the UAP rather than delegated.

Equipment

None (although a pillow is optional for splinting an abdominal or thoracic incision)

Preparation

- Review healthcare provider's orders and patient's nursing plan of care.
- Before starting to teach breathing exercises, determine if a surgical incision prevents deep breathing because of pain. If so, administer analgesic medication 30 minutes prior to implementing deep breathing exercises.

Procedure

1. Introduce self and verify the patient's identity using two identifiers. Explain to the patient you are going to teach them pursed-lip breathing, why it is necessary, and how the patient can participate. Discuss how pursed-lip breathing will help respirations, thus preventing respiratory complications.
2. Perform hand hygiene and observe other appropriate infection control procedures.
3. Provide for patient privacy.
4. Assist the patient to assume a comfortable semi-Fowler or sitting position in bed or on a chair.
5. Teach the patient to inhale through the nose and then, pursing lips as if about to whistle, breathe out slowly and gently, making a slow "whooshing" sound without puffing out their cheeks. **Rationale:** *Pursed-lip breathing creates a resistance to air flowing out of the lungs, increases pressure within the bronchi (main air passages), and minimizes collapse of smaller airways, a common problem for people with chronic obstructive pulmonary disease (COPD).*

6. Teach the patient to blow through a straw that is in a cup of water and see how long a bubbling noise can be made.
7. Instruct the patient to inhale deeply through the nose and count to 3.
8. Have the patient concentrate on tightening the abdominal muscles while breathing out slowly and evenly through pursed lips while counting to 7 or until the patient cannot exhale any more. **Rationale:** *Tightening the abdominal muscles and leaning forward helps compress the lungs and enhances effective exhalation.*
9. Teach the patient how to perform pursed-lip breathing while walking: Inhale while taking two steps, then exhale through pursed lips while taking the next four steps.
10. Instruct the patient to use this exercise whenever feeling short of breath and to increase gradually to 5–10 minutes four times a day. **Rationale:** *Regular practice will help the patient do this type of breathing without conscious effort.*
11. When the procedure is complete, perform hand hygiene and leave patient safe and comfortable.
12. Complete documentation using forms, checklists, or electronic dropdown lists supplemented by nurse's notes or additional comments as appropriate.

SAMPLE DOCUMENTATION

[date] 1312 Sitting in chair watching television. Pursed-lip practice time ×10 min. Able to demonstrate how to do pursed-lip breathing exercise. Tolerated without incident. Encouraged to do pursed-lip breathing every couple of hours. *R. Manly*

Patient Teaching

Promoting Healthy Breathing

- Sit straight and stand erect to permit full lung expansion.
- Exercise regularly.
- Breathe through the nose.
- Breathe in to expand the chest fully.
- Do not smoke tobacco products.
- Eliminate or reduce the use of household pesticides and irritating chemical substances.
- Do not incinerate garbage in the house.
- Avoid exposure to secondhand smoke.
- Make sure furnaces, ovens, and wood stoves are correctly ventilated.
- Support a pollution-free environment.

SKILL 11.7 Thoracentesis: Assisting

Normally, only sufficient fluid to lubricate the pleura is present in the pleural cavity. However, excessive fluid can accumulate as a result of injury, infection, or other pathology. In such a case or in the case of pneumothorax, the healthcare provider may perform a thoracentesis to remove the excess fluid or air to ease breathing. Thoracentesis is also performed to introduce chemotherapeutic drugs intrapleurally.

Delegation or Assignment

Assisting with a thoracentesis is not delegated or assigned to the UAP. However, signs and symptoms of problems may be observed during usual care and may be recorded by individuals other than the nurse. Abnormal findings must be validated and interpreted by the nurse.

Equipment

- Disposable preassembled thoracentesis set or gather supplies for thoracentesis separately:
  - Thoracentesis device (self-assembled)
  - Sterile towels, and fenestrated drape
  - Scalpel blade
  - Gauze pads, 4 × 4
  - Injection needles, 22 gauge, 3.81cm (1.5 in.) and 25 gauge, 2.54 cm (1 in.)
  - Luer-Lok syringes, 5 mL, 10 mL, and 60 mL
  - Tubing set with control device
  - Lidocaine 1% for local anesthetic
  - Antiseptic swabs such as 10% povidone-iodine or 2% chlorhexidine gluconate with alcohol
  - Sterile gauze dressing or transparent semipermeable membrane (TSM) dressing
  - Sterile gloves and clean gloves
  - Specimen vials
  - Drainage bag

Preparation

- Review healthcare provider's orders and patient's nursing plan of care.
- Verify signed informed consent for procedure in front of patient's record.
- Review patient's record for allergies.
- Gather equipment and supplies.

Procedure

1. Introduce self to patient and verify the patient's identity using two identifiers. Explain to the patient you are assisting the healthcare provider to do a thoracentesis, why it is necessary, and how the patient can participate. Discuss how the results will be used in planning further care or treatments.
2. Perform hand hygiene and observe appropriate infection control procedures.
3. Provide for patient privacy.
4. Assess the patient's vital signs including O_2 saturation and breath sounds.
5. Assist the patient to assume a position that allows easy access to the intercostal spaces.
   - This is usually a sitting position with the arms above the head, which spreads the ribs and enlarges the intercostal space.
   - Two commonly used positions are one in which the arm is elevated and stretched forward and one in which the patient leans forward over a pillow ❶.

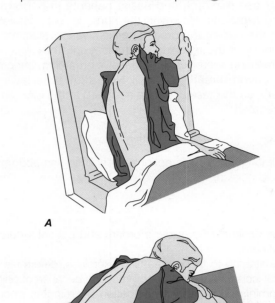

A

B

❶ Two positions commonly used for a thoracentesis: **A,** Sitting on one side with arm held to the front and up; **B,** Sitting and leaning forward over a pillow.

6. To make sure that the needle is inserted below the fluid level when fluid is to be removed (or above any fluid if air is to be removed), the healthcare provider will palpate and percuss the chest and select the exact site for insertion of the needle.
   - A site on the lower chest is often used to remove fluid, ❷ and a site on the upper anterior chest is used to remove air.
   - A chest x-ray prior to the procedure will help pinpoint the best insertion site.
7. The healthcare provider and the assisting nurse follow strict sterile technique.
8. The procedure is as follows:
   - The healthcare provider attaches a syringe and/or stopcock to the aspirating needle. The stopcock must be in the closed position so that no air will enter the pleural space.

SKILL 11.7 Thoracentesis: Assisting (*continued*)

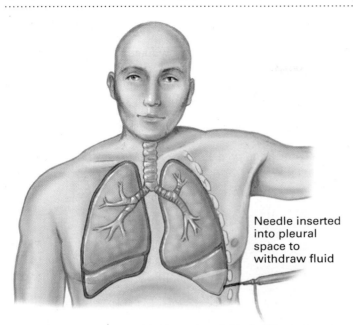

Needle inserted into pleural space to withdraw fluid

Source: From B. Fremgen and S. Frucht. (2013). *Medical Terminology: A Living Language,* 5th ed.

❷ Needle is inserted into the pleural space on the lower posterior chest to withdraw fluid.

- The healthcare provider inserts the needle through the intercostal space to the pleural cavity. In some instances, the healthcare provider threads a small plastic tube through the needle and then withdraws the needle. (The tubing is less likely to puncture the pleura.)
- The nurse monitors the patient for signs of distress.
- If a syringe is used to collect the fluid, the plunger is pulled out to withdraw the pleural fluid as the stopcock is opened.
- If a large container is used to receive the fluid, the tubing is attached from the stopcock to the adapter on the receiving bottle.
- When the adapter and stopcock are opened, gravity allows fluid to drain from the pleural cavity into the container, which should be kept below the level of the patient's lungs.
- After the fluid has been withdrawn, the healthcare provider removes the needle or plastic tubing.
- A small sterile dressing is applied over the puncture site.

- The healthcare provider usually will order a chest x-ray after the procedure.
9. The nurse repositions the patient per facility protocol and continues to monitor the patient.
10. Reassess the patient's vital signs including O_2 saturation and breath sounds.
11. Label the specimen tubes, and send them to the lab with lab request slip.
12. When the procedure is complete, perform hand hygiene and leave patient safe and comfortable.
13. Complete documentation using forms, checklists, or electronic dropdown lists supplemented by nurse's notes or additional comments as appropriate.

SAMPLE DOCUMENTATION

[date] 1335 V/S 134/82, P 88, R 18, T 37.17°C (98.9°F), O_2 saturation 97% room air. Dr. Wick here to do thoracentesis at bedside. Placed in sitting position leaning over bedside table with pillow. Procedure done, tolerated it without complaint, states he can breathe a little easier now. 825 mL light beige-colored slightly cloudy fluid removed, specimen tubes sent to lab. DSD applied to needle insertion site, remains dry and intact. Returned to semi-Fowler position. V/S 142/88, P 86, R 22, T 37.17°C (98.9°F), O_2 saturation 97% room air. Denies pain at this time. *T. Lee*

Lifespan Considerations
OLDER ADULTS

- Some older adults will need help maintaining the proper position due to arthritis, tremors, or weakness.
- Provide support with pillows during the procedure.
- Absence of body fat in older adults can help the healthcare provider locate the intercostal spaces.
- Provide an extra blanket to keep the patient warm during the procedure. Older adults tend to have decreased metabolism and less subcutaneous fat.

» Supplemental Oxygen Therapy

Expected Outcomes

1. Supplemental oxygen is delivered via the most appropriate method to meet individual patient's oxygen needs.
2. Respiratory distress will decrease.
3. Oxygen saturation readings will be stable and appropriate for patient.
4. Patient reports improved sleep pattern when using CPAP/BiPAP.
5. The patient on a mechanical ventilator will not develop ventilator-associated pneumonia.

SKILL 11.8 Oxygen Delivery Systems: Using

Supplemental oxygen is provided to patients who are unable to get enough oxygen from the air they breathe. The oxygen therapy can be delivered in many different ways depending on how much oxygen the patient needs and the physical condition of the patient. There are many respiratory illnesses and diseases throughout all ages that can prevent lungs from being able to supply enough oxygen to meet the patient's needs.

Delegation or Assignment

Initiating the administration of oxygen is considered similar to administering a medication and is not delegated or assigned to the UAP. However, reapplying the oxygen delivery device may be performed by the UAP and observing the patient's response to oxygen therapy can be reported to the nurse. The nurse is responsible for ensuring that the correct amount of oxygen is being delivered to the patient. The nurse collaborates with the respiratory therapist when a patient is receiving oxygen therapy.

Equipment

Nasal Cannula

- Oxygen supply with a flow meter and adapter
- Humidifier with distilled water according to facility protocol if needed
- Nasal cannula and tubing
- Tape (optional)
- Padding for the elastic band (optional)
- Extension tubing and tubing connector (optional)

Face Mask

- Oxygen supply with a flow meter and adapter
- Humidifier with distilled water according to facility protocol
- Prescribed face mask of the appropriate size
- Padding for the elastic band

Face Tent

- Oxygen supply with a flow meter and adapter
- Humidifier with distilled water according to facility protocol
- Face tent of the appropriate size

Preparation

- Review the healthcare provider's orders for oxygen therapy and review patient's nursing plan of care.
- Explain that oxygen is not dangerous when safety precautions are observed. Inform the patient and family about the safety precautions connected with oxygen use.

Procedure

1. Introduce self and verify the patient's identity using two identifiers. Explain to the patient that you (or the respiratory therapist) will start some oxygen, why it is necessary, and how the patient can participate. Discuss how the effects of the oxygen therapy will be used in planning further care or treatments.
2. Perform hand hygiene and observe other appropriate infection control procedures.
3. Provide for patient privacy as needed.

4. Set up the oxygen equipment and the humidifier if needed.
   - Attach the green flow meter to the green oxygen wall outlet or tank ❶. The flow meter should be in the OFF position.
   - If needed, fill the humidifier bottle with tap water per facility policy. (This can be done before coming to the bedside.)
   - Attach the humidifier bottle to the base of the flow meter if used.
   - Attach the prescribed oxygen delivery device and tubing to the flow meter or humidifier.

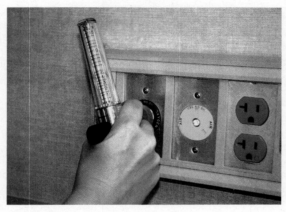

Source: George Draper/Pearson Education, Inc.

❶ Attach the flow meter to the wall outlet.

5. Turn on the oxygen at the prescribed liters per minute (LPM) flow rate, ❷ and ensure proper functioning.
   - Check that the oxygen is flowing freely through the tubing. There should be no kinks in the tubing, and the connections should be airtight. There should be bubbles in the humidifier as the oxygen flows through. You should feel the oxygen at the outlets of the nasal cannula, face mask, or face tent.
6. Apply the oxygen delivery device on the patient.

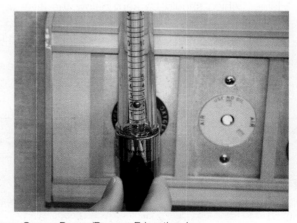

Source: George Draper/Pearson Education, Inc.

❷ This flow meter is set to deliver 2 L/min.

SKILL 11.8 Oxygen Delivery Systems: Using (*continued*)

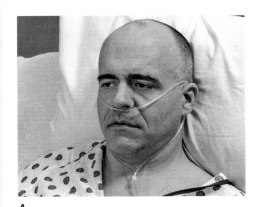

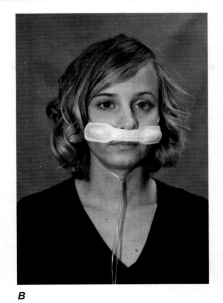

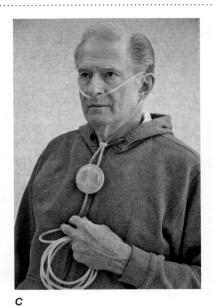

A

B

C

Sources: **A,** Rick Brady/Pearson Education, Inc., **B,** and **C,** Shirlee Snyder

③ *A*, Nasal cannula; *B*, Mustache-style reservoir nasal cannula; *C*, Pendant-style reservoir nasal cannula.

CAUTION! Oxygen is indicated for patients with chronic obstructive pulmonary disease (COPD) but is used conservatively. High levels of oxygen may suppress breathing stimulus, cause hypoventilation and CO_2 retention, and lead to respiratory arrest due to CO_2 narcosis.

NASAL CANNULA

- Adjust the flow meter to 1–6 L/min for low-flow oxygen.
- Put the cannula with the outlet prongs curved downward, fitting into the nares, and the elastic band around the head or the tubing over the ears and under the chin **③**.
- If the cannula will not stay in place, use a short strip of narrow tape to secure it close to the hairline.
- Pad the tubing and elastic band over the ear lobes and cheekbones.
- Assess the patient's nares for encrustations and irritation. Apply a water-soluble lubricant as required to soothe the mucous membranes.
- Assess the top of the patient's ears for any signs of irritation from the cannula strap. If present, padding with a gauze pad may help relieve the discomfort.

CAUTION! Humidification of low-flow oxygen through a nasal cannula is contraindicated because it supports bacterial growth.

- High-flow oxygen nasal cannula
  - A heated humidification system can be added to the high-flow oxygen nasal cannula by the respiratory therapist to prevent upper airways from drying.
  - Assessment of air/oxygen blending in the system ensures that the patient who requires a higher percentage of oxygen has a comfortable and more easily tolerated alternative to a face mask.

SIMPLE FACE MASK

- Covers the patient's nose and mouth. Mask is made of clear, pliable plastic that can be molded to fit the face.
- There are several holes in the sides of the mask (exhalation ports) to allow the escape of exhaled carbon dioxide and intake of room air. To avoid rebreathing of carbon dioxide by the patient while wearing a mask, a minimum 5 L/min oxygen flow rate is required.
- Guide the mask toward the patient's face, and apply it from the nose downward.
- Fit the mask and metal nose bracket to the contours of the patient's face **④**. **Rationale:** *The mask should mold to the face, so that very little oxygen escapes into the eyes or around the cheeks and chin.*

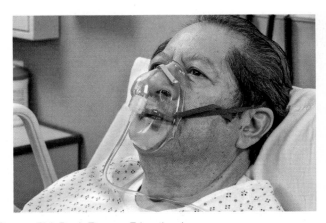

Source: Rick Brady/Pearson Education, Inc.

④ A simple face mask.

(*continued on next page*)

SKILL 11.8 Oxygen Delivery Systems: Using (*continued*)

- Secure the elastic band around the patient's head so that the mask is comfortable but snug.
- Pad the band behind the ears and over bony prominences. **Rationale:** *Padding will prevent irritation from the mask.*

PARTIAL REBREATHER MASK 5

- Delivers oxygen concentrations of 40–60% at liter flows of 6–10 L/min. The oxygen reservoir bag that is attached allows the patient to rebreathe about the first third of the exhaled air in conjunction with oxygen.
- The partial rebreather bag must not totally deflate during inspiration to avoid carbon dioxide buildup. If this problem occurs, the liter flow of oxygen needs to be increased so that the bag remains one third to one half full.

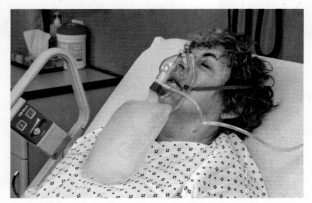

Source: Rick Brady/Pearson Education, Inc.

5 A partial rebreather mask.

NONREBREATHER MASK 6

- Delivers the highest oxygen concentration (95–100%) possible by means other than intubation or mechanical ventilation, at liter flows of 10–15 L/min.

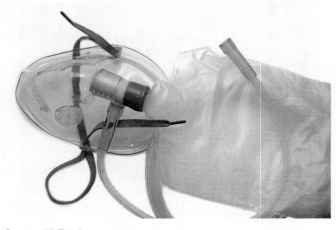

Source: 72/Fotolia

6 A nonrebreather mask.

- Using a nonrebreather mask, the patient breathes only the source gas from the bag.
- One-way valves on the mask and between the reservoir bag and the mask prevent the room air and the patient's exhaled air from entering the bag. In some cases, one of the side valves is removed so that the patient can still inhale room air if the oxygen supply is accidentally cut off.
- To prevent carbon dioxide buildup, the nonrebreather bag must not totally deflate during inspiration. If it does, the nurse can correct this problem by increasing the liter flow of oxygen.

VENTURI FACE MASK 7

- Delivers a prescribed oxygen concentration varying from 24–50% at liter flows of 4–10 L/min.
- The Venturi mask has a section of wide-bore tubing and can have color-coded jet adapters that correspond to a precise oxygen concentration and liter flow. For example, in some cases, a blue adapter delivers a 24% concentration of oxygen at 4 L/min and a green adapter delivers a 35% concentration of oxygen at 8 L/min. However, colors and concentrations may vary by manufacturer, so the equipment must be examined carefully.
- Other manufacturers use a dial for setting the desired concentration. Turning the oxygen source flow rate higher than specified by the equipment manufacturer will not increase the concentration delivered to the patient.

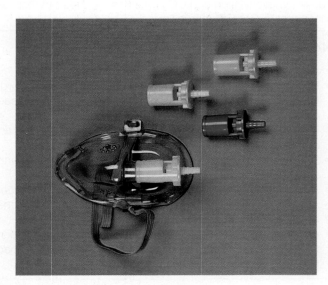

Source: Ronald May/Pearson Education, Inc.

7 Venturi mask with oxygen percent control pieces.

CAUTION!

- Avoid placing SPO_2 clip sensor on the thumb or edematous site. Wrap sensors can be used on the thumb or great toe.
- Avoid extremity with an intra-arterial catheter or noninvasive automatic BP cuff.

SKILL 11.8 Oxygen Delivery Systems: Using (*continued*)

FACE TENT

- Place the tent over the patient's face, and secure the ties around the head.

TRACHEOSTOMY WITH A T-TUBE OR TRACHEOSTOMY COLLAR

- When a patient breathes through a tracheostomy, air is no longer filtered and humidified as it is when passing through the upper airways; therefore, special precautions are necessary.
- Humidity may be provided with a tracheostomy mist collar ⑧. Patients may also wear a stoma protector such as a 4 × 4 gauze held in place with a cotton tie over the stoma or a light scarf to filter air as it enters the tracheostomy.

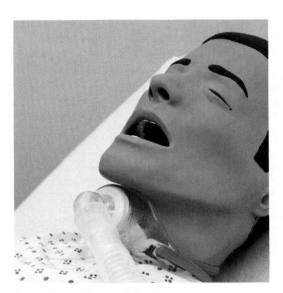

Source: George Draper/Pearson Education, Inc.

⑧ A tracheostomy mist collar.

CONTINUOUS POSITIVE AIRWAY PRESSURE (CPAP) OR BILEVEL POSITIVE AIRWAY PRESSURE (BiPAP)

- CPAP provides a single positive airway pressure to establish a minimal airway value (e.g., 5 mmHg) at the end of exhalation ⑨.
- BiPAP provides two positive airway pressures, one to assist peak pressure on inhalation (e.g., 10 cm H_2O) and a lower one (e.g., 5 cm H_2O) to establish a minimal airway value at the end of exhalation.
- A BiPAP with a rate set feature provides two positive airway pressures and a set respiratory rate to augment breathing for the patient having respiratory insufficiency. This capability qualifies this unit as a *noninvasive mechanical ventilator*. The patient is spared intubation.
- A BiPAP auto-titration device senses and measures the patient's airflow and adjusts its pressure setting automatically to maintain airway patency.

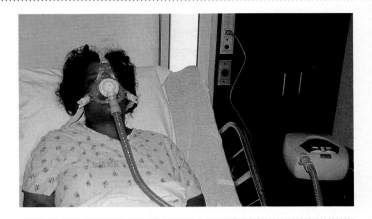

⑨ Patient receiving CPAP via face mask. Machine is capable of CPAP and BiPAP.

- Noninvasive ventilation (NIV) can be used to help some newborns maintain effective breathing with a low expenditure of calories and energy. Continuous positive airway pressure (CPAP) and nasal intermittent positive pressure ventilation (NIPPV) are used in neonate intensive care units (NICUs) as an alternative to intubation and mechanical ventilation.

Safety Considerations

- Patients using CPAP/BiPAP are constantly at risk for aspiration and subsequent respiratory complications. The candidate must be alert and responsive orally, must demonstrate airway protective measures (cough and swallow), and must not be restrained or sedated. Opioids relax the pharynx and contribute further to airway obstruction.
- CPAP/BiPAP should never be used on a sedated patient. There is great danger of aspiration should the patient vomit.

7. When setting up oxygen therapy or just checking it is complete, perform hand hygiene and leave patient safe and comfortable.
8. Complete documentation using forms, checklists, or electronic dropdown lists supplemented by nurse's notes or additional comments as appropriate.

SAMPLE DOCUMENTATION

[date] 0930 Returned from physical therapy c/o SOB. R 26, shallow. P 92, BP 160/98, SPO_2 92% on 3 LPM O_2 via nasal cannula. Skin warm, no cyanosis. Lung sounds clear, no retractions. *P. Isola*

1000 Denies SOB. R 20, P 88, BP 152/92, SPO_2 96% on 3 LPM O_2 via nasal cannula. *P. Isola*

(*continued on next page*)

SKILL 11.8 Oxygen Delivery Systems: Using (*continued*)

Safety Considerations

PATIENT RECEIVING OXYGEN THERAPY

- Inspect the patient's facial skin frequently for dampness or chafing, and dry and treat it as needed.
- Assess the patient regularly.
  - Assess the patient's vital signs (including oxygen saturation), level of anxiety, color, and ease of respirations, and provide support while the patient adjusts to the device.
  - Assess the patient in 15–30 min, depending on the patient's condition, and regularly thereafter.
  - Assess the patient regularly for clinical signs of hypoxia, tachycardia, confusion, dyspnea, restlessness, and cyanosis. Review arterial blood gas results if they are available.
- Inspect the equipment on a regular basis.
  - Check the liter flow and the level of water in the humidifier whenever providing care to the patient.
  - Make sure that safety precautions are being followed.
  - Check the tubing for condensation buildup with humidified oxygen or air. Empty using the trap opening.

Lifespan Considerations

Oxygen Therapy

NEWBORNS AND INFANTS

Oxygen Hood

- An oxygen hood is a rigid plastic dome that encloses a newborn's or infant's head. It provides precise oxygen levels and high humidity.

- The oxygen flow should not be allowed to blow directly into the newborn's or infant's face, and the hood should not rub against the newborn's or infant's neck, chin, or shoulder.

CHILDREN

Oxygen Tent

- An oxygen tent consists of a rectangular, clear, plastic canopy with outlets that connect to an oxygen or compressed air source and to a humidifier that moisturizes the air or oxygen.
- Because the enclosed tent becomes very warm, some type of cooling mechanism such as an ice chamber or a refrigeration unit is provided to maintain the temperature at 20°C–21°C (68°F–70°F).
- Cover the child with a gown or a cotton blanket. Some agencies provide gowns with hoods, or a small towel may be wrapped around the head. **Rationale:** *The child needs protection from chilling and from the dampness and condensation in the tent.*
- Flood the tent with oxygen by setting the flow meter at 15 L/min for about 5 minutes. Then, adjust the flow meter according to orders (e.g., 10–15 L/min). **Rationale:** *Flooding the tent quickly increases the oxygen to the desired level.*
- The tent can deliver approximately 30% oxygen.
- Children may fight having a mask placed on their faces. They are often fearful when placed in oxygen tents or hoods. These are normal responses that vary based on experience, developmental stage, degree of threat to body image, and attachment/abandonment issues. Providing safe toys and a beloved blanket or pillow to hold can help, as can fostering the parent–child bond even though separated by the plastic. Encourage parents to interact with their child around and through the tubing and tent.

SKILL 11.9 Oxygen, Portable Cylinder: Using

Portable O_2 cylinders are green tanks that are pre-filled with oxygen. Because they are small and portable in a small rolling cart, they can supply supplemental oxygen for patients more mobile such as when taking a walk, being transported to another department in the healthcare facility, or anytime patients are away from a wall outlet supply of O_2.

Delegation or Assignment

Changing an empty oxygen cylinder with a full one is usually done by the respiratory therapy department. Some facilities train UAPs to be able to do this task safely. Assisting the patient to ambulate with a portable oxygen tank may be delegated to the UAP. The nurse verifies the correct oxygen flow rate in liters per minute (LPM) and instructs the UAP to report patient observations to the nurse for follow-up. Assessment and evaluation of effectiveness of the exercise remain the responsibility of the nurse. Note that state laws for UAPs vary, so this task might be assigned to the UAP rather than delegated.

Equipment

- Steel cylinder portable oxygen tank
- Regulator/flow meter
- Oxygen delivery tubing

Preparation

- Review healthcare provider's orders and patient's nursing plan of care.
- Take the portable oxygen tank to the patient's room.
- It is a safe practice to check fullness of oxygen tank when preparing to use it to transport a patient or ambulate with the patient needing the oxygen.

Procedure

1. Introduce self to patient and verify the patient's identity using two identifiers. Explain to the patient what you are going to do, why it is necessary, and how the patient can participate. Discuss how the results will be used in planning further care or treatments.
2. Prepare portable oxygen tank by applying the pressure gauge and flowmeter regulating unit ❶.
   - Place oxygen cylinder in carrier in secure upright position ❷. **Rationale:** *If cylinder of compressed air falls accidentally, unit becomes a missile with uncontrollable force and direction.*
   - Using hexagon key, slowly turn cylinder release valve clockwise (left is loose) to crack tank open for a brief

SKILL 11.9 Oxygen, Portable Cylinder: Using (*continued*)

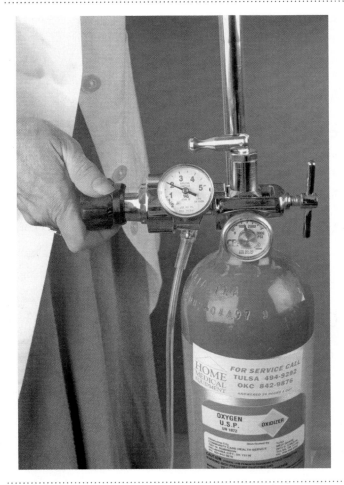

1 Attach regulator to cylinder neck, attach tubing, open cylinder release valve, and adjust oxygen flow rate (LPM) as prescribed.

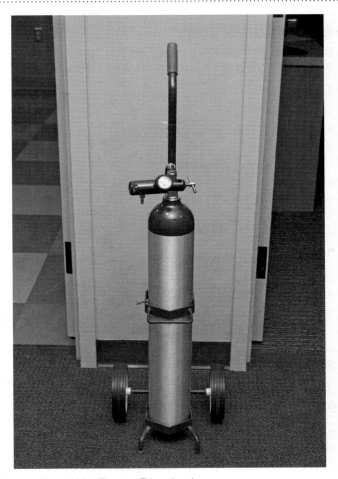

Source: Ronald May/Pearson Education, Inc.

2 Oxygen tank holder with wheels secures oxygen tank, making it portable and easy to maneuver.

period, then close (right to tighten). **Rationale:** *This action removes lint from system.*

- Check pressure gauge on front of tank to determine amount of oxygen pressure in tank. **Rationale:** *Full status is 2200 psi.*
- Attach flowmeter regulator unit over neck of cylinder, aligning pins with green "O" ring openings.
- Use hexagon key to tighten regulator to cylinder neck.
- Connect delivery tubing to "Christmas tree" adapter on regulator unit.
- Open cylinder release valve using hexagon key on top of cylinder. **Rationale:** *This allows oxygen flow.*

3. Perform hand hygiene and observe appropriate infection control procedures.
4. Prepare patient to get up from bed.
5. Slowly open regulator/flowmeter and adjust to prescribed rate of oxygen delivery in liters per minute.
6. Attach oxygen delivery tubing to flowmeter on portable oxygen tank.
7. When patient returns, disconnect oxygen delivery tubing from portable tank flowmeter and connect it back to the wall outlet flowmeter at the ordered LPM oxygen flow rate.

8. When the procedure is complete, perform hand hygiene, leave patient safe and comfortable, and return portable oxygen tank to storage area.
9. Complete documentation using forms, checklists, or electronic dropdown lists supplemented by nurse's notes or additional comments as appropriate.

SAMPLE DOCUMENTATION

[date] 1815 Ready to walk down the hallway and back to room. Portable O_2 tank put on 2 LPM oxygen and patient's oxygen delivery system tubing connected to flowmeter. Walked 30 ft down hallway and back to room. No SOB noted, states she feels tired when returned to room. Tolerated walk with O_2 saturation remaining 95%. Back to bed, delivery system connected back to wall outlet flowmeter at 2 LPM. *W. Jones*

(*continued on next page*)

SKILL 11.9 Oxygen, Portable Cylinder: Using *(continued)*

Safety Considerations

Signs and Symptoms of Hypoxia (SaO$_2$ less than 90% or below desired range for patient's situation)

EARLY SYMPTOMS

- Restlessness
- Headache
- Visual disturbances
- Confusion or change in behavior
- Tachypnea
- Tachycardia
- Hypertension
- Dyspnea
- Anxious face

ADVANCED SYMPTOMS

- Hypotension
- Bradycardia
- Cyanosis
- Metabolic acidosis (production of lactic acid)

CHRONIC HYPOXIA

- Polycythemia
- Clubbing of fingers and toes
- Peripheral edema
- Right-sided heart failure
- Chronic PO$_2$ less than 55 mmHg; O$_2$ saturation less than 87%
- Elevated PCO$_2$ (respiratory acidosis)

SKILL 11.10 Ventilator, Mechanical: Caring for Patient

Safety Note! *During scheduled clinical time, nursing students may have a learning opportunity to observe or assist with this skill only with faculty permission and with direct supervision from faculty or another RN.*

Sometimes patients are unable to mechanically breathe effectively or don't have adequate oxygen available for gas exchange to sufficiently meet the oxygen demands of their bodies to sustain life. Mechanical ventilation can support patients while medical treatments are done to correct the etiology of these conditions or prevent further multiple organ dysfunction.

Delegation or Assignment

UAPs may be delegated or assigned basic care for patients on mechanical ventilation and collect routine data such as vital signs, but they do not adjust ventilator settings or perform sterile procedures such as suctioning. They report any ventilator alarms, but they do not assess the patient or troubleshoot the system. Note that state laws for UAPs vary, so specific tasks might be assigned to the UAP rather than delegated.

Equipment

- Prescribed type of ventilator ❶
- Oxygen source
- Bag–valve–mask (BVM) ventilator system (Ambu bag)
- Suctioning supplies
- Ventilator setting flow sheet and medical record forms or access to the electronic record system
- Stethoscope
- Pulse oximeter and other vital signs monitors
- End-tidal carbon dioxide (ETCO$_2$) colorimetric measuring device, or other system for measuring expired carbon dioxide level

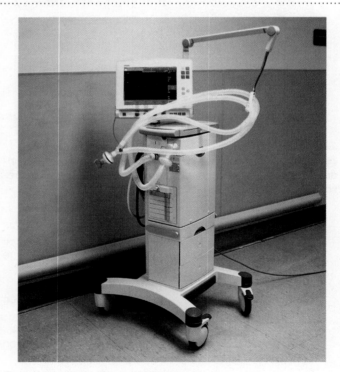

Source: Ronald May/Pearson Education, Inc.

❶ Computerized mechanical ventilator.

Preparation

- Review information about ventilator modes (**Table 11–1 》**).
- Review healthcare provider's orders; review the patient record for serial ABGs results, data indicating the changes that have been made in the patient's ventilator settings over time, and the patient's tolerance of mechanical ventilation.

SKILL 11.10 Ventilator, Mechanical: Caring for Patient *(continued)*

TABLE 11–1 Ventilator Control Modes

Mode	Features
Adaptive support ventilation (ASV)	Inspiratory pressure, inspiratory/expiratory ratio, and mandatory respiratory rate adjusted to maintain target volume and rate
Assist-control (AC)	Set volume with each patient-triggered breath and set rate
Pressure control (PC)	Pressure-limited breath delivered at a set rate
Pressure-regulated volume control (PRVC); adaptive pressure ventilation (APV)	Pressure adjusted to deliver a set tidal volume
Pressure support ventilation (PSV)	Set pressure held during the entire inspiration
Synchronized intermittent mandatory ventilation (SIMV)	Set number of breaths and tidal volume while also allowing the patient to take spontaneous breaths at a patient-determined tidal volume and rate

Procedure

1. Introduce self and verify the patient's identity using two identifiers. Explain to the patient what you are going to do and how the patient can participate. Discuss how the results will be used in planning further care or treatments.
2. Perform hand hygiene and observe other appropriate infection control procedures.
3. Provide for patient privacy as needed.
4. Measure patient temperature, pulse, blood pressure, and oxygen saturation using pulse oximetry. **Rationale:** *Changes in these vital signs may indicate either patient improvement or inadequate ventilation requiring adjustments in ventilator settings.*
5. Arterial blood gases (ABGs) are ordered routinely or only if the patient's condition warrants. Arterial blood may be drawn by the nurse, respiratory therapist, or laboratory technologist, depending on facility policy.
6. Confirm artificial airway tube placement by:
   - Auscultating lungs
   - Measuring ETCO$_2$ at end expiration ❷
   - Checking the most recent chest x-ray for tube position.

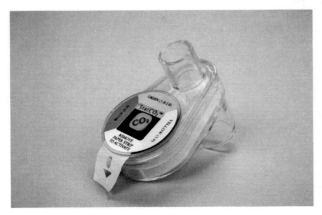

Source: Rick Brady/Pearson Education, Inc.

❷ End-tidal CO$_2$ Colorimetric measuring device.

7. Check the endotracheal tube (ETT) for proper cuff inflation. **Rationale:** *Proper cuff inflation helps prevent ventilator-associated pneumonia (VAP) by ensuring that secretions that collect above the cuff cannot leak down into the lungs.*
8. Suction the patient if indicated. Use the bag–valve–mask (BVM) device to hyperventilate the patient as indicated.
9. Once you have confirmed that the patient's status does not require immediate intervention, examine the ventilator equipment and settings.
   - Tubing from the airway to the ventilator should be secured so it does not pull on the patient's airway. This includes having adequate slack to allow the patient to turn without pulling on the tubing.
   - Verify that ventilator settings are as ordered ❸.
   - Verify that ventilator alarms are set correctly and are active.
   - Check for condensation in the tubing. If condensation is present, empty it appropriately and discard. Never empty fluid back into the humidifier, and use care that the fluid cannot run into the patient's airway. **Rationale:** *Liquid in the tubing may be contaminated.* Refill the humidifier if needed.

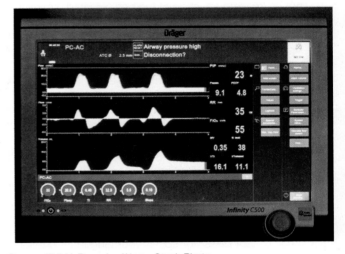

Source: ZUMA Press Inc/Alamy Stock Photo

❸ Verify the ventilator settings and patient data frequently.

10. Provide oral care every 2 hours. Brush the teeth using a toothbrush and toothpaste at least twice per day.
    - Use a Yankauer suction tip to suction the mouth.
    - Some ETTs have a lumen above the cuff to allow for continuous suction of secretions that could collect there.
    - If the patient has an oral endotracheal airway, it can be moved and resecured to the opposite side of the mouth every 24 hours. **Rationale:** *This minimizes pressure on lips and oral mucosa.* Recheck that the tube is correctly positioned after such a move.

(continued on next page)

SKILL 11.10 Ventilator, Mechanical: Caring for Patient (*continued*)

11. Administer medications as ordered to prevent complications of mechanical ventilation. For example, administer histamine receptor inhibitors to prevent gastric ulcers.

12. Administer pain or sedation medications as needed for comfort and to help keep the patient in sync with the ventilator.

Safety Considerations

Paralytic agents have no effect on wakefulness or sensory perception, including perception of pain. With complete paralysis, pain might be manifested as increased heart rate, increased blood pressure, or sweating. Never assume that a patient receiving a paralytic agent is asleep. Continually inform patient about care, offer reassurance, and provide pain relief while the paralyzing effect of the drug persists.

The use of sedatives in mechanically ventilated patients prolongs duration of mechanical ventilation as well as length of hospitalization and ICU stay.

13. Institute actions to decrease complications such as deep venous thrombosis that may result from immobility related to the ventilator.
    - Perform range-of-motion (ROM) exercises.
    - Assist the patient to change positions at least every 2 hours, keeping the head of the bed elevated a minimum of 30 degrees.
    - Assist the patient to stand or sit in a chair as tolerated.
    - Apply sequential compression devices to lower limbs according to facility policy.
    - If the patient has a tracheostomy and is able to eat, encourage adequate intake of fluids and dietary fiber to promote gastrointestinal motility. For patients with an ETT, enteral feedings through a gastric tube are preferred over parenteral nutrition.
    - Administer prophylactic anticoagulant medications according to facility policy.

14. Establish an effective method of communicating with the intubated patient.
    - Explain everything you are doing.
    - If the patient requires eyeglasses, make them available.
    - If the patient does not speak your language, provide a translator.
    - Ask yes/no questions when possible. Ask the patient to nod the head if she agrees. Hand signals can also be used. Be sure to allow adequate time for the patient to respond.
    - If the patient is able to write, provide a writing pad or slate.
    - Be sure that the call light or bell is within reach at all times.
    - Acknowledge signs of frustration and attempt to determine and resolve the cause.

15. When intervention is complete, perform hand hygiene and leave patient safe and comfortable.

16. Document the ventilator settings and patient parameters using checklists, flowcharts, and narrative notes as appropriate. Include results of settings changes, suctioning, activity, physical assessments, and laboratory data.

SAMPLE DOCUMENTATION

(Note that vital signs and ventilator settings would be recorded on flow sheets.)

[date] 1530 ETT remains in place and secured, $ETCO_2$ 3%. Lungs clear to auscultation. Oral care provided. No signs of oral trauma or infection. Skin warm, no cyanosis. Active ROM all extremities. Turned to left side, HOB @ 30 degrees. Skin dry & intact. No bowel sounds. Compression devices in place both calves. Indicates pain is 5 on scale of 0 to 10 by holding up fingers. Medicated IV with immediate reduction to pain level of 3. Family in to visit. *T. Kourza*

Lifespan Considerations

NEWBORNS, INFANTS, AND CHILDREN

- Mechanical ventilation is used for children both in hospitals and in the home. Include the parents and other lay caregivers in all teaching and care instructions.
- When the child's condition is stable, provide age-appropriate activities such as play, art, and educational opportunities.

OLDER ADULTS

- Older patients may be at greater risk for oxygen toxicity, especially if they have chronic lung conditions. As with all patients, the lowest effective oxygen concentration should be used.
- Provide reassurance and emotional support, recognizing that the need for ongoing mechanical ventilation may be viewed by the patient or family as a sign of deteriorating health and movement toward death.

Patient Teaching

Long-term mechanical ventilation in the home is commonplace in many communities.

- Teach caregivers all of the interventions, emergency, and safety measures needed to provide effective patient assistance.
- Ensure caregivers know how to contact local emergency agencies to inform them that a ventilator-dependent patient is in the home.
- Ensure caregivers know what to do if a backup power source is needed to run the ventilator should standard power be interrupted.
- Provide community resources for obtaining needed equipment and disposal of biohazard waste.
- Ensure family has extra supplies that might be needed in an emergency such as a bag and mask system.
- Provide family information about securing a touch-button voice system that allows English or non-English-speaking patients on mechanical ventilation to tap a touch screen that delivers preprogrammed audible words, phrases, or symbols to hold two-way communication with staff.

SKILL 11.10 Ventilator, Mechanical: Caring for Patient (*continued*)

Safety Considerations

Preventing Ventilator-Associated Pneumonia (VAP)

Preventing VAP is an important nursing goal. Patients who develop VAP have a significantly greater mortality rate than those patients who do not develop this infection. The Centers for Disease Control and Prevention (2015) describes interventions that can significantly reduce VAP in the Safe Care Campaign program (CDC, 2015).

Interventions to prevent or decrease VAP include the following:

- Maintain rigorous hand hygiene before and after touching the patient or the ventilator
- Maintain the head of the bed at least at 45 degrees unless contra-indicated
- Check the patient's ability to breathe on his own every day so that the patient can be taken off the ventilator as soon as possible
- Peptic ulcer disease medication prevention
- Prevention measures for deep venous thrombosis.

>> Maintaining a Patent Airway

Expected Outcomes

1. As needed, appropriate artificial airway will be used to maintain patency of patient's airway.
2. Secretions are removed via appropriate suctioning method without complications.
3. The least invasive method of suctioning will be used to meet individual patient's need for a clear airway.

SKILL 11.11 Airway, Nasopharyngeal: Inserting

Safety Note! *During scheduled clinical time, nursing students may have a learning opportunity to observe or assist with this skill only with faculty permission and with direct supervision from faculty or another RN.*

An artificial airway is inserted into the nostril of an unresponsive patient who is not tolerating an oropharyngeal airway because of an active gag reflex or there is an inability to insert the oropharyngeal airway safely. It should not be used in a patient with significant head or facial trauma.

Delegation or Assignment

The initial insertion of a nasopharyngeal airway is not delegated or assigned to the UAP. In some states, a trained UAP may help to maintain the position of the nasopharyngeal airway. Assessment and evaluation of effectiveness of the procedure remain the responsibility of the nurse.

Equipment

- Correct size of flexible nasopharyngeal airway
- Water-soluble lubricant
- Clean gloves
- Pen light
- Suctioning set-up readily available

Preparation

- Review healthcare provider's orders and patient's nursing plan of care.
- Assess patency of patient's airway to determine need for nasopharyngeal airway and state of consciousness.
- Gather equipment and supplies.

Procedure

1. Introduce self and verify the patient's identity using two identifiers. Explain to the patient you are going to insert a nasopharyngeal airway, why it is necessary, and how the patient can participate. Discuss how the results will be used in planning further care or treatments. Patient may be unconscious or semiconscious so verbal explanation about procedure is given to the patient.
2. Select appropriate size tube (length from tip of nose to earlobe and lumen slightly narrower than patient's naris) ❶.

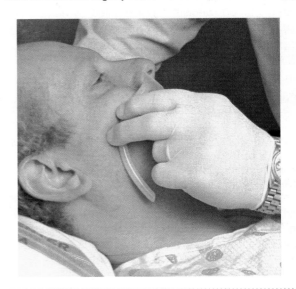

❶ Nasal trumpet protects airway from repeated trauma with upper airway (nasopharyngeal) suctioning.

(*continued on next page*)

SKILL 11.11 Airway, Nasopharyngeal: Inserting (*continued*)

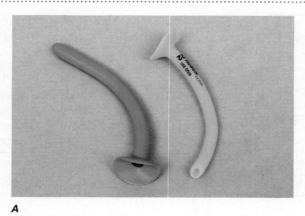
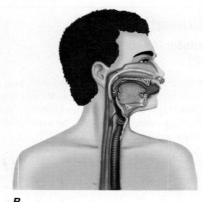

Source: B, George Draper/Pearson Education, Inc.

❷ *A,* Nasopharyngeal airways; *B,* A nasopharyngeal airway in place.

3. Perform hand hygiene and observe other appropriate infection control procedures; don gloves.
4. Provide for patient privacy.
5. Lubricate entire length of tube.
6. Insert entire tube gently through naris, following anatomical line of nasal passage. If obstructed, try other naris.
7. Validate position by
   • Feeling exhaled air through tube opening
   • Inspecting for tube tip behind uvula ❷.
8. Position patient on side to facilitate drainage of secretions.
9. Remove and discard gloves. Perform hand hygiene.
10. Continue to monitor position of airway, airway patency, and patient's response.
11. Suction upper airway PRN using clean technique.
12. When the procedure is complete, perform hand hygiene and leave patient safe and comfortable.
13. Complete documentation using forms, checklists, or electronic dropdown lists supplemented by nurse's notes or additional comments as appropriate.

SAMPLE DOCUMENTATION

[date] 0230 Unresponsive to verbal command, loud snoring noise heard on inspiration and expiration. V/S 126/90, P 76, R 14, O_2 saturation 94% room air. Placed on right side, airway opened with neck slightly hyperextended. Placed on 2 LPM O_2 via nasal cannula per protocol. Nasopharyngeal tube lubricated and inserted into left naris without difficulty. Small amount mucus suctioned from both nares. Snoring noise stopped, patient breathing through nose without assistance at 16 breaths/min, remains on 2 LPM O_2. Dr. Martin notified. *K. Randel*

SKILL 11.12 Airway, Oropharyngeal: Inserting

Safety Note! *During scheduled clinical time, nursing students may have a learning opportunity to observe or assist with this skill only with faculty permission and with direct supervision from faculty or another RN.*

An artificial oral airway is inserted to prevent airway obstruction from the tongue and maintain a patent airway in an unconscious patient. Oropharyngeal suctioning is more easily done to keep the airway clear of secretions or blood.

Delegation or Assignment

The initial insertion of an oropharyngeal airway is not delegated or assigned to the UAP. In some states, a trained UAP may help to maintain the position of the oropharyngeal airway.

Assessment and evaluation of effectiveness of the procedure remain the responsibility of the nurse.

Equipment

- Appropriate size oropharyngeal airway
- Tongue depressor
- Pen light
- Clean gloves
- Suction catheter
- Suction source

Procedure

1. Ensure that patient is unresponsive and has NO gag reflex. **Rationale:** *A conscious patient may vomit and*

SKILL 11.12 Airway, Oropharyngeal: Inserting (*continued*)

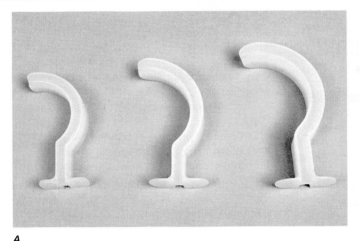

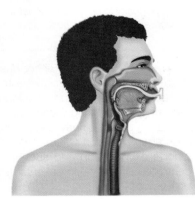

A   *B*

Source: **A,** George Draper/Pearson Education, Inc.

❶ **A,** Oropharyngeal airways; **B,** An oropharyngeal airway in place.

aspirate or develop laryngospasm during airway insertion.

2. Select appropriate size airway—length should be from corner of mouth to corner of ear tragus ❶.
3. Perform hand hygiene and observe other appropriate infection control procedures; don gloves.
4. Provide for patient privacy.
5. Gently open patient's mouth with crossed finger technique, placing your thumb on patient's lower teeth and index finger on the upper teeth and gently pushing them apart. You may need to use modified jaw thrust to insert tube.
6. Perform oral suctioning.
7. Hold tongue down with tongue depressor and advance airway to back of tongue **OR** advance airway upside down (curved upward) and, as airway passes uvula, rotate the airway 180 degrees ❷.
8. Check that concave curve fits over tongue. It should extend from the lips to the pharynx, displacing the tongue anteriorly. **Rationale:** *Proper positioning helps prevent injury to lips, teeth, tongue, and posterior pharynx.*
9. Tape top and bottom of airway in position where flange rests on lips. **Rationale:** *Stabilization of the tube prevents injuries.*
10. Position patient on side to facilitate drainage of secretions out of the mouth.
11. Remove and discard gloves. Perform hand hygiene.
12. Observe position of airway, need for oropharyngeal suctioning, and evaluate quality of patient's spontaneous breathing.
13. When the procedure is complete, perform hand hygiene and leave patient safe and comfortable.
14. Complete documentation using forms, checklists, or electronic dropdown lists supplemented by nurse's notes or additional comments as appropriate.

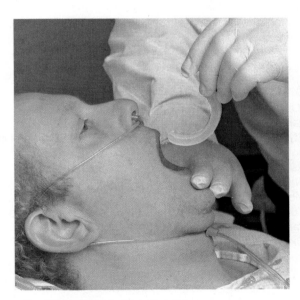

Source: Ronald May/Pearson Education, Inc.

❷ Oropharyngeal airway is initially inserted upside down (curved upward), then rotated 180 degrees.

> **SAMPLE DOCUMENTATION**
>
> [date] 0425 Found unconscious, gurgling sound heard at back of throat. Placed on side with slight hyperextension of neck to open airway. V/S 102/70, P 74, R 14, O₂ saturation 90% room air. O₂ at 4 LPM via face mask applied. Oral airway inserted without difficulty, oropharyngeal suctioning produced large amount of salivary secretions. Dr. Jay notified. *L. Jackson*

SKILL 11.13 Endotracheal Tube: Caring for

Safety Note! *During scheduled clinical time, nursing students may have a learning opportunity to observe or assist with this skill only with faculty permission and with direct supervision from faculty or another RN.*

An endotracheal tube (ETT) is inserted either nasally or orally and advanced into the trachea to just above the carina ❶. Patients are intubated when they are unconscious and unable to breathe on their own either during surgery or because they are unable to maintain a patent airway and are having severe respiratory distress and ventilation failure. The ETT maintains the airway, supports oxygenation and suctioning of secretions, and is a controlled airway when patients need mechanical ventilatory assistance.

Delegation or Assignment

The maintenance and suctioning of an endotracheal tube is not delegated or assigned to the UAP. The routine care and taking vital signs of the patient can be done by the UAP. The nurse can request the UAP to report patient observations to the nurse for follow-up. Assessment and evaluation of effectiveness of the procedure remain the responsibility of the nurse.

Equipment

Only for Inserting ETT

- "Crash cart" (contains most needed supplies)
- Laryngoscope with several blade sizes
- Stylet to guide endotracheal tube (ETT) (ONLY for oral intubation)
- Assortment of various sizes of endotracheal tubes
- Water-soluble lubricant
- McGill forceps
- Suctioning set-up including sterile suction catheters and Yankauer (for oral suctioning)
- Oxygen source
- Bag–valve–mask (BVM) ventilator system

- Twill tape, adhesive tape, Velcro holder, or endotracheal tube stabilizer
- 10-mL syringe for cuff inflation
- Stethoscope
- CO_2 detector (for airway placement validation)
- Oral airway or bite block
- Clean gloves, personal protective equipment including face shield
- Established pulse oximetry and cardiac monitor if available
- Wrist restraints (if ordered)
- Prepared sedative/neuromuscular blocking agent as ordered

Note: Noninvasive positive pressure ventilation methods (CPAP, BiPAP) provide an appropriate alternative to intubation for many patients with ventilator insufficiency.

Only for Extubating ETT

- Suctioning set-up
- Oral suction catheter (or Yankauer)
- Sterile suction catheter set
- Clean gloves
- Sterile gloves
- Personal protective equipment
- Oxygen source
- Postextubation oxygen delivery device
- 10 mL syringe for cuff deflation

Preparation

- Check healthcare provider's order.
- Obtain vital signs, O_2 saturation, assess breath sounds and state of consciousness.

Procedure

1. Introduce self to patient and family and verify the patient's identity using two identifiers. Explain to the patient and family what the healthcare provider will be doing, why it is necessary, and how the patient can participate. Discuss how the results will be used in planning further care or treatments.

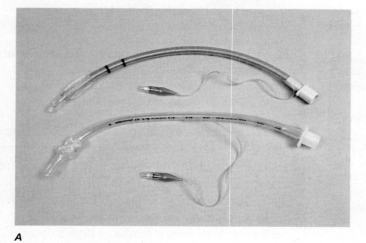

A

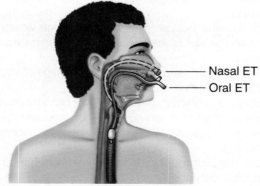

Nasal ET
Oral ET

B

*Source: **A,** George Draper/Pearson Education, Inc.*

❶ **A,** Endotracheal tubes; **B,** An endotracheal tube in place.

SKILL 11.13 Endotracheal Tube: Caring for (continued)

2. Perform hand hygiene and observe appropriate infection control procedures.
3. Provide for patient privacy.

INTUBATING

4. Prepare the patient.
   - Determine that patient has *no protective airway reflexes.*
   - Remove patient's dentures/bridgework and place in labeled container.
   - Place patient in flat supine position with pillow under shoulders to hyperextend neck and help open airway. Position so that mouth, pharynx, and trachea are aligned. **Rationale:** *Proper positioning facilitates intubation.*
   - Restrain patient's wrists only if necessary.
   - Premedicate patient as ordered.
5. Prepare the equipment.
   - Bring crash cart to patient's doorway.
   - Check that all necessary equipment is functioning: oxygen/suction source, and delivery systems, laryngoscope batteries, and heart monitoring system.
   - Inflate and deflate airway cuff to determine if it is intact.
   - Perform hand hygiene and don gloves. Don personal protective equipment.
   - Insert stylet into tube (only for oral intubation); ensure that stylus does not extend beyond tube tip.
   - Lubricate tube.
6. Assist the healthcare provider during procedure.
   - Preoxygenate patient for several minutes, using BVM device. **Rationale:** *This is to create an "oxygen reserve."*

CAUTION!

- Even if spontaneously breathing, the patient should be preoxygenated with 100% O_2 for endotracheal tube placement. Ventilation must not be interrupted for more than 30 seconds.
- Cricoid pressure may be used only if the patient is nonresponsive, is not vomiting, or does not have a cuffed tracheal tube in place.

   - Using thumb and index finger, apply cricoid pressure during tube insertion. **Rationale:** *This facilitates tracheal placement and protects against aspiration of gastric contents.*
   - Maintain cricoid pressure while inflating cuff to "minimal leak" inflation by placing stethoscope at patient's suprasternal notch and noting a slight hissing sound at peak of inspiration.
   - Attach BVM device, provide ventilation, and look for chest to rise. **Rationale:** *If chest does not rise, esophageal intubation is likely.*
   - Check tube placement using CO_2 detector. **Rationale:** *Presence of CO_2 indicates tracheal intubation.*
   - Place stethoscope over epigastrium. **Rationale:** *If gurgling is heard, and abdominal distention noted, esophageal placement is likely.*

- Auscultate lung fields for bilateral breath sounds. **Rationale:** *This ensures that accidental right main stem intubation has not occurred.*
- Mark tube at level of patient's front teeth and tape securely with twill or adhesive tape, Velcro holder, or Endotube stabilizer. **Rationale:** *Secure taping prevents tube displacement.*
- Recheck tube placement with the previous measures.
- Place bite block or oral airway if ETT has been positioned orally.
- Attach O_2 source to ETT.
7. Position patient in position as ordered.
8. Obtain chest x-ray to confirm tracheal placement of ETT.
9. Reposition ETT every 4 hours: right, center, left, then repeat (using Velcro or Endotube stabilizer).
10. Monitor the patient's vital signs, O_2 saturation, breathing pattern, need for suctioning, and patency of airway. Proceed to step 11.

CAUTION!

- The presence of an endotracheal tube bypasses defenses that normally protect the lower airways (filtration, humidification, and hydration of inspired air and epiglottal closure). In addition, mucociliary transport of secretions and trapped pathogens is impaired. These alterations place intubated patients at risk for aspiration pneumonia.
- While cuff pressures are typically maintained at 20–25 mmHg, an individual patient's tracheal capillary pressure cannot be determined and excessive cuff pressure is the best predictor of tracheolaryngeal injury.

---

or

MAINTAINING

4. Monitor breath sounds every 4 hours. Breath sounds should be heard equally throughout lung fields bilaterally.
5. ETT assessment
   - Check marked points on tube at insertion level for tube movement.
   - Inspect positioning and stabilization of tube. **Rationale:** *A change of position can obstruct airway or cause erosion and necrosis of tissues.*
   - Inspect and clean mouth and nose. Observe for pressure areas or ulceration.
   - Reposition ET tube every 4 hours (right, center, left), noting tube depth each time.
6. Support patient's head and tube when turning. **Rationale:** *This prevents tube from becoming dislodged or airway from becoming obstructed.*
7. Provide alternative means of communication when cuffed tube is in place.
8. Support patient by spending extra time, using touch, and anticipating patient's needs.
9. Ensure adequate hydration. **Rationale:** *Artificial airways bypass the humidifying process of normal breathing.*
10. Provide suction toothbrushing every 12 hours, oral swabbing every 2 hours, and oropharyngeal subglottal suctioning

(continued on next page)

SKILL 11.13 Endotracheal Tube: Caring for (continued)

every 6 hours. **Rationale:** *This reduces oropharyngeal bacteria and helps prevent pulmonary infection.*

CAUTION! Even with appropriate cuff inflation, intubated patients receiving gastric/enteral tube feedings are at high risk for aspiration.

---

or

EXTUBATING

4. Assess patient's readiness for extubating.
5. Prepare postextubation oxygen delivery system ordered.
6. Place patient in the Fowler position and perform oral or nasopharyngeal suctioning.
7. Assist the healthcare provider during the procedure.
   - Have patient take several slow deep breaths. **Rationale:** *This hyperoxygenates patient in preparation for extubation.*
   - Deflate tube cuff using syringe.
   - Untie the tracheal tube.
   - Remove gloves, perform hand hygiene, and don sterile gloves.
   - Connect sterile catheter to suction source.
   - Insert sterile suction catheter into airway until resistance is met, then retract slightly.
   - Leave suction catheter in place.
   - Have patient take a deep breath. **Rationale:** *This dilates the vocal cords and makes removal easier and less traumatic.*
   - Apply suction while removing catheter and airway at the same time.

8. Immediately apply supplementary oxygen device. Do a respiratory assessment and obtain vital signs.
9. Monitor patient frequently at first, then regularly. Have an alternate communication method available for patient to use.
10. When the procedure is complete, dispose of equipment, remove protective gear and gloves, perform hand hygiene and leave patient safe and comfortable.
11. Complete documentation using forms, checklists, or electronic dropdown lists supplemented by nurse's notes or additional comments as appropriate.

CAUTION! Do not feed patient orally immediately after extubation. Collaborate with physical therapist for a feeding trial for patients at risk for aspiration.

SAMPLE DOCUMENTATION

[date] 0030 Severe respiratory distress noted, cyanosis noted around mouth, V/S 82/68, P 68, R 8, O_2 saturation 84% on partial rebreather mask, slow to respond to verbal command to open his eyes. Dr. Paul here, size 6 ETT inserted orally, breath sounds checked for placement. Transferred to RICU to be placed on mechanical ventilator. *M. Timely*

SKILL 11.14 Suctioning, Oropharyngeal and Nasopharyngeal: Newborn, Infant, Child, Adult

Oral suctioning of secretions or blood is frequently performed on adults and children using a Yankauer suction tip, which is made of firm plastic that maintains its shape when suctioning. A bulb syringe is used for oral and nasal suctioning of newborns and infants. Suction catheters are used for nasopharyngeal and pharyngeal suctioning.

Delegation or Assignment

Oral suctioning using a Yankauer suction tube can be delegated or assigned to the UAP, but oropharyngeal and nasopharyngeal suctioning is not delegated or assigned to the UAP. The nurse needs to review the procedure and important points, such as not applying suction during insertion of the tube to avoid trauma to the mucous membranes. Oropharyngeal suctioning uses a suction catheter. Although it is not a sterile procedure, oropharyngeal suctioning should be performed by a nurse or respiratory therapist because it can stimulate the gag reflex, hypoxia, and dysrhythmias that may require problem solving. Nasopharyngeal suctioning requires use of a sterile technique and application of

knowledge and problem solving and should be performed by a nurse or respiratory therapist. Note that state laws for UAPs vary, so this task might be assigned to the UAP rather than delegated.

Equipment

Oropharyngeal and Nasopharyngeal Suctioning (Using Sterile Technique)

- Towel or moisture-resistant pad
- Portable or wall suction machine with tubing, collection receptacle, and suction pressure gauge
- Sterile disposable container for fluids
- Sterile normal saline or water
- Goggles or face shield, if appropriate
- Moisture-resistant disposal bag
- Sputum trap, if specimen is to be collected
- Sterile gloves
- Sterile suction catheter kit (#12 to #18 Fr for adults, #8 to #10 Fr for children, #5 to #8 Fr for infants, and #5 to #6 for newborns)

SKILL 11.14 Suctioning, Oropharyngeal and Nasopharyngeal: Newborn, Infant, Child, Adult *(continued)*

- Water-soluble lubricant
- Y-connector

Oral and Oropharyngeal Suctioning (Using Clean Technique)

- Yankauer suction catheter or suction catheter kit
- Clean gloves
- Bulb syringe (for newborn or infant only)

Preparation

- Review healthcare provider's orders and patient's nursing plan of care.
- Assess patient for the need of suctioning.
- Gather equipment and supplies.

Procedure

1. Introduce self and verify the patient's identity using two identifiers. Explain to the patient (or parent) what you are going to do, why it is necessary, and how the patient can participate. Inform the patient (parent) that suctioning will relieve breathing difficulty and, although the procedure is painless, it is noisy and can cause discomfort by stimulating the cough, gag, or sneeze reflex. **Rationale:** *Knowing that the procedure will alleviate breathing problems is often reassuring and engages the patient's cooperation.*
2. Perform hand hygiene and observe other appropriate infection control procedures.
3. Provide for patient privacy.

ORAL AND OROPHARYNGEAL

4. Prepare the patient.
   - Position a conscious person who has a functional gag reflex in the semi-Fowler position with the head turned to one side for oral suctioning or with the neck hyperextended for nasal suctioning. **Rationale:** *These positions facilitate the insertion of the catheter and help prevent aspiration of secretions.*
   - Position an unconscious patient in the lateral position, facing you. **Rationale:** *This position allows the tongue to fall forward, so that it will not obstruct the catheter on insertion. The lateral position also facilitates drainage of secretions from the pharynx and prevents the possibility of aspiration.*
   - Place the towel or moisture-resistant pad over the pillow or under the chin.
5. Turn the suction device on and set to appropriate negative pressure on the suction gauge ❶. The amount of negative pressure should be high enough to clear secretions but not too high. **Rationale:** *Too high of a pressure can cause the catheter to adhere to the tracheal wall and cause irritation or trauma.* A rule of thumb is to use the lowest amount of suction pressure needed to clear the secretions.
6. Perform suctioning procedure.
   - Don clean gloves.

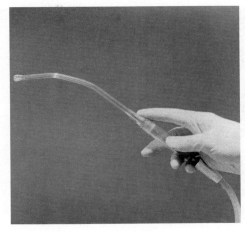

Source: George Draper/Pearson Education, Inc.

❶ Oral (Yankauer) suction tube.

- Moisten the tip of the Yankauer or suction catheter with sterile water or saline. **Rationale:** *This reduces friction and eases insertion.*
- Pull the tongue forward, if necessary, using gauze.
- Do not apply suction (that is, leave your finger off the port) during insertion. **Rationale:** *Applying suction during insertion causes trauma to the mucous membrane.*
- Advance the catheter about 10–15 cm (4–6 in.) along one side of the mouth into the oropharynx. **Rationale:** *Directing the catheter along the side avoids stimulating the gag reflex, which can cause vomiting and compromise the airway.*
- It may be necessary during oropharyngeal suctioning to apply suction to secretions that collect in the vestibule of the mouth and beneath the tongue. Proceed to step 7.

or

ORAL AND NASAL (NEWBORN OR INFANT)

4. A bulb syringe is used to remove secretions from an infant's nose or mouth.
5. Perform suctioning procedure.
   - An assistant may be needed to gently position the newborn, infant, or child, hold the head in midline and keep the child's hands out of the way.
   - Oral suctioning should always be done before nasal suctioning if both areas need to be cleaned of secretions to avoid stimulating a gasp from the newborn or infant which may result in aspiration of secretions in the throat or oral cavity.
   - Don gloves and place saline nose drops in a naris. **Rationale:** *The nose drops loosen dried secretions.*
   - Deflate the bulb. Insert the tip of the bulb syringe into the newborn's or infant's naris ❷. **Rationale:** *Deflating the bulb first prevents pushing the secretions back into the nasopharynx.*

(continued on next page)

SKILL 11.14 Suctioning, Oropharyngeal and Nasopharyngeal: Newborn, Infant, Child, Adult *(continued)*

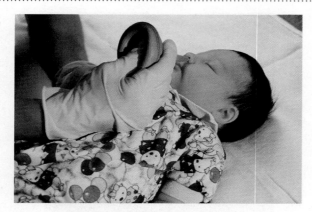

Source: George Draper/Pearson Education, Inc.

2 Insertion of a deflated bulb syringe.

- Release the bulb and remove the syringe from the naris **3**. Expel the secretions into the proper receptacle.
- Repeat the procedure in the other naris.
- Clean the bulb syringe with soap and water and allow to air dry before reuse.

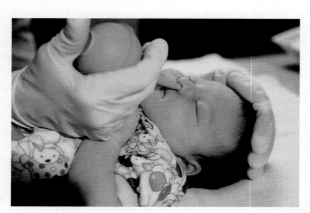

Source: George Draper/Pearson Education, Inc.

3 Removal of a reinflated bulb syringe.

6. Assess the child's ability to breathe easily. Repeat the suctioning as necessary. Proceed to step 7.

NASOPHARYNGEAL

4. Prepare the equipment.
   - Open the lubricant if performing nasopharyngeal/naso-tracheal suctioning.
   - Open the sterile suction package.
     a. Set up the cup or container, touching only the outside.
     b. Pour sterile water or saline into the container.
     c. Apply the sterile gloves, or apply an unsterile glove on the nondominant hand and then a sterile glove on the dominant hand. **Rationale:** *The sterile gloved hand maintains the sterility of the suction catheter,*

and the unsterile glove holds the suction connecting tubing and prevents the transmission of microorganisms to the nurse.

5. Perform suctioning procedure.
   - With your sterile gloved hand, pick up the sterile suction catheter and attach it to the suction unit **4** **5**.

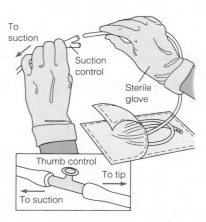

4 Attaching the catheter to the suction unit.

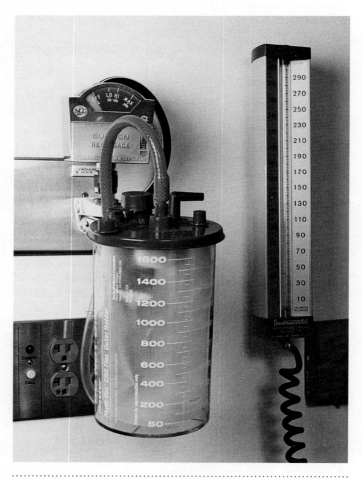

5 A wall suction unit.

SKILL 11.14 Suctioning, Oropharyngeal and Nasopharyngeal: Newborn, Infant, Child, Adult *(continued)*

- Test the pressure of the suction and the patency of the catheter by applying your sterile gloved finger or thumb to the port or open branch of the Y-connector (the suction control) to create suction. If needed, apply or increase supplemental oxygen.
- Lubricate and introduce the catheter.
- Lubricate the catheter tip with sterile water, saline, or water-soluble lubricant. **Rationale:** *This reduces friction and eases insertion.*
- Remove oxygen with the nondominant hand, if appropriate.
- *Without applying suction,* insert the catheter into either naris and advance it along the floor of the nasal cavity. **Rationale:** *This avoids the nasal turbinates.*
- Never force the catheter against an obstruction. If one nostril is obstructed, try the other.
- Apply your finger to the suction control port to start suction, and gently rotate the catheter. **Rationale:** *Gentle rotation of the catheter ensures that all surfaces are reached and prevents trauma to any one area of the respiratory mucosa due to prolonged suction.*
- Apply suction for 5–10 seconds while slowly withdrawing the catheter, then remove your finger from the control and remove the catheter.
- A suction attempt should last only 5–10 seconds. During this time, the catheter is inserted, the suction applied and discontinued, and the catheter removed.

6. Rinse the catheter and repeat suctioning as above.
   - Rinse and flush the catheter and tubing with sterile water or saline.
   - Relubricate the catheter, and repeat suctioning until the air passage is clear.
   - Allow sufficient time between each suction for ventilation and oxygenation. Limit suctioning to 5 minutes total. **Rationale:** *Applying suction for too long may cause secretions to increase or may decrease the patient's oxygen supply.*
   - Encourage the patient to breathe deeply and to cough between suctions. Use supplemental oxygen, if appropriate. **Rationale:** *Coughing and deep breathing help carry secretions from the trachea and bronchi into the pharynx, where they can be reached with the suction catheter. Deep breathing and supplemental oxygen provide oxygen to the alveoli.*
   - Empty and rinse the suction collection container as needed or indicated by protocol. Change the suction tubing and container daily.
   - Ensure that supplies are available for the next suctioning (suction kit, gloves, and water or normal saline).

7. Assess the effectiveness of suctioning.
   - Auscultate the patient's breath sounds to ensure they are clear of secretions. Observe skin color, respiratory rate, heart rate, level of anxiety, and oxygen saturation levels.

8. When the procedure is complete, perform hand hygiene and leave patient safe and comfortable.

9. Complete documentation using forms, checklists, or electronic dropdown lists supplemented by nurse's notes or additional comments as appropriate including the amount, consistency, color, and odor of sputum (e.g., foamy, white mucus; thick, green-tinged mucus; blood-flecked mucus) and the patient's respiratory status before and after the procedure. This may include lung sounds, rate and character of breathing, and oxygen saturation.

SAMPLE DOCUMENTATION

[date] 0830 Producing large amounts of thick, tenacious white mucus to back of oral pharynx but unable to expectorate into tissue. Uses Yankauer suction tube as needed. O_2 sat increased from 89% before suctioning to 93% after suctioning. RR also decreased from 26 to 18–20 after suctioning. Lungs clear to auscultation. Continuous O_2 at 2 LPM via nasal cannula. Will continue to reassess q hour. *L. Webb*

Lifespan Considerations

NEWBORNS AND INFANTS

- A bulb syringe is used to remove secretions from a newborn's or infant's nose and mouth. Care needs to be taken to avoid stimulating the gag reflex.

CHILDREN

- A catheter is used to remove secretions from an older child's mouth or nose.

OLDER ADULTS

- Older adults often have cardiac and/or pulmonary disease, thus increasing their susceptibility to hypoxemia related to suctioning. Watch closely for signs of hypoxemia. If noted, stop suctioning and hyperoxygenate.

Safety Considerations

- Patients and families need to practice frequent hand hygiene to prevent infection.
- Airway suctioning in the home is considered a clean procedure.
- The catheter or Yankauer should be flushed by suctioning recently boiled or distilled water to rinse away mucus, followed by the suctioning of air through the device to dry the internal surface and, thus, discourage bacterial growth. The outer surface of the device may be wiped with alcohol or hydrogen peroxide. The suction catheter or Yankauer should be allowed to dry and then stored in a clean, dry area.
- Suction catheters treated in the manner described above may be reused. It is recommended that catheters be discarded after 24 hours. Yankauer suction tubes may be cleaned, boiled, and reused.

SKILL 11.15 Suctioning, Tracheostomy or Endotracheal Tube

Safety Note! *During scheduled clinical time, nursing students may have a learning opportunity to observe or assist with this skill only with faculty permission and with direct supervision from faculty or another RN.*

Suctioning a tracheostomy or endotracheal tube (ETT) is done to maintain a patent airway and help prevent secretions from collecting within these artificial airways resulting in obstruction of airflow in and out of the lungs. Collecting secretions could also become contaminated and cause an infection in the lungs.

Delegation or Assignment

Suctioning a tracheostomy or endotracheal tube is a sterile, invasive technique requiring application of scientific knowledge and problem solving. This skill is performed by a nurse or respiratory therapist and is not delegated or assigned to the UAP. The nurse can request the UAP to report patient observations to the nurse for follow-up. The nurse remains responsible for the assessment, interpretation of abnormal findings, and determination of appropriate responses.

Equipment

- Bag–valve–mask (BVM) ventilator system connected to an oxygen source
- Pulse oximeter (optional)
- Sterile towel (optional)
- Equipment for suctioning (also see Skill 11.14)
- Goggles and mask if necessary
- Gown (if necessary)
- Sterile gloves
- Moisture-resistant bag

Preparation

- Review healthcare provider's orders and patient's nursing plan of care.
- Gather equipment and supplies.
- Determine if the patient has been suctioned previously and, if so, review the documentation of the procedure. This information can be very helpful in preparing the nurse for both the physiological and psychological impact of suctioning on the patient.

Procedure

1. Introduce self and verify the patient's identity using facility protocol. Explain to the patient (parent) what you are going to do, why it is necessary, and how the patient can participate. Inform the patient (parent) that suctioning usually stimulates the cough reflex and that this assists in removing the secretions.
2. Perform hand hygiene and observe other appropriate infection control procedures (e.g., gloves, goggles).
3. Provide for patient privacy. An assistant or parent may be needed to hold the child gently and to keep hands out of the way. The assistant or parent should maintain the child's head in the midline position.
4. If not contraindicated, place the patient in the semi-Fowler position to promote deep breathing, maximum lung expansion, and productive coughing. Apply pulse oximeter finger clip to monitor oxygen saturation values during procedure (optional). **Rationale:** *Deep breathing oxygenates the lungs,*

counteracts the hypoxic effects of suctioning, and may induce coughing. Coughing helps loosen and move secretions.

OPEN-SUCTION SYSTEM

5. Prepare the equipment.
   - Attach resuscitation apparatus (BVM) to oxygen source ❶. Adjust the oxygen flow to 100%.
   - Open the sterile supplies:
     a. Suction kit or catheter
     b. Sterile basin/container.
   - Pour sterile normal saline or water in sterile basin.
   - Place the sterile towel, if used, across patient's chest below tracheostomy or ETT or on a workspace.
   - Turn on the suction, and set the pressure in accordance with facility policy. For a wall unit, a pressure setting between 80–120 mmHg is normally used for adults, 60 mmHg for children.
   - Apply goggles, mask, and gown if necessary.
   - Apply sterile gloves. Some facilities recommend putting a sterile glove on the dominant hand and an unsterile glove on the nondominant hand. **Rationale:** *The sterile gloved hand maintains the sterility of the suction catheter, and the unsterile glove holds the suction connecting tubing and prevents the transmission of microorganisms to the nurse.*
   - Holding the catheter in the dominant hand and the connector in the nondominant hand, attach the suction catheter to the suction tubing.
   - Using the dominant hand, place the catheter tip in the sterile saline solution.
   - Using the thumb of the nondominant hand, occlude the thumb control and suction a small amount of the sterile solution through the catheter. **Rationale:** *This determines that the suction equipment is working properly and lubricates the outside and the lumen of the catheter. Lubrication eases insertion and reduces tissue trauma during insertion. Lubricating the lumen also helps prevent secretions from sticking to the inside of the catheter.*

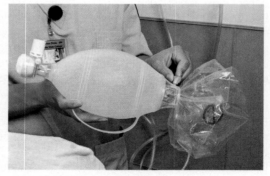

Source: Rick Brady/Pearson Education, Inc.

❶ Attaching the resuscitation apparatus to the oxygen source.

Safety Considerations

- Suction patient's airway PRN. Secretions are usually more copious following the irritation of intubation.
- *Don't* instill normal saline solution into the endotracheal tube in an attempt to promote secretion removal.

SKILL 11.15 Suctioning, Tracheostomy or Endotracheal Tube (*continued*)

- Suction catheter diameter should be no larger than one half the inner diameter of the artificial airway. To determine catheter diameter size, multiply the artificial airway's diameter × 2 (e.g., for 8-mm tube, use a 16-French suction catheter).

- Hyperoxygenate the patient before and after each time the airway is entered for suctioning, and wait 1 minute before suctioning again to prevent severe hypoxemia.

6. If the patient does not have copious secretions, hyperventilate the lungs with a resuscitation bag before suctioning ❷.
   - Summon an assistant, if one is available, for this step.
   - Using your nondominant hand, turn on the oxygen to 12–15 L/min.
   - If the patient is receiving oxygen, disconnect the oxygen source from the tracheostomy tube or ETT using your nondominant hand.
   - Attach the resuscitator to the tracheostomy or ETT.
   - Compress the BVM device 3–5 times as the patient inhales. This is best done by a second person who can use both hands to compress the bag, thus providing a greater inflation volume.
   - Observe the rise and fall of the patient's chest to assess the adequacy of each ventilation.
   - Remove the resuscitation device and place it on the bed or the patient's chest with the connector facing up. Proceed to step 7 below.

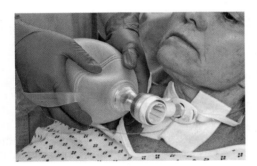

Source: Rick Brady/Pearson Education, Inc.

❷ Attaching the resuscitator to the tracheostomy.

or

CLOSED SUCTION SYSTEM (IN-LINE CATHETER)

5. Prepare the equipment.
   - If a catheter is not attached, don clean gloves, aseptically open a new closed catheter set, and attach the ventilator connection on the T-piece to the ventilator tubing. Attach the patient connection to the endotracheal tube or tracheostomy.
6. Prepare to suction.
   - Attach one end of the suction connecting tubing to the suction connection port of the closed system and the other end of the connecting tubing to the suction device.
   - Turn suction on, occlude or kink tubing, and depress the suction control valve (on the closed catheter system) to set suction to the appropriate level. Release the suction control valve.

- Use the ventilator to hyperoxygenate and hyperinflate the patient's lungs.

7. Suction the tracheostomy tube or ETT.
   - Remove oxygen source or, for closed system, unlock the suction control mechanism if required by manufacturer.
   - With dominant hand, advance the suction catheter or, for closed system, suction catheter in its plastic sheath. Steady the T-piece with the nondominant hand.
   - Depress the suction control valve and apply intermittent suction for no more than 10 seconds and gently withdraw the catheter. Replace oxygen source.
   - Repeat as needed, remembering to provide hyperoxygenation and hyperinflation as needed.

8. Flush and, for closed system, close the system.
   - When suctioning is complete, withdraw catheter or, for closed system, withdraw catheter into its sleeve and close the access valve, if appropriate. **Rationale:** *If the closed system does not have an access valve on the patient connector, the nurse needs to observe for the potential of the catheter migrating into the airway and partially obstructing the artificial airway.*
   - Flush the catheter by instilling normal saline into the irrigation port and applying suction. Repeat until the catheter is clear.
   - For closed system, close the irrigation port and close suction valve.

9. When the procedure is complete, discard disposable supplies in appropriate container, doff gloves, perform hand hygiene, and leave patient safe and comfortable.

10. Complete documentation using forms, checklists, or electronic dropdown lists supplemented by nurse's notes or additional comments as appropriate.

SAMPLE DOCUMENTATION

[date] 0530 Coughing small amount of secretions from tracheostomy tube, but gesturing that he is having trouble coughing up the secretions. Hyperoxygenated with 100% O_2 via BVM device, then suctioned for moderate amount tenacious yellow foul-smelling secretions. States he feels he can get more air in now. T-bar with humidified air replaced on trach tube. Tolerated suctioning without incident. *S. Dallas*

Patient Teaching

- Clear the airway by effective coughing whenever possible.
- Know how to suction the patient's secretions if unable to cough effectively.
- Caregiver needs to use clean gloves when endotracheal suctioning is performed in the home environment.
- Caregiver needs to know how to determine the need for suctioning and the correct process to avoid potential complications of suctioning.
- Reinforce the importance of adequate hydration to thin secretions, which can aid in their removal by coughing or suctioning.

SKILL 11.16 Tracheal Tube: Inflating the Cuff

The tracheal tube with a cuff is used when maintaining a closed airway system between a ventilator and the patient. When the cuff is inflated the patient is not able to speak using the vocal cords. The inflated cuff provides little protection against aspiration. The friction generated around the cuff can cause complications at the cuff site in the trachea.

Delegation or Assignment

Inflating the cuff of a tracheal tube is not delegated or assigned to the UAP. In some states, a trained UAP may help to maintain the inflated tracheal tube. Assessment and evaluation of effectiveness of the procedure remain the responsibility of the nurse.

Equipment

- 10-mL syringe
- Suction equipment
- Stethoscope
- Clean gloves

Note: The foam cuff does not require injected air. Air enters the balloon when the port is open.

Preparation

- Review healthcare provider's orders and patient's nursing plan of care.
- Gather needed equipment and supplies.

Procedure

1. Introduce self to patient and verify the patient's identity using two identifiers. Explain to the patient what you are going to do, why it is necessary, and how the patient can participate. Discuss how the results will be used in planning further care or treatments.
2. Perform hand hygiene and observe appropriate infection control procedures.
3. Provide for patient privacy and don clean gloves.
4. Attach 10-mL syringe to distal end of inflatable cuff port, making sure seal is tight ❶.
5. Inflate cuff for a minimal leak or minimal occlusive volume detected by auscultating over the suprasternal notch for a hissing sound at peak of inspiration. **Rationale:** *This provides an adequate seal without risking tracheal pressure necrosis.*
6. Ask patient to speak—if voice is heard, inflation is inadequate for mechanical ventilation ❷.
7. Connect ventilator or T-piece to tracheal tube opening if indicated. Document relevant information.
8. Assess breath sounds every 2 hours. **Rationale:** *Presence of bilateral breath sounds indicates proper tube position in trachea.*

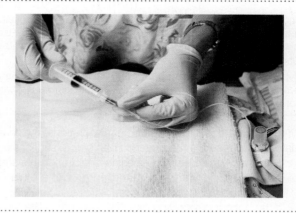

❶ Attach 10-mL syringe to inflate tube cuff.

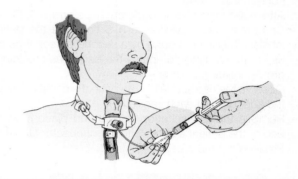

❷ Inflate endotracheal or tracheostomy tube cuff to minimal occlusive volume.

9. Monitor cuff pressure regularly. **Rationale:** *This may detect inadvertent cuff overinflation and prevent potential necrosis of tracheal tissue.* Pressure is usually maintained at 20–25 mmHg to prevent tracheal necrosis. However, an individual patient's tracheal capillary pressure cannot be determined.
10. When the procedure is complete, perform hand hygiene and leave patient safe and comfortable.
11. Complete documentation using forms, checklists, or electronic dropdown lists supplemented by nurse's notes or additional comments as appropriate.

SAMPLE DOCUMENTATION

[date] 0812 Awake and alert. Tracheal tube secured with ties. Small amount beige secretions on trach dressing noted. Tracheal tube cuff inflated with 4 mL air to get breathing treatment. Tolerated without incident. *T. Lee*

CAUTION! Tracheal tube cuff inflation is essential for mechanically ventilated patients. Without cuff inflation, delivered air diverts out through the nose and mouth, and lungs are not ventilated.

SKILL 11.17 Tracheostomy: Caring for

Tracheostomy care includes keeping the skin around the trach stoma and the neck clean and dry, changing the cotton twill ties or Velcro collar that secure the trach tube, and changing as needed the trach stoma dressing when soiled. It is also providing suctioning when the patient is unable to cough up secretions adequately, and maintaining humidification of air or oxygen the patient is breathing into the lungs.

Delegation or Assignment

Tracheostomy care involves application of scientific knowledge, sterile technique, and problem solving. It therefore is not delegated or assigned to the UAP, but needs to be performed by a nurse or respiratory therapist. The nurse can request the UAP to report patient observations to the nurse for follow-up. Assessment and evaluation remain the responsibility of the nurse.

Equipment

- Sterile disposable tracheostomy cleaning kit or supplies including sterile containers, sterile nylon brush and/or pipe cleaners, sterile applicators
- Disposable inner cannula if applicable
- Towel or drape to protect bed linens
- Sterile suction catheter kit (suction catheter and sterile container for solution)
- Sterile normal saline (Some agencies may use a mixture of hydrogen peroxide and sterile normal saline. Check facility protocol for soaking solution.)
- Sterile gloves (Two pairs—one pair is for suctioning if needed)
- Clean gloves
- Moisture-proof bag
- Commercially prepared sterile tracheostomy dressing or sterile 4 × 4 gauze dressing
- Cotton twill ties or Velcro collar
- Clean scissors

CAUTION! An obturator is kept at the bedside for emergency use. If the tracheostomy tube is inadvertently dislodged, it can be reinserted immediately using the obturator.

Preparation

- Review healthcare provider's orders and patient's nursing plan of care.
- Gather equipment and supplies.

Procedure

1. Introduce self and verify the patient's identity using facility protocol. Explain to the patient (parent) you are going to provide tracheostomy care, why it is necessary, and how the patient can participate. Provide for a means of communication, such as eye blinking or raising a finger, to indicate pain or distress. Follow through by carefully observing the patient throughout the procedure. Offer periodic eye contact, caring touch, and verbal reassurance. Some patients respond well to a sense of efficiency and gentle humor, and nurses must decide when to use this approach.

2. Perform hand hygiene and observe other appropriate infection control procedures.
3. Provide for patient privacy.
4. Prepare the patient and the equipment.
   - Assist the patient to a semi-Fowler or Fowler position to promote lung expansion.
   - Suction the tracheostomy tube, if needed.
   - If suctioning was required, allow the patient to rest and restore oxygenation.
   - Open the tracheostomy kit or sterile basins.
   - Establish a sterile field.
   - Open other sterile supplies as needed, including sterile applicators, suction kit, tracheostomy dressing, and, if applicable, the disposable inner cannula.
   - Pour the soaking solution and sterile normal saline into separate containers.
   - Don clean gloves.
   - Remove oxygen source.
   - Unlock the inner cannula (if present) and remove it by gently pulling it out toward you in line with its curvature ❶. Place the inner cannula in the soaking solution. **Rationale:** *This moistens and loosens dried secretions.*
   - Replace oxygen source.
   - Remove the soiled tracheostomy dressing. Place the soiled dressing in your gloved hand and peel the glove off so that it turns inside out over the dressing. Remove and discard gloves and the dressing. Perform hand hygiene.
   - Apply sterile gloves. Keep your dominant hand sterile during the procedure.

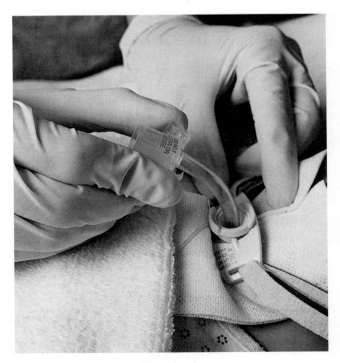

Source: Ronald May/Pearson Education, Inc.

❶ Gently pull inner cannula upward and outward to remove.

(continued on next page)

SKILL 11.17 Tracheostomy: Caring for (continued)

5. Clean the inner cannula. (See the section below for changing a disposable inner cannula.)
   - Remove the inner cannula from the soaking solution.
   - Clean the lumen and entire inner cannula thoroughly using the brush or pipe cleaners moistened with sterile normal saline ❷. Inspect the cannula for cleanliness by holding it at eye level and looking through it into the light.
   - Rinse the inner cannula thoroughly in the sterile normal saline.
   - After rinsing, gently tap the cannula against the inside edge of the sterile saline container. Use a pipe cleaner folded in half to dry only the inside of the cannula; do not dry the outside. **Rationale:** *This removes excess liquid from the cannula and prevents possible aspiration by the patient, while leaving a film of moisture on the outer surface to lubricate the cannula for reinsertion.*

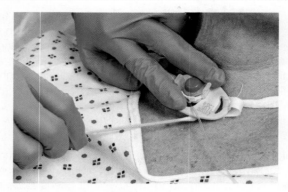

Source: Rick Brady/Pearson Education, Inc.

❸ Using an applicator stick to clean the tracheostomy site.

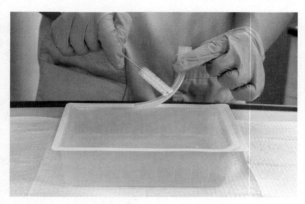

Source: Ronald May/Pearson Education, Inc.

❷ Cleaning the inner cannula with a brush.

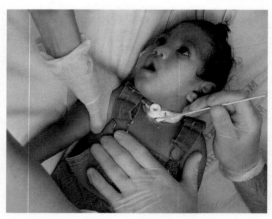

Source: George Dodson/Pearson Education, Inc.

❹ Cleaning the tracheostomy tube.

6. Replace the inner cannula, securing it in place.
   - Remove oxygen source.
   - Insert the inner cannula by grasping the outer flange and inserting the cannula in the direction of its curvature.
   - Lock the cannula in place by turning the lock (if present) into position to secure the flange of the inner cannula to the outer cannula.
   - Replace oxygen source
7. Clean around the trach stoma and tube flange.
   - Using sterile applicators or gauze dressings moistened with normal saline, clean around the trach stoma ❸ ❹. Handle the sterile supplies with your dominant hand. Use each applicator or gauze dressing only once and then discard. **Rationale:** *This avoids contaminating a clean area with a soiled gauze dressing or applicator.*
   - Hydrogen peroxide may be used (usually in a half-strength solution mixed with sterile normal saline; use a separate sterile container if this is necessary) to remove crusty secretions around the tracheostomy site. Do not use directly on the site. Check facility policy. Thoroughly rinse the cleaned area using gauze squares moistened with sterile normal saline. **Rationale:** *Hydrogen peroxide can be irritating to the skin and inhibit healing if not thoroughly removed.*

   - Clean the flange of the tube in the same manner.
   - Thoroughly dry the patient's skin and tube flanges with dry gauze squares.
8. Apply a sterile dressing.
   - Use a commercially prepared tracheostomy dressing ❺ or open and refold a nonraveling 4 × 4 gauze dressing

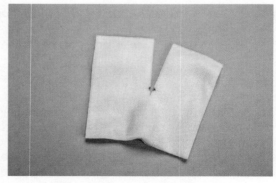

Source: Rick Brady/Pearson Education, Inc.

❺ A commercially prepared tracheostomy dressing of nonraveling material.

SKILL 11.17 Tracheostomy: Caring for (continued)

into a V shape. Avoid using cotton-filled gauze squares or cutting the 4 × 4 gauze. **Rationale:** *Cotton lint or gauze fibers can be aspirated by the patient, potentially creating a tracheal abscess.*
- Place the dressing under the flange of the tracheostomy tube ⑥.
- While applying the dressing, ensure that the tracheostomy tube is securely supported. **Rationale:** *Excessive movement of the tracheostomy tube irritates the trachea.*

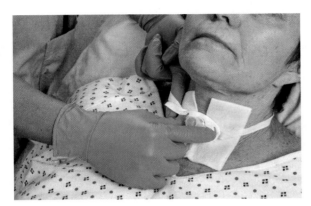

Source: Rick Brady/Pearson Education, Inc.

⑥ A tracheostomy dressing placed under the flange of the tracheostomy tube.

9. Change the tracheostomy ties or Velcro collar.
- Change as needed to keep the skin clean and dry.
- Twill ties and specially manufactured Velcro collars are available. A twill tie is inexpensive and readily available; however, it is easily soiled and can trap moisture that leads to irritation of the skin of the neck. Velcro collars are commonly used ⑦.

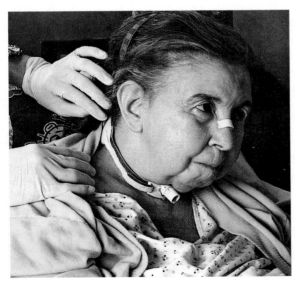

Source: Ronald May/Pearson Education, Inc.

⑦ A Velcro tracheostomy collar.

Safety Considerations

- When a child is admitted with a tracheostomy, ⑧ talk with the parents about the method used for tracheostomy management at home. Develop a nursing care plan for tracheostomy management that integrates home management as well as teaching to enhance home management techniques.

- Remember that the child with an endotracheal tube or tracheostomy tube is unable to talk or cry. Implement other ways of communication. Picture boards that illustrate common activities or requests work for younger children. An electronic tablet or a pad and pencil can be used by older children with normal motor skills.

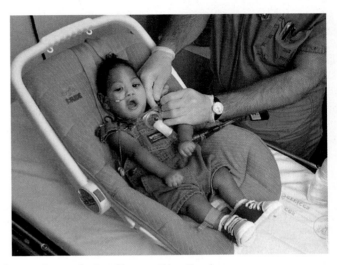

Source: George Dodson/Pearson Education, Inc.

⑧ Infant with a tracheostomy collar.

TWO-STRIP METHOD (TWILL TIES)

- Cut two unequal strips of twill ties, one approximately 25 cm (10 in.) long and the other about 50 cm (20 in.) long. **Rationale:** *Cutting one tape longer than the other allows them to be fastened at the side of the neck for easy access and to avoid the pressure of a knot on the skin at the back of the neck.*
- Cut a 1-cm (0.5-in.) lengthwise slit approximately 2.5 cm (1 in.) from one end of each tie. To do this, fold the end of the tie back onto itself about 2.5 cm (1 in.), then cut a slit in the middle of the tie from its folded edge.
- Leaving the old ties in place, thread the slit end of one clean tie through the eye of the tracheostomy flange from the bottom side; then thread the long end of the tie through the slit, pulling it tight until it is securely fastened to the flange. **Rationale:** *Leaving the old ties in place while securing the clean ties prevents inadvertent dislodging of the tracheostomy tube. Securing ties in this manner avoids the use of knots in the flange area, which can come untied or cause pressure and irritation.*
- If old ties are very soiled or it is difficult to thread new ties onto the tracheostomy flange with old ties in place, have an

(continued on next page)

SKILL 11.17 Tracheostomy: Caring for (*continued*)

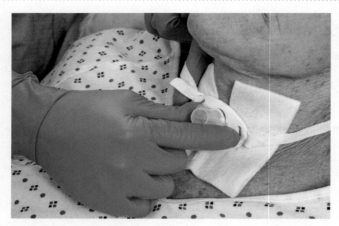

Source: Rick Brady/Pearson Education, Inc.

⑨ Placing a finger underneath the tie tape before tying it.

assistant don a sterile glove and hold the tracheostomy in place while you replace the ties. **Rationale:** *This is very important because movement of the tube during this procedure may cause irritation and stimulate coughing. Coughing can dislodge the tube if the ties are undone.*

- Repeat the process for the second tie.
- Ask the patient to flex the neck. Slip the longer tape under the patient's neck, place a finger between the tape and the patient's neck, and tie the ties together at the side of the neck ⑨. **Rationale:** *Flexing the neck increases its circumference the way coughing does. Placing a finger under the tie prevents making the tie too tight, which could interfere with coughing or place pressure on the jugular veins.*
- Tie the ends of the ties using square knots. Cut off any long ends, leaving approximately 1–2 cm (0.5 in.). **Rationale:** *Square knots prevent slippage and loosening. Adequate ends beyond the knot prevent the knot from inadvertently untying.*
- Once the clean ties are secured, remove the soiled ties and discard.

or

ONE-STRIP METHOD (TWILL TIE)

- Cut a length of twill tie 2.5 times the length needed to go around the patient's neck from one tube flange to the other.
- Thread one end of the tie into the slot on one side of the flange.
- Bring both ends of the tie together. Take them around the patient's neck, keeping them flat and untwisted.
- Thread the end of the tie next to the patient's neck through the slot from the back to the front.
- Have the patient flex the neck. Tie the loose ends with a square knot at the side of the patient's neck, allowing for slack by placing two fingers under the ties as with the two-strip method. Cut off long ends.

10. Tape and pad the tie knot.
    - Place a folded 4 × 4 gauze square under the tie knot, and apply tape over the knot. **Rationale:** *This reduces skin irritation from the knot and prevents confusing the knot with the patient's gown ties.*

11. Check the tightness of the ties.
    - Frequently check the tightness of the tracheostomy ties and position of the tracheostomy tube. **Rationale:** *Swelling of the neck may cause the ties to become too tight, interfering with coughing and circulation. Ties can loosen in restless patients, allowing the tracheostomy tube to extrude from the stoma.*

12. When the procedure is complete, remove and discard sterile gloves. Perform hand hygiene and leave patient safe and comfortable.

13. Complete documentation using forms, checklists, or electronic dropdown lists supplemented by nurse's notes or additional comments as appropriate including suctioning, tracheostomy care, and the dressing change, noting your assessments.

or

DISPOSABLE INNER CANNULA

- Check policy for frequency of changing the inner cannula because standards vary among institutions.
- Open a new cannula package.
- Using a gloved hand, unlock the current inner cannula (if present) and remove it by gently pulling it out toward you in line with its curvature.
- Check the cannula for amount and type of secretions and discard properly.
- Pick up the new inner cannula touching only the outer locking portion.
- Insert new cannula and lock the cannula in place by turning the lock (if present).

SAMPLE DOCUMENTATION

[date] 0900 Respirations 18–20/min. Lung sounds clear. Able to cough up secretions requiring little suctioning. Inner cannula changed. Trach dressing changed. Minimal amount of serosanguineous drainage present. Trach incision area pink to reddish in color 0.2 cm around entire opening. No broken skin noted in the reddened area. Tolerated without incident. J. Garcia

---

Lifespan Considerations

NEWBORNS, INFANTS, AND CHILDREN

- An assistant should always be present while tracheostomy care is performed.
- Always keep a sterile, packaged tracheostomy tube taped to the child's bed so that if the tube dislodges, a new one is available for immediate reintubation.

OLDER ADULTS

- Older adult skin is fragile and prone to breakdown. Care of the skin at the tracheostomy stoma is very important.

SKILL 11.17 Tracheostomy: Caring for (*continued*)

Patient Teaching

- For tracheostomies older than 1 month, ensure caregiver knows, clean technique (rather than sterile technique) is used for tracheostomy care.
- Teach the importance of good hand hygiene to the caregiver.
- Caregiver needs to know tap water may be used for rinsing the inner cannula.
- Observe a return demonstration by the caregiver about tracheostomy care. Periodically reassess caregiver knowledge and/or tracheostomy care technique.

- Ensure the caregiver knows the signs and symptoms that may indicate an infection of the stoma site or lower airway.
- Ensure the names and telephone numbers of healthcare personnel who can be reached for emergencies or advice are available to the patient and/or caregiver.
- Provide contact information for available support groups.

≫ Maintaining Lung Expansion

Expected Outcomes

1. Chest drainage system remains a closed system.
2. Chest tubes remain patent and secured in place.

SKILL 11.18 Chest Tube Drainage: Maintaining

Safety Note! *During scheduled clinical time, nursing students may have a learning opportunity to observe or assist with this skill only with faculty permission and with direct supervision from faculty or another RN.*

The chest tube drainage system must be maintained as a closed system functioning as it was intended and assessed for compromises to the system such as an air leak. Tube connections need to be assessed to ensure they are intact and secure. The insertion site of a chest tube needs to be monitored for drainage and that the chest tube remains secured. If collecting drainage, chest drainage must be monitored for appearance and amount. If monitoring air using a water seal, water level must be maintained. If using wet suction, water in the suction chamber needs to be maintained at a specific level and the suction gauge must be maintained at a constant pressure.

Delegation or Assignment

Care of chest tubes is not delegated or assigned to the UAP. However, aspects of the patient's condition are observed during usual care and may be recorded by individuals other than the nurse. Abnormal findings must be validated and interpreted by the nurse.

Equipment

- Sterile gloves
- Petrolatum gauze (optional)
- Pour bottle of sterile water, 250 mL
- 4 × 4 gauze sponges
- Split drain sponges
- Drainage system ❶
- Skin cleansing solutions (e.g., povidone-iodine)
- Adhesive or foam tape

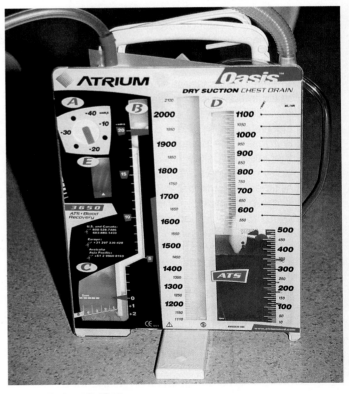

Source: Barbara C. Martin

❶ This dry suction system requires that water be added to the water seal, but does not require water in the suction chamber. The suction is wall regulated. These systems are quieter and easier to use.

(*continued on next page*)

SKILL 11.18 Chest Tube Drainage: Maintaining (*continued*)

Preparation

- Check healthcare provider's orders.
- Determine when the last dressing change was performed.
- Gather needed equipment and supplies.

Procedure

1. Introduce self and verify the patient's identity using two identifiers. Explain to the patient what you are going to do, why it is necessary, and how the patient can participate. Discuss how the results will be used in planning further care or treatments.
2. Perform hand hygiene and observe other appropriate infection control procedures.
3. Provide for patient privacy.
4. Assess the patient.
   - Determine ease of respirations, breath sounds, respiratory rate and depth, oxygen saturation, and chest movements every 2 hours.
   - Observe the dressing site. Inspect the dressing for excessive and abnormal drainage, such as bleeding or foul-smelling discharge. Palpate around the dressing site for crackling indicative of subcutaneous emphysema. **Rationale:** *Subcutaneous emphysema can result from an inadequate seal (air leak) at the chest tube insertion site.*
   - Determine level of discomfort with and without activity.
   - Evaluate the impact of possible changes to the patient's body image that occur when an individual has tubes extending out from the body. The patient may be afraid of pulling them out.
5. Implement all necessary safety precautions.
   - Monitor intactness of closed chest drainage system. Keep a 250-mL pour bottle of sterile water and a sterile occlusive dressing (like a petroleum dressing) at bedside in case of a breech in this system (see step 9 for further information).
   - Keep the drainage system below chest level and upright at all times ❷. **Rationale:** *Keeping the unit below chest level prevents backflow of fluid from the drainage chamber into the pleural space. Keeping the unit upright maintains the water seal.*
6. Maintain the patency of the drainage system.
   - Check that all connections are secured with tape. **Rationale:** *This ensures that the system is airtight.*
   - Inspect the drainage tubing for kinks or loops dangling below the entry level of the drainage system.
   - Coil the drainage tubing and secure it to the bed linen, ensuring enough slack for the patient to turn and move.
   - Inspect the air vent in the system periodically to make sure it is not occluded.
   - Avoid any forceful manipulation of the tube. In some agencies, this includes milking (stripping) the chest tubing. Stripping is compressing the chest tube between fingers and thumb, using a pulling motion down the rest of the tubing away from the chest wall. Milking involves squeezing, kneading, or twisting the tubing to create bursts of suction to move any clots.

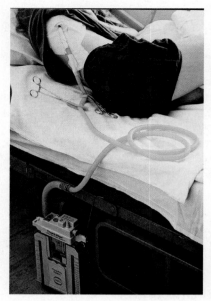

Source: Ronald May/Pearson Education, Inc.

❷ Chest tube drainage system should always be lower than the chest tube insertion site.

CAUTION! Strip and milk chest tubes only with healthcare provider's orders. Excessive negative pressure created by stripping and milking increases negative pressure in the intrapleural space.

7. Assess fluid level fluctuations and bubbling in the drainage system.
   - Check for fluctuation (tidaling) of the fluid level in the water-seal chamber as the patient breathes. **Rationale:** *Tidaling reflects the pressure changes in the pleural space during inhalation and exhalation. The fluid level rises when the patient inhales and falls when the patient exhales. The absence of tidaling may indicate tubing obstruction from a kink, dependent loop, blood clot, or outside pressure (e.g., because the patient is lying on the tubing), or may indicate that full lung re-expansion has occurred.*
   - Check for intermittent bubbling in the water of the water-seal chamber. **Rationale:** *Intermittent bubbling normally occurs when the system removes air from the pleural space, especially when the patient takes a deep breath or coughs. Absence of bubbling may indicate that the drainage system is blocked or that the pleural space has healed and is sealed but this must be verified by x-ray. Continuous bubbling or a sudden change from an established pattern can indicate a break in the system (i.e., an air leak) and should be reported immediately.*
   - Check for gentle bubbling in the suction control chamber in wet systems. **Rationale:** *Gentle bubbling indicates proper suction pressure.*

SKILL 11.18 Chest Tube Drainage: Maintaining (*continued*)

8. Assess the drainage.
   - Inspect the drainage in the collection container at least every 15 minutes during the first 2 hours after chest tube insertion and every 2 hours thereafter.
   - Every 4–8 hr mark the time, date, and drainage level on a piece of adhesive tape affixed to the container, or mark it directly on a disposable container ❸.
   - Note any sudden change in the amount or color of the drainage.
   - If drainage exceeds 100 mL/hr or if a color change indicates hemorrhage, notify the healthcare provider immediately.

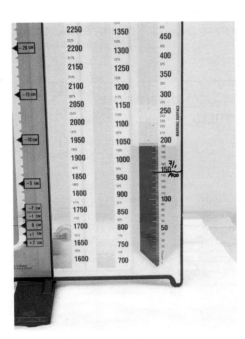

Source: George Draper/Pearson Education, Inc.

❸ Marking the date, time, and drainage level.

9. Watch for dislodgement of the tubes, and remedy the problem promptly.
   - Keep a 250-mL pour bottle of sterile water (or normal saline) and a sterile occlusive dressing (like a petroleum dressing) at the bedside.
   - If the chest tube becomes disconnected from the drainage system or the system breaks or cracks, the end of the chest tube is immediately inserted 2.5–5 cm (1–2 in.) into the sterile pour bottle of water to create a water seal.
   - Another closed drainage system can then be set up and connected to the chest tube.
   - If the chest tube becomes dislodged from the patient, the sterile occlusive dressing would immediately be applied to the insertion site and taped down on three sides.
   - The fourth side is periodically lifted open when the patient exhales to allow air trapped in the pleural space to be expelled.

- The healthcare provider is called to insert another chest tube. **Rationale:** *These actions will prevent the patient from sucking air into the chest on inspiration and allow air trapped in the pleural space to be expelled on expiration. They are important interventions to prevent a tension pneumothorax, which can develop into an emergency situation for the patient.*
- Assess the patient closely for respiratory distress (dyspnea, pallor, diaphoresis, blood-tinged sputum, or chest pain).
- Check vital signs every 10 minutes until stable.
- Document the incident in the patient's medical record or other appropriate records according to the facility's protocol.

10. If bubbling persists in the water-seal collection chamber or air leak chamber, determine its source. Continuous bubbling in the water-seal collection chamber normally occurs for only a few minutes after a chest tube is attached to drainage.

11. Take a specimen of the chest drainage as required.
    - Specimens of chest drainage may be taken from a disposable chest drainage system through the resealable connecting tubing. If a specimen is required:
      a. Use a povidone-iodine swab to wipe the self-sealing tubing below the connection to the chest tube. Allow it to dry.
      b. Attach a sterile 18- or 20-gauge needle to a syringe, and insert the needle into the tubing, being careful not to pass all the way through the opposite side of the tubing.
      c. Aspirate the specimen, discard the needle in the appropriate container, and securely cap the syringe, or transfer the specimen to an appropriate collection tube. Label the syringe or tube while still at the patient's side, matching it to the requisition slip and the patient identification.

12. Ensure essential patient care.
    - Encourage deep breathing and coughing exercises every 2 hr, if indicated (this may be contraindicated in patients with a lobectomy). Premedicate the patient for pain as needed. Have the patient sit upright to perform the exercises, and splint the tube insertion site with a pillow or with a hand to minimize discomfort. **Rationale:** *Deep breathing and coughing help remove accumulations from the pleural space, facilitate drainage, and help the lung to re-expand.*
    - Auscultate the patient's chest every 4 hr. Breath sounds should be symmetric. **Rationale:** *Decreased breath sounds on the side of the chest tube could indicate that air or fluid has reaccumulated in the pleural space. Breath sounds that are louder on the affected side could indicate that fluid has accumulated on the other side of the chest.*
    - Check that the chest tube site dressing is dry and occlusive. The dressing does not need to be changed unless it is loose or wet. In some agencies, chest tube dressings are changed daily. **Rationale:** *A wet dressing could indicate a fluid leak around the tube.*

(*continued on next page*)

SKILL 11.18 Chest Tube Drainage: Maintaining (*continued*)

- Examine the chest tube insertion site for signs of healing, skin irritation, or infection.
- Reposition the patient every 2 hr. When the patient is lying on the affected side, place rolled towels on either side of the tubing. **Rationale:** *Frequent position changes promote drainage, prevent complications, and provide comfort. Rolled towels prevent occlusion of the chest tube by the patient's weight.*
- Assist the patient with ROM exercises of the affected shoulder three times per day to maintain joint mobility.
- Conduct regular pain assessments using a scoring system. If necessary, ask the healthcare provider for more aggressive pain management (possibly patient-controlled analgesia). **Rationale:** *Pain will limit the patient's mobility and will result in shallow breaths and incomplete lung expansion.*
- When transporting and ambulating the patient:
  a. Keep the water-seal unit below chest level and upright.
  b. Disconnect the drainage system from the suction apparatus before moving the patient, and make sure the air vent is open. Or, if ordered, obtain a portable suction device.
13. When the procedure is complete, perform hand hygiene and leave patient safe and comfortable.
14. Complete documentation using forms, checklists, or electronic dropdown lists supplemented by nurse's notes or additional comments as appropriate including patency of chest tubes, type, amount, and color of drainage, presence of fluctuations, appearance of insertion site, respiratory assessments, vital signs, and level of comfort.

SAMPLE DOCUMENTATION

[date] 0800 Awake and alert sitting on side of bed. Denies pain or problem breathing during the night. V/S 132/84, P 78, R 18, T 37.11°C (98.8°F), O_2 saturation 98% room air. Breath sounds remain slightly diminished on right upper lobe. Chest tube on right upper side remains with closed water seal system. Insertion site dressing dry and intact, no crepitus noted around site. Tube connections secured, water seal has small amount of bubbling, tidaling noted with breaths.

States ready to get up to chair for breakfast. *M. Hynes*

Lifespan Considerations
OLDER ADULTS

- Coughing and deep breathing exercises are particularly important because shallow breathing and decreased ability to cough may occur with aging.
- Encourage the patient to take pain medication when needed. Some older adults may be reluctant to take pain medication.
- Take special care of the patient's skin due to the possibility of skin tears from tape and increased risk of skin breakdown over bony prominences as skin becomes thinner and less elastic.
- The older patient is at increased risk for respiratory distress due to increased lung stiffness.

SKILL 11.19 Chest Tube Insertion: Assisting

Safety Note! *During scheduled clinical time, nursing students may have a learning opportunity to observe or assist with this skill only with faculty permission and with direct supervision from faculty or another RN.*

Patients need chest tubes to treat two main conditions, fluid in the pleural space, or air in the pleural space. Air builds up in the pleural space from a pneumothorax, and fluid can build up from pleural effusion or empyema. Chest tubes help to drain the fluid and allow the air to escape from the pleural space.

Delegation or Assignment

Assisting the healthcare provider with insertion of a chest tube is not delegated or assigned to the UAP. However, signs and symptoms of problems may be observed during usual care and may be recorded by individuals other than the nurse. Abnormal findings must be validated and interpreted by the nurse.

Equipment

- Sterile chest tube tray that includes:
  - Drapes
  - 10-mL syringe
  - Gauze sponges
  - #22-gauge needle
  - #25-gauge needle
  - #11 blade scalpel
  - Forceps
- Extra 4 × 4 gauze sponges or other occlusive bandage material
- Split drain sponges
- Chest tube and Kelly clamps
- Suture materials
- Closed drainage system (water or dry seal) ➊
- Suction source, if indicated
- Sterile gloves
- Local anesthetic vial
- Skin cleansing solution (e.g., povidone-iodine)
- Adhesive or foam tape

SKILL 11.19 Chest Tube Insertion: Assisting (*continued*)

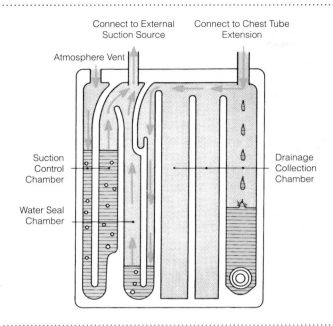

1 Disposable water-seal chest drainage system. The suction control chamber regulates the amount of negative pressure applied to the chest. The water-seal chamber allows air to escape from the intrapleural space and prevents air from re-entering.

- Petrolatum gauze
- Pour bottle of sterile water, 1000 Ml

Preparation

- Unless done as an emergency procedure, signed informed consent is obtained.
- Although the healthcare provider will have already done initial patient and family teaching, the nurse reinforces key elements.
- Confirm with the healthcare provider the desired type and size of chest tubes, suture, or other supplies needed.
- Gather all equipment and supplies.
- Add sterile water into the water-seal chamber to water line mark either by pouring it from the top of the system or injecting it into the self-sealing port using a syringe and needle **2** **3**.
- Add water in the suction control chamber to the correct level if suctioning is ordered by the healthcare provider.

Procedure

1. Introduce self and verify the patient's identity using two identifiers. Explain to the patient what your role will be, why it is necessary, and how the patient can participate. Discuss how the results will be used in planning further care or treatments.
2. Perform hand hygiene and observe appropriate infection control procedures.
3. Provide for patient privacy. Obtain base vital signs and auscultate lung sounds.
4. Premedicate the patient for pain and monitor for change in respirations. Incorporate complementary health stress-reducing strategies as needed.

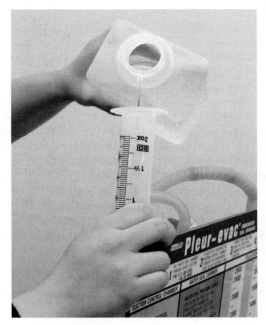

Source: George Draper/Pearson Education, Inc.

2 Filling the water-seal chamber with sterile water.

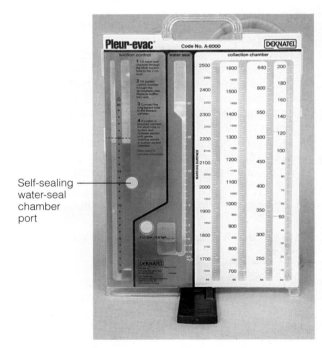

Self-sealing water-seal chamber port

Source: George Draper/Pearson Education, Inc.

3 A three-chamber wet-suction/wet-seal disposable chest drainage system.

5. Position the patient as directed by the healthcare provider.
   - The patient may be placed flat or in semi-Fowler position.
   - Turn the patient laterally so that the area receiving the tube is facing upward.

(*continued on next page*)

SKILL 11.19 Chest Tube Insertion: Assisting (*continued*)

6. Prepare for the insertion.
   - Open the chest tube tray and sterile gloves on the over-bed table.
   - Assist the healthcare provider to clean the insertion site.
   - Assist the healthcare provider to draw up the local anesthetic by holding the anesthetic bottle upside down with the label facing the healthcare provider. The healthcare provider will withdraw the solution.
7. Provide emotional support to the patient during insertion as the healthcare provider makes a small incision through the skin and muscle. Often, the practitioner will probe through the incision with a finger to ensure there are no underlying structures that may be damaged during insertion of the tube. The practitioner will use a Kelly clamp to broaden and deepen the insertion site and then pass the tube into the chest. Monitor the patient's condition, including respiratory rate and effort, pulse, and reaction to the procedure.
8. Dress the site.
   - Don sterile gloves and wrap the petrolatum gauze (if prescribed) around the chest tube at the insertion site.
   - Place split drain gauze around the chest tube, one from the top and one from the bottom.
   - Place several additional gauze squares and tape or occlusive bandage materials over the drain gauze. These form an airtight seal at the insertion site.
9. Secure the tube.
   - Assist with connecting the chest tube to the valve or drainage system.
   - Attach the longer tube from the collection chamber to the patient's chest tube.
   - Remove and discard gloves. Perform hand hygiene.
   - Tape the chest tube to the patient's skin so that any pull on the tubing creates traction on the skin and not on the insertion site.
   - Tape all connections using spiral turns, but do not completely cover the collection tubing with tape ❹. **Rationale:** *Taping prevents inadvertent separation.*

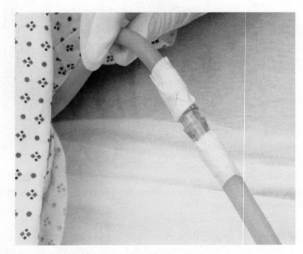

Source: George Draper/Pearson Education, Inc.

❹ Taped tubing connection with the connector exposed for observation of drainage.

- Coil the drainage tubing and secure it to the linen, ensuring slack for the patient to turn and move. **Rationale:** *This prevents kinking of the tubing and impairment of drainage.*
- If suction is ordered, attach the remaining shorter tube from the suction chamber to the suction source and turn it on. If wet suction is used, inspect the suction chamber for bubbling. Gentle bubbling indicates an appropriate suction level.
- If suction has not been ordered, keep the shorter rubber tube unclamped. This maintains negative or equal pressure in the system.
10. When all drainage connections are complete, ask the patient to take a deep breath and hold it for a few seconds, then slowly exhale. These actions facilitate drainage from the pleural space and lung re-expansion.
11. Check vital signs and auscultate lung sounds for changes. Prepare the patient for a chest x-ray to check for placement of the tube and lung expansion.
12. Ensure patient safety.
    - Monitor intactness of closed chest drainage system. Keep a 250-mL pour bottle of sterile water and a sterile occlusive dressing (such as a petroleum dressing) at the bedside in case of a breach in this system. (See Skill 11.18 for information about maintaining chest tube drainage.) **Rationale:** *The bottle of sterile water (or normal saline) would be used as a water seal if the chest tube becomes disconnected from the drainage system or the system breaks or cracks. The sterile occlusive dressing taped down at the chest tube insertion site would prevent sucking air into the chest and also inhibit air from escaping from the chest (which could result in a tension pneumothorax).*
    - Assess the patient for signs of a new or worsening pneumothorax.
    - Assess the patient for signs of subcutaneous emphysema (collection of air under the skin). Palpate around the dressing site for crackling indicative of subcutaneous emphysema.

CAUTION! Subcutaneous emphysema (air in tissue) may be felt around the chest tube insertion site, but should be reported if it extends beyond this.

- Assess drainage and vital signs every 15 min for the first hour and then as ordered. Mark the collection chamber with a line and the date and time. Report bleeding or drainage greater than 100 mL/hr.
13. When the procedure is complete, perform hand hygiene and leave patient safe and comfortable.
14. Complete documentation using forms, checklists, or electronic dropdown lists supplemented by nurse's notes or additional comments as appropriate including the name of the healthcare provider, site of placement, type of tube, type of drainage system, characteristics of the immediate drainage (**Table 11–2 》》**), and other assessment findings.

SKILL 11.19 Chest Tube Insertion: Assisting (*continued*)

TABLE 11–2 Characteristics of Chest Tube Drainage

Description of Fluid	Indication
Blood tinged or bloody	Anticoagulant use
	Pulmonary infarct
	Trauma
	Malignancy
	Inflammation
Cloudy	Infection or inflammation
Purulent (pus)	Empyema
Food particles	Esophageal rupture
Black	*Aspergillus* (fungal) infection
Low pH	Tuberculosis, malignancy

SAMPLE DOCUMENTATION

[date] 0130 32-Fr chest tube inserted into l chest by Dr. Novarty & connected to water-seal drainage unit. Suction at 20 cm H_2O. Immediately drained 120 mL straw-colored fluid. Moderate coughing after insertion, eased in 10 minutes. All connections taped, tubing taped to chest wall & attached to draw sheet. Tidaling c̄ respirations. Patient instructed re: positioning & care of tube & collection device. Expresses understanding. VS - T 38.33°C (101°F), P 100, R 26, BP 170/94, O_2 saturation 97% on 2 LPM O_2 via nasal cannula. *J. Lygas*

SKILL 11.20 Chest Tube Removal: Assisting

Safety Note! *During scheduled clinical time, nursing students may have a learning opportunity to observe or assist with this skill only with faculty permission and with direct supervision from faculty or another RN.*

There are two strong indicators that help the healthcare provider make the decision it is time to remove a chest tube. One indicator is the chest tube drainage is an acceptably small amount or has stopped, and the other indicator is that no more air leak is present.

Delegation or Assignment

Assisting with the removal of a chest tube is not delegated or assigned to the UAP. However, many effects of the removal may be observed during usual care and may be recorded by persons other than the nurse. Abnormal findings must be validated and interpreted by the nurse.

Equipment

- Clean gloves and face mask
- Sterile gloves
- Suture removal set with forceps and scissors
- Sterile petrolatum gauze
- 4 × 4 gauze sponges
- Adhesive or foam tape
- Moisture-proof medical waste bag
- Linen-saver pad
- Sharps container
- Safety goggles

Preparation

- Review healthcare provider's orders and patient's nursing plan of care.
- Gather supplies and equipment needed.

Procedure

1. Introduce self and verify the patient's identity using two identifiers. Explain that the healthcare provider will be removing the chest tube(s) and how the patient can participate. Discuss how the results will be used in planning further care or treatments. The patient should be given the opportunity to discuss and express any concerns.
2. Perform hand hygiene and observe other appropriate infection control procedures.
3. Provide for patient privacy.
4. Prepare the patient.
   - Assist the patient to a side-lying or semi-Fowler position with the chest tube site exposed.
   - Place the linen-saver pad under the patient, beneath the chest tube. **Rationale:** *This protects the bed linens and provides a place for the chest tube after removal.*
   - Instruct the patient that the healthcare provider will ask the patient not to breathe during removal. (i.e., holding a full inhalation, holding a full exhalation, doing the Valsalva maneuver—exhaling against a closed glottis). **Rationale:** *These techniques increase the intrathoracic pressure and prevent air from entering the pleural space.*
5. Prepare the sterile field and supplies. Have the petrolatum gauze opened and ready for quick application.
6. Remove the dressing around the chest tube.
   - Don clean gloves and dispose of the dressing in the moisture-proof bag.
   - Remove and discard gloves. Perform hand hygiene.
7. Assist with removal of the tube ❶.
   - Don face mask and sterile gloves.
   - Assist the patient with the breathing technique and provide emotional support during the healthcare provider's removal of the sutures and tube.

(*continued on next page*)

SKILL 11.20 Chest Tube Removal: Assisting *(continued)*

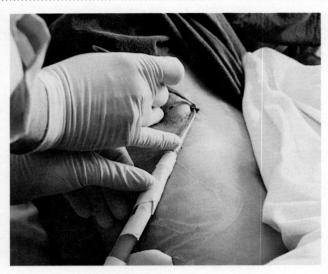

Source: Ronald May/Pearson Education, Inc.

① Sutures anchoring chest tube are cut.

- As the healthcare provider removes the chest tube, either the provider or the nurse immediately applies the petrolatum gauze, and covers it with dry gauze and adhesive tape. **Rationale:** *This forms an airtight bandage.*
- Remove all used equipment and place in appropriate medical waste containers.
- When the procedure is complete, doff gloves and face mask, perform hand hygiene and leave patient safe and comfortable.

8. Assess and monitor the patient's response to tube removal.
   - Obtain vital signs every 15 min for the first hour and, if stable, then as indicated.
   - Auscultate lung sounds every hour for the first 4 hr to determine that the lung is remaining inflated.
   - Observe for signs of pneumothorax.
9. Complete documentation using forms, checklists, or electronic dropdown lists supplemented by nurse's notes or additional comments as appropriate including any drainage noted, and the patient's response to the procedure.
10. Prepare the patient for a chest x-ray 1–2 hr after chest tube removal and possibly again in 12–24 hr.

SAMPLE DOCUMENTATION

[date] 1430 Assisted to left side-lying position. Dr. Wink cut the sutures at the tube insertion site, patient instructed to take a deep breath in and hold it while chest tube was being pulled out in continuous movement. Occlusive dressing with 4 x 4 cover placed on site and taped in place. V/S 128/84, P 82, R 18, O_2 saturation 99% on room air. No drainage noted on dressing removed. No complaints of pain, "just a small catch feeling." Breath sounds clear and equal bil. Tolerated procedure without incident. *H. Morris*

» Life-Threatening Situations

Expected Outcomes

1. Obstructed airway is cleared of foreign body.
2. Rescue breathing or cardiopulmonary resuscitation (CPR) is begun within two minutes after assessment has determined that the patient has a life-threatening need for these actions.
3. Patient's heart rhythm is restored to normal after defibrillation with an automated external defibrillator (AED) or manual defibrillator.
4. Rescue breathing or CPR is continued until rapid-response team arrives.

SKILL 11.21 Airway Obstruction: Clearing

Delegation or Assignment

UAPs usually have certification as basic CPR providers, including procedures for clearing airway obstruction. If they are the first to find an unconscious patient, they should immediately call for a nurse. The nurse is responsible to make an assessment and determine what needs to be done. The nurse can direct UAPs to perform external cardiac compressions. The nurse remains responsible for the assessment, interpretation of abnormal finds, and determination of appropriate actions.

Equipment

- Standard precautions supplies should always be easily accessible: gloves, CPR mask or manual resuscitator (bag–valve–mask [BVM] device), gowns, and protective eyewear.

SKILL 11.21 Airway Obstruction: Clearing (continued)

Preparation

■ Have and maintain Healthcare Provider CPR certification through the American Heart Association or Basic Life Support for Healthcare Providers certification through the American Red Cross.

Procedure

1. Initiate Clearing Airway Obstruction skill steps learned through Healthcare Provider CPR certification.
2. Initiate the following additional actions. Call for help but do not leave the patient until other help arrives. If another individual is present and can participate, have that individual go get help. Tell the individual to return and report that help has been called.
3. Observe appropriate infection control procedures including donning clean gloves as much as possible.
4. Provide for as much privacy as possible without interfering with the necessary individuals and activities. If family members are present, the nurse may request they temporarily leave the room. This option requires policies and procedures to be in place for someone to stay with the family and:
   ● Explain to the family what is happening.
   ● Support the family before, during, and after the event.
   ● Support any family decisions not to be present.
   ● Enforce contraindications for family presence such as extreme emotional behavior or interference with medical procedures.
5. Most healthcare facilities that are clinical sites and allow nursing students to gain clinical experience in their facility require them to be Healthcare Provider CPR certified by the American Heart Association (AHA). Some healthcare facilities accept Basic Life Support for Healthcare Providers certification (BLS) through the American Red Cross which is consistent with AHA guidelines for CPR and emergency cardiovascular care (ECC).
   ● Students must maintain CPR certification throughout the nursing curriculum until graduation from their nursing program. Skill 11.21, Clearing Airway Obstruction, is a skill included in Healthcare Provider CPR certification and the Basic Life Support for Healthcare Providers certification courses. ➊ ➋ ➌

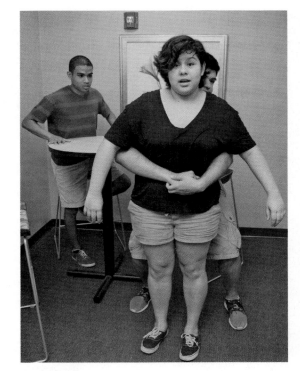

Source: Ronald May/Pearson Education, Inc.

➋ Position hands to perform abdominal thrust making a fist and placing the other hand on top of it.

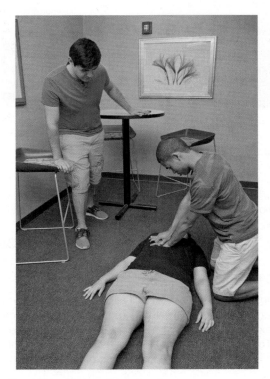

Source: Ronald May/Pearson Education, Inc.

➌ If patient is unresponsive, begin CPR.

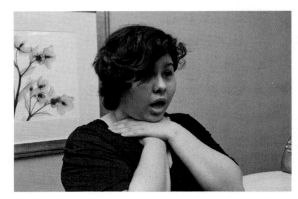

Source: Ronald May/Pearson Education, Inc.

➊ Determine whether patient is choking.

(continued on next page)

SKILL 11.21 Airway Obstruction: Clearing (*continued*)

- The American Heart Association and the American Red Cross utilize current evidence to make periodic changes to the sequential steps of these skills to maintain best practice in performing them. This certification means nursing students have already received the training for this skill, have successfully passed a written test, and correctly demonstrated the ability to perform it. ④ ⑤

- After careful assessment of the patient and situation, the life-saving knowledge and skills acquired through gaining Healthcare Provider CPR certification or Basic Life Support for Healthcare Providers certification would be performed as learned.

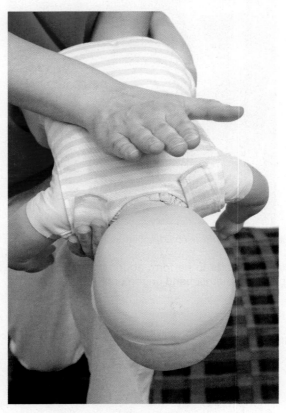

Source: Roman Milert/Alamy Stock Photo

④ Infant back slaps.

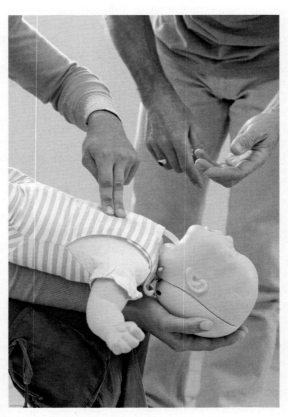

Source: Burger/Phanie/Science Source

⑤ Infant chest thrusts.

SKILL 11.22 Cardiac Compressions, External: Performing

Delegation or Assignment

Although UAPs cannot perform all interventions during a life-threatening situation, they are trained in CPR and can perform external cardiac compressions. If they are the first to find an unconscious patient, the UAP should immediately call for a nurse. The nurse is responsible to make an assessment and determine what needs to be done. The nurse can direct the UAP to perform external cardiac compressions. The nurse remains responsible for the assessment, interpretation of abnormal finds, and determination of appropriate actions.

Equipment

- Standard precautions supplies should always be easily accessible: gloves, CPR mask or manual resuscitator (bag–valve–mask [BVM] device), gowns, and protective eyewear.
- Emergency equipment such as defibrillation and intubation equipment should be centrally located (most units have an emergency cart with supplies, equipment, and medications needed).
- Face mask with one-way valve or mouth shields or a BVM device.

SKILL 11.22 Cardiac Compressions, External: Performing *(continued)*

- A hard surface, such as a cardiac board or the floor, on which to place the individual.

Preparation

- Have and maintain Healthcare Provider CPR certification through the American Heart Association or Basic Life Support for Healthcare Providers certification through the American Red Cross.

Procedure

1. Initiate Basic CPR and Defibrillation skill steps learned through Healthcare Provider CPR certification.
2. Initiate the following additional actions. Call for help but do not leave the patient until other help arrives. If another individual is present and can participate, have that individual go get help. Tell the individual to return and report that help has been called.
3. Observe appropriate infection control procedures including donning clean gloves as much as possible.
4. Provide for as much privacy as possible without interfering with the necessary individuals and activities. If family members are present, the nurse may request they temporarily leave the room. This option requires policies and procedures to be in place for someone to stay with the family and:
   - Explain to the family what is happening.
   - Support the family before, during, and after the event.
   - Support any family decisions not to be present.
   - Enforce contraindications for family presence such as extreme emotional behavior or interference with medical procedures.
5. Most healthcare facilities that are clinical sites and allow nursing students to gain clinical experience in their facility require them to be Healthcare Provider CPR certified by the American Heart Association (AHA). Some healthcare facilities accept Basic Life Support for Healthcare Providers certification (BLS) through the American Red Cross which is consistent with AHA guidelines for CPR/ECC. ❶ ❷ ❸

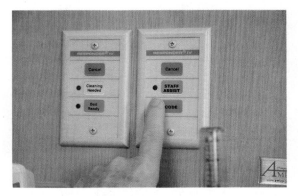

Source: Rick Brady/Pearson Education, Inc.

❷ Call for help and to bring AED.

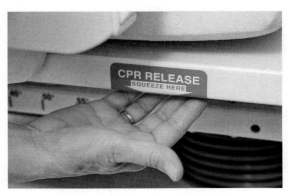

Source: Rick Brady/Pearson Education, Inc.

❸ Place bed in flat position for CPR.

- Students must maintain CPR certification throughout the nursing curriculum until graduation from their nursing program. Skill 11.22, Performing External Cardiac Compressions, is a skill included in Healthcare Provider CPR certification and the Basic Life Support for Healthcare Providers certification courses. ❹ ❺ ❻

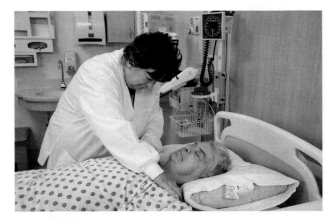

Source: Rick Brady/Pearson Education, Inc.

❶ Check for response: Tap patient, speak loudly and clearly, check for pulse.

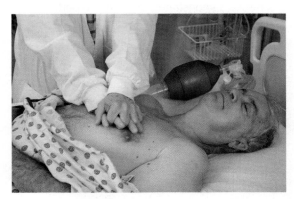

Source: Rick Brady/Pearson Education, Inc.

❹ Begin compressions at 120/min, unless other instructions are provided.

(continued on next page)

SKILL 11.22 Cardiac Compressions, External: Performing (*continued*)

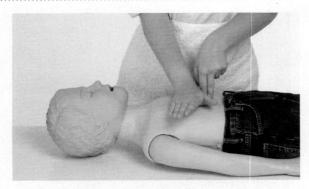

Source: Jules Selmes/Dorling Kindersley/Getty Images

5 Locating the site for chest compressions on a child.

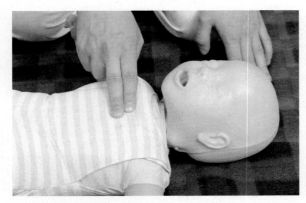

Source: Roman Milert/Alamy Stock Photo

6 CPR on an infant with one healthcare provider.

- The American Heart Association and the American Red Cross utilize current evidence to make periodic changes to the sequential steps of these skills to maintain best practice in performing them. This certification means nursing students have already received the training for this skill, have successfully passed a written test, and correctly demonstrated the ability to perform it. **7 8 9**

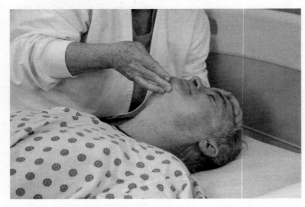

Source: Rick Brady/Pearson Education, Inc.

7 Open airway by using head tilt-chin lift method.

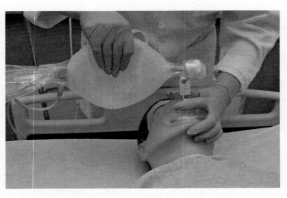

Source: Rick Brady/Pearson Education, Inc.

8 Ventilate with two rescue breaths using bag-valve-mask (BVM) or CPR mask.

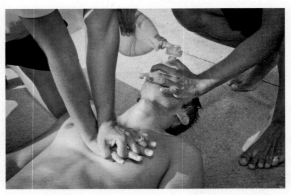

Source: Daviles/Fotolia

9 Arm and hand position for external cardiac compression.

- After careful assessment of the patient and situation, the life-saving knowledge and skills acquired through gaining Healthcare Provider CPR certification or Basic Life Support for Healthcare Providers certification would be performed as learned. **10 11 12**

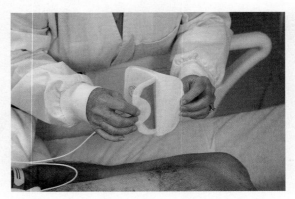

Source: Rick Brady/Pearson Education, Inc.

10 After setting up the AED unit, remove backing and apply pads to patient's chest.

SKILL 11.22 Cardiac Compressions, External: Performing (*continued*)

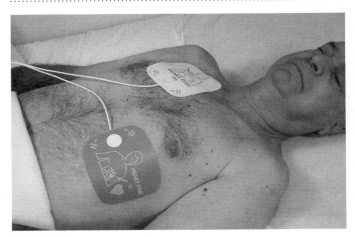

Source: Rick Brady/Pearson Education, Inc.

⑪ Apply pads to chest, one below right clavicle, one below and lateral to heart.

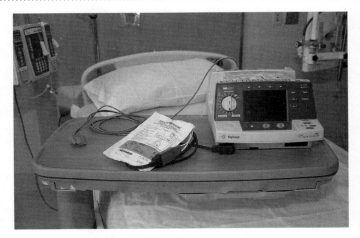

Source: Rick Brady/Pearson Education, Inc.

⑫ If AED indicates need for shock, push SHOCK on AED.

SKILL 11.23 Rescue Breathing: Performing

Delegation or Assignment

Although UAPs cannot perform all aspects of a life-threatening situation, they are trained in CPR and can perform rescue breathing. If they are the first to find an unconscious patient, the UAP should immediately call for a nurse. The nurse is responsible to make an assessment and determine what needs to be done. The nurse can direct the UAP to perform rescue breathing. The nurse remains responsible for the assessment, interpretation of abnormal finds, and determination of appropriate actions.

Equipment

- Standard precautions supplies should always be easily accessible: gloves, CPR mask or manual resuscitator (bag–valve–mask [BVM] device), gowns, and protective eyewear.
- Emergency equipment such as intubation supplies should be centrally located.
- Pocket face mask with one-way valve or mouth shields, or BVM device (often referred to as an Ambu bag).

Preparation

- Have and maintain Healthcare Provider CPR certification through the American Heart Association or Basic Life Support for Healthcare Providers certification through the American Red Cross.

Procedure

1. Determine that the individual is having abnormal breathing.
2. If the individual does not respond, call for help, the rapid response team, or assistance following facility protocol. If

another individual is present and can participate, have that individual go get help. Tell the individual to return and report that help has been called.
3. Observe appropriate infection control procedures including donning clean gloves as much as possible.
4. Provide for as much privacy as possible without interfering with the necessary individuals and activities. If family members are present, the nurse may request they temporarily leave the room. This option requires policies and procedures to be in place for someone to stay with the family and:
   - Explain to the family what is happening.
   - Support the family before, during, and after the event.
   - Support any family decisions not to be present.
   - Enforce contraindications for family presence such as extreme emotional behavior or interference with medical procedures.
5. Most healthcare facilities that are clinical sites and allow nursing students to gain clinical experience in their facility require them to be Healthcare Provider CPR certified by the American Heart Association (AHA). Some healthcare facilities accept Basic Life Support for Healthcare Providers certification (BLS) through the American Red Cross which is consistent with AHA guidelines for CPR/ECC.
   - Students must maintain CPR certification throughout the nursing curriculum until graduation from their nursing program. Skill 11.23, Performing Rescue Breathing, is a skill included in Healthcare Provider CPR certification and the Basic Life Support for Healthcare Providers certification courses. ❶ ❷ ❸

(*continued on next page*)

SKILL 11.23 Rescue Breathing: Performing (*continued*)

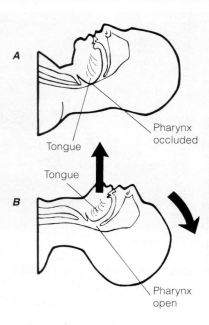

① The position of an unconscious individual's tongue: *A,* Airway occluded; *B,* Airway open.

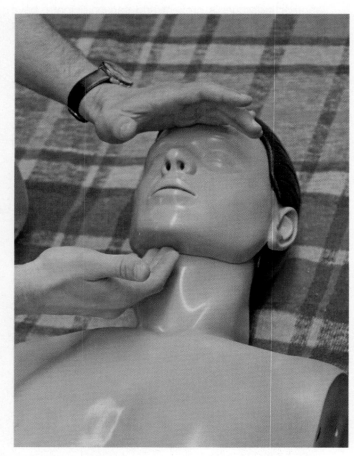

Source: Roman Milert/Fotolia

② Head tilt–chin lift maneuver.

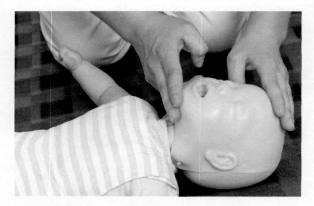

Source: Roman Milert/Alamy Stock Photo

③ Infant head tilt–chin lift maneuver.

- The American Heart Association and the American Red Cross utilize current evidence to make periodic changes to the sequential steps of these skills to maintain best practice in performing them. This certification means nursing students have already received the training for this skill, have successfully passed a written test, and correctly demonstrated the ability to perform it. ④ ⑤ ⑥

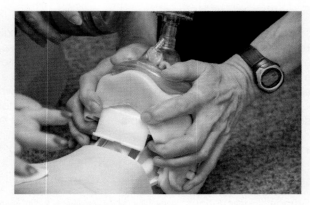

Source: Dr. P. Marazzi/Science Source

④ Jaw-thrust maneuver.

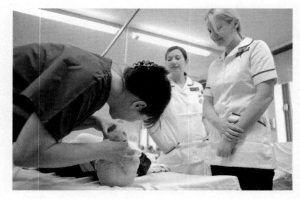

Source: Wunkley/Alamy Stock Photo

⑤ Mouth-to-mask rescue breathing.

SKILL 11.23 Rescue Breathing: Performing (*continued*)

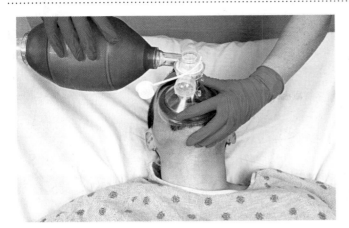

Source: George Draper/Pearson Education, Inc.

6 Bag-to-mask breathing.

- After careful assessment of the patient and situation, the life-saving knowledge and skills acquired through gaining Healthcare Provider CPR certification or Basic Life Support for Healthcare Providers certification would be performed as learned. **7** **8** **9**

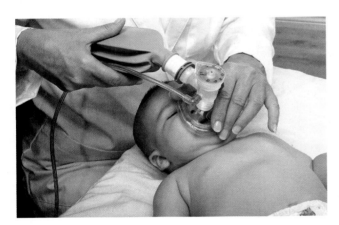

Source: Lee F. Snyder/Science Source

7 Infant bag-to-mask breathing. (Photo Researchers)

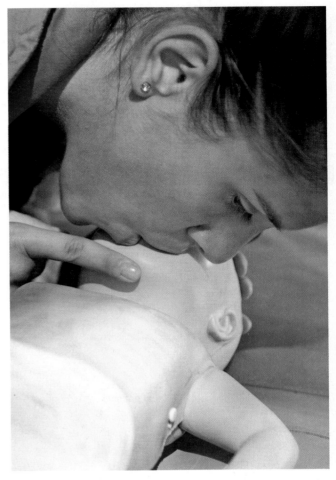

Source: Microgen/Getty Images

8 Infant mouth-to-mouth rescue breathing.

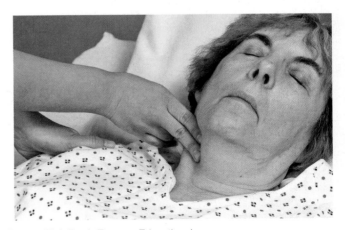

Source: Rick Brady/Pearson Education, Inc.

9 Checking the carotid pulse.

» Critical Thinking Options for Unexpected Outcomes

Not all unexpected outcomes require further nursing intervention; however, many times they do. When the patient demonstrates a change in signs/symptoms indicating an emerging problem, the nurse should immediately assess and troubleshoot what is happening. The assessment data must be processed quickly to formulate a hypothesis so the nurse can make a clinical judgment. The nurse then decides how best to resolve the problem and improve the patient's situation for a better outcome.

EXPECTED OUTCOME	UNEXPECTED OUTCOME	POSSIBLE INTERVENTIONS
Interventions Patient maintains breathing rate and pattern to support oxygen needs adequately. Patient maintains patent airway by using preventative actions, effective coughing and expectoration of secretions, frequent repositioning, periodic deep breathing, maintaining hydration, and ambulating as able. Encourage deep breathing to minimize or reverse atelectasis in the lungs. Prevent pulmonary complications for the immediate postoperative patient.	Patient develops atelectasis.	■ Encourage patient to change position frequently, cough, take deep breaths, and ambulate as healthcare provider orders. ■ Encourage patient to use an incentive spirometer several times each day. ■ Chest physiotherapy may be ordered. ■ Monitor breath sounds.
Supplemental Oxygen Therapy Supplemental oxygen is delivered via the most appropriate method to meet individual patient's oxygen needs. Respiratory distress will decrease. Oxygen saturation readings will be stable. Patient reports improved sleep pattern when using CPAP/BiPAP. The patient on a mechanical ventilator will not develop ventilator-associated pneumonia. Promote gas exchange through the use of a sustained maximal inspiration device (incentive spirometer), controlled breathing to sustain maximal expiration (pursed lips breathing), positioning to support respirations, or chest physiotherapy to mobilize secretions. Maximize COPD patient's ability to maintain airway patency, decrease shortness of breath, control breathing rate, and maximize breathing effectiveness.	Patient remains having difficulty breathing after supplemental oxygen is begun.	■ Place patient in high Fowler position. ■ Check supplemental oxygen setup and that oxygen flow rate is correct. ■ Assess oxygen saturation and lung sounds and compare to previous findings. ■ Ask patient to describe what the patient is experiencing. ■ Conduct actions to increase comfort and decrease anxiety.
Maintaining a Patent Airway Secretions are removed via appropriate suctioning method without complications. The least invasive method of suctioning will be used to meet individual patient's need for a clear airway.	Patient's oxygen saturation decreases and tachycardia develops while suctioning.	■ Suction only as needed. ■ Oxygenate patient before and after suctioning. ■ Limit suctioning time to less than 10 seconds. ■ Use correct catheter diameter (less than half the inner diameter of the airway it enters).
	Frequent suctioning is required due to the amount of secretions.	■ Suction as needed but pre-oxygenate with 100% oxygen. ■ Allow rest period before suctioning again. ■ Maintain adequate hydration. ■ Reposition patient frequently to keep secretions mobile.

EXPECTED OUTCOME	UNEXPECTED OUTCOME	POSSIBLE INTERVENTIONS
As needed, appropriate artificial airway will be used to maintain patency of patient's airway.	Tracheostomy tube becomes dislodged.	■ Quickly use new obturator to insert new tracheostomy tube (both items should be kept at the bedside). ■ Encourage patient to remain calm and take slow deep breaths. ■ Retie tracheostomy ties or secure Velcro tracheostomy collar to secure correct tracheostomy tube position.
Maintaining Lung Expansion Chest drainage system remains a closed system.	Chest tube becomes disconnected from the drainage system or the system breaks or cracks.	■ Immediately insert the end of the chest tube 2.5–5 cm (1–2 in.) into a sterile pour bottle of water to create a water seal (a small pour bottle of sterile water should be kept at the bedside). ■ Then set-up another closed drainage system and connect it to the chest tube.
Chest tubes remain patent and secured in place.	Chest tube becomes dislodged from the patient.	■ Immediately apply a sterile occlusive dressing to the insertion site and tape it down on three sides (a sterile occlusive dressing should be kept at the bedside). ■ Periodically lift open the fourth side when the patient exhales to allow air trapped in the pleural space to be expelled. ■ Call the healthcare provider to insert another chest tube.
Life-Threatening Situations Obstructed airway is cleared of foreign body.	Patient's airway becomes obstructed during a meal.	■ Assess and then follow emergency maneuvers to clear the airway. ■ Call for help. ■ If unable to clear the airway, call for rapid-response team. ■ Begin rescue breathing or CPR as patient needs. ■ Use AED with patient as appropriate. ■ Have emergency cart brought to bedside.
Rescue breathing or CPR is begun within 5 min after assessment has determined that the patient has a life-threatening need for these actions. Patient's heart rhythm is restored to normal after defibrillation with an AED or manual defibrillator. Rescue breathing or CPR is continued until rapid-response team arrives.	Patient suddenly has a condition change that becomes life-threatening.	■ Call for help. ■ Call for rapid-response team. ■ Assess and begin rescue breathing or CPR as patient needs. ■ Use AED with patient as appropriate. ■ Have emergency cart brought to bedside.

REVIEW Questions

1. While collecting a throat culture, the client begins to cough. What action should the nurse take?
   1. Provide the client with water.
   2. Assist the client to perform mouth care.
   3. Wait for coughing to stop and depress the tongue.
   4. Have the client expectorate into a specimen container.

2. The nurse observes a client use an incentive spirometer. Which action indicates that the client would benefit from additional instruction about the use of the device?
   1. Exhales normally
   2. Holds the spirometer upright
   3. Seals lips around the mouthpiece
   4. Takes a brisk low-volume breath

3. A client's chest x-ray shows a large pleural effusion of the right lower lobe. What should the nurse ensure is at the bedside when preparing this client for a thoracentesis?
   1. Gauze pads
   2. 60-mL syringe
   3. Drainage bag
   4. Antiseptic swabs

4. A client is intubated with the ventilator set at synchronized intermittent mandatory ventilation (SIMV). Which finding should the nurse expect when assessing this client?
   1. Spontaneous breaths
   2. Condensation in the tubing
   3. Deflated endotracheal tube cuff
   4. Consistent number of breaths per minute

5. The nurse prepares to insert an oropharyngeal airway into a client. Which measurement should the nurse use to determine the correct size of the airway?
   1. Tip of the nose to the tip of the ear
   2. Corner of the mouth to the tip of the ear
   3. Middle of the mouth to the tip of the chin
   4. Corner of the mouth to the tragus of the ear

6. The nurse is assisting in the removal of a client's endotracheal tube. At which point should the nurse instruct the client to take a deep breath?
   1. Before deflating the cuff
   2. Before removing the tube
   3. Before preparing the suction catheter
   4. Before the endotracheal tube ties are untied

7. After connecting a sterile suction catheter to the suction tubing in preparation for performing nasopharyngeal suctioning, the sterile catheter tip accidentally touches the client's chin. What should the nurse do first?
   1. Relubricate the tip.
   2. Hyperoxygenate the client.
   3. Dip the tip in sterile water.
   4. Obtain another sterile catheter.

8. While the nurse is suctioning an endotracheal tube, the client begins to cough. What should the nurse do?
   1. Hyperoxygenate for 3–5 breaths.
   2. Instill sterile normal saline into the tube.
   3. Continue to suction the loosened secretions.
   4. Stop suctioning until the client stops coughing.

9. The nurse observes the spouse of a client with a 2-month-old permanent tracheostomy performing care of the site at home. Which observation indicates that additional teaching is required?
   1. Tied the ties after having the client flex the neck
   2. Placed the inner cannula in tap water for cleansing
   3. Used full-strength hydrogen peroxide to cleanse around the stoma
   4. Cleansed the hands before donning gloves and after gloves were removed

10. After turning and repositioning a client with a chest tube, the nurse notes that the fluid in the container is not fluctuating. What should the nurse do first?
    1. Milk the tube.
    2. Strip the tube.
    3. Palpate around the tube.
    4. Check the tube for kinks.

11. The nurse reports a moderate amount of cloudy drainage in a client's chest tube collection container. What should the nurse expect to be prescribed for this client?
    1. Hold anticoagulants.
    2. Culture the drainage.
    3. Begin airborne precautions.
    4. Maintain nothing by mouth status.

12. The nurse auscultates diminished breath sounds in a client who had a chest tube removed 30 minutes ago. What should the nurse expect to be prescribed for this client?
    1. Chest x-ray
    2. Incentive spirometry
    3. Reinsertion of the chest tube
    4. Deep breathing and coughing

Note: For answers and rationales for the review questions, go to Appendix A or your Pearson MyLab Nursing and eText.

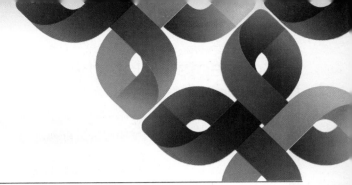

Chapter 12
Perfusion

Chapter at a Glance

❶ Nursing students may observe or assist with the following skills only with faculty permission and while under direct supervision of faculty or another RN.

» The Concept of Perfusion

Perfusion is the immersion of body cells in a fluid. Tissue perfusion refers to the movement of solutes such as oxygen, nutrients, and electrolytes in the blood through the vascular system to capillary networks. Tissue cells are bathed in solutes so they can readily cross cell membranes. Waste products of cellular metabolic activity pass into the interstitial fluid from the cells and are carried away from the cells. When tissue perfusion is diminished or absent, cells do not receive adequate oxygen, nutrients, or electrolytes. This may be manifested by a decrease in blood pressure, restlessness, confusion, cool extremities, pallor or cyanosis of distal extremities, faint peripheral pulses, slowed capillary refill, edema, or life-threatening conditions.

Learning Outcomes

12.1 Give examples of priority safety considerations when preparing and administering a unit of blood to a patient.

12.2 Support the benefits of applying sequential compression devices (SCDs) to promote circulation in the lower legs of an adult patient.

12.3 Summarize priority nursing actions if SCDs are being used on a patient, and the patient complains of numbness and tingling in one leg.

12.4 Explain proper placement of skin electrodes on the patient being monitored on telemetry to avoid artifacts on the monitor screen.

12.5 Differentiate the causes for different waves and intervals, the P wave, the PR interval, the QRS wave, the T wave, and the QT interval when interpreting an electrocardiogram (ECG) pattern.

12.6 Examine the arterial insertion site for signs and symptoms of bleeding, infection, or inflammation.

12.7 Explain why a transcutaneous pacemaker would be applied to a patient with a life-threatening dysrhythmia.

12.8 Explain what a pacemaker spike indicates in an ECG monitor pattern.

The following feature links some, but not all, of the concepts related to assessment. They are presented in alphabetical order.

Concepts Related to
Perfusion

CONCEPT	RELATIONSHIP TO PERFUSION	NURSING IMPLICATIONS
Cognition	Thought processing or mental status is affected if blood volume is decreased.	▪ Monitor oxygen saturation, vital signs, and orientation status ▪ Rule out physical reasons cognition may change
Comfort	Tissues not adequately oxygenated manifest pain.	▪ Monitor pain and for signs of local and systemic hypoxia ▪ Implement oxygen therapy as ordered ▪ Monitor oxygen saturations and vital signs
Fluids and Electrolytes	Excess extracellular fluid volume causes lung congestion and impaired gas exchange.	▪ Monitor fluid intake and output, vital signs, and oxygen saturation ▪ Implement oxygen therapy as ordered ▪ Administer medications as ordered
Intracranial Regulation	Blood flow volume to brain can change intracranial pressure (ICP).	▪ Monitor vital signs, pupils, sensorium, and assess for motor or sensory neuro deficits
Tissue Integrity	Wound healing delayed without adequate perfusion to tissue.	▪ Oxygen is needed for cell metabolism; hyperbaric oxygen therapy can be effective

» Maintaining Blood Volume

Most people in good health give little thought to their cardiovascular function. Changing position frequently, ambulating, and exercising usually maintain adequate cardiovascular functioning. Immobility is detrimental to cardiovascular function.

Expected Outcomes

1. Early detection of bleeding occurs and loss of blood is minimized.
2. Pressure dressing is applied, and bleeding is controlled.

Preventing venous stasis is an important intervention to reduce the risk of complications following surgery, trauma, or major medical problems. The use of antiembolism stockings and sequential compression devices is an additional measure that can help prevent venous stasis.

3. Blood volume and components stabilize after blood product administration as reflected in vital signs and oxygen saturation assessment.

SKILL 12.1 Blood Products: Administering

Safety Note! *During scheduled clinical time, nursing students may have a learning opportunity to observe or assist with this skill only with faculty permission and with direct supervision from faculty or another RN.*

Blood products such as platelets, red blood cells, fresh frozen plasma, and cryoprecipitate are processed components removed from whole blood. Plasma processed components include albumin, coagulation factors, and immunoglobulins. These products are given to patients who only require certain elements of blood for specific treatments such as increasing oxygen-carrying capacity and promoting coagulation.

Delegation or Assignment

Due to the need for sterile technique and technical complexity, administering blood products is not delegated or assigned to the

UAP. The nurse must ensure that the UAP knows what complications or adverse signs can occur and should report these to the nurse. In some states, only RNs can administer blood products.

Equipment

▪ Blood component
▪ IV solution of normal saline, 250 mL
▪ Appropriate IV administration kit
▪ Filter, if indicated
▪ Clean gloves

Preparation

▪ Review healthcare provider's orders and patient's nursing plan of care.
▪ Verify patient has signed informed consent to receive the blood products.

SKILL 12.1 Blood Products: Administering (*continued*)

- Review patient's record for allergies.
- Anticipate results of infusing blood component:
  - Fresh frozen plasma—given to build up clotting factors, albumin, and immune-globulins
  - Platelets—given to improve coagulation and prevent bleeding
  - Red blood cells (RBC)—given to build up red blood cell count for improved oxygenation and treatment of anemia.
- Gather equipment and supplies.

Procedure

1. Introduce self to patient and verify the patient's identity using two identifiers. Explain to the patient you are going to administer a blood product ordered by the healthcare provider, why it is necessary, and how the patient can participate. Discuss how the results will be used in planning further care or treatments.
2. Perform hand hygiene and observe appropriate infection control procedures.
3. Provide for patient privacy.
4. Follow directions for proper administration of the blood product/component.

5. Identify rate at which blood component should infuse.
6. Infusing blood components may produce adverse effects that can range from mild allergic manifestations to fatal reactions (see steps 10 and 11 in Skill 12.2).
7. When the procedure is complete, perform hand hygiene and leave patient safe and comfortable.
8. Complete documentation using forms, checklists, or electronic dropdown lists supplemented by nurse's notes or additional comments as appropriate.

Safety Considerations

In addition to the usual blood components such as platelets and cryoprecipitate, modified blood products are becoming more popular. Washed, irradiated, or leukocyte-removed blood is being used for patients at risk because of multiple transfusions or a weakened immune system. Testing for cytomegalovirus and matching RBC or human leukocyte antigens is also done to ensure safe transfusions.

When infusing a blood product that has undergone leukocyte reduction, remember that it must be filtered again through a standard blood administration set in order to trap cellular debris that may have accumulated since the original filtration.

SKILL 12.2 Blood Transfusion: Administering

Safety Note! *During scheduled clinical time, nursing students may have a learning opportunity to observe or assist with this skill only with faculty permission and with direct supervision from faculty or another RN.*

A blood transfusion transfers blood from a donor to a patient to replace blood volume lost from trauma, medical conditions, or surgical procedure. Whole blood contains red blood cells, white blood cells, platelets, plasma, and electrolytes. The patient's blood type must be compatible with the donor's blood type. Some patients who know they will need blood for a surgical procedure can donate their own blood, have it stored in the healthcare facility's blood bank, and receive it later during surgery. This is called an autologous transfusion.

Delegation or Assignment

Due to the need for sterile technique and technical complexity, blood transfusion is not delegated or assigned to the UAP. The nurse must ensure that the UAP knows what complications or adverse signs can occur and should report these to the nurse. In some states, only RNs can administer blood or blood products.

Equipment

- Unit of whole blood (for packed RBCs, or other blood components, see Skill 12.1)
- Blood administration set
- IV pump (follow facility policy for device and method of controlling flow rate if IV pump not available; see Skill 5.7)

- 250 mL normal saline for infusion
- Venipuncture start kit containing an 18- to 20-gauge needle or catheter (if one is not already in place) or, if the blood is to be administered quickly, a larger catheter
- Alcohol swabs
- Tape
- Clean gloves

Preparation

- Review healthcare provider's orders and patient's nursing plan of care.
- Review patient's record for allergies.
- Verify patient's signed informed consent is in the patient's record.
- Gather equipment and supplies.
- If the patient has an intravenous solution infusing, check the IV catheter size and IV solution running. The only IV solution that is appropriate to use when administering blood is normal saline. The preferred IV catheter size is #18 to #20 gauge.

CAUTION! Dextrose solution (which causes lysis of RBCs), Ringer's solution, medications and other additives, and hyperalimentation solutions are incompatible with blood or blood components.

- If the patient does not have an IV solution infusing, check facility policies. In some facilities an infusion must be running

(*continued on next page*)

SKILL 12.2 Blood Transfusion: Administering (*continued*)

before the blood is obtained from the blood bank. In this case, you will need to perform a venipuncture on a suitable vein and start an IV infusion of normal saline using a blood administration tubing set.

Procedure

1. Introduce self and verify the patient's identity using facility protocol. Explain to the patient you are going to administer a blood transfusion, why it is necessary, and how the patient can participate. Discuss how the results will be used in planning further care or treatments. Instruct the patient to report promptly any sudden chills, nausea, itching, rash, dyspnea, back pain, or other unusual symptoms.
2. Provide for patient privacy and prepare the patient.
   - Assist the patient to a comfortable position, either sitting or lying. Expose the IV site but provide for patient privacy.
3. Perform hand hygiene and observe other appropriate infection control procedures.
4. Prepare the infusion equipment.
   - Ensure that the blood filter inside the drip chamber is suitable for the blood product to be transfused. Attach the blood tubing to the blood filter, if necessary. **Rationale:** *Blood filters have a surface area large enough to allow the blood components through easily but are designed to trap clots.*
   - Don gloves and locate IV pump close to IV insertion site.
   - Close all the clamps on the Y-set: the main flow rate clamp and both Y-line clamps ❶.
   - Insert the piercing spike into the saline solution.
   - Hang the container on the IV pole about 1 m (39 in.) above the venipuncture site.
5. Prime the tubing.
   - Open the upper clamp on the normal saline tubing, and squeeze the drip chamber until it covers the filter and one third of the drip chamber above the filter.
   - Tap the filter chamber to expel any residual air in the filter.
   - Turn IV pump on; open the saline and main flow rate clamps on IV tubing to begin the saline infusion.
   - Close both clamps; thread IV tubing through pump following manufacturer's recommendations; set appropriate flow rate on IV pump.
6. Start the saline solution.
   - If an IV solution incompatible with blood is infusing, stop the infusion and discard the solution and tubing according to facility policy.
   - Attach the blood tubing primed with normal saline to the intravenous catheter.
   - Open the saline and main flow rate clamps and adjust the flow rate. Use only the main flow rate clamp to adjust the rate.
   - Allow a small amount of solution to infuse to make sure there are no problems with the flow or with the venipuncture site. **Rationale:** *Infusing normal saline before initiating the transfusion also clears the IV catheter of incompatible solutions or medications.*
7. Obtain the correct blood to be transfused for the patient ❷.
   - Check the order against the blood bank requisition.

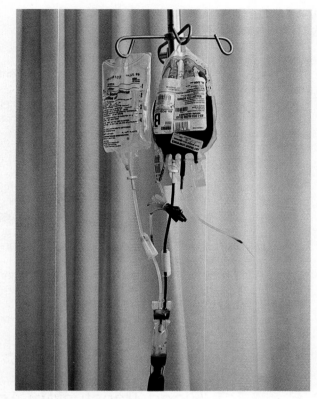

Source: Ronald May/Pearson Education, Inc.

❶ Prime blood administration Y-set tubing with sterile normal saline before starting infusion.

- Check the requisition form and the blood bag label with a blood bank technician or according to facility policy. Specifically, check the patient's name, identification number, blood type (A, B, AB, or O) and Rh group, the blood donor number, and the expiration date of the blood. Observe the blood for abnormal color, clumping, gas bubbles, and extraneous material. Return outdated or abnormal blood to the blood bank.

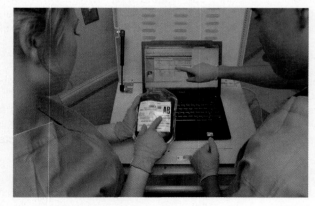

Source: Ronald May/Pearson Education, Inc.

❷ Obtain ordered typed and matched blood/component bag from blood bank.

SKILL 12.2 Blood Transfusion: Administering (*continued*)

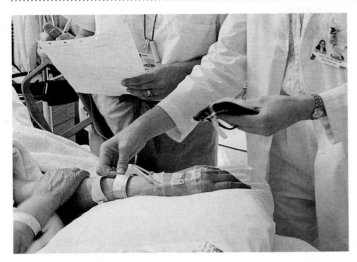

Source: Ronald May/Pearson Education, Inc.

❸ Ascertain that patient's name, ID number, blood group, number/Rh, unit expiration date, and hospital number match the number on the record on the blood bag.

- With another nurse (many agencies require an RN), verify the following before initiating the transfusion:
  - *Healthcare provider's order:* Check the blood against the healthcare provider's written order.
  - *Patient identification:* The name and identification number on the patient's identification band must be identical to the name and number attached to the unit of blood ❸.
  - *Unit identification:* The unit identification number on the blood container, the transfusion form, and the tag attached to the unit must agree.
  - *ABO and Rh type:* The ABO group and Rh type on the primary label of the donor unit must agree with those recorded on the transfusion form.
  - *Expiration:* The expiration date and time of the donor unit should be verified as acceptable.
  - *Compatibility:* The interpretation of compatibility testing must be recorded on the transfusion form and on the tag attached to the unit.
- If any of the information does not match *exactly,* notify the charge nurse and the blood bank. Do not administer blood until discrepancies are corrected or clarified.
- Sign the appropriate form with the other nurse according to facility policy.
- Make sure the unit of blood is left at room temperature for no more than 30 minutes before starting the transfusion. Agencies may designate different times at which the blood must be returned to the blood bank if it has not been started. **Rationale:** *As blood warms, the risk of bacterial growth increases.* If the start of the transfusion is unexpectedly delayed, return the blood to the blood bank within 30 minutes. Do **not** store blood in the unit refrigerator. **Rationale:** *The temperature of unit refrigerators is not precisely regulated and the blood may be damaged.*

8. Prepare the blood bag.
   - Invert the blood bag gently several times to mix the cells with the plasma. **Rationale:** *Rough handling can damage the cells.*
   - Expose the port on the blood bag by pulling back the tabs.
   - Insert the remaining Y-set spike into the blood bag.
   - Suspend the blood bag.
9. Establish the blood transfusion.
   - Close the upper clamp below the IV saline solution container.
   - Open the upper clamp below the blood bag. The blood will run into the saline-filled drip chamber. If necessary, squeeze the drip chamber to re-establish the liquid level with the drip chamber one third full. (Tap the filter to expel any residual air within the filter.)
   - Readjust the flow rate on IV pump to recommended rate of 1-2 mL/min for first 15 minutes of infusion.
   - Remove and discard gloves. Perform hand hygiene.
10. Observe the patient closely for the first 15 minutes ❹.
    - Take a set of baseline vital signs before beginning the unit of blood.
    - It is recommended that transfusions of RBCs be started at 1-2 mL/min for the first 15 minutes of the transfusion to check for a reaction from the patient to the blood. The nurse should stay with the patient during this time to note adverse reactions, such as chilling, nausea, vomiting, dyspnea, headache, vital changes, skin rash, flank pain, or tachycardia. **Rationale:** *The earlier a transfusion reaction occurs, the more severe it tends to be. Promptly identifying such reactions helps to minimize the consequences.*

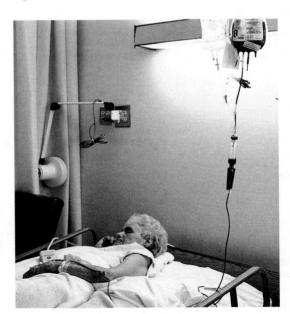

Source: Ronald May/Pearson Education, Inc.

❹ Observe the patient carefully for the first 15 min and frequently throughout the blood transfusion. It is recommended to stay at the patient's side during the first 15 min of the transfusion.

(*continued on next page*)

SKILL 12.2 Blood Transfusion: Administering (*continued*)

- Remind the patient to call a nurse immediately if any unusual symptoms are felt during the transfusion such as chills, nausea, itching, rash, dyspnea, or back pain.
- If one of these reactions occurs, take these immediate actions:
  - Stop and disconnect the transfusion.
  - Using a new IV tubing administration set, keep the IV line open with normal saline solution.
  - Stay with the patient, and call for help.
  - Intervene for reaction signs and symptoms manifested by the patient.
  - Report situation to the nurse in charge, healthcare provider, and blood bank.
11. Monitor the patient.
    - Fifteen minutes after initiating the transfusion (or according to facility policy), check the vital signs. If there are no signs of a reaction, establish the required flow rate. Most adults can tolerate receiving one unit of blood in 1½–2 hr. Do not transfuse a unit of blood for longer than 4 hr.
    - Assess the patient, including vital signs, every 30 minutes or more often, depending on the health status and facility policy. If the patient has a reaction and the blood is discontinued, send the blood bag to the laboratory for investigation of the blood.
12. Terminate the transfusion.
    - Don clean gloves.
    - If no infusion is to follow, clamp the blood tubing. Check facility protocol to determine if the blood component bag needs to be returned or if the blood bag and tubing can be disposed of in a biohazard container. The IV line can be discontinued or capped with an adapter, or a new infusion line and solution container may be added. If another transfusion is to be transfused, follow manufacturer's directions and facility policy regarding changing tubing for multiple units of transfused blood.
    - If the primary IV is to be continued, flush the maintenance line with saline solution. Disconnect the blood tubing system and re-establish the intravenous infusion using new tubing. Adjust IV pump flow rate to prescribed infusion rate. Often a normal saline or other solution is kept running in case of delayed reaction to the blood.
    - Measure vital signs.

13. Follow facility protocol for appropriate disposition of the used supplies.
    - Discard the administration set according to facility practice.
    - Dispose of blood bags.
      a. On the requisition attached to the blood unit, fill in the time the transfusion was completed and the amount transfused.
      b. Attach one copy of the requisition to the patient's record and another to the empty blood bag if required by facility policy.
      c. Facility policy generally involves returning the bag to the blood bank for reference in case of subsequent or delayed adverse reaction.
14. When the procedure is complete, remove and discard gloves. Perform hand hygiene and leave the patient safe and comfortable.
15. Complete documentation using forms, checklists, or electronic dropdown lists supplemented by nurse's notes or additional comments as appropriate.
    - At the beginning of the blood transfusion, record time the blood unit was started, including vital signs, type of blood, blood unit number, sequence number (e.g., #1 of three ordered units), site of the venipuncture, size of the needle, and drip rate.
    - At the completion of the blood transfusion, record the amount of blood absorbed, the blood unit number, and the vital signs. If the primary intravenous infusion was continued, record connecting it. Also record the transfusion on the IV flow sheet and intake and output record.

SAMPLE DOCUMENTATION

[date] 1420 C/o feeling warm, headache, & backache. Skin flushed. T 39.2°C (102.6°F), BP 140/90 mmHg, P-112 bpm, R-28/min. Approximately 50 mL PRBCs infused over past 20 minutes. Infusion stopped. Tubing changed, NS infusing at 15 mL/h. Blood & admin. tubing sent to blood bank. Dr. Riley notified. *C. Jones*

SKILL 12.3 Direct Pressure: Applying

Applying direct pressure is a quick action to control bleeding. Once the flow stops, the blood starts coagulating and forms a clot. Elevating the area will help this process. Use appropriate personal protective equipment (PPE) such as gloves with gauze pad to create a barrier from direct contact with blood.

Delegation or Assignment

The nurse must first assess and evaluate the UAP on performing this skill safely and effectively while calling for help. The nurse may then delegate the skill. The nurse remains responsible for the assessment, interpretation of abnormal findings, and determination of appropriate responses.

Equipment

- Sterile gauze pads if available
- Clean gloves

Preparation

- Observe patient has overt active bleeding.

SKILL 12.3 Direct Pressure: Applying (*continued*)

Procedure

1. Introduce self to patient and verify the patient's identity using two identifiers. Explain to the patient what you are going to do, why it is necessary, and how the patient can participate. Discuss how the results will be used in planning further care or treatments.
2. Perform hand hygiene and observe appropriate infection control procedures immediately. Don gloves.
3. Assess site with active bleeding. Apply direct pressure to the bleeding site with sterile gauze pad over it to control manageable bleeding.

or

3. For a major hemorrhaging situation, identify the closest proximal artery ❶. **Rationale:** *The rapid loss of more than 40% of the total blood volume leads to death if rapid aggressive intervention is not implemented.*
   - Apply direct pressure to artery, using your gloved finger.
   - If towels or 4 × 4 gauze pads are available, apply direct pressure to site.
4. Raise the affected limb about 30 degrees above the level of the heart and call for help. **Rationale:** *This decreases arterial blood flow to the area and promotes venous return.*
5. Maintain direct pressure for 5 minutes to promote clot formation. If still hemorrhaging, continue to hold pressure.

CAUTION! Determine if individual is receiving medications or herbal therapies, which affect blood coagulation (e.g., warfarin [Coumadin]). If so, increase time of applied pressure.

---

6. If bleeding subsides, proceed to clean and dress the wound gently.
7. To control nose bleeds (epistaxis), place patient in sitting position, with head tilted forward. Pinch the soft part of the nose against the bridge of the nose for 5 minutes. Apply ice pack to neck. **Rationale:** *This aids vasoconstriction.*
8. Continue to monitor site post bleeding and patient's response to blood loss.
9. Remove and discard gloves when bleeding subsides.
10. When the procedure is complete, perform hand hygiene and leave patient safe and comfortable.
11. Complete documentation using forms, checklists, or electronic dropdown lists supplemented by nurse's notes or additional comments as appropriate.

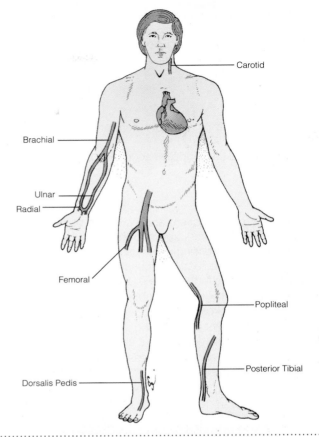

❶ Pulse sites that may be used to control bleeding.

SAMPLE DOCUMENTATION

[date] 1520 Active bleeding noted at IV site, IV catheter pulled out of insertion site at left back of hand. Direct pressure applied with sterile 4 × 4 gauze pad and glove barrier. Arm lifted up, pressure maintained. Bleeding stopped post 2 minutes. Area cleaned and dried, DSD applied. Remained without complaint except for need for another IV stick. Tolerated situation without incident. *R. Agustin*

SKILL 12.4 Pressure Dressing: Applying

A pressure dressing is applied firmly to exert pressure on the wound or area covered to prevent blood or other body fluids from collecting in underlying tissues. It is frequently used to prevent tissue healing disruption caused by edema with burns and skin grafts.

Delegation or Assignment

Due to specific knowledge and skill required, this skill is not delegated or assigned to the UAP. The nurse can request the UAP to report patient observations to the nurse for follow-up. Assessment and evaluation remain the responsibility of the nurse.

Equipment

- Sterile 4 × 4 gauze pad
- Sterile dressings—number and size depends on wound

(*continued on next page*)

SKILL 12.4 Pressure Dressing: Applying (*continued*)

- Sterile gloves or clean gloves as prescribed or stated in facility policy
- Sterile NS or cleansing solution as prescribed or stated in facility policy
- Hypoallergenic tape

Preparation

- Check healthcare provider's orders and patient's nursing plan of care.
- Assemble necessary supplies according to the extent of the wound.

Procedure

1. Introduce self to patient and verify the patient's identity using two identifiers. Explain to the patient you are going to apply a firm dressing, why it is necessary, and how the patient can participate. Discuss how the results will be used in planning further care or treatments.
2. Perform hand hygiene and observe appropriate infection control procedures.
3. Provide for patient privacy. Don sterile gloves.
4. Set up sterile field and prepare cleansing solution.
5. Cleanse wound and apply dressing. Use several layers of 4 × 4 gauze pads.
6. Place tape tightly over entire dressing to provide an occlusive dressing. Do not completely circle an extremity or the body. **Rationale:** *Encircling an extremity with a bandage creates a tourniquet effect and may prevent blood flow.*
7. Check for pulses distal to pressure site. **Rationale:** *This ensures that collateral blood flow is maintained.*
8. Place all soiled material in biohazard bag.
9. When the procedure is complete, doff and discard gloves and perform hand hygiene.

10. Monitor vital signs and observe for signs of shock. Continue to monitor extremity distal to pressure dressing for adequate circulation.
11. Elevate extremity to prevent bleeding.
12. Monitor frequently for signs of bleeding and hematoma. *Note:* Hematomas feel spongy even under bandages.
13. When the procedure is complete, perform hand hygiene, and leave the patient safe and comfortable.
14. Complete documentation using forms, checklists, or electronic dropdown lists supplemented by nurse's notes or additional comments as appropriate, including:
    - Size (in centimeters), location based on anatomical landmark, condition of wound
    - Color, odor, consistency, amount of drainage
    - Type and number of dressings used
    - Approximate amount of blood loss
    - Condition of dressing when removed (e.g., saturated with drainage).

SAMPLE DOCUMENTATION

[date] 1350 Dressing covering third degree burn located left calf changed using sterile technique. Burn cleaned with saline and dried, measures 5 cm (2 in) diameter, small amount eschar tissue noted in middle, white tissue surrounding it with redness noted around burn. Silver burn cream applied as prescribed and pressure dressing firmly applied. Small amount of crying noted, stated it hurt. Comfort and support given to patient by mother. Told him I would return with something to help it hurt less. *T. Moore*

≫ Antiembolism Devices

Expected Outcomes

1. Compression stockings remain wrinkle free and pressure is evenly distributed.
2. Peripheral pulses are present during use of sequential stockings and elastic hosiery.
3. Patient's skin remains intact while using compression stockings.

SKILL 12.5 Antiembolism Stockings: Applying

EVIDENCE-BASED PRACTICE

Compression Stockings—Safe Practice Issues

Compression stockings are generally prescribed as a means of preventing deep venous thrombosis (DVT)—blood clots in the legs. Clots from DVT may travel to the lungs, producing a potentially fatal condition called pulmonary embolism (PE). The current recommendation of the American College of Chest Physicians is ambulation with compression as tolerated, after starting anticoagulation, in patients with acute DVT. However, there are several roadblocks to the correct and consistent use of compression stockings.

Common issues with compression stockings are proper fit, proper use, and patient compliance. Some manufacturers' stockings do not fit patient measurements or are too loose or tight. Effectiveness depends on the appropriate amount of compression for the particular patient's condition, so it is essential to measure the legs and to obtain properly fitting stockings. Also, regular review measurements should be taken to check for changes in leg size and to correct excessive pressure.

SKILL 12.5 Antiembolism Stockings: Applying (*continued*)

Improper use, such as allowing compression stockings to roll down, increases pressure at the ankle and decreases it in the calf or thigh. Improper application or use can create a tourniquet effect.

Patient teaching is important to encourage compliance. Patients should be taught the importance of removing stockings at least once a day and assessing the skin. Nurses should monitor stockings with the patient in a seated, not supine, position to determine whether the stockings are obstructing blood flow. Nurses may need to encourage patients to start or continue to wear compression stockings and explain their purpose, because some patients find compression stockings uncomfortable and simply stop wearing them.

Source: Based on Health Communities. Editors. (2015). *Pulmonary embolism/DVT. Compression stockings & blood clots.* Retrieved from http://www.healthcommunities. com/pulmonary-embolism-dvt/compression-stockings.shtml.

Delegation or Assignment

The UAP frequently removes and applies antiembolism stockings as part of assigned hygiene care. The nurse should stress the importance of removing and reapplying the stockings and reporting to the nurse any changes in the patient's skin. The nurse is responsible for assessment of the skin. Note that state laws for UAPs vary, so this task might be assigned to the UAP or delegated.

Equipment

- Single-use tape measure (to prevent cross-infection)
- Clean knee or thigh antiembolism stockings of appropriate size

Preparation

- Check healthcare provider's order and patient's nursing plan of care.
- Gather supplies needed.
- Take measurements as needed to obtain the appropriate size stockings.
  - Measure the length of both legs from the heel to the gluteal fold (for thigh-length stockings) or from the heel to the popliteal space or bend of the knee (for knee-length stockings).
  - Measure the circumferences of each calf and each thigh at the widest point.
  - Compare measurements to the size chart on the back of the manufacturer's package to obtain stockings of correct

size (**Table 12–1 ≫**). Obtain two sizes if there is a significant difference. **Rationale:** *Stockings that are too large for the patient do not place adequate pressure on the legs to facilitate venous return and may bunch, increasing the risk of pressure and skin irritation. Stockings that are too small may impede blood flow to the feet and cause skin breakdown.*

Procedure

1. Introduce self and verify the patient's identity using two identifiers. Explain to the patient you are going to apply antiembolism stockings, why it is necessary, and how the patient can participate.
2. Perform hand hygiene and observe other appropriate infection control procedures.
3. Provide for patient privacy.
4. Select an appropriate time to apply the stockings.
   - Apply stockings in the morning, if possible, before the patient gets out of bed. **Rationale:** *In sitting and standing positions, the veins can become distended so that edema occurs; the stockings should be applied before this can happen.*
   - Assist the patient who has been ambulating to lie down and elevate legs for 15–30 min before applying the stockings. **Rationale:** *This facilitates venous return, reduces swelling, and facilitates application of the stockings.*
5. Prepare the patient.
   - Assist the patient to a lying position in bed. Raise bed to appropriate height.
   - Wash and dry the legs as needed. Assess legs for skin integrity and circulatory status.
6. Apply the stockings.
   - Reach inside the stocking from the top, and grasping the heel, turn the upper portion of the stocking inside out so the foot portion is inside the stocking leg. **Rationale:** *Firm elastic stockings are easier to fit over the foot and calf when inverted in this manner rather than when they are bunched up.*
   - Ask the patient to point the toes, and then position the stocking on the patient's foot. With the heel of the stocking down and stretching each side of the stocking, ease the stocking over the toes taking care to place

TABLE 12–1 Measuring for Graduated Compression Stockings (Elastic Hosiery)

Thigh-High Measuring		Knee-High Measuring	
Circumference	**Length**	**Circumference**	**Length**
Measure mid-thigh circumference.	Measure leg from bottom of heel to fold of buttocks.	Measure calf at largest circumference.	Measure leg from Achilles tendon to popliteal fold.

(*continued on next page*)

SKILL 12.5 Antiembolism Stockings: Applying (*continued*)

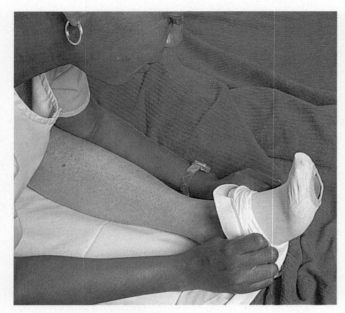

Source: Ronald May/Pearson Education, Inc.

❶ Applying the stocking over the toes.

the toe and heel portions of the stocking appropriately ❶ ❷. **Rationale:** *Pointing the toes makes application easier.*

- Grasp the loose portion of the stocking at the ankle and gently pull the stocking over the leg, turning it right side out in the process. If applying the thigh-length stockings, stretch them over the knee until the top is below the gluteal fold ❸.

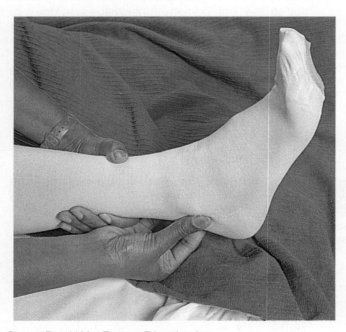

Source: Ronald May/Pearson Education, Inc.

❷ Ensure hose fits properly without wrinkles over toe or heel.

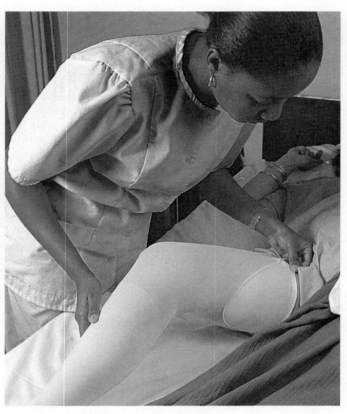

Source: Ronald May/Pearson Education, Inc.

❸ Position support section on inner thigh.

7. When the procedure is complete, return bed to lowest height, perform hand hygiene, and leave patient safe and comfortable.
8. Complete documentation using forms, checklists, or electronic dropdown lists supplemented by nurse's notes or additional comments as appropriate, including the size and length of stockings used.

SAMPLE DOCUMENTATION

[date] 0745 Antiembolism stockings, size L, applied to patient without difficulty while lying in bed. States the stockings feel snug but not too tight. Helped to chair, ready for breakfast. Tolerated without incident. *O. Chu*

CAUTION! Postoperative DVT of the lower extremity is often asymptomatic. In many patients, fatal pulmonary embolism is the first clinical sign of postoperative venous thromboembolism.

SKILL 12.5 Antiembolism Stockings: Applying (*continued*)

Lifespan Considerations
OLDER ADULTS

- Because the elastic is quite strong in antiembolism stockings, older adults may need assistance putting on the stockings. Patients with arthritis may need to have another person put the stockings on for them.
- Many older adults have circulation problems and wear antiembolism stockings. It is important to check for wrinkles in the stockings and to see if the stocking has rolled down or twisted. If so, correct it immediately. *Rationale: The stockings must be evenly distributed over the limb to promote—rather than hinder—circulation.*
- Stockings should be removed at least once a day (check facility policy) so that a thorough assessment can be made of the legs and feet. *Rationale: Redness and skin breakdown on the heels can occur quickly and go undetected if not thoroughly assessed on a regular basis.*
- Provide information about the importance of wearing the elastic stockings, how to wear them correctly, and how to take care of them.

Patient Teaching

Wearing Antiembolism Stockings at Home

- Ensure the patient or caregiver knows how to apply antiembolism stockings.
- Reinforce the importance and the rationales for no wrinkles and no rolling down of the stockings.
- Reinforce the importance of removing the stockings daily and inspecting the skin on the legs.
- Include instructions about:
  - Laundering the stockings (air dry because putting them in a dryer can affect their elasticity.)
  - Needing two pairs of stockings to allow one pair to be worn while the other is being laundered.
  - Replacing the stockings when they lose their elasticity.
- Reinforce knowledge about slipperiness of stockings if worn without slippers or shoes.
  - If the patient is ambulatory, emphasize the need for footwear to prevent falling.

SKILL 12.6 Pneumatic Compression Device: Applying

This device has an air compressor that fills an inflatable sleeve for a period of time, usually positioned over a leg, then allows the air to drain out of the sleeve. The inflating and deflating cycle repeats, applying pressure every time the sleeve is inflated. This treatment, called compression therapy, helps prevent blood clots in deep veins of the legs.

Delegation or Assignment

This skill can be delegated or assigned to the UAP as the pneumatic compression device is frequently removed and reapplied during hygiene care. The nurse should stress the importance of reporting to the nurse any changes in the patient's skin. The nurse is responsible for assessment of the skin. Note that state laws for UAPs vary, so this task might be assigned to the UAP rather than delegated.

Equipment

- Disposable leg sleeve(s), knee-length or thigh-length
- Tubing assembly
- Compression controller (motor)
- Single-use tape measure (to prevent cross-infection)

Preparation

- Review healthcare provider's orders for type of disposable leg sleeve needed.
- Review the patient's nursing plan of care.
- Gather equipment and supplies.
- Assess patient for potential problems and contraindications for use of these devices. *Rationale: Patients on long-term bed rest and patients with ischemic conditions,* *massive edema of the leg, dermatitis, gangrene, or pre-existing DVT within the past 6 months are* not *candidates for these devices.*
- Complete a neurovascular assessment. Include an evaluation of skin color, temperature, sensation, capillary refill, and presence and quality of pedal pulses. Document findings. *Rationale: This assessment provides baseline data for evaluating neurovascular changes while devices are used.*
- Assemble equipment. Read manufacturer's directions for connecting and operating compression controller.
- Read directions for setting sleeve pressure (between 35–45 mmHg). Maximum pressure should not exceed patient's diastolic pressure.
- Locate and identify the indicator lights on the controller for the ankle, calf, and thigh pressure. *Rationale: Light is on when the pressure is applied to the three leg sleeves.*

Procedure

1. Introduce self to patient and verify the patient's identity using two identifiers. Explain to the patient that this device decreases the risk of developing deep venous thrombosis (DVT) for patients following surgery or those on long-term bed rest, why it is necessary, and how the patient can participate. Discuss how the results will be used in planning further care or treatments.
2. Perform hand hygiene and observe appropriate infection control procedures.
3. Provide for patient privacy.
4. Provide comfort and safety for patient and self, including raising bed to appropriate height.

(*continued on next page*)

SKILL 12.6 Pneumatic Compression Device: Applying (continued)

5. Apply the sleeve to the patient's leg.
   - Remove sleeve from plastic bag.
   - Unfold sleeve and follow directions to fit sleeve to patient's leg. Leg is placed on white side (lining) of sleeve. Markings on the lining indicate the ankle and popliteal area.
   - Place patient's leg on sleeve. Position back of knee over popliteal opening.
   - Starting at the side, wrap sleeve securely around patient's leg.
   - Attach Velcro straps securely.
   - Check the fit by placing two fingers between patient's leg and sleeve to determine if sleeve fits properly. Readjust Velcro as needed. **Rationale:** *This is to ensure the sleeve does not constrict circulation.*
6. Turn the device on to begin.
   - Attach tubing and connect to plugs on leg sleeve by pushing ends firmly together.
   - Connect tubing assembly plug to the controller at the tubing assembly connector site.
   - Ensure tubing is free of kinks or twists. **Rationale:** *Kinks and twists can restrict airflow through system.*
   - Plug controller power cable into grounded electric outlet and attach unit to bed frame.
   - Turn controller power switch to ON. Confirm that alarms are audible.
   - Check that pressure indicator lights are functioning properly. Lower bed to lowest height.
7. Monitor that compression cycles are correct.
8. Conduct neurovascular checks every 2–4 hr.
9. Monitor patient's tolerance of device.

10. Turn off machine at prescribed time intervals to assess skin and to provide skin care.

CAUTION!

- Turn machine off immediately if the patient complains of numbness or other signs of DVT.
- Follow hospital policy for amount of time alternating pneumatic compression devices are removed during the day. It is important to keep stockings on most of the day to prevent clot formation.

---

11. To remove sleeve, turn power switch OFF, disconnect tubing assembly from sleeve at connection site. Unwrap sleeve from leg.
12. When the procedure is complete, perform hand hygiene, lower the bed to lowest position, and leave patient safe and comfortable.
13. Complete documentation using forms, checklists, or electronic dropdown lists supplemented by nurse's notes or additional comments as appropriate, including care, assessment, and patient response.

SAMPLE DOCUMENTATION

[date] 0720 Awake and alert, states she is ready for the compression device. Sleeves positioned, connected to compressor pump and turned on. Tolerated without complaint. *R. Ho*

SKILL 12.7 Sequential Compression Devices: Applying

Sequential compression devices (SCDs) operate differently from pneumatic compression devices. SCDs use many inflatable compartments to compress the leg in a graduated sequential fashion. The compartment closest to the foot inflates first and the compartment closest to the thigh inflates last. The amount of pressure also differs in each compartment. The highest pressure is in the first compartment and the lowest in the last one. This creates a "milking" action to empty deeper veins of the lower leg to promote optimal blood flow.

Delegation or Assignment

The UAP often removes and reapplies SCDs when performing assigned or delegated hygiene care. The nurse should check that the UAP knows the correct application process for SCDs. Remind the UAP that the patient should not have SCDs removed for long periods of time because the purpose of the SCDs is to promote circulation. Note that state laws for UAPs vary, so this task might be assigned to the UAP or delegated.

Equipment

- Single-use tape measure (to prevent cross-infection)
- SCDs, including disposable sleeves, air pump, and tubing

Preparation

- Review healthcare provider's orders and the patient's nursing plan of care.
- Gather equipment and supplies.

Procedure

1. Introduce self and verify the patient's identity using two identifiers. Explain to the patient what you are going to do, why it is necessary, and the procedure for applying the sequential compression device. **Rationale:** *The patient's participation and comfort will be increased by understanding the reasons for applying the SCD.*
2. Perform hand hygiene and observe other appropriate infection control procedures.

SKILL 12.7 Sequential Compression Devices: Applying *(continued)*

3. Provide for patient privacy and drape the patient appropriately. Assess legs for skin integrity and neurovascular status.
4. Prepare the patient. Position bed at correct height for procedure.
   - Place the patient in a dorsal recumbent or semi-Fowler position.
   - Measure the patient's legs as recommended by the manufacturer if a thigh-length sleeve is required. **Rationale:** *Foot and knee-length sleeves come in just one size; the thigh circumference determines the size needed for a thigh-length sleeve.*
5. Apply the sequential compression sleeves.
   - Place a sleeve under each leg with the opening at the knee ❶.
   - Wrap the sleeve securely around the leg, securing the Velcro tabs. Allow two fingers to fit between the leg and sleeve ❷. **Rationale:** *This amount of space ensures that the sleeve does not impair circulation when inflated.* Ensure that there is no overlapping or increases in the SCD. **Rationale:** *This prevents skin breakdown.*
6. Connect the sleeves to the control unit and adjust the pressure as needed ❸. Reposition bed to lowest height.
   - Connect the tubing to the sleeves and control unit ensuring that arrows on the plug and the connector are in alignment and that the tubing is not kinked or twisted. **Rationale:** *Improper alignment or obstruction of the tubing by kinks or twists will interfere with operation of the SCD.*

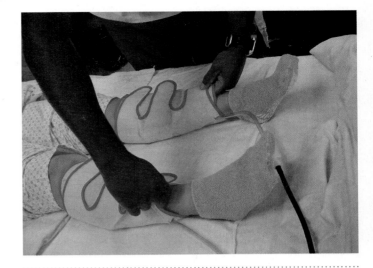

❷ Slip two fingers under wrap to ensure that it is not too tight.

   - Turn on the control unit and adjust the alarms and pressures as needed. The sleeve cooling control and alarm should be on; ankle pressure is usually set at 35–55 mmHg. **Rationale:** *It is important to have the sleeve cooling control on for comfort and to reduce the risk of skin irritation from moisture under the sleeve. Proper pressure settings prevent injury to the patient.*

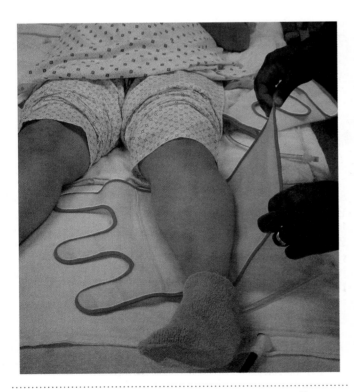

❶ Place inflatable bladder directly behind patient's calf.

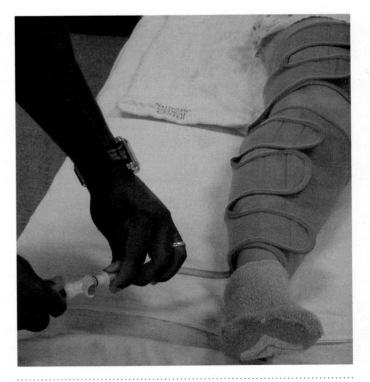

❸ Attach tubing from wrap to tubing connected to pump.

(continued on next page)

SKILL 12.7 Sequential Compression Devices: Applying (*continued*)

7. When the procedure is complete, lower the bed to lowest position, perform hand hygiene and leave patient safe and comfortable.

8. Complete documentation using forms, checklists, or electronic dropdown lists supplemented by nurse's notes or additional comments as appropriate including baseline assessment data and application of the SCD. Note control unit settings. Assess and document skin integrity and neurovascular and peripheral vascular status per facility policy while the SCD is in place.

SAMPLE DOCUMENTATION

[date] 0812 Awake and alert sitting up in bed. SCD active, leg wraps in place and warm to touch. No complaints of pain, numbness, or tingling of toes. Both legs set at 45 mm pressure per SCD device. Tolerating SCD device without incident. *S. Diaz*

CAUTION! Remove the unit and notify the healthcare provider if the patient complains of numbness and tingling or leg pain.

Safety Considerations

CONTRAINDICATIONS TO USE OF SCDs

- Known or suspected acute deep vein thrombosis (DVT), phlebitis, severe atherosclerosis, or ischemic peripheral vascular disease

- DVT within the past 6 months
- Pulmonary embolism
- Any condition in which an increase in venous return to the heart might be detrimental
- Local conditions such as dermatitis, gangrene, recent skin graft, infected leg wound, or ulcer

EVIDENCE-BASED PRACTICE

Recommend Bed Rest for DVT?

Prolonged immobilization has been associated with DVT in critically ill patients. However, the value and safety of mobilizing patients with acute DVT has been a concern, largely because of the potential for venous thromboembolism (dislodging of the clot into the bloodstream) and life-threatening pulmonary embolism (PE).

A number of studies have shown that patients with acute DVT who use compression stockings and begin ambulating early after initiation of anticoagulant therapy experience several benefits from this approach. Benefits include reduced pain level, more rapid reduction in edema, increased strength maintenance, and improved flexibility. Early ambulation in these patients, with careful monitoring for any evidence of PE, resulted in no increase in incidence of PE. Conversely, bed rest and immobilization did not result in any reduction in incidence of PE. Therefore, the current recommendation of the American College of Chest Physicians is ambulation with compression as tolerated, after starting anticoagulation, in patients with acute DVT.

Source: Data from Christakou, A. (2015). *Effectiveness of early mobilization in hospitalized patients with deep venous thrombosis*. Retrieved from http://www.hospitalchronicles.gr/index.php/hchr/article/view/553.

>> Electrical Conduction in the Heart

Any disturbance in the rate or rhythm of the heartbeat is termed *dysrhythmia*. Historically, the term *arrhythmia* has been used in the literature. Although the terms are often used interchangeably, dysrhythmia, which means "a disturbance in cardiac rhythm," is more accurate. Dysrhythmias are classified according to their site of origin: sinus, atrial, junctional, ventricular, and atrioventricular (AV) nodal tissue. A sinus dysrhythmia usually reflects a change in rate or rhythm. An atrial dysrhythmia results from a disturbance with the sinoatrial (SA) node or atria indicated by an abnormality in the P-wave configuration.

A junctional dysrhythmia occurs when there is a problem associated with the AV node as indicated by a change in the PR interval. A ventricular dysrhythmia results from a problem with the ventricle and is indicated by an abnormality in the configuration of the QRS complex. Although many dysrhythmias have no clinical manifestations, many others have serious consequences. A ventricular dysrhythmia is the most life threatening because it compromises cardiac output.

Expected Outcomes

1. AED and its electrodes and cables are applied appropriately to patient.
2. Electrocardiogram (ECG) leads are applied appropriately and without difficulty.
3. Abnormal ECG findings are interpreted accurately.
4. Monitor waveforms are distinct and readable.
5. Patient's cardiac rate is maintained through use of a pacemaker.
6. Patient is prepared psychologically and physically for insertion of the pacemaker.
7. Pacemaker is inserted without complications.

SKILL 12.8 Automated External Defibrillator (AED): Adult, Using

Safety Note! *During scheduled clinical time, nursing students may have a learning opportunity to observe or assist with this skill only with faculty permission and with direct supervision from faculty or another RN.*

This piece of equipment is a portable lightweight easy-to-use automated external defibrillator (AED). Nonmedical people in public places such as airports, sports stadiums, libraries, and shopping malls are being trained to use the AED. Evidence supports this device can save lives when used appropriately for sudden cardiac arrests.

Delegation or Assignment

Any person who has been trained in its use can apply and activate the AED.

Equipment

- AED with all components including the automatic override key, event documentation module or tape, electrodes and cables, and charged battery pack. Brands and models differ in their features.

Preparation

- Assess for unresponsiveness, call for nearby help, assess breathing and pulse simultaneously.
- Start chest compressions immediately, call for more help, the AED, and rapid response team.

Procedure

1. Follow steps for CPR. Traditional CPR must be performed until the AED can be attached.
2. Attach the AED.
   - Turn on the power of the AED (usually a green ON/OFF button).
   - Apply the electrode pads to dry skin: one in the upper right chest near the clavicle, and the other in the lower left chest below the nipple ❶.
   - If the person has heavy chest hair, it may be necessary to remove the hair with pocket scissors or a razor.

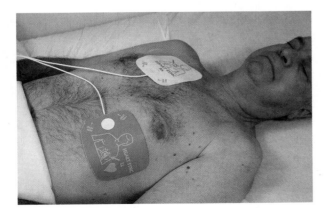

Source: Rick Brady/Pearson Education, Inc.

❶ Apply pads to chest, one below right clavicle, one below and lateral to heart.

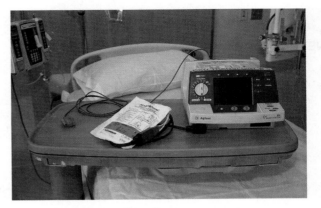

Source: Rick Brady/Pearson Education, Inc.

❷ If AED indicates need for shock, push SHOCK on AED.

Rationale: *Heavy chest hair may prevent the pads from sticking to the chest and may also catch fire during defibrillation.*
   - Attach the cables to the box if necessary.
3. Initiate rhythm analysis. Be sure no one is touching the person. **Rationale:** *This ensures that the AED is reading only the person's cardiac electrical activity.* The analysis may take 5–15 sec. In most models, this also charges the AED.
4. Defibrillate as indicated.
   - Before delivering the shock, state loudly "Clear" and check visually to ensure that no one is touching the person and that nothing is touching the person (e.g., the bed) ❷. **Rationale:** *If a shock is delivered while someone is in contact with the person, that person will also receive the shock.*
   - Press the shock button and observe for the brief contraction of the person's muscles that indicates the shock has been delivered.
5. Resume CPR. The AED will automatically prompt to reanalyze the person at 2-min intervals. Continue the sequence of CPR and defibrillation until the AED specifies that no shock is indicated, the person converts to a functional rhythm (pulse is felt or movement observed), or the rapid response team takes over.
6. Complete documentation using forms, checklists, or electronic dropdown lists supplemented by nurse's notes or additional comments as appropriate including data provided by the AED.
7. Attach ECG strips or other records made by the AED.

SAMPLE DOCUMENTATION

[date] 1050 Found on bathroom floor. Assessed, unresponsive, called for help, not breathing, no pulse, chest compressions begun, called for more help, AED, and rapid response team. Attached to AED. No shock advised. Continued CPR. *R. Lee*

(continued on next page)

SKILL 12.8 Automated External Defibrillator (AED): Adult, Using (continued)

Lifespan Considerations

NEWBORNS AND INFANTS

- Use child-size pads if available and place one on anterior left chest and one on posterior left chest.

- A manual defibrillator is preferred. If a manual defibrillator is not available, an AED with pediatric dose attenuation is desirable. If neither is available, an AED without a dose attenuator may be used.

CHILDREN

- Use child-size pads if available.

- Select a child shock dose (pediatric dose attenuator) on the AED if available. This may require turning a key or switch. If a child dose is not available, an AED without a dose attenuator may be used.

SKILL 12.9 ECG, 12-Lead: Recording

A 12-lead electrocardiogram (ECG) recording is made from electrical activity in the heart muscle. The electrical activity is shown as deflections representing changes in the voltage and polarity magnitude over time and the electrical conduction pathway. The deflections are named the P wave, QRS complex, and T wave (sometimes a U wave, too).

Delegation or Assignment

A lab, respiratory, or ECG technician trained to do an ECG recording usually does this diagnostic test. In some states, the UAP is trained to do an ECG recording. Nurses in special care units can be trained to do an ECG recording. Assessment and evaluation remain the responsibility of the nurse. Note that state laws for UAPs vary, so this task might be assigned to the UAP rather than delegated.

Equipment

- Electrodes
- Skin prep pad or alcohol swab
- ECG machine
- Cable

Preparation

- Review healthcare provider's order for ECG and patient's nursing plan of care.
- Gather ECG machine.

Procedure

1. Introduce self to patient and verify the patient's identity using two identifiers. Explain to the patient what you are going to do, why it is necessary, and how the patient can participate. Discuss how the results will be used in planning further care or treatments. Reassure patient that machine will not cause discomfort or electrical shock.
2. Perform hand hygiene and observe appropriate infection control procedures.
3. Provide for patient privacy. Provide comfort and safety for patient and self, including raising bed to appropriate height.
4. Attach lead electrodes to patient's chest.
   - Assess chest for placement of electrodes.
   - Determine if skin site care is necessary. If so, cleanse areas with skin prep pad or alcohol swab, or clip hair if needed. Allow area to dry thoroughly before placing electrodes.

- Attach lead wires to electrodes before pressing onto patient's chest. **Rationale:** *This prevents excess pressure, especially after open heart surgery or chest trauma.*
- Check the color coding on the manufacturer's directions before placing electrodes to ensure they are correct.
- When placing electrodes, ensure lead wires are all going in the same direction.
- Place electrodes on fleshy areas, avoiding bone and muscle. **Rationale:** *This is to ensure good electrical conduction and clear ECG tracings.*
- Place the four-limb leads, one on each limb, according to the color coding. Three standard leads will be recorded on the 12-lead ECG:
  Lead I: Right arm wrist (negative electrode) white; and left arm (positive electrode) black. Records activity between the two arms.
  Lead II: Right arm (negative electrode) and left leg ankle (positive electrode) red. Records activity between arm and leg. Best for monitoring atrial functioning.
  Lead III: Left arm (negative electrode) black and left leg (positive electrode) green. Records activity between arm and leg.
- Three augmented limb lead tracings are obtained on the ECG as follows:
  aVR: Records activity between the center of the heart and right arm.
  aVL: Records activity between the center of the heart and left arm.
  aVF: Records activity between the center of the heart and the left leg or foot.
- Place the chest leads as follows ❶.
  V_1: Fourth intercostal space, right sternal border. Records activity between the center of the heart and the fourth intercostal space; P wave is shown best here.
  - Palpate the jugular notch above sternum (feels like a depression).
  - Move finger down and palpate the manubrium of sternum (feels solid).
  - Continue to move finger down to the angle of Louis, which is at the top of the sternal body.
  - Move finger to the right of the angle of Louis to the second right rib.
  - Below the rib is the second intercostal space.

SKILL 12.9 ECG, 12-Lead: Recording (*continued*)

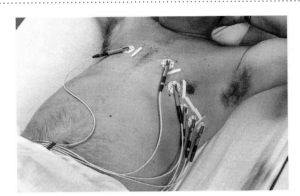

Source: Rick Brady/Pearson Education, Inc.

1 Electrode placement for chest leads V₁ through V₆.

- Move fingers down, palpating the next two ribs. Below the fourth rib and to the right of the sternal body is the fourth intercostal space. Place electrode in this area.
  V_2: Fourth intercostal space, left sternal border.
  V_3: Midway between V_2 and V, between fourth and fifth intercostal space.
  V_4: Fifth intercostal space, left midclavicular line.
  V_5: Fifth intercostal space, anterior axillary line.
  V_6: Fifth intercostal space, left midaxillary line.

5. Once electrodes and leads are attached, ask patient to lie still for recording of ECG according to manufacturer's directions on the machine **2**.
6. Remove electrodes.
7. Place tracing copy in patient's chart **3**.
8. When the procedure is complete, lower bed to lowest position, perform hand hygiene, and leave patient safe and comfortable.
9. Complete documentation using forms, checklists, or electronic dropdown lists supplemented by nurse's notes or additional comments as appropriate.

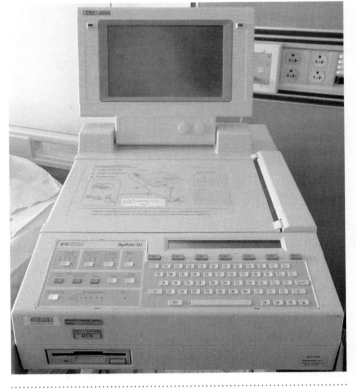

2 Portable ECG machine for taking 12-lead tracing.

SAMPLE DOCUMENTATION
[date] 1810 Lying in semi-Fowler position in bed, awake and alert. 12-lead ECG done. Tolerated without complaint. Placed in sitting position per patient's request. *E. Muck*

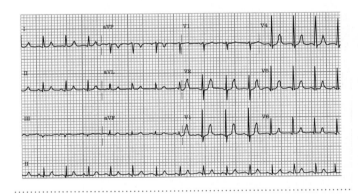

3 Normal 12-lead ECG.

SKILL 12.10 ECG Leads: Applying

To monitor the electrical activity of a patient's heart continuously, the healthcare provider can order telemetry monitoring. A small electronic device is attached to the patient along with electrocardiogram (ECG) leads. The heart rate and rhythm are then displayed on a monitor screen in a room close to the nurse's station. The telemetry ECG system usually has 5-lead electrodes and wires, although some healthcare and other facilities use a 3-lead electrodes and wires system.

Delegation or Assignment

Applying and replacing ECG leads can be done by UAPs who are trained to do this skill. Nurses are responsible for ECG lead placement. Assessment and evaluation remain the responsibility of the nurse. Note that state laws for UAPs vary, so this task might be assigned to the UAP rather than delegated.

(*continued on next page*)

SKILL 12.10 ECG Leads: Applying (*continued*)

Equipment

- Telemetry transmitter box with 9-volt battery ❶

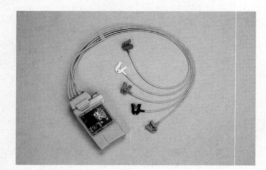

Source: Rick Brady/Pearson Education, Inc.

❶ Transmitter box, cable, and 5-lead electrodes and wires for telemetry.

- Electrode pouch or gown with transmitter pocket
- 5-lead electrode cable and wires, or a 3-lead electrode cable and wires
- Electrodes
- Skin prep pad or alcohol swab

Preparation

- Check healthcare provider's order and patient's nursing plan of care.
- Gather equipment.
- Review the patient's cardiac assessment. **Rationale:** *The choice of monitoring lead is based on the patient's assessment and potential dysrhythmias that could occur.*
- Place a fresh 9-volt battery, if needed, in the telemetry transmitter box.
- Attach lead wire securely into transmitter box, ensuring colors match.

Procedure

1. Introduce self to patient and verify the patient's identity using two identifiers. Explain that you are going to connect a telemetry monitor to the patient, why it is necessary, and how the patient can participate. Discuss how the results will be used in planning further care or treatments. Explain that radio waves transmit the heart's electrical activity to a central monitoring station. This system allows the patient to move around while the heart is constantly being monitored. Explain that the telemetry range is limited; therefore, patient cannot wander out of the range, which is usually the nursing unit. If patient goes off the unit, the nurse must be notified. Instruct the patient to notify the nurse if the electrode falls off.
2. Perform hand hygiene and observe appropriate infection control procedures.
3. Provide for patient privacy.
4. Check the expiration date on the electrode packet. **Rationale:** *This ensures electrode gel is moist.*
5. Select electrode sites according to leads to be used for monitoring. Ensure they are not over bony prominences, muscular areas, joints, breasts, or skin creases.

Note: If patient is overly obese, electrodes may have to be placed on the bones, since a large amount of adipose tissue results in a poor image on the oscilloscope.

6. Assess skin site before placing electrode. Wipe skin areas using alcohol swab. Allow site to dry thoroughly before affixing electrode. **Rationale:** *This removes oily substances and dead skin for better adherence of electrodes.* If patient's chest is hairy, clip the hair. **Rationale:** *This enables electrodes to adhere well to skin and minimizes artifact.*
7. Attach lead wires to chest electrodes. Some healthcare facilities use a 5-lead electrode cable and wires system; others use a 3-lead electrode cable and wires system (see **Table 12–2 ≫**).
8. Apply electrodes to patient's chest ❷: peel off paper backing on electrode disc. Check that sponge pad in center of electrode is moist with conductive jelly. Place electrode on skin with adhesive side down. Press edges down to secure.

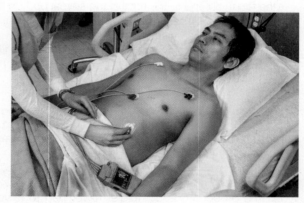

Source: Rick Brady/Pearson Education, Inc.

❷ Color-coded 5-lead electrodes and wires and placement of electrodes for ECG monitoring.

9. Attach wire to transmitter box, matching the color codes of the wires to the telemetry box ❸. **Rationale:** *Mismatch of the colors will cause the patient's rhythm pattern to appear inverted.*

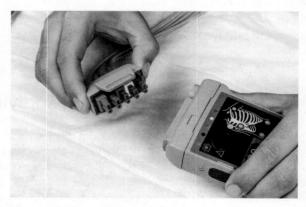

Source: Rick Brady/Pearson Education, Inc.

❸ Insert electrode cable into transmitter box.

SKILL 12.10 ECG Leads: Applying (continued)

TABLE 12–2 Telemetry 3-Lead and 5-Lead Electrode Placement

3-Lead, Standard Electrode Placement

RA (white)

LA (black)

LL (red)

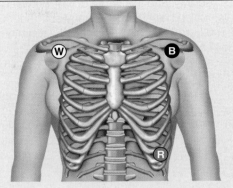

3-lead placement

5-Lead, Standard Electrode Placement

RA (white)

LA (black)

RL (green) (ground electrode)

LL (red)

V1-V6 (brown) chest

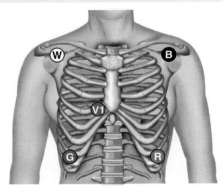

5-lead placement

Telemetry Electrode Placement		
Color	**Lead**	**Electrode Placement**
White	RA - Right Arm	Below right clavicle, mid-clavicular line
Black	LA - Left Arm	Below left clavicle, mid-clavicular line
Green	RL - Right Leg	Right lowest rib cage area
Red	LL - Left Leg	Left lowest rib cage area
Brown	V1-6 - Chest leads	V1 is fourth intercostal space, right sternal border through to V6 at left fifth intercostal space, midaxillary line

Note: Limb leads and any one chest lead can be monitored using these electrode positions.

10. Have base station run an ECG strip to check clarity of transmission.
11. Set HIGH and LOW alarm limits on the monitor. Turn alarm buttons to ON per facility/unit protocol (e.g., 50 low, 100 high).
12. Assess the skin regularly surrounding the electrode for signs of irritation.
13. Check lead placement at least once a shift unless notified by patient or monitoring station that electrodes are not functioning properly.
14. Change electrodes at least every three days or if ECG strip indicates poor conduction of waveform. See Table 12–2 for telemetry 3-lead and 5-lead electrode system placement.
15. When the procedure is complete, return bed to lowest position, perform hand hygiene, and leave patient safe and comfortable.

16. Complete documentation using forms, checklists, or electronic dropdown lists supplemented by nurse's notes or additional comments as appropriate.

SAMPLE DOCUMENTATION

[date] 0503 ECG recording showed straight line pattern. When awakened, stated he had just turned over while sleeping. Chest lead found on bed, replaced with new electrode. ECG recording sinus rhythm with no ectopic beats. Tolerated without incident. *B. Sid*

SKILL 12.11 ECG, Strip: Interpreting

Interpretation of electrocardiogram (ECG) strips can provide information about the heart's rate of contraction, its pattern of rhythm and regularity, and the length of time between impulses and intervals. It also helps to identify any aberrant conduction pathways. The hard copy of the electrical activity of the heart is sometimes called a rhythm strip.

Delegation or Assignment

Due to specific knowledge and skill in interpreting an ECG strip, this skill is not delegated or assigned to the UAP. The nurse remains responsible for the assessment, interpretation of abnormal findings, and determination of appropriate actions.

Equipment

- Calipers (optional)
- ECG rhythm strip

Preparation

- Review healthcare provider's orders and patient's nursing plan of care.
- Obtain a 6-second ECG rhythm strip and calipers.

Procedure

1. Assess ECG grid ❶ ❷.
   - Each small square represents 0.04 second (horizontal measurement).
   - Each large block (5 small squares) represents 0.20 second.
   - 15 large blocks represent 3 seconds.

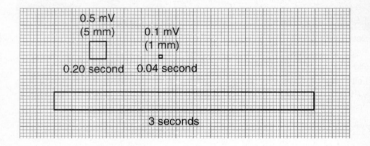

❶ ECG grid.

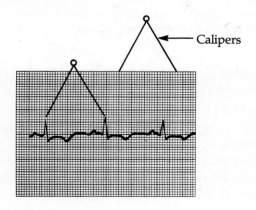

❷ Use calipers to measure heart rate.

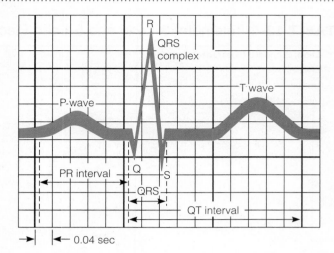

❸ It is important to determine configuration and location of wave pattern to interpret an ECG accurately.

2. Determine heart rate by calculating ventricular rate; normal is 60–100 beats/min.
   - Count the number of R waves in a 6-second period (30 large blocks) and multiply this by 10 to obtain the heart rate.

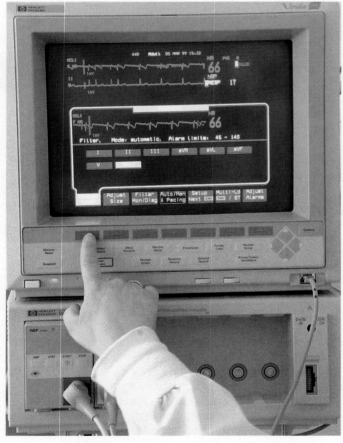

❹ ECG pattern and lead placement are depicted on monitor.

SKILL 12.11 ECG, Strip: Interpreting (*continued*)

- For true accuracy, count patient's apical heart rate for 1 full minute.
3. Determine the regularity of ventricular rhythm (R waves should be equally spaced.)
4. Determine the P-wave rate (atrial depolarizations).
   - There should be one P wave in front of each QRS complex.
   - Note if there are more P waves or fewer P waves than QRS complexes.
5. Determine the regularity of the P waves; are they all equally spaced?
6. Measure the PR interval (beginning of the P wave to the beginning of the QRS complex); represents conduction time through the electrical tissue to the ventricles (from the SA node, through the AV node, bundle of His, bundle branches, and Purkinje fibers); normal is 0.12–0.20 second.
7. Measure the QRS duration from beginning of the Q wave, if present, to end of the S wave; normal is less than 0.12 second ❸ ❹.

8. Interpret the patient's cardiac rhythm (**Table 12–3** ❯❯ and **Table 12–4** ❯❯) and place ECG rhythm sample strip in patient's chart, according to hospital policy.
9. Complete documentation using forms, checklists, or electronic dropdown lists supplemented by nurse's notes or additional comments as appropriate.

Safety Considerations

Always assess patient to determine whether the abnormal rhythm is potentially life threatening and emergency measures should be taken. Signs of hemodynamic instability include:

- Ongoing chest pain
- Shortness of breath
- Change in mental status
- Systolic blood pressure (SBP) less than 90 mmHg
- Heart rate greater than 150 beats/min.

TABLE 12–3 Normal Sinus Rhythm

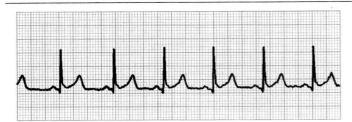

Normal sinus rhythm; regular configuration, uniform P wave precedes each QRS

Atrial rate: 60–100

PR interval: 0.12–0.2 second

QRS width: less than (<) 0.12 second

Ventricular rate: 60–100

TABLE 12–4 Selected Cardiac Rhythms and Dysrhythmias

Sinus Tachycardia	Sinus Bradycardia
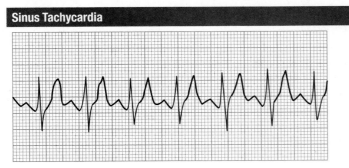	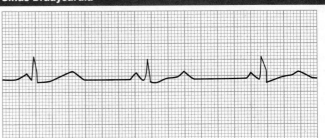
Regular rhythm: more than (>) 100 beats/min	Regular rhythm: less than (<) 60 beats/min
P waves: normal	P waves: normal
Atrial rate: >100 beats/min	Atrial rate: <60 beats/min
PR interval: 0.12–2.0 second	PR interval: 0.20 second
QRS complex width: 0.06–0.08 second usually normal	QRS complex width: 0.08 second usually normal
Note: A moderately faster heart rate can be a physiological normal variant.	*Note:* A slow heart rate can be physiologically normal for some patients.

(continued on next page)

SKILL 12.11 ECG, Strip: Interpreting (*continued*)

TABLE 12–4 Selected Cardiac Rhythms and Dysrhythmias (*continued*)

Sinus Tachycardia	Sinus Bradycardia
Etiology	**Etiology**
Underlying causes such as anxiety, fever, shock, drugs, exercise, electrolyte disturbances	Drugs
	Hypoxia
	Altered metabolic states (hypothyroidism)
	Cardiac diseases
	Athleticism
Initial Treatment	**Initial Treatment**
Immediately initiate cardioversion if unstable	Maintain patent airway; assist breathing as needed
Treatment dependent on elimination of cause	Oxygen
Decreasing anxiety	IV
Pain relief	Atropine 0.5–1 mg bolus IV if patient has signs of poor perfusion
Antipyretics	May repeat to a total dose of 3 mg
O$_2$	Then, epinephrine (2–10 mg/min) or dopamine (2–10 mg/kg/min) infusion while awaiting pacemaker
Medications (e.g., sedatives, tranquilizers, antianxiety)	Transcutaneous pacing for symptomatic bradycardia
Calcium channel blockers and beta-blockers	

Multifocal Premature Ventricular Contraction (PVCs)	Ventricular Tachycardia

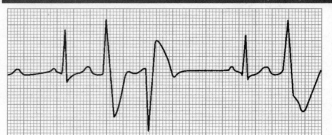

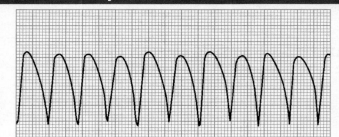

Irregular rhythm	Regular rhythm
P waves: none with premature beat, impulse originates in ventricle	Atrial rate: cannot differentiate
Atrial rate: undetermined	PR interval: none
PR interval: none with premature beat	QRS width: greater than 0.12 second
QRS width: greater than 0.12 second for premature beat	Ventricular rate: 130–250 beats/min
Ventricular rate: varies	*Note:* Ventricular tachycardia is a result of myocardial irritability and is life threatening.
Note: Each PVC has different configuration as foci are from different areas of heart.	
PVCs may be the result of imbalance between oxygen demand versus supply, thereby making the myocardium irritable.	
Etiology	**Etiology**
Heart disease (myocardial infarction [MI])	Acute MI
Hypoxia	Coronary artery disease, cardiomyopathy
Acidosis	Electrolyte imbalance
Electrolyte imbalances	Drug intoxication (digitalis)
Myocardial ischemia	
Drug toxicity (especially digitalis)	
Initial Treatment	**Initial Treatment**
Oxygen	Lidocaine 1.5 mg/kg bolus; may repeat in 3–5 min to maximum dose of 3 mg/kg
Potassium or magnesium if electrolytes dictate	Amiodarone 300 mg IV/IO can be followed by 150 mg
Lidocaine bolus—1–1.5 mg/kg; may repeat doses of 0.5–0.75 mg/kg every 5–10 min up to 3 mg/kg	IV/IO
Refractory to lidocaine: amiodarone or procainamide	Cardioversion if cardiac output is compromised
Continuous lidocaine, amiodarone, or procainamide drip may be started following a bolus of the same medication	Pulseless ventricular tachycardia—follow treatment for ventricular fibrillation (epinephrine)
Correct underlying cause	

SKILL 12.11 ECG, Strip: Interpreting (*continued*)

TABLE 12–4 Selected Cardiac Rhythms and Dysrhythmias (*continued*)

Atrial Fibrillation

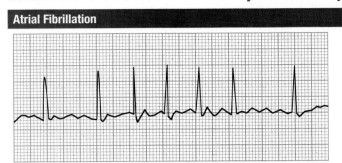

Irregularly irregular rhythm

Disorganized atrial activity: greater than 350 beats/min

P waves: none identifiable

PR interval: not measured

QRS: variable

QRS complex: irregular

Etiology

Heart failure

Rheumatoid heart disease

Coronary heart disease

Hypertension

Hyperthyroidism

Initial Treatment

Cardioversion

Diltiazem

Beta-blocker: carvedilol (Coreg) or metoprolol (Toprol XL)

Digoxin

Quinidine

Procainamide

Amiodarone or dronedarone ibutilide

Anticoagulant to reduce risk of clot formation and stroke, if atrial fibrillation duration new in onset but older than 48 hr

Atrial Flutter

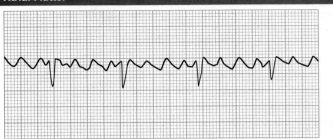

Regular or irregular rhythm (depending on block)

Atrial rate: >250 beats/min

P wave: usually sawtooth pattern; PR interval cannot be calculated

PR interval: regular

Ventricular rate can be irregular

QRS complex: 0.6–0.10 second

Etiology

Sympathetic nervous system stimulation (i.e., anxiety), caffeine, and alcohol intake

Thyrotoxins

Coronary heart disease, MI, pulmonary embolism

Initial Treatment

Cardioversion—if symptomatic

Diltiazem

Calcium channel blocker (Cardizem) or beta-blocking agents to slow ventricular response

Followed by ibutilide, quinidine, procainamide

Ventricular Fibrillation

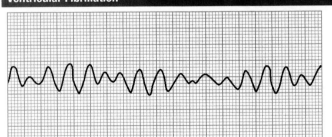

Irregular, totally chaotic rhythm

Atrial rate: cannot differentiate

PR interval: none

QRS width: fibrillating waves only

Ventricular rate: cannot differentiate

Note: Ineffective quivering of ventricles with no audible heartbeat, pulse, or respiration

Third-Degree Heart Block

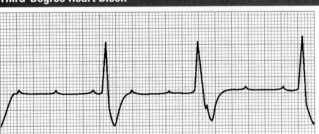

Regular atrial and ventricular rhythm

Atrial rate: greater than ventricular rate

PR interval: varies

QRS width: less than 0.12 second if pacemaker cell in junction; greater than 0.12 second if cell in ventricle

Ventricular rate: 40–60 beats/min if pacemaker is from bundle of His; <40 beats/min if from Purkinje fibers in ventricle

Note: Electrical impulse originates in SA node but is blocked in either the AV node, the bundle of His, or the Purkinje fibers. There is no correlation between the atrial rate and the ventricular rate.

(*continued on next page*)

SKILL 12.11 ECG, Strip: Interpreting (*continued*)

TABLE 12–4 Selected Cardiac Rhythms and Dysrhythmias (*continued*)

Ventricular Fibrillation	Third-Degree Heart Block
Etiology	**Etiology**
Myocardial ischemia, acute MI	Digitalis toxicity
Coronary artery disease	Myocardial infarction, inferior or anterior wall
Cardiomyopathy	Organic heart disease
Acid–base imbalance	
Severe hypothermia	
Electrolyte imbalance	
Initial Treatment	**Initial Treatment**
Immediately defibrillate, shock	Atropine bolus
CPR—100 chest compressions/minute—no cycles	Transcutaneous pacing
Ventricular fibrillation continues—give a vasopressor (epinephrine 1 mg IV push), repeat 3–5 min	Dopamine or epinephrine
Defibrillate again and continue CPR	Prepare for pacemaker insertion
Second-line drugs may be used, such as amiodarone (300 mg IV), lidocaine	

SKILL 12.12 Pacemaker, Insertion: Assisting

Safety Note! *During scheduled clinical time, nursing students may have a learning opportunity to observe or assist with this skill only with faculty permission and with direct supervision from faculty or another RN.*

A pacemaker is a small electronic device that can be implanted just under the skin in the chest if permanent, or it can be worn outside the body if it is temporary. The pacemaker sends electrical signals through one or two wires that connect it to the heart to regulate rate, rhythm, or electrical conduction pathways to sustain necessary heartbeats.

Delegation or Assignment

Assisting with inserting a pacemaker is not delegated or assigned to the UAP. However, signs and symptoms of problems may be observed during usual care and may be recorded by individuals other than the nurse. Abnormal findings must be validated and interpreted by the nurse.

Equipment

- Emergency cart with defibrillator
- External pacemaker pulse generator ① ②
- Pacing catheter electrodes
- ECG monitor
- Patient cable
- Rubber glove
- Sterile antiseptic solution
- Sterile gloves, gown, and mask
- Sterile towels
- Lidocaine, 1–2%
- Alcohol wipes
- Syringe
- Needles

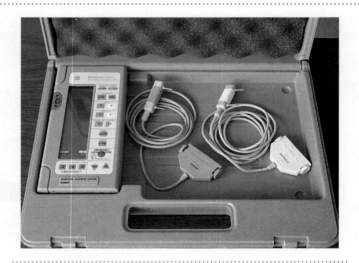

① Type of external pacemaker.

- Suture with attached needle
- Sterile 4 × 4 gauze pads
- Tape
- Venous cutdown tray
- Gloves

Preparation

- Validate that signed informed consent has been obtained for pacemaker insertion.
- Review healthcare provider's orders and patient's nursing plan of care.
- Perform a baseline assessment, including vital signs, sensorium, and heart rhythm.
- Provide sedation as ordered. Diazepam or midazolam is frequently used. Conscious sedation may be used.

SKILL 12.12 Pacemaker, Insertion: Assisting (*continued*)

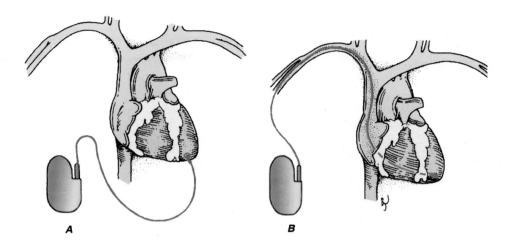

A   **B**

❷ Temporary pacemakers have two parts, the pulse generator and the electrode. The pulse generator is external to the body. **A,** Epicardial ventricular pacemaker; **B,** Transvenous ventricular pacemaker.

- Connect patient to a continuous electrocardiogram (ECG) monitor.
- Have all equipment and supplies gathered.

Procedure

1. Introduce self to patient and verify the patient's identity using two identifiers. Explain to the patient that the healthcare provider is going to insert a pacemaker, why it is necessary, and how the patient can participate. Discuss how the results will be used in planning further care or treatments.
2. Perform hand hygiene and observe appropriate infection control procedures.
3. Provide for patient privacy. Provide comfort and safety for patient.
4. Prepare the patient.
   - Raise bed to appropriate height for procedure.
   - Place the patient in a supine position with head flat or slightly lower than body.
   - If either the subclavian or external jugular vein is to be used, place a towel roll under the patient's shoulders to provide better exposure of the insertion site.
5. Assist healthcare provider as needed.
   - Healthcare provider dons mask, sterile gown, and gloves.
   - Insertion site is cleansed with sterile antiseptic solution.
   - Drape area with sterile towels.
   - Break single-dose vial of lidocaine and hold at angle for healthcare provider's withdrawal.
   - Healthcare provider withdraws lidocaine, using filtered needle, then changes to 25-gauge needle and injects skin.
   - Insertion is accomplished (transvenous method via cutdown or percutaneously). Catheter electrode wires are positioned, and skin sutures are applied.
6. Continuously monitor the ECG and patient status during the insertion.

7. Don gloves to prevent microshock to patient.
8. Assist in the connection of the pacing electrode to the appropriate outlet terminal (unipolar to negative and bipolar to both the positive and negative terminals).
9. Healthcare provider turns on power switch on external pacemaker and sets the rate. The milliamperes (mA) are set by determining threshold. To do this, the ECG is observed while the healthcare provider slowly increases the number of milliamperes from its lowest setting to a point where a QRS complex is captured and preceded by a pacing spike.
10. Healthcare provider sets sensitivity mode (usually 1.5 mV).
11. Secure all connections. The plastic cover is put back over pacemaker controls if required.
12. The external pacemaker and exposed wires are placed in a rubber glove to ensure insulation against electric shock to patient.

Safety Considerations
ELECTRICAL

- Use only grounded equipment; use common ground.
- Remove and tag any defective equipment.
- Maintain environmental humidity at 50–60%.
- Do not roll equipment over electrical cords.
- Avoid placing wet articles on electrical equipment.
- Insulate exposed pacing electrodes at all times.
- Wear rubber gloves when handling pacing electrodes or terminals.
- Do not touch any electric equipment while handling wire or terminals.
- Discharge static electricity by touching faucets or other metal that communicates with ground.

(continued on next page)

SKILL 12.12 Pacemaker, Insertion: Assisting (*continued*)

CAUTION! When temporary transvenous pacemakers are used, the balloon air port is not to be used for IV access.

13. Sterile dressings are applied to insertion site and taped securely.
14. Lower bed to lowest height.
15. Chest x-ray is obtained following insertion to validate lead placement if pacemaker not inserted using fluoroscopy.
16. Obtain 12-lead ECG.
17. When the procedure is complete, perform hand hygiene and leave patient safe and comfortable.
18. Complete documentation using forms, checklists, or electronic dropdown lists supplemented by nurse's notes or additional comments as appropriate including ECG strip and document significant events during the procedure, pacemaker settings, sterile dressing applied, and patient's response to the procedure.

CAUTION! A generic code for antibradycardia pacing was developed jointly by the North American Society of Pacing and Electrophysiology and the British Pacing and Electrophysiology Group and can be found at the National Institutes of Health website.

Safety Considerations

When a nurse observes a shape under the chest skin that looks characteristically like a pulse generator, further information must be obtained from the patient before concluding the patient has an implanted pacemaker. Permanent cardiac pacemakers are not the only implantable electronic device that treats cardiac dysrhythmias. Implantable cardio-

---

SAMPLE DOCUMENTATION

[date] 0730 V/S 112/78, P- 60, R- 16, T 36.8°C (98.2° F), O_2 sat 97% on 2 LPM O_2 via NC, ECG atrial fib. Prepped per orders, signed informed consent on front of patient's record. Scheduled permanent pacemaker inserted by Dr. Podner without difficulty. Tolerated procedure without complication. Pacemaker spikes noted on ECG strip. Resting quietly in room, V/S 114/78, P- 72, R- 16, O_2 sat 98% on 2 LPM O_2 via NC. *K. Vesco*

verter defibrillators (ICDs) are being used more frequently to treat tachycardia and sudden cardiac death from ventricular tachyarrhythmia with defibrillation. Together these two electronic devices are commonly referred to as cardiac implantable electronic devices, or CIEDs.

When asked, some patients may not know what type of CIED they have. To help identify which implantable CIED a patient has, ask to see the CIED information card for the healthcare provider. The healthcare provider can also look at the patient's chest x-ray to identify lead positions. Looking at a 12-lead ECG can also provide information about a paced rhythm.

It is most important to recognize a patient has a CIED before having a surgical procedure due to potential electromagnetic interference, or EMI, on the device function during the surgery. Cardiac device magnets are generally used to provide appropriate and safe CIED management during this period of time to prevent malfunction of the device.

Source: Based on Chia. P. (2015). A practical approach to perioperative management of cardiac implantable electronic devices. *Singapore Med J. 2015 Oct; 56*(10): 538–541. doi: 10.11622/smedj.2015148. Retrieved from http://www.ncbi.nlm.nih.gov/pmc/articles/PMC4613927/.

SKILL 12.13 Pacemaker, Permanent: Teaching

Safety Note! *During scheduled clinical time, nursing students may have a learning opportunity to observe or assist with this skill only with faculty permission and with direct supervision from faculty or another RN.*

Delegation or Assignment

Teaching about a permanent pacemaker is not delegated or assigned to the UAP. However, signs and symptoms of problems may be observed during usual care and may be recorded by individuals other than the nurse. Abnormal findings must be validated and interpreted by the nurse.

Equipment

- Audiovisual aids
- Written material

Preparation

- Review healthcare provider's orders and nursing plan of care.
- Ascertain what patient already knows and understands.

- Determine patient's ability and level of interest in learning about the pacemaker.
- Gather audiovisual and written materials.

Procedure

1. Introduce self to patient and verify the patient's identity using two identifiers. Explain to the patient you will be discussing information about permanent pacemakers, why it is necessary, and how the patient can participate. Discuss how the results will be used in planning further care or treatments.
2. Perform hand hygiene and observe appropriate infection control procedures.
3. Provide for patient privacy.
4. Recognize patient's fears, and provide opportunity to talk about them.
5. Review facts: heart anatomy and physiology and pacemaker information. Use illustrations and audiovisual aids to help clarify misconceptions and allay fears.
6. Provide rationale for any mobility restrictions.
7. Answer questions, and provide additional opportunities to discuss procedure.

SKILL 12.13 Pacemaker, Permanent: Teaching (*continued*)

8. Check pacemaker function regularly per instructions. With new pacemakers, healthcare providers check them on routine visits.
9. Instruct patient in clinical manifestations related to pacemaker failure and when to contact healthcare provider or pacemaker clinic.
10. Provide patient with pacemaker information ID card (provided by manufacturer) and instruct patient to carry in wallet.
11. Suggest a medical alert band be worn at all times.

Safety Considerations

Inform patient of electromagnetic interference restrictions:

- No MRI; do not place cell phone or cardiovert over generator.
- Avoid airport hand wand, high-voltage areas, and diathermy.
- If dizziness is experienced, move away from area.

12. When discussion is complete, perform hand hygiene and leave patient safe and comfortable.
13. Complete documentation using forms, checklists, or electronic dropdown lists supplemented by nurse's notes or additional comments as appropriate.

SAMPLE DOCUMENTATION

[date] 1320 Sitting in chair resting. Discussion about her new permanent pacemaker done including a short video and written materials. Had many questions about lifestyle changes, addressed and stated she appreciated the information. Safety and suggested activity modifications given, received with interest. Expressed feelings with some tearing noted. Support and encouragement given. Agreed to meet again tomorrow shortly for any more questions she may have needing to be answered. Tolerated without incident. *G. Diagos*

Safety Considerations

Many patients use telephone transmission of the generator's pulse rate to determine status of pacemaker function. Special equipment is used to transmit information concerning function of the pacemaker over the telephone to a receiving system in a pacemaker clinic. The equipment converts information to electronic signals that are permanently recorded on an ECG strip. Healthcare providers monitor patient's records and can intervene quickly when abnormalities appear on an ECG strip. This type of clinic is very common in outlying areas where patients are unable to go to a clinic easily.

SKILL 12.14 Pacemaker, Temporary: Maintaining

Safety Note! *During scheduled clinical time, nursing students may have a learning opportunity to observe or assist with this skill only with faculty permission and with direct supervision from faculty or another RN.*

A temporary pacemaker is used for short-term external pacing of the heart for dysrhythmias such as bradycardia and tachycardia, postoperative cardiac surgery, or if the permanent pacemaker stops. Patients stay in the healthcare facility until the temporary pacemaker is not needed or the decision is made to insert a permanent pacemaker.

Delegation or Assignment

Maintaining a temporary pacemaker is not delegated or assigned to the UAP. However, signs and symptoms of problems may be observed during usual care and may be recorded by individuals other than the nurse. Abnormal findings must be validated and interpreted by the nurse.

Equipment

- Battery
- Oscilloscope

Preparation

- Review healthcare provider's orders and patient's nursing plan of care.
- Gather equipment and supplies.

Procedure

1. Introduce self to patient and verify the patient's identity using two identifiers. Explain to the patient what you are going to do, why it is necessary, and how the patient can participate. Discuss how the results will be used in planning further care or treatments.
2. Perform hand hygiene and observe appropriate infection control procedures.
3. Provide for patient privacy. Provide comfort and safety for patient and self.
4. Observe for failure of the pacemaker to sense.
   - Observe the monitor for presence of pacemaker artifact (spikes); artifact before QRS complex in ventricular paced or preceding the P waves and QRS waves in atrioventricular (AV) sequential pacing ❶.
   - Check connections for secure, tight fit.
   - Observe that pace–sense needle deflects to right, indicating pacing is occurring.
   - Check sensitivity dial to determine if sensitivity threshold is set correctly.
5. Observe for failure to pace.
   - Check that external generator is ON.
   - Check battery to ensure it is functioning.
   - Check lead connector sites.
   - Check pace–sense indicator. (Absence of or slight deflection of the pace–sense indicator reveals battery failure.)

(*continued on next page*)

SKILL 12.14 Pacemaker, Temporary: Maintaining *(continued)*

Pacemaker Spike

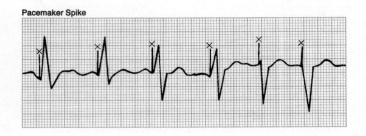

❶ ECG tracing showing pacemaker spike triggering ventricular depolarization (QRS).

6. Observe for failure to capture.
   - Observe for pacing artifact not followed by QRS complex ❷. **Rationale:** *This indicates a failure of the stimulus to trigger a ventricular response.*

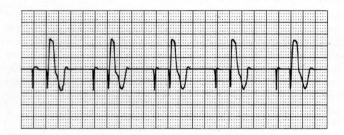

❷ ECG tracing showing pacing spikes not followed by QRS complex.

   - Check the setting of the milliamperes (mA), or output dial, to determine if setting should be increased. **Rationale:** *The myocardial threshold may be altered as a result of disease or drugs.*
   - Check all connector sites for secure, tight fit.
7. Observe that sutures are intact.
8. Assess insertion site for bleeding, hematoma formation, or infection.
9. Obtain chest x-ray postinsertion.
10. Monitor patient's response to therapy.
    - Assess urine output. **Rationale:** *Decreased urine output indicates poor cardiac output.*

   - Observe for dyspnea, crackles, heart rate, decreased blood pressure.
   - Monitor temperature.
   - Observe patient for signs of anxiety. Complete pacemaker teaching as necessary.
11. Obtain and analyze a strip for functioning of pacemaker.
12. Observe for battery failure.
13. Observe for electrical interference and development of microshocks.
    - Ground all electrical equipment in proximity to patient.
    - Cover exposed wires with nonconductive material.
    - Wear gloves when handling generator/lead wires.
14. Complete pacemaker teaching as necessary.
15. When the procedure is complete, perform hand hygiene and leave patient safe and comfortable.
16. Complete documentation using forms, checklists, or electronic dropdown lists supplemented by nurse's notes or additional comments as appropriate.

SAMPLE DOCUMENTATION

[date] 0200 Sleeping quietly, slow even respirations noted. Temporary pacemaker pulse generator at pillow, monitor in sinus rhythm with irregular pacing spikes followed by QRS configurations, no ectopic beats noted, ECG strip posted in patient's chart. Battery indicator light is green. Pacing wire insertion site dressing dry and intact. *T. Munford*

Safety Considerations

Observe for the following signs of pacemaker failure:

- Decreased urine output
- Electrocardiogram (ECG) pattern change
- Decreased blood pressure
- Bradycardia
- Shortness of breath.

SKILL 12.15 Temporary Cardiac Pacing, Transvenous, Epicardial: Monitoring

Safety Note! *During scheduled clinical time, nursing students may have a learning opportunity to observe or assist with this skill only with faculty permission and with direct supervision from faculty or another RN.*

A transvenous pacemaker has the pacing wire inserted into the jugular vein and advanced to the inner wall of the right ventricle. An epicardial pacemaker has the pacing wire placed on the epicardium, or outer layer of the heart muscle, during cardiac surgery.

Delegation or Assignment

Monitoring temporary cardiac pacing, transvenous or epicardial, is not delegated or assigned to the UAP. However, signs and symptoms of problems may be observed during usual care and may be recorded by individuals other than the nurse. Abnormal findings must be validated and interpreted by the nurse.

SKILL 12.15 Temporary Cardiac Pacing, Transvenous, Epicardial: Monitoring (*continued*)

Equipment

- Cardiac monitor
- Transcutaneous: pacing generator, pacing electrodes
- Appropriate temporary pulse generator (select for single- or dual-chamber pacing)
- 9-volt battery for pulse generator (single- or dual-chamber version)
- Bridging cable for epicardial wires
- Clean gloves
- Established continuous cardiac monitoring (also see Skill 12.10)

Preparation

- Check healthcare provider's order. Validate that signed informed consent has been obtained for temporary pacing.
- Reinforce the healthcare provider's explanation of why the temporary pacemaker is necessary by explaining to the patient the rationale for temporary pacing and necessary restrictions/precautions, and provide reassurance of close continuous monitoring.
- Perform a baseline assessment: vital signs, urinary output, level of consciousness (LOC), heart rate, rhythm, and skin color. If life-threatening dysrhythmia is assessed, assist healthcare provider for pacemaker insertion. **Rationale:** *Transcutaneous pacemakers are used for symptomatic bradycardia unresponsive to atropine or high-degree atrioventricular block causing hemodynamic compromise.*
- Assess IV site for patency; if no IV, obtain healthcare provider's order for one. **Rationale:** *IV access is needed for drug administration.*
- Document patient's cardiac rhythm and post a rhythm strip in patient's chart.

Procedure

1. Introduce self to patient and verify the patient's identity using two identifiers. Explain to the patient the healthcare provider is applying a transcutaneous pacemaker, why it is necessary, and how the patient can participate. Discuss how the results will be used in planning further care or treatments.
2. Perform hand hygiene and observe appropriate infection control procedures.
3. Provide for patient privacy.
4. Provide sedation as ordered. **Rationale:** *This procedure causes discomfort.*
5. Clip hair, if necessary. Do not shave under electrode placement. Do not use alcohol or tincture of benzoin because they can cause burns to occur. **Rationale:** *Improve conduction between electrode and skin. Shaving may cause nicks in skin, which may increase discomfort with pacing.*
6. Ensure patient is on cardiac monitoring with either lead I, II, or III. Lead II is customary as it assesses atrial activity.
7. Provide healthcare provider with clean gloves. **Rationale:** *Gloves are worn to prevent microshock to patient.*

TRANSCUTANEOUS PACING (TCP)

8. Assist healthcare provider performing the following actions as needed.
   - Connect electrocardiogram (ECG) cable to input connection on pacing generator.
   - Turn switch selector to MONITOR ON. ECG waveform will appear.
   - Set alarm, press ALARM ON. Ensure alarm parameters are set 20 beats higher and lower than patient's desired rate.
   - Record waveform by pressing START/STOP button.
   - Apply pacing pads as marked, first removing posterior pad covering, then placing posterior (back) pad left of spine between the scapulas. Place anterior "front" pad to left side of lower sternum.
   - Press firmly on and around pacing electrodes. **Rationale:** *This ensures good skin contact.*
   - Attach pacing cable to pace connector on defibrillator/monitor.
   - Select PACER button and green light will appear.
   - Set pacing rate to 60 to 80 beats/min.
   - Assess cardiac rhythm on oscilloscope and observe the QRS for sensing marker.
   - Set milliamperes (mA) threshold initially at 0. **Rationale:** *This prevents pacemaker discharge while setting adjustment.*
   - Activate pacing by depressing START/STOP button.
   - Increase mA slowly, increasing it until capture appears.
9. Assess pulse and blood pressure. Record ECG strip and document pacing parameters, significant events during the procedure, and patient's response to the procedure.
10. Monitor for perfusion. Continually assess patient's need for sedation. **Rationale:** *Pacing causes discomfort.* Proceed to step 11 below.

EPICARDIAL PACING

8. Assist healthcare provider performing the following actions as needed:
   - Locate epicardial pacing wires on patient's chest wall.
   - Securely connect pacing wires to external generator. **Rationale:** *This promotes pacemaker impulse reception from and transmission to the myocardium.*
   - Connect cable to pulse generator (positive to positive, negative to negative). **Rationale:** *Pacing stimulus goes from pulse generator to the negative terminal and back to pulse generator by the positive terminal.*
   - Remove protective cover to dial settings.
   - Select pacing mode (e.g., atrial, ventricular, atrioventricular (AV) synchronous, or demand).
9. Return bed to lowest position.
10. Record ECG strip and document pacing parameters, significant events during the procedure, and patient's response to the procedure.

(*continued on next page*)

SKILL 12.15 Temporary Cardiac Pacing, Transvenous, Epicardial: Monitoring (*continued*)

TRANSVENOUS OR EPICARDIAL PACING

11. Assist healthcare provider performing the following actions as needed:
    - Set dial at prescribed pacing rate (atrial and/or ventricular).
    - Set energy output (mA) on pulse generator to prescribed level (set for both atrial and ventricular pacing). **Rationale:** *Energy output setting ensures that pacemaker stimulates the patient's myocardium.*
    - Return plastic cover to protect generator dial settings and hang generator from pole at patient's bedside.
    - Monitor pacemaker function for sensing (light indicates patient's QRS complexes), capture (pacemaker spike is followed by QRS complex), and pacemaker rate.
12. Monitor patient's heart rhythm, vital signs, and other responses to pacing, including femoral pulsation palpable with captured beats. **Rationale:** *These demonstrate effectiveness of pacemaker support.*
13. Evaluate electrode insertion/exit sites and apply dressing according to facility protocol.
14. When the procedure is complete, perform hand hygiene and leave patient safe and comfortable.
15. Complete documentation using forms, checklists, or electronic dropdown lists supplemented by nurse's notes or additional comments as appropriate including ECG strip and significant events during the procedure, pacemaker settings, sterile dressing applied, and patient's response to the procedure.

Safety Considerations

Transvenous single-chamber (ventricular) pacing is most commonly used as an emergency measure to support ventricular contraction and cardiac output. Epicardial pacing occurs when pacing electrodes are inserted into the epicardium of the right ventricle during cardiac surgery. If the healthcare provider wants to initiate atrioventricular sequential pacing, then the surgeon places an additional electrode in the right atrium. The pacing wires are then pierced through the chest wall and may be attached to the external pulse generator, which is placed on standby mode should pacing become necessary. If no pacing is indicated at this time, the pacing wires are inserted in either a sterile rubber glove or finger cot. Place sterile gauze and occlusive dressing over pacing wires and insertion site to prevent microshock and/or infection. Epicardial pacing electrodes provide either single-chamber atrial pacing, single-chamber ventricular pacing, or dual-chamber pacing, known as A-V sequential pacing, which is used to simulate normal pump function (atrial followed by ventricular stimulation/contraction).

≫ Arterial Line

Expected Outcomes

1. Peripheral perfusion distal to arterial catheter placement site remains adequate.
2. Arterial cannulation is accomplished without complication.
3. Arterial blood pressure monitoring system functions reliably and accurately.
4. Arterial blood samples are obtained.

SKILL 12.16 Allen Test: Performing

The Allen test is used before doing an arterial puncture of the radial artery. It is done to demonstrate adequate collateral blood flow through the ulnar artery due to the potential of thrombus formation after the radial artery puncture that would obstruct blood flow to the hand.

Delegation or Assignment

Assessing arterial flow with the Allen test is not delegated or assigned to the UAP. However, signs and symptoms of problems may be observed during usual care and may be recorded by individuals other than the nurse. Abnormal findings must be validated and interpreted by the nurse.

Equipment

No equipment is needed for this skill.

Preparation

- Review healthcare provider's orders and patient's nursing plan of care.

Procedure

1. Introduce self to patient and verify the patient's identity using two identifiers. Explain to the patient what you are going to do, why it is necessary, and how the patient can participate. Discuss how the results will be used in planning further care or treatments.
2. Perform hand hygiene and observe appropriate infection control procedures.
3. Provide for patient privacy.
4. Perform the modified Allen test to determine distal peripheral perfusion. **Rationale:** *This procedure assesses blood*

SKILL 12.16 Allen Test: Performing (continued)

supply to the patient's hand to determine that the radial and ulnar arteries are functioning before an arterial line is inserted.

- Compress both arteries at patient's wrist for about 1 minute.
- Instruct patient to clench and unclench fist several times. **Rationale:** *This causes blanching in the hand and palm.*
- With patient's hand in open, relaxed position, release pressure on ulnar artery.
- Observe how quickly (7 seconds) the palm color flushes. **Rationale:** *If color returns quickly, good collateral blood supply to the hand exists.* If normal color does not return, there would be insufficient collateral circulation to the hand should radial artery occlusion occur.

5. Repeat procedure with release of the radial artery.

6. Report to healthcare provider if collateral blood flow is insufficient. **Rationale:** *A Doppler flow study may be used to help determine collateral blood flow.*

7. When the procedure is complete, perform hand hygiene and leave patient safe and comfortable.

8. Complete documentation using forms, checklists, or electronic dropdown lists supplemented by nurse's notes or additional comments as appropriate.

SAMPLE DOCUMENTATION

[date] 0822 Awake and alert, sitting on side of bed. Allen test done on arteries of both wrists. Color returned before 5 seconds both wrists. Tolerated without incident. *M. Key*

SKILL 12.17 Arterial Blood Pressure: Monitoring

Safety Note! *During scheduled clinical time, nursing students may have a learning opportunity to observe or assist with this skill only with faculty permission and with direct supervision from faculty or another RN.*

Arterial lines can directly and more accurately measure blood pressures in real time. The most common artery used for an arterial line is usually the radial artery.

Delegation or Assignment

Monitoring arterial blood pressure is not delegated or assigned to the UAP. However, signs and symptoms of problems may be observed during usual care and may be recorded by individuals other than the nurse. Abnormal findings must be validated and interpreted by the nurse.

Equipment

- Disposable pressure transducer, dome, and amplifier
- Flush valve with flush system
- Display monitor (oscilloscope)
- Sterile stopcock cap
- Sterile transparent dressing
- Gloves
- Carpenter's level
- Marker

Preparation

- Review healthcare provider's orders and the patient's nursing plan of care.
- Gather equipment and supplies and go to patient's room.

Procedure

1. Introduce self to patient and verify the patient's identity using two identifiers. Explain to the patient you are going to measure the blood pressure using the arterial line, why it is necessary, and how the patient can participate. Discuss how the results will be used in planning further care or treatments.

2. Perform hand hygiene and observe appropriate infection control procedures.

3. Provide for patient privacy.

4. Level and calibrate (zero out) the system.
   - Calibrate system at beginning of each shift. **Rationale:** *Monitor readings are altered by changes in atmospheric pressure.*
   - Position patient with head of bed flat or at up to a 45-degree elevation.
   - Using a carpenter's level, align stopcock above transducer level with patient's left atrium (phlebostatic axis) and mark patient's chest for future readings. **Rationale:** *Readings will be inaccurately high or low if stopcock above transducer is not level with patient's phlebostatic axis.*
   - To zero ("calibrate") the system, turn stopcock near transducer off to patient. Remove cap from stopcock, opening it to air.
   - Depress ZERO button on monitor, release button, and note monitor reading is zero. **Rationale:** *Zero reading indicates monitor is calibrated to atmospheric pressure.*
   - Replace cap or place new sterile cap on stopcock.
   - Turn stopcock so transducer is open to patient.

5. Observe waveform at eye level for the sharp systolic upstroke, peak, dicrotic notch, and end diastole ❶ ❷.

6. Fast flush the continuous flush system and quickly release. A sharp upstroke followed by a horizontal line, then a brisk downstroke descending below, then returning to baseline indicates that the system requires no adjustment ❸.

7. Ensure pressure bag is maintained at 300 mmHg.

8. Leave cannulated extremity uncovered for easy observation. Assess site at every shift for signs of infection.

(continued on next page)

SKILL 12.17 Arterial Blood Pressure: Monitoring *(continued)*

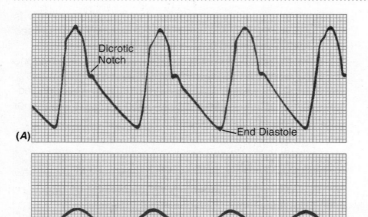

(A)

(B)

1 **A,** Arterial line—normal waveform; **B,** arterial line—flattened waveform. Flattened arterial waveform indicates damping. Damping results from obstruction in arterial line or imbalance of transducer.

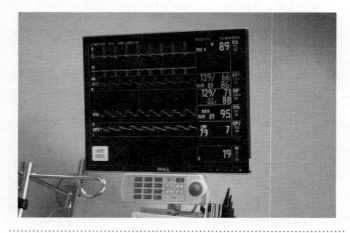

2 Arterial line allows direct measurement of blood pressure and the monitor displays digital and waveform.

9. Assess circulation, motion, and sensation of extremity distal to cannulation site every 2 hr initially, then every 8 hr.
10. Immobilize extremity if necessary.

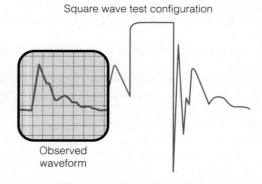

Square wave test configuration

Observed waveform

3 Fast flush the continuous flush system and quickly release. A sharp upstroke, followed by a horizontal line, then a brisk downstroke descending below and then returning to baseline indicates the system requires no adjustment (squarewave test).

11. Change flush solution and tubing every 96 hr (according to facility policy).
12. Change dressing weekly or if it becomes wet, loose, or soiled. **Rationale:** *Loose or soiled dressings increase risk of infection at site.*
    * Don gloves.
    * Remove dressing and discard in biohazard container.
    * Remove gloves and perform hand hygiene.
    * Apply transparent dressing, date, and initials.
13. When the procedure is complete, perform hand hygiene and leave patient safe and comfortable.
14. Complete documentation using forms, checklists, or electronic dropdown lists supplemented by nurse's notes or additional comments as appropriate such as posting an arterial monitor strip, arterial monitor settings, assessment data, and patient's response to the procedure.
15. Monitor site to ensure hemostasis occurs.
16. Monitor extremity distally for adequacy of perfusion.

> **SAMPLE DOCUMENTATION**
>
> [date] 0800 Resting in bed in Fowler position, placed at 45-degree elevation. Arterial line system calibrated to zero. Waveform noted systolic 120 and diastolic 86. Fast flush done. Dressing dry and intact. Tolerated procedure without complaint. *L. Koe*

SKILL 12.18 Arterial Blood Samples: Withdrawing

Safety Note! *During scheduled clinical time, nursing students may have a learning opportunity to observe or assist with this skill only with faculty permission and with direct supervision from faculty or another RN.*

Arterial blood is needed to monitor arterial blood gases (ABGs) and provides valuable data about respiratory and metabolic function in maintaining acid–base balance and oxygenation status in the body. The arterial line allows repeated and frequent arterial blood sampling to monitor for changes in condition.

Delegation or Assignment

Withdrawing arterial blood samples is not delegated or assigned to the UAP. However, signs and symptoms of problems may be

SKILL 12.18 Arterial Blood Samples: Withdrawing (*continued*)

observed during usual care and may be recorded by individuals other than the nurse. Abnormal findings must be validated and interpreted by the nurse.

Equipment

- One 6-mL sterile syringe
- ABG kit with one 3-mL syringe with dry lithium heparin and an air filter device *or* Vacutainer with Luer-Lok adapter cannula and blood specimen tubes
- Gloves
- Face shield
- Container with ice (paper cup, emesis basin)
- Two specimen labels
- Bubble packaging
- Biohazard specimen bag
- Gauze sponges/pads

Preparation

- Review healthcare provider's orders and patient's nursing plan of care.
- Gather equipment and supplies.
- Attach label to specimen syringe with patient's name, hospital number, room number, time, and date. Also add patient's current temperature and fraction of inspired oxygen (FiO_2).
- For arterial blood gases (ABGs) specimen, maintain patient's current oxygen delivery setting for 20 min before obtaining specimen.
- Fill paper cup or emesis basin with ice.

Procedure

1. Introduce self to patient and verify the patient's identity using two identifiers. Explain to the patient you are getting a blood sample from the arterial line, why it is necessary, and how the patient can participate. Discuss how the results will be used in planning further care or treatments.
2. Perform hand hygiene and observe appropriate infection control procedures.
3. Provide for patient privacy.
4. Momentarily disengage arterial alarms.
5. Turn stopcock off to patient.
6. Remove protective cap from open blood sampling port on three-way stopcock closest to arterial line insertion site.
7. Attach syringe or Vacutainer with Luer-Lok adapter cannula to open port of three-way stopcock.
8. Turn stopcock off to flush solution.
9. Attach syringe or blood specimen tube into Vacutainer to establish blood draw ❶.
10. Discard obtained sample. **Rationale:** *This discard ensures that the specimen will be free of heparin or flush solution.*

CAUTION! For an ABGs sample, discard volume should be twice the dead space volume of the catheter and tubing up to the sampling site. For coagulation studies, discard volume should be 6 times the dead space volume.

---

11. Engage ABG specimen tube in Vacutainer.

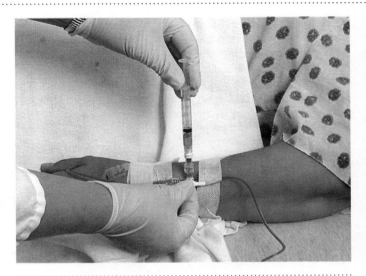

❶ Engage syringe or Vacutainer to sample port to obtain arterial blood.

12. Obtain ABG specimen. See **Table 12–5 》** for ABG values in acid–base imbalances.
13. Turn stopcock off to open port. **Rationale:** *This re-establishes flow between flush solution and patient.*
14. Remove Vacutainers for blood conservatory process.

For Blood Conservation Process

- Don clean gloves.
- Aspirate blood into reservoir tubing.
- Close stopcock to reservoir tubing.
- Access sampling port (closest to patient) using blunt cannula with tube holder (Vacutainer).
- Engage blood collection tubes in tube holder and allow to fill.
- When sampling is complete, remove blunt cannula and tube holder.
- Open stopcock to reservoir tubing and return contents to patient ❷.

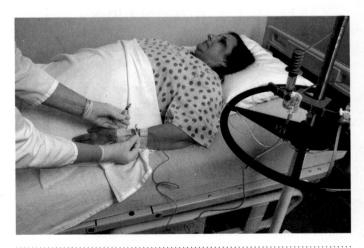

❷ When sampling is complete, open stopcock to reservoir tubing and return contents of blood conservatory system to patient.

(*continued on next page*)

SKILL 12.18 Arterial Blood Samples: Withdrawing (continued)

15. Place ABG specimen tubes in container filled with ice.
16. Fast flush remaining blood onto gauze pad.
17. Reattach protective cap on open port.
18. Validate good arterial waveform on monitor.
19. Reactivate monitor alarms.
20. Wrap syringe/specimen in bubble packaging and place in biohazard bag with ice.
21. Remove and discard gloves.
22. Perform hand hygiene and leave patient safe and comfortable.
23. Send specimens to laboratory immediately and notify lab that tubes are being sent.
24. Complete documentation using forms, checklists, or electronic dropdown lists supplemented by nurse's notes or additional comments as appropriate including amount of blood sample removed.

TABLE 12–5 Arterial Blood Gas Values in Acid–Base Imbalances

Normal ABG Values		
pH	7.35–7.45	
PCO_2	35–45 mmHg	
HCO_3^-	22–28 mEq	
Respiratory Acidosis		**Compensated**
pH: decreased	Less than (<) 7.35	7.35
PCO_2: increased	Higher than (>) 45 mmHg	
HCO_3^-: normal	24	> 26 mEq
Respiratory Alkalosis		**Compensated**
pH: increased	> 7.45	7.45
PCO_2: decreased	< 35 mmHg	
HCO_3^-: normal	24	< 22 mEq
Metabolic Acidosis		**Compensated**
pH: decreased	< 7.35	7.35
PCO_2: normal	40	< 35 mmHg
HCO_3^-: decreased	< 22 mEq	
Metabolic Alkalosis		**Compensated**
pH: increased	> 7.45	7.45
PCO_2: normal	40	> 45 mmHg
HCO_3^-: increased	> 26 mEq	

SKILL 12.19 Arterial Line: Caring for

Safety Note! *During scheduled clinical time, nursing students may have a learning opportunity to observe or assist with this skill only with faculty permission and with direct supervision from faculty or another RN.*

An arterial line, sometimes called an a-line or art-line, is the insertion of a 20-gauge intravenous catheter into an artery by a healthcare provider, for the purpose of obtaining arterial blood for ABGs samples or real time accurate BP readings. It can be inserted in the radial, ulnar, brachial, axillary, or dorsalis pedis arteries, but is commonly inserted in the radial artery.

Delegation or Assignment

Caring for an arterial line is not delegated or assigned to the UAP. However, signs and symptoms of problems may be observed during usual care and may be recorded by individuals other than the nurse. Abnormal findings must be validated and interpreted by the nurse.

Equipment

- 20-gauge Teflon catheter with introducer and flexible guidewire
- 500 mL of normal saline for flush
- Heparin, 1000 units/mL
- 1-mL unit-dose syringe
- Pressure bag for flush infusion
- IV tubing
- Short wide-bore, high-pressure tubing
- Three-way stopcocks with nonvented caps
- Established pressure monitor system
- Clean gloves, sterile gloves
- Personal protective equipment (PPE)
- Sterile towels and drape

SKILL 12.19 Arterial Line: Caring for (continued)

- Skin prep solution (2% chlorhexidine)
- Sterile 4 × 4 gauze sponges
- Lidocaine 1% (without epinephrine)
- 3-mL syringe with 18- and 25-gauge needles for topical anesthetic
- Alcohol wipes
- Silk suture, size 000 (if used)
- Sterile transparent dressing
- Atropine for reversal of bradycardia
- Transparent tape

For Removing the Arterial Line Only Add the Following:

- Suture removal set

Preparation

- Validate that signed informed consent has been obtained and available in the front of the patient's chart.
- Review healthcare provider's orders and the patient's nursing plan of care.
- When inserting the arterial line, determine whether the patient has received anticoagulant therapy. **Rationale:** *Anticoagulants increase the risk of prolonged bleeding.*
- When removing the arterial line, check patient's coagulation lab results (values).
- Gather equipment and supplies.

CAUTION! Arterial catheter alarms should always be enabled to detect disconnection, alterations in blood pressure, or pulseless electrical activity.

Procedure

1. Introduce self to patient and verify the patient's identity using two identifiers. Explain to the patient what you are going to do, why it is necessary, and how the patient can participate. Discuss how the results will be used in planning further care or treatments.
2. Perform hand hygiene and observe appropriate infection control procedures.
3. Provide for patient privacy.

INSERTING

4. Prepare the arterial line set-up.
   - Add heparin to normal saline solution and label bag with additive and date (commonly 2 units of heparin/mL fluid). Follow hospital protocols.
   - Connect IV tubing to solution bag.
   - Remove all air from flush solution bag.
   - Insert flush infusion bag into pressure bag and hang bag on IV pole.
   - Prepare and assemble pressurized monitoring system (transducer, continuous flush device, and stopcocks) following manufacturer's instructions.
   - Level stopcock above transducer to patient's phlebostatic axis (also see Skill 12.17).
   - Inflate pressure bag to 300 mmHg using hand pump on bag.
5. Don gloves and PPE and prepare to assist the healthcare provider as needed.

- Skin is prepped briskly with 2% chlorhexidine for 3 seconds.
- Lidocaine vial is cleansed with alcohol wipe.
- Healthcare provider dons sterile gloves.
- Sterile drape is placed over arterial insertion site.
- Healthcare provider aspirates lidocaine with 18-gauge needle, changes needle, and injects patient's skin with 25-gauge needle. **Rationale:** *This size is used for local anesthesia.*
- Percutaneous insertion is made at arterial insertion site, and arterial catheter is inserted.
- Healthcare provider advances catheter in artery.
- Arterial catheter is sutured in place with 000 silk suture secured with transparent dressing ❶.

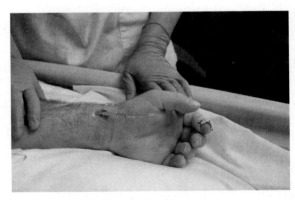

Source: Celina Burkhart/Pearson Education, Inc.

❶ Apply sterile transparent dressing (with date and initials) to the site after the catheter is sutured into place.

6. Assist healthcare provider performing as needed the following actions:
   - Observe for pulsating bright-red blood spurting retrograde into catheter. **Rationale:** *This evidence ensures arterial catheter position.*
   - Attach catheter to primed pressure-monitoring system tubing. Make sure all connections are secure.
   - Press fast flush valve to clear system.
   - Observe oscilloscope for arterial waveform.
   - Apply sterile transparent dressing (with date and initials) to site after catheter is sutured into place.
7. Remove and discard gloves. Perform hand hygiene.
8. Set monitor alarms for both HIGH and LOW parameters. Proceed to step 9 below.

CAUTION!

Mean Arterial Blood Pressure

In general, the mean arterial pressure (MAP) provides a more accurate interpretation of a patient's hemodynamic status than a single blood pressure reading. The MAP is the averaging of blood pressure readings over a single cardiac cycle. The MAP reflects perfusion pressure and is notated on a monitor screen in parentheses by the blood pressure reading; 154/86 (108).

(continued on next page)

SKILL 12.19 Arterial Line: Caring for (continued)

REMOVING

4. Don gloves and PPE.
5. Remove the arterial cannula.
   - Remove the dressing, and discard in appropriate container.
   - Clip retaining sutures if present.
   - Apply finger pressure approximately 2 cm above skin puncture site. **Rationale:** *The artery puncture site is proximal to the skin puncture site.*
   - Place folded 4 × 4 gauze pad over cannula site with nondominant hand, and apply gentle pressure.
   - Pull arterial cannula straight out of artery with quick, even pressure.
   - Apply firm pressure over and just above cannula site for at least 5–10 min. **Rationale:** *This action achieves hemostasis and prevents formation of a hematoma.*

CAUTION! Apply pressure to puncture site for at least 10 minutes if patient is on anticoagulation or antithrombotic therapy.

6. Place folded 4 × 4 gauze pad over puncture site, and tape tightly. **Rationale:** *This provides additional pressure to site to prevent bleeding.*
7. Check cannulation site frequently.
8. Check distal extremity for temperature, circulation, motion, and sensation intermittently for several hours, then routinely after catheter removal. **Rationale:** *Delayed complications (thrombosis) may occur.*
9. When the procedure is complete, lower bed to lowest height. Discard supplies, remove and discard gloves and PPE, and perform hand hygiene. Leave the patient safe and comfortable.
10. Complete documentation using forms, checklists, or electronic dropdown lists supplemented by nurse's notes or additional comments as appropriate including:
    - After inserting the arterial line, posting an arterial monitor strip, significant events during the procedure, arterial monitor settings, sterile dressing applied, and patient's response to the procedure.
    - After removing the arterial line, assessment data, significant events during the procedure, sterile dressing applied, and patient's response to the procedure.

⟫ Critical Thinking Options for Unexpected Outcomes

Not all unexpected outcomes require further nursing intervention; however, many times they do. When the patient demonstrates a change in signs/symptoms indicating an emerging problem, the nurse should immediately assess and troubleshoot what is happening. The assessment data must be processed quickly to formulate a hypothesis so the nurse can make a clinical judgment. The nurse then decides how best to resolve the problem and improve the patient's situation for a better outcome.

EXPECTED OUTCOME	UNEXPECTED OUTCOME	POSSIBLE INTERVENTIONS
Maintaining Blood Volume Transfusion reaction does not occur. Transfusions of blood or blood products will be done utilizing best evidence safety protocols to avoid errors and minimize occurrence of adverse reactions for best patient outcomes.	Transfusion reaction occurs.	■ Stop blood administration and with new IV tubing, begin infusion of normal saline to keep vein open. ■ Check transfusion reaction form for appropriate nursing intervention. ■ Complete all relevant nursing actions.
	Blood does not flow through tubing.	■ Check patient's IV site and gauge of catheter (at least 18 or 20 gauge). ■ Gently agitate blood bag to mix blood cells with the anticoagulant. ■ Raise blood bag higher on IV pole. Squeeze flexible tubing to promote blood flow. ■ Adjust clamp on tubing. As the blood passes over the filter, more blood microaggregates clog the filter and slow drip rate. ■ Replace tubing. ■ Utilize an infusion pump, especially if administering blood through a small catheter.
	Potential circulatory overload occurs.	■ Monitor symptoms: sudden dyspnea, tachypnea, tachycardia, chest discomfort, distended neck veins, moist crackles and rales, restlessness, sudden increase in blood pressure. ■ Stop transfusion and place patient in Fowler position. ■ Start oxygen at 2 L/min per nasal cannula.

EXPECTED OUTCOME	UNEXPECTED OUTCOME	POSSIBLE INTERVENTIONS
Pressure dressing is applied, and bleeding is controlled.	Even with direct pressure and application of pressure dressing, bleeding continues.	■ Reinforce pressure dressing. ■ Maintain IV infusion. ■ Notify healthcare provider, and be prepared to send patient to surgery for wound closure. ■ Monitor closely for signs of shock (level of consciousness [LOC], vital signs, oliguria or anuria, tachycardia, narrow pulse pressure, hypotension). ■ Apply pressure directly or proximal to wound. ■ Place tourniquets proximal to site of hemorrhage to control bleeding if all other actions are unsuccessful.
Antiembolism Devices Compression stockings remain wrinkle free and pressure is evenly distributed.	Graduated compression stockings are loose and do not provide support.	■ Remeasure legs and compare to chart to determine correct size. ■ Hosiery may be old with no elasticity and should be discarded; ensure line drying rather than with electric dryer. ■ Need to order different knit design and elastomeric yarn denier that will increase pressure.
Peripheral pulses are present during use of sequential stockings and elastic hosiery.	While compression device is being used, patient complains of numbness or tingling in leg.	■ Remove devices immediately. ■ Suggest use of foot pulse device as alternate. ■ Complete neurovascular assessment. ■ Notify healthcare provider of assessment findings.
Electrical Conduction in the Heart Monitor waveforms are distinct and readable.	Electrocardiogram (ECG) is not clearly displayed on monitor.	■ Ensure that electrodes are applied in correct position and are securely attached. ■ Observe for electrical interference resulting in a 60-cycle interference on oscilloscope. ■ Observe for excessive patient activity resulting in artifact display on oscilloscope.
	Electrical interference appears on monitor.	■ Check all other electric equipment in the immediate environment. ■ Check for proper grounding of monitor. ■ Change electrodes and cable; poor conduction may cause 60-cycle interference. ■ Check that monitor is calibrated.
	Telemetry signal not picked up at base station.	■ Check that patient hasn't wandered to an area where transmission is not available. ■ Check that transmitter battery is functioning. ■ Check that transmitter is ON. ■ Change wires. ■ Usual cause is a dry electrode. Replace electrodes.
ECG leads applied appropriately and without difficulty. Abnormal ECG findings interpreted accurately.	Electrodes do not adhere to skin, and interference appears on oscilloscope.	■ Change placement of electrodes to another area. Clip hair if needed to improve skin contact. ■ Reclean skin thoroughly using skin prep or alcohol and allow to air dry.
	ECG pattern is abnormal.	■ If patient is asymptomatic, recheck lead placement and ensure cables are attached properly. ■ Check if pattern is a life-threatening arrhythmia (for ventricular tachycardia, call rapid response team; for ventricular fibrillation, call code). ■ Increasing PVCs—notify rapid response team. ■ Notify healthcare provider immediately.
	Asystole displays on monitor.	■ Check patient's LOC, pulse, and electrodes, wires, and cable connection. ■ If the patient has an arterial line, check for an arterial waveform in the absence of an ECG waveform.
Patient's cardiac rate is maintained through use of a pacemaker.	Temporary pacing is ineffective.	■ Check for battery depletion and change if necessary (9-volt batteries). ■ Record rhythm strip and correlate to patient's signs and symptoms. ■ Monitor vital signs, mental status. ■ Check sensitivity setting. (If too high, P or T wave may be sensed; if too low, fixed-rate pacing occurs.) ■ Check milliampere setting (may be too high). ■ Check pace indicator for movement. ■ Check rate setting. ■ Check all connections. ■ Check catheter insertion site for swelling, hematoma.

(continued on next page)

EXPECTED OUTCOME	UNEXPECTED OUTCOME	POSSIBLE INTERVENTIONS
Patient is prepared psychologically and physically for insertion of the pacemaker.	Patient does not understand function of pacemaker.	■ If frightened, reassure the patient that a pacemaker is not dangerous. ■ If patient does not understand pacemaker or procedure, use illustrated learning aids. ■ Allow time for questions and further explanations. ■ Orient your teaching to the patient's intellectual and interest level.
Pacemaker is inserted without complications.	Inflammation occurs at insertion site.	■ Provide daily care using strict aseptic technique. ■ Keep dressing dry at all times. ■ Monitor vital signs. ■ Instruct patient to limit movement of extremities.
Patient's cardiac rate is maintained through use of a pacemaker.	Failure to capture is suspected.	■ Check patient's heart rate. If heart rate is less than the rate set on the generator, and if pace indicator shows firing, suspect failure to capture. ■ Check all connections. ■ Anticipate that pacer wires are dislodged. ■ Check battery. ■ Change position of extremity. ■ Turn patient on left side; catheter may float back to epicardial wall. ■ Increase amperage (mA) after checking threshold. ■ Obtain chest x-ray and 12-lead ECG. ■ Anticipate change of batteries, electrode terminals, or generator.
	Battery depletion occurs.	■ Have atropine and isoproterenol available. ■ Anticipate possible CPR. ■ Turn on power switch, and observe pace indicator. If there is little or no movement, replace battery immediately. ■ Record clock hours of battery usage. (Record should be taped to back of generator.) ■ Determine rate fluctuations. ■ Label each pacemaker with the date battery is inserted. ■ Store extra batteries in refrigerator and put new battery in pacemaker before use. ■ Disconnect catheter from pacemaker before replacing battery. ■ Contact with battery terminal may be dangerous to the patient.
Peripheral perfusion distal to arterial catheter placement site remains adequate.	Cannulated extremity develops diminished distal perfusion.	■ Check periphery for changes in color, temperature, motion, and sensation resulting from possible thrombus occlusion or circulatory "steal." ■ Notify healthcare provider immediately. ■ Prepare for catheter removal.
Arterial Line Care Arterial cannulation is accomplished without complication.	Hematoma or bleeding occurs at arterial insertion site.	■ Apply direct pressure over artery while you check for leaks in the system. ■ Check all stopcocks: check if catheter is inserted in artery as it should be. ■ Keep cannulated extremity exposed for observation. ■ Remove catheter if oozing continues.
	Signs of infection or inflammation appear at insertion site.	■ Use sterile transparent dressings exclusively. ■ Always use aseptic technique with dressing changes; change dressing weekly. ■ Cap open port on stopcock to maintain asepsis. ■ Do not apply ointment to insertion site. ■ Change tubing, flush solution, and transducer every 96 hr or with catheter change using sterile technique. ■ Flush open port after obtaining blood specimens. ■ Prepare for catheter removal if infection is suspected.
Arterial blood pressure monitoring system functions reliably and accurately.	Arterial waveform loses definition and digital pressures drop.	■ Reverse response with atropine administration. ■ Use low-compliance (rigid), short (less than [<] 90–120 cm [< 3–4 ft]) monitor tubing. ■ Check for thrombus formation by aspirating blood through stopcock and then flushing system. ■ Be sure to fast-flush arterial line thoroughly after arterial blood samples are obtained or system is zeroed. ■ Make sure all stopcocks are closed to air. ■ Maintain 300 mmHg of pressure in pressure bag. ■ Ensure secure fit of all stopcocks and connections. Avoid adding stopcocks and line extensions. ■ Change position of extremity in which catheter is placed.

EXPECTED OUTCOME	UNEXPECTED OUTCOME	POSSIBLE INTERVENTIONS
Arterial blood pressure monitoring system functions reliably and accurately.	Direct blood pressure readings vary significantly.	■ Flick tubing system to remove tiny air bubbles escaping the flush solution. ■ Recheck transducer and patient position to ensure accurate data. ■ Recalibrate transducer. ■ Flush system after sampling and zeroing. ■ Keep flush bag adequately filled and cleared of air. ■ Maintain bag external pressure at 300 mmHg. ■ Check that connections are tightly secured.
	Patient has decreased urinary output or develops signs of radial artery occlusion.	■ Suspect balloon migration. ■ Maintain head-of-bed elevation at less than 45 degrees to prevent kinking and migration of catheter. ■ Immobilize cannulated extremity to prevent catheter migration.
Arterial blood samples are obtained.	Arterial blood sample is unobtainable.	■ Suspect arterial spasm; allow spasm of artery to stop, then attempt to aspirate blood with gentle pressure using a 6-mL syringe rather than Vacutainer. ■ Reposition patient's arm, making sure there is no pressure at catheter insertion site. ■ Check that catheter is in artery (note waveform on oscilloscope), flush catheter, then attempt to obtain sample.

REVIEW Questions

1. A client receiving a unit of packed red blood cells begins to vomit 15 minutes into the transfusion. What should the nurse do first?
   1. Call for help.
   2. Stop the transfusion.
   3. Provide an emesis basin.
   4. Increase infusing normal saline.

2. The nurse assigns the UAP to complete morning care for a client with a sequential compression device. What information should the nurse instruct the UAP to report to the nurse?
   1. Presence of pulses in the client's feet
   2. Condition of the skin under the devices
   3. Amount of time the devices were turned off
   4. Sensation and movement of the client's feet

3. A new graduate is using an automated external defibrillator (AED) for a client who was discovered without a pulse. For which reason should the charge nurse intervene?
   1. Resuming CPR after discharging the AED
   2. Loudly stating "Clear" before discharging the AED
   3. Stopping compressions for the AED to analyze the client's rhythm
   4. Placing electrode pads below the right clavicle and above the left nipple

4. The nurse evaluates the ability of the UAP to complete a 12-lead electrocardiogram for a client. Which lead placement should the nurse correct before the measurement is recorded?
   1. Green lead placed on the client's left leg
   2. White lead placed on the client's right wrist
   3. V2 placed at the fourth intercostal space, left sternal border
   4. V6 placed at the fifth intercostal space, left midclavicular line

5. A client is prescribed 3-lead telemetry to monitor atrial fibrillation. Which lead approach should the nurse use to obtain the best assessment of this client's atrial functioning?
   1. Lead I
   2. Lead II
   3. Lead III
   4. Lead aVL

6. The nurse notes the following when analyzing a client's cardiac rhythm strip: atrial rate 60; ventricular rate 42; QRS width 0.10 seconds. Which diagnostic test should the nurse anticipate to determine the best treatment for this client's rhythm?
   1. Digoxin level
   2. T3 and T4 levels
   3. Arterial blood gases
   4. Serum electrolyte levels

7. The nurse visits the home of a client with a newly inserted permanent pacemaker. Which observation indicates that the client would benefit from additional teaching about the device?
   1. Medical alert bracelet on the right wrist
   2. Telephone transmission device installed
   3. Pacemaker information card in the wallet
   4. Cell phone in shirt pocket over the pacemaker

8. A new graduate reports that a client's arterial blood pressure monitor reading is 20 mmHg higher than the measurement from the previous shift. What should the nurse assess *first* to determine the reason for the change in measurement?
   1. Calibration process
   2. Pressure bag setting
   3. Arterial site dressing
   4. Angle of the head of the bed

Note: For answers and rationales for the review questions, go to Appendix A or your Pearson MyLab Nursing and eText.

Chapter 13
Perioperative Care

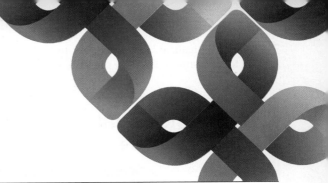

Chapter at a Glance

» The Concept of Perioperative Care

Perioperative care includes three phases of the surgical experience, preoperative, intraoperative, and postoperative. During these three phases, nurses work with safety checklists, technology, equipment, instruments, supplies, and collaborative team guidelines for patient safety. Each phase also has specific nursing assessments, interventions, and evaluations for ongoing improvements and quality service and performance during the patient's surgical experience. Perioperative nurses can be found in many healthcare settings, such as hospital surgery departments, outpatient day-surgery centers, clinics, and healthcare providers' offices. All sites have routines and standardized care for preoperative teaching, support for the patient and family, diagnostic studies, preparation of the surgical patient, evaluation, and follow-up after the surgical procedure. The intraoperative phase takes place in the surgical suite environment. Strict surgical sterile technique must be maintained by everyone to ensure a safe environment during the surgical procedure. There can be scrub nurses, circulating nurses, or nurses assisting the surgeon during the surgery. In the postoperative phase, the patient is transferred to the postanesthesia care unit (PACU) where the patient can safely wake up and become responsive again after anesthesia. PACU nurses monitor patients, assessing airway maintenance, vital signs, sensorium, pain, and surgical sites. They monitor and troubleshoot equipment, tubes, and drains to ensure they are functioning as needed. When patients return to their rooms, they remain in need of support and nursing intervention to remain safe and to prevent postsurgical complications (discussed later in Table 13–1).

Learning Outcomes

13.1   Differentiate patient safety considerations during the three phases of perioperative care, preoperative, intraoperative, and postoperative.

13.2   Give examples of four common perioperative teaching points about preventing complications in the postoperative phase.

13.3   Contrast differences and reasoning for them between performing medical antisepsis hand hygiene and surgical antisepsis hand scrubs.

13.4   Summarize six priority principles in preparing and maintaining a sterile field for a surgical procedure.

13.5   Support the rationale for using a surgical checklist in the preoperative phase.

13.6   Explain common surgical site assessment data to collect when performing a dressing change.

13.7   Give examples of common safety considerations when assisting a postsurgical procedure patient with early ambulation.

13.8   Explain the importance of removing dentures or denture appliances from patients during the preoperative phase.

The following feature links some, but not all, of the concepts related to assessment. They are presented in alphabetical order.

Concepts Related to
Perioperative Care

CONCEPT	RELATIONSHIP TO PERIOPERATIVE CARE	NURSING IMPLICATIONS
Assessment	Note assessment data that could indicate post-operative (post-op) complications.	▪ Monitor vital signs. ▪ Monitor surgical wound site. ▪ Monitor sensorium. ▪ Monitor intake and output.
Comfort	Maintain a post-op level of comfort.	▪ Use nonpharmaceutical measures. ▪ Administer medication for discomfort as ordered.
Infection	Prevent infection of the surgical wound.	▪ Keep wound clean and dry. ▪ Change dressing as appropriate and assess wound for early signs/symptoms of infection.
Mobility	Prevent post-op complications with early mobility as appropriate.	▪ Encourage and support patient to start moving after surgical procedure as appropriate. ▪ Assist patient to be mobile.
Safety	Prevent errors while patient is in the operating room.	▪ Follow safety check protocols of facility with pre-stop checks for right site, right patient, right side, and right procedure.

≫ General Perioperative Care

Expected Outcomes

1. Patient's physical or emotional deviations from normal are identified preoperatively.
2. Preoperative baseline data are obtained.
3. Surgical site is marked and prepared correctly.
4. Patient states expectations regarding intraoperative and postoperative course.

SKILL 13.1 Preoperative Patient Teaching

Preoperative teaching includes preparing the patient for the three phases of the surgical experience, the preoperative, intraoperative, and postoperative. To improve postoperative outcomes (see Evidence-Based Practice under Preparation below), nurses give patients information about what they can expect during each of these phases and teach them what they need to know to avoid postsurgical complications.

Delegation or Assignment

Professional knowledge and critical thinking are required when assessing the learning needs of the patient (and support people) and when determining appropriate teaching content and teaching strategies. For this reason, preoperative teaching is conducted by the nurse and is not delegated or assigned to unlicensed assistive personnel (UAP). The UAP, however, can reinforce teaching, assist the patient with the exercises, and report to the nurse if the patient is unable to perform the exercises.

Equipment

▪ Pillow
▪ Incentive spirometer
▪ Teaching materials (e.g., videotape, written materials) if available at the facility

Preparation

▪ Review healthcare provider's orders and patient's nursing plan of care.
▪ Gather equipment and supplies.
▪ Ensure that potential distracters (e.g., pain, TV, visitors) to teaching are not present. Family and significant others should be included in the teaching plan, if appropriate.

SKILL 13.1 Preoperative Patient Teaching (*continued*)

EVIDENCE-BASED PRACTICE

Presurgery Education Can Make a Difference

A study with over 2500 adult participants was done to determine if presurgery education would make a difference in postsurgical outcomes. Analysis of this study focused on patients who received educational information about their surgery, what they could expect to happen after surgery, and actions they could do to support recovery from the surgery. The study showed that presurgical education made a significant positive difference in satisfaction about the surgical experience. Participants who received presurgical education reported fewer complications and improved recovery.

Source: Data from Ellrich, M. (2015). *The benefits of pre-surgery education.* Retrieved from http://www.gallup.com/businessjournal/183317/benefits-pre-surgeryeducation.aspx

CAUTION! Other patient items commonly removed presurgery and secured until the patient returns from surgery include jewelry items (including body piercing sites), prosthetic body parts, metallic items (such as a bra or barrette), wigs, extremity braces, valuables, sensory assistive devices (such as hearing aid), contact lenses, glasses, and in many cases clothing.

Procedure

1. Introduce self and verify the patient's identity using two identifiers. Explain to the patient that you are going to teach the patient about the importance of the patient's participation in the exercises and actions to do after surgery to prevent complications (**Table 13–1 ≫**). Inform the patient that immediately after surgery and before returning to the patient's own bed, the patient will wake up in the PACU to be monitored during immediate recovery after anesthesia.
2. Perform hand hygiene and observe other appropriate infection control procedures.
3. Provide for patient privacy.
4. Show the patient ways to turn in bed and to get out of bed.
   - Instruct a patient who will have a right abdominal incision or a right-sided chest incision to turn to the left side of the bed and sit up as follows:
   a. Flex the knees.
   b. Splint the wound by holding the left arm and hand or a small pillow against the incision.
   c. Turn to the left while pushing with the right foot and grasping a partial side rail on the left side of the bed with the right hand.

TABLE 13–1 Common Postoperative Complications

Complication	Clinical Manifestations	Supportive Nursing Interventions
Atelectasis	Dyspnea, ↓ breath sounds, restlessness	Encourage using incentive spirometry and taking deep breaths at intervals, O_2 therapy as ordered, and mobility as able.
Deep vein thrombus of calf	Pain with dorsiflexion of foot, swelling in calf area with redness	Maintain on bed rest, anticipate order for heparin therapy, sequential-compression devices, elevation of legs, and pain management.
Hemorrhage	Weak pulse, cool, pale, clammy, ↓B/P	Immediate care: stay with patient, call for help, notify surgeon, start O_2 therapy, monitor V/S and amount of bleeding, anticipate order for IV fluids and possible blood transfusion.
Nausea and vomiting (anesthesia-related)	Unable to eat or drink several hours after surgery	Provide antiemetic as ordered, ice chips, monitor I&O, deep breaths at intervals, IV fluids as ordered.
Ileus	↓Bowel sounds, no stool, abd distention, abdominal pain	Provide pain management as ordered, ambulate, monitor bowel sounds, distention, and V/S.
Partial wound dehiscence	Open section of wound with pain and drainage, broken sutures	Immediate care: stay with patient, call for help, notify surgeon, place sterile moist abdominal pad over incision, monitor V/S and surgical site.
Pneumonia	Shallow, rapid breathing, fever, productive cough, malaise, fatigue	Provide O_2 therapy and antibiotics as ordered, use productive coughing, encourage mobility, monitor I&O sputum, and O_2 saturations.
Pulmonary embolus	Chest pain, dyspnea, ↑anxiety, ↑respirations	Provide anticoagulation therapy, pain management and O_2 therapy as ordered, monitor V/S and O_2 saturations.
Surgical site infection	Redness, drainage, and pain at incision with fever	Provide antibiotics and O_2 as ordered, change dressing PRN, monitor wound site, V/S, diet, and I&O.
Urinary retention	Unable to void, palpable bladder, pain ↓abd, trickle urine output	Insert Foley catheter as ordered, trend I&O, pain management as ordered, encourage mobility and PO fluids unless contraindicated.

Sources: Data from ICD10 Monitor. (2016). *Postoperative complications: It's complicated.* Retrieved from http://www.icd10monitor.com/enews/item/1599-postoperative-complications-it-s-complicated; NetCE. (2015). #90761. *Postoperative complications.* Retrieved from http://www.netce.com/coursecontent.php?courseid=1143; Denu, Z. A., Yasin, M. O., Melekie, T. B., Berhe, A. (2015). *Postoperative pulmonary complications and associated factors among surgical patients.* Retrieved from http://www.omicsonline.org/open-access/postoperative-pulmonary-complications-and-associated-factors-among-surgical-patients-2155-6148-1000554.php?aid=59597; Patient. (2013). *Common postoperative complications.* Retrieved from http://patient.info/doctor/common-postoperative-complications; Brinkley, M. (2015). *Abdominal surgery postoperative complications.* Retrieved from http://www.livestrong.com/article/244440-abdominal-surgery-postoperative-complications/.

(*continued on next page*)

SKILL 13.1 Preoperative Patient Teaching (*continued*)

d. Come to a sitting position on the side of the bed by using the right arm and hand to push down against the mattress and swinging the feet over the edge of the bed.

- Teach a patient with a left abdominal or left-sided chest incision to perform the same procedure but splint with the right arm and turn to the right.
- For patients with orthopedic surgery (e.g., hip surgery), use special aids such as a trapeze, immobilizer, medical lift, walker, crutches, or splint to assist with movement.

5. Teach the patient the following leg exercises:
   - Alternate dorsiflexion and plantar flexion of the feet. **Rationale:** *This exercise is sometimes referred to as calf pumping, because it alternately contracts and relaxes the calf muscles, including the gastrocnemius muscles.*
   - Flex and extend the knees, and press the backs of the knees into the bed while dorsiflexing the feet ❶, providing assistance as needed.
   - Raise and lower the legs alternately from the surface of the bed. Flex the knee of the stable leg and extend the knee of the moving leg ❷. **Rationale:** *This exercise contracts and relaxes the quadriceps muscles.*

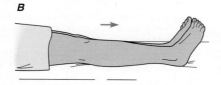

❶ Flexing and extending the knees.

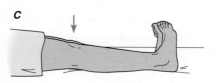

❷ Raising and lowering the legs.

- Encourage patients early postsurgery to ambulate as able and per healthcare provider orders. Make walking aids such as canes, crutches, and walkers available and provide instructions on safely using them.

6. Demonstrate deep breathing (diaphragmatic) exercises as follows:
   - Place your hands palms down on the border of your rib cage, and inhale slowly and evenly through the nose until the greatest chest expansion is achieved ❸.
   - Hold your breath for 2–3 seconds.
   - Then exhale slowly through the mouth.
   - Continue exhalation until maximum chest contraction has been achieved.

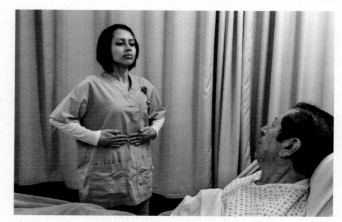

Source: Rick Brady/Pearson Education, Inc.

❸ Demonstrating deep breathing.

7. Help the patient perform deep breathing exercises.
   - Ask the patient to assume a sitting position.
   - Place the palms of your hands on the border of the patient's rib cage to assess respiratory depth.
   - Ask the patient to perform deep breathing, as described in step 6.
   - Encourage patient to use as able the incentive spirometer several times a day.

8. Instruct the patient to cough voluntarily after five deep inhalations.
   - Ask the patient to inhale deeply, hold the breath for a few seconds, and then cough once or twice.
   - Ensure that the patient coughs deeply and does not just clear the throat.

9. If the incision will be painful when the patient coughs, demonstrate techniques to splint the abdomen.
   - Show the patient how to support the incision by placing the palms of the hands on either side of the incision site or directly over the incision site, holding the palm of one hand over the other. **Rationale:** *Coughing uses the abdominal and other accessory respiratory muscles. Splinting the incision may reduce pain while coughing if the incision is near any of these muscles.*

SKILL 13.1 Preoperative Patient Teaching (continued)

- Show the patient how to splint the abdomen with clasped hands and a firmly rolled pillow held against the patient's abdomen ❹.

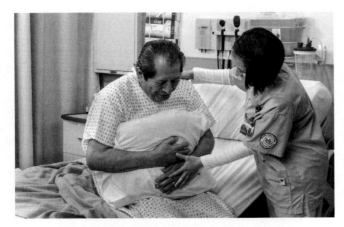

Source: Rick Brady/Pearson Education, Inc.

❹ Splinting an incision with a pillow while coughing.

10. Inform the patient about the expected frequency of these exercises.
    - Instruct the patient to start the exercises as soon after surgery as possible.
    - Encourage patients to carry out deep breathing and coughing at least every 2 hours (depending on their condition), taking a minimum of five breaths at each session. People who are susceptible to pulmonary problems may need deep breathing exercises every hour. People with chronic respiratory disease may need special breathing exercises such as pursed-lip breathing, abdominal breathing, or exercises using various kinds of incentive spirometers (also see Skill 11.5 and Skill 11.6).
11. Emphasize the importance of adequate nutrition to support wound healing and muscle strength. Provide a variety of beverages to ensure adequate fluid intake.
12. Discuss adequate pain control for comfort and encourage movement by the patient.
13. Stress that skin stays clean and dry to prevent skin breakdown while patient is moving less out of bed. Teach that patient should turn frequently and move about in bed.
14. When teaching is complete, perform hand hygiene and leave patient safe and comfortable.
15. Complete documentation of teaching using forms, checklists, or electronic dropdown lists supplemented by nurse's notes or additional comments as appropriate about patient's ability to demonstrate moving, leg exercises, deep breathing, coughing exercises and verbalize key information presented.

SAMPLE DOCUMENTATION

[date] 0900 Instructed how to splint abdomen while deep breathing and coughing. Able to perform correctly. Stated that he will use this technique after surgery. *A. Moore*

Patient Teaching

Preoperative Teaching
Children

- Ensure that parents know what to expect and how to express their concerns.
- Ensure the time of separation from parents is minimized and parents are allowed to interact with the child both immediately preceding and following the surgery.
- Present teaching and communicating with children (both timing and content) to the child's developmental level and cognitive abilities (e.g., "You will have a sore tummy").
- Use therapeutic play as an effective teaching tool with children (e.g., the child can put a bandage on an incision on a doll).

Safety Considerations
OLDER ADULTS AND SURGERY

- Assess hearing ability to ensure the older patient hears the necessary information.
- Assess short-term memory. Presenting one focused idea at a time and repeating or reinforcing information may be necessary.
- Older adults are at greater risk for postoperative complications, such as pneumonia. Reinforce moving and deep breathing and coughing exercises.
- Assess potential postoperative needs at this time. Arrangements can be made preoperatively to obtain necessary items. Examples are medical equipment, such as walkers, raised toilet seats, and bed trapezes; Meals-on-Wheels; and help with transportation.
- If the older adult patient will need to be in extended care for a period of time after surgery, this is the time to initiate these plans.
- Assess the patient for risk of pressure wound development postoperatively, and be extra attentive to use of proper padding and support devices to prevent injury during positioning and transfers in the operating room. Risks include:
  - Older age
  - Poor nutritional status
  - History of diabetes or cardiovascular problems
  - History of taking steroids, which cause increased bruising and skin breakdown.

SKILL 13.2 Surgical Hand Antisepsis and Scrubs

Surgical hand antisepsis scrub refers to performing antiseptic hand washing or an antiseptic hand rub preoperatively to eliminate or reduce transient and resident flora commonly found on hands.

Delegation or Assignment

Due to specific knowledge and skill in performing a surgical hand antisepsis scrub, this skill is not delegated or assigned to the UAP. In some states, a trained UAP may perform surgical hand antisepsis when helping during certain surgical procedures. Assessment and evaluation of effectiveness remain the responsibility of the nurse.

Equipment

- Deep sink with foot, knee, or elbow controls
- Antiseptic hand scrub or hand wash
- Nail-cleaning tool, such as a file or orange stick
- Surgical scrub brush
- Sterile towels for drying the hands

Preparation

- Ensure that the following surgical protective items are in place: shoe covers cap, face mask, and protective eyewear.

Procedure

1. Prepare for the surgical hand antisepsis scrub or rub.
   - Remove wristwatch, bracelets, and all rings. Ensure that fingernails are trimmed. **Rationale:** *Jewelry and long fingernails harbor microorganisms. Removal of jewelry permits full skin contact with the antimicrobial agent.*
   - Clean the nails with a file or orange stick if necessary ❶. Rinse the nail tool after each nail is cleaned. **Rationale:** *Sediment under the nails is removed more readily when the hands are moist.*
   - Turn on the water, using either the foot, knee, or elbow control, and adjust the temperature to lukewarm. **Rationale:** *Warm water removes less protective oil from the skin than hot water. Soap irritates the skin more when hot water is used.*

2. Wash hands.
   - Wet the hands and forearms under running water, holding the hands above the level of the elbows so that the water runs from the fingertips to the elbows. **Rationale:** *The hands will become cleaner than the elbows. The water should run from the least contaminated to the most contaminated area.*
   - Apply 2–4 mL (1 tsp) antimicrobial solution to the hands.
   - Use firm, rubbing, and circular movements to wash the fingers, palms, and backs of the hands.
   - Interlace the fingers and thumbs, and move the hands back and forth ❷. Continue washing for 20–25 seconds. **Rationale:** *Circular strokes clean most effectively, and rubbing ensures a thorough and mechanical cleaning action.*
   - Hold the hands and arms under the running water to rinse thoroughly, keeping the hands higher than the elbows.

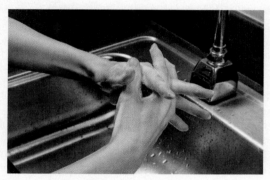

Source: Rick Brady/Pearson Education, Inc.

❷ Interlacing the fingers during hand washing.

HAND WASH SCRUB

3. Perform hand wash antisepsis/scrub (with brush/sponge).
   - Apply antimicrobial agent to wet hands and forearms and lather hands again. Using a scrub brush, scrub each hand. Visualize each finger and hand as having four sides. Wash all four sides effectively ❸. Repeat this process for

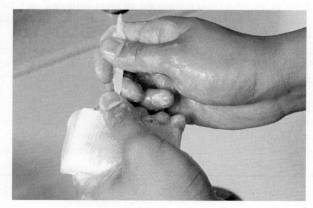

Source: George Draper/Pearson Education, Inc.

❶ Cleaning the fingernails.

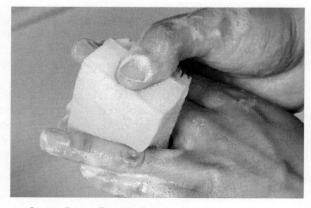

Source: George Draper/Pearson Education, Inc.

❸ Scrubbing side of finger.

SKILL 13.2 Surgical Hand Antisepsis and Scrubs (*continued*)

opposite fingers and hand. **Rationale:** *Scrubbing loosens bacteria, including those in the creases of the hands.*

- Using the scrub sponge, scrub from the wrists to 5 cm (2 in.) above each elbow. Visualize each arm as having four sides. Using facility protocol (e.g., scrubbing by number of strokes or length of time), wash all parts of the arms: lower forearm, upper forearm, and antecubital space to marginal area above elbows. Continue to hold the hands higher than the elbows. **Rationale:** *Scrubbing thus proceeds from the cleanest area (hands) to the least clean area (upper arm).*
- Discard the scrub brush/sponge.
- Rinse hands and arms thoroughly so that the water flows from the hands to the elbows.
- Avoid splashing water onto surgical attire.
- If a longer scrub is required, use a second brush and scrub each hand and arm with the antimicrobial agent for the recommended time.
- Discard second brush, and rinse hands and arms thoroughly.
- Turn off the water with the foot or knee pedal.
- Keeping hands elevated and away from the body, enter the operating room by backing into the room. **Rationale:** *This position of the hands maintains the cleanliness of the hands and backing into the room prevents accidental contamination.*

4. Dry the hands and arms.
- Use a sterile towel to dry one hand thoroughly from the fingers to the elbow ➍. Use a rotating motion. Use a second sterile towel to dry the second hand in the same manner. In some agencies, towels are of a sufficient size that one half can be used to dry one hand and arm and the second half for the second hand and arm.

Rationale: *The nurse dries the hands (the cleanest area) to the least clean area.*
- Discard the towel(s).

5. Keep the hands in front and above the waist. **Rationale:** *This position maintains the cleanliness of the hands and prevents accidental contamination.*

ALCOHOL-BASED HAND RUB

3. Perform hand antisepsis alcohol-based rub.
- Dry hands and forearms thoroughly with a paper towel.
- Always follow the manufacturer's directions for use of the waterless surgical hand antisepsis product. Following is an example of how to use one waterless product.
- Using a foot pump, dispense one pump (2 mL) of the surgical hand rub product into the hand ➎. **Rationale:** *A foot pump avoids contamination of the hands.*
- Dip fingertips of the opposite hand into the hand-rub product and work under fingernails ➏. Spread

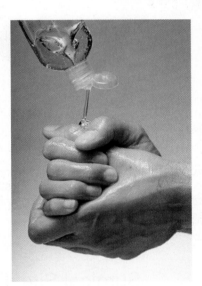

Source: Belmonte/BSIP SA/Alamy Stock Photo

➎ Dispensing hand rub.

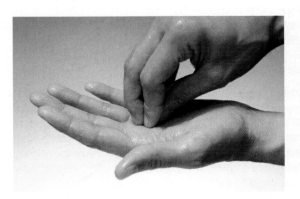

Source: Belmonte/BSIP SA/Alamy Stock Photo

➏ Dip fingers into hand prep.

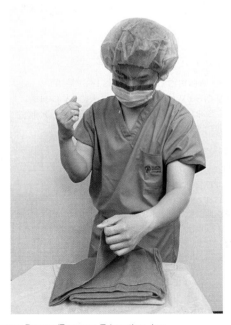

Source: George Draper/Pearson Education, Inc.

➍ Picking up sterile towel to dry hands and arms.

(continued on next page)

SKILL 13.2 Surgical Hand Antisepsis and Scrubs *(continued)*

remaining hand-rub product over the hand and up to just above the elbow.

- Dispense another pump (2 mL) of the surgical hand-rub product into the palm of the opposite hand and repeat procedure.
- Dispense a final pump (2 mL) of hand-rub product into either hand and reapply to all aspects of both hands up to the wrists ⑦.

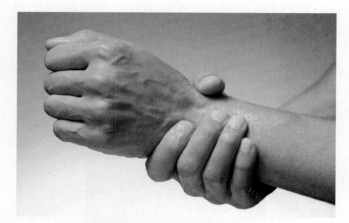

Source: Belmonte/BSIP SA/Alamy Stock Photo

⑦ Reapply hand rub to both hands up to wrists.

4. Rub thoroughly until dry. Do not use towels.
5. Keep the hands in front and above the waist. **Rationale:** *This position maintains the cleanliness of the hands and prevents accidental contamination.*

EVIDENCE-BASED PRACTICE

Surgical Hand Antisepsis

Problem

One of the more common healthcare-associated infections for surgical patients is surgical site infection (SSI). Pathogens can be transmitted to the patient's surgical wound during surgery. A major preventive measure against SSI is surgical hand antisepsis.

Evidence

A review of 14 studies was done, comparing different methods for surgical hand antisepsis. The two used most frequently were a hand washing scrub of either chlorhexidine gluconate or povidone iodine, and a hand rub consisting of an alcohol solution with additional antiseptic ingredients. After cleansing, both groups donned surgical gloves. The data was analyzed (1) by measuring the difference in the number of patient SSI and (2) by determining the number of colonized pathogens on the hands of the surgeon before and after surgery. Further scrutiny and improved quality research studies are needed to define more specific conclusions from evidence.

Implications

The review of studies supports the need for surgical hand antisepsis. The data did not support one method of surgical hand antisepsis over another in lessening the incidence of SSI. Both the hand washing scrub using chlorhexidine gluconate or povidone iodine and the hand rub using an alcohol solution with additional antiseptic ingredients reduced pathogens.

Source: Data from Tanner, J. (2016). *Surgical hand antisepsis to reduce surgical site infection.* Retrieved from http://www.cochrane.org/CD004288/WOUNDS_surgical-hand-antisepsis-reduce-surgical-site-infection; Association of periOperative Registered Nurses (AORN). (2015). *Hand hygiene.* Retrieved from https://www.aorn.org/guidelines/clinical-resources/clinical-faqs/hand-antisepsis-hygiene; Centers for Disease Control and Prevention (CDC). (2016). *Hand hygiene guideline.* Retrieved from http://www.cdc.gov/handhygiene/providers/guideline.html

SKILL 13.3 Surgical Site: Preparing

Preparation of a skin site that will become the surgical incision wound can include antiseptic cleaning, hair removal, and other preoperative preparations. These skin preparations are used to reduce the number of transient and resident microorganisms found frequently on the skin.

Delegation or Assignment

Certain surgical site preparations may be delegated or assigned to the UAP. The nurse can assess and evaluate the UAP's ability to complete this skill safely and, if needed, additional instruction may be given. Assessment and evaluation of effectiveness of the preparation remain the responsibility of the nurse. Note that state laws for UAPs vary, so this task might be assigned to the UAP rather than delegated.

Equipment

- Absorbent pad
- Bath blanket or drape

- Scissors or electric clippers (as needed)
- Depilatory cream (as ordered or facility policy)
- Antiseptic solution (as ordered or facility policy)
- Disposable prep kit

If Kit Is Not Available

- 2 sterile bowls
- 4 × 4 gauze pads
- Emesis basin
- Cotton applicator sticks
- Cleansing solution
- Sterile water
- Clean gloves

Preparation

- Review healthcare provider's orders for specific operative site area preparation needed. Always check with the surgeon about hair removal at surgical site. If hair removal is to be done before the patient goes to the surgery department,

SKILL 13.3 Surgical Site: Preparing (*continued*)

scissors, clippers, or depilatory cream are used following facility policy. Razors are not used because of increased risk for surgical site infection (SSI).

- Review patient's nursing plan of care.
- Gather equipment and supplies to perform needed preparation.

Procedure

1. Introduce self to patient and verify the patient's identity using two identifiers. Explain to the patient that the UAP (or nurse) is going to prepare the surgical site, why it is necessary, and how the patient can participate. Discuss how the results will be used in planning further care or treatments.
2. Perform hand hygiene and observe appropriate infection control procedures.
3. Provide for patient privacy and adjust light to ensure good visualization.
4. Position patient for maximum comfort and site exposure and have bed positioned at correct height.
5. Drape patient for comfort and to prevent undue exposure.
6. Protect bed with absorbent pad.
7. Arrange equipment for your convenience.
8. Don clean gloves.
9. Assess surgical site before skin preparation for moles, warts, rash, and other skin conditions. **Rationale:** *Inadvertent removal of lesions traumatizes skin and may contribute to infection*.
10. If hair removal of surgical site is ordered, it is commonly done in the preoperative area outside of the procedure room of the surgery department or according to facility policy. Use the following steps when hair removal is done before patient goes to the surgery department:
    - Follow healthcare provider's orders or facility policy concerning any removal of hair from the surgical site and other surgical preparations to the area.
    - Remove hair immediately before the surgery. **Rationale:** *Hair removal immediately before surgery is associated with a lower risk of infection*.
    - Use electric clippers or depilatory cream to remove hair, according to facility policies. An electric clipper with a disposable head that can be changed between patients or disposable battery-powered clippers should be used.
    - Wash skin with antiseptic soap, removing all hair with washing; dry area thoroughly. **Rationale:** *This provides clean, smooth skin, free of abrasions and cuts*.
    - Wipe all residual hair off site with 4 × 4 gauze pads or use sticky mitt or tape to remove remaining hair.

EVIDENCE-BASED PRACTICE

Presurgery Hair Removal in Surgical Department

A literature review of 15 studies was done to determine best evidence to decrease surgical site infections (SSIs) by comparing hair removal at the surgical site before surgery using three methods: shaving, clipping, and using depilatory cream. The results showed that use of clippers or depilatory cream was preferred, and shaving with razors should be avoided. SSIs were reduced when using depilatory cream or clippers. The evidence also suggested that hair removal was not always necessary but that, when done, it should be done as close to the time of the surgical procedure as possible.

Source: Data from Al Maqbali. M. (2016). International Journal of Nursing & Clinical Practices. Pre-operative Hair Removal: A Literature Review. *Al Maqbali, Int J Nurs Clin Pract* 2016, 3:163 http://dx.doi.org/10.15344/2394-4978/2016/163.

11. After removing hair, apply antiseptic solution with 4 × 4 pads or use disposable prep kit.
12. Begin at incision site and, with light friction, make ever-widening circles, moving outward from the center to the most distant line of area. **Rationale:** *Working from most clean to least clean area prevents contamination*. Scrub area for 2–3 min.
13. Rinse area with warm water and blot dry with 4 × 4 gauze pads.
14. Remove and dispose of equipment; scissors are disposed of in sharps container. Return bed to lowest height.
15. Remove gloves and discard.
16. Assist patient to put on clean gown.
17. When the procedure is complete, perform hand hygiene and leave patient safe and comfortable.
18. Complete documentation using forms, checklists, or electronic dropdown lists supplemented by nurse's notes or additional comments as appropriate.

SAMPLE DOCUMENTATION

[date] 0630 Awake and alert. Right lower abdominal quadrant cleansed with antisepsis solution per Dr. Dingue's order. No hair growth noted in area. Area dried, clean gown put on. Tolerated procedure without complaint. *T. Quen*

≫ Using Sterile Technique

Expected Outcomes

1. Infection is prevented in patients during surgical procedures.
2. Surgical asepsis is maintained during surgical procedure.
3. Sterile field is maintained on instrument tray during surgical procedure.

SKILL 13.4 Sterile Field: Maintaining

A sterile field is an area that is microorganism-free, including absence of spores. It is maintained by using only sterile gloves to move items or remove items on the sterile field. Sterile on sterile is the only method to maintain a sterile field. The opened and setup sterile field needs to be in constant direct vision and used within 2 hours (or according to facility policy) to be considered safe from contamination.

Delegation or Assignment

Due to the need for sterile technique and technical complexity, the maintaining of a sterile field is not delegated or assigned to the UAP. The UAP may care for patients after the procedure. The nurse must ensure that the UAP knows what complications or adverse signs should be reported to the nurse. The nurse remains responsible for the assessment, interpretation of abnormal finds, and determination of appropriate actions.

Equipment

- Packaged supplies
- Pour container of sterile water or normal saline
- Small sterile container for water

Preparation

- Review healthcare provider's orders and patient's nursing plan of care.
- Review patient's record for allergies.
- Gather equipment and supplies.

Procedure

1. Introduce self to patient and verify the patient's identity using two identifiers. Explain to the patient what you are going to do, why it is necessary, and how the patient can participate. Discuss how the results will be used in planning further care or treatments.
2. Perform hand hygiene and observe appropriate infection control procedures.
3. Provide for patient privacy.
4. Ensure working surface is clean and dry. Patient's over-bed table is frequently used as preparation area. **Rationale:** *This prevents contamination of sterile package*.
5. Remove outer plastic wrap or open pour container.

OPENING PACKAGING

6. Place package in center of work area and position so that you first open package flap away from you. **Rationale:** *This prevents reaching across the sterile field as you continue to open package*.
7. Grasp edge of the first flap of the wrapper, move it away from you, and place it on the working surface ❶.
8. Grasp the first side flap, lift it up; grasp the second side flap and together move both hands out toward the sides.
9. Place the flaps down on the working surface.
10. Grasp the last flap of the wrapper and open it toward you, taking care not to touch the inside of the flap or any of the contents of the package ❷. **Rationale:** *This prevents contamination of the supplies*. Proceed to step 11 below.

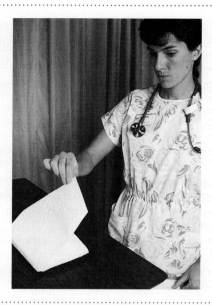
❶ Grasp edge of top flap of wrapper and lift it away from you.

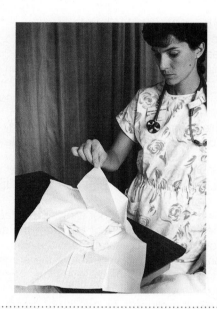
❷ Open last flap toward you—do not cross over sterile field.

POURING LIQUIDS

6. Place container on firm surface and take cap off the bottle and invert the cap before placing it on a firm surface. **Rationale:** *This keeps the cap sterile*.
7. Hold the bottle with the label facing up. Pour a small amount of liquid into a nonsterile container ❸. **Rationale:** *This action cleans the lip of the bottle*.
8. Pour the liquid into the sterile container while keeping the label facing up and not touching the container with the bottle ❹. Do not reach over a sterile field if the container has been placed on one. **Rationale:** *Crossing over a sterile field can lead to contamination of the field*.

SKILL 13.4 Sterile Field: Maintaining (*continued*)

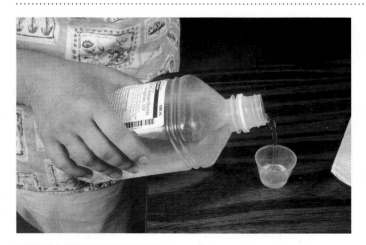

③ First pour a small amount of liquid into a nonsterile container.

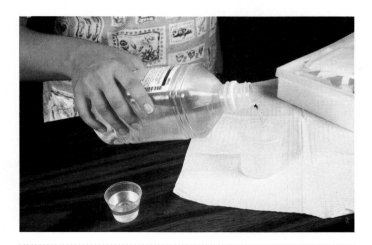

④ Pour liquid by placing container close to edge of sterile area.

9. Replace the cap if liquid remains in the bottle. If total contents have been used, dispose of bottle in trash.
10. Date and initial bottle if reusing. If using a partially filled bottle, check the label and pour off some of the solution in a waste container before pouring solution into container on sterile field. Leave partially filled bottle in patient's room if it is to be reused.
11. When the procedure is complete, discard disposable supplies in proper waste container, perform hand hygiene, and leave patient safe and comfortable. (For information about wound irrigation, see Skill 16.19, and changing a sterile dressing, see Skill 16.5.)
12. Complete documentation using forms, checklists, or electronic dropdown lists supplemented by nurse's notes or additional comments as appropriate.

Safety Considerations

MAINTAINING SURGICAL ASEPSIS

- Items that are sterile become contaminated unless touched only by other sterile items.

Sterile to Sterile = Sterile	Sterile to Contaminated = Contaminated
Sterile to Clean = Contaminated	Sterile to Questionable = Contaminated

- Sterile items out of range of vision or below the waist level of the nurse are considered contaminated.
- Sterile objects are contaminated by airborne sources, so minimize air movement or control its direction.
- Moist or damp sterile fields are considered contaminated if the surface below them is not sterile or if the surface has been exposed to the air for a short amount of time.
- Objects are rendered sterile by the processes of dry and moist heat, chemicals, and radiation.
- Fluids flow in the direction of gravity.
- The edges of a sterile field are considered contaminated, so keep sterile objects within a 2-cm (1-in.) margin from the edges.
- Conscientiousness, alertness, and honesty are necessary in maintaining surgical asepsis.
- Check sterility indicators, expiration dates, and package integrity prior to placing supplies on a sterile field.
- Keep unsterile objects, including your own arms, from being placed over a sterile field.
- Keep sterile objects at a distance from unsterile ones to prevent the transfer of microorganisms.
- When an item becomes contaminated or when in doubt about the sterility of any item, consider it unsterile and take corrective action.

SURGICAL ASEPSIS AT HOME

- Clean and wipe dry a flat surface for the sterile field.
- Keep pets and noninvolved small children out of the area when setting up for and performing sterile procedures.
- Dispose of all soiled materials in a waterproof bag. Check with the facility as to how to dispose of medical refuse.
- Remove all instruments from the home or other setting where others might accidentally find them. **Rationale:** *New instruments can be sharp or capable of causing injury and used instruments may transmit infection.*

SKILL 13.5 Sterile Gown and Gloves: Donning (Closed Method)

The closed method of donning a sterile gown and then gloves maintains a sterile front surface of the gown worn during surgical procedures. Closed gloving is used when the individual wears a sterile surgical gown during the aseptic procedure.

Delegation or Assignment

Donning a sterile gown and sterile gloves is performed by members of the surgical team. It can be, however, delegated or assigned to a UAP in some agencies. The UAP often assists the nurse or scrub person by preparing the sterile pack containing the sterile gown and gloves. Note that state laws for UAPs vary, so this task might be assigned to the UAP rather than delegated.

Equipment

- Sterile pack containing a sterile gown and sterile gloves

Preparation

- Gather sterile pack and ensure its sterility.

Procedure

1. Perform surgical hand antisepsis/scrub or rub (see Skill 13.2).

STERILE GOWN

2. Don the sterile gown.
   - Touching only the inside of the gown, grasp the sterile gown at the crease near the neck, hold it away from you, and permit it to unfold freely without touching anything, including the uniform. **Rationale:** *The gown will not be sterile if its outer surface touches any unsterile objects.*
   - Put the hands inside the shoulders of the gown without touching the outside of the gown.
   - Work the hands down the sleeves only to the beginning of the cuffs ❶.

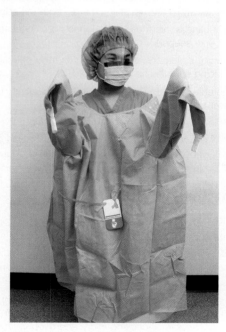

Source: George Draper/Pearson Education, Inc.

❶ Working the hands down the sleeves of a sterile gown.

- Have a coworker wearing a hair cover and mask reach inside arm seams and pull gown over shoulders.
- The coworker grasps the neck ties without touching the outside of the gown and pulls the gown upward to cover the neckline of the scrub person's uniform in front and back ❷.

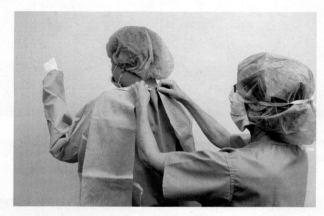

Source: George Draper/Pearson Education, Inc.

❷ Coworker ties the neck ties of the sterile gown.

STERILE GLOVES (CLOSED METHOD)

3. Open the sterile glove wrapper ❸.
4. Put the glove on the nondominant hand.
   - With the dominant hand, pick up the opposite glove with the thumb and index finger, handling it through the sleeve.
   - Position the dominant hand palm upward inside the sleeve. Lay the glove on the opposite gown cuff, thumb side down, with the glove opening pointed toward the fingers.
   - Use the nondominant hand to grasp the cuff of the glove through the gown cuff, and firmly anchor it.
   - With the dominant hand working through its sleeve, grasp the upper side of the glove's cuff, and stretch it

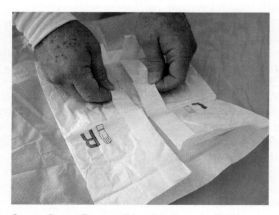

Source: George Draper/Pearson Education, Inc.

❸ Opening the sterile glove wrapper. If no assistant is present, keep hands inside sleeves of gown to open wrapper.

SKILL 13.5 Sterile Gown and Gloves: Donning (Closed Method) *(continued)*

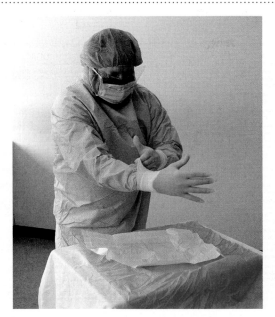

Source: George Draper/Pearson Education, Inc.

④ Pulling on the first sterile glove and letting wrist portion snap into place.

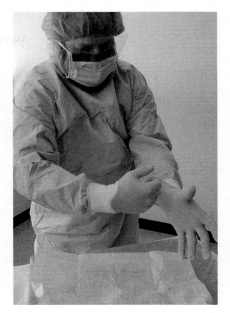

Source: George Draper/Pearson Education, Inc.

⑤ Extending the fingers into the second glove of the dominant hand.

over the cuff of the gown while extending the fingers of the nondominant hand into the glove's fingers ④.

5. Put the glove on the dominant hand.
   - Place the fingers of the gloved hand under the cuff of the remaining glove.
   - Place the glove over the cuff of the second sleeve.
   - Extend the fingers into the glove as you anchor the cuff with the nondominant hand ⑤.
   - Unfold the second cuff and adjust as for the first hand. Keep gloved hands above the sterile field ⑥.

COMPLETION OF GOWNING

6. Complete gowning as follows:
   - Have a coworker hold the waist tie of your gown, using sterile gloves or a sterile forceps or drape. **Rationale:** *This approach keeps the ties sterile.*
   - Make a three-quarter turn, then take the tie and secure it in front of the gown.

   or

   - Have a coworker take the two ties at each side of the gown and tie them at the back of the gown, making sure that the scrub person's uniform is completely covered.
   - When worn, sterile gowns should be considered *sterile* in front from the waist to the shoulder. Once the nurse approaches a table, the gown is considered contaminated from the waist or table down, whichever is higher. The sleeves should be considered sterile from the cuff to 5 cm (2 in.) above the elbow, since the arms of a scrubbed person must move across a sterile field.

Moisture collection and friction areas such as the neckline, shoulders, underarms, back, and sleeve cuffs should be considered unsterile.

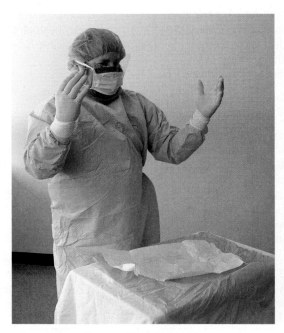

Source: George Draper/Pearson Education, Inc.

⑥ Sterile gloved hands must remain above waist level or the level that defines the sterile field.

SKILL 13.6 Surgical Patient: Preparing

CAUTION! The Association of periOperative Registered Nurses (AORN) recommends that the preop skin preparation should be an antimicrobial agent that has a broad germicidal range and is nontoxic. The most common antiseptic agents used for preoperative skin preparation and surgical scrubs include alcohol, chlorhexidine, and iodine, and iodophors.

- **Alcohol** has the most rapid microbial action, which denatures proteins and is effective against both gram-positive and gram-negative bacteria, viruses, and fungi. However, it is not often used as a surgical skin prep because it does not stay on the skin.
- **Chlorhexidine** has an intermediate rapidity of action, disrupting the cell membrane. It should not be used on mucous membranes, eyes, or brain tissue (neurotoxic). It works well against gram-positive bacteria, and less well against gram-negative bacteria.
- **Iodine/iodophors** has an intermediate action and is acceptable for use against a wide range of bacteria, fungi, and viruses.

Delegation or Assignment

Some interventions to prepare the surgical patient may be delegated or assigned to the UAP. The nurse can assess and evaluate the UAP's ability to complete this skill safely and, if needed, additional instruction may be given. Assessment and evaluation of effectiveness of the preparation remain the responsibility of the nurse. Note that state laws for UAPs vary, so this task might be assigned to the UAP rather than delegated.

Equipment

- Preoperative checklist
- Specific equipment needed to provide physical care as ordered, such as enema equipment, nasogastric tube, Foley catheter
- Antiseptic agent for shower (as ordered)

Preparation

- Review healthcare provider's orders and patient's nursing plan of care.
- Verify patient's signed informed consent is in the front of the patient's record ❶.
- Ensure the preoperative checklist is completed.
- Ensure the preanesthesia evaluation form is signed by the patient.
- Review patient's record for allergies.
- Gather equipment and supplies.

CAUTION! Guidelines and expectations to prevent mistakes in surgery are included in the 2016 Hospital National Patient Safety Goals, UP.01.01.01, UP.01.02.01, and UP.01.03.01 (Joint Commission, 2016).

Procedure

1. Introduce self to patient and verify the patient's identity using two identifiers. Explain to the patient what you are going to do, why it is necessary, and how the patient can

❶ Surgical consent form.

participate. Discuss how the results will be used in planning further care or treatments.

2. Perform hand hygiene and observe appropriate infection control procedures.
3. Provide for patient privacy.
4. Verify preoperative checklist has been completely filled in with no blank areas and is in the front of the patient's record ❷.

Safety Considerations

The World Health Organization (WHO) developed the Safe Surgery Initiative which includes the WHO Surgical Safety Checklist to enhance the communication and collaboration of the surgical team. The checklist includes 19 items used to identify and avoid potential safety hazards before anesthesia has been initiated, before the skin incision has been made, and before the patient leaves the surgical arena during the intraoperative phase. Many countries around the world have adopted this initiative and are currently using this safety checklist. (WHO, 2016).

5. Assist patient to complete anesthesia questionnaire if required and be sure it is located in the front of the patient's record ❸.
6. Assess if bowel prep was completed at home. **Rationale:** *Most patients complete bowel prep before admission to a facility. Administer an enema if ordered.*

SKILL 13.6 Surgical Patient: Preparing *(continued)*

PREOPERATIVE CHECKLIST

Date ⏷

PATIENT INFORMATION   Time ⏷

Name

Age   Gender

Allergies

Current medications

Procedure planned   ☐ Location confirmed   ☐ Consent obtained

SYSTEMS ASSESSMENT   ☐ General appearance   ☐ Cardiovascular
                         ☐ Head and neck   ☐ GI
                         ☐ Integumentary   ☐ Genitourinary
                         ☐ Chest and lungs   ☐ Neurologic

PREOPERATIVE SCREENING   ☐ Urinalysis   Results
                         ☐ Chest x-ray   Results
                         ☐ ECG   Results
                         ☐ CBC   Results
                         ☐ Blood type and cross-match Results
                         ☐ Serum electrolytes   Results
                         ☐ Fasting blood glucose   Results
                         ☐ BUN and creatinine   Results
                         ☐ ALT, AST, LDH, bilirubin Results
                         ☐ Serum albumin, total protein Results

TYPE(S) OF ANESTHESIA   ☐ Local   ☐ Epidural block
PLANNED   ☐ Nerve block (specify)   ☐ Spinal anesthesia

Anesthesia history   ☐ General anesthesia   ☐ Last record included
                         ☐ Complications (specify)
                         Route   IM ☐ IV ☐ PO ☐ Other ☐ (specify)

PERSONAL ITEMS   ☐ Cell phone   ☐ Wallet
                         ☐ Purse   ☐ Pager
                         ☐ Jewelry (specify)

Surgeon

Attending anesthesiologist

② Preoperative checklist.

7. Assist patient to shower if not completed at home. Instruct on how to shower and specific time guidelines according to facility guidelines.
8. Complete skin prep, if ordered. Follow facility guidelines for skin prep.
9. Assess for latex allergy. If present, ensure allergy band is applied, healthcare provider is notified, and operating room (OR) personnel are notified. **Rationale:** *All latex products must be removed from OR and patient must be scheduled for first case in morning.*

10. Enquire for symptoms and observe for signs of cold or upper respiratory infection.
11. Explain need for patient to be NPO for 8–10 hr preoperatively.
12. Remove lipstick and nail polish if required by hospital policy.
13. Insert Foley catheter if ordered.
14. Take and record vital signs.
15. Remove earrings, necklaces, medals, watch, rings and keep jewelry secured by locking it up. (Ring may be taped to finger or

(continued on next page)

SKILL 13.6 Surgical Patient: Preparing (continued)

PREANESTHESIA EVALUATION FORM

Date [▼]   Time [▼]

Patient name [_____]

Age [_____]   Sex [_____]

Ethnicity [_____]

Procedure [_____]   Confirmed [_____]

Consent obtained [_____]

Systems review [_____]

Pulse [_____]   BP [_____]

Temp [_____]   Wt [_____]

Heart [_____]   Ht [_____]

Lungs [_____]   CNS [_____]

Allergies [_____]

Current medications [_____]

Anesthesia history
General anesthesia   Y ☐   N ☐
Last record included   Y ☐   N ☐
Complications   Y ☐   N ☐

Anesthesia plan [_____]

Route   IM ☐ IV ☐ PO ☐ Other ☐ (specify) [_____]

Examiner [_____]

Attending anesthesiologist [_____]

❸ Preanesthesia evaluation form.

toe in some facilities.) If possible, remove body piercing jewelry. Cover with tape if not possible to remove. **Rationale:** *Protect skin from possible burns from electrical arcing generated by electrical cautery machines.*

16. Remove contact lenses, glasses, hairpieces, and dentures. Some hospitals/anesthesiologists allow full dentures to remain if using a mask.
17. Assist patient to void if catheter not inserted, and record time and amount.
18. Check patient's identity, blood band, and allergy bracelet. During this stage the patient must be identified by at least two identifiers (e.g., medical record number, birth date, name, charge number).
19. Put antiembolism stockings on patient as ordered.
20. Administer preoperative medications.
21. Observe that the operative site is verified, both site and side, and has been marked by the surgeon while the patient was awake.
22. Place side rails in UP position and bed in LOW position following administration of medications.
23. Darken room, and provide quiet environment following administration of medications.
24. When the procedure is complete, perform hand hygiene and leave patient safe and comfortable.

25. Complete documentation using forms, checklists, or electronic dropdown lists supplemented by nurse's notes or additional comments as appropriate.
26. Check patient 15 minutes after medication administered to observe for possible side effects.

Safety Considerations

UNIVERSAL PROTOCOL FOR PREVENTING WRONG SITE, WRONG PROCEDURE, AND WRONG PERSON SURGERY (SPEAK UP™)

The Joint Commission (2016) has issued guidelines for preventing wrong site, wrong procedure, and wrong person surgery as discussed here.

Preoperative validation of the right patient, procedure, and site should occur while the patient is awake, aware, and still in the preoperative area before entering the surgical suite.

■ The marking should be made by an individual who is familiar with the patient and is involved with the patient's procedure. This individual is encouraged to be the surgeon or (1) individuals permitted through a residency program to participate in the procedure or (2) a licensed individual who performs duties in collaboration with the surgeon (i.e., nurse practitioners and physician assistants).

■ Incision site must be marked, using a marker that is not easily removed, at or near the incision site.

■ DO NOT MARK any nonoperative site(s) unless necessary for some other aspect of care.

■ Use initials, word "yes," or a line indicating proposed incision site to prevent ambiguous marks.

■ Mark must be visible after patient is prepped and draped and before the procedure begins.

■ Final verification of site mark must take place in the location where the procedure will take place. This time is identified as the "time-out" period. Nothing happens until this final check has occurred. The entire team must be present during this check.

■ Verification must include:
  a. Correct patient identity.
  b. Correct site and side.
  c. Agreement on procedure to be done.
  d. Correct patient position.

e. Availability of any special documentation, diagnostic and radiology tests results, blood products, equipment or implants needed for procedure.

EXEMPTIONS FROM MARKING PROCEDURE

■ Single-organ cases (e.g., larynx surgery, cardiac surgery).

■ Interventional cases: insertion site of instrument/catheter not pre-determined.

■ Premature newborns or infants: for whom the mark may become a permanent mark.

■ Teeth—BUT indicate operative tooth name(s) on documentation or mark the operative tooth (teeth) on the dental radiographs or dental diagram.

Sources: Data from The Joint Commission. (2016). *Universal protocol. Wrong site surgery.* Retrieved from https://www.jointcommission.org/standards_information/up.aspx; Trichak, A. (2016). *Are you practicing proper pre-op skin preparation?* Retrieved from http://mkt.medline.com/advancing-blog/are-you-practicing-properpre-op-skin-preparation/

≫ Critical Thinking Options for Unexpected Outcomes

Not all unexpected outcomes require further nursing intervention; however, many times they do. When the patient demonstrates a change in signs/symptoms indicating an emerging problem, the nurse should immediately assess and troubleshoot what is happening. The assessment data must be processed quickly to formulate a hypothesis so the nurse can make a clinical judgment. The nurse then decides how best to resolve the problem and improve the patient's situation for a better outcome.

EXPECTED OUTCOME	UNEXPECTED OUTCOME	POSSIBLE INTERVENTIONS
General Perioperative Care Preoperative baseline data are obtained.	Factors that can affect the postoperative course are identified during the preoperative care (e.g., arthritic changes in patient's back, history of thrombophlebitis).	■ Place information in patient's plan of care and inform charge nurse and surgeon about findings. ■ Write a note in patient's chart and alert the operating room and PACU staff of the findings so that they can assess for the problems.
Patient's physical or emotional deviations from normal are identified preoperatively.	Patient refuses to go to operating room without dentures.	■ Explain to patient that dentures are likely to be lost, broken, or inadvertently pushed to back of mouth if not removed. ■ If patient refuses to remove dentures, alert anesthesiologist that dentures are in place.
	Patient is abnormally stressed.	■ Explore feelings and reasons for patient's or family's stressed behaviors. ■ Explore more effective methods to reduce stress for patient and family. ■ Clarify misconceptions and inappropriate perceptions. ■ Have healthcare provider speak to patient and answer questions.
Surgical site is marked and prepared correctly.	Patient refuses surgery site marking.	■ Patient has right to refuse; document patient refusal on appropriate forms. ■ Procedure may be performed without marking. ■ Provide patient with information regarding safety aspects for marking procedure. ■ Discuss rationale for patient's refusal to determine whether insufficient information was provided regarding marking procedure.

(continued on next page)

EXPECTED OUTCOME	UNEXPECTED OUTCOME	POSSIBLE INTERVENTIONS
Using Sterile Technique Infection is prevented in patients during surgical procedures.	Patient's skin is cut during hair clipping.	■ Notify healthcare provider and operating room (OR) staff of patient's condition. ■ Follow specific directions; surgery may be canceled as infection could occur as a result of break in skin integrity.
Surgical asepsis is maintained during surgical procedure.	A hole develops in a glove while performing sterile technique.	■ Discard gloves and replace with sterile gloves. ■ Examine hands for cuts if the hole was caused by sharp object. ■ If hands are cut, scrub hands and replace sterile gloves.
Sterile field is maintained on instrument tray during surgical procedure.	Sterile field becomes wet or damp.	■ Discard supplies on sterile field. ■ Set up new sterile field.

REVIEW Questions

1. The nurse schedules preoperative teaching sessions for an older client having bowel surgery. What should the nurse reinforce during every teaching session with this client?
   1. Signs of a wound infection
   2. Use of a splint for breathing exercises
   3. Indications of postoperative hemorrhaging
   4. Actions to prevent lower extremity venous stasis

2. The nurse performs surgical hand scrub antisepsis prior to entering the operating room. What should the nurse do *next* after cleaning the broad surfaces of the hands, wrists, and forearms with circular movements?
   1. Scrub each finger of both hands with a brush.
   2. Hold the hands and arms under running water.
   3. Check the nails and clean them with a file or orange stick.
   4. Interlace the fingers and thumbs and move the hands back and forth.

3. The nurse prepares the site for a client's surgery. What should the nurse do first after removing the hair from the surgical area?
   1. Rinse the area with warm water.
   2. Assist the client to put on a clean gown.
   3. Apply antiseptic solution in circular strokes.
   4. Wash the area with antimicrobial gel and allow to air dry.

4. The charge nurse observes a new graduate opening a sterile package for a procedure to be conducted at a client's bedside. For which action should the charge nurse intervene?
   1. Grasps the two side flaps at once
   2. Opens the closest flap first
   3. Opens the flap farthest away first
   4. Extends the two side flaps together

5. While preparing a sterile field on a client's over-the-bed table, a small amount of sterile water splashes on the sterile field. What should the nurse do?
   1. Leave the area alone to air dry.
   2. Blot the water with sterile gauze.
   3. Consider the field contaminated and start over.
   4. Place the container with the poured sterile water at the edge of the field.

6. During a bedside surgical procedure, the tip of a sterile catheter brushes the cuff of the nurse's sterile gown. What should the nurse do?
   1. Remove and reapply sterile gloves.
   2. Hand the catheter to the healthcare provider for use.
   3. Ask someone to bring another sterile catheter to the bedside.
   4. Drop the catheter onto the sterile field and apply another sterile gown.

7. A surgical time out occurs for a client having lumbar spinal fusion surgery. Which aspect of the verification is waived for this client?
   1. Client name
   2. Surgical site and side
   3. Name of the procedure
   4. Body position to be placed

8. A client scheduled for surgery refuses to remove the wedding band on the left ring finger. What should the nurse do?
   1. Suggest that the ring be pinned to the client's gown.
   2. Explain that no jewelry is to be worn in the operating room.
   3. Apply a piece of tape that covers the entire ring on the finger.
   4. Ask the surgeon to discuss with the client the need to remove the ring.

Note: For answers and rationales for the review questions, go to Appendix A or your Pearson MyLab Nursing and eText.

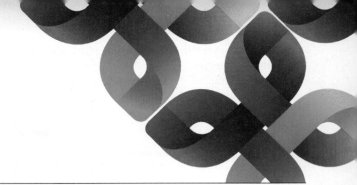

Chapter 14
Reproduction

Chapter at a Glance

❶ Nursing students may observe or assist with the following skills only with faculty permission and while under direct supervision of faculty or another RN.

» The Concept of Reproduction

Reproduction includes three stages of pregnancy: antepartum, intrapartum, and postpartum, and nurses perform assessments, interventions, and evaluations specific for each stage. There are many opportunities during these stages for nurses to provide education to women so they can understand the physical changes in their bodies and recognize signs and symptoms of potential complications. Nurses must know normal, abnormal, and danger signs during prenatal care for the woman and the developing fetus. During labor, there are two individuals who depend on the knowledge and skills of nurses monitoring for expected progression but alert for unexpected events in preparing for delivery. After delivery, nurses are responsible for postpartum care for the woman and her newborn. Many of these skills include special assessment techniques, equipment, and safety concerns for the woman's well-being and the newborn's transition during delivery.

Learning Outcomes

14.1 Give examples of common changes in the body of a woman during the antepartum phase.

14.2 Demonstrate how to assess deep tendon reflexes and clonus to gain information about central nervous system irritability in the woman with diagnosed pre-eclampsia.

14.3 Differentiate the purposes of performing abdominal assessment in the three phases of pregnancy: antepartum, intrapartum, and postpartum.

14.4 Summarize using a Doppler device in auscultating fetal heartbeat rate and how to differentiate it from the woman's pulse.

14.5   Show the steps to apply external electronic fetal monitoring equipment.

14.6   Give examples of priority safety considerations when oxytocin is used to induce labor in the intrapartum phase.

14.7   Explain why, how, and how often to assess the uterine fundus following a vaginal birth.

14.8   Summarize assessment characteristics for each of the five criteria to determine an Apgar score: heart rate, respiratory effort, muscle tone, reflex irritability, and color.

The following feature links some, but not all, of the concepts related to assessment. They are presented in alphabetical order.

Concepts Related to
Reproduction

CONCEPT	RELATIONSHIP TO REPRODUCTION	NURSING IMPLICATIONS
Assessment	Specific assessment needed during the three phases of pregnancy.	■ Be familiar with special monitoring equipment and assessment devices and potential meaning of results. ■ Assess the newborn.
Comfort	Increased need during labor progression.	■ Administer nonpharmaceutical measures and medications to provide comfort as ordered.
Elimination	Change in bladder and bowel habits during pregnancy.	■ Teach patient how to cope with bladder urgency and frequency. ■ Teach patient dietary foods to promote regular bowel movements.
Oxygenation	Breathing may become more difficult during late antepartum phase.	■ Teach patient breathing techniques, posture, and to rest more to assist with shortness of breath.
Perfusion	Complications during delivery may result in large amount of blood loss.	■ Monitor vital signs for changes postpartum. ■ Monitor amount of lochia on perineal pads postpartum. ■ Maintain intravenous fluid infusion as ordered.

For more information about the Reproduction Concept in addition to the skills included in this chapter, go to Module 33, the Reproduction Concept, in Volume 2.

Nursing assessment of the obstetrical patient is a major responsibility for any nurse, whether she or he works in an office setting or in an acute care facility. The nurse-midwife and nurse practitioners have become integral members of the interdisciplinary team that provides care for the family during the birthing process. More advanced practice nurses, such as certified nurse midwives and nurse practitioners, have in-depth education and skill in performing assessment responsibilities with the healthcare provider. While performing the antepartum physical assessment (described in Table 14–1 in Skill 14.2), the nurse should establish an environment in which the woman feels comfortable and free to discuss any concerns. This is also an opportunity to establish rapport with the patient to support her during the intrapartum assessment and care. The last phase of the patient relationship includes postpartum maternal assessment and care, in addition to newborn assessment and care. The information collected during the antepartum (prenatal), intrapartum, postpartum, and newborn assessments can be used to identify needed areas for teaching.

›› Antepartum Care

Expected Outcomes

1. Patient is psychologically prepared for a pelvic examination.
2. Patient experiences no discomfort throughout assessment of fetal well-being nonstress testing.
3. Patient exhibits no signs of side effects or allergic responses at the injection site of administered Rh immune globulin.
4. An amniocentesis is completed without complication.
5. Patient experiences no physical problems during pregnancy.

SKILL 14.1 Amniocentesis: Assisting

Safety Note! *During scheduled clinical time, nursing students may have a learning opportunity to observe or assist with this skill only with faculty permission and with direct supervision from faculty or another RN.*

During amniocentesis, a needle is inserted into the amniotic sac and a sample of amniotic fluid is collected for a variety of tests between 14 and 20 weeks, such as determination of fetus gender, genetic testing to detect chromosomal abnormalities (e.g., sickle cell anemia, cystic fibrosis), and screening for neural tube defects such as Down syndrome and spina bifida. If the mother goes into premature labor in the third trimester, amniocentesis testing can determine the lung maturity.

Delegation or Assignment

Assisting with amniocentesis is not delegated or assigned to the UAP. The nurse can request the UAP to report patient observations to the nurse for follow-up. The nurse remains responsible for the assessment, interpretation of abnormal findings, and determination of appropriate responses.

Equipment

- Real-time ultrasound machine
- Sterile gloves
- 22-gauge spinal needle with stylet
- 10- and 20-mL syringes
- 1% lidocaine (Xylocaine)
- Chlorhexidine gluconate (CHG) and isopropyl alcohol sterile pads
- Three 10-mL test tubes with tops (amber colored or covered with tape) **Rationale:** *Amniotic fluid must be protected from the light to prevent breakdown of bilirubin.*

Preparation

- Review healthcare provider's orders and patient's nursing plan of care.

- Verify a signed informed consent is in the patient's record. **Rationale:** *It is the healthcare provider's responsibility to obtain informed consent. The woman's signature indicates her awareness of the risks and gives her consent to the procedure.*
- Review patient's record for allergies.
- Gather equipment and supplies.

Procedure

1. Introduce self to patient and verify the patient's identity using two identifiers. Explain to the patient what an amniocentesis procedure is, why it is necessary, and how she can participate. Discuss how the results will be used in planning further care or treatments.
2. Perform hand hygiene and observe appropriate infection control procedures.
3. Provide for patient privacy.
4. Provide comfort and safety for patient and self, including raising bed to appropriate height for procedure.
5. Obtain baseline vital signs, including maternal blood pressure (BP), pulse, respirations, temperature, and fetal heart rate (FHR) before the procedure begins; then monitor BP, pulse, respirations, and FHR every 15 minutes during the procedure.
6. Provide gel for the real-time ultrasound and assist as needed with the procedure to assess needle insertion during the procedure. **Rationale:** *Amniocentesis is usually performed laterally in the area of fetal small parts, where pockets of amniotic fluid are often seen. Real-time ultrasound will identify fetal parts, locate the placenta, and locate pockets of amniotic fluid.*
7. Cleanse the woman's abdomen with CHG sterile pads. **Rationale:** *Cleansing the abdomen prior to needle insertion helps decrease the risk of infection.*
8. The healthcare provider dons gloves, inserts the needle into the identified pocket of fluid, and withdraws a sample ❶.

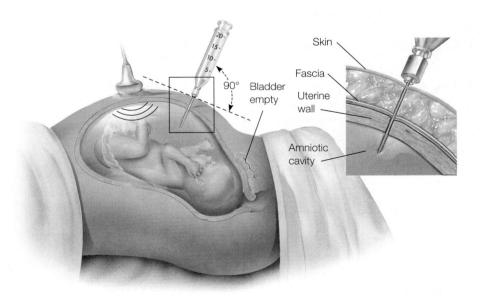

❶ Amniocentesis.

(continued on next page)

SKILL 14.1 Amniocentesis: Assisting (*continued*)

9. Obtain the test tubes from the healthcare provider. Label the tubes with the woman's correct identification and send to the lab with the appropriate lab slips.
10. Monitor the woman and reassess her vital signs.
    * Determine the woman's BP, pulse, respirations, and the FHR.
    * Palpate the woman's fundus to assess for uterine contractions.
    * Monitor her using an external fetal monitor for 20– 30 min after the amniocentesis.
    * Assist with treatment course to counteract any supine hypotension and to increase venous return and cardiac output. **Rationale:** *Monitoring maternal and fetal status postprocedure provides information about response to the procedure and helps detect any complications such as inadvertent fetal puncture.*
11. Assess the woman's blood type and determine any need for Rh immune globulin.
12. Administer Rh immune globulin if indicated. **Rationale:** *To prevent Rh sensitization in a Rh-negative woman, Rh immune globulin is administered prophylactically following amniocentesis.*

CAUTION! Have the woman lie on her left side to ensure adequate placental perfusion.

---

13. Instruct the woman to report any of the following changes or symptoms to her healthcare provider:
    * Unusual fetal hyperactivity or, conversely, any lack of fetal movement
    * Vaginal discharge—either clear drainage or bleeding
    * Uterine contractions or abdominal pain
    * Fever or chills.
14. Encourage the woman to engage only in light activities for 24 hours and to increase her fluid intake. **Rationale:** *A decrease in maternal activity will decrease uterine irritability and increase uteroplacental circulation. Increased hydration helps replace amniotic fluid through the uteroplacental circulation.*
15. When the procedure is complete, return bed to lowest height. Perform hand hygiene and leave the patient safe and comfortable.
16. Complete documentation using forms, checklists, or electronic dropdown lists supplemented by nurse's notes or additional comments as appropriate including the type of procedure and the name of the healthcare provider who performed the procedure. Also record the maternal–fetal response, disposition of the specimen, and discharge teaching.

SAMPLE DOCUMENTATION

[date] 1115 V/S 124/78, 84, 18, T 37.11°C (98.8°F) oral, FHR 142. Amniocentesis done by Dr. Wick, real-time ultrasound used for needle insertion. 32 mL amniotic fluid collected and put in specimen tubes, labeled and sent to lab with lab request slips. Tolerated procedure without incident. V/S 128/82, 88, 18, FHR 146, fundus soft. *K. Mills*

SKILL 14.2 Antepartum, Maternal and Fetal: Assessing

Assessment examinations are scheduled throughout the antepartum phase of pregnancy. These assessments can include lab tests, screening tests, and physical examinations. Teaching is a part of all the phases of pregnancy.

Delegation or Assignment

Assisting with antepartum examination is not delegated or assigned to the UAP. The nurse can request the UAP to report patient observations to the nurse for follow-up. The nurse remains responsible for the assessment, interpretation of abnormal findings, and determination of appropriate responses.

Equipment

* Need for appropriate equipment according to which assessment is being done.

Preparation

* Review healthcare provider's or certified nurse-midwife's (MD/CNM) orders and patient's nursing plan of care.
* Review patient's record for allergies.
* Gather equipment and supplies.

Procedure

1. Introduce self to patient and verify the patient's identity using two identifiers. Explain to the patient that the healthcare provider is going to perform a maternal and fetal assessment, why it is necessary, and how she can participate. Discuss how the results will be used in planning further care or treatments.
2. Perform hand hygiene and observe appropriate infection control procedures.
3. Provide for patient privacy.
4. Provide comfort and safety for patient and self, including raising bed to appropriate height for procedure.
5. Perform a systematic assessment (see **Table 14–1 》**).
6. When procedure is complete, lower bed to lowest position, perform hand hygiene, and leave patient safe and comfortable.
7. Complete documentation using forms, checklists, or electronic dropdown lists supplemented by nurse's notes or additional comments as appropriate.

SKILL 14.2 Antepartum, Maternal and Fetal: Assessing (*continued*)

TABLE 14–1 Antepartum Assessment

Assessment	Normal Findings During Pregnancy	Abnormal Findings During Pregnancy
Take vital signs, blood pressure (BP), temperature, pulse, and respiration (TPR).	Temperature: 36.6°C–37.2°C (98°F–99°F) Pulse: 80–90 bpm (pulse rates can increase 10 beats during pregnancy) Respirations: 16–24 breaths/min (pregnancy may induce a mild form of hyperventilation and thoracic breathing) BP: less than 120/80 mmHg	Elevated temperature—infection Increased pulse rate—anxiety or excitement; cardiac disorder Marked tachypnea—assess for respiratory distress Increased: possible anxiety (patient should rest 20–30 min before you take BP again) Systolic >130 or diastolic <80: sign of preeclampsia Decreased: sign of supine hypotensive syndrome. If lying on back, turn patient on left side and take BP again.
Evaluate weight to assess maternal health and nutritional status and growth of fetus.	Minimum weight gain during pregnancy: 10 kg (24 lb) If underweight: 11.7–17.5 kg (28–42 lb) If obese: 6.25 kg (15 lb or more) Normal weight gain: 10.4–16.7 kg (25–40 lb)	Inadequate weight gain: possible maternal malnutrition Excessive weight gain: if sudden at onset, may indicate preeclampsia; if gradual and continual, may indicate overeating
Skin ■ Color	Nail beds are pink; color of skin is consistent with racial background. *Striae* (reddish-purple lines) on breasts, hips, and thighs; after pregnancy, faint silvery-gray *Spider nevi* common in pregnancy	Pallor—anemia; yellowish—liver disease or some form of jaundice Dark-skinned individuals with anemia may have bluish, reddish, mottled skin; dusty or pale appearance of the palms and nail beds Petechiae, multiple bruises, ecchymosis (hemorrhage; abuse)
■ Condition	Absence of edema (slight edema in lower extremities normal); usually no rashes	Edema could be suggestive of pregnancy-induced hypertension (PIH). Presence of rash could indicate dermatitis; allergic reaction. Ulcerations could indicate varicose veins or decreased circulation.
■ Edema	In lower extremities	In upper extremities and face may indicate PIH.
Nose, mouth, and neck	Nasal mucosa redder than oral; nasal mucosa edematous due to increased estrogen resulting in nasal stuffiness and nosebleeds; gingival tissue hypertrophy related to increase in estrogen	Pallor in mucosa may be anemia; edema in mucosa tissue may be inflammation or infection.
Chest and lungs	Should be no difference during pregnancy	
Breasts and nipples ■ Contour and size ■ Presence of lumps ■ Secretions	Size increases are noticeable during first 20 weeks; become nodular; tingling sensation may be felt during first and third trimester; breasts feel heavy; darker pigmentation of nipple and areola Colostrum appears in late first trimester or early second trimester. Secondary areola appears at 20 weeks, characterized by series of washed-out spots surrounding primary areola. Old striae marks may be present in multiparas.	Redness, heat, tenderness, cracked or fissured nipples (infection); "pigskin" or orange-peel appearance, nipple retraction, swelling, hardness (carcinoma) Secretions other than colostrum
Heart	Palpitations during pregnancy may occur due to sympathetic nervous system disturbance. Short systolic murmurs that increase in held expiration are normal due to increased volume.	Enlargement, thrills, thrusts, gross irregularity or skipped beats, gallop rhythm or extra sounds could indicate cardiac disease.
Abdomen	Flat, rounded abdomen; progressive enlargement due to pregnancy Primiparas: coincidentally with growth *Linea nigra* (black line of pregnancy along midline of abdomen) Primiparas: coincidentally with growth of fundus Multiparas: after 13–15 weeks' gestation	Distention with discomfort due to constipation or gas, enlarging uterus pain, urinary tract infection, early preeclampsia, or distention of abdomen due to polyhydramnios (too much amniotic fluid)
Fundal height in centimeters (fingerbreadths less accurate): measure from symphysis pubis to top of fundus	Fundus palpable just above symphysis at 8–10 weeks Halfway between symphysis and umbilicus at 16 weeks Umbilicus at 20–22 weeks	Large measurements: expected date of confinement or delivery (EDC) is incorrect; tumor; ascites; multiple pregnancy; polyhydramnios; hydatidiform mole Less than normal enlargement: fetal abnormality; oligohydramnios; placental dysmaturity; missed abortion; fetal death

(*continued on next page*)

SKILL 14.2 Antepartum, Maternal and Fetal: Assessing *(continued)*

TABLE 14–1 Antepartum Assessment *(continued)*

Assessment	Normal Findings During Pregnancy	Abnormal Findings During Pregnancy
Fetal heart rate by quadrant, location, and rate	120–160 bpm (in utero) 110–160 bpm (at term) May be heard with Doppler at 10–12 weeks' gestation; with fetoscope at 17–20 weeks	Decreased: indicates fetal distress with possible cord prolapse or cord compression Accelerated: initial sign of fetal hypoxia Absent: may indicate fetal demise
Fetal movement	Trained examiner should be able to feel fetal movement after 18th week.	Fewer fetal movements may indicate a fetal health problem, no movement in response to maternal eating or active activity, or absence of movements after 20 weeks.
Ballottement	Tapping the uterus sharply during the 4th or 5th month results in the fetus rising and then returning to the original position.	No rebound felt against wall of uterus from fetus falling back with ballottement maneuver.
Determine fetal position using Leopold maneuvers: Complete external palpations of the abdomen to determine fetal position, lie, presentation, and engagement. First maneuver: to determine part of fetus in fundus Second maneuver: to locate the back, arms, and legs: fetal heart heard best over fetal back Third maneuver: to determine part of fetus presenting into pelvis Fourth maneuver: to determine degree of cephalic flexion and engagement ❶	Vertex presentation	Breech presentation or transverse lie

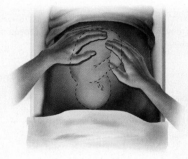 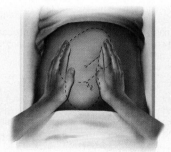 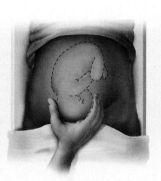 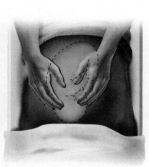

A. First maneuver   *B.* Second maneuver   *C.* Third maneuver   *D.* Fourth maneuver

❶ Steps of Leopold maneuvers.

Pelvis and perineum	1–4 weeks: enlargement in anteroposterior diameter	Absence of Goodell sign: inflammatory condition, carcinoma
	4–8 weeks: softening of cervix (Goodell sign); softening of isthmus of uterus (Hegar sign); cervix takes on bluish color (Chadwick sign)	
	8–12 weeks: vagina and cervix appear bluish-violet in color (Chadwick sign)	
	External genital: in multiparas labia majora loose and pigmented; urinary and vaginal orifices visible and appropriately located	
	Vagina: in multiparas, vaginal folds smooth and flattened; may have episiotomy scar	
	Cervix: in multiparas, cervical os allows insertion of one fingertip	
	Pelvic Measurements:	Deviations in pelvic measurements may indicate that vaginal birth may not be possible.
	Internal measurements:	
	Diagonal conjugate at least 11.5 cm	Disproportion of pubic arch
	Obstetric conjugate estimated by subtracting 1.5–2 cm from diagonal conjugate	Fixed or malposition of coccyx
	Mobility of coccyx: external intertuberosity diameter greater than 9 cm	

SKILL 14.2 Antepartum, Maternal and Fetal: Assessing (*continued*)

TABLE 14–1 Antepartum Assessment (*continued*)

Assessment	Normal Findings During Pregnancy	Abnormal Findings During Pregnancy
Reflexes	Normal and symmetrical	Hyperactivity, clonus would be present in PIH
Assessment of Pregnant Woman Evaluate lab findings: Complete blood count (CBC) Hemoglobin (Hgb) Hematocrit (Hct)	12–16 g/dL 38–47%; physiological anemia (pseudoanemia) may occur	Less than 10.5 g/dL indicating anemia (commonly iron deficient anemia)
White blood cell (WBC) count: 5000–12,000/μL	Elevations in pregnancy and labor are normal.	Need to find out why it is elevated; may be sign of infection if other symptoms present, or WBC count higher than expected with pregnancy.
Red blood cell (RBC) count	No alteration	4.0–6.0 million/μL
Urinalysis: sugar, protein, albumin	Normal color and specific gravity Negative for protein, RBCs, WBCs, casts	Positive for sugar: may indicate subclinical or gestational diabetes Proteinuria between 300 mg/L and 1 g (1+ – 2+ dipstick indicates mild PIH)
Glucose	Negative or small amount of glycosuria may occur in pregnancy.	May develop hyperglycemia problems or gestational diabetes
Rubella titer	Hemagglutination: inhibition (HAI) test 1:10 indicates immunity	HAI test 1:8 or less indicates little or no immunity to rubella.
Hepatitis B screen	Negative	Positive: maternal treatment and prevention of mother-to-child transmission
HIV	Negative	Positive
Syphilis test	Nonreactive	Reactive
Gonorrhea culture	Negative	Positive
Illicit drug screen	Negative	Positive
Sickle cell screen	For those of African descent—negative	For those of African descent—positive
Pap smear	Negative	Positive
Blood type and Rh factor	A variety of blood groupings Rh positive Does not require RhoGAM	If Rh negative, father's blood should be typed. If Rh positive, titers should be followed. Possible RhoGAM at termination of pregnancy
Group B *Streptococcus* test Either cultured (35–37 weeks' gestation) or FDA-approved IDI-Strep B provides results in 1 hr	Strep not present	If strep present, woman is given IV antibiotic treatment every 4 hr during labor (penicillin or ampicillin) until delivery.
Assess for Signs of Labor Lightening and dropping (the descent of the presenting part into the pelvis)	Several days to 2 weeks before onset of labor Multipara: may not occur until onset of labor Relief of shortness of breath and increase in frequency	No lightening or dropping: may indicate disproportion between fetal presenting part and maternal pelvis
Check if mucus plug has been expelled from cervix. Assess for bloody show.	Usually expelled from cervix prior to onset of labor Clear, pinkish, or blood-tinged vaginal discharge that occurs as cervix begins to dilate and efface	Mucus plug comes out in tiny pieces instead of all at once, no color noted or pinkish color discharge noted.
Assess for ruptured membranes. ■ Time water breaks	Before, during, or after onset of labor	Breech presentation: frank meconium or meconium staining
■ Color of amniotic fluid	Clear, straw color	Greenish-brown: indicates meconium has passed from fetus, possible fetal distress Yellow-stained: fetal hypoxia 36 hr or more prior to rupture of membrane possible sign of hemolytic disease
■ Quantity of amniotic fluid	Normal is 500–1000 mL of amniotic fluid, rarely expelled at one time	Polyhydramnios—excessive amniotic fluid (over 2000 mL) Observe newborn for congenital anomalies: craniospinal malformation, orogastrointestinal anomalies, Down syndrome, and congenital heart defects Oligohydramnios—minimal amniotic fluid (less than 500 mL) Observe newborn for malformation of ear, genitourinary tract anomalies, and renal agenesis
■ Odor of fluid	No odor	Odor may indicate infection: deliver within 24 hr.

(*continued on next page*)

SKILL 14.2 Antepartum, Maternal and Fetal: Assessing (*continued*)

TABLE 14–1 Antepartum Assessment (*continued*)

Assessment	Normal Findings During Pregnancy	Abnormal Findings During Pregnancy
Assessment of fetal well-being	Appropriate fetal movement counts, FHR in response to fetal movement, amount of amniotic fluid, reactive nonstress test, ultrasound measurements, movements, appearance	Hypertensive disorder, diabetes, and renal or heart disease are among conditions that may warrant diagnostic testing for fetal well-being in the third trimester: amniocentesis; nonstress testing (NST), contraction stress test (CST), biophysical profile scoring
Evaluate fundal height	Drop around 38th week: sign of fetus engaging in birth canal Primipara: sudden drop Multipara: slower, sometimes not until onset of labor	Large fundal growth: may indicate wrong dates, multiple pregnancy, hydatidiform mole, polyhydramnios, tumors Small fundal growth: may indicate fetal demise, fetal anomaly, retarded fetal growth, abnormal presentation or lie, decreased amniotic fluid

SKILL 14.3 Antepartum Pelvic Examination: Assisting

Safety Note! *During scheduled clinical time, nursing students may have a learning opportunity to observe or assist with this skill only with faculty permission and with direct supervision from faculty or another RN.*

An antepartum pelvic examination is usually done at the first appointment when lab tests are done to determine that the woman is pregnant. The exam includes assessing for sexually transmitted infections, evaluating the size of the woman's pelvis, and assessing the uterine cervix. A Pap smear may be done if the woman has not had this test for a long period of time.

Delegation or Assignment

Assisting with antepartum examination is not delegated or assigned to the UAP. The nurse can request the UAP to report patient observations to the nurse for follow-up. The nurse remains responsible for the assessment, interpretation of abnormal findings, and determination of appropriate responses.

Equipment

- Examination table with stirrup attachments
- Vaginal specula of various sizes, warmed with water or on a heating pad prior to insertion
- Sterile gloves
- Water-soluble lubricant
- Materials for Pap smear or liquid-based Pap test method and cultures
- Good light source

CAUTION! Lubricant may alter the results of tests and cultures and is not used during the speculum examination. Its use is reserved for the bimanual examination.

Preparation

- Review healthcare provider or certified nurse-midwife's (MD/CNM) orders and patient's nursing plan of care.
- Review patient's record for allergies.
- Gather equipment and supplies.
- Ensure that the room is sufficiently warm by checking the room temperature and adjusting the thermostat if necessary.
- Have padding on the stirrups. If stirrups are not padded, the woman may prefer to leave her shoes on during the procedure.

Procedure

1. Introduce self to patient and verify the patient's identity using two identifiers. Explain to the patient that she is going to have a pelvic examination done by her healthcare provider, why it is necessary, and how she can participate. Discuss how the results will be used in planning further care or treatments. Explain the procedure to the woman. If she has never had a pelvic examination, show her the equipment to be used as part of the explanation. **Rationale:** *Explaining the procedure helps reduce anxiety and increase cooperation.*

2. Perform hand hygiene and observe appropriate infection control procedures.

3. Provide for patient privacy.

4. Provide comfort and safety for patient and self, including raising bed to appropriate height for procedure. Ask the woman to empty her bladder and remove clothing below her waist.

5. Perform a pelvic examination.
   - Ask the woman to sit at the end of the examining table with the drape across her lap.
   - Position the woman in the lithotomy position with her thighs flexed and adducted. Place her feet in the stirrups. Her buttocks should extend slightly beyond the edge of the examining table.
   - Drape the woman with the sheet, leaving a flap so that the perineum can be exposed. **Rationale:** *The drape helps preserve the woman's sense of dignity and privacy.*
   - The examiner dons clean gloves for the procedure. Explain each part of the procedure as the healthcare provider performs it.

SKILL 14.3 Antepartum Pelvic Examination: Assisting (continued)

- Let the woman know that the examiner begins with an inspection of the external genitalia. The speculum is then inserted to allow visualization of the cervix and vaginal walls and to obtain specimens for testing. After the speculum is withdrawn, the examiner performs a bimanual examination of the internal organs using the fingers of one hand inserted in the woman's vagina while the other hand presses over the woman's uterus and ovaries. The final step of the procedure is generally a rectal examination.
- Ask the woman to breathe slowly and regularly and to use any method she finds effective in helping her to remain relaxed.
- Let her know when the examiner is ready to insert the speculum and ask her to bear down. **Rationale:** *Relaxation helps decrease muscle tension. Bearing down helps open the vaginal orifice and relaxes the perineal muscles.*
- After the speculum is withdrawn, lubricate the examiner's fingers prior to the bimanual examination.
6. After the examiner has completed the examination and moved away from the woman, move to the end of the examination table and face the woman. Cover her with the drape. Apply gentle pressure to her knees and encourage her to move toward the head of the table. Assist her to remove her feet from the stirrups, then offer your hand to her and assist her to sit up.
7. Provide her with tissues to wipe the lubricant from her perineum. **Rationale:** *Vaginal secretions and lubricant may be discharged from the vagina when the woman sits upright.*
8. Provide the woman with privacy while she dresses. Be sure that she is not dizzy and that she is standing or sitting safely before leaving the room.
9. Complete documentation using forms, checklists, or electronic dropdown lists supplemented by nurse's notes or additional comments as appropriate.

SAMPLE DOCUMENTATION

[date] 1512 V/S 118/76, 78, 16, T 37.11°C oral (98.8°F). Pelvic exam done via Dr. Manes. PAP smear done, specimen labeled and to lab. Tolerated procedure without complaint. M. Hayes

---

SKILL 14.4 Deep Tendon Reflexes and Clonus: Assessing

Assessing deep tendon reflexes (DTRs) is done to test for the presence of hyperreflexia and clonus. Hyperreflexia indicates a stronger than normal reflexive response with continued twitching or purposeful movements. Clonus is a sustained involuntary muscular contraction and relaxation tremor caused by a passive stretch of the muscle and tendon. Either of these may indicate central nervous system irritability and preeclampsia or eclampsia for the pregnant woman. Monitoring DTRs can help determine the need for magnesium therapy to be started, adjusted, or stopped.

Delegation or Assignment

Assessing DTRs and clonus is not delegated or assigned to the UAP. The nurse can request the UAP to report patient observations to the nurse for follow-up. The nurse remains responsible for the assessment, interpretation of abnormal findings, and determination of appropriate responses.

Equipment

■ Percussion hammer

CAUTION! If a percussion hammer is not available, you may use the side of your hand to elicit DTRs.

Preparation

■ Review physician's or certified nurse-midwife's (MD/CNM) orders and patient's nursing plan of care.

■ Explain the procedure, the indications for its use, and the information that will be obtained.
■ Most nurses check the patellar reflex and one other such as the biceps, triceps, or brachioradialis. **Rationale:** *DTRs are assessed to gain information about CNS irritability secondary to preeclampsia and to assess the effects of magnesium sulfate if the woman is receiving it.*

Procedure

1. Introduce self to patient and verify the patient's identity using two identifiers. Explain to the patient that you are going to assess deep tendon reflexes, why it is necessary, and how she can participate. Discuss how the results will be used in planning further care or treatments.
2. Perform hand hygiene and observe appropriate infection control procedures.
3. Provide for patient privacy.
4. Elicit reflexes.
   - Patellar reflex. Position the woman with her legs hanging over the edge of the bed (feet should not be touching the floor) ❶. Briskly strike the patellar tendon, which is located just below the patella. Normal response is extension or a thrusting forward of the foot. **Rationale:** *In an inpatient setting, the patellar reflex is often assessed while the woman lies supine. Flex her knees slightly and support them.*

(continued on next page)

SKILL 14.4 Deep Tendon Reflexes and Clonus: Assessing *(continued)*

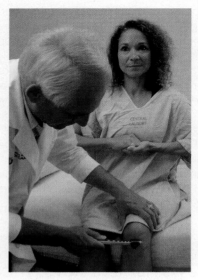

Source: Patrick Watson/Pearson Education, Inc.

❶ Correct sitting position for eliciting the patellar reflex.

- Biceps reflex. Flex the woman's arm 45 degrees at the elbow and place your thumb on the biceps tendon. Allow your fingers to hold the biceps muscle. Strike your thumb in a slightly downward motion and assess the response. Normal response is flexion of the arm.
- Triceps reflex. Flex the woman's arm up to 90 degrees and allow her hand to hang against the side of her body. Using the percussion hammer, strike the triceps tendon just above the elbow. Normal response is contraction of the muscle, which causes extension of the arm.
- Brachioradialis reflex. Flex the woman's arm slightly and lay it on your forearm with her hand slightly pronated. Using the percussion hammer, strike the brachioradialis tendon, which is found about 2.5–5 cm (1–2 in.) above the wrist. Normal response is pronation of the forearm and flexion of the elbow. **Rationale:** *The correct*

position causes the muscle to be slightly stretched. Then when the tendon is stretched, with a tap the muscle should contract. Correct positioning and technique are essential to elicit the reflex.

5. Grade reflexes. Reflexes are graded on a scale of 0 to 4+, as follows:
   - 4+   Hyperactive; very brisk, jerky, or clonic response; abnormal
   - 3+   Brisker than average; may not be abnormal
   - 2+   Average response; normal
   - 1+   Diminished response; low normal
   - 0   No response; abnormal

   Rationale: *Normally reflexes are 1+ or 2+. With CNS irritation, hyperreflexia may be present; with high magnesium levels, reflexes may be diminished or absent.*

6. Assess for clonus. With the woman's knee flexed and the leg supported, vigorously dorsiflex the foot, maintain the dorsiflexion momentarily, and then release. With a normal response, the foot returns to its normal position of plantar flexion. Clonus is present if the foot "jerks" or taps against the examiner's hand. If so, record the number of taps or beats of clonus. **Rationale:** *Clonus occurs with more pronounced hyperreflexia and indicates CNS irritability.*

7. When the procedure is complete, return bed to lowest height. Perform hand hygiene and leave patient safe and comfortable.

8. Complete documentation using forms, checklists, or electronic dropdown lists supplemented by nurse's notes or additional comments as appropriate.

SAMPLE DOCUMENTATION

[date] 1640 Sitting on side of bed. Bilateral patellar deep tendon reflexes assessed. Left leg – DTRs 2+, no clonus, right leg – DTRs 4+, 2 beats clonus. *M. Tiny*

SKILL 14.5 Fetal Well-Being, Nonstress Test and Biophysical Profile: Assessing

Safety Note! *During scheduled clinical time, nursing students may have a learning opportunity to observe or assist with this skill only with faculty permission and with direct supervision from faculty or another RN.*

The biophysical profile is an ultrasound scan to assess fetal breathing movement, fetal movement of body or limbs, fetal extension and flexion of extremities, amniotic fluid volume, and reactive nonstress test. The nonstress test assesses fetal well-being by monitoring fetal activity and concurrent fetal heart rate (FHR) response to it.

Delegation or Assignment

Assessing fetal well-being, nonstress test and biophysical profile is not delegated or assigned to the UAP. The nurse can request the UAP to report patient observations to the nurse for follow-up. The nurse remains responsible for the assessment, interpretation of abnormal findings, and determination of appropriate responses.

Equipment

- External fetal heart rate and contraction monitors (ultrasound transducer and tocodynamometer)

SKILL 14.5 Fetal Well-Being, Nonstress Test and Biophysical Profile: Assessing (*continued*)

- Ultrasonic gel

For Biophysical Profile Only
- Ultrasound equipment

Preparation

- Review physician's or certified nurse-midwife's (MD/CNM) orders and patient's nursing plan of care.
- Gather necessary equipment and supplies.

Procedure

1. Introduce self to patient and verify the patient's identity using two identifiers. Explain to the patient and her support person what you are going to do, why it is necessary, and how the patient can participate. Discuss how the results will be used in planning further care or treatments. Allow time for and encourage any questions the woman and her support person may have. Reinforce any teaching as necessary.
2. Perform hand hygiene and observe appropriate infection control procedures.
3. Provide for patient privacy.

NONSTRESS TEST

4. Have the woman empty her bladder before the procedure begins.
   - Have the woman lie comfortably in a left-tilted semi-Fowler sitting position or in the left lateral position with pillows for support if needed. **Rationale:** *These positions displace the uterus to prevent compression of the vena cava and/or aorta. These positions also promote more fetal movement and are more likely to have a reactive tracing.*
5. Apply fetal heart rate and contraction monitors. Apply the ultrasonic gel to the diaphragm of the ultrasound transducer to improve contact.
   - Monitor the fetal heart rate and any contraction activity for at least 20 minutes. Note any fetal movement. **Rationale:** *Accelerations in fetal heart rate should occur spontaneously and in response to fetal movement.*
   - If there are no accelerations in 20 minutes, continue monitoring 20 more minutes. **Rationale:** *The fetus may be in a sleep cycle, during which there are usually no heart rate accelerations.*

- If there are no accelerations or fetal movement during the testing period, stimulation of the fetus may be necessary (e.g., acoustic stimulation, maternal intake of cold liquids) **①**.

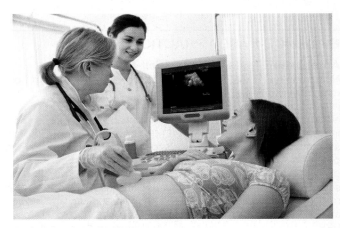

Source: Alexander Raths/Fotolia

① Fetal acoustic stimulation testing.

Test Interpretation

Reactive NST (normal): Shows at least two accelerations of FHR with fetal movements of 15 beats per minute, lasting 15 seconds or more, over 20 minutes.

Nonreactive NST: Accelerations are not present or do not meet the reactive criteria. For example, the accelerations do not meet the requirements of 15 beats per minute or do not last 15 minutes. If the test is considered nonreactive (nonreassuring), further testing may be needed. Proceed to step 6 below.

BIOPHYSICAL PROFILE

4. A nonstress test is performed using either an external fetal monitor or ultrasound equipment.
5. A score of 2 is given to each normal finding and a score of 0 is given to each abnormal finding for a maximum total score of 10. Scores of 8–10 are considered normal (see **Table 14–2 》**).

TABLE 14–2 Criteria for Biophysical Profile Scoring

Component	Normal (Score = 2)	Abnormal (Score = 0)
Fetal breathing movements	≥1 episode of rhythmic breathing lasting ≥ 30 sec within 30 min	≤30 sec of breathing in 30 min
Gross body movements	≥3 discrete body or limb movements in 30 min (episodes of active continuous movement considered as single movement)	≤2 movements in 30 min
Fetal tone	≥1 episode of extension of a fetal extremity with return to flexion, or opening or closing of hand	No movements or extension/flexion
Amniotic fluid volume	Single vertical pocket > 2 cm amniotic fluid index (AFI) > 5 cm	Largest single vertical pocket ≤ 2 cm AFI < 5 cm
Nonstress test	≥2 accelerations of ≥15 bpm for ≥15 sec in 20–40 min	0 or 1 acceleration in 20–40 min

(*continued on next page*)

SKILL 14.5 Fetal Well-Being, Nonstress Test and Biophysical Profile: Assessing (continued)

6. Document the procedure, results, any intervention(s) needed, or any need for further testing in the patient's medical record and notify the ordering healthcare provider of the results of the assessment of fetal well-being per facility policy.

EVIDENCE-BASED PRACTICE

Antepartum Tests for Fetal Well-Being

Numerous tests exist to determine fetal well-being, ranging from maternal reporting of fetal movements ("count to 10" method) to invasive procedures like amniocentesis. However, limited definitive evidence exists about the benefit of antenatal testing in decreasing the perinatal mortality rate (PMR). Despite the lack of clear evidence, testing is widely used for various indications during pregnancy.

For example, the biophysical profile (BPP) is a commonly used set of tests of fetal well-being. BPP includes ultrasound monitoring of fetal movement, fetal tone, and fetal breathing; ultrasound assessment of amniotic fluid volume; and assessment of fetal heart rate. Studies of BPP to date have found no significant differences between the BPP and non-BPP groups in perinatal deaths or Apgar scores of less than 7 at 5 minutes, but they do suggest an increased risk of caesarean section. Furthermore, no studies have addressed the impact of BPP on factors like neonatal morbidity, length of hospital stay, or parental satisfaction.

Of all antenatal assessment methods, Doppler ultrasound has been tested most rigorously. Studies indicate that routine umbilical artery Doppler screening has no apparent benefit in low-risk pregnancies (no significant difference in PMR, neonatal morbidity, Apgar scores under 7 at 5 minutes, cesarean section, labor induction, or resuscitation). However, for high-risk pregnancies, use of Doppler ultrasound to evaluate the fetal umbilical artery was associated with a significant reduction in perinatal deaths.

Given that most antenatal tests have not been proven effective in preventing incidence of PMR, obstetricians should be cautious in recommending their use in high-risk patients. They are not recommended for pregnancies at low risk of intrauterine fetal demise. Informed consent should always be obtained from the woman before ordering an invasive test.

Source: Data from American College of Radiology. L. Simpson. (2016). Assessment of Fetal Well-Being.

SKILL 14.6 Rh Immune Globulin: Administering

Safety Note! *During scheduled clinical time, nursing students may have a learning opportunity to observe or assist with this skill only with faculty permission and with direct supervision from faculty or another RN.*

To prevent an immune response when the newborn is Rh positive, Rh immune globulin is a blood product given as an intramuscular injection to a pregnant woman who is Rh negative. Without Rh immune globulin, the mother's Rh negative blood makes antibodies to destroy the fetus's Rh positive blood cells. Firstborn infants may be affected if the mother has had past miscarriages or abortions. All later infants that are Rh-positive may be affected.

Delegation or Assignment

Administration of Rh immune globulin is not delegated or assigned to the UAP. The nurse can request the UAP to report patient observations to the nurse for follow-up. The nurse remains responsible for the assessment, interpretation of abnormal findings, and determination of appropriate responses.

Equipment

- Rh immune globulin, which is obtained from the blood bank or pharmacy according to facility protocol (Lot numbers for the drug and the crossmatch should be the same.)
- Syringe and IM needle

Preparation

- Review physician's or certified nurse-midwife's (MD/CNM) orders and patient's nursing plan of care.
- Confirm that Rh immune globulin is indicated by checking the patient's prenatal record to verify that she is Rh negative. Then confirm that alloimmunization has not occurred—maternal indirect Coombs test is negative. Postpartum, confirm that the newborn is Rh positive but not sensitized (direct Coombs negative) and that the mother's indirect Coombs is negative. Rh immune globulin is not indicated if the baby is Rh negative. **Rationale:** *Rh immune globulin is only indicated for an Rh-negative, unsensitized woman who gave birth to an Rh-positive baby.*
- Review patient's record for allergies to confirm that the woman does not have a history of allergies to immune globulin preparations by checking entries on medication allergies in her chart and by asking her whether she has ever had any allergic reactions to medications, globulins, or blood products. **Rationale:** *Rh immune globulin is made from the plasma portion of blood. Allergic reactions are possible.*
- Verify a signed informed consent form is in the patient's record, if required by facility policy. **Rationale:** *Many agencies require separate consent for the administration of Rh immune globulin because it is a blood product.*
- Gather appropriate medication and supplies.

SKILL 14.6 Rh Immune Globulin: Administering *(continued)*

Procedure

1. Introduce self to patient and verify the patient's identity using two identifiers. Explain to the patient you are going to give an injection of Rh immune globulin. Discuss how the results will be used in planning further care or treatments. The woman should clearly understand the purpose of the Rh immune globulin, its rationale, the administration procedure, and any related risks. Common side effects are redness and tenderness at the injection site and allergic responses.
2. Perform hand hygiene and observe appropriate infection control procedures.
3. Provide for patient privacy.
4. Provide comfort and safety for patient and self, including raising bed to appropriate height for procedure.
5. Administer prefilled syringe of 1500 international units (300 mcg) Rh immune globulin IM in the deltoid muscle.
6. An immune globulin microdose is used after miscarriage, elective abortion, ectopic pregnancy, or molar pregnancy occurring within the first 12 weeks of gestation. Antepartum, the Rh immune globulin is generally given within 3 hr but not more than 72 hr after the event.
7. If a larger bleed is suspected at birth (as in cases of severe abruptio placentae), additional doses may be administered at one time using multiple sites or at regular intervals as long as all doses are given within 72 hr of childbirth. **Rationale:** *The normal 300-mcg dose provides passive immunity following exposure of up to 15 mL of transfused RBCs or 30 mL of fetal blood.*
8. Provide opportunities for the woman to ask questions and express concerns.

CAUTION! Many women, especially primigravidas, are not aware of the risk for Rh-positive fetus of a sensitized Rh-negative mother. They need to understand the importance of receiving Rh immune globulin for each pregnancy to ensure continued protection.

9. When the procedure is complete, return bed to lowest height. Perform hand hygiene and leave patient safe and comfortable.
10. Complete documentation using forms, checklists, or electronic dropdown lists supplemented by nurse's notes or additional comments as appropriate. Most agencies chart lot number, route, dose, and patient education.

SAMPLE DOCUMENTATION

[date] 0745 V/S 132/88, 82, 16, T 37.11°C (98.8°F) oral. Rh immune globulin 300 mcg given IM left deltoid. Tolerated without incident. Monitored × 4 hours without significant change in V/S; no allergic reaction noted. *T. Goose*

CAUTION! In most cases, Rh immune globulin is administered in the deltoid muscle. However, in an extremely thin woman, or in the case of a larger-than-normal dose, consider administering the medication in the ventrogluteal site. You may also divide the dose into multiple injections. Some Rh immune globulin medications are administered intravenously as ordered.

» Intrapartum Care

Expected Outcomes

1. Ongoing fetal heartbeat documentation occurs with external electronic fetal monitoring.
2. Induction of labor with Pitocin progresses without evidence of fetal distress.
3. The epidural injection is completed as painlessly as possible.

SKILL 14.7 Amniotomy (Artificial Rupture of Membranes): Assisting

Safety Note! *During scheduled clinical time, nursing students may have a learning opportunity to observe or assist with this skill only with faculty permission and with direct supervision from faculty or another RN.*

An amniotomy is a procedure to intentionally rupture the amniotic sac with an amnio hook to release amniotic fluid. It is usually performed to induce labor or encourage the progression of labor.

Delegation or Assignment

Assisting with an amniotomy is not delegated or assigned to the UAP. The nurse can request the UAP to report patient

(continued on next page)

SKILL 14.7 Amniotomy (Artificial Rupture of Membranes): Assisting (*continued*)

observations to the nurse for follow-up. The nurse remains responsible for the assessment, interpretation of abnormal findings, and determination of appropriate responses.

Equipment

- Sterile vaginal exam glove for healthcare provider or certified nurse-midwife (MD/CNM)
- Sterile gloves (for nurse)
- Sterile amnio hook
- Sterile water-soluble lubricant
- Doppler or monitor (external or internal)
- Waterproof linen
- Towels

Preparation

- Review healthcare provider's (MD/CNM) orders and patient's nursing plan of care.
- Ensure informed signed consent has been obtained from patient.
- Gather equipment and supplies.

Procedure

1. Introduce self to patient and verify the patient's identity using two identifiers. Explain to the patient that the healthcare provider is going to perform an amniotomy, why it is necessary, and how the patient can participate. Discuss how the results will be used in planning further care or treatments. Encourage and answer any questions the woman or her support person(s) may have at this time. Reassure the woman that amniotic fluid is constantly produced, because she may worry about a "dry birth."
2. Perform hand hygiene and observe appropriate infection control procedures.
3. Provide for patient privacy.
4. Provide comfort and safety for patient and self, including raising bed to appropriate height for procedure. Assist the woman to the lithotomy position, maintaining privacy.

CAUTION! Assess fetal heart rate (FHR) prior to, during, and following amniotomy because rupturing the amniotic membranes changes the pressure inside the uterus and causes risk of a prolapsed cord.

---

5. Don sterile gloves.
6. Using sterile technique, apply sterile lubricant to the healthcare provider's sterile gloved hand, and open the package containing the amnio hook for the healthcare provider to grasp. **Rationale:** *Lubricant decreases friction*

between the gloved hand and vaginal wall during the procedure. Sterile technique is essential during amniotomy to prevent potential contamination and decrease the risks of maternal and fetal infection.

7. Once the membranes are ruptured and fluid is seen, note the color, amount, odor, and presence of meconium or blood. **Rationale:** *Amniotic fluid should be clear or slightly cloudy and without any odor. Meconium-stained or bloody amniotic fluid indicates or places the fetus at risk for complications. Foul-smelling fluid may indicate infection. Absent, decreased, or increased amounts of amniotic fluid may indicate fetal stress.*
8. Assess FHR immediately before and after the rupture of membranes. **Rationale:** *Fetal well-being must be confirmed prior to and after amniotomy to assess fetal tolerance to the procedure.*
9. Maternal temperature should be assessed every 2 hr or more frequently if febrile and/or ordered. **Rationale:** *A rise in maternal temperature might indicate an intrauterine infection (chorioamnionitis).*
10. While wearing disposable gloves, cleanse the perineum with a warm washcloth, dry the perineal area, and change the waterproof linen pads as needed. **Rationale:** *A dry underpad enhances maternal comfort.*
11. Keep vaginal examinations to a minimum. **Rationale:** *This is to prevent introducing ascending infections.*
12. Assist the woman to a comfortable position.
13. When the procedure is over, return bed to lowest position. Perform hand hygiene and leave patient safe and comfortable.
14. Complete documentation using forms, checklists, or electronic dropdown lists supplemented by nurse's notes or additional comments as appropriate including time of ruptured membranes, color, amount and odor (if applicable), who performed the procedure, cervical exam results, fetal heart rate, and how the patient tolerated the procedure.

SAMPLE DOCUMENTATION

[date] 0230 V/S 136/88, 88, 20, T 37.28°C (99.1°F) oral FHR 146. D. Holmes, CNM, here. Membranes ruptured with amniotic hook per D. Holmes, CNM. Large gush amniotic fluid noted, clear with slight amount meconium-colored streaks, no odor or blood noted. FHR 172. Procedure tolerated without complaint. Perineum cleaned and dried, linen changed. V/S 132/86, 84, 20, FHR 150. Husband with woman at this time. *G. Hosea*

SKILL 14.8 Epidural: Assisting and Caring for Patient

Safety Note! *During scheduled clinical time, nursing students may have a learning opportunity to observe or assist with this skill only with faculty permission and with direct supervision from faculty or another RN.*

Epidural anesthesia is used to lessen sensation in the lower body by blocking nerve impulses from the lower spine. This is a popular method of relieving pain during labor.

Delegation or Assignment

Assisting with administering an epidural anesthesia is not delegated or assigned to the UAP. The nurse can request the UAP to report patient observations to the nurse for follow-up while the UAP provides care to the patient. The nurse remains responsible for the assessment, interpretation of abnormal findings, and determination of appropriate responses.

Equipment

- Fetal heart rate (FHR) and contraction monitoring equipment as ordered
- IV fluid and apparatus as ordered and per hospital policy
- Epidural administration set
- Anesthetic medications per anesthesia department protocol, if certified registered nurse anesthetist (CRNA) or anesthesiologist does not provide it
- High-pressure volumetric pump if epidural will be a continuous infusion
- Ephedrine syringe, dosage according to hospital protocol

Preparation

- Review the healthcare provider's or certified nurse-midwife's (MD/CNM) order for epidural.
- Notify anesthesia personnel per hospital policy.
- Verify the correct procedure for the correct patient.
- Verify patient's signed informed consent form is in the patient's record. Ensure potential side effects, such as headache, and complications, such as hypotension, have been explained to patient and the importance of telling the nurse about the onset of a headache.
- Explain the procedure and interventions that may be required because of the epidural: continuous intravenous infusion, continuous fetal monitoring, complete bed rest, indwelling or intermittent urinary catheterization, frequent blood pressure assessments, and other interventions according to hospital policy. **Rationale:** *The woman may be focused on pain relief and not aware of further interventions that will be required due to epidural infusion.*
- Gather equipment and supplies.

Procedure

1. Introduce self to patient and verify the patient's identity using two identifiers. Explain to the patient the anesthesiologist (or CRNA) will administer an epidural anesthesia, why it is necessary, and how the patient can participate. Discuss how the results will be used in planning further care or treatments. Throughout the procedure and following, allow time to answer any questions the woman or her support person may have. Follow up with further teaching regarding any matter that may have been unforeseen or out of the ordinary.

2. Perform hand hygiene and observe appropriate infection control procedures.

3. Provide for patient privacy.

4. Provide comfort and safety for patient and self, including raising bed to appropriate height for procedure. Obtain maternal baseline vital signs, fetal heart rate, and variability. The fetal heart rate tracing should show a reassuring tracing before starting the epidural process.

5. Administer an IV fluid bolus per hospital protocol before the epidural is begun (usually 500–1000 mL lactated Ringer solution). **Rationale:** *This is to avoid maternal hypotension associated with the vasodilation common with epidurals.*

6. Assist and support the woman in position per anesthesia personnel request (usually side-lying with knees flexed or sitting up on side of bed with back flexed) ❶. **Rationale:** *This will assist the anesthesia personnel in locating the correct vertebrae between which to administer the epidural.*

7. The BP, heart rate, and fetal heart rate is assessed before the test dose, often every 5 min during the test dose, at the end of the test dose, and frequently thereafter according to facility policy.

8. Return bed to lowest height. Perform hand hygiene.

9. Have ephedrine at bedside in case of hypotensive or fetal bradycardia episode. Administer according to unit protocol and MD/CNM orders.

10. Assess the bladder for distention every 30 min. Catheterize with intermittent catheter if birth is imminent or indwelling if not. **Rationale:** *A full bladder can slow the descent of the fetus, as well as risk damage to the bladder.*

11. Assess maternal position (from side to side) and body alignment frequently, changing position at least every hour. **Rationale:** *Changing positions frequently maximizes uteroplacental blood flow, increases circulation, promotes comfort, and avoids a one-sided block.*

12. Assess the level of anesthesia and pain control as prescribed or following facility policy. Notify anesthesia personnel as needed for changes in epidural infusion.

13. Change syringes as needed per hospital policy.

14. After birth, per hospital policy, a qualified RN may remove the epidural catheter.

15. When the procedure is complete, perform hand hygiene and leave patient safe and comfortable.

16. Complete documentation using forms, checklists, or electronic dropdown lists supplemented by nurse's notes or additional comments as appropriate, including procedure throughout administration of the epidural and removal of the catheter. Document time of removal, condition of epidural puncture site, catheter condition (intact), any dressing applied (if applicable), and how the woman tolerated the procedure.

(continued on next page)

SKILL 14.8 Epidural: *Assisting and Caring for Patient* (continued)

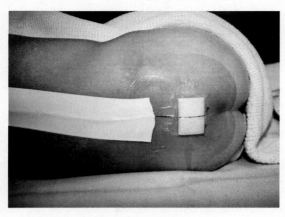

Source: Roy Ramsey/Pearson Education, Inc.

❶ Epidural pain block taped into place and wrapped securely.

SKILL 14.9 Fetal External Electronic: Monitoring

The fetal external electronic monitoring device is used to listen to, see visual configurations, and record or print rhythm strips of the fetal heartbeat through the abdomen of the mother.

Delegation or Assignment

Fetal external monitoring is not delegated or assigned to the UAP. The nurse can request the UAP to report patient observations to the nurse for follow-up. The nurse remains responsible for the assessment, interpretation of abnormal findings, and determination of appropriate responses.

Equipment

- Monitor
- Two elastic monitor belts
- Tocodynamometer ("toco")
- Ultrasound transducer
- Ultrasound gel

Preparation

- Check healthcare provider's or certified nurse-midwife's (MD/CNM) orders.
- Gather equipment and supplies.

Procedure

1. Introduce self to patient and verify the patient's identity using two identifiers. Explain to the patient you are going to place monitor belts that will connect to the monitoring device around the woman's abdomen, why it is necessary, and how the patient can participate. Discuss how the results will be used in planning further care or treatments.
2. Perform hand hygiene and observe appropriate infection control procedures.
3. Provide for patient privacy. Provide comfort and safety for patient and self, including raising bed to appropriate height for procedure.
4. Have the woman empty her bladder.
5. Turn on the monitor and place the two elastic belts around the woman's abdomen.
6. Place the toco over the uterine fundus off the midline on the area palpated to be firmest during contractions. Secure it with one of the elastic belts. **Rationale:** *The uterine fundus is the area of greatest contractility.*
7. Note the uterine contraction (UC) tracing. The resting tone tracing (that is, without a UC) should be recording on the 10 or 15 mmHg pressure line. Adjust the line to reflect that reading.
8. Apply the ultrasonic gel to the diaphragm of the ultrasound transducer. **Rationale:** *Ultrasonic gel is used to maintain contact with the maternal abdomen.*
9. Place the diaphragm on the maternal abdomen in the midline between the umbilicus and the symphysis pubis.
10. Listen for the FHR, which will have a whip-like sound. Move the diaphragm laterally if necessary to obtain a stronger sound ❶.
11. When the FHR is located, attach the second elastic belt snugly to the transducer ❷.

CAUTION! Evaluating the FHR tracing provides information about fetal status and response to the stress of labor. The presence of reassuring characteristics is associated with good fetal outcomes. Rapid identification of nonreassuring characteristics allows prompt interventions and the opportunity to determine the fetal response to the interventions.

---

12. Place the following information on the beginning of the fetal monitor paper: date, time, woman's name, gravida, para, membrane status, and name of healthcare provider. **Rationale:** *Each birthing unit may have specific guidelines about additional information to include.*

SKILL 14.9 Fetal External Electronic: Monitoring (*continued*)

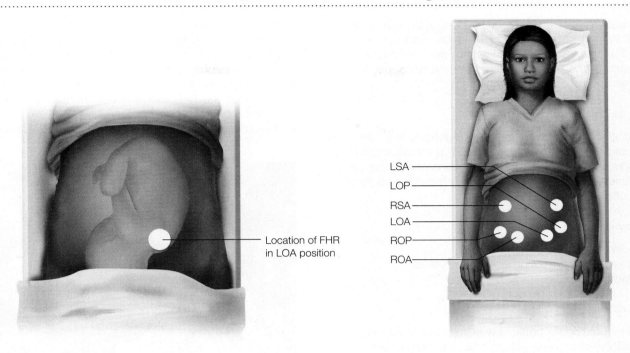

Location of FHR
in LOA position

LSA
LOP
RSA
LOA
ROP
ROA

❶ Location of the fetal heart rate (FHR) in relation to the more commonly seen fetal positions.

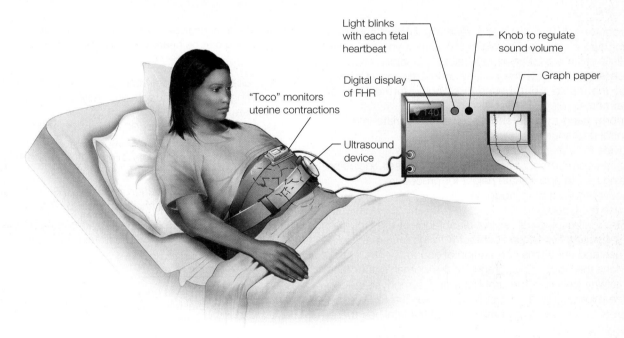

Light blinks
with each fetal
heartbeat

Knob to regulate
sound volume

Digital display
of FHR

Graph paper

"Toco" monitors
uterine contractions

140

Ultrasound
device

❷ External electronic fetal monitoring.

13. When the procedure is complete, return bed to lowest height. Perform hand hygiene and leave patient safe and comfortable.
14. Complete documentation using forms, checklists, or electronic dropdown lists supplemented by nurse's notes or additional comments as appropriate. Ongoing documentation should provide information about FHR, including baseline rate in beats per minute (bpm), presence of variability, response to uterine contractions (accelerations or decelerations), procedures performed, changes in position and the like, as well as any therapy initiated.

SKILL 14.10 Fetal Heart Rate: Auscultating

Fetal heart rate (FHR) can be heard using a Doppler at 10–12 weeks. When using an ultrasound device, FHR can be heard at 8–10 weeks. Auscultating FHR provides information about the health of the fetus and also how the fetus responds to changes in the uterus environment.

Delegation or Assignment

Auscultating is not delegated or assigned to the UAP. The nurse can request the UAP to report patient observations to the nurse for follow-up. The nurse remains responsible for the assessment, interpretation of abnormal findings, and determination of appropriate responses.

Equipment

- Doppler device
- Ultrasound device (during visits to the office)
- Ultrasonic gel

Preparation

- Review healthcare provider's or certified nurse-midwife's (MD/CNM) orders and patient's nursing plan of care.
- Gather equipment and supplies.

Procedure

1. Introduce self to patient and verify the patient's identity using two identifiers. Explain to the patient you are going to listen to the fetal heart rate using a Doppler, why it is necessary, and how the patient can participate. Discuss how the results will be used in planning further care or treatments.
2. Perform hand hygiene and observe appropriate infection control procedures.
3. Provide for patient privacy.
4. Provide comfort and safety for patient and self, including raising bed to appropriate height for procedure.
5. Uncover the woman's abdomen.
6. To use the Doppler:
   - Place ultrasonic gel on the diaphragm of the Doppler. Gel is used to maintain contact with the maternal abdomen and enhances conduction of sound.
   - Place the Doppler diaphragm on the woman's abdomen halfway between the umbilicus and symphysis and in the midline. You are most likely to hear the FHR in this area. Listen carefully for the sound of the fetal heartbeat.

7. Check the woman's pulse against the fetal sounds you hear. If the rates are the same, reposition the Doppler and try again. **Rationale:** *If the rates are the same, you are probably hearing the maternal pulse and not the FHR.*
8. If the rates are not similar, count the FHR for 1 full minute. Note that the FHR has a double rhythm and only one sound is counted.
9. If you do not locate the FHR, move the Doppler laterally ❶.

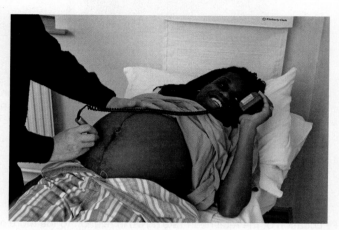

Source: Jennie Hart/Alamy Stock Photo

❶ When the fetal heartbeat is picked up by the electronic monitor, the sound can be heard by everyone in the room.

10. Auscultate the FHR between, during, and for 30 seconds following uterine contractions. Frequency recommendations are as follows:
    - *Low-risk women:* Every 30 minutes in the first stage and every 15 minutes in the second stage.
    - *High-risk women:* Every 15 minutes in the first stage and every 5 minutes in the second stage.

    Rationale: *This evaluation provides the opportunity to assess the fetal status and response to labor.*
11. Document FHR data (rate and rhythm), characteristics of uterine activity, and any actions taken as a result of the FHR.

CAUTION! The FHR is heard most clearly through the fetal back. Locate the fetal back using the Leopold maneuvers.

SKILL 14.11 Fetal Internal Scalp Electrode Placement: Monitoring

Safety Note! *During scheduled clinical time, nursing students may have a learning opportunity to observe or assist with this skill only with faculty permission and with direct supervision from faculty or another RN.*

For better electronic monitoring of the fetal heart rate (FHR), a fetal scalp electrode may be placed internally after the amniotic sac has ruptured and the cervix has opened during labor.

SKILL 14.11 Fetal Internal Scalp Electrode Placement: Monitoring (*continued*)

Delegation or Assignment

Placement of fetal internal scalp electrode or monitoring afterward is not delegated or assigned to the UAP. The nurse can request the UAP to report patient observations to the nurse for follow-up. The nurse remains responsible for the assessment, interpretation of abnormal findings, and determination of appropriate responses.

Equipment

- Sterile exam glove
- Sterile water-soluble lubricant
- Spiral fetal scalp electrode apparatus
- Fetal monitor
- Scalp electrode cable
- Grounding pad (usually found in electrode packaging)

Preparation

- Review physician's or certified nurse-midwife's (MD/CNM) orders and patient's nursing plan of care.
- Verify correct procedure for correct patient.
- Ensure informed signed consent has been obtained from patient.
- Woman's membranes must have already ruptured spontaneously or been ruptured by the healthcare provider. **Rationale:** *Fetal scalp electrode cannot be applied to the scalp if the membranes are covering the scalp, and generalist RNs are not allowed to rupture membranes.*
- Gather equipment and supplies.

Procedure

1. Introduce self to patient and verify the patient's identity using two identifiers. Explain to the patient that you are going to place a fetal scalp internal electrode for monitoring. Explain the procedure, purpose, and implications of using a fetal scalp electrode to patient and support person. Discuss how the results will be used in planning further care or treatments.
2. Perform hand hygiene and observe appropriate infection control procedures.
3. Provide for patient privacy.
4. Assist the woman into lithotomy position; provide for safety and comfort.
5. Using sterile technique, open lubricant package, don a sterile glove on the dominant hand, and with nondominant hand, apply lubricant to the glove. **Rationale:** *Sterile technique is essential to decrease the risk of intrauterine infection.*
6. Perform vaginal exam to determine dilation and presentation of the fetus. Ensure presenting part is vertex.

CAUTION! Contraindications for the fetal scalp electrode to be placed on the fetal occiput include the following: the membranes are not ruptured, the cervix is not dilated at least 2 cm, there is a reason a cervical examination cannot be done, there is a diagnosed infectious risk to the fetus, the presenting part isn't known, and the presenting part is not down against the cervix.

7. Apply fetal scalp electrode on a firm area of the fetal vertex according to package directions, avoiding fontanelles, face, genitals, etc. This usually involves inserting the electrode within the firm plastic guide. Place end of the guide/electrode against firm area of the scalp, and rotate electrode end clockwise until resistance is met. Release the guide according to package directions and discard. **Rationale:** *Care must be taken to avoid attaching the monitor to soft tissue, which could result in fetal trauma.*
8. Following package instructions, connect spiral electrode wire to a leg plate, commonly secured by a self-adhesive grounding pad to the mother's inner thigh. This in turn is attached to the electronic fetal monitor ❶.
9. Verify fetal heart rate is tracing before discontinuing the intermittent or continuous external monitor.
10. To remove fetal scalp electrode, disconnect the electrode wire from the cable and rotate the lead counterclockwise. Once removed, visually examine the electrode to ensure it is intact. If unable to remove before going for a cesarean birth, tape electrode wire to the mother's thigh and notify the surgeon.
11. When the procedure is complete, return bed to lowest height. Perform hand hygiene and leave patient safe and comfortable.
12. Complete documentation using forms, checklists, or electronic dropdown lists supplemented by nurse's notes or additional comments as appropriate.

SAMPLE DOCUMENTATION

[date] 0424 Awake but trying to rest between contractions. Cervix dilated to 4 cm, membranes ruptured at 0355. Fetal scalp electrode applied per order for better contact. Vertex visualized, electrode placed firmly against area, guide released and removed. FHR rhythm on monitor, rate 148. Tolerated without complaint. *T. Jewels*

(*continued on next page*)

SKILL 14.11 Fetal Internal Scalp Electrode Placement: Monitoring (*continued*)

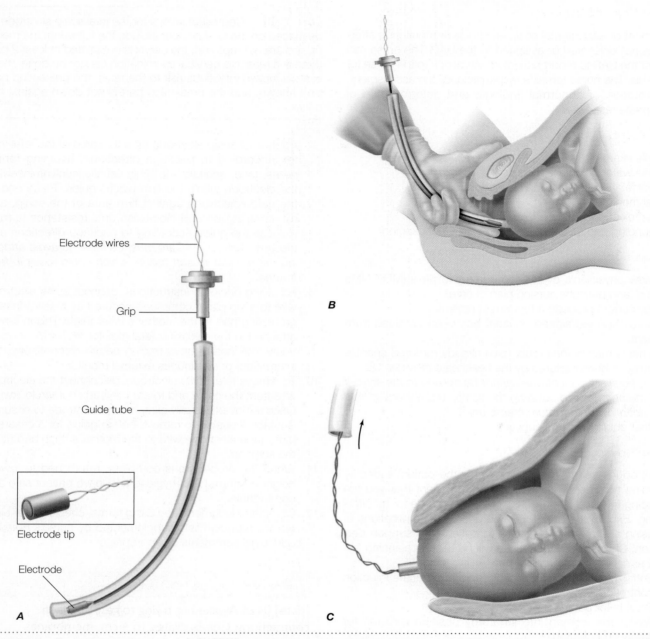

Electrode wires

Grip

Guide tube

Electrode tip

Electrode

A

B

C

❶ Technique for internal, direct fetal monitoring. *A,* Spiral electrode; *B,* Attaching the spiral electrode to the scalp; *C,* Attached spiral electrode with the guide tube removed.

SKILL 14.12 Induction of Labor with Oxytocin and Other Agents: Assisting and Caring for Patient

Safety Note! *During scheduled clinical time, nursing students may have a learning opportunity to observe or assist with this skill only with faculty permission and with direct supervision from faculty or another RN.*

Inducing labor for medical reasons is done for a variety of reasons to protect the woman and or fetus from complications or potential life-threatening conditions. Medical high risks include gestational diabetes or hypertension, preeclampsia, heart dysrhythmias, placenta abruption, bleeding, membranes rupture

SKILL 14.12 Induction of Labor with Oxytocin and Other Agents: Assisting and Caring for Patient (continued)

without onset of labor within 24 hours, gestation time greater than 42 weeks, and slow onset or progression of labor.

Delegation or Assignment

Administering medications, monitoring the effects of medications on the patient during induction of labor is not delegated or assigned to the UAP. The UAP can provide care for the patient within scope of practice. The nurse can request the UAP to report patient observations to the nurse for follow-up. The nurse remains responsible for the assessment, interpretation of abnormal findings, and determination of appropriate responses.

Equipment

- Fetal and contraction monitoring equipment
- IV fluids per facility policy, or healthcare provider (includes certified nurse-midwife) orders
- IV administration sets for oxytocin infusion
- IV infusion pump (two if available) for oxytocin infusion
- Appropriate induction medications ordered by healthcare provider
- Sterile exam gloves, sterile lubricant (cervical ripening)

Preparation

- Review healthcare provider's or certified nurse-midwife's (MD/CNM) orders and patient's nursing plan of care.
- Review patient's record for allergies.
- Verify correct procedure as ordered by healthcare provider for the correct patient.
- Explain the procedure, purpose, and implications of the procedure to the woman and her support person.

CAUTION! The mother and her family need to be aware that induction of labor may take longer than spontaneous labor. They also need to know there may be limitations on food intake and activity and that continuous fetal monitoring and frequent assessments may be necessary due to the method of induction.

- Obtain oxytocin premixed bag from pharmacy or mix 10 units oxytocin per 1000 mL secondary fluid. Obtain cervical ripening medication.
- Gather equipment and supplies.

EVIDENCE-BASED PRACTICE

Possible Side Effects of Oxytocin

The body of a pregnant woman entering labor typically produces oxytocin, a hormone that increases the intensity and duration of contractions and aids delivery. When this normal process does not occur within 2 weeks of the due date or in the presence of signs like oligohydramnios (insufficient fluid surrounding the fetus), synthetic oxytocin is often administered to initiate the birthing process and provide a more positive outcome for mother and newborn. Side effects of oxytocin for

mothers are generally fairly minor and include irritation at the injection site, appetite loss, nausea, vomiting, and cramping. Effects on the fetus have not generally been noted.

A 2013 study, reported at a conference of the American Congress of Obstetricians and Gynecologists (ACOG), examined the effect of oxytocin on 3000 full-term infants delivered between 2009 and 2011. The study showed an association between use of oxytocin and Apgar scores lower than 7 at 5 minutes. Oxytocin also was an independent risk factor for unexpected admission to the NICU lasting more than 24 hours for full-term infants.

The study concluded that more research is warranted to examine the risk of oxytocin's side effects on newborns and to define a systematic process for determining when oxytocin is medically necessary to induce labor.

Source: Data from American Congress of Obstetricians and Gynecologists (ACOG) (2013), Siddique (2013), and Lewis (2016).

Procedure

1. Introduce self to patient and verify the patient's identity using two identifiers. Explain to the patient and support person what you are going to do, why it is necessary, and how the patient can participate. Discuss how the results will be used in planning further care or treatments. Allow time for and encourage any questions the woman and her support person may have. Reinforce any teaching as necessary.
2. Perform hand hygiene and observe appropriate infection control procedures.
3. Provide for patient privacy, comfort, and safety.
4. Apply fetal and contraction monitors per unit policy. Assess for reactive or reassuring fetal heart rate tracing.

CAUTION! A baseline of fetal well-being and uterine activity should be established before medication is administered so that the nurse will recognize complications associated with the medication given, such as uterine hyperstimulation and fetal distress.

---

5. Start IV infusion using aqueous solution at 125 mL/hr. **Rationale:** *This is done to keep the woman hydrated and to have an intravenous line available if needed.*
6. Assess maternal vital signs and hydration status.

OXYTOCIN (PITOCIN)

7. Attach secondary line to an infusion pump. **Rationale:** *An intravenous infusion pump must be used during oxytocin induction to ensure that accurate volume and dosage of oxytocin are administered to the woman.*
8. Start oxytocin infusion per facility policy and increase accordingly. One suggested method is to begin at 1–2 milliunits/min and increase by 1–2 milliunits/min every 30–40 min. Low dosage is less than 4 milliunits/min.
9. Evaluate fetal heart rate pattern, contraction pattern, and maternal vital signs before each increase in oxytocin.

(continued on next page)

SKILL 14.12 Induction of Labor with Oxytocin and Other Agents: Assisting and Caring for Patient (continued)

CAUTION! Accurate monitoring of uterine contraction frequency, duration, and intensity and uterine resting tone is essential to evaluate the effect of each oxytocin dosage level and determine the need to increase the infusion rate.

10. Increase oxytocin rate until adequate labor is established and then maintain at the current rate. Decrease oxytocin if hypersystole occurs, per facility policy. Proceed to step 11 below.

CAUTION! Because the half-life of oxytocin is very short (1–6 min), stopping an oxytocin infusion may quickly reverse the effects of excessive uterine activity and improve fetal oxygenation.

MISOPROSTOL (CYTOTEC)

7. Don sterile glove. Have the woman empty her bladder prior to insertion of cervical ripening agent.
8. Perform sterile vaginal exam, establishing the cervix is "unfavorable" for induction using oxytocin only (1 cm or less, little to no effacement).
   - Remove glove, wash hands, don sterile glove, apply minimal lubricant, and insert two fingers (second and third digits) into the vagina with low dose, 25 micrograms (1/4 tablet), misoprostol at end of fingers. It is placed in the posterior vaginal fornix.
   - Have the woman remain in bed for 30 min following insertion and then may allow up to void.
   - This process may be repeated every 3–6 hr for up to 24 hr. The healthcare provider should be notified if hyperstimulation occurs or if there is no onset of labor.

9. Oxytocin should not be administered less than 4 hr after the last misoprostol dose.
10. The fetal heart rate/contraction pattern should be evaluated for 3 hr following the insertion of misoprostol. Monitor closely for uterine hyperstimulation. Proceed to step 11 below.

DINOPROSTONE (PGE2) (CERVIDIL OR PREPIDIL)

7. Don sterile glove. Have the woman empty her bladder prior to insertion of cervical ripening agent.
8. Perform sterile vaginal exam, establishing the cervix is "unfavorable" for induction using oxytocin only (1 cm or less, little to no effacement).
   - Cervidil (10 mg): Administer as vaginal insert, × 1 dose. Monitor for 2 hr after insertion.
   or
   - Prepidil (0.5 mg): Administer intracervically. Monitor for 1–2 hr. May repeat after 6 hr. No more than 3 doses in 24 hr. If hypersystole occurs, remove medication by gently pulling attached string out of vagina.
9. Oxytocin should not be administered less than 4 hr after the last dose.
10. The fetal heart rate/contraction pattern should be evaluated for 3 hr following the insertion of these drugs. Monitor closely for uterine hyperstimulation.
11. When medication administration is complete, perform hand hygiene and monitor patient.
12. Complete documentation using forms, checklists, or electronic dropdown lists supplemented by nurse's notes or additional comments as appropriate, including the procedures, results, vital signs, fetal heart rate/contraction patterns, and labor progress in the patient's medical record, including date and times of administration of medication and any complications.

SKILL 14.13 Intrapartum, Maternal and Fetal: Assessing

Assessment examinations are done throughout the intrapartum phase of pregnancy. These assessments can include physical examinations through all stages of labor. Teaching is a part of all the phases of pregnancy.

Delegation or Assignment

Assisting with intrapartum examination is not delegated or assigned to the UAP. The nurse can request the UAP to report patient observations to the nurse for follow-up. The nurse remains responsible for the assessment, interpretation of abnormal findings, and determination of appropriate responses.

Equipment

- Need for appropriate equipment according to which assessment is being done

Preparation

- Review healthcare provider's or certified nurse-midwife's (MD/CNM) orders and patient's nursing plan of care.
- Review patient's record for allergies.
- Gather equipment and supplies.

Procedure

1. Introduce self to patient and verify the patient's identity using two identifiers. Explain to the patient you are going to monitor and perform maternal and fetal assessments, why it is necessary, and how she can participate. Discuss how the results will be used in planning further care or treatments.
2. Perform hand hygiene and observe appropriate infection control procedures.
3. Provide for patient privacy.

SKILL 14.13 Intrapartum, Maternal and Fetal: Assessing (*continued*)

4. Provide comfort and safety for patient and self, including raising bed to appropriate height for procedure.
5. Perform a systematic assessment (see **Table 14–3 》》**).
6. When the procedure is complete, lower bed to lowest position, perform hand hygiene, and leave patient safe and comfortable.
7. Complete documentation using forms, checklists, or electronic dropdown lists supplemented by nurse's notes or additional comments as appropriate.

TABLE 14–3 Intrapartum Assessment

Assessment	Normal Intrapartum Findings	Abnormal Intrapartum Findings
Take vital signs (TPR): ■ Temperature	Temperature: 36.6°C–37.2°C (98°F–99°F)	Elevated temperature: infection
■ Pulse	Pulse: 80–90 bpm (pulse rates can increase 10 beats)	Increased pulse rates (excitement or anxiety; early shock; cardiac disease; drug use)
■ Respiration	Respirations: 16–24 breaths/min (pregnancy may induce a mild form of hyperventilation and thoracic breathing)	Hyperventilation: anxiety/pain Hyperventilation expected in transition phase Decreased respirations with use of narcotics for pain Marked tachypnea with respiration distress
■ Blood pressure (BP)	BP: 119/79 mmHg	Low BP with supine hypotension, hemorrhage, hypovolemia, shock, or drugs High BP with pregnancy-induced hypertension (PIH); pain
Pulse oximeter	95% or greater	<90% hypoxia, hypotension, hemorrhage
Fetal heart rate	120–160 bpm	<120 or >160 bpm
Weight	25–35 lb > than prepregnancy weight	>16 (35 lb) could be fluid retention, obesity, large baby, diabetes mellitus, PIH <6.8 kg (15 lb) could be a small-for-gestational-age (SGA) baby, substance abuse, psychosocial problems
Fundus	40 weeks: just below xiphoid process	Uterine size not compatible with estimated date of birth: SGA; large for gestational age (LGA); hydramnios; multiple pregnancy; placental/fetal anomalies; malpresentations
Edema	Slight amount of dependent edema in lower extremities expected	Pitting edema of face, hands, legs, abdomen, sacral area indicative of PIH
Hydration	Normal skin turgor	Poor skin turgor with dehydration
Perineum	Same as antepartum	Varicosities of vulva, herpes lesions/genital warts
Uterine contractions	Frequency: from start of one contraction to start of next Duration: from beginning of contraction to time uterus begins to relax; 50–90 sec Intensity (strength of contraction): measured with monitoring device; Peak 25 mmHg End of labor may reach 50–75 mmHg	Irregular contractions with long intervals between: indicates false labor >90 sec: uterine tetany; stop oxytocin if running >75 mmHg: uterine tetany or uterine rupture
Cervical dilation (progressive cervical dilation from size of fingertip to 10 cm) **First stage** Latent phase (0–4 cm dilation) Active phase (4–8 cm)	0–4 cm; average 6.4 hr	Failure to dilate could be cervical rigidity, failure of presenting part to engage; cervical edema (pushing effort by woman before full dilation and effacement of the cervix) Prolonged time in any phase: may indicate poor fetal position, incomplete fetal flexion, cephalopelvic disproportion, or poor uterine contractions
Transitional phase (8–10 cm) Assess for bloody show Observe for presence of nausea or vomiting Evaluate urge to bear down	Length of time varies—may be 1–2 hr Beginning to bulge	Often uncontrolled multipara can cause precipitous delivery "Panting" (helps control process until safe delivery area established)

(continued on next page)

SKILL 14.13 Intrapartum, Maternal and Fetal: Assessing (continued)

TABLE 14–3 Intrapartum Assessment (continued)

Assessment	Normal Intrapartum Findings	Abnormal Intrapartum Findings
Cervical effacement (progressive thinning of cervix)	Occurs faster than dilation; 0–100%	Failure to efface could indicate cervical rigidity, infections, scar tissue, failure of presenting part to engage, cephalopelvic disproportion
Fetal descent (progressive descent of fetal presenting part from station −5 to + 4)	The head is the presenting part that descends from floating position above the pelvis (−5), through engaged position at bottom of pelvis, and ends with emerging position from the birth canal, or crowning (+4)	The presenting part of fetus is the buttocks, shoulder, arm, foot, forehead, or trunk
Membranes	Ruptured; if ruptured more than 12–24 hr before onset of labor	If not ruptured, healthcare provider may perform amniotomy
Fetal status	Fetal heart rate (FHR) 110–160 bpm Auscultation of fetal heart rate	<110 or >160 bpm may indicate fetal distress with cord compression or prolapse of cord; abnormal fetal patterns on fetal monitor (decreased variability, late decelerations, variable decelerations, absence of accelerations with fetal movement)
Evaluate FHR tracing	Short-term variability is present Long-term variability ranges from 3–5 cycles/min	Absence of variability (no short term or long term present) Severe variable decelerations (FHR < 70 for longer than 30–45 sec with decreasing variability)
Deceleration	Early deceleration (10–20 beat drop) Recovery when acme contraction passes—often not serious	Monitor closely—distinguish from decrease with hypertonic contraction; leads to fetal distress
Variable deceleration; decrease in FHR, below 120 bpm	Mild; may be within normal parameters—continue to monitor	Cord compression—may result in fetal difficulty
Loss of beat-to-beat variation	If lasts less than 15 min, no problem is apparent	Late deceleration pattern occurs—monitor for hypertonic contraction; leads to total distress
Evaluate pain and anxiety	Medication required after dilated 4–5 cm unless using natural childbirth methods	Severe pain early in first stage of labor: inadequate prenatal teaching, backache due to position in bed, uterine tetany
Second stage (10 cm to delivery)	Primipara: up to 2 hr Multipara: several minutes to 2 hr	>2 hr: increased risk of fetal brain damage and maternal exhaustion
Assess for presenting part	Vertex with right occiput anterior (ROA) or left occiput anterior (LOA) presentation	Occiput posterior, breech, face, or transverse lie
Assess caput (baby's head) Multipara: move to delivery room when caput size of dime Primipara: move to delivery room when caput size of half dollar	Visible when bearing down during contraction	"Crowns" in room other than delivery room: delivery imminent (do not move patient)
Assess fetal heart rate Bradycardia, drop of 20 bpm below baseline (↓ less than 120 bpm) Tachycardia, increase in FHR over 160 bpm for 10 min	120–160 bpm	Decreased: may indicate supine hypotensive syndrome (turn patient on side and take again) Hemorrhage (check for other signs of bleeding; notify healthcare provider) Increased or decreased: may indicate fetal distress secondary to cord compression or prolapsed cord
Third stage (from delivery of newborn to delivery of placenta)	Placental separation occurs within 30 min (usually 3–5 min)	Failure of placental separation Abnormality of uterus or cervix, weak, ineffectual uterine contraction, titanic contractions causing closure of cervix > 3 hr: indicates retained placenta
Fourth stage (first hour postpartum) Assess vital signs every 15 min for 1 hr, every 30 min for 1 hr, every hour	Vital signs are stable, O_2 saturation is >98% room air, fundus solid and hard, small amount of bleeding noted vaginally	Mother in unstable condition (hemorrhage usual cause) Highest risk of hemorrhage in first postpartum hour
Temperature	36.5°C–37.5°C (97.7°F–99.5°F)	>37.5°C (99.5°F): may indicate infection Slight elevation: due to dehydration from mouth breathing and NPO
Pulse	60–100 bpm	Increased may indicate pain or hemorrhage

SKILL 14.13 Intrapartum, Maternal and Fetal: Assessing (*continued*)

TABLE 14–3 Intrapartum Assessment (*continued*)

Assessment	Normal Intrapartum Findings	Abnormal Intrapartum Findings
Respirations	Respirations: 12–20 breaths/min	Respirations less than 12 or greater than 20 breaths/min
Blood pressure	Blood pressure: 120–140/80 mmHg	Increased: may indicate anxiety, pain, or postpartum pre-eclampsia Decreased: hemorrhage
Uterine assessment	Fundus firm, midline	Displaced to right indicates full bladder.
Lochia assessment	Large amount, bright red	Excessive amounts may be caused by retained placental fragments.
Comfort	Shivering response (tremors)	May have low back pain, afterpains, leg pain, chest pain, vaginal pain, anal pain
Apgar scoring	Newborns who score 7–10 are considered free of immediate danger.	Newborns who score 4–6 are moderately depressed. Newborns who score 0–3 are severely depressed.

SKILL 14.14 Intrapartum Pelvic Examination: Assisting

Safety Note! *During scheduled clinical time, nursing students may have a learning opportunity to observe or assist with this skill only with faculty permission and with direct supervision from faculty or another RN.*

A digital exam helps determine the cervix being in an anterior or posterior position and the degree of dilatation from 0–10 cm of the cervix. Effacement, or the cervical length, can be determined as well as its consistency of being firm or soft. The station of the fetus can be determined by palpating the presenting part of the fetus and comparing this distance to the maternal ischial spines.

Delegation or Assignment

This skill is not delegated or assigned to the UAP. The nurse can request the UAP to report patient observations to the nurse for follow-up. The nurse remains responsible for the assessment, interpretation of abnormal findings, and determination of appropriate responses.

Equipment

- Clean, disposable gloves if membranes not ruptured (use nonlatex gloves if the woman has a latex allergy)
- Sterile gloves if membranes ruptured
- Lubricant
- Nitrazine test tape
- Glass slide
- Sterile cotton-tipped swab (Q-tip)

Preparation

- Review physician's or certified nurse-midwife's (MD/CNM) orders and patient's nursing plan of care.
- Review patient's record for allergies, including latex allergies.
- Gather equipment and supplies.

Procedure

1. Introduce self to patient and verify the patient's identity using two identifiers. Explain to the patient that you are going to perform a pelvic exam, explain the procedure, the indications for the exam, what the exam may feel like, and that it may cause discomfort. Discuss how the results will be used in planning further care or treatments.
2. Perform hand hygiene and observe appropriate infection control procedures.
3. Provide for patient privacy, safety, and comfort.
4. Position the woman with her thighs flexed and abducted. Instruct her to put the heels of her feet together. Drape the woman with a sheet, leaving a flap to access the perineum.
5. Encourage the woman to relax her muscles and legs. Inform the woman prior to touching her.
6. Test for fluid leakage
   - If fluid leakage has been reported or noted, use Nitrazine test tape and a Q-tip with a slide for the fern test before performing the exam.
   - The fern test is done by inserting the swab in the pool of fluid in the posterior vagina and then applying the fluid to a slide. Nitrazine tape registers a change in pH if amniotic fluid is present.
7. Vaginal examination
   - Pull glove on dominant hand. **Rationale:** *A single glove is worn when membranes are intact. If a sterile exam is needed, both hands will be gloved with sterile gloves.*
   - Using your gloved hand, position the hand with the wrist straight and the elbow tilted downward. Insert your well-lubricated second and index fingers of the gloved hand gently into the vagina until they touch the cervix. Use care when positioning your hand.

(*continued on next page*)

SKILL 14.14 Intrapartum Pelvic Examination: Assisting (*continued*)

- If the woman expresses discomfort, pause for a moment and allow her to relax before progressing.
- To determine the status of labor progress, perform the vaginal examination during and between contractions.
- Palpate for the opening, or a depression, in the cervix. Estimate the diameter of the depression to identify the amount of dilation ❶. **Rationale:** *This allows determination of effacement and dilation.*
- Determine the status of the fetal membranes by observing for leakage of amniotic fluid. If fluid is expressed, test for amniotic fluid (see step 6 above).
- Palpate the presenting part ❷. **Rationale:** *This is done to assess the position of the fetus and evaluate fetal descent.*
- Assess the fetal descent and station by identifying the position of the fetal presenting part in relation to the ischial spines. Station progresses from −5 to +4 ❸.

8. When the procedure is complete, perform hand hygiene and leave patient safe and comfortable.

9. Complete documentation using forms, checklists, or electronic dropdown lists supplemented by nurse's notes or additional comments as appropriate, including fetal monitor strip if being used.

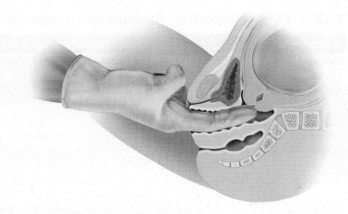

❶ To gauge cervical dilation, place the index and middle fingers against the cervix and determine the size of the opening. Before labor begins, the cervix is long (approximately 2.5 cm [1 in.]), the sides feel thick, and the cervical canal is closed, so an examining finger cannot be inserted. During labor, the cervix begins to dilate, and the size of the opening progresses from 1–10 cm (0.4–4 in.) in diameter.

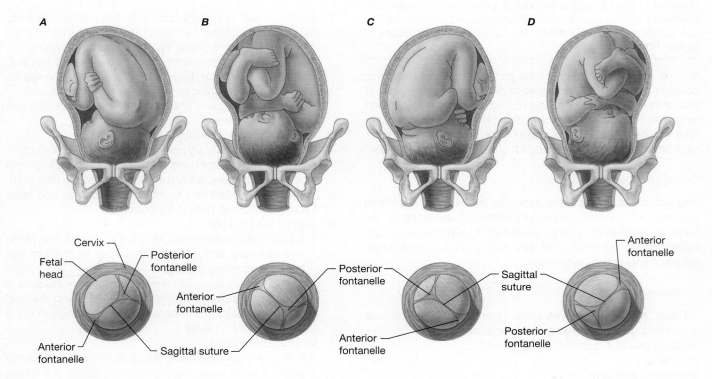

❷ Palpating the presenting part (portion of the fetus that enters the pelvis first). **A,** Left occiput anterior (LOA). The occiput (area over the occipital bone on the posterior part of the fetal head) is in the left anterior quadrant of the woman's pelvis. When the fetus is LOA, the posterior fontanelle (located just above the occipital bone and triangular in shape) is in the upper left quadrant of the maternal pelvis; **B,** Left occiput posterior (LOP). The posterior fontanelle is in the lower left quadrant of the maternal pelvis; **C,** Right occiput anterior (ROA). The posterior fontanelle is in the upper right quadrant of the maternal pelvis; **D,** Right occiput posterior (ROP). The posterior fontanelle is in the lower right quadrant of the maternal pelvis.

Note: The anterior fontanelle is diamond shaped. Because of the roundness of the fetal head, only a portion of the anterior fontanelle can be seen in each of the views, so it appears to be triangular in shape.

SKILL 14.14 Intrapartum Pelvic Examination: Assisting (*continued*)

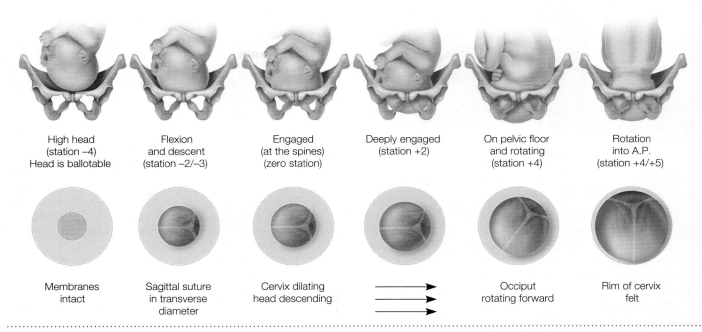

High head (station –4) Head is ballotable	Flexion and descent (station –2/–3)	Engaged (at the spines) (zero station)	Deeply engaged (station +2)	On pelvic floor and rotating (station +4)	Rotation into A.P. (station +4/+5)
Membranes intact	Sagittal suture in transverse diameter	Cervix dilating head descending	→ → →	Occiput rotating forward	Rim of cervix felt

❸ The fetal head progressing through the pelvis. *Bottom*: The changes that will be detected on palpation of the occiput through the cervix while doing a vaginal examination.

SKILL 14.15 Prolapsed Cord: Caring for Patient

Safety Note! *During scheduled clinical time, nursing students may have a learning opportunity to observe or assist with this skill only with faculty permission and with direct supervision from faculty or another RN.*

A prolapsed cord means the umbilical cord precedes the fetus in the vagina or out of the mother's body usually in a loop or coil. This results in a high risk for cord compression, which would compromise the flow of oxygen to the fetus and quickly become life-threatening to the fetus.

Delegation or Assignment

This skill is not delegated or assigned to the UAP. The nurse can request the UAP to report patient observations to the nurse for follow-up. The nurse remains responsible for the assessment, interpretation of abnormal findings, and determination of appropriate responses.

Equipment

- Sterile exam glove
- Sterile lubricant
- Sterile gauze pad moistened with saline solution, if cord is outside of vagina
- Oxygen and mask
- Fetal monitor/Doppler

Preparation

- Review physician's or certified nurse-midwife's (MD/CNM) orders.
- A prolapsed cord is an unexpected event and an emergency.
- Ask for help of another nurse during this emergency situation.

Procedure

1. Introduce self to patient and verify the patient's identity using two identifiers. Calmly explain the rationale for interventions, what to expect, and the plan of care to the woman and her support person. Discuss how the results will be used in planning further care or treatments. Allow time for questions from the laboring woman, her support person, and any other family that may be present. Another RN may need to answer questions if the patient's RN is busy with the patient's care.
2. Perform hand hygiene and observe appropriate infection control procedures.
3. Although difficult at times with this particular situation, privacy and safety are priorities.
4. Don sterile gloves.
5. If the cord is visualized extending through the vagina, a sterile gauze moistened with sterile saline must be placed

(continued on next page)

SKILL 14.15 Prolapsed Cord: Caring for Patient (continued)

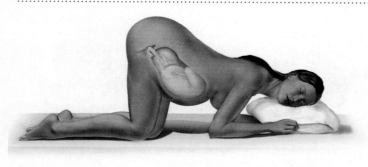

❶ The knee–chest position is used to relieve cord compression during cord prolapse emergency.

on the cord immediately to prevent the cord from drying. Do not handle the cord to help prevent spasms of it.

6. Notify healthcare provider immediately.
7. Place woman in the knee–chest position to use gravity to relieve umbilical cord pressure ❶.
8. If the cord is palpated during vaginal exam (using sterile glove and lubricant), place two fingers on either side of the cord or both fingers on one side of the cord to avoid

compressing it. Exert upward pressure against the presenting part to relieve pressure on the cord.

9. Continue assessing fetal heart rate to determine if interventions and position of fingers are successful in keeping fetal heart rate between 110–160 bpm. **Rationale:** *A fetal heart rate in this range indicates that fetal well-being has not been compromised by cord compression.*
10. Start oxygen via face mask at 10 L/min.
11. Examiner must keep fingers on the presenting part until baby is born, usually via cesarean. This may require examiner to travel to the operating room (OR) on the bed with the mother to maintain the position of fingers and presenting part. The woman's position must be maintained until birth or arrival at OR and placement on the OR table. Although difficult, privacy and safety should be maintained during transport to surgery. This may require extra personnel and sheets to cover the woman.
12. Complete documentation using forms, checklists, or electronic dropdown lists supplemented by nurse's notes or additional comments as appropriate, including the course of events, interventions, and maternal and fetal response to interventions. If there is a poor fetal outcome, further quality assurance documentation may be necessary.

≫ Postpartum Care

Expected Outcomes

1. Complications are prevented during the postpartum period.
2. Patient has progressively less lochia every day.
3. Engorgement of breasts is relieved with breastfeeding.

SKILL 14.16 Breastfeeding: Assisting

Breastfeeding provides newborns and infants with immunological, nutritional, and psychosocial advantages. It also promotes involution in women who have just given birth. Babies who are put to breast soon after birth benefit from the physical warmth of their mother's body, from the stimulation of sucking and swallowing, from replenishment of nutrients, and from the opportunity to interact intimately with their mother. As long as the mother is tolerating the birth well and her newborn is adjusting to extrauterine life without complication, breastfeeding can be promoted in the first 1 hour of life when the newborn is usually alert and ready to nurse.

Delegation or Assignment

Teaching the mother about breastfeeding and helping her learn how to engage the newborn to breastfeed is not delegated or assigned to the UAP. The nurse can request the UAP to report patient observations to the nurse for follow-up. The

nurse remains responsible for the assessment, interpretation of abnormal findings, and determination of appropriate responses.

Equipment

None

Preparation

- Review healthcare provider's or certified nurse-midwife's (MD/CNM) orders and patient's nursing plan of care.
- Gather supplies.

Procedure

1. Introduce self to patient and verify the patient's identity using two identifiers. Explain to the patient that

SKILL 14.16 Breastfeeding: Assisting *(continued)*

you are going to help her learn about breastfeeding her newborn. Discuss how the results will be used in planning further care or treatments. Many facilities have lactation consultants available to assist patients learn breastfeeding techniques and provide support during breastfeeding.

2. Perform hand hygiene and observe appropriate infection control procedures.

3. Provide for privacy, safety, and comfort for mother and newborn.

4. Assist the mother to a comfortable position. Support her head, shoulders, and arms as necessary for comfort.

Rationale: A position of comfort allows the new mother to focus on breastfeeding.

5. Help the mother to wash her hands using a washcloth with soap and water, then rinse well and dry. **Rationale:** *Hands carry a variety of organisms that are common causes of breast infections.*

6. Provide warmed bath blankets to wrap around the mother and newborn together.

7. Help the mother to place the newborn skin to skin against her body. Encourage a position that is comfortable for the mother ➊. **Rationale:** *The mother should hold the baby in a way that feels natural and provides her with a free hand.*

A **Modified cradle.**

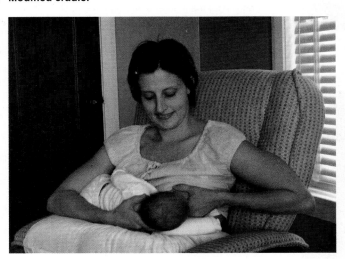

- Have the mother sit comfortably in an upright position using good body alignment. Use pillows for support (may use Boppy, body pillow, or standard bed pillows). Lap pillow should help bring the baby up to breast level so the mother does not lean over baby.
- Place the baby on the mother's lap and turn the baby's entire body toward the mother (the baby is in side-lying position). Position the baby's body so that the baby's nose lines up to the nipple. Maintain the baby's body in a horizontal alignment.
- To feed at left breast, the mother supports the baby's head with her right hand at nape of the baby's neck (allow head to slightly lag back); the mother's right thumb by the baby's left ear, and right forefinger near the baby's right ear.
- With the mother's free left hand, she can offer her left breast.

B **Cradling.**

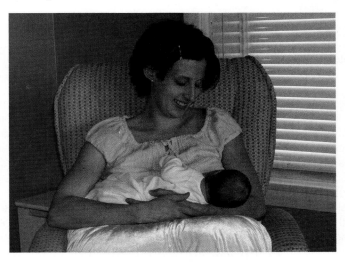

- Position as for modified cradle.
- If feeding from the left breast, have the mother cradle the baby's head near the crook of her left arm while supporting her baby's body with her left forearm.
- With the mother's free right hand, she can offer her left breast.

*Sources: **A,** and **B,** Courtesy of Brigitte T. Hall, MSN, RNC, IBCLC.*

➊ Four common breastfeeding positions: **A,** Modified cradle; **B,** cradling. *(continued)*

(continued on next page)

SKILL 14.16 Breastfeeding: Assisting *(continued)*

C Football (or clutch) hold.

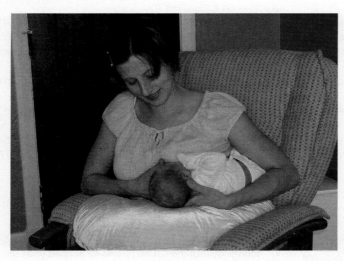

- Have the mother sit comfortably and use pillows to raise the baby's body to breast level. If using a Boppy and the Boppy is in "normal" position on the mother's lap, turn it counterclockwise slightly (if feeding at left breast) to provide extended support for the baby's body resting along the mother's left side and near the back of the mother's chair.
- If feeding at the left breast, place the baby on the left side of the mother's body, heading the baby into position feet first. The baby's bottom should rest on the pillow near the mother's left elbow.
- Turn the baby slightly on her side so that she faces the breast.
- The mother's left arm clutches the baby's body close to the mother's body. The baby's body should feel securely tucked in under the mother's left arm.
- Have the mother support the baby's head with her left hand. With the mother's free right hand, she can offer her breast. (Good position for the mother with a c-section.)

D Side-lying position.

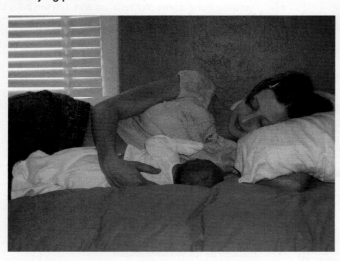

- Have the mother rest comfortably lying on her side (left side for this demonstration). Use pillows to support the mother's head and back, and provide support for the mother's hips by placing a pillow between her bent knees.
- Place the baby in side-lying position next to the mother's body. The baby's body should face the mother's body. The baby's nose should line up to the mother's nipple. Place a roll behind the baby's back, if desired.
- With the mother's free right hand, she can offer her left breast. After the baby is securely attached, mom can rest her right hand anywhere that is comfortable for her.

*Sources: **C**, and **D**, Courtesy of Brigitte T. Hall, MSN, RNC, IBCLC*

❶ Four common breastfeeding positions: **C**, Football (or clutch) hold; **D**, Side-lying position.

8. Instruct the mother to use the thumb and first two fingers of her dominant hand to make a C-shape around her breast with the nipple in the center of the C-shape and to steadily support her breast ❷. **Rationale:** *This C-hold hand position enables the mother to position the breast correctly in the baby's mouth.*

9. Help the mother hold her newborn so that the mouth is in alignment with her breast at the level of the nipple. She then lightly tickles the newborn's mouth with the nipple until the baby opens the mouth. She then brings the baby closely in to her breast. It is important for the baby to take the whole nipple into the mouth so that the gums are on the areola. Provide firm steady support as the baby begins to suckle. If sucking does not begin, stroke the cheek gently to elicit the suck–search

response and then offer the breast again. Instruct the mother to be sure that the breast tissue does not occlude the baby's nares. **Rationale:** *The baby's gums need to be positioned over the areola because as the newborn suckles, this allows the baby's jaws to compress the milk ducts located directly beneath the areola.*

10. If the newborn is sufficiently responsive, have the baby suckle at both breasts. Initially some babies suck well; others may simply lick or nuzzle the nipple. Reassure the mother that this is a positive interaction. **Rationale:** *Breast stimulation promotes the release of oxytocin, which aids uterine involution and lactation.*

11. When teaching is complete, perform hand hygiene and leave mother and newborn safe and comfortable.

SKILL 14.16 Breastfeeding: Assisting *(continued)*

C-hold hand position.

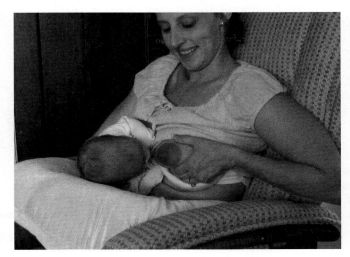

To be ready to draw the baby's mouth onto the mother's breast, as soon as the baby opens the mouth widely enough, the mother needs to have her hand supporting her breast in the ready position. She can use various hand holds, but she needs to keep her fingers well behind the areola. One such hand position is called the "C-hold." In this hold, the thumb is placed on top of the breast near the 12:00 position and the other four fingers are placed on the underside of the breast near the 6:00 position (depends on mother's hand size and length of fingers). The key point is to keep the fingers at least 1½ inches back from the base of the nipple as the fingers support the breast. Mothers are not often aware of where they place their fingers especially on the underside of the breast. If the fingers are too far forward (too close to the nipple), then the infant cannot grasp a large amount of areola in her mouth and this results in a "shallow" latch. A shallow latch is associated with nipple pain and ineffective drainage of the breast. An alternate handhold not shown is a "U-hold" hand position. The thumb and forefinger are near the 3 and 9 position on the breast again with fingers at least 1½ inches back from the base of the nipple; the body of the hand rests on the lower portion of the breast. Using this handhold, the mother's arm position is down at her side rather than sticking outward as it is when supporting the breast using the C-hold position.

Source: Courtesy of Brigitte T. Hall, MSN, RNC, IBCLC

❷ C-hold hand position.

12. Complete documentation using forms, checklists, or electronic dropdown lists supplemented by nurse's notes or additional comments as appropriate, including time and duration of the breastfeeding, the quality of the latch, and interaction between the mother and newborn. Note any difficulties such as flat or inverted nipples, and initiate referral to a lactation consultant.

SKILL 14.17 Lochia: Evaluating

During the postpartum phase, the vaginal discharge that occurs is called *lochia*. This discharge contains uterus lining tissue, blood, and microorganisms. Right after birth, the discharge contains a large amount of blood, so it is very red. Over the next few days, the discharge has less blood in it, so the color lightens up to pink and finally a light yellow to white.

Delegation or Assignment

Evaluating lochia is not delegated or assigned to the UAP. The nurse can request the UAP to save perineal pads and report patient observations to the nurse for follow-up. The nurse remains responsible for the assessment, interpretation of abnormal findings, and determination of appropriate responses.

Equipment

- Clean perineal pad
- Clean gloves

Preparation

- Review healthcare provider's orders and patient's nursing plan of care.
- Gather equipment and supplies.

Procedure

1. Introduce self to patient and verify the patient's identity using two identifiers. Explain to the patient you are going to assess the lochia on the perineal pad and assess uterine fundal height and firmness. Explain why lochia occurs, why it is assessed, how it is assessed, and how it changes during the postpartum. Discuss how the results will be used in planning further care or treatments.
2. Perform hand hygiene and observe appropriate infection control procedures.
3. Ask the woman to void.

(continued on next page)

SKILL 14.17 Lochia: Evaluating *(continued)*

4. Provide comfort and safety for patient and self, including raising bed to appropriate height for procedure.

5. Complete the assessment of uterine fundal height, measured in fingerbreadths (*fb*) or centimeters (cm), and firmness. **Rationale:** *This practice provides a more thorough assessment.*

6. If she has not already done so for the fundal assessment, ask the woman to flex her legs. Then ask her to spread her legs apart. Use the bed sheet as a drape to preserve her modesty.

7. Don gloves.

8. Lower the perineal pad and observe the amount of lochia on the pad. Because women's pad-changing practices vary, ask her about the length of time the current pad has been in use, whether the amount of lochia is changed, and whether any clots were passed before this examination, such as during voiding.

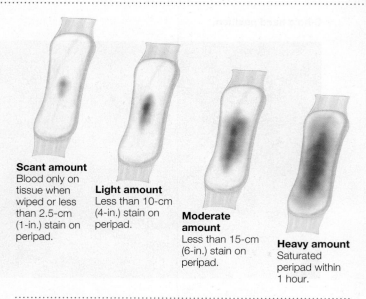

Scant amount
Blood only on tissue when wiped or less than 2.5-cm (1-in.) stain on peripad.

Light amount
Less than 10-cm (4-in.) stain on peripad.

Moderate amount
Less than 15-cm (6-in.) stain on peripad.

Heavy amount
Saturated peripad within 1 hour.

① Suggested guidelines for assessing lochia volume.

CAUTION! During the first 1–3 days, the woman's lochia should be rubra, or dark red. A few small clots are normal and occur as a result of pooling of blood in the vagina when the woman is lying down. The passage of large clots is abnormal, and the cause should be investigated immediately.

---

9. If the woman reports heavy bleeding or clots, ask her to put on a clean perineal pad and then reassess the pad in 1 hour. Also ask her to call you before flushing any clots she passes into the toilet during voiding.

10. When the uterine fundus is firm and stabilized with the nondominant hand, press down on it with the dominant hand while watching to see if any clots are expelled.

11. Determine the amount of lochia, using the following guide **①**:
    * Heavy amount—Perineal pad has a stain larger than 15 cm (6 in.) in length within 1 hour; 30–80 mL lochia.
    * Moderate amount—Perineal pad has a stain less than 15 cm (6 in.) in length within 1 hour; 25–50 mL lochia.
    * Small amount—Perineal pad has a stain less than 10 cm (4 in.) in length after 1 hour; 10–25 mL lochia.
    * Scant amount—Perineal pad has a stain less than 2.5 cm (1 in.) in length after 1 hour or lochia is only on tissue when the woman wipes.

12. In most cases, a woman is discharged while her lochia is still rubra. Provide her with information about assessing her lochia serosa and lochia alba when at home and when to contact her healthcare provider.

13. When the procedure is complete, assist patient in cleaning peritoneal area and applying clean perineal pad.

14. Return bed to lowest height, perform hand hygiene, and leave patient safe and comfortable.

15. Complete documentation using forms, checklists, or electronic dropdown lists supplemented by nurse's notes or additional comments as appropriate.

SAMPLE DOCUMENTATION

[date] 0630 Awake and alert. Uterus firm, 1 finger breadth below uterus. Lochia moderate rubra, no clots passed. Tolerated procedure without complaint. Up to take shower. *W. Mass*

CAUTION! Lochia should never exceed a moderate amount, such as 4–8 partially saturated perineal pads daily. Using a consistent standard for measuring lochia improves the accuracy of the information charted and conveyed to others.

CAUTION! If blood loss exceeds the guidelines given in this chapter, weigh the perineal pads and the chux pads to more accurately estimate the blood loss. Typically, 1 g = 1 mL blood. Because blood can pool below the woman on the chux or peri pad, the pads are included in your assessment.

SKILL 14.18 Postpartum, Maternal: Assessing

Assessment examinations are done throughout the postpartum phase of pregnancy. These assessments can include physical examinations. Teaching is a part of all the phases of pregnancy.

Delegation or Assignment

Assisting with postpartum examination is not delegated or assigned to the UAP. The nurse can request the UAP to report patient observations to the nurse for follow-up. The nurse remains responsible for the assessment, interpretation of abnormal findings, and determination of appropriate responses.

Equipment

- Need for appropriate equipment according to which assessment is being done

Preparation

- Review healthcare provider's or certified nurse-midwife's (MD/CNM) orders and patient's nursing plan of care.
- Review patient's record for allergies.
- Gather equipment and supplies.

Procedure

1. Introduce self to patient and verify the patient's identity using two identifiers. Explain to the patient you are going to monitor and perform assessments, why they are necessary, and how she can participate. Discuss how the results will be used in planning further care or treatments.
2. Perform hand hygiene and observe appropriate infection control procedures.
3. Provide for patient privacy.
4. Provide comfort and safety for patient and self, including raising bed to appropriate height for procedure.
5. Perform a systematic assessment (see **Table 14–4 ≫**).
6. When the procedure is complete, lower the bed to the lowest position, perform hand hygiene, and leave patient safe and comfortable.
7. Complete documentation using forms, checklists, or electronic dropdown lists supplemented by nurse's notes or additional comments as appropriate.

TABLE 14–4 Postpartum (PP) Maternal Assessment

Assessment	Normal PP Findings	Abnormal PP Assessment
Assess vital signs every hour for 4 hr, every 8 hr, and as needed	Pulse may be 45–60 bpm in stage 4 Pulse to normal range about third day	Decreased BP and increased pulse: probably postpartum hemorrhage. Elevated temperature >38°C (100.4°F) indicates possible infection. Temperature elevates when lactation occurs.
Assess breasts and nipples daily	Days 1–2: soft, intact, secreting colostrum Days 2–3: engorged, tender, full, tight, painful Days 3+: secreting milk Increased pains as newborn sucks: common in multiparas	Tenderness, heat, edema indicate engorgement. Sore or cracked (clean and dry nipples); decrease breastfeeding time; apply breast shield between feedings. If milk does not "let down," help patient relax and decrease anxiety by giving glass of wine or beer, if not culturally, religiously, or otherwise contradicted. Reddened area could indicate mastitis. Palpable mass indicates mastitis. Engorgement indicates venous stasis.
Nipples	Pigmented, intact, become erect when stimulated	Fissures, cracks, soreness can be caused by poor breastfeeding techniques. Inverted nipples will cause nipples not to erect when stimulated.
Assess fundus every 15 min for 1 hr, every 8 hr for 48 hr, then daily	Firm (like a grapefruit) in midline and at or slightly above umbilicus Return to prepregnant size in 6 weeks: descending at rate of 1 fingerbreadth/day	Boggy fundus: immediately massage gently until firm; report to healthcare provider and observe closely; empty bladder; medicate with oxytocin if ordered. Fundus misplaced 1–2 fingerbreadths from midline: indicates full bladder (patient must void or be catheterized).
Assess lochia every 15 min for 1 hr, every 8 hr for 48 hr, then daily	Scant to moderate amount, earthy odor, no clots	Clots indicate hemorrhage.
■ Color	3 days postpartum: dark red (rubra) 4–10 days postpartum: clear pink (serosa) 10–21 days postpartum: white, yellow brown (alba)	Failure to progress from rubra to serosa to alba indicates subinvolution.

(continued on next page)

SKILL 14.18 Postpartum, Maternal: Assessing (continued)

TABLE 14–4 Postpartum (PP) Maternal Assessment (continued)

Assessment	Normal PP Findings	Abnormal PP Assessment
■ Quantity	Moderate amount, steadily decreases	No lochia: may indicate clot occluding cervical opening (support fundus; express clot)
		Heavy, bright red: indicates hemorrhage (massage fundus, give medication on order, notify healthcare provider)
		Spurts: may indicate cervical tear
■ Odor	Minimal	Foul: may indicate infection
Assess perineum daily	May have slight edema and bruising	Swelling or bruising: may indicate hematoma
■ Episiotomy	Episiotomy intact, no swelling, no discoloration	Redness, ecchymosis, discharge, or gaping stitches may indicate infection
■ Hemorrhoids	None present; could have a few small, nontender	Full, tender, red could indicate inflammation
Assess bladder every 4 hr	Voiding regularly with no pain	Not voiding: bladder may be full and displaced to one side, leading to increased lochia (catheterization may be necessary)
		Symptoms of urgency, frequency, and dysuria could be infection.
Assess bowels	Spontaneous bowel movement 2–3 days after delivery	Fear associated with pain from hemorrhoids, episiotomy, or perineal trauma; no bowel movement could be constipation
Evaluate Rh-negative status	Patient does not require RhoGAM.	RhoGAM administered
Assess mother–newborn bonding	Touching newborn, talking to newborn, talking about newborn	Refuses to touch or hold baby
Assess extremities	Negative Homans sign; no pain with palpation	Positive findings indicate thrombophlebitis.
Material History: Definition of Terms		
Abortion: pregnancy loss before fetus is viable (usually <20 weeks or 500 g)	Multigravida: refers to second or any subsequent pregnancy	Nullipara: refers to female who has never carried pregnancy to viable age for fetus
Gravida: any pregnancy, including present one	Para: past pregnancies that continued to viable age (20 weeks); babies may be alive or dead at birth	Multipara: refers to female who has given birth to two or more viable babies; either alive or dead
Primigravida: refers to first-time pregnancy	Primipara: refers to female who has delivered first viable baby; born either alive or dead	

SKILL 14.19 Postpartum, Perineum: Assessing

The woman's postpartum perineum may have bruising and tenderness. If she had an episiotomy or a tissue tear, this area is assessed for healing process and hardened areas or hematomas. The anus is assessed for hemorrhoids, noting size and number.

Delegation or Assignment

Assessment of the postpartum perineum is not delegated or assigned to the UAP. The nurse can request the UAP to save perineal pads and report patient observations to the nurse for follow-up. The nurse remains responsible for the assessment, interpretation of abnormal findings, and determination of appropriate responses.

Equipment

- Clean perineal pad, clean ice pack if desired/needed
- Small light source such as a penlight may be necessary
- Clean gloves

Preparation

- Review healthcare provider's or certified nurse-midwife's (MD/CNM) orders and patient's nursing plan of care.
- Gather needed supplies.

Procedure

1. Introduce self to patient and verify the patient's identity using two identifiers. Explain to the patient you are going to perform an assessment of her perineum, why it is necessary, and how the patient can participate. Discuss how the results will be used in planning further care or treatments.
2. Perform hand hygiene and observe appropriate infection control procedures.
3. Ask the patient to empty her bladder before beginning the physical exam.
4. Provide for patient privacy, safety, and comfort. Raise bed to appropriate height for procedure.
   - Complete the assessment of fundal height and lochia with the woman lying on her back with her knees flexed.
   - Ask her to turn onto her side with her upper knee drawn forward and resting on the bed (Sims position).
5. Use a systematic approach to assessment.
   - Complete the assessment of fundal height and lochia with the woman lying on her back with her knees flexed. In evaluating the perineum, begin by asking the woman to describe her discomfort. Does it seem excessive to her? Has it become worse since the birth?

SKILL 14.19 Postpartum, Perineum: Assessing (*continued*)

- Assess the condition of the tissue. Ask the woman to lift the knee of her upper leg to expose her perineum more fully. Note any swelling (edema) or bruising (ecchymosis), and use the REEDA scale to recall what to assess (see **CAUTION!** below). **Rationale:** *Excessive bruising may indicate a hematoma is developing.*
- Evaluate the episiotomy, if there is one, or any repaired laceration for its state of healing. Is it reddened? Note the edges of the incision. Are they well approximated? Tell the woman that you are going to palpate the incision gently, then do so. Note any areas of hardness. Note whether the incision is warmer to the touch than the surrounding tissue. **Rationale:** *Redness, warmth, or areas of hardness may suggest infection. Typically, within 24 hours the edges of the incision should be well approximated.*

CAUTION! In evaluating the perineum, use the REEDA scale as a quick reminder of what to assess.

Specifically:
R = redness
E = edema or swelling
E = ecchymosis or bruising
D = drainage
A = approximation (how well the edges of an incision—the episiotomy—or a repaired laceration seem to be holding together)

- During the assessment, be alert for odors. Typically the lochia has an earthy, but not unpleasant, smell that is easily identifiable. **Rationale:** *A foul odor often indicates infection.*
- Assess for hemorrhoids. To visualize the anal area, lift the upper buttocks 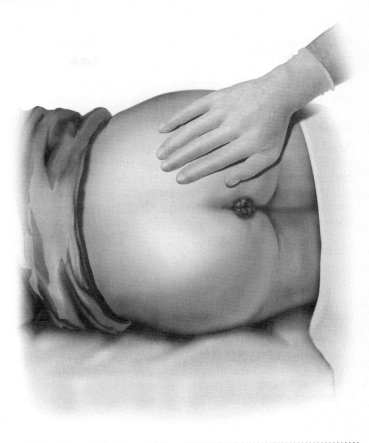. If hemorrhoids are present, note the size, number, and pain or tenderness.
6. During the assessment, talk to the woman about the effectiveness of comfort measures being used. Provide teaching about care of the episiotomy, hemorrhoids, and about good healthcare practices in both the short and long term.
7. Provide the woman with a clean perineal pad. Replenish the ice pack for the perineum if necessary.
8. When the procedure is complete, return bed to lowest height. Perform hand hygiene and leave patient safe and comfortable.
9. Complete documentation using forms, checklists, or electronic dropdown lists supplemented by nurse's notes or additional comments as appropriate.

❶ Intact perineum with hemorrhoids. Note how the nurse's hand raises the upper buttocks to expose fully the anal area.

SAMPLE DOCUMENTATION

[date] 1316 Midline episiotomy, no edema, ecchymosis, or tenderness. Skin edges well approximated. States pain relief measures are controlling discomfort. Ice pack to perineum with clean peri-pad. Tolerated assessment without incident. *B. Viper*

SKILL 14.20 Uterine Fundus, After Vaginal or Cesarean Birth: Assessing

Safety Note! *During scheduled clinical time, nursing students may have a learning opportunity to observe or assist with this skill only with faculty permission and with direct supervision from faculty or another RN.*

Typically, the uterine fundus returns to its prepregnancy state in a few weeks which includes being well contracted and eventually returning to approximately the size of a fist. Its location returns to midline of the abdomen, will be firm when

(*continued on next page*)

SKILL 14.20 Uterine Fundus, After Vaginal or Cesarean Birth: Assessing (*continued*)

palpated, and will return to a low position in the abdomen, receding approximately one fingerbreadth (FB) per day. Assessment of the uterine fundus is important to monitor frequently for abnormal assessment data that can be characteristic of a variety of complications that need to be treated.

Delegation or Assignment

Assessment of the uterine fundus is not delegated or assigned to the UAP. The nurse can request the UAP to save perineal pads and report patient observations to the nurse for follow-up. The nurse remains responsible for the assessment, interpretation of abnormal findings, and determination of appropriate responses.

Equipment

- A clean perineal pad
- Clean gloves

Preparation

- Review physician's or certified nurse-midwife's (MD/CNM) orders and consider recommending to premedicate 30–45 min before assessing the fundus, especially if the patient has had a cesarean section.
- Gather needed equipment and supplies.

Procedure

1. Introduce self to patient and verify the patient's identity using two identifiers. Explain the procedure, the information it provides, and what it might feel like. Discuss how the results will be used in planning further care or treatments.
2. Perform hand hygiene and observe appropriate infection control procedures.
3. Provide for patient privacy, safety, and comfort. Raise bed to appropriate height for procedure.
4. Ask the patient to empty her bladder before the procedure begins.
5. Have the woman lie flat in bed with her head on a pillow or with her legs flexed. Flexing the legs and providing support under them with folded pillows is especially helpful to patients after a cesarean section.
6. Gently place one hand on the lower segment of the uterus for support. Using the side of the other hand, palpate the abdomen until you locate the top of the fundus. **Rationale:** *Support of the uterus prevents stretching of the ligaments that support the uterus.*
7. Determine whether the fundus is firm. If it is, it will feel hard and round like a firm grapefruit in the abdomen. If it is not firm, massage the abdomen lightly until it becomes firm, then check for bleeding. **Rationale:** *A firm fundus indicates that the uterine muscles are contracted and bleeding will not occur.*
8. Use a systematic approach to perform the assessment.
   - Measure the top of the fundus in fingerbreadths (FB) above, below, or at the umbilicus ❶. **Rationale:** *Fundal height gives information about the progress of involution.*

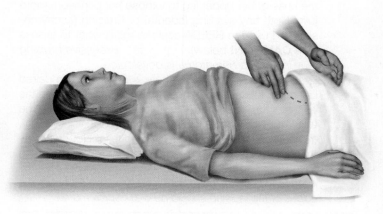

❶ Measuring the descent of the fundus in the woman with a vaginal birth. In this case, the fundus is located two fingerbreadths below the umbilicus.

- Determine the position of the fundus in relation to the midline of the body. If it is not in the midline, locate it and then evaluate the bladder for distention. **Rationale:** *The fundus may deviate from the midline when the bladder is full.*
- If the bladder is distended, use nursing measures to help the woman void. If she is not able to void after a specified period of time, catheterization may be necessary.
- Measure urine output for the next few hours until normal elimination is established. **Rationale:** *During the postpartum period, the bladder may fill more rapidly. (A diminished tone of the uterus may cause loss of the urge to void.)*
- Don gloves to assess the lochia on the peri-pad and at the vaginal opening.
9. During the first few hours postpartum, if the fundus becomes boggy frequently or is located high above the umbilicus and the woman's bladder is empty, the uterine cavity may be filled with clots of blood. In this case, don gloves and do the following:
   - Release the front of the perineal pad and lay it back so that you can see the perineum and the pad lying between the woman's legs.
   - Massage the uterine fundus until it is firm.
   - Keep one hand in position stabilizing the lower portion of the uterus. With the hand you used to massage the fundus, put steady pressure on the top of the now-firm fundus and see if you are able to express any clots. (Watch the pad between her legs for clots to pass from the vagina.) **Rationale:** *Blood clots act as an irritant and the uterus will not remain contracted. When the muscle fibers relax, bleeding results. Pushing on a uterus that is not firm is dangerous because it is possible to cause the uterus to invert, a true emergency.*
10. Provide the woman with a clean perineal pad.

SKILL 14.20 Uterine Fundus, After Vaginal or Cesarean Birth: Assessing (*continued*)

11. When the procedure is complete, return bed to lowest height. Perform hand hygiene and leave patient safe and comfortable.
12. Complete documentation using forms, checklists, or electronic dropdown lists supplemented by nurse's notes or additional comments as appropriate. Fundal height is recorded in fingerbreadths. If fundal massage was necessary, note that fact.

> **SAMPLE DOCUMENTATION**
>
> [date] 0645 Uterine fundus is 2 finger breadths below umbilicus. Uterus soft and boggy, light massage applied and firmed up. Tolerated without incident. *R. Lois*

» Newborn Care

Expected Outcomes

1. The newborn's Apgar score 5 minutes after birth is 8–10.
2. The newborn's cord is kept clean and dry.
3. There are no signs of infection at the circumcision site.

SKILL 14.21 Apgar Score: Assessing

The Apgar score is an assessment of the newborn's ability to breathe, move, respond, and survive outside the uterus without medical assistance. The newborn is evaluated 1 minute after birth and then again at 5 minutes.

Delegation or Assignment

Assessing the Apgar score is not delegated or assigned to the UAP. The nurse can request the UAP to report patient observations to the nurse for follow-up. The nurse remains responsible for the assessment, interpretation of abnormal findings, and determination of appropriate responses.

Equipment

- Apgar or digital timer that counts seconds or a watch with a second hand
- Newborn radiant warmer with skin temperature control (ISC) and probe preheated
- Clean gloves
- Stethoscope (neonatal or pediatric if available)
- Sterile baby blankets

Preparation

- Review healthcare provider's orders and patient's nursing plan of care.
- Identify the individual responsible for assigning the Apgar score.
- Preheat the radiant warmer to 36.5°C (97.7°F).
- Prewarm blankets under the warmer.

CAUTION! A newborn is wet with amniotic fluid, vernix, and secretions. Consequently, universal precautions are indicated when handling the baby until the initial bath is completed.

Procedure

1. Perform hand hygiene and don gloves.
2. Provide comfort, safety, and stimulation (if needed) during the procedure.
3. The Apgar scoring system is a method of evaluating a newborn's condition at 1 minute and 5 minutes after birth (see **Table 14–5 »**). Use the five criteria to determine a

TABLE 14–5 Apgar Scoring

Criterion	Score – 0	Score – 1	Score – 2
1. Heart rate Palpate the pulse at the base of the umbilical cord for 6 seconds and multiply by 10, or use the stethoscope to auscultate the heart rate.	No heart rate detected	Heart rate less than 100 bpm	Heart rate more than 100 bpm
2. Respiratory effort Observe respirations and cry.	No respiratory effort; no cry	Slow, irregular, breathing; weak cry	Good respiratory effort; robust cry
3. Muscle tone Assess flexion of extremities and quality of muscle tone.	Flaccid; none	Some flexion of extremities	Active motion; extremities well flexed
4. Reflex irritability Assess response to noxious stimuli, such as vitamin K injection.	No response	Grimace	Vigorous cry
5. Color Assess skin color.	Generally poor color; pale or blue	Body pink, extremities and area around mouth pale or blue	Completely pink

(*continued on next page*)

SKILL 14.21 Apgar Score: Assessing (*continued*)

score for each, and assign an Apgar score at 1 minute to *provide a quick indication of the baby's physical adaptation to the extrauterine environment.*

4. The Apgar scores for each criterion are totaled and interpreted as follows:
   - Newborns who score 7–10 are considered free of immediate danger.
   - Newborns who score 4–6 are considered moderately depressed.
   - Newborns who score 0–3 are considered severely depressed.

When the total score at 5 minutes is less than 7, repeat every 5 minutes for 20 minutes. The newborn may be intubated unless two successive total scores of 7 or more take place.

5. Complete the documentation using forms, checklists, or electronic dropdown lists supplemented by nurse's notes or additional comments as appropriate.

CAUTION! Heart rate and respirations are the two most significant categories to evaluate.

SKILL 14.22 Circumcision: Caring for

Circumcision is the surgical removal of the foreskin that covers the glans of the penis. This can be done as a cultural or religious practice or parental choice for the newborn male.

Delegation or Assignment

Assessing and providing care for the circumcision site of a newborn is the nurse's responsibility and is not delegated or assigned to the UAP. The UAP may provide care to the newborn within the scope of practice. The nurse can request the UAP to report patient observations to the nurse for follow-up. The nurse remains responsible for the assessment, interpretation of abnormal findings, and determination of appropriate responses.

Equipment

- Newborn radiant warmer
- Circumcision board
- Iodine skin prep
- Circumcision tray
- Analgesia medications as ordered
- Pacifier
- Sucrose solution
- Petroleum gauze or ointment (as prescribed by healthcare provider or facility policy)
- Clean diaper
- Sterile gloves

Preparation

- Review healthcare provider's orders.
- Verify a signed informed consent is in the front of the patient's record.
- Medicate the newborn for pain if ordered.
- Plan for distraction and safe positioning.
- Obtain necessary supplies.
- Coordinate timing to avoid performing the procedure within 3–4 hr after feeding following healthcare provider's preference.

Procedure

CIRCUMCISION

1. Introduce self to parent and verify the patient's identity, comparing the ID number on the newborn's band with the number in the medical record with the circumcision order. Explain to the parent the healthcare provider is going to circumcise the patient and how the parent can participate. Answer any questions the parent or guardian may have.
2. Perform hand hygiene and observe appropriate infection control procedures.
3. Provide for patient privacy.
4. Confirm that the newborn has been NPO following healthcare provider's instructions.
5. Have equipment and medications available for medicating the newborn for pain as ordered.
6. Assist the healthcare provider during the procedure. Don sterile gloves.
7. Provide comfort and safety for newborn, including securing the baby to the circumcision board using Velcro straps or other restraint devices; restrain only the legs.
8. Apply warm blankets to the upper body. Provide sucrose as ordered for comfort.
9. Offer a pacifier for nonnutritive sucking. Lightly stroke the baby's head.

POST CIRCUMCISION CARE

10. Apply petroleum gauze or ointment to the head of the penis to avoid trauma to the surgical site ❶.
11. Apply a clean diaper. Fasten diaper over penis snugly enough so that it does not move and rub the tender glans.
12. Assess the ability to void. **Rationale:** *Swelling or damage may obstruct the urethral opening.*
13. Return the newborn to his parents. Explain the procedure.
14. Dispose of waste items in appropriate container, perform hand hygiene, and leave the newborn clean and dry, warm, safe, and comfortable with parent or guardian.

SKILL 14.22 Circumcision: Caring for (*continued*)

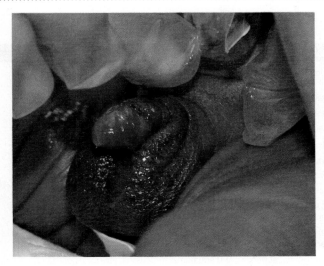

Source: George Dodson/Pearson Education, Inc.

❶ Following circumcision, petroleum ointment may be applied to the site for the next few diaper changes.

15. Teach parents to apply petroleum gauze to the site and use A&D ointment to prevent adherence of the diaper to the surgical site (unless a circumcision device is in place). Teach them that the glans is sensitive and to avoid placing the newborn on his stomach for the first day after the procedure. Explain the need to contact their healthcare provider for sustained swelling of the circumcised site or blood in the urine.

16. Monitor temperature.

17. Check the site hourly for signs of complications until discharge.

18. Complete documentation using forms, checklists, or electronic dropdown lists supplemented by nurse's notes or additional comments as appropriate, including any bleeding, discharge, abnormal temperature, urination following procedure, or inability to void in the medical record.

SAMPLE DOCUMENTATION

[date] 1540 Mother verifies newborn has been NPO as ordered. Dr. Diaz here, patient placed on circumcision board, Velcro straps applied to legs, warmed blanket applied to chest and arms. Circumcision procedure completed, small amount bleeding noted, offered sucrose for comfort per order. Petroleum gauze applied to head of penis, clean diaper applied. Removed from circumcision board and given to mother. No urine noted at this time. *V. Ham*

SKILL 14.23 Newborn: Assessing

Assessment examinations are scheduled throughout the time the newborn is in the healthcare facility and then every few months the first year. These assessments include a physical examination. Teaching provided to parents or guardian is a part of this process.

Delegation or Assignment

Assisting with newborn assessment is not delegated or assigned to the UAP. The nurse can request the UAP to report patient observations to the nurse for follow-up. The nurse remains responsible for the assessment, interpretation of abnormal findings, and determination of appropriate responses.

Equipment

- Need for appropriate equipment according to which assessment is being done

Preparation

- Review healthcare provider's orders and patient's nursing plan of care.
- Gather equipment and supplies.

Procedure

1. Introduce self to parents or guardian and verify the patient's identity using two identifiers. Explain to the parents or guardian you are going to perform an assessment examination on the patient and why it is necessary. Discuss how the results will be used in planning further care or treatments and always allow time for any questions.

2. Perform hand hygiene and observe appropriate infection control procedures.

3. Provide for patient privacy.

4. Provide comfort and safety for patient and self, including raising bed to appropriate height for procedure.

5. Perform a systematic assessment (see **Table 14–6 》》**).

6. When the procedure is complete, lower bed to lowest position, perform hand hygiene, and leave patient safe and comfortable.

7. Complete documentation using forms, checklists, or electronic dropdown lists supplemented by nurse's notes or additional comments as appropriate.

(*continued on next page*)

SKILL 14.23 Newborn: Assessing (continued)

TABLE 14–6 Newborn Assessment

Assessment	Normal	Abnormal
Vital Signs Temperature	Rectal 36.6°C–37.2°C (97.8°F–99°F) Axilla 36.4°C–37.2°C (97.5°F–99°F)	Elevated temperatures may be related to high ambient temperature or too much clothing. Subnormal temperatures may be related to cold, sepsis, or brainstem involvement. Differences of 2° in either direction could indicate infection.
Pulse	120–160 bpm; will go higher if crying	Bradycardia (< 120 bpm) is indicative of severe asphyxia or cardiac arrhythmia. Weak pulse is related to decreased cardiac output. Tachycardia (>160 bpm) indicates infection, arrhythmia, central nervous system problems.
Respirations	Respiration rate 30–50 breaths/min; transient tachypnea Respiration movement irregular in rate and depth Resonant chest (hollow sound on percussion) Abdominal respirations	Tachypnea indicates pneumonia, respiratory distress syndrome (RDS). Rapid, shallow breathing may occur if mother is given large doses of magnesium sulfate during labor for pregnancy-induced hypertension (hypermagnesemia). Respirations below 30 breaths/min are indicative of maternal anesthesia or analgesia during labor and delivery. Expiratory grunting, subcostal and substernal retractions, flaring of nostrils are indicative of respiratory distress, apnea, or respiratory disorder.
Blood pressure	At birth: 80–60/45–40 Day 10: 100/50	Low BP indicates hypovolemia or shock.
Assess cry (see also Table 14–5 on Apgar scoring)	Lusty cry	Weak, groaning cry: possible neurological abnormality High-pitched cry: newborn drug withdrawal (may occur 6–12 months after birth); hoarse or crowing inspirations, catlike cry: possible neurological or chromosomal abnormality
Assess weight	2.5–3.7 kg (5.5–8.14 lb) Normal weight loss during first 3 days: up to 5–10%	Birthweights below 2.5 kg (5.5 lb) indicates small for gestational age (SGA) or preterm newborn. Birthweights above 3.7 kg (8.14 lb) indicates large for gestational age (LGA) baby or baby born to a mother with diabetes. Greater loss indicates feeding problems, decreased fluid intake, or losses due to meconium expulsion or urination.
Skin Assessment Note skin color, pigmentation, turgor, and lesions	Pink Mongolian spots may occur over buttocks in dark-skinned babies Erythema	Cyanosis, pallor, beefy red petechiae, ecchymoses, or purpuric spots: signs of possible hematologic disorder or clotting disorders Impetigo (group A beta-hemolytic *Streptococcus* or *Staphylococcus*)
	Capillary hemangiomas on face or neck	Café au lait spots (patches of brown discoloration): possible sign of congenital neurological disorder Raised capillary hemangiomas on areas other than face or neck
	Localized edema in presenting part	Edema of peritoneal wall Poor skin turgor: indicates dehydration
	Cheesy white vernix Desquamation (peeling off)	Yellow discolored vernix (meconium stained)
	Milia (small white pustules over nose and chin)	Impetigo neonatorum (small pustules with surrounding red areas)
	Jaundice after 24 hr; gone by second week	Jaundice at birth or within 12 hr Dermal sinuses (opening to brain) Holes along spinal column Low hairline posteriorly: possible chromosomal abnormality Sparse or spotty hair: congenital goiter or chromosomal abnormality
Note color of nails	Pink	Yellowing of nail beds (meconium stained)
Note muscle strength/tone	Strong, tremulous	Flaccid, convulsions Muscular twitching, hypertonicity
Head and Neck Assessment Note shape of head	Fontanels: anterior open until 18 months; posterior closed shortly after birth; is 3–4 cm long and 2–3 cm wide; diamond shaped Posterior fontanel is 1–2 cm at birth and triangle shaped	Depressed fontanels indicate dehydration; closed or bulging indicate congenital anomalies; full or bulging indicate edema or increased intracranial pressure (ICP). Cephalohematoma that crosses the midline Microcephaly and macrocephaly

SKILL 14.23 Newborn: Assessing (continued)

TABLE 14–6 Newborn Assessment (continued)

Assessment	Normal	Abnormal
	Circumference is ¼ size of body and 2 cm larger than the chest circumference. Breech and cesarean newborns' heads are rounded and well-shaped.	Cephalohematoma trauma from birth lasts up to 3 weeks. Caput succedaneum occurring from a long labor and birth will disappear in about 1 week.
Assess eyes	Slight edema of lids	Purulent discharge indicates infection. Lateral upward slope of eye with an inner epicanthal fold in babies not of Asian heritage Exophthalmos (bulging of eyeball): may be congenital anomaly, sign of congenital glaucoma or thyroid abnormality Enophthalmos (recession of eyeball): may indicate damage to brain or cervical spine
	Pupils equal and reactive to light by 3 weeks of age Intermittent strabismus (occasional crossing of eyes) Conjunctival or scleral hemorrhages Symmetrical light reflex (light reflects off each eye in the same quadrant): sign of conjugate gaze Blink reflex in response to light stimuli Corneal reflex present Vision: tracks objects to midline; fixed focus on objects at a distance; prefers faces and black and white to color Cry usually tearless	Constricted pupil, unilateral dilated; unequal pupils due to CNS damage Fixed pupil, nystagmus (rhythmic nonpurposeful movement of eyeball): continuous strabismus Haziness of cornea Absence of red reflex; asymmetrical light reflex Blink reflex absent indicates CNS injury Ulceration indicates herpes infection Cataracts from congenital infection Excessive tearing from plugged tear ducts; could be narcotic withdrawal
Note placement of ears, shape and position	The top of the ear should be on an imaginary line from the edge of the eye.	Low-set ears: may indicate chromosomal or renal system abnormality
Assess nose	Sneezes to clear nasal passageways Nose breathers	Flat or broad bridge of nose seen in Down syndrome Flaring nostrils indicates respiratory distress Blockage of nares due to mucus or secretions Thick, bloody nasal discharge if infection present
Assess mouth	Gag, swallowing, sucking reflexes present	Absent of reflexes
	Hard and soft palates intact	Cleft lip, palate Flat, white nonremovable spots (thrush)
	Esophagus intact; drooling in newborns	Frequent vomiting: may indicate pyloric stenosis; esophageal atresia Vomitus with bile: fecal vomiting Profuse salivation: may indicate tracheoesophageal fistula
	Tongue moves freely in all directions; pink color; noncoated	Lack of movement indicates neurological damage. White cheesy coating indicates thrush.
Assess neck	Short, straight, extra skinfolds Tonic neck reflex (Fencer position)	Short neck in Turner syndrome Distended neck veins Fractured clavicle Unusually short neck Excess posterior cervical skin Resistance to neck flexion
Chest and Lung Assessment Assess chest	2 cm smaller than head; wider than long; lower end of sternum may protrude Bilateral expansion with no retractions	Funnel chest with congenital problems Depressed sternum Retractions, asymmetry of chest movements: indicates respiratory distress and possible pneumothorax

(continued on next page)

SKILL 14.23 Newborn: Assessing (*continued*)

TABLE 14–6 Newborn Assessment (*continued*)

Assessment	Normal	Abnormal
Assess respirations/lungs	Breath sounds louder in newborns Bronchial breath sounds bilaterally Rales may indicate normal newborn atelectasis Cough reflex absent until second day	Thoracic breathing, unequal motion of chest, rapid grasping or grunting respirations, flaring nares Deep sighing respirations Grunt on expiration: possible respiratory distress
Breasts	Flat with symmetrical nipples Engorgement occurs third day; may have liquid discharge in full-term babies (both sexes)	SGA babies lack breast tissue.
Heart Assessment Assess the rate, rhythm, and murmurs of the heart.	Rate: 100–160 bpm at birth; stabilizes at 120–140 bpm Regular rhythm Murmurs: significance cannot usually be determined in newborn	Heart rate > 200 or < 100 bpm Irregular rhythm Dextrocardia, enlarged heart
Abdomen and Gastrointestinal Tract Assessment Assess the abdomen.	Prominent No protrusion of umbilicus; however, protrusion may be seen in babies of African descent.	Distention of abdominal veins: possible portal vein obstruction Umbilical hernia
	Umbilical cord with one vein and two arteries; soft granulation tissue at umbilicus; no bleeding	One artery present in umbilical cord: may indicate other anomalies Bleeding, redness, or exudate indicates infection
Assess the gastrointestinal tract.	Bowel sounds present Liver 2–3 cm below right costal margin Spleen tip palpable	Visible peristaltic waves Increased pitch or frequency: intestinal obstruction Decreased sounds: paralytic ileus Distention of abdomen Enlarged liver or spleen Midline suprapubic mass: may indicate Hirschsprung disease
Femoral pulses	Palpable No bulges in inguinal area	Absent or diminished in coarctation of aorta Inguinal hernia
Genitourinary Tract Assessment Assess kidneys and bladder.	May be able to palpate kidneys Bladder percussed 1–4 cm above symphysis pubis Voids at birth or within 3 hr	Enlarged kidney Distended bladder; presence of any masses Failure to void within 24–48 hr
Assess the genitalia.	Edema and bruising after delivery Unusually large clitoris in females a short time after birth Vaginal mucoid or bloody discharge may be present in the first week	Ambiguous genitalia (chromosomal abnormality) Excessive vaginal bleeding indicates coagulation defect
Urethral orifice	Urethra opens on ventral surface of penile shaft Uncircumcised foreskin tight for 2–3 months	Hypospadias (urethra opens on the inferior surface of the penis) Epispadias (urethra opens on the dorsal surface of the penis) Ulceration of urethral orifice
Testes	Testes in scrotal sac or inguinal canal	Hydroceles in males Phimosis if still tight after 3 months Enlarged testes indicate tumor Small testes indicate Klinefelter syndrome or adrenal hyperplasia
Spine and Extremities Assessment Assess the spine.	Straight spine; slight lordosis; full-term newborn should hold head at 45-degree angle	Spina bifida, pilonidal sinus; scoliosis Unable to hold head or floppy trunk indicates neurological problems
Assess extremities.	Soft click with thigh rotation; should abduct to more than 60 deg Skin creases Feet in straight line; flat feet normal for first 3 months; some newborns may have a positional clubfoot from position in utero	Asymmetry of movement Sharp click with thigh rotation: indicates possible congenital hip dislocation Uneven major gluteal folds: indicates possible congenital hip dislocation Polydactyly (extra digits on a hand or foot); syndactyly (webbing or fusion of fingers or toes) Talipes equinovarus (clubfoot)

SKILL 14.23 Newborn: Assessing (*continued*)

TABLE 14–6 Newborn Assessment (*continued*)

Assessment	Normal	Abnormal
Assess anus and rectum.	Patent anus; passage of meconium within 48 hr after birth	Closed anus: no meconium
Reflexes	Rooting and sucking (turns in direction of stimulus to cheek or mouth)—disappears about fourth to seventh month	Poor sucking or fatigability in preterm
		Absence of reflex in preterm, neurologic involvement or depressed newborns
		Neurologic problems if response is asymmetrical
	Palmar grasp (fingers grasp adult finger when palm is stimulated); goes away about third to fourth month	Unilateral indicates fractured clavicle or nerve injury; complete absence suggests damage to the brain or spinal cord
		Neurologic problems if asymmetrical
		Low spinal cord defects if no response
	Moro reflex (an involuntary startle response to stimulation; arms extend with palms up and thumbs flexed); normally disappears after 3–4 months	
	Stepping (will step alternatively when held upright and one foot is touching a flat surface); disappears about 4–5 months	
	Babinski (fanning and extension of toes when sole of foot is stroked from heel across ball of foot); disappears at about 12 months	

SKILL 14.24 Newborn, Initial Bathing

Safety Note! *During scheduled clinical time, nursing students may have a learning opportunity to observe or assist with this skill only with faculty permission and with direct supervision from faculty or another RN.*

The initial bathing of a newborn occurs at different times in various healthcare and home settings. Sometimes the bath is given soon after the baby begins to regulate its body temperature, and sometimes the bath is given several days after birth. Amniotic fluid, meconium, and blood can be removed, but the vernix caseosa keeps the baby's skin moist and protected against infection.

Delegation or Assignment

Assessment done during the initial bath of the newborn is the nurse's responsibility and is not delegated or assigned to the UAP. The UAP may provide additional care to the baby within the scope of practice. The nurse can request the UAP to report patient observations to the nurse for follow-up. The nurse remains responsible for the assessment, interpretation of abnormal findings, and determination of appropriate responses.

Equipment

- Clean gloves
- Warm water
- Washcloths
- Blankets or towels for drying

Preparation

- Review healthcare provider's orders and patient's nursing plan of care.
- The newborn should be resting in a radiant warmer or an incubator.
- Prewarm all baby blankets to be used.
- Gather equipment and supplies.

Procedure

1. Introduce self to parent and verify the patient's identity using two identifiers. Explain to the parent you are going to bathe the patient, why it is necessary, and how the parent can participate. Discuss how the results will be used in planning further care or treatments.
2. Perform hand hygiene and observe appropriate infection control procedures.
3. Provide for patient privacy, safety, warmth, and comfort.
4. Assess newborn's temperature by axillary or rectal route. The rectal route is used when precision and accuracy is needed for core temperature. Once the baby has demonstrated the ability to maintain a stable temperature greater than 36.6°C (97.9°F), a first bath can be given. **Rationale:** *Temperature instability introduces a threat to newborn adaptation that can lead to serious complications, including respiratory distress, hypoglycemia, and acidosis.*
5. Bathe the newborn under the radiant warmer. If feasible, position the warmer close to a sink for a source of warm

(*continued on next page*)

SKILL 14.24 Newborn, Initial Bathing (continued)

water. Alternatively, fill a basin with warm water. **Rationale:** *Newborns need protection against heat loss by using warm, dry blankets and hats, or an external heat source such as the warmth of the mother's body or a warmer.*

6. Using a clean, warm, wet washcloth, clean the eyes, washing from the inner to outer canthus of each eye, moving to a clean portion of the washcloth for each eye.

7. Wash the remainder of the face, cleaning the washcloth after each use.

8. A mild soap may be used for the remainder of the bath. Wash the folds of skin in the neck and axilla. Wash between the fingers and toes.

CAUTION! Use only a small amount of soap. Excessive soap and lather can be difficult to rinse off.

---

9. Wash the abdomen, extremities, and back. Wash the groin and diaper area. Dry the newborn after each area is washed.

10. Complete cord care according to facility policy.

11. The hair and scalp can be washed using a mild shampoo, typically at a sink. To do so, wrap the newborn in a warm blanket with arms tucked inside the blanket out of the way. Hold the baby in a football hold with head extended over the sink. Use the free, cupped hand to bring water from the faucet to the baby's head. Wet the scalp, apply a small quantity of shampoo, lather, and rinse, again using a cupped hand to bring water to the newborn's head. Dry the head thoroughly and apply a cap. (*Note:* The head may also be shampooed over a basin.) **Rationale:** *It is important to work quickly and to dry the head thoroughly. The cap helps retain heat.*

12. Repeat assessment of temperature. If the temperature is normal and stable, dress the newborn in a shirt, diaper, and cap. Wrap the baby and return to parents in an open crib. If the newborn's axillary temperature is below 36.4°C (97.5°F), return the baby to the radiant warmer.

13. When the procedure is complete, perform hand hygiene and leave patient safe and comfortable with parent or guardian.

14. Complete documentation using forms, checklists, or electronic dropdown lists supplemented by nurse's notes or additional comments as appropriate, including any significant findings, and temperature in the medical record.

SAMPLE DOCUMENTATION

[date] 0900 Placed in radiant warmer, T 36.8°C (98.3°F) (A). Bath given, small amount meconium, blood, and vernix caseosa removed. Cord care provided. Cap applied to head. T 36.7°C (98.1°F) (A). Placed in warmed blanket and given to mother. C. Yin

---

SKILL 14.25 Newborn Thermoregulation: Assisting

Safety Note! *During scheduled clinical time, nursing students may have a learning opportunity to observe or assist with this skill only with faculty permission and with direct supervision from faculty or another RN.*

Thermoregulation is a way to minimize heat loss of the newborn, especially after birth and the weeks afterward. Equipment like the incubator and radiator warmer provide a warm environment for the newborn when care is provided. Towels and blankets are warmed before wrapping the newborn in them.

Delegation or Assignment

Making adjustments to newborn thermoregulation is the nurse's responsibility and not delegated or assigned to the UAP. The UAP may provide assistance in preparing warmed towels or blankets and turning on the incubator or radiant warmer. The nurse can request the UAP to report patient observations to the nurse for follow-up. The nurse remains responsible for the assessment, interpretation of abnormal findings, and determination of appropriate responses.

Equipment

- Incubator or radiant warmer
- Prewarmed towels or blankets
- Newborn stocking cap
- Servo control probe
- Newborn T-shirt and diaper
- Open crib
- Clean gloves

Preparation

- Review healthcare provider's orders and patient's nursing plan of care.
- Prewarm the incubator or radiant warmer. Make sure warm towels and/or lightweight blankets are available.
- Maintain the temperature of the birthing room at 22°C (71°F), with a relative humidity of 60–65%. **Rationale:** *The change from a warm, moist intrauterine environment to a cool, dry, drafty environment stresses the newborn's immature thermoregulation system.*

CAUTION! Gloves are worn whenever there is the possibility of contact with body fluids—in this case, a newborn wet with amniotic fluid, vernix, and maternal blood.

SKILL 14.25 Newborn Thermoregulation: Assisting (*continued*)

Procedure

1. Introduce self to parent and verify the patient's identity using two identifiers. Explain to the parent that the newborn is placed in an incubator or radiant warmer to help maintain body temperature, why it is necessary, and how the patient can participate. Discuss how the results will be used in planning further care or treatments.
2. Perform hand hygiene and observe appropriate infection control procedures.
3. Provide for patient privacy, safety, warmth, and comfort. Don gloves.
4. Place the newborn under the radiant warmer. Wipe the newborn free of blood, fluid, and excess vernix, especially from the head, using prewarmed towels. **Rationale:** *Drying is important to prevent the loss of body heat through evaporation*. Discard gloves and perform hand hygiene.
5. If the newborn is stable, wrap the baby in a prewarmed blanket and apply a stocking cap.
   - Carry the baby to the mother. The mother and her support person can hold and enjoy the baby together.
   or
   - Carry the wrapped newborn to the mother, loosen the blanket, and place the baby skin to skin on the mother's chest under a warmed blanket. **Rationale:** *Use of a prewarmed blanket reduces convection heat loss and facilitates maternal–newborn baby contact without compromising the newborn's thermoregulation*.
6. After the newborn has spent time with the parents, return the baby to the radiant warmer. Leave the newborn uncovered (except for the cap and diaper) under the radiant warmer. **Rationale:** *Radiant heat warms the outer skin surface, so the skin needs to be exposed*.
7. Tape a servo control probe on the newborn's anterior abdominal wall, with the metal side next to the skin. Do not place it over the ribs. Secure the probe with porous tape or a foil-covered aluminum heat deflector patch. The figure shows a newborn with a skin probe ❶. Note that in this picture, the newborn is no longer wearing a stocking cap.

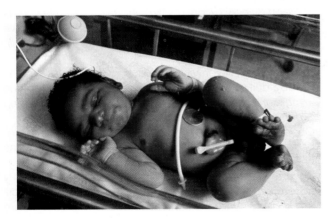

Source: Tom McCarthy/PhotoEdit, Inc.

❶ Temperature monitoring for the newborn. A skin thermal sensor is placed on the newborn's abdomen, upper thigh, or arm and secured with porous tape or a foil-covered foam pad.

CAUTION! The servo control is an electronic device that communicates with the incubator or radiant warmer to regulate heat produced. It functions as a thermostat to maintain a constant skin temperature for the newborn.

8. Turn the heater to servo control mode so that the abdominal skin is maintained at 36.0°C–36.5°C (96.8°F–97.7°F).

Safety Considerations

Take action to help the newborn maintain a stable temperature.

- Keep the newborn's clothing and bedding dry.
- Double-wrap the newborn and put a stocking cap on the baby.
- Use the radiant warmer during procedures.
- Reduce the newborn's exposure to drafts.
- Warm objects that will be in contact with the newborn (e.g., stethoscopes).
- Encourage the mother to snuggle with the newborn under blankets, or to breastfeed the baby with hat and light cover on.

9. Monitor the newborn's axillary and skin probe temperatures per facility protocol. **Rationale:** *The temperature indicator on the radiant warmer continually displays the newborn's probe temperature. The axillary temperature is checked to ensure that the machine is accurately recording the newborn's temperature*.
10. When the newborn's temperature reaches 37°C (98.6°F), add a T-shirt, double-wrap the baby (two blankets), and place the baby in an open crib.
11. Recheck the baby's temperature in 1 hour and regularly thereafter according to facility policy.
12. If the newborn's temperature drops below 36.1°C (97°F), rewarm the baby gradually. Place the newborn (unclothed except for a diaper) under the radiant warmer with a servo control probe on the anterior abdominal wall.
13. Recheck the newborn's temperature in 30 minutes, then hourly.
14. When the temperature reaches 37°C (98.6°F), dress the newborn, remove from the radiant warmer, double-wrap, and place in an open crib. Check the temperature hourly until stable, then regularly according to facility policy.
   Note: A newborn who repeatedly requires rewarming should be observed for other signs and symptoms of illness, and the healthcare provider should be notified, because it may warrant screening for infection.
15. When the procedure is complete, perform hand hygiene and leave patient safe and comfortable.
16. Complete documentation using forms, checklists, or electronic dropdown lists supplemented by nurse's notes or additional comments as appropriate.

SAMPLE DOCUMENTATION

[date] 1010 Tolerated assessment without incident. T 36.61°C (97.9°F) (A). Remains in radiant warmer wearing diaper and T-shirt. Mother at side of warmer. D. Brook

SKILL 14.26 Phototherapy, Newborn, Infant: Providing

Safety Note! *During scheduled clinical time, nursing students may have a learning opportunity to observe or assist with this skill only with faculty permission and with direct supervision from faculty or another RN.*

Phototherapy is light therapy to treat certain medical conditions, such as when the newborn has too much bilirubin in the blood and may have jaundice, called *hyperbilirubinemia.* Special light therapy helps break down the bilirubin for the body to remove.

Delegation or Assignment

Monitoring the newborn during phototherapy is the nurse's responsibility and is not delegated or assigned to the UAP. The UAP may provide assistance in preparing warmed towels or blankets. The nurse can request the UAP to report patient observations to the nurse for follow-up. The nurse remains responsible for the assessment, interpretation of abnormal findings, and determination of appropriate responses.

Equipment

- Bank of phototherapy lights
- Eye patches
- Small scale to weigh diapers

Preparation

- Review healthcare provider's orders and patient's nursing plan of care.
- Be sure that recent serum bilirubin levels are available.
- Gather equipment and supplies.

Procedure

1. Introduce self to parent and verify the patient's identity using two identifiers. Explain to the parent the purpose of phototherapy, the procedure itself (including the need to use eye patches), and possible side effects, such as dehydration. Discuss how the results will be used in planning further care or treatments.
2. Perform hand hygiene and observe appropriate infection control procedures.
3. Provide for patient privacy, safety, and comfort.
4. Obtain vital signs, including the axillary temperature. Assess for jaundice in the skin, sclera, and mucous membranes (in newborns or infants with darkly pigmented skin). **Rationale:** *The most recent assessment results prior to starting therapy serve as a baseline to evaluate the effectiveness of therapy.*
5. Phototherapy
   - Remove all of the newborn's or infant's clothing except the diaper. **Rationale:** *Best results with exposure of the newborn or infant to high-intensity light are obtained when there is maximum skin surface exposure.*
   - Apply eye coverings (eye patches or a bili mask) to the newborn or infant according to facility policy.

Rationale: *Eye coverings are used to protect delicate eye structures, particularly the retina, from injures.*
   - Place the newborn or infant in an open crib or isolette (more commonly used in preterm newborns or infants and babies who are sicker) about 45–50 cm (18–20 in.) below the bank of phototherapy lights.
   - Reposition newborn or infant every 2 hr. **Rationale:** *Repositioning exposes different areas of skin to the lights, prevents the development of pressure areas on the skin, and varies the stimulation the newborn or infant receives.*
   - Monitor vital signs every 4 hr with axillary temperatures. **Rationale:** *Temperature assessment is indicated to detect hypothermia or hyperthermia. Deviation in pulse and respirations may indicate developing complications.*
   - Check the lights using a bilimeter to ensure safe effective treatment.
   - Cluster care activities. **Rationale:** *Care activities are clustered to help ensure that the baby has maximum time under the lights.*
   - Discontinue phototherapy and remove eye patches at least once per 8-hr shift. Also, discontinue phototherapy and remove patches when feeding the newborn or infant and when the parents visit. **Rationale:** *Eye patches are removed to assess for signs of complications such as excessive pressure, discharge, or conjunctivitis. Patches are also removed to provide some social stimulation and to promote parental attachment.*

CAUTION! If the area of jaundice about the eyes begins to disappear, it is probable that the eye patches are allowing light to enter and better eye protection is needed.

6. Maintain adequate fluid intake and monitor urinary output and diarrheal stools. Evaluate the need for IV fluids.
   - Weigh diapers before discarding. **Rationale:** *Newborns or infants undergoing phototherapy treatment have increased water loss and loose stools as a result of bilirubin excretion.*
   - Assess specific gravity with each voiding and weigh the baby daily. **Rationale:** *Specific gravity provides one measure for urine concentration, a sign of developing dehydration, and weight loss is another sign.*
7. Observe the newborn or infant for signs of perianal excoriation, and implement appropriate skin therapy as needed.
8. Ensure that serum bilirubin levels are drawn regularly according to orders or facility policy. Turn the phototherapy lights off while the blood is drawn. **Rationale:** *Serum bilirubin levels provide the most accurate indication of the effectiveness of phototherapy. They are generally drawn every 12 hr, but at least once daily. The phototherapy lights are turned off to ensure accurate serum bilirubin levels.*

SKILL 14.26 Phototherapy, Newborn, Infant: Providing *(continued)*

9. Examine the baby's skin regularly for signs of developing pressure areas, bronzing, maculopapular rash, and changes in degree of jaundice. **Rationale:** *Pressure areas may develop if the newborn or infant lies in one position for an extended period. A benign, transient bronze discoloration of the skin may occur with phototherapy when the newborn or infant has elevated direct serum bilirubin levels or liver disease. A maculopapular rash is another transient side effect of phototherapy that develops occasionally.*

10. Avoid using lotion or ointment on the exposed skin during phototherapy. **Rationale:** *These may cause skin burns.*

11. Provide parents with opportunities to hold the newborn or infant and assist in the newborn's or infant's care. Answer their questions accurately and keep them informed of developments or changes. **Rationale:** *Information helps them deal with their anxiety. They have a right to be kept informed of their baby's status to be able to make informed decisions as needed.*

12. When the procedure is complete, perform hand hygiene and leave patient safe, warm, and comfortable.

13. Complete documentation using forms, checklists, or electronic dropdown lists supplemented by nurse's notes or additional comments as appropriate.

SAMPLE DOCUMENTATION

[date] 0530 Small amount light brown watery stool noted on diaper with small amount urine. Skin cleaned and dried, no signs of redness noted. Tolerated cleaning without crying. Resting quietly at this time.
P. Smith

Safety Considerations

Phototherapy can be provided by using lightweight fiberoptic blankets ("bili blankets").

- With fiberoptic blankets, the newborn is readily accessible for care, feedings, and diaper changes.
- The baby does not get overheated, and fluid and weight loss are not complications of this system.
- The baby is accessible to the parents, and the procedure seems less alarming to parents than standard phototherapy.
- A combination of a fiberoptic light source in the mattress under the baby and a standard phototherapy light source above is also used by some agencies.
- Many agencies and pediatricians use fiberoptic blankets for home care.

SKILL 14.27 Umbilical Cord Clamp: Caring for

After birth, the newborn no longer needs the umbilical cord to connect to the placenta. An umbilical cord clamp is applied to the umbilical cord just before cutting away the excess cord distal to the clamp. Care of the cord is to keep it clean and dry and prevent injury or infection to this area while it is drying. This clamp is removed after the cord has dried and ready to fall off.

Delegation or Assignment

Assisting with the application and removing the umbilical cord clamp is the nurse's responsibility and is not delegated or assigned to the UAP. The UAP may provide care of the newborn baby as trained. The nurse can request the UAP to report patient observations to the nurse for follow-up. The nurse remains responsible for the assessment, interpretation of abnormal findings, and determination of appropriate responses.

Equipment

- Disposable umbilical cord clamp
- Prescribed preparations: triple dye or bacitracin ointment for initial cord care
- Cord clamp remover or scissors
- Gloves

Preparation

- Review healthcare provider's orders and patient's nursing plan of care.
- Verify signed informed consent is available in the patient's record if required by facility.
- Gather equipment and supplies.

Procedure

APPLICATION (to prevent bleeding and promote adaptation to extrauterine circulation)

1. Assist healthcare provider as needed to perform the following actions:
   - Places a disposable clamp at the base of the cord about 2.5 cm (1 in.) distal to the skin demarcation line
   - Secures the clamp by pressing until it clicks and locks
   - Cuts away excess cord distal to the disposable clamp
   - Examines the cord and counts the vessels (one vein and two arteries)
   - Applies antimicrobial agent over the base of the cord and on 2.5 cm (1 in.) of surrounding skin. **Rationale:** *Antimicrobial ointments may be used for initial cord care in an attempt to minimize microorganisms and promote drying.*

(continued on next page)

SKILL 14.27 Umbilical Cord Clamp: Caring for (continued)

2. Documents status of the clamp and cord using forms, checklists, or electronic dropdown lists supplemented by nurse's notes or additional comments as appropriate.

CARE (promotes drying and sloughing of the cord and prevents infection)

1. Apply diapers so that they are folded below the umbilical cord and do not dampen the cord with urine.
2. Change the diaper frequently to prevent urine from soaking the diaper and cord.
3. Keep the site clean and dry per facility protocol ❶. **Rationale:** *Wetness and moistness promote growth of microorganisms.*

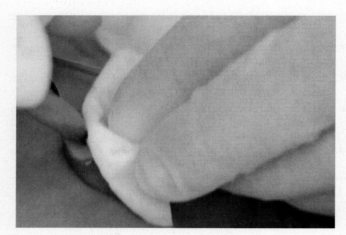

Source: George Dodson/Pearson Education, Inc.

❶ The umbilical cord base is carefully cleaned.

4. Assess the cord for signs and symptoms of infection (foul smell, redness, and greenish-yellow drainage, localized heat and tenderness) or bleeding.

CAUTION! The healthcare provider should be called for signs or symptoms of infection (step 4 above) or continuous bleeding from the umbilical cord stump.

5. Document the condition of the cord in the medical record as part of routine assessment.

REMOVAL (cord should look dark and dried up before falling off before discharge)

1. Verify that the stump is thoroughly dry.
2. Apply the cord clamp removal device or insert scissors into the loop at the base of the clamp.
3. Cut through the loop, directing the tool away from the cord and baby.
4. Observe for any oozing or bleeding.
5. Instruct parents regarding care of the site. Advise them to contact their healthcare provider if bleeding, oozing, or odor is noticed.

6. Complete documentation using forms, checklists, or electronic dropdown lists supplemented by nurse's notes or additional comments as appropriate, including the condition of the cord and teaching.

SAMPLE DOCUMENTATION

[date] 1420 Umbilical cord stump continues to remain dry without drainage. Site cleaned with normal saline and dried, no odor, redness, or bleeding noted. Clamp remains intact. Demonstrated how to clean with Dad observing. Tolerated site care without incident. *C. Pines*

EVIDENCE-BASED PRACTICE

Problem

Years ago, it was believed that the umbilical cord of a newborn should be clamped immediately after birth (within 15 seconds) to prevent the mother from losing too much blood. A few years later, evidence showed there was no significant blood loss. The question now is when is the best time to clamp the umbilical cord for the newborn after vaginal or caesarean birth—before 1 minute (sometimes referred to as *early clamping*), or 1–3 min (sometimes referred to as *late clamping*)?

Evidence

After evaluation and analysis of evidence, the WHO guideline development group included vaginal and caesarean births and preterm and term births in their recommendations for umbilical cord clamping. Evidence showed delaying cord clamping 1–3 min after birth is the best timing for this procedure. The exception to this recommendation is if the newborn requires positive-pressure ventilation or other resuscitative measures, then the cord should be clamped so as not to impede emergency measures.

Evidence is increasing in support of the benefits from the newborn receiving extra blood from the placenta at birth. There are now long-range studies supporting benefits in children who had delayed cord clamping. Evidence for delayed cord clamping for preterm babies is more accepted because of benefits such as more red blood cell volume, higher iron level, and improved circulation transition. There is support for delaying cord clamping to collect umbilical cord blood for banking. Complications for the term newborn with delayed cord clamping might include polycythemia resulting in the need for phototherapy.

Implications

There is currently not enough strong evidence to definitively decide the correct time for all newborns to have the cord clamped. WHO recommends that delayed umbilical cord clamping of over 1 minute from birth is the most advantageous time unless resuscitative measures are required or there are other complications of placental abnormalities or high-risk conditions of maternal health. As a partner with the healthcare provider, the mother needs to have a discussion about this topic with the healthcare provider before the birthing process begins.

Sources: Society for Maternal-Fetal Medicine (SMFM), (2014); World Health Organization (WHO), (2014); American Congress of Obstetricians and Gynecologists (ACOG), (2017); and Public Radio News Network (NPR), (2015).

›› Critical Thinking Options for Unexpected Outcomes

Not all unexpected outcomes require further nursing intervention; however, many times they do. When the patient demonstrates a change in signs or symptoms indicating an emerging problem, the nurse should immediately assess and troubleshoot what is happening. The assessment data must be processed quickly to formulate a hypothesis so the nurse can make a clinical judgment. The nurse then decides how best to resolve the problem and improve the patient's situation for a better outcome.

EXPECTED OUTCOME	UNEXPECTED OUTCOME	POSSIBLE INTERVENTIONS
Antepartum Care There are no signs of side effects or allergic responses at the injection site of administered Rh immune globulin.	Patient complains about tenderness at the injection site.	■ Monitor for temperature elevation. ■ Apply local warmth to the injection site. ■ Monitor for signs and symptoms of infection of site. ■ Notify physician or certified nurse-midwife (MD/CNM) if needed.
Patient experiences no physical problems during pregnancy.	Patient complains of constipation in the second trimester.	■ Encourage patient to drink adequate fluids. ■ Encourage patient to eat fibrous foods. ■ Ask healthcare provider (MD/CNM) about medication interventions like stool softeners, laxatives, or enemas.
Patient experiences no physical problems during pregnancy (cont.).	Patient has a urinary tract infection.	■ Take antibiotics and medication for discomfort as ordered by healthcare provider (MD/CNM). ■ Encourage patient to drink adequate fluids. ■ Reinforce good perineal hygiene practices, like wearing panty liners. ■ Perform Kegel exercises. ■ Maintain bladder emptying pattern.
Intrapartum Care Induction of labor with Pitocin progresses without evidence of fetal distress.	Fetal distress is noted with a patient receiving Pitocin during intrapartum care.	■ Stop the Pitocin infusion. ■ Stay with the patient, and help her reposition to her side. ■ Administer supplemental oxygen following facility guidelines. ■ Monitor maternal vital signs and fetal heartbeat. ■ Monitor contractions. ■ Notify healthcare provider (MD/CNM).
Ongoing fetal heartbeat documentation occurs with external electronic fetal monitoring.	The electronic fetal monitoring system stops producing fetal heartbeat strips.	■ Manually check fetal heartbeat rate. ■ Check monitoring system for available recording paper, and replace empty roll with new roll if needed. ■ Check placement of transducer and belt. ■ Continue monitoring with printed documentation of fetal heartbeat rate and rhythm.
Postpartum Care The patient has progressively less lochia every day.	Lochia remains bright red with heavier flow.	■ Assess vital signs and tenderness. ■ Assess for recent activity of patient (may indicate patient has increased activities too much and too soon). ■ Notify healthcare provider (MD/CNM) if patient states there has not been an increase in activity and the flow remains heavy and bright red (may indicate postpartum hemorrhage, which is a medical emergency).
Newborn Care The newborn's cord is kept clean and dry.	The newborn's umbilical cord is moist with a reddened base.	■ This response is indicative of infection. ■ Antibiotic ointment may be prescribed. ■ Clean area periodically and keep it dry. ■ Monitor for any bleeding or drainage until cord is dried and occluded.

REVIEW Questions

1. During an assessment, the nurse palpates a pregnant client's abdomen. What should the nurse do once the fetal back is identified?
   1. Palpate the feet for edema.
   2. Auscultate the fetal heartbeat.
   3. Measure the client's blood pressure.
   4. Estimate the number of weeks gestation.

2. A pregnant client is concerned about swelling around the eyes and bracelets and rings being too tight. What should the nurse assess to help determine if the client is experiencing eclampsia?
   1. Fundal height
   2. Fetal heart rate
   3. Deep tendon reflexes
   4. Capillary blood glucose

3. During her first prenatal visit, a pregnant client relates having an elective abortion 3 years ago. What information should the nurse obtain to determine if the client needs Rh immune globulin?
   1. Rh factor
   2. Blood type
   3. Fundal height
   4. Weeks of gestation

4. The nurse notes that the blood pressure of a client receiving epidural anesthesia during labor has dropped to 98/60 mmHg. What should the nurse prepare to administer to this client?
   1. Naloxone
   2. Ephedrine
   3. Intravenous fluids
   4. Magnesium sulfate

5. The fetus of a client in labor is demonstrating signs of distress. What must the nurse ensure prior to placing an internal fetal scalp electrode?
   1. Cervix is dilated 1 cm.
   2. Amniotic sac has ruptured.
   3. Client is in a side-lying position.
   4. Monitoring cables are connected.

6. While examining the amount of cervical dilation, a client in labor is diagnosed with a prolapsed umbilical cord. What action should the nurse take?
   1. Hold the cord gently.
   2. Assist the client out of bed to a chair.
   3. Apply oxygen 10 L/min via face mask.
   4. Place the client in a side-lying position.

7. The nurse instructs a postpartum client on the type of lochia to expect after discharge. Which client statement indicates that additional teaching is required?
   1. "The amount of drainage should gradually change from red to pink to clear."
   2. "I should call my healthcare provider if the drainage changes to clear in a week."
   3. "Clots associated with heavy bleeding should be reported to my healthcare provider."
   4. "I should call my healthcare provider if I saturate more than 4 to 8 perineal pads each day."

8. The nurse prepares to assess the perineal tissue of a postpartum client with an episiotomy. What should be included in this assessment?
   1. Lochia
   2. Pain level
   3. Fundal height
   4. Approximation

9. Four hours after delivery, a client's uterus is three fingerbreadths above the umbilicus and feels soft. What should the nurse do **first**?
   1. Ask the client to void.
   2. Remove the perineal pad.
   3. Massage the uterine fundus.
   4. Apply pressure to the top of the fundus.

10. The nurse cares for a newborn who was just circumcised. What should the nurse instruct the parents to do to protect the surgical site?
    1. Apply petroleum gauze to the site.
    2. Fasten a diaper loosely over the penis.
    3. Position the newborn on the abdomen.
    4. Wrap the head of the penis with dry gauze.

11. A newborn's temperature is 36°C (96.9°F). What action should the nurse take **first**?
    1. Place the newborn under the radiant warmer.
    2. Remove all clothing except for the diaper.
    3. Apply the control probe on the anterior abdominal wall.
    4. Remeasure the newborn's temperature and double-wrap with blankets.

12. The nurse notes that a newborn receiving phototherapy is scheduled to have a bilirubin blood level drawn at 0800 hours. What should the nurse do to prepare the newborn for this laboratory test?
    1. Turn off the lights.
    2. Weigh the newborn.
    3. Remove the eye patches.
    4. Reposition under the lights.

Note: For answers and rationales for the review questions, go to Appendix A or your Pearson MyLab Nursing and eText.

Chapter 15
Safety

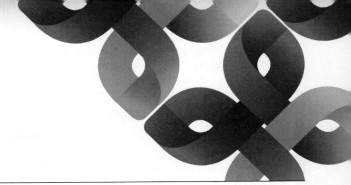

Chapter at a Glance

Patient Safety

Environmental Safety

Immobilizers and Restraints

» The Concept of Safety

To avoid accidents, injuries, infections, and errors, safety is an essential element for all nursing interventions, in all healthcare settings, for all patients' significant others, and all healthcare personnel. When safety is not a priority, safety records show an increase in accidents and errors. Many daily routines of patient care include preventive safety measures to provide safe quality care. There are many situations that require nurses to be alert and able to recognize possible hazards that could lead to accidents, injuries, infections, and errors. These include specific safety hazards associated with age groups across the lifespan, potential environmental hazards such as fire or dangerous weather conditions, and specific safety concerns associated with interventions like use of restraints. They also include interventions using aseptic technique and completing other safety steps to protect patients, others, and themselves.

Learning Outcomes

15.1 Summarize significant cues that would lead you to suspect abuse of an older adult.

15.2 Give examples of interventions to implement for fall prevention with the older adult.

15.3 Support safety preparations for a patient with a history of seizures.

15.4 Explain why environmental safety involves everyone participating in a Safety Program.

15.5 Show how to prevent electrical injuries from electrical devices brought in from home by the patient.

15.6 Summarize four top priorities to do when you see a fire in the patient's waste receptacle.

15.7 Demonstrate the correct way to apply a wrist restraint.

15.8 Differentiate between using an immobilizer to stabilize a child for a procedure and using a restraint to keep the patient safe from injuring himself or herself.

The following feature links some, but not all, of the concepts related to assessment. They are presented in alphabetical order.

Concepts Related to
Safety

CONCEPT	RELATIONSHIP TO SAFETY	NURSING IMPLICATIONS
Accountability	Zero tolerance for intentional neglect or knowingly providing wrong patient care.	▪ Nurses are responsible to provide the standard of nursing care. ▪ Due process should be followed with consequences by state Boards of Nursing.
Caring Interventions	Consideration for the safety of patient when providing care. Safe medication administration.	▪ Be vigilant in observations for safety issues when providing care to patients. ▪ Diligently follow rights of safe medication administration every time.
Clinical Decision Making	Make clinical judgments based on safety for patients, others, and self.	▪ Maintain prevention measures for a safe environment without injury, accident, or illness hazards.
Evidence-Based Practice	Remain current in evidence-based best safety practices.	▪ Modify actions and utilize current evidence when caring for patients for better patient outcomes.
Professional Behaviors	There is a duty to provide current quality care that is consistently safe to all patients.	▪ Stay current as lifetime learner with evidence-based best practices. ▪ Provide same level of care to all patients.

≫ Patient Safety

Expected Outcomes

1. Patient's safety is maintained during the entire healthcare facility stay.
2. All personal articles and call light are within easy reach of the patient.
3. If oxygen is used, appropriate safety measures are in effect.
4. Appropriate care is provided every 2 hr for the patient with restraints.
5. Patient is safely repositioned or transferred without injury to patient or caregiver.
6. Appropriate assistive devices are utilized to transfer patient.
7. Caregiver is able to manage turning, repositioning, and assistive devices.
8. Appropriate body mechanics are utilized by caregiver.

SKILL 15.1 Abuse: Newborn, Infant, Child, Older Adult, Assessing for

Newborns, infants, and children from their birth to 17 years and adults age 65 years or older endure abuse, neglect, and exploitation in many forms from family, friends, and caregivers. According to the Centers for Disease Control and Prevention (CDC), approximately one out of every seven children experience some form of abuse and neglect (CDC, 2016). There are federal and state laws protecting these age groups as well as others who are not able to take care of themselves and who depend on family or caregivers to provide for their basic needs.

Delegation or Assignment

Due to specific knowledge and skill in performing an assessment for an abused newborn, infant, child, or older adult, this skill is not delegated or assigned to the UAP. The nurse can request the UAP to report patient observations to the nurse for follow-up. The nurse remains responsible for the assessment, interpretation of abnormal finds, and determination of appropriate actions.

Preparation

▪ Review healthcare provider's orders and patient's nursing plan of care.

▪ If assisting with the initial assessment of a known abused patient, be familiar with policies and procedures for chain-of-custody to protect and preserve any forensic evidence.

▪ If doing an assessment on an unknown abused patient and discover indications of physical or mental abuse, be familiar with state laws about reporting newborn, infant, child, and older adult abuse. By law, when nurses suspect abuse of any individual, they are mandated to report it to the appropriate authorities. Follow healthcare facility policies and procedures.

▪ Provide a safe environment for the patient ❶.

▪ Gather supplies.

SKILL 15.1 Abuse: Newborn, Infant, Child, Older Adult, Assessing for *(continued)*

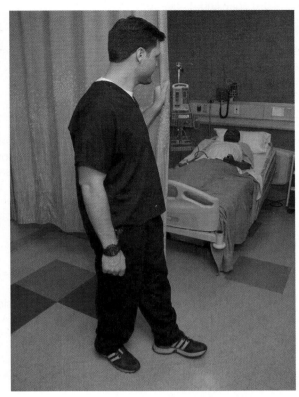

Source: Rick Brady/Pearson Education, Inc.

❶ The abused patient should feel safe and comfortable while in the healthcare facility.

Procedure

1. Introduce self to patient and verify the patient's identity using two identifiers. Explain to the patient you are going to do an assessment, why it is necessary, and how the patient can participate. Discuss how the results will be used in planning further care or treatments. Provide support and build rapport and trust in the nurse-patient relationship.
2. Perform hand hygiene and observe appropriate infection control procedures.
3. Provide for patient privacy, safety, and comfort.
4. Assess the patient for indications of neglect: failure to have adequate food, clothing, medical assistance, or assistance with activities of daily living (ADLs) provided. Check body for signs of cleanliness. Determine if emotional abuse is present. Ask about threats, intimidation, or isolation.
5. For an adult patient, identify if financial abuse has occurred, such as misuse of finances or personal and tangible property.
6. For all patients, assess for signs of physical abuse.
   - Signs of passive restraining or bilateral bruises, or parallel injuries, may indicate forceful restraining; shaking may cause parallel injuries of upper arms.
   - Contusions may appear on trunk, abdomen, buttocks, upper thighs (some black and blue; others yellow, green, or beige).

- Multiple scars and wounds or abrasions may appear in different stages of healing.
- Sexual abuse may cause edema, bruising, or tearing in the genital or anal area.
- Usually, accidental injuries affect knees, back of hands, forehead, and elbows.
- Check skin for tissue breakdown, such as pressure ulcers.
- Note signs of sprains, dislocations, or fractures from pulling or pushing the patient.
7. Assess for signs of malnourishment or dehydration.
8. Ask about visits to the hospital emergency department (ED). (If the patient is a child, ask the parent.) Ask why patient sought medical care, and how much time elapsed between injury and visit to ED.
9. Assess for signs of emotional abuse. Observe if patient is fearful of strangers, becomes quiet when caregiver enters room, refuses to answer if caregiver is present, or craves attention and socialization.
10. When the procedure is complete, perform hand hygiene and leave patient safe and comfortable.
11. Complete documentation using forms, checklists, or electronic dropdown lists supplemented by nurse's notes or additional comments as appropriate.

SAMPLE DOCUMENTATION

[date] 1930 Laying on her side in semi-Fowler position in bed, awake and looking around room. During toileting assistance, bruising noted bilateral buttocks, 5 cm (2 in.) wide by 15 cm (6 in.) long, black, blue contusion noted with reddened area, tender to touch. Patient crying as she stated, "My daughter hit me with a belt when I couldn't make it to the bathroom this afternoon." Stayed with patient, charge nurse called to come to room via call bell. Discussion with patient, charge nurse, and myself concerning the noted bruising injury. *T. May*

Safety Considerations
QUESTIONS TO ASK IF ABUSE IS SUSPECTED

- Who cares for you at home?
- Did someone hurt you?
- Are you happy with where you live?
- Tell me about your daily routine.
- Who assists you with everyday activities?
- Do you feel safe living here?
- Adult patient: Who manages your money?
- How did the injury (or bruises) occur?
- Did you receive medical attention?
- Has this type of injury happened before?

SKILL 15.2 Fall Prevention: Assessing and Managing

Fall prevention includes interventions implemented to prevent the occurrence of falls. For adults age 65 and older, falls are the leading cause of injury (NCOA, 2016). According to a report from The Joint Commission, hundreds of thousands of patients in hospitals fall each year, and approximately half of them sustain injuries (The Joint Commission, 2015). Assessment for the risk for falls is included in the initial admission assessment to determine the need for fall prevention interventions.

Delegation or Assignment

Due to specific knowledge and skill in performing an assessment on the patient for having a high risk for falls, this skill is not delegated or assigned to the UAP. The nurse can request the UAP to assist in setting up preventive measures and to report patient observations to the nurse for follow-up. The nurse remains responsible for the assessment, interpretation of abnormal finds, and determination of appropriate actions.

Equipment

- Have patient's assistive device for walking kept close to bed (if patient uses one)
- Chair alarm as needed
- Tracking electronic device as needed
- Bed alarm activated as needed

Preparation

- Review healthcare provider's orders and patient's nursing plan of care.
- Review patient's record for history of falls.
- Gather equipment and supplies.

Procedure

1. Introduce self to patient and verify the patient's identity using two identifiers. Explain to the patient you are going to do an assessment of risks for falls, why it is necessary, and how the patient can participate. Discuss how the results will be used in planning further care or treatments.
2. Perform hand hygiene and observe appropriate infection control procedures.
3. Provide for patient privacy, safety, and comfort.
4. Assess patient for indications of a risk for falling ❶:
   - Balance or posture instability, abnormal gait, use of assistive devices for walking
   - Altered sensorium or cognition such as confusion, dementia, or medication-induced
   - Frequency of toileting needs

FALL RISK ASSESSMENT FORM

PATIENT INFORMATION

Name _____

Age _____

Allergies _____

Current medications _____

ASSESSMENT* (check if applicable; add specifics as indicated)

Gait

- ☐ Normal length   ☐ Symmetrical
- ☐ Lifts feet   ☐ Maintains direction
- ☐ Outside normal limits (describe) _____

Balance

- ☐ Standing   ☐ Sitting
- ☐ Outside normal limits (describe) _____
- ☐ Cognition (describe) _____

HISTORY*

- ☐ History of falls in past 3 months   ☐ Orthostatic hypotension
- ☐ Dehydration   ☐ Hypoglycemia
- ☐ Cardiac dysrhythmia   ☐ Anemia
- ☐ Seizures   ☐ TIA or stroke
- ☐ Delirium
- ☐ Arthritis
- ☐ Joint replacement (specify) _____
- ☐ Neurologic disorder (specify) _____
- ☐ UTI or other infection (specify) _____
- ☐ Osteoporosis and fracture (describe) _____
- ☐ Effects of medication (specify) _____

ENVIRONMENTAL/EXTRINSIC RISK FACTORS*

- ☐ Use of assistive device (specify) _____
- ☐ IV/heparin lock
- ☐ Absence of grab bars and assistive devices   ☐ Poorly lit environment
                                                    ☐ Clutter and trip hazards in environment

* NOTE: Existence of multiple risk factors requires review and possible use of facility's Fall Risk Protocol.

❶ Fall Risk Assessment Form.

SKILL 15.2 Fall Prevention: Assessing and Managing (*continued*)

- History of seizures or episodes of syncope
- Any sensory deficits such as blurring of vision
- Musculoskeletal disorders or deficits of mobility
- History of previous falls
- Postural hypotension when standing up

5. Implement preventive measures.
   - Per facility policy, identify high risk patients with a color-coded armband, safety socks, sign on door, or other visual cues for staff to recognize patient has a risk of falling.
   - Use bed alarms and electronic tracking devices.
   - Ask family members to stay with patient, or provide sitters to observe patient and assist patient to prevent falls.
   - Have staff do safety rounds and offer toileting assistance more frequently on patients at risk for falls to ensure safety measures remain active.
   - Call for help when getting up out of bed or walking as needed.
   - Have pharmacist review patient's medication profile.
   - Place patient items within easy reach.
   - Wear nonskid socks or slippers.
   - Have good lighting in the room.
   - Use handrails in hallways and bathrooms as needed ❷ ❸ ❹.
   - Involve all disciplines taking care of the patient in fall prevention strategies.
   - Keep patient's room clutter-free with furniture out of walkway to bathroom.
   - Observe patient using assistive devices when walking to ensure proper technique.
   - Assist patient in planning physical activities to build strength, coordination, and balance as able to do.

Safety Considerations

WHAT HEALTHCARE FACILITIES CAN DO

- Involve all employees in a falls prevention program, including safety training to help patients and others avoid falls.
- Use signage to mark wet floor areas.
- Use a team approach with all departments to provide fall prevention for patients.
- Complete a risk for falls assessment on patients on admission.
- Include safety interventions specific for patient in nursing plan of care.
- Teach patient and family about personal safety actions to prevent falls.
- Use evidence-based fall prevention measures during patient's stay in the healthcare facility.
- Do a root-cause analysis of all falls resulting in injuries to identify contributing factors, such as communication breakdown, not following routine safety practices, or inadequate staffing.

6. Managing patients after a fall.
   - Notify charge nurse of patient's fall.
   - Do a systematic assessment for injury or complication before moving patient.
     - Check for spinal injury or signs or symptoms of a bone fracture; stabilize and immobilize if needed.

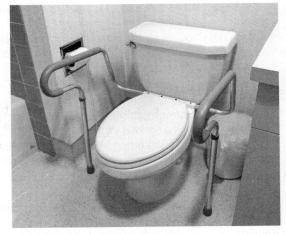

Source: Ronald May/Pearson Education, Inc.

❷ Rails next to the toilet assist in preventing patient falls.

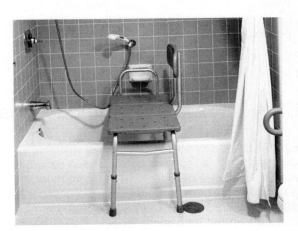

Source: Ronald May/Pearson Education, Inc.

❸ Shower chairs provide for patient safety.

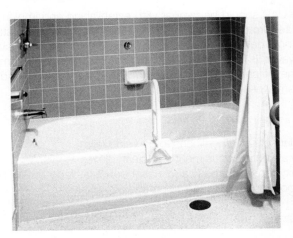

Source: Ronald May/Pearson Education, Inc.

❹ Safety features such as handrails on bathtubs assist in preventing patient falls.

(*continued on next page*)

SKILL 15.2 Fall Prevention: Assessing and Managing *(continued)*

- Check for active bleeding; apply local pressure if needed.
- Check neurological status if head injury has occurred; orientation to person, time, place, pupils, sensorium, and motor/sensory deficits.
- Check vital signs and O_2 saturation.
- Injury needs to be evaluated by healthcare provider within a reasonable amount of time depending on the injury. If patient has a serious injury, patient can be evaluated and treated by the emergency department healthcare provider until primary healthcare provider arrives.
- Documentation is done in patient's record and by completing an incident report.
- Fall prevention measures may need to be enhanced to include increasing frequency of safety rounds, assigning staff to stay with patient until family can arrange a sitter, moving patient closer to the nurses' station, and reviewing patient's medication profile.

7. When assessment is complete, perform hand hygiene. Leave patient safe and comfortable, and keep bed in low position with wheels locked.

8. Complete documentation using forms, checklists, or electronic dropdown lists supplemented by nurse's notes or additional comments as appropriate.

SAMPLE DOCUMENTATION

[date] 0320 Discovered on floor by bathroom door in room. States he slipped and fell when walking from the bathroom back to bed. Awake and alert, denies pain anywhere, no active bleeding noted, denies hitting head or discomfort of neck. No tenderness or deformity noted all 4 extremities, denies dizziness or change in moving. PERRLA noted. Helped to get back up and walk to bed, tolerated without complaint. States he just wants to go back to sleep. V/S 114/82, 78, 18, O_2 saturation 98% room air. Encouraged to put call light on to ask for assistance next time he needs to go to the bathroom. *A. Nixon*

SKILL 15.3 Seizure Precautions: Implementing

A seizure is caused by the sudden burst of electrical activity in the brain and lasts a short amount of time. A seizure is not a disease, but rather a disorder resulting from medical conditions that affect the brain. There are chemical changes in nerve cells that result in surges of electrical activity and seizures. This skill focuses on the tonic-clonic seizure (previously called a *grand mal* seizure).

Delegation or Assignment

The UAP should be familiar with establishing and implementing seizure precautions and methods of obtaining assistance during a patient's seizure. Care of the patient during a seizure, however, is the responsibility of the nurse due to the importance of careful assessment of respiratory status and the potential need for intervention.

Equipment

- Blankets or other linens to pad side rails
- Oral suction equipment and clean gloves
- Oxygen equipment and nasal cannula, face mask, head hood, or tent depending on age of patient

Preparation

- Review healthcare provider's orders and patient's nursing plan of care.
- Review patient's record for history of seizure activity in the past and current history.
- Gather equipment and supplies.

Procedure

1. Introduce self to patient and verify the patient's identity using two identifiers. Explain to the patient (and parent) what a seizure is, why it happens, and how family can keep the patient safe during a seizure. Discuss how the results will be used in planning further care or treatments.
2. Perform hand hygiene and observe appropriate infection control procedures.
3. Provide for patient privacy.

SEIZURE PRECAUTIONS

4. Create a safety plan before a seizure:
   - Maintain patient's bed in lowest position with top side rails up and wheels locked. **Rationale:** *This is to help prevent injury from fall or trauma.*
   - Provide helmets for children who have frequent seizures.
   - Pad the bed of the older child or adult patient who might have a seizure. Secure blankets or other linens around the head, foot, and side rails of the bed ❶.
   - Put oral suction equipment in place and test to ensure that it is functional. **Rationale:** *Suctioning may be needed to prevent aspiration of oral secretions.*
   - Assemble oxygen setup with flowmeter and test to ensure that it is functional. **Rationale:** *Oxygen may be needed to oxygenate patient.*
   - If seizure triggers are known, determine changes that might be made in patient's scheduled tests or treatments. **Rationale:** *This is to avoid possible seizure activity.*

SKILL 15.3 Seizure Precautions: Implementing (*continued*)

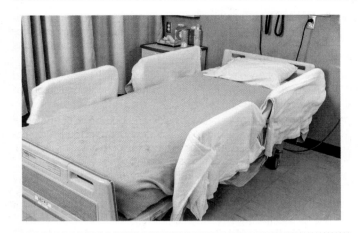

① Padding a bed for seizure precautions.

- Assign the patient to a room located close to the nurses' station.
- Keep unnecessary equipment out of the patient's room.

SEIZURE ACTIVITY

CAUTION! If the patient is experiencing an aura before a seizure begins, have the patient lie down to prevent falling or hitting head on side rail.

5. Follow safety procedures when a seizure occurs.
   - Remain with the patient and call for assistance. Do not restrain the patient.
   - If the patient is not in bed, assist patient to the floor and protect the patient's head from injury. Loosen any clothing around the neck and chest.
   - Turn the patient to a lateral position if possible. **Rationale:** *Turning to the side allows secretions to drain out of the mouth, decreasing the risk of aspiration, and helps keep the tongue from occluding the airway.*
   - Move items in the environment to ensure the patient does not experience an injury.
   - Do not insert anything into the patient's mouth.
   - Time the seizure duration.
   - Observe the progression of the seizure, noting the sequence and type of limb involvement. Observe skin color. When the seizure allows, check pulse and respirations.
   - Don gloves and use equipment to suction the mouth if the patient vomits or has excessive oral secretions.
   - Apply oxygen via mask or nasal cannula to an older child or adult. Apply oxygen to a newborn, infant, or child via head hood, tent, nasal cannula, or face mask, depending on the age and size of the child.
   - Administer anticonvulsant medications as ordered.
6. Follow safety procedures when a seizure ends.
   - This is the postictal phase, when the patient has an altered state of consciousness, commonly with drowsiness and confused behaviors for a short period of time.
   - Continue to protect the patient and assist patient to a comfortable position.
   - Reorient the patient, explain what happened, and reassure the patient.
   - Sometimes the patient may lose bladder or bowel control during seizure activity. Don gloves and assist the patient with hygiene and change linen as necessary.
   - Allow the patient to verbalize feelings about the seizure.
7. If applied, remove and discard gloves. Perform hand hygiene and leave patient safe and comfortable. Notify healthcare provider of seizure.
8. Complete documentation using forms, checklists, or electronic dropdown lists supplemented by nurse's notes or additional comments as appropriate.

SAMPLE DOCUMENTATION

[date] 1815 Observed generalized muscle spasms/contractions of arms and legs lasting 25 seconds. Seizure padding previously placed on bed. Incontinent of urine. Cyanotic. Placed on left side. Oral suctioning done. Airway clear. Respirations 14/min with irregular pattern. O_2 applied at 4 LPM via face mask. O_2 saturation 90% on 4 LPM O_2. Not currently responding to verbal or painful stimuli. Dr. Smith notified. Diazepam 10 mg given IV per order. VS taken every 15 min. See neuro flow sheet. *M. Faustino*

1835 Respirations 15/min, regular. Responding to verbal stimuli, oriented to person, place, and time. O_2 saturation 95% on O_2. O_2 discontinued per healthcare provider's order. VS taken every 15 min. See neuro flow sheet. *M. Faustino*

Lifespan Considerations

NEWBORNS

- Newborns have seizures very differently than children, so are difficult to recognize as a seizure. They often do not have jerking, stiffness, or twitching but instead are more focal such as smacking their lips, or having their eyes straying in different directions, or having short periods of apnea.
- Seizure activity is caused by a variety of conditions including neurologic dysfunction.

INFANTS AND CHILDREN

- For many children, there may be no discernible cause for a seizure, but sometimes the seizure is triggered by an injury or disease.
- As children grow up, their brains develop and seizure activity can change.

(*continued on next page*)

SKILL 15.3 Seizure Precautions: Implementing *(continued)*

- Febrile seizures (temperatures above 39°C [102°F]) are associated with acute infections, occur in children, and are usually preventable through the use of antipyretics and tepid baths.
- Certain neurologic conditions with learning and behavior impairments may be associated with seizure activity.
- Children on anticonvulsant medications should wear a medical identification tag (bracelet or necklace).

Safety Considerations
SEIZURE PREPAREDNESS AT HOME

- Discuss with the patient and family the factors that may precipitate a seizure.

- Ensure if patient has frequent or recurrent seizures or takes anticonvulsant medications, a medical identification tag (bracelet or necklace) should be worn and a card delineating any medications taken should be carried.
- Ensure family periodically inspects anticonvulsant medications and confirms that patient is taking them correctly. Blood level measurements may need to be scheduled.
- Discuss safety precautions for inside and outside of the home. If seizures are not well controlled, activities that may require restriction or direct supervision by others include tub bathing, swimming, cooking, using electric equipment or machinery, and driving.
- Assist patient in determining which individuals in the community should be informed of his or her seizure disorder (e.g., employers, healthcare providers such as dentists, motor vehicle department if driving, companions).

SKILL 15.4 Suicide: Caring for Suicidal Patient

Suicide is ranked as the tenth leading cause of death in the United States and includes ages that range from 10 years old to 64 years old (CDC, 2015). When suicide occurs in an acute healthcare facility, it is categorized as a sentinel event. The staff who have taken care of the patient are often devastated and blame themselves. Early identification of a potentially suicidal patient can make a difference, allowing safety interventions to be implemented to prevent and protect the patient from suicidal behaviors.

Delegation or Assignment

Assessment of a patient is the nurse's responsibility and is not delegated or assigned to the UAP. The UAP may provide routine care of the patient as trained. The nurse can delegate certain safety interventions to the UAP and can have them report patient observations to the nurse for follow-up. The nurse remains responsible for the assessment, interpretation of abnormal findings, and determination of appropriate responses.

Equipment

No equipment, such as restraints, is required for a suicidal patient unless determined necessary for preventing injury to him- or herself or others.

Preparation

- Review healthcare provider's orders and patient's nursing plan of care.
- Review patient's record for history of suicide attempts, depression, and other risk factors.

CAUTION! Use a standardized suicide assessment tool for evaluation of the patient's risk factors to help determine appropriate safety interventions. One such tool is the Suicide Assessment Five-step Evaluation and Triage (SAFE-T) for Mental Health Professionals. This tool is currently available as an app through SAMHSA (SAMHSA, 2015).

Procedure

1. Introduce self to patient and verify the patient's identity using two identifiers. Explain to the patient you are going to do an assessment for suicidal ideation and then discuss safety interventions for the patient while in the hospital, why they are necessary, and how the patient can participate. Discuss how the results will be used in planning further care or treatments.
2. Perform hand hygiene and observe appropriate infection control procedures.
3. Provide for patient privacy and comfort.
   - Assess for current risk factors. Does the patient have any thoughts of killing or harming him- or herself? If the patient says yes, assess the nature of the thoughts and determine if the patient has a plan and the means to carry out the plan.
     - Access to means such as knives, medications, or firearms
     - Recent search of internet for way to commit suicide
     - Development of suicide plan, practice of the plan, attitude of just waiting for the right time
     - Frequent thoughts about ending life to escape, avoid, or try something new
     - Patient history of suicide attempt, or suicide in family history
     - Diagnosed history of psychiatric condition, substance abuse, depression, traumatic brain injury, conduct disorders, or psychosis
     - Diagnosis of chronic illness, terminal disease, or chronic pain without relief
     - Hopelessness, inability to sleep throughout the night, anxiety, voice command hallucination, or expressing feelings of being a burden to others and a failure
     - Recent life-altering change, recent trauma experience, recent loss of relationship and feelings of love, or change in behaviors and thoughts

SKILL 15.4 Suicide: Caring for Suicidal Patient (*continued*)

- Poor coping strategies for protecting self; feeling of being disconnected from spiritual higher power; expressing a desire to die

4. Provide safety interventions for appropriate risk level.
   - Low risk (Patient exhibits mild depression or has thoughts of death with no plan, intent, or behavior.)
     - Place patient in a room close to the nurse's station.
     - Keep the door to the patient's room open unless providing care or doing a procedure.
     - Do safety check every 2 hours, or follow facility policy and procedure.
     - Set up patient appointments for within a week of discharge from the healthcare facility for follow-up care with a mental health resource.
     - Give patient telephone number of a suicide prevention help-line available 24/7 (National Suicide Prevention Lifeline: 800-273-8255).
     - Keep patient in a safe environment. Reduce environmental stimuli.
     - Actively listen if patient would like to talk with you.
   - Moderate risk (Patient expresses suicidal intent, has a plan, but has not taken any action.)
     - Depending on risk factors, patient may need to be admitted to a behavioral health facility.
     - Remove objects and materials that could be used for self-harm by the patient.
     - Give patient telephone number of a suicide prevention help-line available 24/7.
     - Place patient in a room close to the nurse's station.
     - Keep patient in a safe environment. Reduce environmental stimuli.
     - Use plastic utensils, plates, cups, bowls, and so on, on meal trays, and check tray for return of all items when picking tray up.
     - Ask patient to stay in public areas; do frequent checks with patient as facility dictates or at 15-minute time intervals.
     - Keep the door to the patient's room open unless providing care or doing a procedure.
   - High risk (Patient has made a suicide attempt or is experiencing persistent ideation with strong intent or rehearsal.)
     - Have someone stay with patient at all times (one-to-one observation).
     - Keep patient in a safe environment. Reduce environmental stimuli.
     - Ensure that patient is transferred and admitted to a behavioral health facility when discharged from healthcare facility.
     - Remove objects and materials that could be used for self-harm by the patient, including hanging materials such as telephone cords, clothes hooks, shower curtain rods, coat hangers, medications, laptops, and exposed pipes. Monitor medical supplies, such as intravenous tubing, gloves, used needles, or nasogastric tubes. Remove personal items such as belts, razors, nail clippers, tweezers, shoe laces, bathrobe cords, bras, knee high hosiery, scarves, or mirrors.

- As needed, provide staff supervision with toileting, use of personal hygiene items, cigarettes and matches, and cleaning supplies.
- Follow facility policies and procedures for restraints as determined necessary.
- Use plastic utensils, plates, cups, bowls, and so on, on meal trays, and check tray for return of all items when picking tray up.
- Monitor any items brought by visitors that could be used to injure self or others.

5. When assessment or procedure is complete, perform hand hygiene and leave patient safe and comfortable.

6. Complete documentation using forms, checklists, or electronic dropdown lists supplemented by nurse's notes or additional comments as appropriate, including safety interventions implemented, patient's reaction to them, and evaluation of them. All decisions about care of the patient should be well documented in the record, as well as instructions and prevention information given to the patient on discharge and follow-up appointments with behavioral health resources.

SAMPLE DOCUMENTATION

[date] 0400 Admission assessment form completed. Stated, "If I was dead, I would be able to get such good sleep, I'm so tired." I stated, "So, you're thinking if you were dead, you would be able to get good sleep because you are so tired?" Stated, "Oh, I'm just so busy and tired all the time, I just want to sleep a long time." I stated, "Can you clarify what you mean when you say you want to sleep a long time?" "You know what I mean, if I took a really big sleeping pill, I would sleep a long time." I said, "So you would sleep a long time." Stated, "Oh, don't misunderstand me, I don't want to kill myself or anything, I just want a good night's sleep, you know, having the new baby and all, never enough time to rest." I said, "OK, let's talk more about this in the morning, but for now, maybe you could get a little sleep before the morning begins." Stated, "I hope *so*, it's so nice and quiet here." *R. Rodrezo*

Safety Considerations
STAFF RECOVERY FROM A PATIENT SUICIDE

- Maintain quality of care and provide normalcy for staff performing care of unit patients.

- Decide on appropriate actions to support the patient's family during this time.

- Provide annual training for staff to identify suicide risk factors. Nursing staff need to know how to recognize a troubled patient having suicidal thoughts.

(*continued on next page*)

SKILL 15.4 Suicide: Caring for Suicidal Patient (*continued*)

- If a patient successfully commits suicide in the healthcare facility, it deeply affects all healthcare personnel, especially those who were part of the team providing care and treatment for the patient. The event may leave them feeling guilty, in shock, or having a sense of not doing enough to stop it. Many nurses feel unprepared for losing a patient to suicide.

- A staff meeting for the unit staff involved can be organized to answer appropriate questions, inform all staff about what has happened, and give everyone an opportunity to vent feelings and thoughts.

- Suicide in a healthcare facility is a sentinel event that is investigated on many levels, following facility policies and procedures, county medical examiner guidelines, and state and federal laws.

- Based on root cause analysis by healthcare facility risk management, gaps in safety may result in changing staffing patterns, reporting guidelines, or the suicide precaution policy.

- Many healthcare facilities offer counseling services to all affected staff, and some larger healthcare facilities have stress debriefing teams of peers, counselors, and clergy who manage debriefings for those who would like to participate.

- For individual emotional help, many healthcare facilities have employee assistance programs to work with staff members.

- Legal and ethical actions are completed.

- Staff needs the opportunity to ask questions about fear of legal action from family and must be given information about expectations if a lawsuit does happen.

>> Environmental Safety

Expected Outcomes

1. Patient is acclimated to home environment and is able to provide safe self-care after a period of support from facility staff.
2. Patient is provided appropriate home care modalities.
3. Patient's environment is safe from potential mechanical, chemical, fire, and electrical hazards.
4. All electrical equipment is intact and operating safely.
5. Safe environment provides for patient safety in home.

SKILL 15.5 Environmental Safety: Healthcare Facility, Community, Home

In healthcare settings such as an acute facility, a long-term facility, or a community facility, or when providing patient care in the patient's home, environmental safety is everybody's responsibility. Facilities may have Safety Programs, Risk Management Departments, safety cultures, Safety Teams, or Hazard Teams. However, it is the active participation of all employees in keeping patients, visitors, and themselves safe from injury and illness that will make the difference in the safety efforts being successful.

Delegation or Assignment

Environmental safety is not a delegated or assigned task; it is part of safety programs in all healthcare settings, and the responsibility of all healthcare personnel. The UAP would be expected to immediately notify appropriate personnel about safety hazards they may observe. The UAP may be delegated or assigned specific tasks to prevent injury or provide safety measures for patients and others.

Equipment

- Appropriate supplies and equipment for patient, others, and personal safety when performing job expectations in the healthcare setting

Preparation

- Be familiar with the policies and procedures regarding safety behaviors and appropriate response to safety hazards to avoid injuries and illnesses.

- Be familiar with manufacturer's instructions and follow safety guidelines when using equipment.
- Participate in annual safety training and review of facility emergency disaster plans.
- Build awareness of your surroundings and potential safety hazards to avoid.

Procedure

1. Introduce self to patient and parent and let the patient know you are there for the patient's safety. Follow policies and procedures to maintain a safe environment for patients, visitors, others, and yourself.
2. Evaluate patient safety.
   - Cognitive abilities: level of consciousness, orientation, ability to make appropriate judgments, ability to follow commands and directions.
     - Knowledge of medication times and doses to be taken
     - Knowledge of how to call for help: healthcare provider, nurse, fire, police
   - Sensory and motor function
     - Hearing and vision acuity
     - Ability to ambulate with assistance
     - Need for assistive devices or support in ambulation
   - Patient's ability to manage self-care
     - Bathing, grooming, and dressing
     - Preparing food and feeding
     - Toileting

SKILL 15.5 Environmental Safety: Healthcare Facility, Community, Home (*continued*)

- Need for type of transfer assist devices for safe patient handling
  - Gait belts provide secure grip without holding onto patient's clothes or limbs. **Rationale:** *This prevents caregiver strain because patient weight is closer to caregiver and the patient can assume upright position.*
  - Small slide/transfer board is used for seated lateral transfers, such as between bed and wheelchair or commode. **Rationale:** *Caregiver does not need to lift patient manually.*
  - Turning discs are used to pivot seated patients who can bear weight and stand. The patient is guided to a standing position without adjusting the feet. The patient must be able to stand or the caregiver will have to exert excessive force in an awkward position.
  - Mechanical lift devices such as the lean–stand assist lift and sling-type full lift are used for patients who cannot support their own weight.
  - Repositioning devices mechanically pull the patient up in bed without need for caregiver to assist patient.
  - Trapeze lifts are a bar device suspended above the bed that allows patients with upper body strength to reposition.
- Need for alternatives to physical restraints
  - Install bed check system or alarm device.
  - Decrease auditory and visual stimuli.
  - Place supplies close to bed or chair (e.g., tissues, water).
- Most effective type of restraint, if absolutely necessary
  - Determine that less restrictive methods have been attempted.
  - Assess purpose of restraint to determine most appropriate type.

3. Evaluate facility and home safety.
   - Any pollutants that are present in the environment
   - Exterior of the building
     - Condition of sidewalks and steps
     - Presence of railings on steps
     - Barriers that prevent easy access to the building
     - Adequacy of lighting
     - Visible security guards stationed close to entrances
   - Interior of the building
     - Uncluttered pathways throughout the building
     - All throw rugs are removed or secured to floor
     - Adequacy of lighting
     - Doorways wide enough to permit assistive devices
     - Presence of insects, rodents, or infective agents
     - Presence of functioning smoke detectors
     - Adequate heating and cooling systems
   - Hazardous materials (safely stored if present)
   - Medications, supplies, and equipment (safe storage)
   - Stairway and halls
     - Adequacy of light
     - Adequate lighted signage for stairway
     - Handrails that are securely fastened to wall
     - Carpeting (if any) in good repair

- Kitchen area
  - Properly functioning microwave oven and refrigerator
  - Adequacy of light surrounding counters and sink
  - Dated and current food and drink items in refrigerator
  - No nonfood or nonbeverage items stored in refrigerator
  - Adequate disposable waste containers with covers
- Patient bathrooms
  - Skidproof strips or mat in tub or shower
  - Handrails around toilet and tub or shower
  - Adequate space if wheelchairs or walkers are used
  - Temperature of hot water from faucets in sink, tub, or shower
- Patient bedroom
  - Ease in getting into and out of bed
  - Adequate space, if commode or wheelchair is required
  - Accessibility of personal items and water on nightstand or bedside table
  - Calling system or telephone functional to call for assistance
  - Functional electronic equipment, such as an electric bed

4. Evaluate healthcare staff safety in the patient's home.
   - Determine if household pets are present; if so, ask that they be secured during visit.
   - Check neighborhood to determine need for assistance from police to make home visit.
   - Wear identifying name badge. Most agencies request that the nurse wear a lab coat.
   - Maintain personal safety while traveling in the car.
   - Have cell phone available and charged at all times.
   - Keep car doors locked and windows up at all times.
   - Park in full view of neighbors, preferably directly in front of home.
   - Lock all equipment, personal items, and valuables in trunk of the car before leaving home or office.
   - If you feel personal safety is in question, do not make a visit or stay in the residence.
   - Use common walkways or hallways.
   - Knock on the door and wait for permission to enter.
   - Keep a clear pathway to the door if the situation is potentially unsafe.
   - Observe home environment for safety hazards (e.g., weapons, unsanitary conditions).
   - Make visit in the morning when good visual support exists if neighborhood is unsafe.
   - Evaluate healthcare staff safety in the facility.
     - Plans are in place for external disasters and internal disasters and are practiced annually ❶.
     - Personal protective equipment is available for use.
     - Postexposure evaluation and follow-up is provided.
     - Maintenance schedules for safety equipment are followed.
     - Security is able to respond to disruptive behavior and weapons in the building.
     - There is annual safety training for all employees.

(*continued on next page*)

SKILL 15.5 Environmental Safety: Healthcare Facility, Community, Home (*continued*)

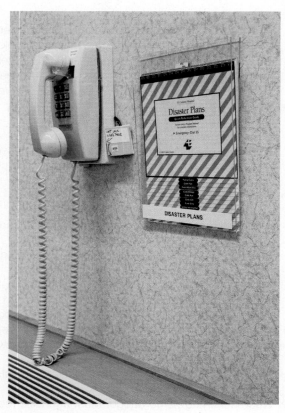

Source: Ronald May/Pearson Education, Inc.

❶ Be familiar with the internal disaster plan in your healthcare facility.

- There is an active attempt to develop a safety culture for everyone.
- Assistive devices and adequate staff are provided for moving and lifting patients.
- There are systems to avoid exposure to infectious and contagious diseases, bloodborne pathogens and body fluids, needle sticks, chemicals, hazardous medications, and radiation.
- Adequate safety precautions are in place to prevent musculoskeletal injuries, violence and physical assault from a patient or visitor, victimization by a co-worker, and a hospital-acquired illness.

5. If safe practice requires it, report the need for change.
- Report all unsafe hazards to appropriate departments to remedy the hazard and maintain a safe environment.
- Identify high-risk areas that have high incidence of injuries so they can be changed.
- Report intimidation and bullying of co-workers, following the chain of command.
- Use assistive moving devices and appropriate staff numbers to move or lift patients.
- Follow correct and safe steps in doing procedures and administering medications, to help avoid errors.
- Take an active role in modeling safety behaviors for employees.
- When safety hazards are found, be part of the solution.
- Let someone know about safety hazards; you might be the first person to notice them.
- Be safe for yourself, so you can provide safe care to patients.

SKILL 15.6 Fire Safety: Healthcare Facility, Community, Home

Fire continues to be a common safety hazard for healthcare facilities even with local, state, and federal regulations and guidelines. Electrical equipment, which provides a high potential for electrical fires, is located throughout these facilities. Additional potential hazards are found in the kitchen departments. Cigarette smoking remains a common fire-starting hazard. Oxygen and other gases under pressure can provide fuel for fires.

Delegation or Assignment

This is not a delegated or assigned task; it is part of fire safety policies and procedures in all healthcare facilities and community facilities, and a responsibility of all healthcare personnel. The UAPs are expected to immediately notify other staff about a fire and help move patients or others from the immediate area. The UAPs may be delegated or assigned specific tasks to prevent the fire from spreading or provide

safety to patients and others. All staff should be oriented to where fire extinguishers, fire pulls, and gas controls are located on each unit.

Equipment

- Appropriate extinguisher for fire:
  - Water type
  - Soda-acid type
  - Foam type
  - Dry chemical type
  - ABC extinguisher

Preparation

- Annual participation in fire safety training.
- Be familiar with fire safety policies and procedures, including the evacuation plan for facility.
- Stay alert for the smell of smoke and investigate its origin.

SKILL 15.6 Fire Safety: Healthcare Facility, Community, Home (*continued*)

Safety Considerations
RACE: **PRIORITIES FOR FIRE SAFETY**

Rescue and remove all patients in immediate danger.

Activate fire alarm.

Confine the fire; close doors and windows, turn off oxygen supplies and electrical equipment.

Extinguish fire when possible.

Procedure

1. Introduce self to patient and explain you are going to help them move away from a safety hazard. Provide safety for patient and self. Follow hospital policies and procedures for type of fire safety program and for ringing the fire alarm to summon help.
2. Remove all patients from the immediate area to a safe place. Be familiar with fire exits and facility evacuation plan.
3. To remove a patient safely from the fire, use carrying method that is most comfortable for you and safe for patient.
   - Place blanket (or bedspread) on floor. Lower patient onto blanket. Lift up head end of blanket and drag patient out of danger.
   - Use two-person swing method. Place patient in sitting position. Form a seat by having two people clasp forearms or shoulders. Lift patient into "seat" and carry out of danger.
   - Carry patient using "back-strap" carry method. Step in front of patient. Place patient's arms around your neck. Grasp patient's wrists and hold tight against your chest. Pull patient onto your back and carry to safety.
4. Activate fire alarm.
5. Secure the burning area by closing all doors and windows.
6. Shut off all possible oxygen sources and electrical appliances in the fire area.
7. If evacuating from the building, NEVER use the elevator to get to the ground floor. Always use the stairs.
8. If possible, employ the appropriate extinguishing method without endangering yourself. Fire extinguishers should not be used directly on an individual.
9. Be familiar with the different types of fire extinguishers and their locations ❶.

CLASS A

- Water-under-pressure type or soda-acid type.
- Use on cloth, wood, paper, plastic, rubber, or leather.
- Never use on electrical or chemical fires due to danger of shock.

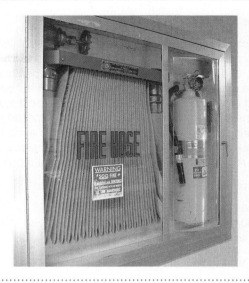

❶ Become familiar with the location and use of fire extinguishers in your healthcare facility.

CLASS B

- Foam, dry chemical type.
- Use on fires such as gasoline, alcohol, acetone, oil, grease, or paint thinner and remover.
- Class A extinguisher is never used on Class B fires.

CLASS C

- Dry chemical or carbon dioxide types.
- Use on electrical wiring, electrical equipment, or motors.
- Class A or Class B extinguishers are never used on Class C fires.

CLASS ABC COMBINATION

- Contains graphite.
- Use on any type of fire.
- Most common extinguisher in use.

10. Keep fire exits clear at all times.

Safety Considerations
PASS: **USING A FIRE EXTINGUISHER**

Pull the pin.

Aim at the base of the fire.

Squeeze the trigger.

Sweep the fire side to side.

SKILL 15.7 Thermal and Electrical Injuries: Preventing

Thermal hazards that alter normal body heat can result in hyperthermia or hypothermia and could become life threatening. These hazards can be found in departments with hot sterilization rooms or in storage areas with extremely low temperature freezers. Electrical hazards include faulty wires, nongrounded electrical devices, exposed electrical cords, and multiple electrical plugs in inappropriate outlets. Thermal and electrical hazards can cause thermal burns and other injuries.

(*continued on next page*)

SKILL 15.7 Thermal and Electrical Injuries: Preventing (*continued*)

Delegation or Assignment

This is not a delegated or assigned task; it is part of safety policies and procedures in all healthcare facilities and community facilities, and a responsibility of all healthcare personnel. The UAPs are expected to follow the healthcare facilities' safety policies and procedures in regard to thermal and electrical hazard environments or equipment. Any equipment, exposed electrical cords, ungrounded electrical devices, and damaged electrical plugs and outlets need to be reported to the charge nurse and the item reported to or taken to maintenance for repair.

Equipment

- Fire extinguishers
- Electrical equipment found on unit
- Thermal equipment found on unit

Preparation

- Build awareness of electrical equipment, electrical cords, plugs, and so on, for maintenance issues.
- Be familiar with the reporting process to have electrical equipment repaired.
- Follow safety guidelines when using thermal equipment.

Procedure

1. Check to verify that all electrical plugs, cords, outlets, coils, thermostats, and other electrical equipment are routinely checked and maintained. Look for safety inspection expiration dates on biomedical equipment.
2. As allowed by facility, have all electrical appliances brought to the hospital by the patient (radios, electric razors, hair dryers, etc.) inspected by hospital maintenance staff (follow facility policy). It is best to discourage use of non-hospital equipment.
3. Verify water in the tub or shower is not more than 43°C (110°F) (or 35°C [95°F] for those with circulatory insufficiency).
4. When heating pads, sitz bath, or hot compresses are used, check the patient frequently for redness. Maximum temperature should not exceed 41°C (105°F) (or 35°C [95°F] for those with circulatory insufficiency).
5. Healthcare facilities do not allow the use of tobacco products or smoking in the facility. Sometimes there may be designated smoking areas outside the building, but many facilities do not allow smoking on their premises, including the parking lots. Inform patients and visitors about smoking regulations. Do not allow confused, sedated, or severely incapacitated patients to smoke in designated smoking areas without direct supervision.
6. Store all combustible materials securely to prevent spontaneous combustion.
7. Make sure that all staff and employees participate in training and understand fire safety measures, such as extinguishing fires, and the plan for evacuating patients.
8. Report and do not use any apparatus that produces a shock, has a broken plug or ground pin, or has a frayed cord.
9. Never apply direct heat (e.g., heating pad) to ischemic tissue—doing so increases the tissue's need for oxygen.
10. Turn equipment off before unplugging it. **Rationale:** *This prevents sparks that can cause a fire.*
11. Plug devices that require a high current (i.e., ventilators or radiant warmers) into separate outlets. **Rationale:** *This prevents overloading the circuit, which could lead to a fire.*
12. Use only three-pronged grounded plugs.

» Immobilizers and Restraints

Expected Outcomes

1. Patient is prevented from injuring self or others.
2. Restraints are applied appropriately.
3. Patient does not develop complications due to restraint use (e.g., agitation, pressure ulcers, circulatory disturbance).
4. Child is prevented from reaching an incision site, IVs, or tubes.
5. Patient remains in restraints for a limited amount of time.
6. Patient does not endure undue psychological stress while being placed in restraints.

SKILL 15.8 Bed or Chair Alarm, Exit Monitor Device: Applying

Bed and chair alarms are used to help prevent falls by alerting staff that the patient is trying to get up out of bed. The exit monitor device can be part of the bed itself or an attachment on the patient. The alarm system is an addition to other preventive measures to keep the patient safe from falls.

Delegation or Assignment

The nurse is responsible for assessing the patient and confirming that there is a risk of the patient falling when getting out of a chair or bed unassisted. The use of a safety monitoring device may be delegated or assigned to the UAP who has been trained in its application and monitoring. The nurse remains responsible for the assessment, interpretation of abnormal findings, and determination of appropriate actions. Note that state laws for UAPs vary, so this task might be assigned to the UAP rather than delegated.

Equipment

- Alarm and control device
- Sensor
- Connection to nurse call system

SKILL 15.8 Bed or Chair Alarm, Exit Monitor Device: Applying (continued)

Preparation

- Review healthcare provider's orders and patient's nursing plan of care.
- Review patient's record for verification that the patient is a high risk for fall.
- Gather equipment.

Procedure

1. Introduce self to patient and verify the patient's identity using two identifiers. Explain to the patient and family the purpose and procedure for using a safety monitoring device. Explain that the device does not limit mobility in any manner; rather, it alerts the staff when the patient is about to get out of the bed or a chair. Explain that the nurse must be called when the patient needs to get out of the bed or a chair.
2. Perform hand hygiene and observe other appropriate infection control procedures.
3. Provide for patient privacy.
4. Test the battery device and alarm sound every shift. **Rationale:** *Testing ensures that the device is functioning properly prior to use.*
5. Apply the leg band or sensor pad.
   - Place the leg band according to the manufacturer's recommendation. Place the patient's leg in a straight horizontal position. **Rationale:** *The alarm device is position sensitive; that is, when it approaches a near-vertical position (such as in walking, crawling, or kneeling as the patient attempts to get out of bed), the audio alarm will be triggered.*
   - For the bed or chair device, the sensor is usually placed under the buttocks area. Follow manufacturer's recommendations on how often this sensor pad should be changed.
   - For a bed or chair device, set the time delay to 1–12 seconds for determining the patient's movement patterns.
   - Connect the sensor pad to the control unit and the nurse call system.
6. Instruct the patient to call the nurse when the patient wants or needs to get up, and assist as required.
   - When assisting the patient up, deactivate the alarm.
   - Assist the patient back to the bed or chair, and reattach the alarm device.
7. Ensure patient safety with additional safety precautions.
   - Place call light within patient reach, lift top side rails per healthcare facility policy, and lower the bed to its lowest position. **Rationale:** *The alarm device is not a substitute for other precautionary measures.*
   - Place fall risk or fall precaution signs on the patient's door, chart, and other relevant locations.
8. When the procedure is complete, perform hand hygiene and leave patient safe and comfortable.
9. Document the type of alarm used, where it was placed, and its effectiveness in the patient record using forms, checklists, or electronic dropdown lists supplemented by narrative notes when appropriate. Record all additional safety precautions and interventions discussed and employed.

SAMPLE DOCUMENTATION

[date] 1130 Found out of bed despite frequent verbal reminders to use call light for assistance. Explained about using a magnetic box mobility alarm to ensure own safety from possible fall. Verbalized agreement. Alarm device applied. Reminded again of importance to call the nurse for assistance. Call light placed within patient's reach. *J. Wallace*

Safety Considerations

When a monitoring device is used in the home, instruct caregivers to:

- Test the monitoring device every 12–24 hr to ensure that it is working.
- Check the volume of the alarm to ascertain they can hear it.
- Investigate all alarms, and not to assume a false alarm, although these devices are sensitive and alarms can be triggered by normal movement. They may adjust the alarm controls.
- Provide proper supervision of patient at risk for falling in addition to the monitoring device.

SKILL 15.9 Immobilizer, Mummy: Applying

The mummy immobilizer is used to hold a child still during many procedures. A baby blanket can be used for newborns and infants and a larger blanket used for the small child. The blanket is wrapped around the child in such a way as to immobilize the arms on each side of the child.

Delegation or Assignment

The nurse applying the mummy immobilizer may ask the UAP to assist in holding the child as it is wrapped and secured around the child's body. The nurse remains responsible for the assessment, interpretation of abnormal findings, and determination of appropriate actions.

Equipment

- Soft blanket or sheet two to three times larger than the child

Preparation

- Review healthcare provider's orders and nursing plan of care.
- Have the UAP (or the parent) available to help position and hold the child if needed. **Rationale:** *The mummy immobilizer is used when the nurse does not have an*

(continued on next page)

SKILL 15.9 Immobilizer, Mummy: Applying (*continued*)

assistant available or a parent willing to restrain the child for a procedure.

■ Gather appropriate size blanket.

Procedure

1. Introduce self to child and parent and verify patient's identity using two identifiers. Explain to the child and parent the reason for immobilization and how long it will be needed. Tell the child how the restraint will feel, why it is necessary, and how the patient can participate. *Rationale: Young children will be less anxious if the explanation about what they will feel is placed in non-threatening, developmentally appropriate terms.*

2. Perform hand hygiene and observe appropriate infection control procedures.

3. Provide for patient privacy, safety, and comfort.

4. Put the blanket (or sheet) on the bed or examination table. Fold down one corner until it reaches the middle of the blanket.

NEWBORN AND INFANT

5. Place the newborn or infant in a diagonal position with the neck on the folded edge.

6. Bring one side of the blanket over the newborn's or infant's arm and then under the back. Tuck that edge under and over the other arm and around the back. It may be helpful to roll the newborn or infant on the side to smooth the blanket behind the back, and then roll the newborn or infant onto the back over the smoothed section of blanket.

7. Bring the other side of the blanket around the body and tuck underneath the body.

8. Bring the bottom corner of the blanket up and over the abdomen. Proceed to step 9 below.

CHILD

5. Place the child on the blanket, positioning so that there is sufficient material to wrap the knees and lower legs.

6. If necessary, fold down the top edges of the blanket to the shoulders.

7. Bring one side of the blanket over the arm, body, and legs, and tuck it under the other arm and around the back and legs ❶.

8. Bring the other side of the blanket up and around the body, and tuck underneath the back and legs. *Rationale: The child should not be able to flex the knees and kick, or it may be impossible to perform the procedure.*

9. During the procedure, monitor the patient's airway and circulation. When the procedure is complete, unwrap the blanket to allow the newborn, infant, or child to move arms and legs. Perform hand hygiene and leave patient safe and comfortable.

10. Complete documentation using forms, checklists, or electronic dropdown lists supplemented by nurse's notes or additional comments as appropriate.

SAMPLE DOCUMENTATION

[date] 0915 Dad in room playing with patient. Placed in mummy immobilizer during eye exam per Dr. Harper. After exam, removed from immobilizer and held by Dad. Tolerated procedure without distress or crying. Returned to playing with puzzle. *L. Meric*

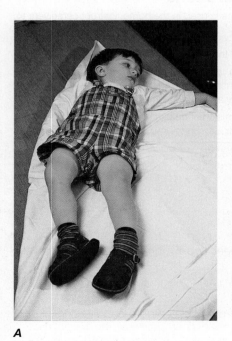
A

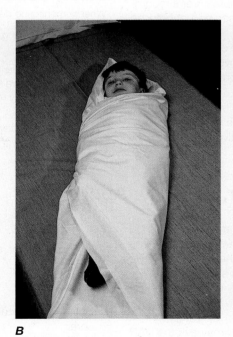
B

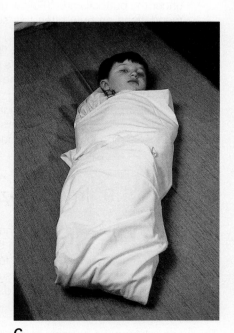
C

❶ Steps in applying mummy immobilization *A, B, C.*

SKILL 15.10 Immobilizer, Papoose Board: Applying

The papoose board comes in a variety of sizes and is used to immobilize a child up to the age of 12. It stabilizes the child during treatments or procedures and enhances safety from injury by restraining movement.

Delegation or Assignment

The nurse applying the papoose board immobilizer may ask the UAP to assist in holding the child as it is wrapped and secured around the child's body. The nurse remains responsible for the assessment, interpretation of abnormal findings, and determination of appropriate actions.

Equipment

- Papoose board immobilizer to fit the child's size
- Sheet

Preparation

- Review healthcare provider's orders and patient's nursing plan of care.
- Have the UAP (or the parent) available to help position and hold the child if needed. **Rationale:** *The papoose board is most often used when the nurse does not have an assistant available or a parent willing to restrain the child for a procedure.* Parents can provide emotional support to child by staying near, stroking, providing distractions, and talking softly to the child.
- Gather equipment and supplies for the procedure. **Rationale:** *Having supplies prepared reduces the time the child spends in temporary restraint devices and reduces the anxiety felt by the child.*

Procedure

1. Introduce self to patient and parent. Verify the patient's identity using two identifiers. Explain the reason for immobilization to the child and parent and how long it will be needed. Tell the child how the restraint will feel. **Rationale:** *Young children will be less anxious if the explanation about what they will feel is placed in nonthreatening, developmentally appropriate terms.*
2. Perform hand hygiene and provide privacy, comfort, and safety for patient.
3. Place a towel or sheet over the board.

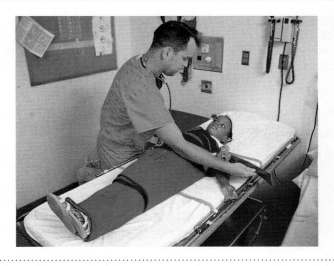

1 Child on a papoose board.

4. Have the child lie supine on the board, with the head at the top **1**.
5. Place the fabric wrappings around the child and secure the Velcro fasteners. To be most effective, the fabric wrappings should be secure over the elbows, hips, and knees to prevent flexion. **Rationale:** *This action prevents the child from pulling apart the wrappings or from kicking.*
6. When the procedure is complete, release the child and allow the parents to provide comfort. Perform hand hygiene and leave patient safe and comfortable.
7. Complete documentation using forms, checklists, or electronic dropdown lists supplemented by nurse's notes or additional comments as appropriate.

SAMPLE DOCUMENTATION

[date] 1430 Mom in room with patient. Papoose board immobilizer applied and secured around child. Dr. Wicker removed 2 small lima beans from patient's right naris without complication. Released from immobilizer, sat on Mom's lap, and stopped crying. No bleeding noted from right naris. Tolerated procedure without incident. *R. Seller*

SKILL 15.11 Restraints and Alternatives: Caring for

Restraints are designed to safely and effectively limit the movement of patients to prevent injury to themselves or others. There is a variety of physical restraints, different sizes and styles that are made of fabric materials, straps, mitts, or leather to accommodate all ages and circumstances. Restraints are indicated only as a last resort available to protect the patient, and then they are implemented only when alternatives have failed and the patient is assessed and evaluated by an appropriate Licensed Independent Practitioner (LIP).

Delegation or Assignment

The nurse assesses the patient for the need to apply appropriate restraint(s). The application of the restraint(s) can be delegated or assigned to the UAP trained to safely apply the restraint(s). The UAP may care for patients after the procedure. The nurse must ensure that the UAP knows what complications or adverse signs should be reported to the nurse. The

(continued on next page)

SKILL 15.11 Restraints and Alternatives: Caring for (continued)

nurse remains responsible for the assessment, interpretation of abnormal findings, and determination of appropriate responses. Note that state laws for UAPs vary, so this task might be assigned to the UAP rather than delegated.

Equipment

- Appropriate restraint and size of restraint: limb, torso

Preparation

- Review healthcare provider's orders and patient's nursing plan of care.
- Follow facility policies and procedures in utilizing restraints.
- Identify and validate less restrictive measures have been explored before the patient is placed in restraints.
- Ensure that a face-to-face assessment is completed on the patient within 8 hr for a nonbehavioral health patient, and 1 hr for a behavioral (psychiatric) health patient. **Rationale:** *Frequent assessments prevent complications.*
- Ensure that restraint orders are renewed every 24 hr or sooner according to facility policy for nonbehavioral health patients, or every 2–4 hr for behavioral health patients. Children from ages 12–17 must have orders renewed every 2 hr, for a maximum of 24 hr. **Rationale:** *Restraints should be discontinued as soon as possible.*
- Establish and implement a plan of care for the patient to eliminate the need for restraints.
- Three types of restraints used in clinical practice include:
  - *Chemical:* Sedating psychotropic drugs to manage or control behavior. Psychoactive medication used in this manner is an inappropriate use of medication.
  - *Physical:* Direct application of physical force to a patient, without the patient's permission, to restrict the patient's freedom of movement.
  - *Seclusion:* Involuntary confinement of a patient in a locked room. Physical force may be applied by individuals, mechanical devices, or a combination of any of them.

Procedure

1. Introduce self to patient and verify the patient's identity using two identifiers. Explain to the patient what you are going to do, why it is necessary, and how the patient can participate. If possible, elicit the support of the family or use sitters to stay with the patient rather than place the patient in restraints. Discuss the use of restraints with the patient and family members.
2. Perform hand hygiene and observe appropriate infection control procedures.
3. Provide for patient privacy, safety, and comfort.
4. Alternative options before using restraints include:
   - Have a family member stay with patient, or ask family to arrange for a sitter.
   - Use distractions or diversional activity appropriate for the patient.
   - Use a calm quiet voice.
   - Explore why the patient may be trying to get out of bed: need for bathroom, hungry, thirsty, looking for an object, and so on.
   - Use bed and chair alarms.

- Reorient patient frequently to location and time.
- Decrease noise, lights, movement in the patient's room.
- Have patient do a physical activity or task.
- Make sure patient can call for assistance.
- Move the patient closer to the nurse's station.

CAUTION! Restraints are never written as a PRN order or used for discipline, convenience, intimidation, or punishment.

5. Apply restraints.
   - Explain the restraints being applied to patient and how they will function.
   - Follow manufacturer's guidelines for applying and using the restraint.
   - Avoid application of force on long bone joints and pad bony prominences beneath restraint. **Rationale:** *This reduces pressure on skin.*
   - In acute medical and postsurgical care, a restraint may be necessary to ensure that an IV or feeding tube is not removed.
6. Care of restrained patient.
   - Patient is assessed every 15 min. Documentation includes observations about behaviors, safety measures applied, and how well patient is tolerating restraints.
   - At least every 2 hr:
     - Toileting is offered.
     - Something to eat or drink is offered.
     - Range of motion to all joints, particularly those in restraints.
     - Check skin integrity under restraint, padding applied as needed.
     - Circulation at extremity restraint and distal to it is checked.
     - Any hygiene needed is performed.
     - Body alignment is checked.
   - The patient is positioned as comfortable as possible.
   - Restraints must be removed as soon as feasible. Changes in patient behaviors are assessed for safety of removing restraints. Obtain a healthcare provider's order and discontinue restraints as soon as it is clinically indicated.
7. When the procedure is complete, perform hand hygiene and leave patient safe and comfortable.
8. Complete documentation using forms, checklists, or electronic dropdown lists supplemented by nurse's notes or additional comments as appropriate.

SAMPLE DOCUMENTATION

[date] 0615 Awake and states needs to go to the bathroom. Bilateral wrist restraints loosened and Velcro undone. Assisted to stand up and walk to bathroom. Voided moderate amount clear straw-colored urine. Assisted back to bed. Wrists restraints reapplied. Room for one fingerbreadth underneath restraints. No redness noted at wrists, radial pulses full bilateral. Closing eyes, resting quietly. Tolerated walking to bathroom without respiratory distress. G. Yan

SKILL 15.12 Restraints, Torso and Belt: Applying

The belt restraint is applied to the patient's torso to keep the patient safely in bed, chair, or stretcher. Patient can move to sides, but cannot get up out of the bed or chair.

Delegation or Assignment

The nurse assesses the patient for the need to apply a torso or belt restraint as ordered. The application of these restraints can be delegated or assigned to the UAP trained to use the torso and belt restraint. The nurse remains responsible for the assessment, interpretation of abnormal findings, and determination of appropriate responses. Note that state laws for UAPs vary, so this task might be assigned to the UAP rather than delegated.

Equipment

- Safety belt restraint (usually 2-in. soft webbing material) with waist and side belts (for bed)
- Vest restraint

Preparation

- Review the healthcare record and the patient's nursing plan of care.
- Check healthcare provider's order. If no order, call healthcare provider or licensed independent practitioner (LIP) for restraint order before applying restraints. If restraints must be placed before the order is obtained, ensure the order is obtained within 1 hr for either a nonbehavioral health patient or a behavioral health patient. **Rationale:** *Healthcare provider's order is required to apply restraints*. Follow guidelines for obtaining restraint orders and updating orders according to hospital policy.
- Have the UAP available to help position and secure torso or belt restraint if needed.
- Apply restraint according to manufacturer's specific directions.
- Gather belt restraint.

Procedure

1. Introduce self to patient and verify the patient's identity using two identifiers. Explain the necessity for safety belt to patient and family, and seek the patient's cooperation with restraint procedure, if possible. Discuss how the results will be used in planning further care or treatments.
2. Perform hand hygiene and observe appropriate infection control procedures.
3. Provide for patient privacy, safety, and comfort.
4. Apply torso restraint as follows:
   - Slip waist belt through flat buckle, adjusting to patient's size. Belts usually have a key-locked buckle ❶. The key must be readily available so restraint may be released immediately in emergency situations (follow facility policy for designated location). **Rationale:** *This prevents slipping and provides a snug fit.*
   - Snap hinged plate shut by hooking plain end of key over cross bar and lifting upward.
   - Attach side belts to bed frame in similar manner.
   - Release restraint by hooking green end of key over cross bar from below and pulling downward.
   - The vest restraint fits around the upper torso with the patient's arms through armholes, then wraps around to the back to be secured while the patient is in the bed or a chair ❷ ❸.

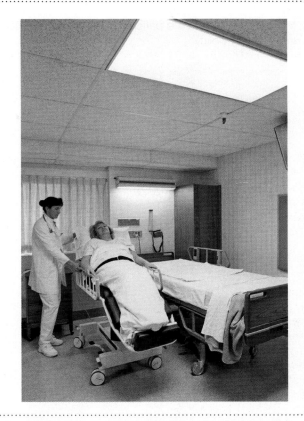

❶ Some belts have a key-locked buckle to prevent slipping and to provide a snug fit.

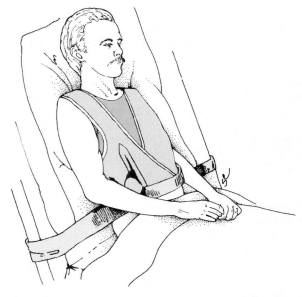

Source: Clinical Nursing Skills: Basic to Advanced Skills, 9e by Sandra F. Smith, Donna J. Duell, Barbara C. Martin, Michelle Aebersold, and Laura Gonzalez. Copyright © 2017 by Pearson Education.

❷ Vest restraint can be used for patient on bed rest or patient sitting in chair.

(continued on next page)

SKILL 15.12 Restraints, Torso and Belt: Applying (*continued*)

5. Monitor and assess the patient every 15 min, or according to facility policy.

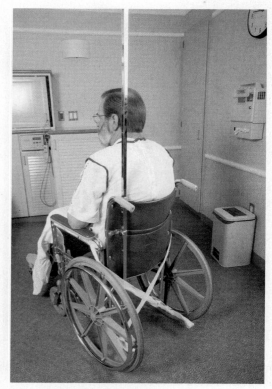

Source: Ronald May/Pearson Education, Inc.

❸ Check patient every 15 min while in restraint.

6. Release restraint at least every 2 hr or sooner (per The Joint Commission). **Rationale:** *Releasing restraints allows the patient to be provided with the following:*
   • Toileting
   • Fluids and food
   • Hygiene care such as brushing teeth or washing face and hands
   • Circulation checked; skin care provided
   • Body alignment checked
   • Range of motion to all joints, particularly those in restraints.
7. When the procedure is complete, perform hand hygiene and leave patient safe and comfortable.
8. Complete documentation using forms, checklists, or electronic dropdown lists supplemented by nurse's notes or additional comments as appropriate, including time, rationale, and type of safety belt used in nurse's notes, along with patient monitoring, patient response, frequency of care measures, and time and rationale for discontinuing restraint. Documentation must be done every 15 min.

SAMPLE DOCUMENTATION

[date] 0120 Found out of bed for 4th time tonight wandering down hallway, confused about what he was doing. Dr. Banks notified, torso belt restraint ordered. Belt restraint applied to patient in bed. Resting quietly at this time. Tolerated procedure without incident. *R. Mays*

SKILL 15.13 Restraints, Wrist and Ankle: Applying

Wrist and ankle restraints can also be used on elbows and knees to inhibit their movement and protect them from potential injury or harming others. Confused patients and small children may have their arms loosely restrained to keep them from scratching lesions, pulling out IV catheters, touching a dressed wound, or other actions of possible self-harm.

Delegation or Assignment

The nurse must make the determination that restraints are appropriate in specific situations, select the proper type of restraints, evaluate the effectiveness of the restraints, and assess for potential complications from their use. Application of ordered restraints and their temporary removal for skin monitoring and care may be delegated or assigned to the UAP trained in their use. Note that state laws for UAPs vary, so this task might be assigned to the UAP rather than delegated.

Equipment

■ Appropriate type and size of extremity restraints

Preparation

■ Review the patient's medical record as well as the nursing plan of care.
■ Check healthcare provider's order. If no order, call healthcare provider or licensed independent practitioner (LIP) for restraint order before applying restraints. If restraints must be placed before the order is obtained, ensure the order is obtained within 1 hr for either a nonbehavioral health patient or a behavioral health patient. **Rationale:** *Healthcare provider's order is required to apply restraints.* Follow guidelines for obtaining restraint orders and updating orders according to hospital policy.
■ Apply restraint according to manufacturer's specific directions.
■ Have the UAP available to help position and secure extremity restraints if needed.
■ Gather extremity restraints.

Procedure

1. Introduce self to patient and verify the patient's identity using two identifiers. Explain to the patient what you are

SKILL 15.13 Restraints, Wrist and Ankle: Applying *(continued)*

going to do, why it is necessary, and seek the patient's cooperation with restraint procedure, if possible. Discuss how the results will be used in planning further care or treatments. Allow time for the patient to express feelings about being restrained. Provide needed emotional reassurance that the restraints will be used only when absolutely necessary and that there will be close contact with the patient in case assistance is required.

2. Perform hand hygiene and observe appropriate infection control procedures.

3. Provide for patient privacy, safety, and comfort.

4. Apply the extremity restraint(s) as follows:
   - Pad bony prominences on the wrist or ankle if needed to prevent skin breakdown.
   - Apply the padded portion of the restraint around the ankle or wrist ❶.
   - Pull the tie of the restraint through the slit in the wrist portion or through the buckle and ensure the restraint is not too tight ❷.

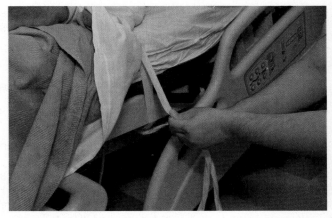

Source: Ronald May/Pearson Education, Inc.

❸ Secure restraint to movable part of bed frame.

- Using a half-bow knot, attach the other end of the restraint to the movable portion of the bed frame ❸ ❹. **Rationale:** *If the ties are attached to the movable portion, the wrist or ankle will not be pulled when the bed position is changed.*

5. Monitor and assess the patient every 15 min, or according to facility policy.

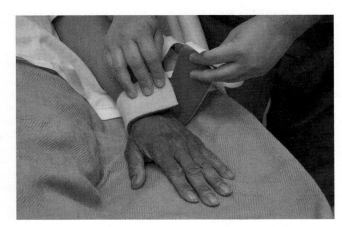

Source: Ronald May/Pearson Education, Inc.

❶ First, apply padded portion of restraint around wrist or ankle.

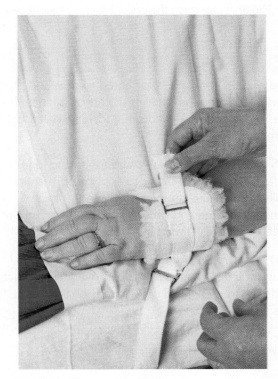

Source: Ronald May/Pearson Education, Inc.

❹ An alternate type of soft restraint. Slide strap through slit in restraint, and tighten strap, leaving fingerbreadth space between restraint and patient's limb.

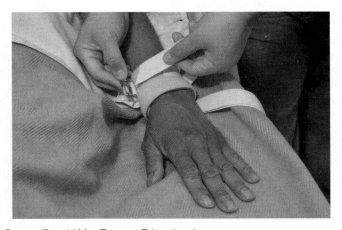

Source: Ronald May/Pearson Education, Inc.

❷ Secure restraint by pinching long-pronged adapter and inserting into buckle end of restraint, leaving fingerbreadth space between restraint and patient's limb.

(continued on next page)

SKILL 15.13 Restraints, Wrist and Ankle: Applying (continued)

6. Release restraint at least every 2 hr or sooner (per The Joint Commission). **Rationale:** *Releasing restraints allows the patient to be provided with the following:*
   - Toileting
   - Fluids and food
   - Hygiene care such as brushing teeth or washing face and hands
   - Circulation checked; skin care provided
   - Body alignment checked
   - Range of motion to all joints, particularly those in restraints.

7. When the procedure is complete, perform hand hygiene and leave patient safe and comfortable.

8. Complete documentation using forms, checklists, or electronic dropdown lists supplemented by nurse's notes or additional comments as appropriate, including behavior(s) indicating the need for the restraint, all other interventions implemented in an attempt to avoid the use of restraints and their outcomes, and the time the healthcare provider was notified of the need for restraint. Also record:
   - The type of restraint applied, the time it was applied, and the goal for its application
   - The patient's response to the restraint
   - The times that the restraints were removed and skin care given
   - Any other assessments and interventions
   - Explanations given the patient and significant others.

SAMPLE DOCUMENTATION

[date] 1200 Confused, disoriented to time and place. Reoriented frequently. Pulling at central IV line, NG tube, and chest tube. Medicated for pain relief. Lights dimmed. *M. Murray*

1245 Continues to pull at IV and tubes. Dr. Jones notified. Received an order to apply mitt restraints. Family notified and situation explained. Family member to come and sit with patient. Mitt restraints applied, relaxation music initiated. *M. Murray*

1330 Son arrived and sitting with patient. Calm though still disoriented. Mitts removed, skin intact, hands warm with good color and mobility. Vital signs stable. *M. Murray*

Lifespan Considerations
CHILDREN

- A UAP or willing parent can immobilize an infant or child during intramuscular injections.
- An elbow restraint keeps children from bending their elbows and reaching for tubes, IV tubing, and equipment ⑤.

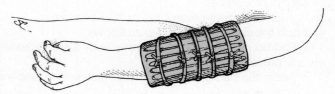

Source: Clinical Nursing Skills: Basic to Advanced Skills, 9e by Sandra F. Smith, Donna J. Duell, Barbara C. Martin, Michelle Aebersold, and Laura Gonzalez. Copyright © 2017 by Pearson Education.

⑤ **Elbow restraints keep children from reaching tubes, IV tubing, and equipment.**

- A papoose board immobilizer can be used for toddlers and larger children.
- A crib net is simply a device placed over the top of a crib to prevent active young children from climbing out of the crib. At the same time, it allows them freedom to move about in the crib. The crib net or dome is not attached to the movable parts of the crib so that the caregiver can have access to the child without removing the dome or net.
  - Place the net over the sides and ends of the crib.
  - Secure the ties to the springs or frame of the crib. The crib sides can then be freely lowered without removing the net.
  - Test with your hand that the net will stretch if the child stands against it in the crib.

Safety Considerations
RESTRAINTS IN THE HOME

While other measures should always be tried first, restraints may be necessary for patients in wheelchairs in the home. Safety guidelines apply in all cases. Assess the knowledge and skill of all caregivers in the use of restraints and educate as indicated.

- Use means other than restraints as much as possible, and stay with the patient. Remember that the goal is a restraint-free environment.
- Pad bony prominences, such as wrists and ankles, if needed before applying a restraint over them.
- Tie restraints with half-bow (quick release) knots that will not tighten when pulled, and to parts of the wheelchair that do not move and release quickly in case of emergency. Tie to parts of the wheelchair that do not move.
- Assess restrained limbs for signs of impaired blood circulation.
- Always stay with a patient whose restraint is temporarily removed.

Many institutions use a restraint monitoring and intervention flow sheet to ensure careful documentation.

>> Critical Thinking Options for Unexpected Outcomes

Not all unexpected outcomes require further nursing intervention; however, many times they do. When the patient demonstrates a change in signs or symptoms indicating an emerging problem, the nurse should immediately assess and troubleshoot what is happening. The assessment data must be processed quickly to formulate a hypothesis so the nurse can make a clinical judgment. The nurse then decides how best to resolve the problem and improve the patient's situation for a better outcome.

EXPECTED OUTCOME	UNEXPECTED OUTCOME	POSSIBLE INTERVENTIONS
Patient Safety All personal articles and call light are within easy reach of the patient.	Patient with history of falling has developed acute cognitive changes.	■ Alert all personnel that patient is high risk for fall. ■ Review medication regimen (e.g., Demerol and psychoactive drugs can cause acute confusion). ■ Assess for physiological causes (e.g., hypoxemia, infection, pain) and address alterations. ■ Place bedside commode away from bed and remove all obstacles; provide good lighting as well as night-light. ■ Reduce environmental stimuli (e.g., television). ■ Reorient patient with each encounter. ■ Move patient closer to nurses' station for better surveillance. ■ Employ monitoring alarm/device or engage family attendance. ■ Request floor mattress or recliner chair.
Patient does not have a seizure.	Patient has a tonic-clonic seizure.	■ Remain with patient. Do not restrain the patient. ■ Turn patient to lateral position if possible. ■ Perform oral suctioning after seizure episode to protect airway. ■ Note time length of seizure activity. ■ Provide oxygen via nasal cannula.
Patient is safely repositioned or transferred without injury to patient or caregiver.	Unable to transfer patient from bed to wheelchair due to excess weight.	■ Determine if wheelchair without arms or transfer board can aid in transfer. ■ Contact social services to obtain bariatric assist devices. ■ Determine if other family members can assist with transfer. ■ May need home health aide services to assist with transfer.
Caregiver is able to manage turning, repositioning, and assistive devices.	Injury occurs to patient when caregiver attempts transfer to wheelchair.	■ Do not continue to reposition patient; place in bed. ■ Conduct a complete sensory, motor, and pain assessment. ■ Notify healthcare provider. ■ Document findings.
Environmental Safety Patient is acclimated to home environment and is able to provide safe self-care after a period of support from facility staff.	Patient is noncompliant with treatments, safety procedures, and taking medications at home.	■ Explain rationale for following home care plan. ■ Discuss reason with patient, caregiver, and family members to determine whether change in plan would increase compliance. ■ Remind patient that if refusing to follow plan, the result will be removal from services. ■ Document appropriately on all forms, indicating noncompliance issues. ■ Notify healthcare provider.
Patient's environment is safe from potential mechanical, chemical, fire, and electrical hazards.	The patient, nurse, or visitor experiences an accident or injury related to mechanical, chemical, or thermal trauma.	■ Provide immediate first aid or care. ■ Assess vital signs and notify healthcare provider. ■ Report the incident according to facility procedure. Unusual occurrence forms are used to protect the injured individual, the nurse, and the facility. ■ Review safety procedures to ensure a safe environment. ■ Report all malfunctioning equipment immediately to the proper department.
	Unfamiliarity with facility fire and disaster protocol results in poor performance.	■ Review protocols frequently to update knowledge base. ■ Participate in fire and disaster drills to become familiar with protocols.

(continued on next page)

EXPECTED OUTCOME	UNEXPECTED OUTCOME	POSSIBLE INTERVENTIONS
Immobilizers and Restraints Patient does not develop complications due to restraint use (e.g., agitation, pressure ulcers, circulatory disturbance).	Skin abrasion, maceration, or rash occurs after application of restraints.	■ Reassess absolute need for restraint. ■ Reassess application method. ■ Increase padding of soft restraints before application. ■ Keep restraints off as much as possible and have staff or family member stay with patient.
	Impaired circulation or edema evidenced by change in color, sensation, movement, and blanching of nail beds.	■ On observation of signs of neurovascular changes, immediately release restraints. ■ Massage area gently to increase circulation. ■ If extremity is edematous, elevate extremity above level of heart. Encourage range-of-motion movements. ■ Request order for different type of restraint.
Restraints are applied appropriately.	Patient unties restraints.	■ Camouflage restraint to decrease patient's awareness. ■ Reassess need for restraint. ■ Offer diversional activities to promote safety. ■ Anticipate and attend to patient's needs.
Child is prevented from reaching an incision site, IVs, or tubes.	Child is able to reach incision site even with elbow restraints in place.	■ Make sure the elbow restraints are tight enough and extend over the elbow. ■ Tie the one elbow restraint to the opposite elbow restraint by placing the tie under the child's back and securing the tie with the upper tie on the opposite restraint. ■ Check that the restraint is large enough to completely immobilize the elbow. If not, obtain a larger size or use two restraints and tie them together securely.

REVIEW Questions

1. The nurse determines that a client is at a high risk for falling. What information in the health history did the nurse use to make this clinical determination?
   1. Wears eyeglasses
   2. Walks with a cane
   3. Diagnosed with diabetes
   4. Treated for hypertension

2. A new graduate nurse prepares the room for a client with a known seizure disorder. Which item should the nurse discuss with the graduate before the client arrives from the emergency department?
   1. Oxygen
   2. Padded side rails
   3. Suction equipment
   4. Padded tongue blade

3. The nurse arrives to visit the home of a client recovering from knee replacement surgery. Which environmental issue should the nurse address to reduce the client's risk of injury in the home?
   1. Throw rug on the floor next to the bed
   2. Handrails around the toilet and bathtub
   3. Double banisters mounted along the stairways
   4. Functioning telephone in each room of the home

4. The nurse manager examines client rooms in anticipation of a regulatory body visit over the next few days. Which situation should the manager address to reduce the risk of a fire?
   1. Suction machine plugged into an extension cord
   2. Equipment with frayed cords tagged for removal
   3. No Smoking signs prominently displayed in each room
   4. Three-pronged plug for the beds placed directly into an outlet

5. A client with confusion has a safety monitoring device with a leg band. What should the nurse do **first** after receiving a report on the status of this client?
   1. Test the battery and alarm system.
   2. Make sure that all side rails are raised.
   3. Check the location and position of the leg band.
   4. Remind the client to call for help to get out of bed.

6. A client demonstrating aggressive behavior is prescribed wrist restraints. What should the nurse do to ensure this client's safety?
   1. Assess the client every hour.
   2. Apply restraint directly over the wrist joint.
   3. Offer food and fluids every 3 hr.
   4. Perform range of motion to each wrist every 2 hr.

7. A client with severe confusion is prescribed a vest restraint. Where should the nurse affix the ties of the restraint when the client is in bed?
   1. The bed frame
   2. The bed wheels
   3. The upper side rail
   4. The lower side rail

8. The nurse notes that the hand of a client in wrist restraints is edematous. What action should the nurse take **first**?
   1. Remove the restraint.
   2. Massage the extremity.
   3. Elevate the extremity on a pillow.
   4. Request a different type of restraint.

Note: For answers and rationales for the review questions, go to Appendix A or your Pearson MyLab Nursing and eText.

Chapter 16
Tissue Integrity

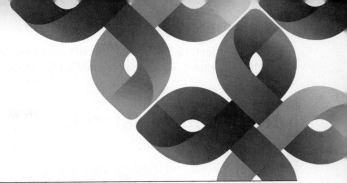

Chapter at a Glance

❶ Nursing students may observe or assist with the following skills only with faculty permission and while under direct supervision of faculty or another RN.

❯❯ The Concept of Tissue Integrity

Skin integrity, which includes the dermis and epidermis, provides the body a strong defense against temperature extremes, secretions, excretions, chemicals, pathogens, and other external environmental conditions and substances. Tissue integrity includes mucous membrane or corneal, integumentary, or subcutaneous tissue that is intact. When there is damage to the skin, tissue integrity can become impaired or damaged also.

Impaired tissue integrity may be the result of a chronic wound, ulcerated lesion, decubitus, or serious burn. Surgical wounds include impairment of both skin and tissue integrity. Understanding the etiology of a wound, the treatment options of wound care, the healing process, and the potential complications of a wound will assist the nurse in managing wound care interventions safely and effectively.

Learning Outcomes

16.1 Give examples of safety considerations when cleaning a surgical wound to prevent transferring microorganisms to other wound and skin areas.

16.2 Show appropriate application of a spiral elastic bandage that is firm but not tight on an extremity.

16.3 Differentiate characteristics of the methods used to debride a wound: autolytic, chemical, and mechanical.

16.4 Explain the importance of inspecting all skin areas for skin breakdown on admission and at least once a shift.

16.5 Summarize the evaluation process done to determine if patient is a candidate and wound is appropriate to implement negative pressure wound therapy.

16.6 Contrast and compare the steps in safely removing staples and sutures from a surgical wound.

The following feature links some, but not all, of the concepts related to assessment. They are presented in alphabetical order.

Concepts Related to
Tissue Integrity

CONCEPT	RELATIONSHIP TO TISSUE INTEGRITY	NURSING IMPLICATIONS
Caring Interventions	Hygiene habits can help protect skin and underlying tissue from dryness, soiling, and cracking.	■ Provide wound care using medical asepsis. ■ Assess skin and tissue at least daily. ■ Use lotion on skin and lip balm.
Elimination	Bowel and bladder incontinence is a high risk for tissue damage.	■ Keep perineal and rectal areas clean and dry. ■ Monitor for skin irritation. ■ Offer toileting to patient at regular intervals.
Infection	Introduction of pathogens for tissue damage with skin breakdown.	■ Implement standard precautions and further infectious control measures as appropriate. ■ Use medical asepsis with wound care or sterile technique as appropriate. ■ Monitor temperature.
Mobility	Shearing, friction, and pressure forces during movement of patient can result in weakened reddened skin areas that can become pressure injuries.	■ Have appropriate help when moving patient in bed and chair. ■ Assess for irritated or reddened skin areas, especially at bony prominences. ■ Encourage patient to reposition frequently or help them to reposition every 2 hr.
Teaching and Learning	Family can learn how to promote protection and healing of skin of home patient.	■ Educate family about how to care for impaired skin. ■ Provide support and encouragement to family.

The skin serves a variety of functions, including protecting the individual from injury. Impaired skin integrity is not a frequent problem for most healthy people, but it is a threat to older adults and patients with restricted mobility, chronic illness, or trauma, and to those undergoing invasive procedures. When the skin or underlying tissues are damaged, the inflammatory process of the individual's immune response acts to eliminate any foreign material, if possible, and to prepare the injured area for healing. This injured body area is called a **wound**. The nurse plays an important role in assessing patient risk for developing wounds, preventing wounds, and treating various types of wounds (**Table 16–1 »**).

TABLE 16–1 Types of Wounds

Type	Cause	Description and Characteristics
Incision	Sharp instrument (e.g., knife, scalpel)	Open wound; deep or shallow
Contusion	Blunt force injury to the soft tissue	Closed wound; skin appears ecchymotic (bruised) because of damaged blood capillaries
Abrasion	Surface scrape, either unintentional (e.g., scraped knee from a fall) or intentional (e.g., dermal abrasion to remove pockmarks)	Open wound involving the skin
Puncture	Penetration of the skin and often the underlying tissues by a sharp instrument, either intentional or unintentional	Open wound with small entry hole
Laceration	Tissues torn apart, often from accidents (e.g., with machinery)	Open wound; edges are often jagged
Penetrating wound	Penetration of the skin and the underlying tissues, usually unintentional (e.g., from a bullet or metal fragments)	Open wound

>> General Assessment

Expected Outcomes

1. Patient's wound does not become infected.
2. Patient's wound remains intact following staple and/or suture removal.
3. Wound care is provided for contaminated wound, and healing occurs.
4. Drainage system functions without obstructions.
5. Wound irrigation is completed using sufficient pressure to cleanse wound bed.
6. Patient maintains adequate fluid and nutrition.
7. Patient's buttocks and perineal area remain free from urine and stool.
8. Patient is periodically repositioned.

SKILL 16.1 Wound Drainage Specimen: Obtaining

Safety Note! *During scheduled clinical time, nursing students may have a learning opportunity to observe or assist with this skill only with faculty permission and with direct supervision from faculty or another RN.*

Drainage from a wound usually indicates infection, especially when there is also increased local pain of the area, redness, and edema, and the patient has an increased temperature. A wound culture is done to diagnose the type of microorganisms causing the infection and how many colonies of the pathogen there are in the wound. When a culture is done in the lab, the healthcare provider commonly orders a sensitivity to be done also. This information is used to determine the appropriate antibiotic treatment and help to prevent antibiotic-resistant microorganisms.

Delegation or Assignment

Obtaining a wound culture is an invasive procedure that requires the application of sterile technique, knowledge of wound healing, and potential problem solving to ensure patient safety. Therefore, the nurse needs to perform this skill and does not delegate or assign it to the UAP. The nurse can request the UAP to report patient observations to the nurse for follow-up. Assessment and evaluation remain the responsibility of the nurse.

Equipment

- Clean gloves
- Protective eyewear, if appropriate
- Moisture-resistant bag
- Disposable sterile dressing kit
- Short disposable measuring ruler with inches and centimeters marked
- Normal saline in a pour bottle and irrigating syringe
- Culture tube with swab and culture medium (aerobic and anaerobic tubes are available) or sterile syringe with needle for anaerobic culture
- Completed lab labels for each container
- Completed lab requisition to accompany the specimens to the laboratory

Preparation

- Review healthcare provider's orders to determine if the specimen is to be collected for an **aerobic** (growing only in

the *presence* of oxygen) or **anaerobic** (growing only in the *absence* of oxygen) culture. Aerobic organisms are generally found on the surface of the wound, whereas anaerobic organisms would be found in deep wounds, tunnels, and cavities.
- Review nursing plan of care for wound care and type of dressing to be applied.
- Administer an analgesic 30 minutes before the procedure if the patient is complaining of pain at the wound site to prevent unnecessary discomfort during the procedure.

Procedure

1. Introduce self to patient and verify the patient's identity using two identifiers. Explain to the patient that you are going to obtain a wound swab for the lab to do a culture test, why it is necessary, and how the patient can participate. Discuss how the results will be used in planning further care or treatments.
2. Perform hand hygiene and observe other appropriate infection control procedures.
3. Provide for patient privacy, comfort, and safety.
4. Remove any dressing that covers the wound.
   - Don clean gloves.
   - Remove the dressing, and observe any drainage on the dressing. Hold the dressing so that the patient does not see the drainage. **Rationale:** *The appearance of the drainage could upset the patient.*
   - Determine the amount, color, consistency, and odor of the drainage. For example, "one 4 × 4 gauze saturated with yellow-greenish, thick, malodorous drainage."
   - Discard the dressing in the moisture-resistant bag. Handle it carefully so that the dressing does not touch the outside of the bag. **Rationale:** *Touching the outside of the bag will contaminate the bag.*
   - Remove and discard gloves. Perform hand hygiene.
5. Open the sterile dressing set using sterile technique.
6. Assess the wound.
   - Don clean gloves.
   - Assess the appearance of the tissues in and around the wound and the drainage. Infection can cause reddened tissues with a thick discharge, which may be foul smelling, whitish, or colored.
   - Measure the wound while it is uncovered. Using the disposable ruler, place the ruler over the wound and

(continued on next page)

SKILL 16.1 Wound Drainage Specimen: Obtaining (*continued*)

measure length and width in centimeters. **Rationale:** *The size of the wound is indicative of the wound healing and getting smaller or of the wound extending and getting larger.*

7. Clean the wound.
   - Using gauze swabs or irrigation, clean the wound with normal saline until all visible exudates have been removed.
   - After cleaning, apply a sterile gauze pad to the wound. **Rationale:** *This absorbs excess saline.*
   - If a topical antimicrobial ointment or cream is being used to treat the wound, use a swab to remove it. **Rationale:** *Residual antiseptic must be removed prior to culture.*
   - Remove and discard gloves. Perform hand hygiene.

AEROBIC CULTURE

8. Obtain the aerobic culture (microorganisms that only grow in the presence of oxygen).
   - Don clean gloves.
   - Open a specimen tube and place the cap upside down on a firm, dry surface so that the inside will not become contaminated, or if the swab is attached to the lid, twist the cap to loosen the swab. Hold the tube in one hand and take out the swab with the other.
   - Rotate the swab back and forth over clean areas of granulation tissue from the sides or base of the wound. **Rationale:** *Microorganisms most likely to be responsible for a wound infection reside in viable tissue.*
   - Do not collect pus or pooled exudates to culture. **Rationale:** *These secretions contain a mixture of contaminants that are not the same as those causing the infection.*
   - Avoid touching the swab to intact skin at the wound edges. **Rationale:** *This prevents the introduction of superficial skin organisms into the culture.*
   - Return the swab to the culture tube, taking care not to touch the top or the outside of the tube ❶. **Rationale:** *The outside of the container must remain free of pathogenic microorganisms to prevent their spread to others.*
   - Crush the inner ampule containing the medium for organism growth at the bottom of the tube. **Rationale:** *This ensures that the swab with the specimen is surrounded by culture medium.*
   - Twist the cap to secure.

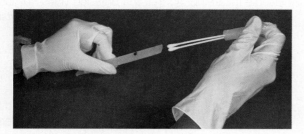

Source: Ronald May/Pearson Education, Inc.

❶ Push applicator stick into specimen tube, being careful not to contaminate stick.

ANAEROBIC CULTURE

8. Obtain the anaerobic culture (microorganisms that only grow in the absence of oxygen).
   - Don clean gloves.
   - Use an anaerobic culture swab system in which the swab is immediately placed into a tube filled with an oxygen-free gas or gel environment ❷.

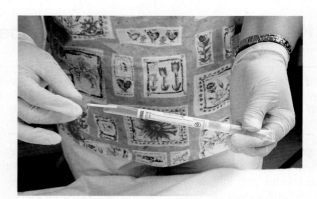

Source: Ronald May/Pearson Education, Inc.

❷ Push tip of swab into a culture medium.

9. If a specimen is required from another site, repeat the steps. Specify the exact site (e.g., inferior drain site or lower aspect of incision) on the label of each container. Be sure to put each swab in the appropriately labeled tube.
10. Dress the wound.
    - Apply any ordered medication to the wound.
    - Cover the wound with a sterile transparent wound dressing.
11. When the procedure is complete, remove and discard gloves. Perform hand hygiene and leave the patient safe and comfortable.
12. Arrange for the specimen(s) to be transported immediately to the laboratory. Be sure to include the completed requisition(s).
13. Complete documentation using forms, checklists, or electronic dropdown lists supplemented by nurse's notes or additional comments as appropriate, including obtaining the specimen and source, the appearance of the wound; the color, consistency, amount, and odor of any drainage; the type of culture collected; and any discomfort experienced by the patient.

SAMPLE DOCUMENTATION

[date] 1000 Obtained specimen from right hip wound for anaerobic culture. Pressure injury 3 × 3 cm, 2 cm deep, minimal amt. thick, yellow drainage. No odor. Skin around wound reddened. Rates pain at 0 on 0–10 scale. *N. Jamaghani*

>> Dressings and Binders

Expected Outcomes

1. Patient's wound heals without complications.
2. Abdominal binder supports patient's abdominal wound.
3. Compression dressing is applied to vascular ulcer site.

SKILL 16.2 Abdominal Binder: Applying

An abdominal binder is made of elastic material that supports the abdominal muscles and keeps incisional dressings in place postsurgical abdominal or pelvic surgery.

Delegation or Assignment

Applying an abdominal binder and assessing the patient with the binder in place is the nurse's responsibility and not delegated or assigned to the UAP. The UAP may provide routine care of the patient as trained. The nurse can request the UAP to report patient observations to the nurse for follow-up. The nurse remains responsible for the assessment, interpretation of abnormal findings, and determination of appropriate responses.

Equipment

▪ Abdominal binder: woven-cotton, synthetic, or elasticized material with Velcro closures

Preparation

▪ Review healthcare provider's order and review nursing plan of care.
▪ Gather binder.

Procedure

1. Introduce self to patient and verify the patient's identity using two identifiers. Explain to the patient you are going to apply a binder around the abdomen, why it is necessary, and how the patient can participate. Discuss how the results will be used in planning further care or treatments.
2. Perform hand hygiene and observe other appropriate infection control procedures.
3. Place patient in supine position.
4. Ask patient to raise hips, and then slide the binder under patient's hips at level of gluteal fold. Place top of binder at patient's waist.
5. Bring ends of binder around patient, ❶ and secure by pressing Velcro surfaces together.
6. Observe for wrinkles in binder. Apply padding over the iliac crests if the patient is thin. **Rationale:** *Wrinkles can cause pressure areas especially over the iliac crest.*
7. Assess patient's ability to move freely, breathe deeply, and feel secure pressure over abdominal incision ❷. **Rationale:** *A binder that is too tight or too high may compromise breathing or place pressure on incisional area. A binder placed too low interferes with elimination and walking.*

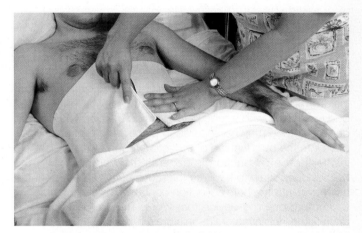

Source: Ronald May/Pearson Education, Inc.

❶ Bring end of binder around patient and secure Velcro surfaces.

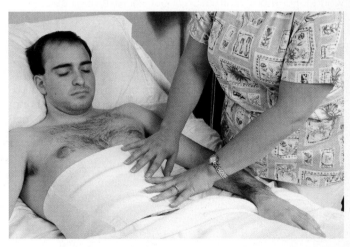

Source: Ronald May/Pearson Education, Inc.

❷ Assess effectiveness of binder (secure pressure over incision, ability to move freely and breathe deeply). Reassess every 4 hr.

(continued on next page)

SKILL 16.2 Abdominal Binder: Applying *(continued)*

8. When the procedure is complete, perform hand hygiene and leave patient safe and comfortable.
9. Complete documentation using forms, checklists, or electronic dropdown lists supplemented by nurse's notes or additional comments as appropriate.
10. Assess effectiveness of binder every 4 hr. Many patients use this binder only when ambulating.

SAMPLE DOCUMENTATION

[date] 1004 Assisted to supine position in bed. Abdominal binder applied and secured with Velcro closures. Denies any pain or problem with breathing. Binder smooth without wrinkles. Tolerated procedure without incident. States she feels better supported now. *H. Hernandez*

SKILL 16.3 Closed Wound Drains: Maintaining

The Jackson-Pratt drain is a device used to collect fluids from inside a surgical area. The bulb-shaped device outside the body connects with a tube placed inside the body during surgery. The tube may be secured in place with a suture. Fluids drain into the bulb instead of collecting around the surgical site inside the body. Suction is generated by compressing the bulb-shaped drain to facilitate the movement of fluid out of the body and into the bulb collection container.

Another draining device that works like the Jackson-Pratt drain is the Hemovac drain. This drain has a larger fluid capacity collection circular container. It also is placed inside a surgical area and connected to the Hemovac by a tube. Like the Jackson-Pratt drain, the Hemovac is compressed to create suction in the tube to aid fluid movement out of the body and into the collection container.

A Penrose drain is used to facilitate open drainage of fluid from inside a wound to collect in the dressing covering the wound. For more information about Penrose drain care, go to Skill 16.9 in this chapter.

Delegation or Assignment

Assessment of the wound, wound drainage, and patency of the wound suction require application of knowledge and problem solving and is the responsibility of the nurse and is not delegated or assigned to the UAP. The UAP, however, can empty the drainage unit, measure the drainage, and record the amount on the intake and output record. The nurse must ensure that the UAP knows how to empty the unit without contaminating it.

Equipment

- Clean gloves
- Calibrated drainage receptacle
- Moisture-proof pad
- Alcohol sponge
- Closed wound drainage system (e.g., Jackson-Pratt, Hemovac)

Preparation

- Check healthcare provider's orders and nursing plan of care.

- Determine the type and placement of the patient's closed wound drain.
- Gather supplies.

Procedure

1. Introduce self and verify the patient's identity using two identifiers. Explain to the patient what you are going to do, why it is necessary, and how the patient can participate. Discuss how the results will be used in planning further care or treatments.
2. Perform hand hygiene and observe other appropriate infection control procedures.
3. Provide for patient privacy.
4. Empty the drainage unit.
   - Don clean gloves.
   - Place the Jackson-Pratt device or Hemovac device on the waterproof pad.
   - Open the plug of the drainage unit.
   - Observe the color, odor, consistency, and amount of drainage.
   - Invert the unit and empty it into the collecting receptacle ❶.
5. Re-establish suction.

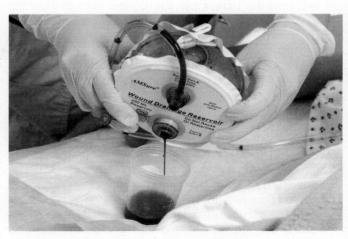

Source: Rick Brady/Pearson Education, Inc.

❶ Emptying drainage from Hemovac drainage system.

SKILL 16.3 Closed Wound Drains: Maintaining (*continued*)

JACKSON-PRATT DRAIN

- Compress the bulb flat between the fingers with the port open.
- While maintaining tight compression on the bulb, clean the ends of the emptying port.
- Insert the plug into the emptying port. **Rationale:** *This re-establishes the vacuum necessary for the closed drainage system to work.*

HEMOVAC

- Place the unit on a solid, flat surface with port open.
- Place palm of hand on unit and press the top and the bottom together.
- While holding the top and bottom together, clean the opening and the plug with an alcohol swab.
- Replace the drainage plug before releasing hand pressure. **Rationale:** *This re-establishes the vacuum necessary for the closed drainage system to work.*

6. Secure the unit to the patient's gown or position the suction unit on the bed.
   - Ensure that the unit is below the level of the wound ❷. **Rationale:** *This facilitates drainage.*

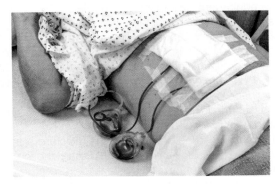

Source: Rick Brady/Pearson Education, Inc.

❷ Two Jackson-Pratt devices compressed to facilitate collection of exudates.

7. When the procedure is complete, remove and discard gloves. Perform hand hygiene and leave patient safe and comfortable.
8. Complete documentation using forms, checklists, or electronic dropdown lists supplemented by nurse's notes or additional comments as appropriate including the amount and type of drainage on the intake and output record.

SAMPLE DOCUMENTATION

[date] 1830 Jackson-Pratt drain intact, insertion site dressing dry. 45 mL dark rusty-colored drainage with few small clots noted, faint smell of blood noted when drain emptied. Plug area cleaned with alcohol, bulb compressed, and plug inserted. Tolerated procedure without incident. *C. Milkadon*

Patient Teaching

Drain Care at Home
- Provide community home care resources for family to schedule regular nursing visits to teach wound care and to observe the drainage site.
- Ensure the patient or a caregiver can empty, measure, and record the drainage at least once daily.
- Ensure the caregiver knows how to observe the wound daily for signs of infection, such as redness, edema, tenderness, or purulent drainage.
- Ensure the patient's temperature will be measured twice daily. **Rationale:** *Elevated temperature can indicate infection.*
- Ensure that the patient has the proper supplies and knows where to obtain new items as needed.
- Verify the patient or caregiver has the healthcare provider's telephone number to call the healthcare provider for excess drainage, signs of infection, or occlusion of the tube.
- Determine when the healthcare provider plans to remove the drain, and assist the patient in making an appointment.

SKILL 16.4 Dressing, Dry: Changing

There is a wide range of dressings used to cover wounds and protect them from contamination that can result in an infection during the healing process. A dry dressing can be made with gauze pads or may be clear and transparent. The type of dry dressing depends on the type and size of the wound. The type of dressing to use can be ordered by the healthcare provider, the wound care nurse, or by observing the type of dressing already applied to cover the wound.

Delegation or Assignment

Due to the need for aseptic technique and assessment skills, most dressing changes are not delegated or assigned to the UAP. In some states, the UAP may apply dry dressings to clean,

chronic wounds. The UAP should observe an exposed wound or dressing during usual care and must report abnormal findings to the nurse. In some agencies, the UAP may be permitted to reinforce the dressing (apply additional dry dressings over a saturated bandage), but this must be reported to the nurse as soon as possible. Assessment of the wound and abnormal findings must be validated and interpreted by the nurse.

Equipment

- Clean gloves
- Sterile gloves (optional)
- Sterile 4 × 4 gauzes

(*continued on next page*)

SKILL 16.4 Dressing, Dry: Changing (continued)

- Hypoallergenic tape, tie tapes, or binder
- Bath blanket (if necessary)
- Moisture-proof bag
- Mask (optional)
- Adhesive removal solution or pads
- Sterile dressing set; if none is available, gather the following sterile items:
  - Drape or towel
  - Gauze squares
  - Container for the cleaning solution
  - Antimicrobial solution
  - Forceps.
- Additional supplies required for the particular dressing (e.g., extra gauze dressings and ointment or powder, if ordered)

CAUTION! Only use sterile supplies, dressing materials, and instruments when changing a dry dressing, even if doing a clean dressing change to protect the wound while healing. Use sterile gloves when handling dressing materials that will be inserted into the wound. Always use hand hygiene when removing and replacing gloves.

Preparation

- Review healthcare provider's order and patient's nursing plan of care.
- Administer prescribed analgesic at least 45 minutes before scheduled dressing change if needed and requested by patient for pain management during procedure.
- Acquire assistance for changing a dressing on a restless or confused adult. **Rationale:** *The person might move and contaminate the sterile field or the wound.*
- Make a cuff on the moisture-proof bag for disposal of the soiled dressings, and place the bag within reach. **Rationale:** *Making a cuff keeps the outside of the bag free from contamination by the soiled dressings. Placement of the bag within reach prevents the nurse from reaching across the sterile field and the wound.*
- Gather supplies.

Procedure

1. Introduce self and verify the patient's identity using two identifiers. Explain to the patient what you are going to do, why it is necessary, and how the patient can participate. Discuss how the results will be used in planning further care or treatments.
2. Perform hand hygiene and observe other appropriate infection control procedures.
3. Provide for patient privacy. Assist the patient to a comfortable position in which the wound can be readily exposed. Expose only the wound area, using a bath blanket to cover the patient, if necessary. **Rationale:** *Undue exposure is physically and psychologically distressing to most people.*
4. Don a face mask, as indicated. **Rationale:** *A mask may be worn for surgical dressing changes to prevent contamination of the wound by droplet spray from the nurse's respiratory tract.*
5. To remove the outer dressing:
   - Don clean gloves.

- If adhesive tape was used, remove it by holding down the skin and pulling the tape gently but firmly toward the wound. **Rationale:** *Pressing down on the skin provides countertraction against the pulling motion. Tape is pulled toward the incision to prevent strain on the sutures.*
- Use a solvent if required to loosen tape. **Rationale:** *Moistening the tape with a solvent lessens the discomfort of removal.*
- Lift the dressing so that the underside is away from the patient's face. **Rationale:** *The appearance and odor of the drainage may be upsetting to the patient.*
- Assess the soiled dressing for type and odor of wound drainage while placing it in the moisture-proof bag; do not touch the outside of the bag. **Rationale:** *Contamination of the outside of the bag is avoided to prevent the spread of microorganisms to the nurse and others.*
- Remove gloves, dispose of them in the moisture-proof bag, and perform hand hygiene.
6. To remove the inner dressings:
   - Open the sterile dressing set, using aseptic technique (see Skill 13.4, p. 576).
   - Place the sterile drape beside the wound or on the bedside table to form a sterile field. Open the individual sterile equipment and place on the field. Don gloves (or sterile gloves, depending on wound).
   - Remove the wound dressings with forceps or sterile gloves. **Rationale:** *Forceps or gloves are used to prevent contamination of the wound by the nurse's hands and contamination of the nurse's hands by wound drainage.*
   - Assess the location, type (color, consistency), amount, and odor of wound drainage.
   - Discard the soiled dressings in the moisture-proof bag.
   - After the dressings are removed, discard the forceps, or set them aside from the sterile field. **Rationale:** *These are now contaminated by the wound drainage.*
   - Remove and discard sterile gloves (if applied). Perform hand hygiene.
7. Assess wound characteristics and measurements including length, width, and depth following facility procedures.
8. To clean the wound:
   - Don clean gloves, using a new pair of forceps and moistened swabs.
   - Keep the forceps' tips lower than the handles at all times. **Rationale:** *This prevents their contamination by fluid traveling up to the handle and nurse's wrist and back to the tips.*
   - Clean with strokes from the top to the bottom, starting at the center and continuing to the outside ❶.
   or
   - Clean outward from the wound ❷. **Rationale:** *The wound is cleaned from the least to the most contaminated area.*
   - Use a separate swab for each stroke, and discard each swab after use. **Rationale:** *This prevents the introduction of microorganisms to other wound areas.*
   - Repeat the cleaning process until all drainage is removed.
   - Remove and discard gloves. Perform hand hygiene.

SKILL 16.4 Dressing, Dry: Changing (*continued*)

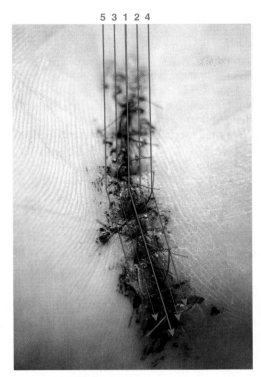

5 3 1 2 4

Source: Samuel Ashfield/Science Source

❶ Cleaning a wound from top to bottom.

Safety Considerations

Normal saline in a pour bottle is widely used for cleaning and irrigating wounds. When using an already opened normal saline pour bottle, check the date on the container. It is only good for 24 hr from time opened (follow facility policy). In severely infected wounds, antimicrobial irrigations may be used as ordered. Povidone-iodine and hydrogen peroxide are not used on acute wounds. They are drying agents and, as such, dry the wound bed. They have also been shown to be cytotoxic to beneficial healthy cells in the wound bed area. Wounds maintained in a moist environment have a lower infection rate than dry wounds.

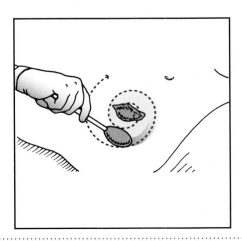

❷ Cleaning a wound from the center outward.

9. Apply sterile dressings.
   - Apply sterile dressings one at a time over the wound, using sterile forceps or sterile gloves. Start at the center of the wound and move progressively outward. The final abdominal dressing can be picked up by gloved hand, touching only the outside, which is often marked by a blue line down the center.
   - Remove and discard gloves if used. Perform hand hygiene.
10. Secure the dressing with tape, tie tapes, or a binder.
    - Place the tape so that the dressing cannot be folded back to expose the wound. Place strips at the ends of the dressing, and space the tape evenly in the middle ❸.
    - Ensure that the tape is long and wide enough to adhere to the skin but not so long or wide that it loosens with activity.
    - Place the tape in the opposite direction from the body action; for example, across a body joint or crease, not lengthwise ❹.

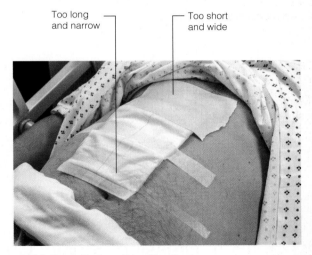

Too long and narrow Too short and wide

Source: Rick Brady/Pearson Education, Inc.

❸ Taping the dressing.

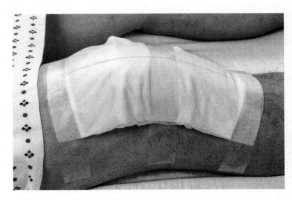

Source: Rick Brady/Pearson Education, Inc.

❹ Dressings over moving parts taped at right angle to the joint movement.

(*continued on next page*)

SKILL 16.4 Dressing, Dry: Changing (*continued*)

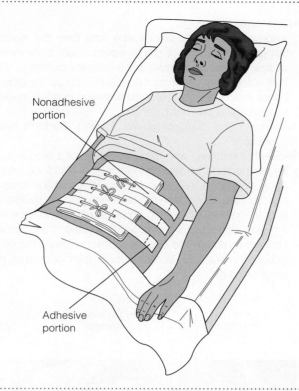

Nonadhesive portion

Adhesive portion

⑤ Montgomery straps, or tie tapes, are used to secure large dressings that require frequent changing.

- Montgomery straps (tie tapes) are commonly used for wounds requiring frequent dressing changes ⑤. **Rationale:** *These straps prevent the skin irritation and*

discomfort caused by removing the adhesive each time the dressing is changed.
  - For patients with tape allergies or other conditions in which tape should not be applied directly to the skin, wrap over the dressing and around the body part with rolled gauze, and tape only the gauze.
11. When the procedure is complete, perform hand hygiene and leave patient safe and comfortable.
12. Complete documentation using forms, checklists, or electronic dropdown lists supplemented by nurse's notes or additional comments as appropriate.

SAMPLE DOCUMENTATION

[date] 0740 Surgical site dressing on lower abdomen remains intact with scant amount pink-tinged drainage on dressing. Dressing removed, inner side has small amount pink-beige drainage, no odor, no clots noted. Old gloves removed, hand hygiene performed, new clean gloves applied. Incision site intact with five sutures, small amount of redness along incision, no tenderness or drainage noted. Old gloves removed, hand hygiene performed, new clean gloves applied. Sterile gauze pad placed along suture line with ABD pad placed on top of them, and secured with plastic tape. Tolerated procedure without complaint, resting quietly. *H. Durch*

SKILL 16.5 Dressing, Sterile: Changing

Safety Note! *During scheduled clinical time, nursing students may have a learning opportunity to observe or assist with this skill only with faculty permission and with direct supervision from faculty or another RN.*

Sterile gloves, sterile technique, and sterile supplies are used to change a sterile dressing. Sterile dressings are commonly used to cover post-op surgical sites to protect the incision from contamination. Sterile gloves are used to place supplies and dressings on a sterile field for use during the dressing change. Normal saline is poured into a sterile container on the sterile field to be used for cleaning the wound or around the wound as needed.

Delegation or Assignment

Due to the need for sterile technique and technical complexity, changing a sterile dressing is not delegated or assigned to the UAP. The UAP may care for patients after the procedure. The nurse must ensure that the UAP knows what complications or

adverse signs should be reported to the nurse. The nurse remains responsible for the assessment, interpretation of abnormal findings, and determination of appropriate responses.

Equipment

- Disposable sterile dressing kit, or gather needed sterile supplies
- Sterile gloves
- Clean gloves
- Antiseptic wipes
- Mask, if needed
- Gown
- Disposal bag for used dressings
- Dressing supplies, as needed
- Plastic tape
- Sterile normal saline in pour bottle
- Package sterile cotton swabs or 4 × 4 pads
- Disposable ruler marked with inches and centimeters to measure the wound
- Bath blanket or sheet

SKILL 16.5 Dressing, Sterile: Changing (*continued*)

Preparation

- Check healthcare provider's orders and patient's nursing plan of care.
- Administer prescribed analgesic at least 45 minutes before scheduled dressing change if needed and requested by patient for pain management during procedure.
- Verify sterile dressing change is required for the wound.
- Gather supplies.

Procedure

1. Introduce self to patient and verify the patient's identity using two identifiers. Explain to the patient you are going to change the dressing, why it is necessary, and how the patient can participate. Discuss how the results will be used in planning further care or treatments.
2. Perform hand hygiene and observe appropriate infection control procedures.
3. Provide privacy. Provide comfort and safety for patient and self, including raising bed to appropriate height.
4. Prepare a sterile field for the sterile dressing supplies:
   - Clean off overbed table, wipe with antiseptic pad, and allow to air dry.
   - Place sterile supplies on overbed table.
   - Place bag for soiled dressings near incision site.
   - Fanfold linen to expose incision area.
   - Cover patient with bath blanket or sheet, leaving incision area exposed.
   - Create a sterile field with a drape or packaging from sterile dressing kit. Open sterile packages by pulling flap back and away from sterile area, and place on overbed table. Arrange packages to ensure you do not cross over the sterile field when reaching for dressings. **Rationale:** *Commercially prepared sterile packages can be opened and used for the sterile field because the inside of the package is sterile.*
   - Cut tape into appropriate length strips.
5. To remove old dressing:
   - Remove tape slowly by pulling tape toward the wound ❶. **Rationale:** *Pulling toward the wound decreases the pain of tape removal by not putting pressure on the incision line.*

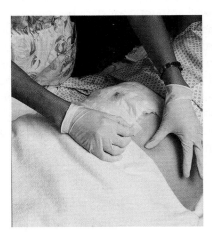

❶ Remove tape by gently lifting toward wound.

- Don clean gloves.
- Remove soiled dressing and dispose of in the proper bag ❷ ❸. Wet dressing with sterile normal saline if it adheres to the suture line.

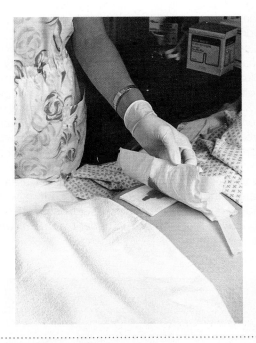

❷ Remove soiled dressing carefully.

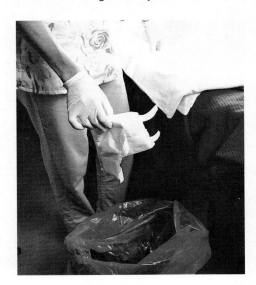

❸ Dispose of dressing in appropriate container.

- Assess area surrounding the incision for erythema, edema, or drainage. **Rationale:** *Persistent drainage, edema, or temperature above 38°C (100.4°F) 2 days postop indicates a complication is occurring.*
- Assess color of incision. (A healing incision looks pink or red.) **Rationale:** *Redness that does not fade 48 hr after surgery may indicate impaired healing.*

(*continued on next page*)

SKILL 16.5 Dressing, Sterile: Changing (*continued*)

- Measure the length and width of the wound, and depth if present.
- Remove clean gloves, discard, and perform hand hygiene.

6. Move overbed table next to working area.
7. Clean the wound and apply a new dressing.
   - Don sterile gloves.
   - Cleanse incision area with sterile swabs or 4 × 4 pads soaked in normal saline, according to facility policy. Clean from incision line outward, cleaning from top to bottom, using the swab only once. Discard swabs or 4 × 4 pads in disposal bag. **Rationale:** *Cleaning outward from incision cleans from least to most contaminated area. Cleaning from top to bottom prevents contamination from secretions that accumulate at the bottom of the wound.*
   - Place 4 × 4 gauze pads over incision area, being careful not to touch incision or patient with your gloves ❹. Reglove if this should occur. **Rationale:** *Touching the incision or patient contaminates the gloves.*

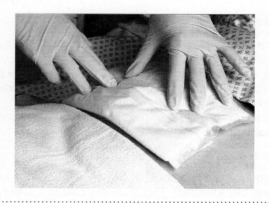

❺ Place abdominal pad over center of incision.

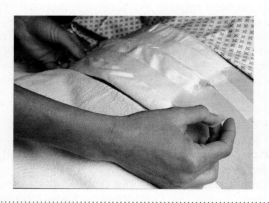

❻ Tape dressing securely to prevent slipping.

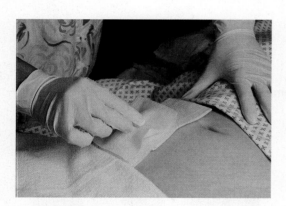

❹ Do not touch incision when applying dressing.

   - Place abdominal (ABD) pad over incision, being careful not to contaminate the gloves ❺.
   - Remove gloves and discard.
   - Tape dressing securely ❻.
   - Discard trash in appropriate receptacle.

8. When the procedure is complete, return bed to lowest height, perform hand hygiene, and leave the patient safe and comfortable.
9. Complete documentation using forms, checklists, or electronic dropdown lists supplemented by nurse's notes or additional comments as appropriate, including assessment of wound, incision area cleaned with saline, dry sterile dressing applied, and patient tolerance of procedure.

SAMPLE DOCUMENTATION

[date] 1643 Found lying on right side, assisted to supine position for dressing change of abdominal incision site. Sterile supplies set-up on bedside table. Old dressing removed using adhesive removal pads. Outer side of dressing had no drainage noted, inner side had small amount clear dark beige-colored stain. Incision has 6 intact staples. Incision is 8 cm long. Light redness around staples, no drainage noted from wound, no tenderness around incision site, slight amount of swelling noted. Area around wound cleaned with normal saline. Sterile gauze placed over wound with abdominal dressing placed to cover the gauze. Plastic tape applied to secure dressing. Tolerated dressing change without complaint. *D. Tutor*

SKILL 16.6 Dressing, Venous Ulcer: Changing

Safety Note! *During scheduled clinical time, nursing students may have a learning opportunity to observe or assist with this skill only with faculty permission and with direct supervision from faculty or another RN.*

A venous ulcer can develop when an individual has poor venous circulation in the legs. Pressure inside the veins increases and over time there is damage to the capillaries. This causes the skin to become weak and more vulnerable to minor bumps, which can result in a skin integrity breakdown or tear. Because the leg venous circulation is impaired, healing of the venous wound or ulcer can take 3–4 months, even with appropriate compression therapy.

Delegation or Assignment

Changing a venous ulcer dressing is the nurse's or wound care nurse's responsibility and not delegated or assigned to the UAP. The UAP may provide routine care of the patient as trained. The nurse can request the UAP to report patient observations to the nurse for follow-up. The nurse remains responsible for the assessment, interpretation of abnormal findings, and determination of appropriate responses.

Equipment

- Cleansing solution
- Sterile normal saline solution in a pour bottle
- Sterile 4 × 4 gauze pads
- Moisture-retentive dressings (hydrocolloid, transparent film, or foam for light-to-moderate drainage)
- Absorbent dressings (foams, alginates, and absorptive dressings) for moderate to heavy exudate
- Compression dressing
- Clean gloves
- Sterile gloves
- Biohazard bag
- Ruler marked in inches and centimeters
- Scissors
- Absorbent pad

Preparation

- Review healthcare provider's orders and patient's nursing plan of care.
- Gather equipment and supplies ❶.

Procedure

1. Introduce self to patient and verify the patient's identity using two identifiers. Explain to the patient you are going to change the dressing on the leg, why it is necessary, and how the patient can participate. Discuss how the results will be used in planning further care or treatments.
2. Perform hand hygiene and observe appropriate infection control procedures.
3. Provide for patient privacy. Raise bed to appropriate height.
4. Clear and clean overbed table. Open sterile packages, and arrange on overbed table.
5. Don clean gloves.

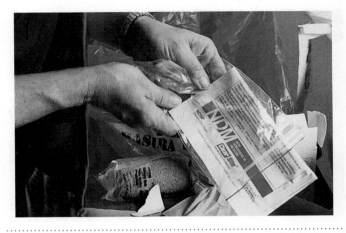

❶ Obtain appropriate wound dressing kit, if available.

6. Place absorbent pad under wound.
7. Remove compression bandage and old dressing, and place in biohazard bag ❷. Compression dressings may be left in place for 3–7 days depending on amount of drainage and type of dressing.

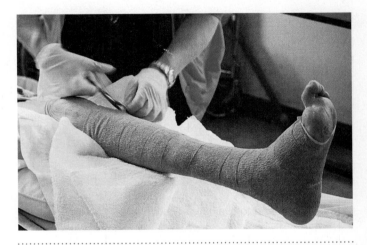

❷ Remove compression dressing, being careful not to cut skin.

8. Assess and measure the wound ❸ ❹. **Rationale:** *This determines effectiveness of treatment.*
9. Clean and debride wound as ordered.
   - Clean off debris by pouring cleansing solution over wound.
   - Rinse wound with sterile normal saline ❺ ❻.

CAUTION! The wound bed should be kept moist to promote granulation and re-epithelialization and to reduce pain. Ointments provide the most occlusive moisturizer because they contain oil and water.

(continued on next page)

SKILL 16.6 Dressing, Venous Ulcer: Changing *(continued)*

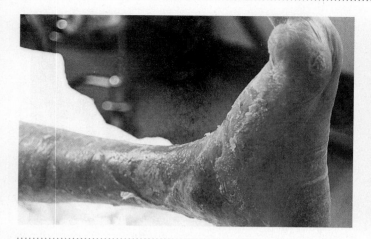

③ Assess wound healing and evaluate progress (stage II).

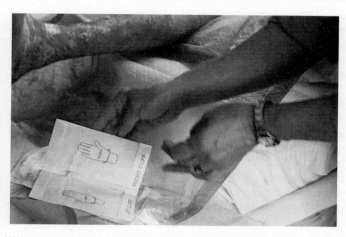

⑥ Don sterile gloves before cleaning wound with 4 × 4 gauze pads.

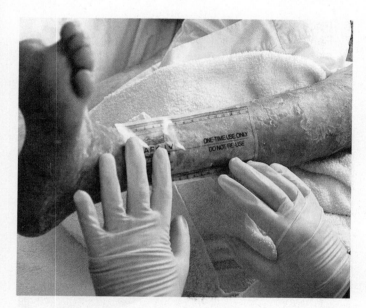

④ Measure wound to evaluate effectiveness of treatment.

- Debride wound, if ordered, using one of the following methods:
  - *Autolytic:* Apply occlusive dressings that assist in maintaining a moist wound environment, therefore promoting re-epithelialization. **Rationale:** *Autolytic dressings use the body's own enzymes and moisture to rehydrate, moisten, and slough tissue.*
  - *Chemical:* Apply enzyme debriding agents (Accuzyme, collagenase, papain, etc.). *Note:* The major disadvantage of this method is that viable tissue is removed with necrotic tissue.
  - *Mechanical:* Apply wet-to-dry dressings, use hydrotherapy, irrigation.
- Dry wound using sterile 4 × 4 gauze pads ⑦. Place in biohazard bag.
- Remove gloves, perform hand hygiene, and don sterile gloves.
10. Provide wound care, apply sterile dressing, and outer compression dressing.
  - Apply medicated moisturizer over wound, if ordered ⑧. **Rationale:** *This keeps wound area moist.*

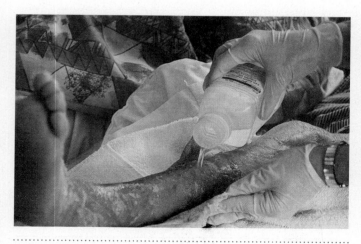

⑤ Pour normal saline solution over wound to clean off debris.

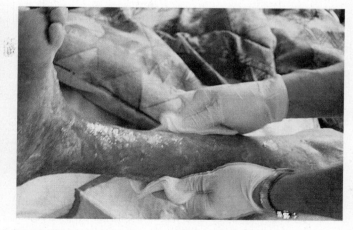

⑦ Dry with 4 × 4 gauze pad after cleansing.

SKILL 16.6 Dressing, Venous Ulcer: Changing (*continued*)

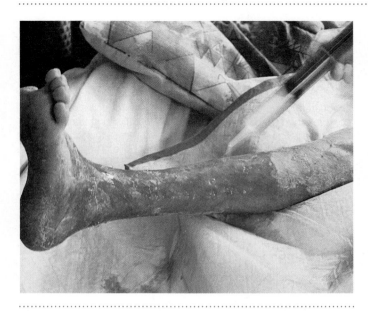

⑧ Apply medicated moisturizer over wound, if ordered.

- Remove backing on moisture-retentive dressing and place over open wound site **⑨**. These dressings prevent entry of bacteria from surface of dressing.
- Palpate arterial system; dorsalis pedis, posterior, or tibial pulse. If pulses are nonpalpable obtain an ankle–brachial index (ABI) reading.

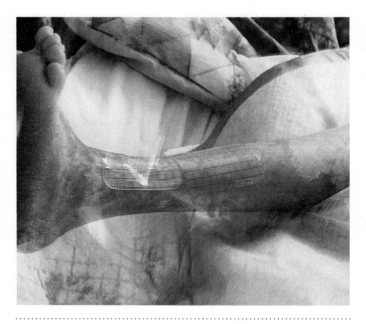

⑨ Apply moisture-retentive dressing over wound site.

CAUTION! If the leg systolic pressure is lower than the brachial systolic pressure, it indicates peripheral arterial disease, which increases one's risk for arterial circulation problems. The ABI index is a ratio comparing the patient's ankle systolic pressure with the brachial artery systolic pressure.

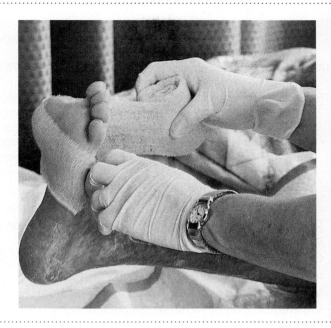

⑩ Apply compression dressing for venous or lymphatic conditions.

- Apply compression dressing if ABI is greater than 0.6 **⑩ ⑪**. **Rationale:** *Effective compression bandages generate 40–70 mmHg pressure. If arterial insufficiency is present, another ulcer can occur.*

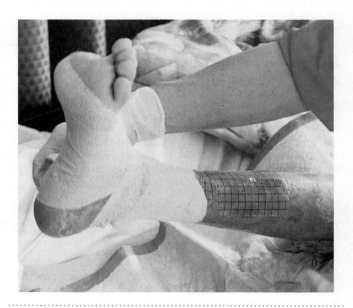

⑪ Cover entire area with compression dressing.

11. Reposition leg in elevated position. Leg should be elevated 18 cm (7 in.) above the heart for 2–4 hr during the day and night. **Rationale:** *This prevents edema and venous stasis, and promotes healing.*
12. Remove gloves, place in biohazard bag, and place biohazard bag in appropriate receptacle.

(continued on next page)

SKILL 16.6 Dressing, Venous Ulcer: Changing (continued)

13. When the procedure is complete, lower bed to lowest position, perform hand hygiene, and leave patient safe and comfortable.
14. Assess peripheral circulation every 4 hr. **Rationale:** *This ensures compression dressing is not too tight.*
15. Complete documentation using forms, checklists, or electronic dropdown lists supplemented by nurse's notes or additional comments as appropriate including appearance of the wound; the color, consistency, amount, and odor of any drainage; the type of dressing applied; and how the patient responded.

SAMPLE DOCUMENTATION

[date] 1410 Compression dressing and inner dressing on left lower leg removed. Wound measures 11 cm. Ordered cleansing solution applied and rinsed with normal saline. Area dried. No debridement ordered today. Medicated ointment applied to wound area followed by applying moisture retention dressing. Dorsalis pedis pulse 74 and weak. Compression dressing applied. Left leg elevated with pillows. Tolerated procedure without incident. *M. Baker*

CAUTION! Use of semiocclusive dressings reduces the incidence of wound infections by more than 50%. They maintain a moist environment, reduce airborne bacteria, and provide a mechanical barrier for bacterial entry.

Safety Considerations
Compression Therapy

INELASTIC SYSTEM

An Unna boot is frequently used to control edema in lower extremities. An inelastic bandaging system is applied to the lower extremity. As it dries it becomes rigid and when calf muscles press against the rigid bandage they pump blood more effectively. This system can be used for both mobile and immobile patients. Patient should seek immediate medical care if toes tingle, change color, or feel numb, there is increased pain with standing, or edema is noted above or below the boot. As edema subsides, the boot becomes less effective.

ELASTIC THERAPY

Graduated compression and multilayer compression stockings and compression pumps are more effective in increasing venous return. Both mobile and immobile patients can use these stockings, although it is more difficult for the patient who is mobile. The stockings are available in different pressures.

Safety Considerations
Arterial Ulcers

ASSESSMENT

- Assess arterial flow; dorsalis pedis, femoral, popliteal, or posterior tibial.
- Use Doppler to assess pulses if necessary.
- Assess ABI; below 0.5 indicates severe arterial insufficiency.
- Assess temperature of skin.
- Observe color of extremities.
- Assess for presence of pain when patient resting.

TREATMENT

- Debride the wound.
- Provide pain control.
- Use occlusive dressings, which reduce pain, protect the wound from infection, control exudates, enhance autolytic debridement, and maintain moist wound environment.
- Secure dressing with gauze; do not use tape as skin is fragile and tears easily.
- Provide management of the disease process (e.g., BP, eliminate smoking, control blood glucose).
- Surgical intervention may be done to improve circulation.
- Negative pressure wound therapy (see Skill 16.14) or hyperbaric oxygen therapy may be used to support wound healing.

SKILL 16.7 Dressing, Wet-to-Moist: Applying

Safety Note! *During scheduled clinical time, nursing students may have a learning opportunity to observe or assist with this skill only with faculty permission and with direct supervision from faculty or another RN.*

These dressings function as osmotic dressings. Normal saline is isotonic. As water evaporates from a saline dressing, the dressing becomes hypertonic and fluid from wound tissue is drained into the dressing.

Delegation or Assignment

Due to specific knowledge and skill in applying, monitoring, and changing a wet-to-moist dressing, this skill is not delegated or assigned to the UAP. The nurse can request the UAP to report patient observations to the nurse for follow-up. The nurse remains responsible for the assessment, interpretation of abnormal finds, and determination of appropriate actions.

Equipment

- Sterile 4 × 8 noncotton gauze dressings
- Semiocclusive dressing, optional
- Sterile gloves
- Clean gloves
- Tape
- Plastic bag or receptacle for contaminated dressings
- Sterile normal saline solution

SKILL 16.7 Dressing, Wet-to-Moist: Applying *(continued)*

- Sterile receptacle (round basin or emesis basin) if dressing not in commercial pack
- Montgomery straps, if desired

Preparation

- Review healthcare provider's orders and patient's nursing plan of care.
- Gather equipment and supplies.

Procedure

1. Introduce self to patient and verify the patient's identity using two identifiers. Explain to the patient what you are going to do, why it is necessary, and how the patient can participate. Discuss how the results will be used in planning further care or treatments.
2. Perform hand hygiene and observe appropriate infection control procedures.
3. Provide for patient privacy.
4. Remove old dressing.
   - Remove tape by pulling it toward the wound. **Rationale:** *This action prevents injury to newly formed tissue.*
   - Don clean gloves.
   - Remove wound packing by gently grasping the gauze without touching the wound and tear it away at a right angle from the wound surface. **Rationale:** *Touching only the gauze prevents contamination of the wound.*
   - Place soiled dressings in disposable bag.
   - Remove gloves, and dispose of them in bag.
   - Perform hand hygiene
5. Cleanse wound and apply new dressing.
   - Cleanse the wound with sterile normal saline following Step 8 of Skill 16.4 on page 666; follow facility policy.
   - Open packages of dressings making sure sterility is maintained ❶.
   - Pour sterile normal saline solution over dressings ❷.
   - Don sterile gloves.
   - Pick up sterile gauze dressings one at a time.
   - Fluff each dressing, and place over wound ❸. **Rationale:** *If packed tightly, dressing can prevent wound edges from contact with capillaries.*
   - Place gauze in the wound, covering all exposed surfaces. Press gauze lightly into depressions or cracks. **Rationale:** *Necrotic tissue is more prevalent in these areas.*

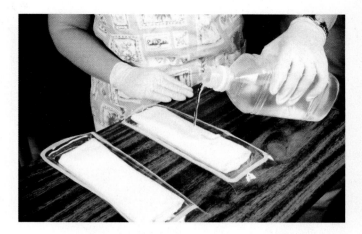

❷ Pour sterile saline solution over dressings to moisten.

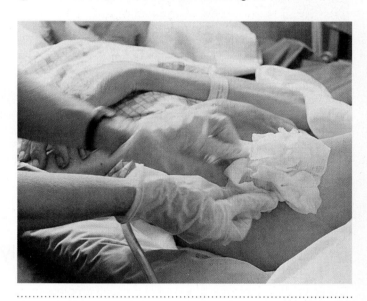

❸ Fluff dressings and apply over wound, covering all exposed surfaces.

   - Unfold a moist, sterile, 4 × 8 (ABD pad) dressing into a single layer and place it on top of wet dressings covering the wound area (not on skin) ❹.
   - Place a dry 4 × 8 pad over the dressing to hold it in place. Some protocols call for semi-occlusive dressing in place of pad.
   - Remove gloves and place in plastic bag.
   - Tape only the edges of the dressing. Montgomery tapes may be used to prevent excessive skin irritation and damage due to frequent dressing changes.
6. Position patient and lower bed. Discard soiled material in appropriate container.
7. When the procedure is complete, perform hand hygiene and leave patient safe and comfortable.
8. Complete documentation using forms, checklists, or electronic dropdown lists supplemented by nurse's notes or additional comments as appropriate, including the appearance of the wound; the color, consistency, amount,

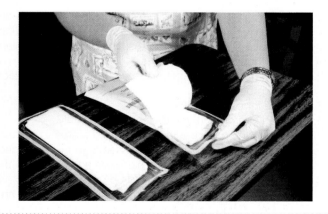

❶ Open sterile packages before beginning dressing change.

(continued on next page)

SKILL 16.7 Dressing, Wet-to-Moist: Applying (*continued*)

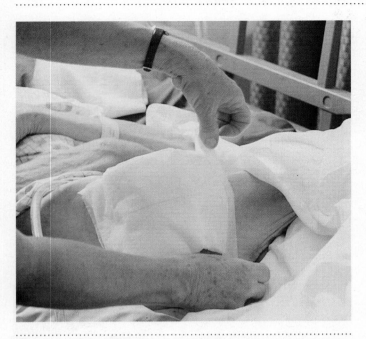

④ Place moist ABD pad over dressings, then cover with dry pad.

and odor of any drainage; the type of dressing applied; and how the patient responded.

9. Observe wound for excessive drainage or drying out of dressing between dressing changes. Remoisten dressing if dry. **Rationale:** *Unless excessive drainage occurs or* *dressing dries out, dressings are usually changed every 8 hours.*

SAMPLE DOCUMENTATION

[date] 1840 Sitting in chair reading. Old dressing and old packing removed from right hand wound. Area around wound cleaned. Wound measures 2.5 cm × 1 cm × 0.5 cm. Wound bed has small amount yellow purulent foul-smelling drainage. Granulating bottom of wound bed noted. Saline-soaked 4 × 4 gauze pad placed in wound and covered with dry 4 × 4 gauze pad and secured with tape. Tolerated without complaint. *V. Shultz*

Safety Considerations

- Wet-to-dry dressings are used only to debride wounds because they can cause tissue damage.
- Maceration of healthy tissue can occur with dressings that are always wet.
- Dry dressings cause damage to granulating tissue if removed without first soaking the gauze.
- Heat lamps should not be used to treat pressure injuries. Preferred wound care is to promote a clean, moist environment.

SKILL 16.8 Elastic Bandage: Applying

Elastic bandages provide localized and even compression to minimize swelling and decrease pain in an extremity area that has been bruised, sprained, or strained. They come in a variety of widths, are washable, and retain elasticity. Most elastic bandages now do not contain latex. Elastic wraps can also be used for other purposes, such as holding a splint in place and for venous conditions like lymphedema.

Delegation or Assignment

Application of elastic bandages can be delegated or assigned to the UAP or family members or caregivers after the nurse has performed initial assessment that these persons can perform this skill safely. The nurse can request the UAP to report patient observations to the nurse for follow-up. The nurse remains responsible for the assessment, interpretation of abnormal findings, and determination of appropriate responses. Note that state laws for UAPs vary, so this task might be assigned to the UAP rather than delegated.

Equipment

- Clean elastic bandage of the appropriate material and size
- Tape, clips, or Velcro

Preparation

- Review healthcare provider's orders and patient's nursing plan of care.
- Gather equipment and supplies.

Procedure

1. Introduce self to patient and verify the patient's identity using two identifiers. Explain to the patient what you are going to do, why it is necessary, and how the patient can participate. Discuss how the results will be used in planning further care or treatments.
2. Perform hand hygiene and observe appropriate infection control procedures.
3. Provide for patient privacy.
4. Position and prepare the patient appropriately.
   - Provide the patient with support for the area to be bandaged. For example, if a hand needs to be bandaged, ask the patient to place the elbow on a table so that the hand does not have to be held up unsupported.
   - Make sure that the area to be bandaged is clean and dry. Wash and dry the area if necessary. Perform wound

SKILL 16.8 Elastic Bandage: Applying (*continued*)

care as indicated. **Rationale:** *Washing and drying remove microorganisms, which flourish in dark, warm, moist areas.*

- Align the part to be bandaged with slight flexion of the joints, unless this is contraindicated. **Rationale:** *Slight flexion places less strain on the ligaments and muscles of the joint.*

5. Apply the bandage. Apply the beginning of the bandage to the most distal part of the body to be bandaged first. **Rationale:** *Wrapping from distal to proximal facilitates venous return and diminishes swelling.*

CIRCULAR TURNS

- Hold the bandage in your dominant hand, keeping the roll uppermost, and unroll the bandage about 8 cm (3 in.). **Rationale:** *This length of unrolled bandage allows good control for placement and tension.*
- Hold the end down with the thumb of the other hand ❶.

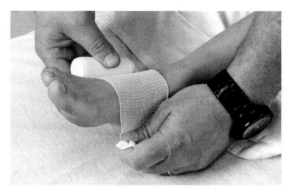

Source: Rick Brady/Pearson Education, Inc.

❶ Starting a bandage with circular turns.

- Encircle the body part a few times or as often as needed, making sure that each layer overlaps one half to two thirds of the previous layer. This provides even support to the area.
- The bandage should be firm, but not too tight. Ask the patient if the bandage feels comfortable. A tight bandage

can interfere with blood circulation, whereas a loose bandage does not provide adequate compression.

- Secure the end of the bandage with tape or clips if there is no Velcro fastener.

SPIRAL TURNS

- Make two circular turns. **Rationale:** *Two circular turns anchor the bandage.*
- Continue spiral turns at about a 30-degree angle, each turn overlapping the preceding one by two thirds the width of the bandage ❷.
- Terminate the bandage with two circular turns, and secure the end as described for circular turns.

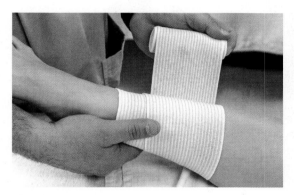

Source: Rick Brady/Pearson Education, Inc.

❷ Applying spiral turns.

SPIRAL REVERSE TURNS

- Anchor the bandage with two circular turns, and bring the bandage upward at about a 30-degree angle.
- Place the thumb of your free hand on the upper edge of the bandage ❸. **Rationale:** *The thumb will hold the bandage while it is folded on itself.*
- Unroll the bandage about 15 cm (6 in.), and then turn your hand so that the bandage falls over itself.
- Continue the bandage around the limb, overlapping each previous turn by two thirds the width of the bandage.

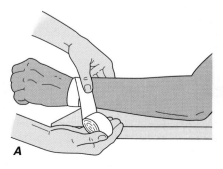

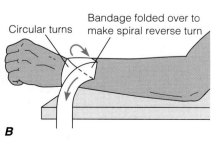

Circular turns

Bandage folded over to make spiral reverse turn

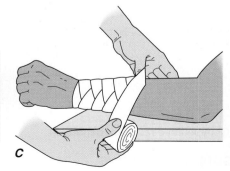

A   B   C

❸ Applying spiral reverse turns.

(*continued on next page*)

SKILL 16.8 Elastic Bandage: Applying (*continued*)

Make each bandage turn at the same position on the limb so that the turns of the bandage will be aligned.
- Terminate the bandage with two circular turns, and secure the end as described for circular turns.

RECURRENT TURNS

- Anchor the bandage with two circular turns.
- Fold the bandage back on itself, hold it with the thumb of the other hand, and bring it centrally over the distal end to be bandaged ④.

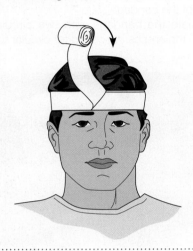

④ Start a recurrent bandage.

- Bring the bandage back over the end to the right of the center bandage but overlapping it by two thirds the width of the bandage.
- Bring the bandage back on the left side, also overlapping the first turn by two thirds the width of the bandage.
- Continue this pattern of alternating right and left until the area is covered. Overlap the preceding turn by two thirds the bandage width each time.
- Terminate the bandage with two circular turns ⑤. Secure the end appropriately.

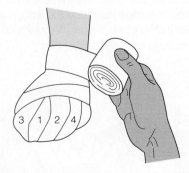

⑤ Completing a recurrent bandage.

FIGURE-EIGHT TURNS

- Anchor the bandage with two circular turns.
- Carry the bandage above the joint, around it, and then below it, making a figure eight ⑥.

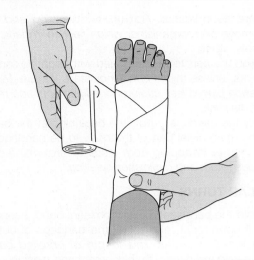

⑥ Applying a figure-eight bandage.

- Continue above and below the joint, overlapping the previous turn by two thirds the width of the bandage.
- Terminate the bandage above the joint with two circular turns, and then secure the end appropriately.

ARM SLING

- Ask the patient to flex the elbow to an 80-degree angle or less, depending on the purpose. The thumb should be facing upward or inward toward the body. **Rationale:** *An 80-degree angle is sufficient to support the forearm, to prevent swelling of the hand, and to relieve pressure on the shoulder joint (e.g., to support the paralyzed arm of a stroke patient whose shoulder might otherwise become dislocated). A more acute angle is preferred if there is swelling of the hand.*
- If a triangle is used, place one end of the unfolded binder over the shoulder of the uninjured side so that the binder falls down the front of the chest of the patient with the point of the triangle (apex) under the elbow of the injured side ⑦.

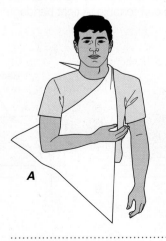
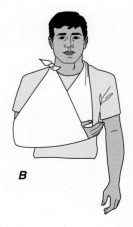

A   *B*

⑦ A triangle arm sling.

SKILL 16.8 Elastic Bandage: Applying (*continued*)

- Take the upper corner, and carry it around the neck until it hangs over the shoulder on the injured side.
- Bring the lower corner of the binder up over the arm to the shoulder of the injured side. Using a square knot, secure this corner to the upper corner at the side of the neck on the injured side. **Rationale:** *A square knot will not slip. Tying the knot at the side of the neck prevents pressure on the bony prominences of the vertebral column at the back of the neck.*
- Fold the sling neatly at the elbow, and secure it with safety pins or tape. It may be folded and fastened at the front.
- If a commercial sling is used, it may also include a second strap that goes around the back of the patient's chest from the finger end of the sling to the elbow ❽. **Rationale:** *This strap holds the arm close to the body at all times, providing shoulder immobilization such as is used following a shoulder dislocation or surgery.*
- Make sure the wrist is supported. **Rationale:** *This maintains alignment.*
- Remove the sling periodically to inspect the skin for indications of irritation, especially around the site of the knot.

6. When the procedure is complete, perform hand hygiene and leave patient safe and comfortable.

7. Complete documentation using forms, checklists, or electronic dropdown lists supplemented by nurse's notes or additional comments as appropriate.

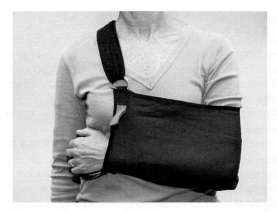

Source: George Draper/Pearson Education, Inc.

❽ A commercial arm sling.

SAMPLE DOCUMENTATION

[date] 1900 c/o severe sharp and cramping pain in shoulder when moving it. Commercial sling with shoulder immobilizer applied to left arm with elbow flexed 60°. Upper extremity warm, no wounds or lesions, peripheral pulses strong, brisk capillary refill. Able to move fingers and wrist's pain. Patient verbalizes understanding of need to request assistance with ADLs. *L. Morris*

SKILL 16.9 Surgical Wound: Caring for

A surgical wound is the cut or incision made in the skin and through tissue by a surgical scalpel during surgery. Surgical wounds vary in size and location depending on the site of surgery.

Delegation or Assignment

Cleaning a newly sutured wound, especially one with a drain, requires application of knowledge, problem solving, and aseptic technique. As a result, this procedure is not delegated or assigned to the UAP. The nurse can ask the UAP to report soiled dressings that need to be changed or if a dressing has become loose and needs to be reinforced. The nurse is responsible for the assessment and evaluation of the wound.

Equipment

- Bath blanket (if necessary)
- Moisture-proof biohazard bag
- Mask (optional)
- Clean gloves
- Sterile gloves
- Sterile normal saline in pour bottle

- Sterile dressing set; if none is available, gather the following sterile items:
  - Drape or towel
  - Gauze squares
  - Container for the cleaning solution
  - Two pairs of forceps
  - Gauze dressings and abdominal pad
  - Applicators or tongue blades to apply ointments as ordered
- Additional supplies required for the particular dressing (e.g., extra gauze dressings and ointment, if ordered)
- Tape, tie tapes, or binder

Preparation

- Review healthcare provider's orders and patient's nursing plan of care.
- Acquire assistance for changing a dressing on a restless or confused patient. **Rationale:** *The person might move and contaminate the sterile field or the wound.*
- Gather equipment and supplies.

(*continued on next page*)

SKILL 16.9 Surgical Wound: Caring for (continued)

Procedure

1. Introduce self and verify the patient's identity using two identifiers. Explain to the patient what you are going to do, why it is necessary, and how the patient can participate. Discuss how the results will be used in planning further care or treatments.

2. Perform hand hygiene and observe other appropriate infection control procedures.

3. Provide for patient privacy. Assist the patient to a comfortable position in which the wound can be readily exposed. Expose only the wound area, using a bath blanket to cover the patient, if necessary. **Rationale:** *Undue exposure is physically and psychologically distressing to most people.*

4. Make a cuff on the moisture-proof bag for disposal of the soiled dressings, and place the bag within reach. It can be taped to the bedclothes or bedside table. **Rationale:** *Making a cuff helps keep the outside of the bag free from contamination by the soiled dressings and prevents subsequent contamination of the nurse's hands or of sterile instrument tips when discarding dressing or sponges.*

5. Don a face mask, if required. **Rationale:** *Some facilities require that a mask be worn for surgical dressing changes to prevent contamination of the wound by droplet spray from the nurse's respiratory tract.*

6. Remove and dispose of soiled dressings appropriately.
   - Don clean gloves and remove the outer abdominal dressing.
   - Lift the outer dressing so that the underside is *away* from the patient's face. **Rationale:** *The appearance and odor of the drainage may be upsetting to the patient.*
   - Place the soiled dressing in the moisture-proof bag without touching the outside of the bag.
   - Remove the under-dressings, taking care not to dislodge any drains. If the gauze sticks to the drain, support the drain with one hand and remove the gauze with the other.
   - Assess the location, type (color, consistency), and odor of wound drainage, and the number of gauze pads saturated or the diameter of drainage collected on the dressings.
   - Discard the soiled dressings in the bag as before.
   - Remove and discard gloves in the moisture-proof bag. Perform hand hygiene.

7. Set up the sterile supplies.
   - Open the sterile dressing set, using surgical aseptic technique.
   - Place the sterile drape beside the wound.
   - Open the sterile cleaning solution and pour it over the gauze sponges in the plastic container.
   - Don sterile gloves.

8. Clean the wound, if indicated.
   - Clean the wound, using your gloved hands or forceps and gauze swabs moistened with cleaning solution.
   - If using forceps, keep the forceps' tips lower than the handles at all times. **Rationale:** *This prevents their contamination by fluid traveling up to the handle and nurse's wrist and back to the tips.*
   - Use the cleaning methods illustrated as described ❶ or one recommended by facility protocol.

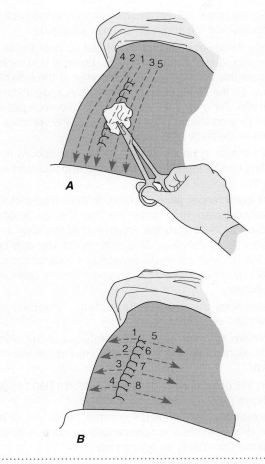

A

B

❶ Methods of cleaning surgical wounds: *A,* Cleaning the wound from top to bottom, starting at the center; *B,* Cleaning a wound outward from the incision. For all methods, a clean sterile swab is used for each stroke.

   - Use a separate swab for each stroke, and discard each swab after use. **Rationale:** *This prevents the introduction of microorganisms to other wound areas.*
   - A Penrose drain may be inserted into the surgical wound. The Penrose drain is a thin, flat, soft latex tube that helps to facilitate open drainage of fluid from inside the wound to collect in the dressing covering the wound. A sterile safety pin is commonly put at the end of the Penrose drain on the outside of the wound to prevent it from advancing into the wound. This type of drain may be placed in a wound when small amounts of drainage are expected.
   - If a Penrose drain is present, clean it next, taking care to avoid reaching across the cleaned incision. Clean the skin around the Penrose drain site by swabbing in half or full circles from around the drain site outward, ❷ using separate swabs for each wipe.
   - Support and hold the Penrose drain erect while cleaning around it. Clean as many times as necessary to remove the drainage.
   - Dry the surrounding skin with dry gauze swabs as required. Do not dry the incision or wound itself. **Rationale:** *Moisture facilitates wound healing.*

SKILL 16.9 Surgical Wound: Caring for (continued)

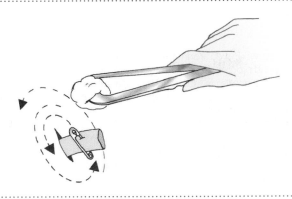

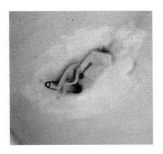

2 Clean the Penrose drain site, using a circular motion (unless using chlorhexidine) from the inside to the periphery of the wound. With chlorhexidine, use a back-and-forth motion.

9. Apply dressings to the Penrose drain site and the incision.
   - Place a precut 4 × 4 gauze snugly around the drain **3**, or open a 4 × 4 gauze to 4 × 8, fold it lengthwise to 2 × 8, and place the 2 × 8 gauze around the drain so that the ends overlap. **Rationale:** *This dressing absorbs the drainage and helps prevent it from excoriating the skin. Using precut gauze or folding it as described, instead of cutting the gauze, prevents any threads from coming loose and getting into the wound, where they could cause inflammation and provide a site for infection.*

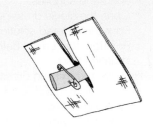

A   **B**

*Source: **A,** Ronald May/Pearson Education, Inc.*

3 Place **A,** folded gauze or **B,** a precut sterile 4 × 4 gauze dressing around the drain site to prevent skin excoriation.

- Apply the sterile dressings one at a time over the Penrose drain and the incision. Place the bulk of the dressings over the drain area and below the drain, depending on the patient's usual position. **Rationale:** *Layers of dressings are placed for best absorption of drainage, which flows by gravity.*
- Apply the final abdominal pad. Secure the dressing with tape or ties.
10. When the procedure is complete, perform hand hygiene and leave patient safe and comfortable.
11. Complete documentation using forms, checklists, or electronic dropdown lists supplemented by nurse's notes or additional comments as appropriate.

Patient Teaching

Wound Care at Home
- Provide pain medication approximately 30 minutes before the procedure if the wound care causes pain or discomfort.
- Wash hands thoroughly and dry prior to handling wound care supplies and providing wound care.
- Clean and wipe dry a flat surface for the sterile field.
- Keep pets out of the area when setting up for and performing sterile procedures.
- Acquire all needed supplies before starting a sterile procedure.
- Maintain sterile or clean technique as instructed.
- Ensure the patient's or caregiver's ability and willingness to perform the bandaging procedure.
- Handle all sterile supplies from the outside of the wrapper or the edges.
- Avoid touching the parts of supplies or equipment that will touch the patient.
- Avoid skin injury by using paper tape or Montgomery straps instead of adhesive tape.
- Report any increasing wound drainage, pain, or redness, increasing swelling, or opening or gaping of wound edges.
- Check for adequate peripheral circulation after applying the bandage.
- Place any soiled dressing materials in a waterproof bag and dispose of it according to public health recommendations.

Lifespan Considerations

CHILDREN
- Allow the child to help with the procedure by holding supplies, opening boxes, counting turns, and so on.
- If a young patient is apprehensive, demonstrate the procedure on a doll or stuffed animal.
- Encourage the child to decorate her or his bandage.
- Teach the caregivers to apply bandages safely.

OLDER ADULTS
- Older patients may need extra support during the procedure, especially if arthritis, contractures, or tremors are present.
- Avoid constricting the patient's circulation with a tight bandage. Observe skin and bony prominences frequently for signs of impaired circulation. The risk for skin breakdown increases with age.

❯❯ Wound Care

Expected Outcomes

1. Stage of pressure injury is accurately accessed.
2. Pressure injury is treated effectively according to stage of ulcer formation.
3. Pressure injury heals within usual time frame.
4. Skin remains free of breakdown in surrounding areas of pressure injury.
5. Absence of additional pressure injury formation.
6. Granulation tissue is evident using adjunctive therapy.
7. Periwound (tissue that surrounds wound) area remains healthy without evidence of maceration.
8. Moist wound environment is maintained.
9. Wound progresses through usual phases with electrical stimulation.
10. Wound healing is facilitated by radiant heat dressing.
11. Exudate is removed and wound healing occurs using negative pressure wound therapy.
12. Hyperbaric oxygen therapy is effective in treating the leg ulcers of patients with diabetes.
13. Patient's stump wound heals without complication.
14. Patient's stump maintains functional alignment.
15. Patient's stump is prepared for prosthesis use.

SKILL 16.10   Dressing, Alginate: Applying

Safety Note! *During scheduled clinical time, nursing students may have a learning opportunity to observe or assist with this skill only with faculty permission and with direct supervision from faculty or another RN.*

Alginate dressings come from seaweed and are effective in maintaining a moist environment to promote healing with hydrophilic gel formation. When applied to a wound, they can clean secreting lesions. Alginates can be rinsed out of the wound with saline irrigation, which does not interfere with healing tissue.

Delegation or Assignment

Due to the need for aseptic technique and assessment skills, alginate dressing changes are not delegated or assigned to the UAP. However, the UAP may observe the dressing during usual care and must report abnormal findings to the nurse. Abnormal findings must be validated and interpreted by the nurse.

Equipment

- Alginate dressing
- Sterile dressing equipment and secondary dressing materials
- Solution for irrigation (e.g., sterile saline or water)
- Irrigating syringe
- Bowl
- Basin to collect irrigation
- Ruler with inches and centimeters marked
- Forceps or cotton-tipped applicators (optional)
- Moisture-proof bag
- Clean gloves
- Sterile gloves (optional)

Preparation

- Review healthcare provider's orders and patient's nursing plan of care.
- Gather equipment and supplies.

Procedure

1. Introduce self to patient and verify the patient's identity using two identifiers. Explain to the patient what you are going to do, why it is necessary, and how the patient can participate. Discuss how the results will be used in planning further care or treatments.
2. Perform hand hygiene and observe appropriate infection control procedures.
3. Provide for patient privacy.
4. Assist the patient to a comfortable position in which the wound can be readily exposed. Expose only the wound area, using a bath blanket to cover the patient, if necessary. **Rationale:** *Undue exposure is physically and psychologically distressing to most people.*
5. Prepare the supplies.
   - Open the sterile dressing set and supplies.
   - Pour the ordered solution into the solution container.
   - Position the basin below the wound to receive the irrigating fluid.
6. Remove the existing dressing and alginate.
   - Don clean gloves, remove and discard the outer secondary dressing in the moisture-proof bag.
   - Irrigate the wound with the prescribed solution until all of the alginate dressing has been removed.
   - If the alginate dressing does not remove easily with irrigation, either the secondary dressing is not maintaining a moist environment or the wound is no longer producing enough exudate to warrant alginate dressing.
7. Assess the wound.
8. Clean the wound if indicated.
   - Remove and discard gloves. Perform hand hygiene.
9. Pack the wound with the alginate.
   - Don sterile gloves.
   - Pack the alginate into all depressions and grooves of the wound. Cover all exposed surfaces.
10. Dress the wound.
    - Cover the alginate with petrolatum gauze, foam, or other secondary dressing that will keep the alginate in place and provide a moist wound environment.
11. When the procedure is complete, perform hand hygiene and leave patient safe and comfortable.
12. Complete documentation using forms, checklists, or electronic dropdown lists supplemented by nurse's notes or additional comments as appropriate.

SKILL 16.10 Dressing, Alginate: Applying *(continued)*

[date] 1310 Sitting in chair with legs elevated. Old dressing removed from left dorsum of foot. Wound irrigated to remove alginate. Surrounding skin cleaned with saline. Measures 1 cm × 1 cm × 0.5 cm, tissue healing, no signs infection. Fresh alginate applied in wound and covered with gauze dressing. Tolerated without incident. *W. Keys*

Patient Teaching

Promoting and Maintaining Healthy Skin

- Discuss relationship between adequate nutrition (especially fluids, protein, vitamins B and C, iron, and calories) and healthy skin.
- Demonstrate appropriate positions for pressure relief.
- Establish a turning or repositioning schedule.
- Demonstrate application of appropriate skin protection agents and devices.
- Instruct to report persistent reddened areas.
- Identify potential sources of skin trauma and means of avoidance.

Wound Care

- Instruct the patient and family about hygiene and medical asepsis, hand cleaning before and after dressing changes, and using a clean area for storage of dressing supplies.
- Instruct the patient and family on where to obtain needed supplies. Be sensitive to the cost of dressings (e.g., transparent barriers are costly) and suggest less expensive alternatives if necessary. Be creative in the use of household items for padding pressure areas.
- Provide information about signs of wound infection and other complications to report.
- Reinforce appropriate aspects of pressure injury prevention.
- Demonstrate wound care techniques such as wound cleaning, dressing change.
- Discuss pain control measures, if needed.
- Instruct the patient and family in proper disposal of contaminated dressings. All contaminated items should be double bagged in moisture-proof bags.

Lifespan Considerations

NEWBORNS AND INFANTS

- The skin of newborns and infants is more fragile than that of older children and adults, and more susceptible to infection, shearing from friction, and burns. Keep skin hydrated by applying lotion daily.

CHILDREN

- *Staphylococcus* and fungus are two major infectious agents affecting the skin of children. Abrasions or small lacerations, commonly experienced by children, provide an entry in the skin for these organisms. Minor wounds should be cleaned with warm, soapy water, and covered with a sterile bandage.
- With more serious skin lesions, remind the child not to touch the wound, drains, or dressing. Cover with an appropriate bandage that will remain intact during the child's usual activities. Cover a transparent dressing with opaque material if viewing the site is distressing to the child. Restrain only when all alternatives have been tried and when absolutely necessary.
- For younger children, demonstrate wound care on a doll. Reassure that the wound will not be permanent and that nothing will fall out of the body.

OLDER ADULTS

- Hold wrinkled skin taut during application of a transparent dressing. Obtain assistance if needed.
- Skin of older adults is more fragile and can easily tear with removal of tape (especially adhesive tape). Use paper tape and tape remover as indicated, keeping tape use to the minimum required. Use extreme caution during tape removal. If possible, use conforming gauze bandage to hold the dressing in place.
- Older adults who are in long-term care facilities often have the following factors: immobility, malnutrition, and incontinence, all of which increase the risk for development of skin breakdown.
- Skin breakdown can occur as quickly as within 2 hours, so assessments should be done with each repositioning of the patient.
- A thorough assessment of a patient's heels should be done every shift. The skin can break down quickly from friction of movement in bed. Whenever possible, heels should be suspended off the mattress using pillows or other mechanisms.

SKILL 16.11 Dressing, Hydrocolloid: Applying

Safety Note! *During scheduled clinical time, nursing students may have a learning opportunity to observe or assist with this skill only with faculty permission and with direct supervision from faculty or another RN.*

These dressings are a combination of adhesive and gelling polymers that are impermeable to oxygen, water, and water vapor (**Table 16–2** ›› and **Table 16–3** ››). They promote a moist wound environment, aid in autolytic debridement, and have no toxic components. They are waterproof and bacteria proof. These dressings are best used in patients who have partial- to full-thickness wounds, such as pressure injuries, skin tears, surgical wounds, and burns, with minimal to moderate exudates.

(continued on next page)

SKILL 16.11 Dressing, Hydrocolloid: Applying (continued)

TABLE 16–2 Additional Moist Wound Dressings

Type of Alternative	Use	Outcome of Treatment	Considerations
Hydrogel sheet	■ Interacts with aqueous solutions ■ Used with minor wounds with light to moderate drainage ■ Absorbs minimal to heavy exudates ■ Is nonadherent	Softens necrotic tissue Creates moist environment	Use outer dressing to prevent wounds from drying out Change dressing every 1–2 days
Impregnated gauze dressing	■ Absorbs minimal to moderate exudates ■ Is nonadherent	Conforms to irregular surfaces Eliminates dead space Creates moist environment	Requires outer dressing Change daily Is nonabsorptive
Alginates*	■ Absorbs heavy exudates ■ Converts to gel when comes in contact with wound drainage ■ Is easily removed from wound ■ Is nonadherent ■ Absorbs up to 20 times its weight in fluid ■ Can be used in infected and uninfected wounds	Maintains moist environment Promotes fast healing of wound	Not to be used on dry wounds It dehydrates wound, delays healing eschar-covered wounds, third-degree burns, or surgical wounds
Foams	■ Absorbs minimal to heavy exudates ■ Is highly absorbent ■ Used for deep cavity wounds	Maintains moist environment Decreases tissue trauma when removed Increases time between dressing changes (3–4 days)	Requires external dressing Can cause drying effect on wound
Hydrophilic	■ Is a type of foam dressing ■ Is nonadherent ■ Is very absorbent	Cushions wound Traps exudate	Used in wounds with moderate to heavy drainage
Hydrophobic	■ Is a nonadherent flexible dressing ■ Used with minimal or no necrotic tissue ■ Used with lightly to moderately exudating wounds	Resists fluid penetration into wound Is used on lightly draining wounds Provides cushion to irritated skin	
Medical hydrolysate of collagen	■ Soluble and degrades in wound site ■ Absorbs wound exudates ■ Is interactive with wound site to provide mechanical protection against physical and bacterial insult	Absorbs up to 30 times own weight Used in stage I through IV pressure injuries Accelerates tissue remodeling and reduces scarring	Cover with nonstick dressing Soak dressing in warm water before removing
Anticoat 7 silver-coated contact dressing	■ Used for wounds with moderate to heavy exudates ■ Has antimicrobial barrier to protect against bacterial contamination and infection ■ Calcium in the dressing provides antimicrobial to protect against bacterial contamination and infection ■ Kills bacteria faster than other forms of silver dressing	Use for leg, pressure, and diabetic foot ulcers and for burns	Stays in place for up to 3 days to provide moist environment

Note: *Alginates are made from acids that are obtained from brown seaweed. The calcium salts of alginic, mannuronic, and guluronic acids are processed into nonwoven, biodegradable fibers. When the fibers come into contact with fluids, sodium, and calcium ions, a soluble sodium gel forms.

Delegation or Assignment

Due to the need for aseptic technique and assessment skills, most dressing changes are not delegated or assigned to the UAP. In some states, the UAP may apply dry dressings to clean, chronic wounds. The UAP should observe an exposed wound or dressing during usual care and must report abnormal findings to the nurse. In some agencies, the UAP may be permitted to reinforce the dressing (apply additional dry dressings over a saturated bandage), but this must be reported to the nurse as soon as possible. Assessment of the wound and abnormal findings must be validated and interpreted by the nurse.

Equipment

- Sterile normal saline pour bottle
- Hydrocolloid dressing ❶

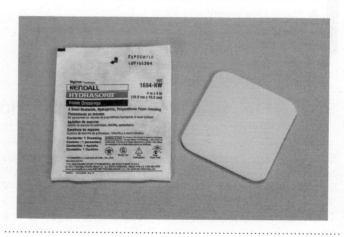

❶ Hydrocolloid dressing.

SKILL 16.11 Dressing, Hydrocolloid: Applying *(continued)*

TABLE 16–3 Comparisons of Moisture-Retentive Dressings

	Transparent	Hydrocolloid
Common brands	Tegaderm OpSite Bioclusive	Tegasorb DuoDERM Comfeel Plus Restore
Characteristics	Provides a sterile, semipermeable membrane with hypoallergenic adhesive Is permeable to oxygen and moisture vapor Allows oxygen exchange Is impermeable to bacteria and prevents contamination	Is impermeable to oxygen Dressing gel maintains moist environment that promotes autolysis Is impermeable to external bacteria and contamination Is minimally to moderately absorptive
Function	Provides moist environment Promotes autolysis and protects newly formed tissue Assists with debridement	Dressing contains hydroactive particles that absorb exudates to form a hydrated gel over wound When dressing is removed, gel separates from dressing, which protects newly formed tissue
Use	Easy assessment of wound; dressing is transparent Is nonabsorbable Used for nondraining or minimally draining wounds only; pressure injuries, stage I and some stage II; and minor burns and lacerations	Absorbs exudates while preserving moist environment needed for autolysis of slough Irrigate gel with saline to allow for assessing wound Used for pressure injuries, some stage III and some clean stage IV; wounds with mild or moderate exudates; wounds with necrosis or slough
Contraindications	Infected wounds Wounds with fragile surrounding skin	Wounds that need frequent assessment, not transparent Wounds with heavy exudate

- Hydrogel, if needed
- Sterile 4 × 4 gauze pads
- Ruler with inches and centimeters marked
- Hypoallergenic tape
- Clean gloves
- Skin prep, optional

Preparation

- Review healthcare provider's orders and the patient's nursing plan of care.
- Select dressing size to ensure coverage 3 cm (1¼ in.) beyond ulcer margin. (Dressing available in 4 × 4 to 8 × 8 sizes.) **Rationale:** *This ensures complete covering of wound. Use for small ulcers and in stages II and III.*
- Gather equipment and supplies.

Safety Considerations

These dressings can be used for dry wounds because they contain 95% water. They are occlusive and do not allow water or bacteria into the wound. Hydrocolloid causes the pH of the wound surface to drop, and this acidic environment can inhibit bacterial growth.

Procedure

1. Introduce self to patient and verify the patient's identity using two identifiers. Explain to the patient what you are going to do, why it is necessary, and how the patient can participate. Discuss how the results will be used in planning further care or treatments.
2. Perform hand hygiene and observe appropriate infection control procedures. Don gloves.
3. Provide for patient privacy. Assist the patient to a comfortable position in which the wound can be readily exposed. Expose only the wound area, using a bath blanket to cover the patient, if necessary. **Rationale:** *Undue exposure is physically and psychologically distressing to most people.*
4. Cleanse skin with gauze pad moistened with sterile normal saline and pat dry with gauze pad.
5. Measure wound using ruler.
6. Apply skin prep to surrounding skin to protect, if ordered.
7. Fill ulcer area with Hydrogel if ordered (usually used with stages III or IV pressure injury of the hip when exudate is present). Do not overfill with gel. **Rationale:** *Facilitates autolytic debridement of devitalized tissue.*
8. Warm dressing by holding in hands. **Rationale:** *This increases activity of adhesive and makes the dressing more pliable.*
9. Remove silicone release paper backing from dressing. Minimize finger contact with adhesive surface. **Rationale:** *Dressing is sterile and contamination should be avoided.*
10. Place dressing over affected area and extend at least 2.5 cm (1 in.) onto periwound skin ❷. Gently roll dressing over pressure injury—do not stretch dressing. **Rationale:** *Stretching the dressing may cause wrinkling of the dressing, which allows air to enter the wound.*
11. Placing dressing one third above wound and two thirds below wound maximizes time between dressing changes. **Rationale:** *This increases the absorption capacity of the dressing.*
12. Mold the dressing gently to skin, and hold down with hand for approximately 1 minute.
13. Apply skin prep to area that is to be covered by tape if ordered. Allow to dry. Do not apply skin prep under

(continued on next page)

SKILL 16.11 Dressing, Hydrocolloid: Applying (*continued*)

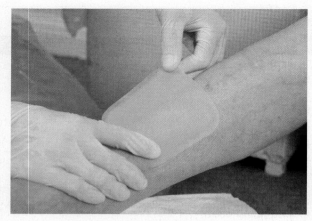

Source: Rick Brady/Pearson Education, Inc.

....

② Applying a hydrocolloid dressing.

hydrocolloid dressing. **Rationale:** *Hydrocolloid dressings are placed over broken skin; skin prep may cause damage to skin.*

14. Use silk or hypoallergenic tape to "window frame" the sides of the hydrocolloid dressing.
15. Check dressing each shift for impaired integrity.
16. Change dressing at first sign of impaired integrity. Dressings should not be left on longer than 7 days; they are usually left in place for 3–4 days.

CAUTION! DuoDERM is removed when exudate seeps from edges of dressing or white blister appears under dressing. Comfeel Plus is changed when dressing becomes transparent or there is leakage.

17. Remove dressing by pressing hand down on adjacent skin surface while carefully lifting edge of dressing from skin. Continue lifting dressing around periphery until all edges are released, then lift dressing carefully away from wound.
18. Remove and discard gloves. Perform hand hygiene and leave patient safe and comfortable.
19. Complete documentation using forms, checklists, or electronic dropdown lists supplemented by nurse's notes or additional comments as appropriate including stage, size, and appearance of ulcer and reason for removal of hydrocolloid dressing.

SAMPLE DOCUMENTATION

[date] 1110 Sitting on side of bed, assisted to right side-lying position. Wound on left buttocks measures 3 cm × 2 cm × 1 cm. Wound has no infectious odor or drainage, tissue deep rusty colored, cleaned with saline and dried. Skin around wound cleaned and dried. Hydrocolloid dressing applied over wound and pressed to secure, edges taped down. Tolerated procedure without incident. Assisted back to sitting position. *Z. O'Malley*

Safety Considerations

Although frequently listed as wound care alternatives, topical disinfectant agents such as iodine and silver sulfadiazine are very controversial in wound care. Iodine is cytotoxic to fibroblasts and can impair wound healing. Silver solutions are sometimes used to prevent bacterial colonization in infection-prone areas. They do not eliminate existing infections.

SKILL 16.12 Dressing, Transparent: Applying

Safety Note! *During scheduled clinical time, nursing students may have a learning opportunity to observe or assist with this skill only with faculty permission and with direct supervision from faculty or another RN.*

Transparent dressings are made of see-through material, generally polyurethane. These dressings allow wound inspection while protecting the skin, especially at pressure spots. They are used for wounds that have scant to no drainage, and they generally remain in place for 5–7 days. They work well to protect IV catheter sites. The dressings are adhesive and permeable to moisture, vapor, and atmospheric gases, allowing one-way movement of excess moisture vapor and carbon dioxide away from the wound. They are also bacteria proof and waterproof, so they cannot absorb wound fluids. They are available in a variety of sizes and shapes, including thin sheets to cover larger wound areas.

Delegation or Assignment

Due to specific assessment knowledge and skill in applying, monitoring, and changing a transparent dressing, this skill is not delegated or assigned to the UAP. The nurse can request the UAP to report patient observations to the nurse for follow-up. The nurse remains responsible for the assessment, interpretation of abnormal finds, and determination of appropriate actions.

Equipment

- Sterile normal saline
- Transparent dressing (e.g., OpSite, Tegaderm, Bioclusive) of appropriate size to cover wound
- Wound-cleaning solution ordered or facility policy (e.g., sterile saline)
- Sterile 4 × 4 gauze pads

SKILL 16.12 Dressing, Transparent: Applying (*continued*)

- Scissors
- Hypoallergenic tape
- Ruler with inches and centimeters marked
- Clean gloves
- Sterile gloves (optional)
- Moisture-proof bag
- Plasticizing agent (e.g., skin prep) (optional)
- Syringe with 26-gauge needle, if needed

Preparation

- Review healthcare provider's orders and patient's nursing plan of care.
- Check type of dressing ordered and frequency of changing it. **Rationale:** *These dressings are very important in preventing pressure injuries; they prevent friction and shear over bony prominences when moving patients.*
- If possible, schedule the dressing change at a time convenient for the patient.
- Gather supplies ❶.
- Obtain appropriately sized transparent dressing ❷. Dressing can be applied to flat surface. (Coccyx area cannot be treated with this type of dressing.)

CAUTION! It is imperative to observe the wound daily to determine if a large amount of secretions or serous fluids accumulate under the dressing. If fluid has increased, aspirate with a 26-gauge needle. These dressings are not used for infected areas.

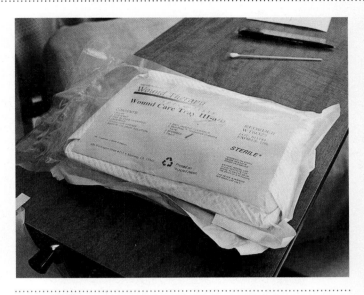

❷ Obtain specific dressing tray for ordered treatment.

Procedure

1. Introduce self to patient and verify the patient's identity using two identifiers. Explain to the patient what you are going to do, why it is necessary, and how the patient can participate. Discuss how the results will be used in planning further care or treatments.
2. Perform hand hygiene and observe appropriate infection control procedures.
3. Provide for patient privacy.
4. Assist the patient to a comfortable position in which the wound can be readily exposed. Expose only the wound area, using a bath blanket to cover the patient, if necessary. **Rationale:** *Undue exposure is physically and psychologically distressing to most people.*
5. Don clean gloves.
6. Remove old dressing. "Walk off" dressing from one edge to the other and discard in appropriate receptacle.
7. Remove gloves. Dispose of them and perform hand hygiene. Don sterile gloves or follow facility policy.
8. Wash wound with sterile gauze pads moistened with sterile normal saline.
9. Dry thoroughly with sterile gauze pad.
10. Measure wound using ruler ❸. **Rationale:** *Measurement determines appropriate size dressing and allows comparison measurements, which assists in determining effectiveness of treatment.*
11. Remove gloves. Dispose of them and perform hand hygiene. Don new clean gloves.
12. Apply plasticizing agent (skin prep, skin gel) over surrounding tissue if ordered. Do not apply directly on wound area, **Rationale:** *This agent contains alcohol.* Alternate treatment: If skin is irritated, apply No Sting barrier film spray to area surrounding tissue. **Rationale:** *This barrier protects from/prevents skin breakdown.*

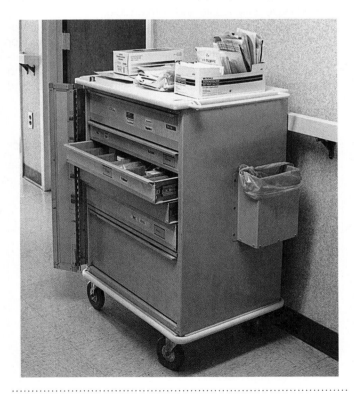

❶ Dressing carts may be used to keep supplies closer to patient area.

(*continued on next page*)

SKILL 16.12 Dressing, Transparent: Applying (continued)

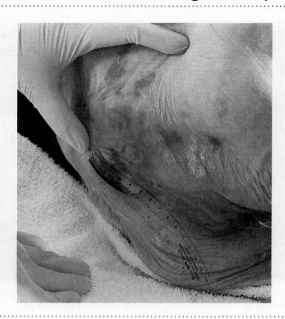

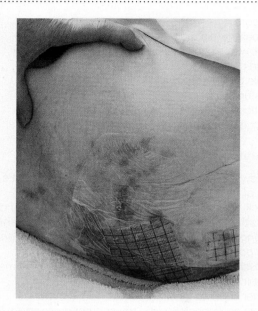

3 Assess size of wound to determine appropriate size of transparent dressing.

5 Apply transparent adhesive dressing over wound.

13. Apply transparent dressing.
    - Loosen transparent dressing from one side of backing paper **4**.
    - "Walk on" dressing: Start at one edge of site and gently lay the dressing down, keeping it free of wrinkles. Allow at least a 4-cm (1.5-in.) margin of dressing beyond the wound margin **5**. **Rationale:** *This ensures coverage of entire wound area.*
    - Cut off tabs if present after wound is completely covered.
14. Tape edges with hypoallergenic tape. **Rationale:** *This assists in preventing frequent dressing changes due to*

loose dressings. These dressings can remain in place for 1 week.
15. Remove gloves and discard in appropriate receptacle.
16. Position patient for comfort. Remove and discard equipment.
17. When the procedure is complete, perform hand hygiene and leave patient safe and comfortable.
18. Complete documentation using forms, checklists, or electronic dropdown lists supplemented by nurse's notes or additional comments as appropriate including the appearance of the wound; the color, consistency, amount, and odor of any drainage; the type of dressing applied; and how the patient responded.

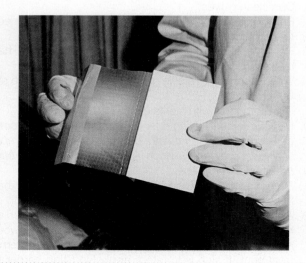

4 Remove backing from transparent dressing before applying.

SAMPLE DOCUMENTATION

[date] 1020 Sitting on side of bed. Old transparent dressing on left shoulder removed. Wound measures 2 cm in diameter. Wound moist with no odor noted or signs of infection. Skin around wound intact and without redness. Wound cleaned with saline gauze pads then dried. Area around wound cleaned with saline gauze pads and then skin protective solution applied per order. Area dried. New transparent dressing applied without incident. Tolerated dressing change without complaint. *D. Hosea*

SKILL 16.13 Electrical Stimulation: Using

Safety Note! *During scheduled clinical time, nursing students may have a learning opportunity to observe or assist with this skill only with faculty permission and with direct supervision from faculty or another RN.*

Electrical stimulation is a treatment to promote healing of chronic wounds using electrical current from electrodes placed on the skin located close to the wound. The electrical current can be varied according to which phase of healing the wound is in: the inflammatory, proliferative, or remodeling phases.

Delegation or Assignment

Due to the need for technical complexity, this skill is managed by the nurse or wound care nurse and not delegated or assigned to the UAP. Assisting the patient with daily care can be delegated or assigned to the UAP. The nurse must ensure that the UAP knows what complications or adverse signs should be reported to the nurse. The nurse remains responsible for the assessment, interpretation of abnormal findings, and determination of appropriate responses.

Equipment

- Normal saline solution
- Bag for soiled dressings
- Gauze pads
- Two sterile basins
- Hydrogel sheets
- Electrode
- Bandage tape
- Alligator clip
- Stimulator
- Clean gloves, 2 pairs
- Sterile gloves

Preparation

- Review healthcare provider's order. Review patient's nursing plan of care.
- Determine if patient is candidate for electrical stimulation.
  - Pressure injuries, stages I–IV
  - Diabetic ulcers
  - Venous ulcers, ischemic ulcer
  - Traumatic wounds
  - Surgical wounds
  - Wound flap
  - Donor site, burn wound
- Determine phase of wound healing. **Rationale:** *This determines the correct treatment protocol.*
- Set the stimulator settings according to manufacturer's directions, based on patient's phase in wound healing. The settings include polarity, pulse rate, intensity, duration, and frequency.
- Gather equipment.

Procedure

1. Introduce self to patient and verify the patient's identity using two identifiers. Explain the electrical stimulation device and how it will help the wound to heal. Explain why it is necessary, and how the patient can participate. Discuss how the results will be used in planning further care or treatments.
2. Perform hand hygiene and observe appropriate infection control procedures.
3. Provide for patient privacy.
4. Provide wound care.
   - Place patient in position to enable staff to work with wound area and equipment. (Placement depends on wound site.)
   - Place supplies on overbed table, near working area.
   - Open all supply packages, maintaining sterility.
   - Pour sterile normal saline into one basin.
   - Don clean gloves.
   - Place disposal bag near wound. **Rationale:** *This provides ease in disposing of soiled dressings.*
   - Remove dressing carefully to avoid interfering with granulation tissue.
   - Remove clean gloves; place in disposal bag. Don sterile gloves.
   - Place sterile basin next to wound to catch irrigation solution as wound is cleansed.
   - Pour sterile normal saline into wound to clean wound. **Rationale:** *This is to remove exudates, slough, and petrolatum products. Current will not be conducted into wound tissue if petrolatum products remain in the wound.*
   - Remove excess irrigation solution using sterile gauze pads.
   - Place fluffed gauze pads into normal saline solution, squeeze out excess liquid.
   - Fill wound cavity with gauze including any undermined/tunneled spaces. Pack gently.
   - Place surface (active) electrode in wound bed, over gauze packing. **Rationale:** *This transfers electrical energy into wound bed, producing positive effects on necessary components for wound healing (i.e., blood flow, oxygen uptake, DNA, and protein synthesis).*
   - Cover with dry gauze pad.
   - Tape dry pad securely.
5. Apply electrical stimulation device.
   - Connect alligator clip to foil.
   - Connect to stimulator lead.
   - Place a wet washcloth over area where dispersive electrode will be placed.

CAUTION! Hydrogel sheets or amorphous hydrogel-impregnated gauze can be used to conduct current. If hydrogel gauze is the conductor, it is changed BID.

   - Select a dispersive pad that is larger than the sum of areas of active electrodes and wound packing.
   - Place dispersive electrode proximal to wound, over soft tissue, avoiding bony prominences.
   Note: The greater the separation between two electrodes, the deeper the current path. Larger separation space is used to treat deep and undermined wounds. Closer

(continued on next page)

SKILL 16.13 Electrical Stimulation: Using (continued)

separation space is used for shallow or partial-thickness wounds. Ensure electrodes do not touch.

- Ensure all edges of electrode are in good contact with skin. Hold electrode in place with nylon elasticized strap.
- Place patient in position of comfort. Electrical stimulation treatments usually last 60 minutes.
- Remove gloves and discard. Perform hand hygiene.

6. Remove electrical stimulation device.
   - Perform hand hygiene.
   - Don clean gloves.
   - Remove electrode from wound following treatment.
   - Remove saline-soaked gauze and cover wound with occlusive dressing.

7. When the procedure is complete, perform hand hygiene and leave patient safe and comfortable.

8. Complete documentation using forms, checklists, or electronic dropdown lists supplemented by nurse's notes or additional comments as appropriate.

SAMPLE DOCUMENTATION

[date] 1530 Sitting in chair with right leg elevated. Dressing on wound at right outer ankle removed. Wound irrigated with saline, area around wound cleaned with saline. Wound measures 2 cm × 1 cm × 0.5 cm, slight reddening area around wound, wound bed contains granulating tissue, no infectious drainage noted. Wound cavity filled with soaked saline gauze and covered with dry gauze pad. Electrodes applied to skin and secured. Tolerated treatment without incident. *G. Bart RN*

EVIDENCE-BASED PRACTICE

Bee Sting Venom Therapy (Apitherapy)

Venom from bee stings has been used as complementary therapy for many years. People who believe in its value as a complementary therapy have used bee sting venom and other bee hive products to treat many illnesses and to help pain from chronic and acute conditions. It has been used in the treatment of such wide-ranging conditions as multiple sclerosis, tendonitis, chronic musculoskeletal pain, and arthritis. However, any reports of its success for these purposes have been anecdotal. Individuals tolerate multiple bee stings at a time, up to 40 to 60 stings, for the bee sting venom to reduce anti-inflammatory pain of joints, muscles, and tendons. The danger from this therapy is the risk of allergic reaction to the bee sting venom, which could happen on the first or the fortieth bee sting. An anaphylactic reaction could be life threatening.

Purified bee venom for intradermal injection is an FDA-approved product that is also now available for individuals who believe that bee venom will help their musculoskeletal inflammation and pain. Bee venom injections are also used for immunotherapy to reduce intensity of allergic reactions to bee stings. Injections are given serially over a period of time.

There have been cases in which bee venom immunotherapy has been effective in providing protection against severe bee sting allergic reactions. However, there have been no studies of bee stings that provide scientific evidence of its therapeutic value. Further empirical research needs to be done to show a role for bee sting venom (e.g., in the treatment of pain). The National Multiple Sclerosis Society and the American Cancer Society both specifically caution the public that evidence does not support use of bee stings as treatment for multiple sclerosis or cancer.

Source: Data from the American Apitherapy Society Inc. (2016); WebMD. (2015); Woolston, C. (2016).

SKILL 16.14 Negative Pressure Wound Therapy: Using

Safety Note! *During scheduled clinical time, nursing students may have a learning opportunity to observe or assist with this skill only with faculty permission and with direct supervision from faculty or another RN.*

Negative pressure wound therapy (commonly called vacuum-assisted closure, V.A.C. or wound VAC) is a wound therapy for treating acute and chronic wounds that requires special training for application, monitoring, and removal. The system includes a vacuum pump, connecting tubing for drainage, a foam dressing, and a clear dressing that covers and seals the wound with adhesive edges. Negative pressure is created inside the wound to assist in removing fluids, infectious by-products, and tissue exudates to support wound healing and closure.

Delegation or Assignment

Applying, monitoring, and removing a wound V.A.C. system is the nurse's or wound care nurse's responsibility and not delegated or assigned to the UAP. The UAP may provide routine care of the patient as trained. The nurse can request the UAP to report patient observations to the nurse for follow-up. The nurse remains responsible for the assessment, interpretation of abnormal findings, and determination of appropriate responses.

Equipment

- Foam, black or white V.A.C. kit ❶
- Gauze pads
- Sterile normal saline
- Irrigating syringe
- Moisture-proof pad or sterile basin
- Skin prep agent (optional)
- Clean gloves
- Sterile gloves
- Disposal bag
- Sterile scissor

SKILL 16.14 Negative Pressure Wound Therapy: Using *(continued)*

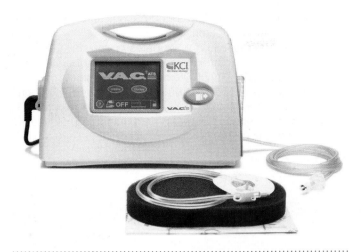

① *V.A.C. unit.*

Preparation

▪ Review healthcare provider's orders and patient's nursing plan of care.

▪ Evaluate if patient is a candidate for V.A.C. therapy: nutritionally stable, able to use device 22 hr each day, and can use a pressure support surface if wound is over bony prominence. **Rationale:** *If therapy is turned off longer than 2 hr, the dressing must be removed and replaced with a traditional dressing.*

▪ Assess wound to determine if therapy can be implemented.
  a. Wound surrounded by at least 2 cm (¾ in.) of intact periwound tissue to maintain airtight seal.
  b. Wound open enough to insert foam dressing that touches all edges.
  c. Wound debrided.
  d. Sufficient circulation to assist in healing process.

▪ Select correct foam dressing according to size and type of wound. Black foam has larger pores and is used to stimulate granulation tissue and wound contraction. White (soft) foam is used when granulation tissue needs to be restricted or patient cannot tolerate pain associated with black foam. White foam is used with superficial wounds, shallow chronic ulcers, and tunneling or undermining wounds.

CAUTION! Average length of treatment is 4–6 weeks. Home systems are available to continue therapy.

▪ Gather equipment and supplies.

Procedure

1. Introduce self to patient and verify the patient's identity using two identifiers. Explain the wound V.A.C. system to the patient and allow time for any questions from the patient or family. Determine patient's willingness to use this therapy. Explain why it is necessary, and how the patient can participate. Discuss how the results will be used in planning further care or treatments.

2. Perform hand hygiene and observe appropriate infection control procedures.

3. Provide for patient privacy and comfort. Don clean gloves.

APPLICATION

4. Prepare the wound area.
   ● Place disposal bag near wound.
   ● Open supplies and place on overbed table. Open kit while maintaining sterility.
   ● Draw up normal saline irrigating solution in syringe.
   ● Place moisture-proof pad or sterile basin under wound. **Rationale:** *This protects skin and bed during irrigation.*
   ● Clean wound using aggressive irrigation. If debridement is to be done, only a trained professional can perform the skill. Notify the appropriate person. **Rationale:** *Devitalized tissue should be removed as areas of soft or stringy slough delays the healing process.*
   ● Remove and discard gloves. Perform hand hygiene.

Safety Considerations
V.A.C.® GRANUFOAM® SILVER

▪ Provides continuous delivery of silver directly to wound bed.

▪ Provides a protective barrier to reduce aerobic, gram-negative, and gram-positive bacteria, yeast, and fungi, and it may reduce infections in wounds.

▪ Indicated for patients with chronic, acute, traumatic, and dehisced wounds, partial-thickness burns, and pressure injuries.

Source: Data from V.A.C. GranuFoam Silver®

---

5. Activate the wound V.A.C. system.
   ● Don sterile gloves.
   ● Dry wound and prepare periwound tissue with skin preparation agent if necessary. **Rationale:** *This is to promote an airtight seal.*
   ● Cut the V.A.C. foam to fit the shape and entire wound cavity, including tunneling or undermined areas **②**. White foam is used for tunneled wounds.

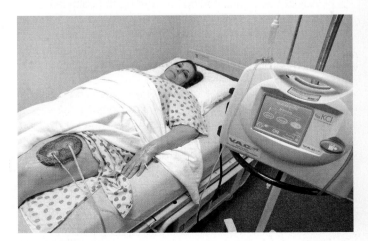

② *V.A.C. foam cut to fit shape and wound cavity, with tubing attached to vacuum pump.*

(continued on next page)

SKILL 16.14 Negative Pressure Wound Therapy: Using (*continued*)

- Size and trim drape to cover foam dressing, leaving a 3.5-cm (1½ in.) border per wound area.
- Gently place the foam into wound, ensuring entire wound is covered.

CAUTION! Do not pack foam into any areas of the wound. Forcing foam dressings in a compressed manner into any wound may lead to risk of adverse health issues.

For deep wounds, reposition tubing to minimize pressure on wound edges every 2 hours. Excess foam can be used to cushion skin under tubing.

- Apply tubing to foam. Tubing can be laid on top of foam or placed inside foam dressing. Keep tubing away from bony prominences.
- Cover foam and 3.5 cm (1½ in.) per wound area with drape.
- Do not stretch drape or compress foam with drape. **Rationale:** *This ensures a tight seal without causing tension or a shearing force on periwound tissue.*
- Lift tubing and place on drape that has been bunched up to protect skin from pressure of tube.
- Secure tubing with additional piece of drape or tape several centimeters away from dressing. **Rationale:** *This prevents pulling on the dressing, leading to a leak.*
- Remove gloves and discard.
- Remove canister from sterile package and push it into the V.A.C. unit until you hear it click in place. Alarm will sound if canister is not properly inserted into unit.
- Connect dressing tubing to canister tubing.
- Open both clamps, one on the dressing tubing and the other on the canister tubing.
- Place V.A.C. unit on level surface or hang from footboard.
- Press power button ON.
- Adjust V.A.C. unit settings according to healthcare provider's orders or Guidelines for Treating Wound Types in the reference manual that comes with the unit. Target pressure should be set for 5 minutes on and 2 minutes off (intermittent therapies on machine). Intensity of setting sets the negative pressure.
- Assess dressing in 1 minute. **Rationale:** *The dressing should collapse unless air leak is present.*

6. When the procedure is complete, perform hand hygiene and leave patient safe and comfortable.
7. Complete documentation using forms, checklists, or electronic dropdown lists supplemented by nurse's notes or additional comments as appropriate, including the appearance of the wound; the color, consistency, amount, and odor of any drainage; and how the patient responded.
8. Dressing changes must be completed every 48 hr unless wound is infected, then change every 12–24 hr.
   - Raise tube connector above level of pump unit.
   - Tighten clamp on dressing tube.

- Separate canister tube and dressing tubes by disconnecting the connector.
- Allow pump unit to pull exudates in canister tube into canister; then tighten clamps on canister tube.
- Press Therapy ON/OFF to deactivate pump.
- Stretch drape horizontally and slowly pull up from skin. Gently remove it from skin. Do not peel it off skin ❸.
- Discard disposable equipment including gloves in appropriate bag or container.

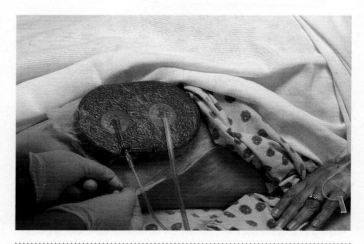

❸ Remove adhesive drape by gently pulling away from skin.

9. When the procedure is complete, perform hand hygiene and leave patient safe and comfortable.
10. Complete documentation using forms, checklists, or electronic dropdown lists supplemented by nurse's notes or additional comments as appropriate.

SAMPLE DOCUMENTATION

[date] 1315 Stage 3 pressure injury of right buttocks has full thickness skin loss, necrosis noted in wound bed, crater-like appearance, length 4 cm, width 3 cm, depth 2 cm. Small amount serosanguineous exudate noted with moderate purulent yellow foul-smelling draining. Small amount eschar noted right side wound bed. Surrounding tissue slightly reddened, small amount edema, firm, and intact. Denies pain of area. Wound bed irrigated with sterile saline and dried. Skin prep cream applied around wound per order. V.A.C. foam cut to fit wound and cover cut to fit area. Foam placed in wound, tubing applied, cover applied. Drainage tube connected to collection canister, unit placed on bedside table. No problems noted after 1 minute of turning V.A.C. on. Tolerated without incident, resting on right side. *T. Niret*

SKILL 16.14 Negative Pressure Wound Therapy: Using (*continued*)

Safety Considerations

- Disconnecting V.A.C. unit:
  - Turn the unit to OFF.
  - Clamp both clamps on tubing.
  - Press quick-release connector to separate dressing tubing from canister tubing.
  - Cover ends of tubing with gauze and secure.
  - Document cessation of therapy and assessments.
- Reconnecting V.A.C. unit:
  - Remove gauze from ends of tubing.
  - Connect tubing.
  - Unclamp clamps.
  - Press V.A.C. green power button to ON.

- Select NO at new patient prompt. Unit will resume previous settings.
- Press therapy to ON. Document reinitiating therapy.
- Changing canister:
  - Don clean gloves.
  - Assess that canister unit is full. Unit will alarm when full.
  - Tighten clamps on canister tubing from dressing tubing.
  - Pull back on release knob on V.A.C. unit at same time as you pull canister from slot.
  - Put canister in biohazard disposable bag and place in designated area for disposal.
  - Remove and discard gloves. Perform hand hygiene. Document canister change.

SKILL 16.15 Pressure Injury: Preventing and Caring for

Individuals that have limited mobility, are immobilized, have impaired sensation, or are unable to turn and reposition themselves have a high risk of developing a pressure injury. Skin breakdown usually occurs over a bony prominence as a result of pressure, friction, wetness, or shear force. A pressure injury can be deep enough to cause tissue destruction extending from the skin layers down to the patient's bone. Surgical interventions such as skin grafts are sometimes necessary.

Delegation or Assignment

Determining preventive measures or providing care of a pressure injury is the nurse's or wound care nurse's responsibility and not delegated or assigned to the UAP. The UAP may provide routine care of the patient as trained. The nurse can request the UAP to report patient observations to the nurse for follow-up. The nurse remains responsible for the assessment, interpretation of abnormal findings, and determination of appropriate responses.

Equipment

- Cleansing solution
- Sterile normal saline solution in a pour bottle
- Sterile 4 × 4 gauze pads
- Clean gloves
- Sterile gloves, as needed
- Biohazard bag
- Ruler marked in inches and centimeters
- Scissors
- Absorbent pad
- Additional supplies required for the particular dressing (e.g., extra gauze dressings and ointment or powder, if ordered)
- Sterile dressing set as needed; if none is available, gather the following sterile items:
  - Drape or towel
  - Gauze squares
  - Container for the cleaning solution
  - Antimicrobial solution
  - Forceps.

Preparation

- Review healthcare provider's orders and patient's nursing plan of care.
- Review patient's record for documentation on wound care and dressings.
- Gather equipment and supplies.

Safety Considerations

Wounds are measured in centimeters, in the order of Length × Width × Depth.

- Length is the direction of head to toe.
- Width is the direction of hip to hip.
- Depth is the deepest part of visible wound bed.

Procedure

1. Introduce self to patient and verify the patient's identity using two identifiers. Explain to the patient what you are going to do, why it is necessary, and how the patient can participate. Discuss how the results will be used in planning further care or treatments.
2. Perform hand hygiene and observe appropriate infection control procedures.
3. Provide for patient privacy.

PREVENTION

4. Inspect skin at least on admission and once a shift, particularly over bony prominences. Heels and sacrum are most common areas for skin breakdown.
   - Use the Braden Risk Assessment Scale to evaluate a patient's risk for skin breakdown and developing a pressure injury. There are six categories assessed: nutrition status, ability to be mobile, activity level, sensory perception, skin moisture, and friction/shear. Total score ranges from 6–23. The lower score indicates the

(*continued on next page*)

SKILL 16.15 Pressure Injury: Preventing and Caring for (*continued*)

higher risk. The level of risk helps the nurse make decisions about preventive intervention strategies (BCPNSWC, 2014).

- The National Pressure Ulcer Advisory Panel (NPUAP) provides a pressure injury staging system which includes wound definitions and descriptions to indicate the extent of tissue damage ❶–❻. There are four stages of pressure injuries plus four additional definitions now available (NPUAP, 2016).
- Document assessment findings.

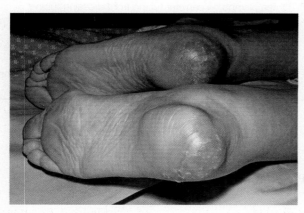

Source: Mike Devlin/Science Source

❶ Stage 1 pressure injury.

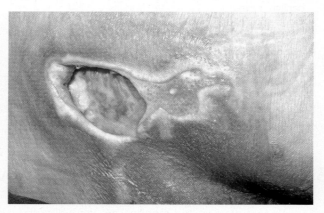

Source: Mediscan/Alamy Stock Photo

❹ Stage 4 pressure injury.

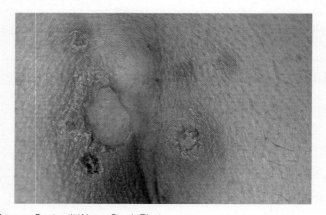

Source: CaptureIt/Alamy Stock Photo

❷ Stage 2 pressure injury.

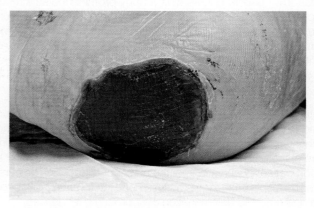

Source: Matt Meadows/Photolibrary/Getty Images

❺ Eschar must be removed by debridement before staging is done.

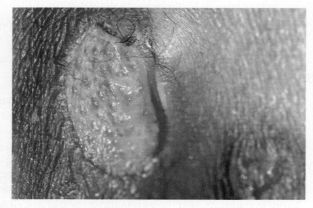

Source: CaptureIt/Alamy Stock Photo

❸ Stage 3 pressure injury.

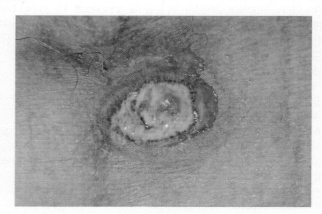

Source: Dr P. Marazzi/Science Source

❻ Clinical signs of infection.

SKILL 16.15 Pressure Injury: Preventing and Caring for (*continued*)

Safety Considerations

- If skin is red or skin breakdown is evident on admission and documented, Medicare and other third party payers will reimburse for treatment.
- If skin is red or skin breakdown is evident but not documented on admission, treatment costs will not be reimbursed.
- If not evident on admission, treatment costs will not be reimbursed.

5. Individualize patient's bathing schedule. Daily baths are not essential. **Rationale:** *Daily cleansing can destroy the skin's natural barrier, making it more susceptible to external irritants.*
   - Avoid hot bath water. **Rationale:** *Tepid water prevents injury to skin.*
   - Use mild cleansing agents to minimize dryness.
   - Clean skin immediately if urine, fecal incontinence, or wound drainage seeps onto skin.
   - Provide humidity to prevent drying of skin.
   - Use cream or thin layer of corn starch to protect skin if facility policy.
6. Avoid massaging bony prominences. **Rationale:** *Massaging can lead to deep tissue trauma.*
   - Keep bony prominences from direct contact with one another.
   - Use pillow, foam wedges, or other positioning devices.
   - Use elbow pads and heel elevators.
7. Promote adequate dietary intake of protein, calories, nutrients, and fluid intake. Protein should be approximately 1.2–1.5 g/kg body weight daily. **Rationale:** *Adequate protein intake in addition to vitamins and minerals helps prevent pressure injury formation.*

Safety Considerations

Be alert to altered skin integrity when pressure is reduced in one anatomical area by turning and repositioning, because the newer location may be placed at risk for pressure injury formation.

AIR-FLUIDIZED BED

Air-fluidized beds and low-air-loss beds are recommended to manage pressure injuries, especially in patients with large or multiple pressure injuries. Warm, pressurized air circulates through beads in the bed and creates a support surface. A polyester sheet allows for moisture and air to pass through, keeping skin dry. Treatment can take several months. Use of this bed is very expensive.

LOW-AIR-LOSS BED

Head and foot of bed can be elevated. Bed is a modified standard bed frame, lighter and more portable than an air-fluidized bed. The bed circulates cool air. Urine and feces do not pass through fabric on the bed. Bed is portable and lightweight.

8. Reposition bedridden patient every 1–2 hr.
   - Do not position directly on trochanter.
   - Do not turn more than a 30-degree angle.
   - Raise heels off bed by placing pillows under legs; allow heels to hang over edges.
   - Use trapeze or turning sheet to reposition patient.

9. Encourage mobility or range-of-motion (ROM) exercises. **Rationale:** *ROM exercises promote activity and reduce effects of pressure on tissue.*
10. Minimize force and friction on skin when turning or moving patient. Use turning sheets or mechanical lift devices. Have adequate staff to assist in moving and lifting patients.
11. Maintain head of bed at lowest degree of elevation consistent with medical problem; below 30 degrees if possible. Place at-risk patients on pressure-reducing devices, in both bed and chair, such as foam, static-air, alternating gel, water mattress, or air-fluidized mattress.
12. Place patient on specialty bed or mattress if the patient already has a pressure injury or is at high risk for ulcer formation. Encourage chair-fast patients to shift position every 15 minutes. Proceed to step 13 below.

CARE

4. Monitor patient's overall condition daily. **Rationale:** *Patients who are confined to bed will have the tendency to develop new skin breakdown (skin failure) as other organs fail. Existing pressure injuries of lesser staging (I and II) almost always worsen over time and become at least stage III.*
5. Differentiate type of wound, pressure versus nonpressure.
6. Determine stage of pressure injury.
7. Monitor and assess pressure injury characteristics daily.
   - Observe dressing to determine if dry, intact, and not leaking.
   - Observe pressure injury bed, if appropriate, and document findings.
8. Assess pain level of patient and provide adequate pain relief.
9. Photograph pressure injury according to facility policy. **Rationale:** *This is to determine progress of ulcer healing.*
   - Monitor progress toward healing and for potential complications.
   - Measure pressure injury size weekly using a pressure injury scale. Usual healing time is 2–4 weeks.
10. If healing is not progressing or has not healed in usual time frame, re-evaluate treatment plan and patient's condition.
    - Maintain turning and positioning schedule to promote healing and prevent additional ulcer formation.
    - Complete a nutritional assessment. Positive nitrogen balance and protein intake are necessary for healing.
11. Complete a psychosocial assessment to determine patient's adherence to pressure injury treatment regimens.
12. Complete dressing change according to facility policy and type of dressing used. Follow manufacturer's guidelines for performing dressing changes. **Rationale:** *Dressing changes are based on a combination of factors, such as manufacturer suggested use, pressure injury characteristics, and goals for healing.*
13. When the procedure is complete, perform hand hygiene and leave patient safe and comfortable.

(*continued on next page*)

SKILL 16.15 Pressure Injury: Preventing and Caring for (continued)

14. Complete documentation using forms, checklists, or electronic dropdown lists supplemented by nurse's notes or additional comments as appropriate including turning and repositioning, how the patient responded, and any skin changes in color, texture, or integrity. Document with photos if facility policy. If the patient has a wound, document the appearance of the wound; the color, consistency, amount, and odor of any drainage; the type of dressing applied; and how the patient responded.

SAMPLE DOCUMENTATION

[date] 0645 Stage I pressure injury on left heel remains reddened and dry but without breakdown of skin at this time. Measures 3 centimeters in diameter. Area cleaned and dried, moisturizer cream applied to area. Repositioned to right side, supported with pillows. Left heel remains supported with pillow without heel touching bed. Denies tenderness to area. Tolerated repositioning and heel care without incident. *L. Wong*

CAUTION! Patients have the right to refuse wound care. However, the staff should provide quality pressure injury prevention or treatment. The Centers for Medicare and Medicaid Services has indicated that long-term care facilities must implement evidence-based protocols of prevention and care for pressure injuries.

EVIDENCE-BASED PRACTICE

Pressure Injury Formation

There has been no definitive research on whether pressure injuries begin to form from the skin down or from deep tissue up. However, there is agreement that pressure injuries form most commonly over bony prominences, often affect deep tissue, and are associated with prolonged immobility and inadequate perfusion of cells. At times skin breakdown may begin superficially, either from friction (as in sliding the patient up in bed) or from shearing forces (movement of deep tissue in one direction while skin is pulled in the opposite direction). Most often, sustained pressure that traps deep tissue between bone and a hard surface (e.g., a wheelchair) is implicated in pressure injury formation. Moisture of the skin (from sweat, urine, etc.) and poor nutrition (especially lack of protein) are also associated factors.

Pressure injuries are difficult and costly to treat. The best strategy is to prevent formation of pressure injuries by moving patients carefully, repositioning regularly, and keeping skin clean and dry.

Sources: Data from MedlinePlus, 2016, WebMD, 2014, National Pressure Ulcer Advisory Panel, 2016.

SKILL 16.16 Staple and Suture: Removing

Safety Note! *During scheduled clinical time, nursing students may have a learning opportunity to observe or assist with this skill only with faculty permission and with direct supervision from faculty or another RN.*

Medical staples and sutures are used to close wounds. Staples are inserted in wound edges by a stapling device and sutures require a needle and suture material for stitching using surgical instruments.

Delegation or Assignment

Removing staples or sutures and assessing the site is the nurse's responsibility and not delegated or assigned to the UAP. The UAP may provide routine care of the patient as trained. The nurse can request the UAP to report patient observations to the nurse for follow-up. The nurse remains responsible for the assessment, interpretation of abnormal findings, and determination of appropriate responses.

Equipment

- Sterile staple remover or sterile suture removal set
- Disposal bag
- Clean gloves, 2 pairs (1 pair optional)
- Dressings
- Tape or butterfly tape
- Antiseptic solution

Preparation

- Review healthcare provider's orders and patient's nursing plan of care.
- Gather equipment and supplies.

Procedure

1. Introduce self to patient and verify the patient's identity using two identifiers. Explain to the patient what you are going to do, why it is necessary, and how the patient can participate. Discuss how the results will be used in planning further care or treatments.
2. Perform hand hygiene and observe appropriate infection control procedures.
3. Provide for patient privacy. Raise the bed to appropriate height for procedure. Expose wound area, using a bath blanket to cover patient as needed ❶.
4. Don clean gloves.
5. Remove dressing, and discard in disposal bag. Perform hand hygiene.

SKILL 16.16 Staple and Suture: Removing *(continued)*

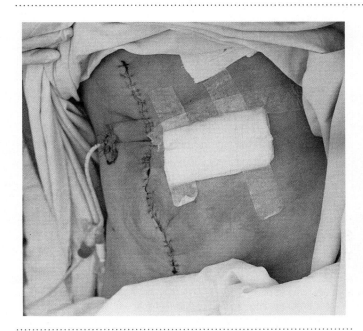

1 Large abdominal wound with staples closing incision.

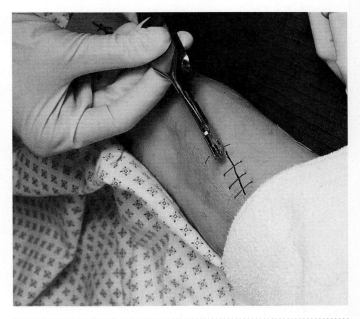

3 Lift staple remover device upward and away from incision.

REMOVE STAPLES

6. Open sterile staple remover. Don gloves if necessary.
7. Place lower tip of staple remover under staple.
8. Press handles together to depress center of staple **2**.
9. Lift staple remover upward, away from incision site when both ends of staple are visible **3**.
10. Place staple removal device over disposal bag and release handles to release staple.

11. Remove all staples or as directed by healthcare provider's order or facility policy. Some policies indicate every other staple is removed with remaining staples done at a later time. **Rationale:** *This prevents wound dehiscence.*
12. Clean incision area with antiseptic solution, if ordered.
13. Remove gloves, and place in disposal bag.
14. Place dressing over incision and secure with tape, or place butterfly tape over incision. Proceed to step 18.

CAUTION! Butterfly closure-strips, or surgical strips, may be applied over incision site to protect it after staples have been removed.

REMOVE SUTURES

6. Open suture removal set, and don gloves, if needed.
7. Pick up forceps with nondominant hand.
8. Grasp suture at the knot with forceps and lift away from skin **4**.
9. Pick up suture scissors with dominant hand.
10. Place curved tip of suture scissors under suture, next to knot.
11. Cut suture and, with forceps, pull suture through skin with one movement **5**.
12. Discard suture into disposal bag.
13. Check that entire suture is removed.
14. Continue to remove remaining sutures according to healthcare provider's order or facility policy. Some policies state that every other suture is removed and then remaining sutures are removed at a later time. **Rationale:** *This prevents wound dehiscence.*
15. Clean suture site with antiseptic solution.

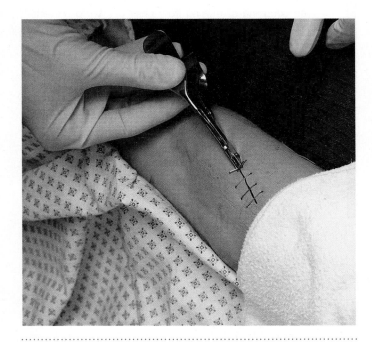

2 With lower tip of staple removal device under staple, press handle together to depress center of staple.

(continued on next page)

SKILL 16.16 Staple and Suture: Removing (*continued*)

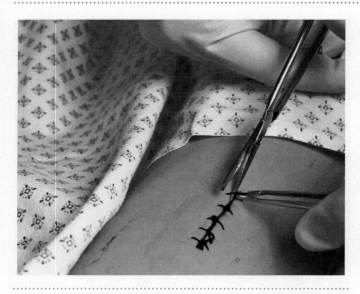

④ Grasp suture at the knot with forceps and lift away from skin.

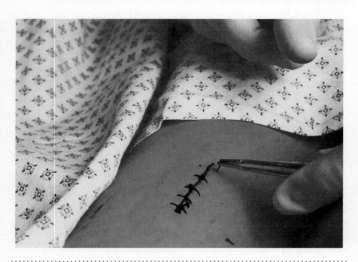

⑤ After cutting suture, grasp suture at knot and pull through skin.

16. Remove gloves and place in disposal bag.
17. Place dressing or butterfly tape over incision area, if ordered.
18. Discard disposal bag into contaminated waste container.
19. When the procedure is complete, perform hand hygiene and leave patient safe and comfortable.
20. Complete documentation using forms, checklists, or electronic dropdown lists supplemented by nurse's notes or additional comments as appropriate.

SAMPLE DOCUMENTATION

[date] 0730 Dressing removed from sutures left arm incision site. Wound edges well-healed with no opened area noted, no redness, drainage, or tenderness. 4 sutures removed per Dr. Ware's order. Complete suture removed on all 4 sutures. Incision site cleaned with sterile normal saline and dried. Adhesive strips applied the length of incision and covered with large band aide. Tolerated without incident. *V. Chau*

Safety Considerations
TOPICAL GLUE FOR WOUND CLOSURE

A product to replace sutures and staples (used in many procedures annually) was approved by the FDA after proving itself in clinical trials. This superglue acting product is a tissue cyanoacrylate adhesive. It is a synthetic, noninvasive glue that mitigates trauma and post-procedure inflammation, while providing a waterproof seal and protecting underlying tissue without the need for bandages. Best used on short, straight low-tension wounds. Tissue adhesive is painless, fast and simple to apply, and naturally sloughs off in 7–10 days.

Patient Teaching

Wound Care at Home

- Ensure patient knows to eat foods high in protein, carbohydrates, vitamins, and minerals to promote wound healing.
- Verify patient knows how to splint the wound with a pillow when coughing or moving from chair or bed to prevent separation of wound edges.
- Ensure patient or caregiver can recognize signs and symptoms of wound infection or delayed healing, and when to notify the healthcare provider.
- Encourage the use of daily showers; water may run over wound.
- Reinforce to patient not to use soap, lotions, or vitamin creams on incision.
- Ensure patient or caregiver knows how to change the dressing safely.
- Verify patient knows not to lift heavy objects (anything over 4.5 kg [10 lb]).
- Ensure patient knows measures to promote elimination.

SKILL 16.17 Stump: Positioning and Exercising

A stump, also referred to as a residual limb, is the body part that remains after a surgical amputation procedure. Positioning and exercising are included in postsurgical rehabilitation of the patient with a stump to help the patient gain muscular strength, control, joint range of motion (ROM), and become as independent as able. Positioning and exercising can help prevent complications such as contractions, phantom sensation, pain, and edema due to fluid in the stump tissue.

SKILL 16.17 Stump: Positioning and Exercising (*continued*)

Delegation or Assignment

Due to the need for technical complexity, initial teaching about positioning and exercising a residual limb is done by the nurse or physical therapist. Assisting the patient to reposition and do exercises with the residual limb can be delegated or assigned to the UAP. The nurse must ensure that the UAP knows what complications or adverse signs should be reported to the nurse. The nurse remains responsible for the assessment, interpretation of abnormal findings, and determination of appropriate responses. Note that state laws for UAPs vary, so repositioning or exercises might be assigned to the UAP rather than delegated.

Equipment

- Pillows

Preparation

- Review healthcare provider's orders and patient's nursing plan of care.
- Gather needed supplies.

Procedure

1. Introduce self to patient and verify the patient's identity using two identifiers. Explain to the patient what you are going to do, why it is necessary, and how the patient can participate. Discuss how the results will be used in planning further care or treatments.
2. Perform hand hygiene and observe appropriate infection control procedures.
3. Provide for patient privacy.

PREOPERATIVE CARE

4. Evaluate nutritional status and request nutritional consult if indicated. **Rationale:** *Adequate protein is necessary to promote wound healing.*
5. Recruit assistance of occupational therapist, physical therapist, and social worker for early multidisciplinary care planning.
6. A prosthetist explains future prosthetic care to the patient and possibly organizes amputee peer visit, because this helps lessen anxiety about living with an amputation.
7. Explain importance of exercises to patient.
8. Tell patient that because flexor muscles are stronger than extensors, the stump position will be permanently flexed and abducted unless the patient practices extension and adduction exercises. **Rationale:** *Exercises increase muscle strength and improve mobility of amputated extremity. Both are necessary for optimal ambulation with a prosthesis.*
9. Teach patient quadriceps-setting exercises with a below-the-knee amputation.
   - Extend leg and try to push back of knee into bed; try to move patella proximally.
   - Contract quadriceps and hold contraction for 10 seconds.
   - Repeat this procedure four or five times.
   - Repeat the exercise at least four times a day.

10. Teach use of ambulatory aids. **Rationale:** *Prepares patient for postsurgery mobility.*
11. Explain phantom limb sensation; the patient may continue to "feel" the lost limb post-surgery.
12. Counsel families, for they also mourn the loss of a visible body part. **Rationale:** *They too need psychological support and education about rehabilitation and necessary skills for self-care.* Proceed to step 13.

POSTOPERATIVE CARE

4. Monitor for complications: hemorrhage, infection, unrelieved pain, wound that will not heal. Assess for excessive wound drainage. Keep tourniquet at bedside. **Rationale:** *If excessive bleeding occurs, tourniquet must be applied, because hemorrhage is a potentially life-threatening complication.*
5. Administer ordered pain medication and continually assess to determine if pain is controlled.

CAUTION! Adequate pain management in the preoperative period can reduce the occurrence of phantom limb pain postoperatively.

---

6. Do not place stump on pillow, but elevate foot of bed for first 24 hours ONLY to reduce stump edema and pain. **Rationale:** *Elevation on a pillow can promote flexion contracture of stump.*
7. Turn patient to prone or supine position for at least 1 hour every 4 hours. **Rationale:** *This promotes hip extension and helps counteract possible flexion contracture formation.*
8. Avoid dependent positioning of stump. **Rationale:** *This prevents edema and discomfort. Edema may be present for up to 4 months after amputation.* Encourage appropriate use of trapeze: Use both hands to pull up with trapeze; place foot flat on mattress to lift body. Do not use heel to push in the mattress.
9. While washing the stump, tap and massage the stump skin toward the incision line. **Rationale:** *This prevents development of painful adhesions.*
10. Teach stump extension exercises.
    - Lie in a prone position with foot hanging over the end of the bed.
    - Keep stump next to intact leg to extend stump and to contract gluteal muscles.
    - Hold the contraction for 10 seconds.
    - Repeat this exercise at least four times a day.
11. Teach adduction exercise.
    - Place a pillow between the patient's thighs.
    - Squeeze the pillow for 10 seconds and then relax for 10 seconds.
    - Repeat this exercise at least four times a day.
12. Have the patient keep track of time spent with the stump flexed and then spend an equal amount of time with the stump extended. After stump incision heals, have patient begin to bear weight on stump, initially pressing

(*continued on next page*)

SKILL 16.17 Stump: Positioning and Exercising (continued)

into padded surface (pillow on chair seat). **Rationale:** *This reduces pain and helps prepare the stump for prosthesis.*

Safety Considerations

- Keep a tourniquet nearby in the event of excessive stump incision bleeding.
- Amputees use more energy in ambulation than nonamputees.
- Older adults with an above-the-knee amputation (AKA) should be encouraged to put forth the extra effort they may need to walk at a slow pace.
- The longer the residual limb, the less energy the patient must expend for ambulation.

13. When the procedure is complete, perform hand hygiene and leave patient safe and comfortable.

14. Complete documentation using forms, checklists, or electronic dropdown lists supplemented by nurse's notes or additional comments as appropriate, including exercising, care, and teaching in the patient's record. Document any stump changes, incision site appearance, and how the patient responded.

SAMPLE DOCUMENTATION

[date] 0813 Noted exercising stump using adduction exercise maneuver. States it tires him out but he knows it will pay off. Discussed periodic rest periods may help him. Dressing on stump remains intact, little edema noted. Denies stump pain at this time. *P. Zerste*

SKILL 16.18 Stump: Shrinking and Molding

Safety Note! *During scheduled clinical time, nursing students may have a learning opportunity to observe or assist with this skill only with faculty permission and with direct supervision from faculty or another RN.*

A stump, also referred to as a residual limb, is the body part that remains after a surgical amputation procedure. The stump is initially kept covered with a soft dressing. An elastic bandage is applied over the soft dressing to control the amount of swelling in the stump. The stump is measured for appropriate size of a shrinker sock, which will help control swelling and begin molding the stump. Further shrinking and molding the stump is done with more rigid dressings that protect the stump and prepare it for weight bearing and prosthetic devices.

Delegation or Assignment

Applying an elastic bandage and assessing the patient's stump is the nurse's responsibility and is not delegated or assigned to the UAP. The UAP may provide routine care of the patient as trained. The nurse can request the UAP to report patient observations to the nurse for follow-up. The nurse remains responsible for the assessment, interpretation of abnormal findings, and determination of appropriate responses.

Equipment

- Two elastic bandages: 10 cm (4 in.) for below-the-knee amputation (BKA), 15 cm (6 in.) for above-the-knee amputation (AKA)
- Tape or safety pins
- Commercial stump shrinker sock

Preparation

- Review healthcare provider's orders to determine date and type of amputation.

- Review patient's nursing plan of care.
- Gather equipment.

Procedure

1. Introduce self to patient and verify the patient's identity using two identifiers. Explain to the patient what you are going to do, why it is necessary, and how the patient can participate. Discuss how the results will be used in planning further care or treatments.
2. Perform hand hygiene and observe appropriate infection control procedures.
3. Provide for patient privacy.
4. Wash stump with soap and water and allow to dry for at least 10 minutes before bandaging. Do not use lotions, powders, or alcohol.
5. Inspect and encourage patient to assess stump for circulatory status, pressure areas, wound healing, and edema.
6. Explain that purpose of wrap is to form a conical AKA stump to prepare for prosthesis use ❶.
7. Explain that the wrap is to be worn at all times except during bathing or when wearing a prosthesis.
8. Begin wrapping by placing the outer surface of the bandage end at the distal stump. **Rationale:** *The pressure gradient of the bandage should be greatest at the distal stump.*
9. Wrap bandage medially and diagonally around stump. Have patient assist by holding turns. Stretch bandages to two thirds of the limit of the elastic.
10. Continue to wrap smoothly up the stump with medially directed spirals or figure eight turns (not circular). Progress up the stump and well into the groin area. **Rationale:** *Circular turns constrict circulation. Medial turns help correct stump tendency toward abduction.*

SKILL 16.18 Stump: Shrinking and Molding *(continued)*

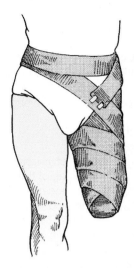

Source: From Pressure Ulcer Treatment: Quick Reference Guide for Clinicians, No. 15. Published by U.S. Department of Health and Human Services.

❶ Compression bandage may be used following amputation to mold and shrink stump in preparation for prosthesis.

11. Finish bandaging with a "spica" turn over and around the patient's pelvis, then back down to stump. **Rationale:** *Large spica turn prevents bandage from slipping.*
12. Secure the bandage with tape or (cautiously) with safety pins. Do not use bandage clips. **Rationale:** *Clips can pierce the skin, or easily come loose.*
13. Reapply elastic bandage every 4–6 hr, or when loose. **Rationale:** *It must never be in place for more than 12 hours without being rewrapped.*
14. If patient has a stump "shrinker sock," roll down and stretch the sock using plastic ring. Fit onto stump end and apply, making sure there are no wrinkles **❷**.
15. Teach patient home care of residual limb and prosthesis (washing; assessing for redness, pressure points, irritation, swelling skin breakdown; socket, stump, socks, liners, mechanical parts, etc.).
16. When the procedure is complete, perform hand hygiene and leave patient safe and comfortable.
17. Complete documentation using forms, checklists, or electronic dropdown lists supplemented by nurse's notes or

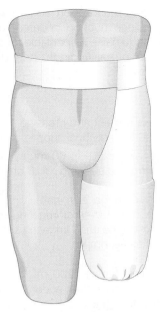

Source: From Pressure Ulcer Treatment: Quick Reference Guide for Clinicians, No. 15. Published by U.S. Department of Health and Human Services.

❷ "Commercial shrinkers" may be used for above-the-knee amputations. They help shape the stump, support healing, and control edema.

additional comments as appropriate, including actions performed, type of dressing applied, and how the patient responded.

SAMPLE DOCUMENTATION

[date] 0810 Suture line of stump cleaned with sterile normal saline and dried. 8 sutures intact, small amount redness around sutures, no drainage noted, no tenderness observed. Dry sterile dressing applied without difficulty; 15-cm (6-in.) elastic wrap applied up to groin with pressure, secured with tape. Denies wrap feels too tight. Encouraged to do exercises as shown by physical therapist. *T. Garrhare*

SKILL 16.19 Wound: Irrigating

Safety Note! *During scheduled clinical time, nursing students may have a learning opportunity to observe or assist with this skill only with faculty permission and with direct supervision from faculty or another RN.*

Wound irrigation is used to help debride a wound, cleanse it, apply antimicrobial solution that has been ordered, or help clear the wound for better visualization. Wound irrigation can be done using an irrigation syringe or a pulsating pressure device using normal saline.

Delegation or Assignment

Due to the need for aseptic technique and assessment skills, wound irrigations are not delegated or assigned to the UAP. However, the UAP may observe the wound and dressing

(continued on next page)

SKILL 16.19 Wound: Irrigating *(continued)*

during usual care and must report abnormal findings to the nurse. Abnormal findings must be validated and interpreted by the nurse. The nurse remains responsible for the assessment, interpretation of abnormal findings, and determination of appropriate responses.

Equipment

- Sterile dressing equipment and dressing materials
- Sterile irrigation set or individual supplies, including:
  - Sterile syringe (e.g., a 30- to 60-mL syringe) with a catheter of an appropriate size (e.g., #18 or #19) or an irrigating tip syringe
  - Splash shield for syringe (optional)
  - Sterile graduated container for irrigating solution
  - Basin for collecting the used irrigating solution
  - Moisture-proof sterile drape
  - Moisture-proof bag
  - Irrigating solution, usually 200 mL (6.5 oz) of solution warmed to body temperature, according to the facility's or healthcare provider's choice
  - Goggles, gown, and mask
  - Clean gloves
  - Sterile gloves (optional).

Safety Considerations

Although a wound may already be contaminated, sterile equipment and supplies are used during irrigation to prevent the possibility of adding new nonresident microorganisms to the site. When doing wound care at home, some reusable supplies such as irrigating syringes or basins may be cleaned and used again with the same wound.

Preparation

- Review healthcare provider's orders and patient's nursing plan of care.
- Verify type of irrigation solution to use for wound irrigation.
- Check that the irrigating fluid is at the proper temperature.
- Gather equipment and supplies.

Procedure

1. Introduce self to patient and verify the patient's identity using two identifiers. Explain to the patient you are going to irrigate the patient's wound, why it is necessary, and how the patient can participate. Discuss how the results will be used in planning further care or treatments.
2. Perform hand hygiene and observe other appropriate infection control procedures.
3. Provide for patient privacy.
4. Prepare the patient.
   - Assist the patient to a position in which the irrigating solution will flow by gravity from the upper end of the wound to the lower end and then into the basin.
   - Place the waterproof drape under the wounds and over the bed.
   - Don clean gloves and remove and discard the old dressing.

5. Measure and assess the wound and drainage.
   - If indicated, clean the wound.
   - Remove and discard gloves. Perform hand hygiene.
6. Prepare the equipment.
   - Open the sterile dressing set and supplies.
   - Pour the ordered solution into the solution container.
   - Position the basin below the wound to receive the irrigating fluid.
7. Irrigate the wound.
   - Don clean gloves.
   - Instill a steady stream of irrigating solution into the wound. Make sure all areas of the wound are irrigated.
   - Use either a syringe with a catheter attached or with an irrigating tip to flush the wound ❶.
   - If you are using a catheter to reach tracts or crevices, insert the catheter into the wound until resistance is met. Do not force the catheter. **Rationale:** *Forcing the catheter can cause tissue damage.*
   - Continue irrigating until the solution becomes clear (no exudate is present).
   - Dry the area around the wound. **Rationale:** *Moisture left on the skin promotes the growth of microorganisms and can cause skin irritation and breakdown.*
   - Remove and discard gloves. Perform hand hygiene.

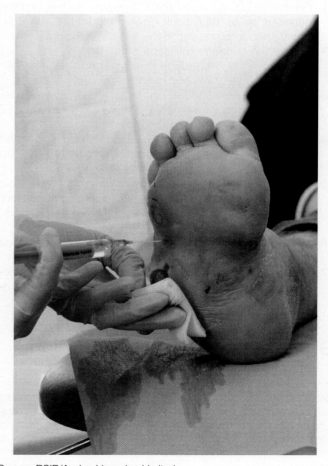

Source: BSIP/Avalon Licensing Limited

❶ Irrigating an open wound.

SKILL 16.19 Wound: Irrigating (*continued*)

8. Assess and dress the wound.
   - Assess the appearance of the wound again, noting in particular the type and amount of exudate still present and the presence and extent of granulation tissue.
   - Using sterile technique, don gloves and apply a sterile dressing to the wound based on the amount of drainage expected.
   - Remove and discard sterile gloves.
9. When the procedure is complete, perform hand hygiene and leave patient safe and comfortable.
10. Complete documentation using forms, checklists, or electronic dropdown lists supplemented by nurse's notes or additional comments as appropriate, including the irrigation and the patient's response. Many agencies use a designated wound/skin documentation sheet.

SAMPLE DOCUMENTATION

[date] 1000 Wound on (R) hip 3 × 3 cm, 6 mm deep, draining minimal amt. thick yellow. No odor. Skin around wound erythematous. Pain 0 on 0–10 scale. Irrigated c̄ NS until clear. Redressed using sterile technique. Tolerated without incident. *N. Jamaghani*

›› Critical Thinking Options for Unexpected Outcomes

Not all unexpected outcomes require further nursing intervention; however, many times they do. When the patient demonstrates a change in signs or symptoms indicating an emerging problem, the nurse should immediately assess and troubleshoot what is happening. The assessment data must be processed quickly to formulate a hypothesis so the nurse can make a clinical judgment. The nurse then decides how best to resolve the problem and improve the patient's situation for a better outcome.

EXPECTED OUTCOME	UNEXPECTED OUTCOME	POSSIBLE INTERVENTIONS
General Assessment Patient's wounds do not become infected.	Wound drainage increases.	■ Decrease time between dressing changes. Change every 4 hr. ■ Obtain order for culture and sensitivity to determine whether different microorganisms are present or antibiotic medication is not sensitive to microorganism.
Moist wound environment is maintained.	Dressings dry between dressing changes.	■ Moisten dressing with sterile normal saline before removing to prevent debridement of granulation tissue. ■ Ensure that dressing is moist when applied to wound, and cover with moist dressing. ■ Moisten and change dressing more frequently. ■ Semiocclusive dressing should be considered.
Patient maintains adequate fluid and nutrition.	Nutritional or hydration deficit occurs.	■ Monitor nutritional and fluid intake accurately. ■ Obtain order for vitamin supplements if patient is not already on vitamins. ■ Increase protein intake by supplementing with high-protein drinks.
Patient's buttocks and perineal area remain free from urine and stool.	Skin is exposed to moisture.	■ Establish bowel or bladder program and select absorbent products for wound area that wick the moisture from skin. ■ Clean skin with pH-balanced cleansers, avoiding friction and dry skin after each incidence of incontinence and dry thoroughly. ■ Apply skin barrier product. ■ Consider use of fecal management system or urinary catheter.
Patient is repositioned using scheduled times.	Shearing and friction occur secondarily related to immobility or reduced activity.	■ Keep head of bed at lowest position possible to prevent patient from sliding down in bed. ■ Have other staff assist in using lifting devices to move patient up in bed or out of bed to prevent friction on skin. ■ Instruct patient on use of trapeze bar to assist in repositioning.

(*continued on next page*)

EXPECTED OUTCOME	UNEXPECTED OUTCOME	POSSIBLE INTERVENTIONS
Dressings and Binders Wound heals without complications.	Patient's wound does not heal with traditional types of treatments.	■ In patient care conference discuss the following: ● Is everyone following same treatment? ● Are causative agents preventing healing? ● Should treatment be adjusted or changed? ● Would use of a support surface be effective? ● Is surgical debridement and grafting necessary for healing?
	Foam is not collapsed in wound bed.	■ Ensure therapy is on. Ensure clamps are open and tubing is not kinked. ■ Check for leaks and patch.
Wound Care Exudate is removed and wound healing occurs with negative wound therapy.	Wound is too large for VAC kit.	■ Use more than one foam piece. ■ Place pieces so they touch each other. ■ Use only one tubing piece to one of the foam pieces.
Periwound area remains healthy without evidence of maceration.	Periwound skin is fragile.	■ Use skin prep prior to applying drape. ■ Frame wound with skin barrier, wound barrier dressing, or Montgomery straps. ■ Cut drape large enough to enclose foam dressing and skin barrier layer.
Moist wound environment is maintained.	Dressing adheres to wound with negative pressure system or gauze packed dressing.	■ Instill sterile water or normal saline into dressing, let sit for 15–20 min, then gently remove dressing from wound.
Hyperbaric oxygen therapy (100% oxygen at a pressure greater than normal) is effective in treating diabetic leg ulcers.	Patient exhibits signs of anxiety when providing education regarding use of hyperbaric chamber.	■ Place patient in pressurized chamber where nurse can explain the value of increasing the oxygen to the wound to promote healing to assess patient with anxiety-reducing interventions.
Patient is repositioned using scheduled times.	Patient sits in chair most of day and keeps stump elevated on a pillow while in bed.	■ Discuss hip and knee contracture complications that occur with prolonged flexion positioning of the stump. ■ Review and reinforce exercises that promote stump adduction and extension to prevent contractures and facilitate prosthesis use.
Stump swelling is controlled and molding begins.	Stump edema occurs in spite of compression bandage application.	■ Evaluate wrapping procedure. ■ Ensure that wraps are applied with pressure greater at distal stump and reapplied several times a day. ■ Instruct patient to avoid prolonged dependent positioning of stump. ■ Consult prosthetist for possible rigid shrinker use. ■ Apply shrinker before patient gets out of bed.
Wound care is provided for contaminated wound and healing occurs.	Patient expresses fear of losing other leg.	■ Teach patient to care for the remaining extremity. ■ Inspect for lesions; wash and dry daily; use lotion for dry skin (not between toes); keep nails trimmed straight across; avoid mechanical, chemical, or thermal injury; wear shoes that are wide and deep enough for toes. ■ Exercise daily and avoid smoking. ■ Consult podiatrist for individual foot care or shoe orthotic adaptations, especially if patient has diabetes. ■ Consult healthcare provider for management of diabetes or atherosclerosis.

REVIEW Questions

1. The report of a culture sent on a client's leg wound states "contaminated specimen." Which nursing action most likely caused the outcome of this wound culture?
   1. Swab included pooled exudate.
   2. Sample was collected from the wound base.
   3. Inner ampule at the bottom of the tube was crushed.
   4. Specimen tube cap was placed upside down on a firm dry surface.

2. The nurse observes a new graduate nurse emptying a client's Jackson-Pratt drain. For which action should the nurse intervene?
   1. Inserts the plug into the emptying port
   2. Cleans the ends of the emptying port
   3. Secures the bulb above the wound level
   4. Compresses the bulb with the port open

3. The nurse prepares to care for a client's wound. Which approach should be used to clean this wound?
   1. Clean from the center outward.
   2. Use a swab for cleaning the entire wound.
   3. Use swabs moistened with hydrogen peroxide.
   4. Don clean gloves before picking up the forceps.

4. The nurse prepares to change a client's sterile wound dressing. Which approach should the nurse use if the old dressing is sticking to the site?
   1. Moisten the dressing with normal saline.
   2. Gently pull on the old dressing toward the wound.
   3. Pick the old dressing off with a pair of sterile forceps.
   4. Gently pull on the old dressing away from the wound.

5. A client is prescribed a wet-to-moist dressing for a leg wound. What technique should the nurse use when changing this dressing?
   1. Tape the entire surface of the dressing.
   2. Press moistened fluffed gauze lightly into wound depressions.
   3. Apply a clean dry 4 × 8 pad over the wet fluffed gauze.
   4. Apply fluffed gauze to the wound bed and saturate with sterile normal saline.

6. The nurse instructs a spouse on how to apply an elastic bandage to the client's ankle at home. Which observation should the nurse correct during the spouse's return demonstration of the skill?
   1. Anchors the bandage with two circular turns
   2. Carries the bandage above the joint and then below it
   3. Terminates the bandage at the joint with two circular turns
   4. Overlaps the previous turn by two thirds the width of the bandage

7. A client has a hydrocolloid dressing over the right greater trochanter area. Which observation indicates to the nurse that the dressing needs to be changed?
   1. Dressing changed 1 day ago
   2. Presence of a white blister under the dressing
   3. Silk tape applied to window frame the dressing
   4. Dressing located one third above the wound and two thirds below the wound

8. A client is prescribed a transparent dressing to be applied over skin tears. Which technique should the nurse use when changing this dressing?
   1. Apply skin prep over the wound area.
   2. "Walk" the dressing over the area, avoiding wrinkles.
   3. Trim the dressing to 1.3-cm (½-in.) margin of the wound.
   4. Cleanse the wound with half-strength hydrogen peroxide.

9. The nurse is caring for a client with a wound V.A.C. with black foam on the left heel. For what should the nurse assess when changing this client's dressing?
   1. Improvement in tunneling
   2. Healing of superficial wound
   3. Amount of wound contraction
   4. Boundary of a shallow chronic ulcer

10. A newly admitted client has a 3 cm × 5 cm reddened area over the coccyx. What should the nurse do **first** for this client?
    1. Massage the area.
    2. Clean the area with hot water.
    3. Position the client off this area.
    4. Raise the head of the bed to 45 degrees.

11. A client with an above-the-knee amputation is developing a hip contracture. What teaching should the nurse reinforce with this client?
    1. Press the stump into a padded surface.
    2. Lie prone and contract the gluteal muscles.
    3. Place the stump on a pillow when seated.
    4. Squeeze a pillow placed between the thighs.

12. While introducing a catheter into a client's wound to irrigate tunneled tracks, resistance is met. What action should the nurse take **first**?
    1. Flush the wound.
    2. Remove the catheter.
    3. Pour irrigation solution over the wound.
    4. Advance the catheter through the obstruction.

Note: For answers and rationales for the review questions, go to Appendix A or your Pearson MyLab Nursing and eText.

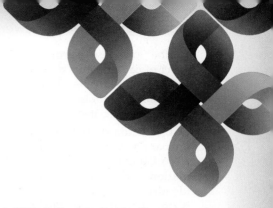

Appendix A
Answers to Review Questions

Chapter 1

1. **2.** The correct answer is option 2. When measuring abdominal circumference, the measurement should be recorded to the nearest 0.6 cm (¼ in.). The measuring tape should be wrapped around the abdomen at the level of the umbilicus, not the bladder. Measurements are recorded to the nearest 0.3 cm (⅛ in.) when measuring the head and chest circumference, not the abdomen. The nipple line is used as a landmark when measuring chest, not abdominal, circumference.

   QSEN Standard: I.B.3. Provide patient-centered care with sensitivity and respect for the diversity of human experience; ANA Standard: 1.1. Collects comprehensive data including but not limited to physical, functional psychosocial, emotional, mental, sexual, cultural, age-related, environmental, spiritual/transpersonal, and economic assessments in a systematic and ongoing process while honoring the uniqueness of the person; Cognitive Level: Applying; Client Need: Health Promotion and Maintenance; Nursing/Integrated Concepts: Nursing Process: Assessment

2. **4.** The first measurement determines the palpated systolic pressure; when taking the second measurement, the palpated systolic pressure is used as a guide for inflating the cuff. The second measurement is not done to validate the first; the first measurement locates the systolic blood pressure level, which is a palpated measurement. It is inaccurate to say that all blood pressure measurements need to be done twice. The question stem does not suggest that the child moved. The first measurement establishes the palpated systolic blood pressure level.

   QSEN Standard: I.B. 15. Communicate care provided and needed at each transition in care; ANA Standard: 1. 8. Uses appropriate evidence-based assessment techniques and instruments and tools; Cognitive Level: Applying; Client Need: Health Promotion and Maintenance; Nursing/Integrated Concepts: Nursing Process: Implementation

3. **1.** A sheet or towel should be used to block large amounts of light, such as from bilirubin lights, because the bright light sensed by the photodetector could alter the measurement. For a neonate, the sensor is applied to the forehead, not the great toe. The location of an adhesive sensor should be changed every 4 hours, not hourly. For a neonate, the high and low settings should be 95% and 80%, not 100% and 85%.

   QSEN Standard: III.B. 3. Base individualized care plan on patient values, clinical expertise, and evidence; ANA Standard: 5. 4. Utilizes technology to measure, record and retrieve patient data, implement the nursing process and enhance nursing practice; Cognitive Level: Applying; Client Need: Health Promotion and Maintenance; Nursing/Integrated Concepts: Nursing Process: Implementation

4. **1.** Increased bowel sounds may indicate a person that has recently eaten or has not eaten for a long time. This assessment finding is expected. Bowel sounds will be hypoactive or nearly absent if a paralytic ileus is developing. A late bowel obstruction would lead to hypoactive, not hyperactive, bowel sounds. Hyperactive bowel can be associated with an early bowel obstruction. However, the length of time since the client ate suggests the sounds are a normal finding.

   QSEN Standard: III.A. 1. Demonstrate knowledge of basic scientific methods and processes; ANA Standard: 5. 4. Utilizes technology to measure, record and retrieve patient data, implement the nursing process and enhance nursing practice; Cognitive Level: Analyzing; Client Need: Health Promotion and Maintenance; Nursing/Integrated Concepts: Nursing Process: Assessment

5. **2.** It is important to detect significant differences in visual acuity of the eyes of children under 5 years of age. When one eye has poorer vision than the other, the brain may decide to stop using the eye with poor vision, leading to further vision deterioration. Corrective lenses are required to enable the child to use both eyes and to preserve vision. A CT scan of the head is not indicated for this finding, which indicates reduced vision in the left eye. The child does not need medication to dilate the pupil. This will not improve the child's vision. The child does not need medication to constrict the pupil. This will not improve the child's vision.

   QSEN Standard: I. B. 10. Engage patients or designated surrogates in active partnerships that promote health, safety and well-being, and self-care management; ANA Standard: 4. 12. Includes strategies for health, wholeness, and growth from infancy through old age; Cognitive Level: Analyzing; Client Need: Physiological Integrity; Client Need Sub: Reduction of Risk Potential; Nursing/Integrated Concepts: Nursing Process: Planning

6. **2.** Carotid sinus massage can precipitate bradycardia, which would cause the continuous cardiac monitor to

trip the "low pulse" alarm. Palpitations are not an adverse effect of carotid sinus massage. Carotid sinus massage does not cause a pulse deficit. Displacement of the point of maximum impulse indicates an enlarged left ventricle. This is not associated with carotid sinus massage.

QSEN Standard: III. B. 3. Base individualized care plan on patient values, clinical expertise, and evidence; ANA Standard: 1. 9. Synthesizes available data, information and knowledge relevant to the situation to identify patterns and variances; Cognitive Level: Analyzing; Client Need: Physiological Integrity; Client Need Sub: Reduction of Risk Potential; Nursing/Integrated Concepts: Nursing Process: Assessment

7. **3.** Shoulder shrug is used to assess trapezius muscle function; a grade 3 indicates normal movement against gravity, but not against any resistance. Shoulder shrug is not used to assess grip strength; a grade 5 indicates normal full movement against gravity and against full resistance. Shoulder shrug is not used to assess deltoid muscle function; a grade 2 indicates full muscle movement against gravity, with support. Shoulder shrug is not used to assess sternocleidomastoid muscle function; a grade 4 indicates normal full movement against gravity and against minimal resistance.

QSEN Standard: III. A. 1. Demonstrate knowledge of basic scientific methods and processes; ANA Standard: 1. 10. Documents relevant data in a retrievable format; Cognitive Level: Analyzing; Client Need: Safe and Effective Care Environment; Client Need Sub: Management of Care; Nursing/Integrated Concepts: Nursing Process: Evaluation/Communication and Documentation

8. **3.** Hooking the index and third fingers over the clavicle lateral to the sternocleidomastoid muscle is a way to assess the supraclavicular nodes. The client's head needs to be bent forward to relax anterior neck and shoulders so clavicles drop. Bending the fingers around the sternocleidomastoid muscle is used to assess the deep cervical nodes, not supraclavicular nodes. Placing the fingertips under the mandible and pulling the skin and subcutaneous tissue laterally is used to assess the submental and submandibular nodes. Moving the fingertips in a forward circular motion against the sternocleidomastoid and trapezius muscles is used to assess the anterior and posterior cervical nodes.

QSEN Standard: III. B. 1. Participate effectively in appropriate data collection and other research activities; ANA Standard: 1. 8. Uses appropriate evidence-based assessment techniques and instruments and tools; Cognitive Level: Applying; Client Need: Health Promotion and Maintenance; Nursing/Integrated Concepts: Nursing Process: Assessment

9. **4.** Anesthesia is a term used to describe a loss of sensation, which is what the nurse assessed. Hypoesthesia is a term used to describe less than normal sensation, not lack of sensation. Paresthesia is a term used to describe an abnormal sensation such as burning, pain, or an electric shock. Hyperesthesia is a term used to describe more than normal sensation.

QSEN Standard: III. A. 1. Demonstrate knowledge of basic scientific methods and processes; ANA Standard: 1. 10. Documents relevant data in a retrievable format; Cognitive Level: Analyzing; Client Need: Safe and Effective Care Environment; Client Need Sub: Management of Care; Nursing/Integrated Concepts: Nursing Process: Evaluation/Communication and Documentation

10. **4.** Brown hyperpigmentation of the lower legs and edema of the ankles are manifestations of chronic venous insufficiency. Dusky red lower legs and cool skin are manifestations of arterial, not venous, insufficiency. Mild ankle edema and thin shiny skin are manifestations of arterial, not venous, insufficiency. Pallor with limb elevation is a manifestation of arterial, not venous, insufficiency. Muscle atrophy can have many causes; however, it is not associated with chronic venous insufficiency.

QSEN Standard: III. B. 3. Base individualized care plan on patient values, clinical expertise, and evidence; ANA Standard: 1. 9. Synthesizes available data, information, and knowledge relevant to the situation to identify patterns and variances; Cognitive Level: Analyzing; Client Need: Physiological Integrity; Client Need Sub: Physiological Adaptation; Nursing/Integrated Concepts: Nursing Process: Assessment

11. **3.** Low-pitched continuous snoring heard over the trachea describes gurgles. This sound is created by air passing through narrowed air passages as a result of secretions, swelling, or tumors. This sound should be reported to the healthcare provider. High-pitched, loud sounds heard over the trachea describes bronchial sounds. This is an expected finding and does not need to be reported. Soft-intensity, low-pitched sounds heard at the lung base describes vesicular sounds. This is an expected finding and does not need to be reported. Moderate-pitched blowing sounds heard between the scapulae describe bronchovesicular sounds. This is an expected finding and does not need to be reported.

QSEN Standard: II. B. 9. Communicate with team members, adapting own style of communicating to needs of the team and situation; ANA Standard: 2. 2. Validates the diagnoses or issues with the patient, family, and other healthcare providers when possible and appropriate; Cognitive Level: Analyzing; Client Need: Physiological Integrity; Client Need Sub: Reduction of Risk Potential; Nursing/Integrated Concepts: Nursing Process: Assessment/Communication and Documentation

12. **2.** Measurement of the client's brachial pulse is within the scope of practice of the UAP and can be safely delegated. The apical pulse is not a peripheral pulse, so this answer is incorrect. Measurement of the femoral pulse requires knowledge and expertise that would be beyond the scope of practice of the UAP. Measurement of the popliteal pulse requires knowledge and expertise that would be beyond the scope of practice of the UAP.

QSEN Standard: II. A. 2. Describe scopes of practice and roles of health care team members; ANA Standard:

12. 3. Oversees the nursing care given by others while retaining accountability for the quality of care given to the client; Cognitive Level: Applying; Client Need: Safe and Effective Care Environment; Client Need Sub: Management of Care; Nursing/Integrated Concepts: Nursing Process: Planning/Communication and Documentation

Chapter 2

1. **3.** A surgical bed is used for the client who is having surgery and will return to bed for the postoperative phase. When making a surgical bed, the linens are horizontally fan-folded to facilitate transfer of the client into the bed. Moving the pillow to the clean side of the bed is appropriate when making an occupied bed, but this client needs to have a surgical bed prepared. Fanfolding the dirty linen towards the center of the bed is appropriate when making an occupied bed, but this client needs to have a surgical bed prepared. Making a fold in the sheet that is perpendicular to the foot of the bed is a vertical toe pleat. This is appropriate for an occupied bed.

   QSEN Standard: I.B.3. Provide patient-centered care with sensitivity and respect for the diversity of human experience; ANA Standard: 4. 9. Integrates current scientific evidence, trends and research affecting care in planning; Cognitive Level: Applying; Client Need: Physiological Integrity; Client Need Sub: Basic Care and Comfort; Nursing/Integrated Concepts: Nursing Process: Assessment

2. **1.** Toe nails should be filed and not cut to prevent injury. Feet should be washed every day. Shoes or foot covering should be worn at all times. The client should not go barefoot. When the feet are cold, extra blankets and warm socks should be used. Heating pads or hot water bottles may burn the skin.

   QSEN Standard: I.B. 15. Communicate care provided and needed at each transition in care; ANA Standard: 5.B. 3. Seeks opportunities for feedback and evaluation of the effectiveness of the strategies used; Cognitive Level: Analyzing; Client Need: Physiological Integrity; Client Need Sub: Basic Care and Comfort; Nursing/Integrated Concepts: Nursing Process: Evaluation/Teaching/Learning

3. **3.** Beginning at about 18 months of age, the child's teeth should be brushed with a soft toothbrush moistened with water. The head of the bed should be lowered if providing mouth care to an unconscious client. The side-lying position is used when providing mouth care to an unconscious client. Using a syringe to apply mouthwash is appropriate if providing mouth care to an unconscious client.

   QSEN Standard: I.A. 1. Integrate understanding of multiple dimensions of patient centered care: physical comfort and emotional support; ANA Standard: 5. 6. Provides holistic care that addresses the needs of diverse populations across the lifespan; Cognitive Level: Applying

Client Need: Physiological Integrity; Client Need Sub: Basic Care and Comfort; Nursing/Integrated Concepts: Nursing Process: Implementation

4. **1.** To ensure that the right dose has been prepared, the nurse should have another nurse double-check the preparation of insulin because it is a Joint Commission high-alert drug. Digoxin is not a Joint Commission high-alert drug and does not need to be checked by another nurse. Penicillin is not a Joint Commission high-alert drug and does not need to be checked by another nurse. Furosemide is not a Joint Commission high-alert drug and does not need to be checked by another nurse.

   QSEN Standard: V.B. 2. Demonstrate effective use of strategies to reduce risk of harm to self or others; ANA Standard: 5. 14. Implements the plan of care in a safe and timely manner in accordance with the National Patient Safety Goals; Cognitive Level: Analyzing; Client Need: Physiological Integrity; Client Need Sub: Pharmacological/Parenteral Therapies; Nursing/Integrated Concepts: Nursing Process: Planning

5. **2.** Dose desired is required when calculating an oral medication dose. Quantity is needed to calculate a liquid or parenteral medication. Weight in pounds is required when calculating a medication for infants and children. Body surface area is required when calculating a medication for infants and children.

   QSEN Standard: V.C. 3. Value own role in preventing errors; ANA Standard: 5. 14. Implements the plan of care in a safe and timely manner in accordance with the National Patient Safety Goals; Cognitive Level: Applying; Client Need: Physiological Integrity; Client Need Sub: Pharmacological/Parenteral Therapies; Nursing/Integrated Concepts: Nursing Process: Planning

6. **2.** After withdrawing the required amount of medication from the second vial, the nurse should attach a new sterile needle to the syringe. Inserting the required amount of air into the first vial is done before withdrawing the medication from the second vial. Drawing the medication into two separate syringes is a step if following the alternative method to prepare medications from two vials. Pulling back the syringe plunger to allow space for the volume of second medication to be added is a step if following the alternative method to prepare medications from two vials.

   QSEN Standard: V.C. 3. Value own role in preventing errors; ANA Standard: 5. 14. Implements the plan of care in a safe and timely manner in accordance with the National Patient Safety Goals; Cognitive Level: Applying; Client Need: Physiological Integrity; Client Need Sub: Pharmacological/Parenteral Therapies; Nursing/Integrated Concepts: Nursing Process: Implementation

7. **3.** The nurse needs to first flush the tube with 15 mL of water. Then between medications one and two, 15 mL of water is used to flush the tube. Then between medications two and three, 15 mL of water is used to flush the tube. After the third medication is provided,

15 mL of water is used to flush the tube. This equals 60 mL of water.

QSEN Standard: I.B. 3. Provide patient-centered care with sensitivity and respect for the diversity of human experience; ANA Standard: 5. 14. Implements the plan of care in a safe and timely manner in accordance with the National Patient Safety Goals; Cognitive Level: Applying; Client Need: Physiological Integrity; Client Need Sub: Pharmacological/Parenteral Therapies; Nursing/Integrated Concepts: Nursing Process: Implementation

8. **2.** Further teaching is needed, because when using a metered-dose inhaler with a spacer, after delivering the medication, the breath should be held for at least 10 seconds (or as long as possible) before exhaling. When using a metered-dose inhaler with a spacer, breath should be inhaled for 3–5 seconds. When using a metered-dose inhaler with a spacer, the canister should be pressed down once. When using a metered-dose inhaler with a spacer, the breath should be exhaled slowly through pursed lips.

QSEN Standard: I.B. 15. Communicate care provided and needed at each transition in care; ANA Standard: 5.B. 3. Seeks opportunities for feedback and evaluation of the effectiveness of the strategies used; Cognitive Level: Analyzing; Client Need: Physiological Integrity; Client Need Sub: Pharmacological/Parenteral Therapies; Nursing/Integrated Concepts: Nursing Process: Evaluation/Teaching/Learning

9. **1.** When applying a transdermal patch medication, the nurse should select a skin area that is clean, dry, hairless, and intact. Alternate skin areas should be used with each dose of medication to prevent skin irritation. After removing the previous patch, the skin should be cleansed with soap and water and not alcohol. The medication should be applied to the paper and then the paper applied to the skin. The medication should not be directly applied to the skin and covered with the paper.

QSEN Standard: I.B. 3. Provide patient-centered care with sensitivity and respect for the diversity of human experience; ANA Standard: 5. 14. Implements the plan of care in a safe and timely manner in accordance with the National Patient Safety Goals; Cognitive Level: Applying; Client Need: Physiological Integrity; Client Need Sub: Pharmacological/Parenteral Therapies; Nursing/Integrated Concepts: Nursing Process: Implementation

10. **4.** One approach to address leak-back after a subcutaneous injection is to apply pressure to the injection site for 10 seconds with a gauze pad. Massaging will encourage more leak-back to occur. An additional dose of the medication is not administered. It is beyond the nurse's scope of practice to do so. A pressure dressing is not necessary.

QSEN Standard: I.B. 3. Provide patient-centered care with sensitivity and respect for the diversity of human experience; ANA Standard: 5. 14. Implements the plan

of care in a safe and timely manner in accordance with the National Patient Safety Goals; Cognitive Level: Applying; Client Need: Physiological Integrity; Client Need Sub: Pharmacological/Parenteral Therapies; Nursing/Integrated Concepts: Nursing Process: Implementation

11. **2.** When providing an injection using the Z-track approach, the syringe should be at a 90-degree angle. When providing an injection using the Z-track approach, the tissue should be displaced laterally. When providing an injection using the Z-track approach, pressure should be applied to the site with a gauze pad after the needle is removed. When providing an injection using the Z-track approach, the nurse should wait 10 seconds before removing the needle.

QSEN Standard: I.B. 3. Provide patient-centered care with sensitivity and respect for the diversity of human experience; ANA Standard: 5. 14. Implements the plan of care in a safe and timely manner in accordance with the National Patient Safety Goals; Cognitive Level: Analyzing; Client Need: Physiological Integrity; Client Need Sub: Pharmacological/Parenteral Therapies; Nursing/Integrated Concepts: Nursing Process: Evaluation

12. **2.** After the nurse injects the medication through the injection port, the needle and syringe should be removed. Aspirating for a blood return would be done prior to administering the intravenous push medication. After injecting the medication through the injection port, a saline flush is provided. The use of heparin for a flush will depend upon the medication provided and organizational policy. The injection port should be cleansed with an antiseptic swab before providing the medication and before providing a saline flush.

QSEN Standard: I.B. 3. Provide patient-centered care with sensitivity and respect for the diversity of human experience; ANA Standard: 5. 14. Implements the plan of care in a safe and timely manner in accordance with the National Patient Safety Goals; Cognitive Level: Applying; Client Need: Physiological Integrity; Client Need Sub: Pharmacological/Parenteral Therapies; Nursing/Integrated Concepts: Nursing Process: Implementation

Chapter 3

1. **2.** A small amount of lotion should be poured onto the palms of the hands and held for a minute to warm the solution and facilitate client comfort. The massage should begin at the sacral area. Pressure should be applied to the client's skin without breaking contact. Circular motions are to be used when massaging over the scapulae.

QSEN Standard: II.C. 5. Respect the unique attributes that members bring to a team, including variations in professional orientations and accountabilities; ANA Standard: 5. 11. Collaborates with healthcare providers from diverse backgrounds to implement the plan; Cognitive Level: Analyzing; Client Need: Physiological Integrity; Client Need Sub: Basic Care and Comfort; Nursing/Integrated Concepts: Nursing Process: Evaluation

2. **1.** Quiet, full, slow breathing that emphasizes prolonged exhalation elicits a parasympathetic response that is the opposite of the fight-or-flight response. The heart rate would be slower while still being within normal limits. A rapid respiratory rate at the conclusion of the exercise might indicate that the exercise was not effective in reducing tension and producing relaxation. An elevated blood pressure does not indicate relaxation. A pulse oximetry measurement of 88% on room air is dangerously low. The slow deep breaths performed during the progressive relaxation exercise have compromised the client's oxygenation status which could heighten anxiety and create air hunger.

QSEN Standard: I.A. 1. Integrate understanding of multiple dimensions of patient centered care: physical comfort and emotional support; ANA Standard: 6. 3. Evaluates, in partnership with the person, the effectiveness of the planned strategies in relation to the person's responses and the attainment of the expected outcomes; Cognitive Level: Analyzing; Client Need: Physiological Integrity; Client Need Sub: Basic Care and Comfort; Nursing/Integrated Concepts: Nursing Process: Evaluation

3. **3.** A TENS unit stimulates the skin with a mild electric current and relieves pain by blocking pain impulses to the brain. Vibration, not TENS, is an electrical form of a massage. Acupressure is based on an ancient method that uses specific points located on meridians throughout the body. Biofeedback uses an electronic monitoring device that provides information about behavior to control internal processes.

QSEN Standard: I.A. 1. Integrate understanding of multiple dimensions of patient centered care: physical comfort and emotional support; ANA Standard: 5. 5. Utilizes evidence-based interventions and treatments specific to the diagnosis or problem; Cognitive Level: Applying; Client Need: Physiological Integrity; Client Need Sub: Basic Care and Comfort; Nursing/Integrated Concepts: Nursing Process: Implementation/Teaching/Learning

4. **4.** Since the client is complaining of pain, the first action should be to assess when the client delivered the last dose through the pump. The dose volume limit is prescribed by the healthcare provider and cannot be changed without an appropriate order. The UAP must not administer a dose (push the button) for the client. Assessing for volume of medication remaining in the pump can be done after the client is assessed.

QSEN Standard: I.A. 1. Integrate understanding of multiple dimensions of patient centered care: physical comfort and emotional support; ANA Standard: 1. 8. Uses appropriate evidence-based assessment techniques and instruments and tools; Cognitive Level: Applying; Client Need: Physiological Integrity; Client Need Sub: Pharmacological and Parenteral Therapies; Nursing/Integrated Concepts: Nursing Process: Assessment

5. **4.** Since the pack is only applied for 10 minutes and the client is experiencing stinging, the pack does not need to be removed. The nurse should explain that stinging is expected and encourage the client to keep the pack on the site. The client will experience four stages of cold progression: cold, stinging, burning, and then numbness. Therapy should be discontinued when the client experiences numbness. A protective wrap should remain around the ice pack to protect the client's skin. It is inaccurate to say that the client is refusing the treatment.

QSEN Standard: I.A. 1. Integrate understanding of multiple dimensions of patient centered care: physical comfort and emotional support; ANA Standard: 5. 5. Utilizes evidence-based interventions and treatments specific to the diagnosis or problem; Cognitive Level: Applying; Client Need: Physiological Integrity; Client Need Sub: Basic Care and Comfort; Nursing/Integrated Concepts: Nursing Process: Implementation

6. **2.** The heating pad should be kept in place for only the designated time, which is usually 30 minutes, to avoid the rebound phenomenon. Since the client used the heating pad for an hour, this could be the reason why more pain is experienced. The heating pad cover should be used and is intact. This would not cause the area to be more painful. Using the pad at the prescribed temperature would not cause the area to be more painful. Gauze ties should be used to hold the pad in place; they would not cause the area to be more painful.

QSEN Standard: I.A. 1. Integrate understanding of multiple dimensions of patient centered care: physical comfort and emotional support; ANA Standard: 6. 3. Evaluates, in partnership with the person, the effectiveness of the planned strategies in relation to the person's responses and the attainment of the expected outcomes; Cognitive Level: Analyzing; Client Need: Physiological Integrity; Client Need Sub: Basic Care and Comfort; Nursing/Integrated Concepts: Nursing Process: Evaluation

7. **3.** When using a radiant warmer, the skin probe should be applied to an area of fatty tissue and not an area of bony tissue. The probe is over the elbow, which is bony. The probe should be moved to an area over the upper thigh or abdomen. When using a radiant warmer, the bed should be set to skin control mode. When using a radiant warmer, the gel patch should be applied over the skin probe. When using a radiant warmer, the temperature probe should be plugged into the bed.

QSEN Standard: I.A. 1. Integrate understanding of multiple dimensions of patient centered care: physical comfort and emotional support; ANA Standard: 6. 3. Evaluates, in partnership with the person, the effectiveness of the planned strategies in relation to the person's responses and the attainment of the expected outcomes; Cognitive Level: Analyzing; Client Need: Physiological Integrity; Client Need Sub: Basic Care and Comfort; Nursing/Integrated Concepts: Nursing Process: Evaluation

8. **2.** Cyanosis indicates slowing of the circulation. Because of this, pain medication should be administered through the intravenous route instead of the subcutaneous or intramuscular routes. Relaxation of the jaw causes the mouth to be open and indicates weakening of muscles. This would not influence the route for administering pain medication. Abdominal distention is an indication of weakening muscles; however, this condition would not influence the route for administering pain medication. Mouth breathing causes dry oral mucous membranes; however, this condition would not influence the route to administer pain medication.

QSEN Standard: I.A. 1. Integrate understanding of multiple dimensions of patient centered care: physical comfort and emotional support; ANA Standard: 1. 8. Uses appropriate evidence-based assessment techniques and instruments and tools; Cognitive Level: Applying; Client Need: Physiological Integrity; Client Need Sub: Pharmacological and Parenteral Therapies; Nursing/Integrated Concepts: Nursing Process: Assessment

Chapter 4

1. **2.** If the client has had a hysterectomy, MALE MODE should be selected on the scanner in order to obtain an accurate reading. The client's pregnancy history does not impact the setting to use for a bladder scan. Lithotripsy does not affect the setting to use for a bladder scan. History of urinary tract infections does not affect the setting to use for a bladder scan.

QSEN Standard: III.A. 2. Describe EBP to include the components of research evidence, clinical expertise, and patient/family values; ANA Standard: 1. 8. Uses appropriate evidence-based assessment techniques and instruments and tools; Cognitive Level: Applying; Client Need: Physiological Integrity; Client Need Sub: Reduction of Risk Potential; Nursing/Integrated Concepts: Nursing Process: Assessment

2. **4.** Clamping the drainage tubing below the port has to be done first to ensure that a fresh sample of urine will be obtained. A specimen for a urine culture is not obtained from the collection bag. The urine in the bag could be contaminated. Swabbing the resealing port would occur before inserting a needle through the port to obtain the specimen, but it is not the first action. Inserting the needle at a 45-degree angle would be done after swabbing the port; it is not the first action.

QSEN Standard: III.A. 2. Describe EBP to include the components of research evidence, clinical expertise, and patient/family values; ANA Standard: 5. 5. Utilizes evidence-based interventions and treatments specific to the diagnosis or problem; Cognitive Level: Applying; Client Need: Physiological Integrity; Client Need Sub: Reduction of Risk Potential; Nursing/Integrated Concepts: Nursing Process: Implementation

3. **2.** Immediately report bright red urine outflow. Because this could indicate an arterial bleed, it must be reported immediately. Dark red (not bright red) drainage contains tissue or blood clots; increasing the drip rate will clear the drainage and flush out debris and clots. Raising the height of the pole with the irrigation fluid will increase the rate of flow, but it will not address the change in drainage or the presence of bright red blood in the outflow. Hand-flushing the bladder requires a healthcare provider's order. Breaking the integrity of the closed urinary drainage system could increase the client's risk of infection.

QSEN Standard: III.A. 2. Describe EBP to include the components of research evidence, clinical expertise, and patient/family values; ANA Standard: 5. 5. Utilizes evidence-based interventions and treatments specific to the diagnosis or problem; Cognitive Level: Applying; Client Need: Physiological Integrity; Client Need Sub: Reduction of Risk Potential; Nursing/Integrated Concepts: Nursing Process: Implementation

4. **3.** The opening on the skin barrier should not be more than 0.3 cm (1/8 in.) larger than the stoma. This allows space for the stoma to expand while minimizing the risk of urine contacting the skin around the stoma. Cutting the skin barrier opening larger than the area of excoriation would encourage urine to collect on the skin around the stoma. This would exacerbate the area already excoriated. Skin prep liquid should not be used on irritated skin. A gauze dressing will absorb any urine leaking from around the stoma. This dressing would be damp and could contribute to skin excoriation.

QSEN Standard: I.A. 1. Integrate understanding of multiple dimensions of patient centered care: physical comfort and emotional support; ANA Standard: 5. 5. Utilizes evidence-based interventions and treatments specific to the diagnosis or problem; Cognitive Level: Applying; Client Need: Physiological Integrity; Client Need Sub: Reduction of Risk Potential; Nursing/Integrated Concepts: Nursing Process: Implementation

5. **3.** The irrigation solution should be no higher than 46 cm (18 in.) above the stoma. The shower curtain rod is much higher than the recommended height. The solution should be instilled over 5 to 10 minutes. The irrigation cone should be held firmly against the stoma. The irrigation container should be filled with 1000 mL of warm tap water.

QSEN Standard: I.B. 1. Elicit patient values, preferences, and expressed needs as part of clinical interview, implementation of care plan, and evaluation of care; ANA Standard: 5b. 3. Seeks opportunities for feedback and evaluation of the effectiveness of the strategies used; Cognitive Level: Analyzing; Client Need: Physiological Integrity; Client Need Sub: Reduction of Risk Potential; Nursing/Integrated Concepts: Nursing Process: Evaluation/Teaching/Learning

6. **1.** Because older adults may be more susceptible to fluid and electrolyte imbalances, tapwater enemas should be used with caution. Since the client is to receive the enemas "until clear," a large number of

enemas might be required. It would be wise for the nurse to question the use of tap water for these enemas. The client should be permitted to have a dinner meal prior to having the enemas until clear. Waiting an hour between each enema permits the solution and enema work to clear the bowel. The enemas should be provided the evening before the test. Waiting until the morning of the test might not be sufficient time to clear the bowel.

QSEN Standard: V.B. 8. Use national patient safety resources for own professional development and to focus attention on safety in care settings; ANA Standard: 11.13. Questions the rationale supporting routine approaches to care processes and decisions when they do not appear to be in the best interest of the patient; Cognitive Level: Applying; Client Need: Safe and Effective Care Environment; Client Need Sub: Safety and Infection Control; Nursing/Integrated Concepts: Nursing Process: Assessment/Communication and Documentation

7. **3.** The presence of a white gelatin-like material indicates shredding of the peritoneal lining's old skin. This material could indicate potential peritonitis and should cause the nurse to be concerned. The drainage bag should be placed on a stool below the level of the client's abdomen. It may take up to 10 minutes for the solution to drain from the abdomen. The drainage bag should be removed and the tubing capped after draining is completed.

QSEN Standard: III.A. 1. Demonstrate knowledge of basic scientific methods and processes; ANA Standard: 6. 7. Actively participates in assessing and assuring the responsible and appropriate use of interventions in order to minimize unwarranted or unwanted treatment and patient suffering; Cognitive Level: Analyzing; Client Need: Physiological Integrity; Client Need Sub: Reduction of Risk Potential; Nursing/Integrated Concepts: Nursing Process: Evaluation

8. **3.** If the hand of the arm with the arteriovenous fistula feels cold and numb, the nurse should first assess for a thrill and bruit. The healthcare provider should be notified after assessment of the fistula occurs. The healthcare provider will decide which intervention is required. This may include a radiologic procedure. The arm with the fistula should not be constricted in any way for any procedures such as venipuncture, intravenous fluid infusions, or blood pressures. A tourniquet could cause further damage to the arteriovenous fistula.

QSEN Standard: III.A. 1. Demonstrate knowledge of basic scientific methods and processes; ANA Standard: 6. 7. Actively participates in assessing and assuring the responsible and appropriate use of interventions in order to minimize unwarranted or unwanted treatment and patient suffering; Cognitive Level: Applying; Client Need: Physiological Integrity; Client Need Sub: Reduction of Risk Potential; Nursing/Integrated Concepts: Nursing Process: Implementation

Chapter 5

1. **1.** Hourly urine output of less than 0.5–1 mL/kg/hr or 24-hour urine output of less than 500 mL can indicate dehydration for an average-size healthy adult. This 55-kg (121-lb) client's urine output needs to be more than 220–440 mL over 8 hr. A urine output of 110 mL over 8 hours means the client has been producing urine at the rate of 0.25 mL/kg/hr. This urine output should be reported. The 132-lb client is producing adequate urine at the rate of 1 mL/hr (132 lb/2.2 × 1 mL = 60 mL/hr × 8 hr = 480 mL). The 143-lb client is producing adequate urine at the rate of 1.25 mL per hour (143 lb/2.2 × 1.5 mL = 81.25 mL/hr × 8 hr = 650 mL). The 154-lb client is producing adequate urine at the rate of 1.75 mL/hr (154 lbs/2.2 × 2 mL = 122.5 mL × 8 hr = 980 mL).

QSEN Standard: I.A. 1. Integrate understanding of multiple dimensions of patient centered care: information, communication, and education; ANA Standard: 1. 9. Synthesizes available data, information, and knowledge relevant to the situation to identify patterns and variances; Cognitive Level: Analyzing; Client Need: Physiological Integrity; Client Need Sub: Reduction of Risk Potential; Nursing/Integrated Concepts: Nursing Process: Assessment

2. **2.** Although there is a discrepancy in the catheter length, the site needs to cleansed and protected with a sterile dressing first. Adjusting the catheter location is beyond the nurse's scope of practice and should not be done. After the dressing change is complete, the nurse would notify the healthcare professional to report the change in catheter length. Documentation should occur last and should include the current catheter length measurement.

QSEN Standard: V.B. 2. Demonstrate effective use of strategies to reduce risk of harm to self or others; ANA Standard: 5. 14. Implements the plan of care in a safe and timely manner in accordance with the National Patient Safety Goals; Cognitive Level: Applying; Client Need: Physiological Integrity; Client Need Sub: Reduction of Risk Potential; Nursing/Integrated Concepts: Nursing Process: Implementation

3. **1.** To minimize pressure on the catheter during injection, never use less than a 10-mL syringe for central lines. The central venous catheter (CVC) and tubing has a volume of 1–3 mL. About 5 mL of solution in a 10-mL syringe should be used to flush the catheter thoroughly. Clamping the catheter before removing the syringe is a correct action to prevent aspiration of blood into the lumen and decrease risk of catheter occlusion. Clean gloves should be applied after performing hand hygiene. The access port should be cleansed before attaching a syringe to flush the catheter.

QSEN Standard: V.B. 2. Demonstrate effective use of strategies to reduce risk of harm to self or others; ANA Standard: 5. 14. Implements the plan of care in a safe and timely manner in accordance with the National Patient Safety Goals; Cognitive Level: Analyzing; Client

Need: Physiological Integrity; Client Need Sub: Pharmacological and Parenteral Therapies; Nursing/Integrated Concepts: Nursing Process: Evaluation

4. **4.** If a capped lumen used for medication has been flushed with heparin solution, aspirate and discard or flush the line with 5 mL of normal saline according to facility protocol before giving the medication because many medications are incompatible with heparin. Lowering the head of the bed would be appropriate if an air embolism is suspected. Changing the cap on the port would be completed during routine central venous catheter care. If facility policy dictates, heparin flush would be provided after the medication is administered.

QSEN Standard: V.B. 2. Demonstrate effective use of strategies to reduce risk of harm to self or others; ANA Standard: 5. 14. Implements the plan of care in a safe and timely manner in accordance with the National Patient Safety Goals; Cognitive Level: Applying; Client Need: Physiological Integrity; Client Need Sub: Pharmacological and Parenteral Therapies; Nursing/Integrated Concepts: Nursing Process: Implementation

5. **4.** The blood should be placed in a biohazard waste container for appropriate removal and incineration. Blood should not be placed with regular trash. A syringe full of blood should not be placed in a sharps container. The initial blood specimen may be diluted with saline and heparin from previous flushes and should be discarded.

QSEN Standard: III.A. 1. Demonstrate knowledge of basic scientific methods and processes; ANA Standard: 5. 14. Implements the plan of care in a safe and timely manner in accordance with the National Patient Safety Goals; Cognitive Level: Applying; Client Need: Safe and Effective Care Environment; Client Need Sub: Safety and Infection Control; Nursing/Integrated Concepts: Nursing Process: Implementation

6. **2.** Typical signs and symptoms of infiltration include a damp dressing. At the first sign of phlebitis or infiltration of an older client's intravenous infusion, remove the IV and restart it in a new site. The first thing to do when removing the intravenous catheter is to clamp the infusion tubing. The dressing would be removed after the intravenous infusion tubing is clamped and gloves are applied. Lowering the infusion container is a technique to check for a blood return. Since the older client is demonstrating signs of infiltration, time should not be taken to assess for a blood return. The catheter should be removed. Applying sterile gauze would occur after the intravenous infusion tubing is clamped, gloves applied, and the wet dressing removed.

QSEN Standard: I.B. 3. Provide patient-centered care with sensitivity and respect for the diversity of human experience; ANA Standard: 5. 14. Implements the plan of care in a safe and timely manner in accordance with the National Patient Safety Goals; Cognitive Level: Applying; Client Need: Safe and Effective Care

Environment; Client Need Sub: Safety and Infection Control; Nursing/Integrated Concepts: Nursing Process: Implementation

7. **42 gtts/min.** First, determine the amount of fluid the client should receive per hour by dividing the total amount of fluid by 24 hours or 3000 mL/24 = 125 mL/hr. Then, use the equation mL/hr × drop factor/60 min to determine gtt/min or 125 mL/hr × 20 gtts/mL/60 min = 41.6 or 42 gtts/min.

QSEN Standard: III.A. 1. Demonstrate knowledge of basic scientific methods and processes; ANA Standard: 5. 14. Implements the plan of care in a safe and timely manner in accordance with the National Patient Safety Goals; Cognitive Level: Applying; Client Need: Physiological Integrity; Client Need Sub: Pharmacological and Parenteral Therapies; Nursing/Integrated Concepts: Nursing Process: Implementation

8. **2.** The larger the catheter diameter is, the faster the flow rate. Cold fluids drip more slowly than warm fluids. The longer the catheter is, the slower the flow rate is because of resistance. The higher the bag is above the insertion site, the faster the infusion. Placing the bag at the level of the side rail will slow the infusion rate.

QSEN Standard: III.A. 1. Demonstrate knowledge of basic scientific methods and processes; ANA Standard: 5. 14. Implements the plan of care in a safe and timely manner in accordance with the National Patient Safety Goals; Cognitive Level: Applying; Client Need: Physiological Integrity; Client Need Sub: Pharmacological and Parenteral Therapies; Nursing/Integrated Concepts: Nursing Process: Implementation

9. **2.** Although the Centers for Disease Control and Prevention (CDC) has not established a recommendation for hang time, common hang time is 24 hours. The fluid and tubing should be changed at 1400 hours the next day; 0800 hours would be too soon; 2200 hours would be too soon; 2400 hours would be too soon.

QSEN Standard: III.A. 1. Demonstrate knowledge of basic scientific methods and processes; ANA Standard: 5. 14. Implements the plan of care in a safe and timely manner in accordance with the National Patient Safety Goals; Cognitive Level: Applying; Client Need: Physiological Integrity; Client Need Sub: Pharmacological and Parenteral Therapies; Nursing/Integrated Concepts: Nursing Process: Implementation

10. **2.** The clinical signs of phlebitis include burning pain along the course of the vein. If phlebitis is detected, discontinue the infusion. Applying a tourniquet will not reduce the pain or burning associated with phlebitis. Repositioning the catheter will not help reduce phlebitis. Lowering the infusion bag checks for a blood return; however, it will not help reduce phlebitis.

QSEN Standard: III.A. 1. Demonstrate knowledge of basic scientific methods and processes; ANA Standard: 5. 14. Implements the plan of care in a safe and timely manner in accordance with the National Patient Safety Goals; Cognitive Level: Applying; Client Need: Safe and Effective Care Environment; Client Need Sub: Safety and Infection Control; Nursing/Integrated Concepts: Nursing Process: Implementation

11. **2.** Typical signs and symptoms of infiltration are erythema and swelling. The catheter needs to be discontinued and another one inserted. Because the pump does not depend on gravity pressure, it can be placed at any level. Eye level is convenient for checking its functioning. Flushing a catheter before starting the infusion depends upon whether the catheter has been locked or newly inserted. Infusion tubing should be coiled to prevent it from catching on bedding or clothing. However, this is not a reason to discontinue the pump and remove the intravenous catheter.

QSEN Standard: III.A. 1. Demonstrate knowledge of basic scientific methods and processes; ANA Standard: 5. 14. Implements the plan of care in a safe and timely manner in accordance with the National Patient Safety Goals; Cognitive Level: Analyzing; Client Need: Safe and Effective Care Environment; Client Need Sub: Safety and Infection Control; Nursing/Integrated Concepts: Nursing Process: Assessment

12. **3.** A rolled towel or blanket between the shoulder blades helps extend the client's neck and upper chest and improves access to the subclavian vein. The Trendelenburg, not a left side-lying, position is used because it prevents air embolism and helps distend subclavian veins. Turning the client's head to the left, away from the side of venipuncture, prevents contamination. As the healthcare provider inserts the catheter, the client should perform the Valsalva maneuver, not deep breathe and cough. The Valsalva maneuver helps prevent the formation of an air embolism.

QSEN Standard: III.A. 1. Demonstrate knowledge of basic scientific methods and processes; ANA Standard: 5. 14. Implements the plan of care in a safe and timely manner in accordance with the National Patient Safety Goals; Cognitive Level: Applying; Client Need: Safe and Effective Care Environment; Client Need Sub: Safety and Infection Control; Nursing/Integrated Concepts: Nursing Process: Implementation

13. **1.** After using swabs of antimicrobial solution to cleanse the site, allow 30 seconds for the solution to dry. The action does not take effect until the solution is dry. The securement device is placed after the antimicrobial solution is dry. The dressing is applied after the antimicrobial solution dries and the securement device is in place. The insertion site is assessed after the old dressing is removed and prior to cleansing with antimicrobial swabs.

QSEN Standard: III.A. 1. Demonstrate knowledge of basic scientific methods and processes; ANA Standard: 5. 14. Implements the plan of care in a safe and timely manner in accordance with the National Patient Safety Goals; Cognitive Level: Applying; Client Need: Safe and Effective Care Environment; Client Need Sub: Safety and Infection Control; Nursing/Integrated Concepts: Nursing Process: Implementation

Chapter 6

1. **3.** For effective cleaning, hands soiled with organic matter require soap or detergents that contain antiseptic and water. The gloves do not need to be rinsed before removing them. An antiseptic gel can be used if there is no threat of organic material being on the hands, but since the nurse was removing feces, there is a possibility of organic material being on or near the hands. A waterless agent does not need to be applied after the hands are washed correctly with soap and water.

QSEN Standard: V. B. 2. Demonstrate effective use of strategies to reduce risk of harm to self or others; ANA Standard: 17. 1. Works to reduce or eliminate environmental health risks in the healthcare setting; Cognitive Level: Applying; Client Need: Safe and Effective Care Environment; Client Need Sub: Safety and Infection Control; Nursing/Integrated Concepts: Nursing Process: Implementation

2. **2.** Client care items such as a stethoscope should not be used with a client in enteric contact precautions and then used with other clients. It needs to be properly cleaned and disinfected before reuse. For the client in enteric contact precautions, healthcare personnel is correct to perform soap-and-water hand washing, not just an alcohol-based hand rub, because alcohol is not effective in removing the pathogens from the hands. The UAP is correct to apply and remove appropriate isolation attire each time the isolation room is entered or exited. The UAP is expected to dispose of used PPE items in a red biohazard waste plastic bag after completing care.

QSEN Standard: V. B. 2. Demonstrate effective use of strategies to reduce risk of harm to self or others; ANA Standard: 17. 1. Works to reduce or eliminate environmental health risks in the healthcare setting; Cognitive Level: Analyzing; Client Need: Safe and Effective Care Environment; Client Need Sub: Safety and Infection Control; Nursing/Integrated Concepts: Nursing Process: Assessment

3. **1.** A client with bacterial meningitis will be in droplet precautions. The face mask should be removed after the gown is removed. The gloves are removed before removing the gown. The mask should not be removed before the gown is removed. The mask should not be removed before the gloves are removed.

QSEN Standard: V. B. 2. Demonstrate effective use of strategies to reduce risk of harm to self or others; ANA Standard: 17. 1. Works to reduce or eliminate environmental health risks in the healthcare setting; Cognitive Level: Applying; Client Need: Safe and Effective Care Environment; Client Need Sub: Safety and Infection Control; Nursing/Integrated Concepts: Nursing Process: Implementation

4. **2.** Linen that is soiled with blood or body fluids should be washed separately with very hot water, detergent, and bleach. Linen that is soiled with blood or body fluids should be washed with very hot, not cool, water.

Soaking linen soiled with blood or body fluids in a half-strength solution of hydrogen peroxide before washing is not the recommended method of cleaning. Linen that is soiled with blood or body fluids should be washed separately.

QSEN Standard: V. B. 2. Demonstrate effective use of strategies to reduce risk of harm to self or others; ANA Standard: 17. 1. Works to reduce or eliminate environmental health risks in the healthcare setting; Cognitive Level: Applying; Client Need: Safe and Effective Care Environment; Client Need Sub: Safety and Infection Control; Nursing/Integrated Concepts: Nursing Process: Implementation/Teaching/Learning

5. **3.** Dispose of body wastes by flushing them down the toilet; wound drainage is a body waste. Used gloves should be placed in a plastic biohazard waste bag. The soiled dressing should be placed in a plastic biohazard waste bag. Since the syringe was used for irrigation, it most likely did not have a needle attached; this syringe can be placed in a plastic biohazard waste bag.

QSEN Standard: V. B. 2. Demonstrate effective use of strategies to reduce risk of harm to self or others; ANA Standard: 17. 1. Works to reduce or eliminate environmental health risks in the healthcare setting; Cognitive Level: Applying; Client Need: Safe and Effective Care Environment; Client Need Sub: Safety and Infection Control; Nursing/Integrated Concepts: Nursing Process: Implementation

6. **1.** The specimen should be placed in a clean plastic biohazard bag outside of the client's room; a clear plastic bag is used so that laboratory personnel can see the specimen easily. The container does not need to be cleansed with an antiseptic solution. The specimen container should be labeled with the client's name and personal identification information before taking it into the client's room to collect the specimen. The specimen container should be labeled with "isolation" before taking it into the client's room to collect the specimen.

QSEN Standard: V. B. 2. Demonstrate effective use of strategies to reduce risk of harm to self or others; ANA Standard: 17. 1. Works to reduce or eliminate environmental health risks in the healthcare setting; Cognitive Level: Applying; Client Need: Safe and Effective Care Environment; Client Need Sub: Safety and Infection Control; Nursing/Integrated Concepts: Nursing Process: Implementation

7. **3.** If the transportation vehicle is soiled, it should be wiped down with an antimicrobial solution. Antimicrobial gel is used to cleanse the hands, not equipment. The soiled linen should be placed in a biohazard receptacle inside in the client's room, not outside. Soap and water are not used to cleanse a transportation vehicle.

QSEN Standard: V. B. 2. Demonstrate effective use of strategies to reduce risk of harm to self or others; ANA Standard: 17. 1. Works to reduce or eliminate environmental health risks in the healthcare setting; Cognitive

Level: Applying; Client Need: Safe and Effective Care Environment; Client Need Sub: Safety and Infection Control; Nursing/Integrated Concepts: Nursing Process: Implementation

8. **1.** A new pair of gloves should be donned after hand hygiene when anticipating contact with blood or another body fluid. The hands are not washed with the gloves on. Because drainage from the wounds can be on the linen or other items around the client's bed, gloves should be worn whether or not the wounds are touched. The nurse most likely will not touch a seeping wound when providing the client with oral pain medication.

QSEN Standard: V. B. 2. Demonstrate effective use of strategies to reduce risk of harm to self or others; ANA Standard: 17. 1. Works to reduce or eliminate environmental health risks in the healthcare setting; Cognitive Level: Applying; Client Need: Safe and Effective Care Environment; Client Need Sub: Safety and Infection Control; Nursing/Integrated Concepts: Nursing Process: Implementation

Chapter 7

1. **1.** Abnormal findings must be validated and interpreted by the nurse. This is the first thing that the nurse should do. Assessment of neurologic sensory and motor functions is not delegated to the UAP; the nurse should not document another caregiver's finding. Notification to the healthcare provider may need to be done after the nurse completes a reassessment of the client and validates the UAP's finding. The nurse has no way of knowing if the client is sleeping; the client needs to be assessed by the nurse to validate what the UAP reported.

QSEN Standard: II. B. 4. Function competently within own scope of practice as a member of the health care team; ANA Standard: 1. 7. Prioritizes data collection activities based on the patient's immediate condition, or anticipated needs of the patient or situation; Cognitive Level: Applying; Client Need: Physiological Integrity; Client Need Sub: Reduction of Risk Potential; Nursing/Integrated Concepts: Nursing Process: Assessment

2. **2.** The Glasgow Coma Scale cannot be used to assess neurologic signs in clients who are unable to respond orally because of sedation; diazepam causes sedation; the assessment using this scale can be delayed until the client regains consciousness. Asking for something to eat may indicate that the client can talk spontaneously; however, eye opening and motor response can still be assessed. The Glasgow Coma Scale can be used for a client who is reporting pain. The client can be assessed after the telephone call is made.

QSEN Standard: II. B. 4. Function competently within own scope of practice as a member of the health care team; ANA Standard: 1. 7. Prioritizes data collection activities based on the patient's immediate condition, or anticipated needs of the patient or situation;

Cognitive Level: Analyzing; Client Need: Physiological Integrity; Client Need Sub: Reduction of Risk Potential; Nursing/Integrated Concepts: Nursing Process: Assessment

3. **3.** Balancing the intracranial pressure (ICP) transducer to zero for calibration when the client's position changes ensures the accuracy of pressure readings and waveforms by the transducer system. The head of the bed should be elevated 15–30 degrees, or according to healthcare provider's order, to prevent compression of blood vessels in the neck and obstruction of venous blood flow, which will cause ICP to increase. Current blood pressure is needed to calculate cerebral perfusion pressure (CPP) but not ICP. The transducer system should be placed and maintained at the level of the foramen of Monro or the line between the top of the ear and the outer canthus of the eye; the midaxillary line is used as a landmark to assess central venous pressure.

QSEN Standard: II. B. 4. Function competently within own scope of practice as a member of the health care team; ANA Standard: 1. 8. Uses appropriate evidence-based assessment techniques and instruments and tools; Cognitive Level: Applying; Client Need: Physiological Integrity; Client Need Sub: Reduction of Risk Potential; Nursing/Integrated Concepts: Nursing Process: Assessment

4. **3.** Cerebral perfusion pressure (CPP) is calculated by subtracting the intracranial pressure (ICP) from the mean arterial pressure (MAP). MAP is calculated by $[(2 \times \text{diastolic}) + \text{systolic}]/3$. This client's MAP is $[(2 \times 90) + 178/3] = [180 + 178/3] = 358/3 = 119.3$. The CPP is calculated by the MAP $-$ ICP, or $119.3 - 25 = 94.3$. This pressure would be 94 mmHg rounded to the nearest whole number, 94. All other options are incorrect.

QSEN Standard: II. B. 4. Function competently within own scope of practice as a member of the health care team; ANA Standard: 1. 8. Uses appropriate evidence-based assessment techniques and instruments and tools; Cognitive Level: Applying; Client Need: Physiological Integrity; Client Need Sub: Reduction of Risk Potential; Nursing/Integrated Concepts: Nursing Process: Assessment

5. **4.** Manifestations of an intracranial pressure (ICP) between 20–50 mmHg include varying respiratory patterns. Readings of 5, 10, and 19 mmHg are normal ICP pressure measurements.

QSEN Standard: II. B. 4. Function competently within own scope of practice as a member of the health care team; ANA Standard: 1. 8. Uses appropriate evidence-based assessment techniques and instruments and tools; Cognitive Level: Applying; Client Need: Physiological Integrity; Client Need Sub: Reduction of Risk Potential; Nursing/Integrated Concepts: Nursing Process: Planning

6. **3.** A high-pitched catlike cry is an additional sign of increased intracranial pressure (ICP) in an infant. Thumb sucking is an expected newborn behavior.

Newborns have a more rapid respiratory rate than adults. Opened eyes and looking at the mother is an expected newborn behavior.

QSEN Standard: I. B. 4. Assess presence and extent of pain and suffering; ANA Standard: 1. 7. Prioritizes data collection activities based on the patient's immediate condition, or anticipated needs of the patient or situation; Cognitive Level: Applying; Client Need: Physiological Integrity; Client Need Sub: Reduction of Risk Potential; Nursing/Integrated Concepts: Nursing Process: Assessment

7. **2.** If leaking after a lumbar puncture persists, the healthcare provider may prescribe that the client be placed in the Trendelenburg position to prevent a headache. A pressure dressing will not stop the flow of cerebral spinal fluid after a lumbar puncture. The semi-Fowler position may encourage the development of a headache after a lumbar puncture. Intravenous fluid replacement is not indicated for leaking from a lumbar puncture site.

QSEN Standard: I. A. 1. Integrate understanding of multiple dimensions of patient centered care: coordination and integration of care; ANA Standard: 2. 4. Identifies actual or potential risks to the patient's health and safety or barriers to health, which may include but are not limited to interpersonal, systematic, or environmental circumstances; Cognitive Level: Applying; Client Need: Physiological Integrity; Client Need Sub: Reduction of Risk Potential; Nursing/Integrated Concepts: Nursing Process: Planning

8. **4.** The fetal position is used during an adult lumbar puncture because in this position, the back is arched, increasing the spaces between the vertebrae so that the spinal needle can be inserted readily. Spreading the vertebrae apart prior to a lumbar puncture eases the placement of the needle; however, the client may still experience pain when the needle is inserted. Spreading the vertebrae apart for a lumbar puncture will not help the procedure to be completed faster. Spreading the vertebrae apart for a lumbar puncture will not affect the results of the procedure.

QSEN Standard: I. A. 1. Integrate understanding of multiple dimensions of patient centered care: information, communication, and education; ANA Standard: 14. 2. Communicates with patient, family, and healthcare providers regarding patient care and the nurse's role in the provision of that care; Cognitive Level: Applying; Client Need: Physiological Integrity; Client Need Sub: Reduction of Risk Potential; Nursing/Integrated Concepts: Nursing Process: Implementation/Teaching/Learning

Chapter 8

1. **3.** For serum thyroid tests, the client should avoid eating shellfish for several days before the test. Smoking cigarettes does not affect the results of serum thyroid tests. Lying supine for 1 hour does not affect the results of serum thyroid tests. Fasting does not need to be done before serum thyroid tests.

QSEN Standard: II. B. 4. Function competently within own scope of practice as a member of the health care team; ANA Standard: 1. 7. Prioritizes data collection activities based on the patient's immediate condition, or anticipated needs of the patient or situation; Cognitive Level: Analyzing; Client Need: Physiological Integrity; Client Need Sub: Reduction of Risk Potential; Nursing/Integrated Concepts: Nursing Process: Assessment

2. **1.** Yoga is identified as a complementary and alternative therapy approach for Addison disease. Yoga is not identified as a complementary and alternative therapy approach for myxedema coma, Cushing syndrome, or Hashimoto thyroiditis.

QSEN Standard: II. B. 4. Function competently within own scope of practice as a member of the health care team; ANA Standard: 5b. 1. Provides health teaching that addresses such topics as healthy lifestyles, risk-reducing behaviors, developmental needs, activities of daily living, and preventive self-care; Cognitive Level: Analyzing; Client Need: Health Promotion and Maintenance; Nursing/Integrated Concepts: Nursing Process: Planning

3. **3.** Normally about 1500 mL is the maximum amount of fluid drained at one time and it is drained very slowly. Limiting the amount and speed of fluid withdrawal prevents hypovolemic shock; a low blood pressure could indicate that the client is experiencing an adverse effect from the procedure. Warm, dry skin does not indicate an adverse effect from this procedure. A heart rate of 94 bpm is within normal limits and does not indicate an adverse effect from this procedure. A respiratory rate of 18/min and unlabored could indicate an improvement in respiratory functioning after this procedure, not an adverse effect.

QSEN Standard: II. B. 7. Clarify roles and accountabilities under conditions of potential overlap in team member functioning; ANA Standard: 6. 3. Evaluates, in partnership with the person, the effectiveness of the planned strategies in relation to the person's responses and the attainment of the expected outcomes; Cognitive Level: Analyzing; Client Need: Physiological Integrity; Client Need Sub: Reduction of Risk Potential; Nursing/Integrated Concepts: Nursing Process: Evaluation

4. **2.** Urate crystals are found in urine and are precursors to the development of gout. If these crystals were present in a paracentesis sample, the bladder was most likely punctured. Urate crystals are not found in paracentesis fluid. Urate crystals do not indicate an electrolyte imbalance. Urate crystals do not indicate an insufficient amount of fluid was sent as a sample for testing.

QSEN Standard: I. A. 1. Integrate understanding of multiple dimensions of patient centered care: information, communication, and education; ANA Standard: 1. 9. Synthesizes available data, information, and knowledge relevant to the situation to identify patterns and

variances; Cognitive Level: Analyzing; Client Need: Physiological Integrity; Client Need Sub: Reduction of Risk Potential; Nursing/Integrated Concepts: Nursing Process: Assessment

5. **2.** If the UAP received a reading of insufficient sample size, it is possible that the skill is not being performed correctly. The best way to evaluate competency and obtain an accurate reading would be for the nurse to observe the UAP perform the skill on the client again. Having another UAP perform the skill does not help evaluate the original UAP's competency to perform capillary blood glucose measuring. The nurse is responsible for the assessment, interpretation of abnormal findings, and determination of appropriate responses for the capillary glucose measurement. The nurse needs to investigate why an insufficient sample was obtained. It could be due to the UAP's technique. The nurse needs to obtain an accurate capillary blood glucose measurement prior to contacting the healthcare provider for the insulin dose.

QSEN Standard: II. B. 4. Function competently within own scope of practice as a member of the health care team; ANA Standard: 1. 8. Uses appropriate evidence-based assessment techniques and instruments and tools; Cognitive Level: Applying; Client Need: Safe and Effective Care Environment; Client Need Sub: Management of Care; Nursing/Integrated Concepts: Nursing Process: Implementation

6. **4.** The client should be instructed to gently squeeze proximal to, but not to touch, the puncture site until a large drop of blood forms. The site should be cleansed with an antiseptic swab and allowed to dry completely; alcohol can affect accuracy, and the site burns when punctured if wet with alcohol. The skin should be punctured with a lancet using a darting motion. Wrapping the finger in a warm cloth before puncturing the skin increases the blood flow to the area, ensuring an adequate specimen and reducing the need for a repeat puncture.

QSEN Standard: II. B. 4. Function competently within own scope of practice as a member of the health care team; ANA Standard: 5b. 1. Provides health teaching that addresses such topics as healthy lifestyles, risk-reducing behaviors, developmental needs, activities of daily living, and preventive self-care; Cognitive Level: Analyzing; Client Need: Health Promotion and Maintenance; Nursing/Integrated Concepts: Nursing Process: Evaluation/Teaching/Learning

7. **1.** People with diabetes mellitus have a high incidence of problems with their feet and subsequent amputations. Guidelines for foot care management in the client with diabetes include never going barefoot. A client with diabetes should be instructed on smoking cessation. Using an ashtray for spare change and house keys indicates that the ashtray is not being used for smoking. Having a list of daily capillary glucose levels next to the monitor indicates that blood glucose levels are being monitored regularly. A glass of water placed near the client indicates that the client is attempting to have an adequate fluid intake.

QSEN Standard: II. B. 4. Function competently within own scope of practice as a member of the health care team; ANA Standard: 5b. 1. Provides health teaching that addresses such topics as healthy lifestyles, risk-reducing behaviors, developmental needs, activities of daily living, and preventive self-care; Cognitive Level: Analyzing; Client Need: Health Promotion and Maintenance; Nursing/Integrated Concepts: Nursing Process: Evaluation/Teaching/Learning

8. **3.** The nurse's plan of care should reflect sick-day management guidelines, which include drinking 240–360 mL of fluid each waking hour. The nurse's plan of sick-day management for the client with type 2 diabetes mellitus (T2DM) includes monitoring blood glucose at least 4 times a day. Sick-day management guidelines would include a small amount of carbohydrate being offered every 1–2 hr; there is no need to restrict the total amount of carbohydrates. The nurse's plan of care should reflect sick-day management guidelines; the nurse should provide the usual insulin dose or oral antidiabetic agent.

QSEN Standard: II. B. 4. Function competently within own scope of practice as a member of the health care team; ANA Standard: 4. 9. Integrates current scientific evidence, trends, and research affecting care in planning; Cognitive Level: Applying; Client Need: Physiological Integrity; Client Need Sub: Reduction of Risk Potential; Nursing/Integrated Concepts: Nursing Process: Planning

Chapter 9

1. **1.** The ankle is not rotated. Ankle range of motion is flexion and extension. The limb should be supported above and below the joint being exercised. A head-to-toe approach is recommended. Rolling the foot and leg inward and then outward provides internal and external range of motion of the hip.

QSEN Standard: I. B. 10. Engage patients or designated surrogates in active partnerships that promote health, safety and well-being, and self-care management; ANA Standard: 5B. 1.Provides health teaching that addresses such topics as healthy lifestyles, risk-reducing behaviors, developmental needs, activities of daily living, and preventive self-care; Cognitive Level: Analyzing; Client Need: Physiological Integrity; Client Need Sub: Reduction of Risk Potential; Nursing/Integrated Concepts: Nursing Process: Evaluation/Teaching/Learning

2. **1.** Since the client is starting to fall forward, the nurse should first widen his or her own stance to increase the base of support. Separating the feet allows the nurse to rock backward and use the femoral muscles when supporting the client's weight. It also lowers the center of gravity to prevent back strain. Pulling on the client's arm could cause an injury to both the client and the nurse. Tightening the grip on the gait belt will not be sufficient if the client is falling forward. Having the client look down on the floor may cause the client to fall forward faster.

QSEN Standard: V. B. 2. Demonstrate effective use of strategies to reduce risk of harm to self or others; ANA Standard: 5. 5. Utilizes evidence-based interventions and treatments specific to the diagnosis or problem; Cognitive Level: Applying; Client Need: Safe and Effective Care Environment; Client Need Sub: Safety and Infection Control; Nursing/Integrated Concepts: Nursing Process: Implementation

3. **4.** The client's entire body should be moved in unison to the side of the bed. Moving the upper body then the lower body does not keep the spine in alignment. The client's arms are crossed over the chest to ensure that the arms are not injured or trapped under the body when the client is turned. Pillows between the legs prevent adduction of the upper leg and keep the legs parallel and aligned. Placing a pillow where it will support the client's head after the turn prevents lateral flexion of the neck and ensures alignment of the cervical spine. QSEN Standard: V. B. 2. Demonstrate effective use of strategies to reduce risk of harm to self or others; ANA Standard: 11. 11. Identifies problems that occur in day to day work routines and participates in deriving solutions to inefficiencies; Cognitive Level: Analyzing; Client Need: Safe and Effective Care Environment; Client Need Sub: Safety and Infection Control; Nursing/Integrated Concepts: Nursing Process: Assessment

4. **4.** Once the draw sheet is in place, it should be grasped at the shoulders and hips because it draws the client's weight closer to the nurse's center of gravity for balance and stability. Lowering the head of the bed is the first action the nurse should take; it would be done before placing the draw sheet. Raising the height of the bed is the second action that the nurse should take; it would be done before placing the draw sheet. A pillow should be placed against the head of the bed after the bed is flat and raised to the appropriate height; this would also be done before placing the draw sheet.

QSEN Standard: V. B. 2. Demonstrate effective use of strategies to reduce risk of harm to self or others; ANA Standard: 5. 6. Provides holistic care that addresses the needs of diverse populations across the lifespan; Cognitive Level: Applying; Client Need: Safe and Effective Care Environment; Client Need Sub: Safety and Infection Control; Nursing/Integrated Concepts: Nursing Process: Implementation

5. **2.** The client has a left leg injury, so the chair should be parallel to the bed on the client's right (unaffected) side. If the wheelchair is facing the bed, the client would have to turn around completely to sit. The wheelchair should be placed so the client can move toward the uninjured lower extremity. Placing the wheelchair at a 45-degree angle is appropriate for the client who has difficulty walking. This is not the case for this client situation.

QSEN Standard: V. B. 2. Demonstrate effective use of strategies to reduce risk of harm to self or others; ANA Standard: 5. 6. Provides holistic care that addresses the needs of diverse populations across the lifespan;

Cognitive Level: Applying; Client Need: Safe and Effective Care Environment; Client Need Sub: Safety and Infection Control; Nursing/Integrated Concepts: Nursing Process: Implementation

6. **1.** Since the client should never be pulled across the bed in the prone position, the best way to ensure proper positioning is to start over. Placing pillows against the left raised side rail does not ensure proper positioning. This could also be unsafe. Never pull a client across the bed while the client is in the prone position. Doing so can injure a woman's breasts or a man's genitals. Moving the body in segments toward the center of the bed could be harmful and cause injury to the client.

QSEN Standard: V. B. 2. Demonstrate effective use of strategies to reduce risk of harm to self or others; ANA Standard: 5. 6. Provides holistic care that addresses the needs of diverse populations across the lifespan; Cognitive Level: Applying; Client Need: Safe and Effective Care Environment; Client Need Sub: Safety and Infection Control; Nursing/Integrated Concepts: Nursing Process: Implementation

7. **3.** After moving the cane forward, the client should move the weak leg to the level of the cane. Moving the weak leg ahead of the cane can throw the client off balance and precipitate a fall. The weak leg should be moved first.

QSEN Standard: V. B. 2. Demonstrate effective use of strategies to reduce risk of harm to self or others; ANA Standard: 5. 6. Provides holistic care that addresses the needs of diverse populations across the lifespan; Cognitive Level: Applying; Client Need: Safe and Effective Care Environment; Client Need Sub: Safety and Infection Control; Nursing/Integrated Concepts: Nursing Process: Implementation/Teaching/Learning

8. **4.** When moving down a step, the crutches and the affected leg should be moved together. Then the unaffected leg is moved down to the step. The elbows should be flexed at a 30-degree angle. The client's body weight should be supported by the hands on the hand bar. The client should start by assuming the tripod position at the top of the stairs.

QSEN Standard: V. B. 2. Demonstrate effective use of strategies to reduce risk of harm to self or others; ANA Standard: 5. 6. Provides holistic care that addresses the needs of diverse populations across the lifespan; Cognitive Level: Analyzing; Client Need: Safe and Effective Care Environment; Client Need Sub: Safety and Infection Control; Nursing/Integrated Concepts: Nursing Process: Evaluation/Teaching/Learning

9. **2.** If one leg is weaker than the other, the walker and the weak leg should be moved ahead together. The walker should be moved ahead first before moving either of the feet. Moving the right leg up to the walker first would be appropriate if both legs are equally weak. Moving the strong leg and the walker together could cause the client to become unstable and fall.

QSEN Standard: V. B. 2. Demonstrate effective use of strategies to reduce risk of harm to self or others; ANA Standard: 5. 6. Provides holistic care that addresses the needs of diverse populations across the lifespan; Cognitive Level: Applying; Client Need: Safe and Effective Care Environment; Client Need Sub: Safety and Infection Control; Nursing/Integrated Concepts: Nursing Process: Implementation/Teaching/Learning

10. **1.** Complaints of severe pain could indicate compartment syndrome. The first thing that the nurse should do is apply ice to reduce inflammation. The nurse needs to apply ice and notify the healthcare provider before providing pain medication. The healthcare provider should be notified after ice is applied to the limb and the limb is placed in a neutral position. Elevating the limb on two pillows is not a neutral position. This position is not recommended if compartment syndrome is suspected.

QSEN Standard: V. B. 2. Demonstrate effective use of strategies to reduce risk of harm to self or others; ANA Standard: 5. 6. Provides holistic care that addresses the needs of diverse populations across the lifespan; Cognitive Level: Applying; Client Need: Physiological Integrity; Client Need Sub: Reduction of Risk Potential; Nursing/Integrated Concepts: Nursing Process: Implementation

11. **1.** When the cast is removed, the underlying skin is usually macerated and encrusted. Oil should be applied before soaking the leg in warm water. Vigorous rubbing can cause bleeding or excoriation of fragile skin. Vigorous rubbing with a dry washcloth can cause bleeding or excoriation of fragile skin. Antibiotic ointment does not need to be applied to open areas.

QSEN Standard: V. B. 2. Demonstrate effective use of strategies to reduce risk of harm to self or others; ANA Standard: 5. 6. Provides holistic care that addresses the needs of diverse populations across the lifespan; Cognitive Level: Applying; Client Need: Physiological Integrity; Client Need Sub: Basic Care and Comfort; Nursing/Integrated Concepts: Nursing Process: Implementation

12. **3.** If purulent drainage is present, notifying the healthcare provider is the priority. After the drainage has been reported and cultured, pin care can be performed as prescribed. Sterile ointment may or may not be prescribed. The ointment may hinder the drainage. If purulent drainage is present, obtain specimens after notifying the healthcare provider.

QSEN Standard: V. B. 2. Demonstrate effective use of strategies to reduce risk of harm to self or others; ANA Standard: 5. 6. Provides holistic care that addresses the needs of diverse populations across the lifespan; Cognitive Level: Applying; Client Need: Safe and Effective Care Environment; Client Need Sub: Safety and Infection Control; Nursing/Integrated Concepts: Nursing Process: Implementation

Chapter 10

1. **45 grams** First convert the client's weight into grams by dividing weight in lb by 2.2, or 165 lb/2.2 = 75 kg. Then, multiply the amount of protein prescribed by the weight or 75 kg × 0.6 = 45 grams.

   QSEN Standard: I. B. 10. Engage patients or designated surrogates in active partnerships that promote health, safety, and well-being, and self-care management; ANA Standard: 5B. 1. Provides health teaching that addresses such topics as healthy lifestyles, risk-reducing behaviors, developmental needs, activities of daily living, and preventive self-care; Cognitive Level: Applying; Client Need: Physiological Integrity; Client Need Sub: Basic Care and Comfort; Nursing/Integrated Concepts: Nursing Process: Implementation/Teaching/Learning

2. **2.** Cream of mushroom soup has cream and milk, which should be restricted on a low-fat diet. Almonds contain monounsaturated fats and are permitted on a low-fat diet. Whole wheat products and margarine are permitted on a low-fat diet. Green leafy vegetables are permitted on a low-fat diet. Olive oil is a monounsaturated fat which is permitted on a low-fat diet.

   QSEN Standard: I. B. 10. Engage patients or designated surrogates in active partnerships that promote health, safety, and well-being, and self-care management; ANA Standard: 5B. 1. Provides health teaching that addresses such topics as healthy lifestyles, risk-reducing behaviors, developmental needs, activities of daily living, and preventive self-care; Cognitive Level: Applying; Client Need: Physiological Integrity; Client Need Sub: Basic Care and Comfort; Nursing/Integrated Concepts: Nursing Process: Evaluation/Teaching/Learning

3. **1.** For the client with dysphagia, swallowing takes concentration; talking increases risk of aspiration. For the client with dysphagia, sitting upright assists with proper bolus movement to the stomach. A towel under the tray stabilizes it for eating or feeding. The use of a straw increases the risk of aspiration because the client with dysphagia has less control over the amount of fluid intake.

   QSEN Standard: II. A. 4. Recognize contributions of other individuals and groups in helping patient/family achieve health goals; ANA Standard: 5. 1. Partners with the person/family/significant others/ caregiver to implement the plan in a safe, realistic, and timely manner; Cognitive Level: Analyzing; Client Need: Physiological Integrity; Client Need Sub: Reduction of Risk Potential; Nursing/Integrated Concepts: Nursing Process: Assessment

4. **4.** After the feeding, the tube should be flushed with water to maintain patency. Clamping the feeding tube will not ensure that it remains patent. Sterile normal saline is not used to flush a gastrostomy tube. Maintaining an upright position for 30 minutes after the feeding prevents aspiration; it does not guarantee patency.

   QSEN Standard: V. B. 2. Demonstrate effective use of strategies to reduce risk of harm to self or others; ANA Standard: 5. 5. Utilizes evidence-based interventions and treatments specific to the diagnosis or problem; Cognitive Level: Applying; Client Need: Physiological Integrity; Client Need Sub: Basic Care and Comfort; Nursing/Integrated Concepts: Nursing Process: Implementation

5. **3.** Diabetes mellitus, as well as physiological changes associated with aging, may result in increased amount of time to empty the stomach. Heart failure is not identified as a health problem that adversely affects absorption of enteral feedings. Diverticulitis is not identified as a health problem that adversely affects absorption of enteral feedings. Parkinson disease is not identified as a health problem that adversely affects absorption of enteral feedings.

   QSEN Standard: V. B. 2. Demonstrate effective use of strategies to reduce risk of harm to self or others; ANA Standard: 5. 5. Utilizes evidence-based interventions and treatments specific to the diagnosis or problem; Cognitive Level: Analyzing; Client Need: Physiological Integrity; Client Need Sub: Physiological Adaptation; Nursing/Integrated Concepts: Nursing Process: Assessment

6. **2.** If the signs do not indicate placement in the lungs or the stomach, advance the tube 5 cm (2 in.) and repeat the test. The client would be gagging and coughing if the tube is coiled in the throat. Placing the end of the tube in a container of water is not an appropriate method to assess for placement. There is no reason to remove the tube. It might not be advanced enough to reach the stomach.

   QSEN Standard: V. B. 2. Demonstrate effective use of strategies to reduce risk of harm to self or others; ANA Standard: 5. 5. Utilizes evidence-based interventions and treatments specific to the diagnosis or problem; Cognitive Level: Applying; Client Need: Physiological Integrity; Client Need Sub: Reduction of Risk Potential; Nursing/Integrated Concepts: Nursing Process: Implementation

7. **4.** Having the client take a deep breath and hold it closes the glottis and prevents accidental aspiration of gastric contents. Instilling air into the tube clears the tube of contents and prevents dragging drainage through the esophagus and nasopharynx. It does not prevent coughing. Flushing the tube will not prevent the client from coughing. The side-lying position is not recommended when removing a nasogastric tube. This position may encourage aspiration of tube contents.

   QSEN Standard: V. B. 2. Demonstrate effective use of strategies to reduce risk of harm to self or others; ANA Standard: 5. 5. Utilizes evidence-based interventions and treatments specific to the diagnosis or problem; Cognitive Level: Analysis; Client Need: Physiological Integrity; Client Need Sub: Reduction of Risk Potential; Nursing/Integrated Concepts: Nursing Process: Evaluation

8. **2.** For 500 mL, first subtract 15 mL for the first 15 min of the infusion. Then divide the remaining amount of 485 mL by 2 since the rate will increase to 2 mL/min. Take this value of 242.5 and divide it by 60 minutes (60 minutes = 1 hour). It will take approximately 4 hours for the intralipids to infuse. If the infusion started at 1000 hours, it should conclude at 1400 hours. Two hours is not enough time to infuse the intralipids properly. Six hours is too much time to infuse the intralipids properly. Eight hours is too much time to infuse the intralipids properly.

QSEN Standard: V. C. 3. Value own role in preventing errors; ANA Standard: 5. 5. Utilizes evidence-based interventions and treatments specific to the diagnosis or problem; Cognitive Level: Applying; Client Need: Physiological Integrity; Client Need Sub: Pharmacological and Parenteral Therapies; Nursing/Integrated Concepts: Nursing Process: Planning

9. **3.** Capillary blood glucose should be measured to determine if the excess infusion has had an adverse effect on the client's metabolism of glucose. Never interrupt or discontinue a TPN infusion abruptly because the client could develop rebound hypoglycemia. A change in weight would reflect fluid volume; however, weighing the client is not the first action that the nurse should take. If the prescribed TPN solution is temporarily unavailable, a solution containing at least 5–10% dextrose would be infused. An infusion of normal saline could cause rebound hypoglycemia.

QSEN Standard: V. B. 4. Communicate observations or concerns related to hazards and errors to patients, families, and the health care team; ANA Standard: 5. 5. Utilizes evidence-based interventions and treatments specific to the diagnosis or problem; Cognitive Level: Applying; Client Need: Physiological Integrity; Client Need Sub: Pharmacological and Parenteral Therapies; Nursing/Integrated Concepts: Nursing Process: Implementation

Chapter 11

1. **3.** Coughing could indicate that the nurse used inappropriate technique to obtain the culture. The nurse should wait for the client to stop coughing and start the procedure again, using correct technique. Water may cause exudate in the throat to be flushed down the esophagus and alter the results of the culture. Mouth care may cause exudate in the throat to be cleansed away and alter the results of the culture. The nurse is collecting a throat culture, and not a sputum culture.

QSEN Standard: V C. 3. Value own role in preventing errors; ANA Standard: 5. 1. Partners with the person/family/significant others/caregiver to implement the plan in a safe, realistic, and timely manner; Cognitive Level: Applying; Client Need: Physiological Integrity; Client Need Sub: Reduction of Risk Potential; Nursing/Integrated Concepts: Nursing Process: Implementation

2. **4.** The client should take a slow deep breath and not a brisk low-volume breath. Slow deep breaths ensure maximum ventilation to achieve greater lung expansion. The client should exhale normally. The spirometer should be held in the upright position. The lips should be sealed around the mouthpiece.

QSEN Standard: V. B. 2. Demonstrate effective use of strategies to reduce risk of harm to self or others; ANA Standard: 5B. 3. Seeks opportunities for feedback and evaluation of the effectiveness of the strategies used; Cognitive Level: Analyzing; Client Need: Physiological Integrity; Client Need Sub: Reduction of Risk Potential; Nursing/Integrated Concepts: Nursing Process: Evaluation/Teaching/Learning

3. **3.** Since the x-ray showed a large pleural effusion, a drainage bag should be at the bedside prior to the beginning of this procedure. The use of gauze pads would not depend on the size of the pleural effusion. Since the x-ray showed a large pleural effusion, a 60-mL syringe may not be large enough. The use of antiseptic swabs does not depend on the size of the pleural effusion.

QSEN Standard: V. B. 2. Demonstrate effective use of strategies to reduce risk of harm to self or others; ANA Standard: 4. 3. Includes strategies in the plan of care that address each of the identified diagnoses or issues. These strategies may include, but are not limited to, strategies for promotion and restoration of health and prevention of illness, injury, and disease, the alleviation of suffering and provision of supportive care for those who are dying; Cognitive Level: Applying; Client Need: Physiological Integrity; Client Need Sub: Reduction of Risk Potential; Nursing/Integrated Concepts: Nursing Process: Planning

4. **1.** With synchronized intermittent mandatory ventilation (SIMV), the ventilator is set to deliver a predetermined number of breaths and tidal volume while also allowing the client to take spontaneous breaths at a self-determined tidal volume and rate. Condensation would not be an expected finding; it would need to be cleared from the tubing. The endotracheal tube cuff needs to be inflated to prevent the development of pneumonia. With adaptive support ventilation (ASV), not SIMV, inspiratory pressure, inspiratory/expiratory ratio, and mandatory respiratory rate are set to maintain a specific target volume and respiratory rate.

QSEN Standard: V. B. 2. Demonstrate effective use of strategies to reduce risk of harm to self or others; ANA Standard: 1. 9. Synthesizes available data, information, and knowledge relevant to the situation to identify patterns and variances; Cognitive Level: Applying; Client Need: Physiological Integrity; Client Need Sub: Reduction of Risk Potential; Nursing/Integrated Concepts: Nursing Process: Assessment

5. **4.** To select the correct size of the oropharyngeal airway, the nurse should measure from the corner of the mouth to the tragus of the ear. The tip of nose to tip of ear is used as partial measurement for nasogastric, not oropharyngeal, tube insertion. The tip of the ear is not used when measuring the length of an oropharyngeal

airway. Middle of mouth to tip of chin would not provide an adequate length for an oropharyngeal airway.

QSEN Standard: III. A. 1. Demonstrate knowledge of basic scientific methods and processes; ANA Standard: 1. 8. Uses appropriate evidence-based assessment techniques and instruments and tools; Cognitive Level: Applying; Client Need: Physiological Integrity; Client Need Sub: Reduction of Risk Potential; Nursing/Integrated Concepts: Nursing Process: Planning

6. **2.** When removing the endotracheal tube, have the client take a deep breath to dilate the vocal cords and make removal easier and less traumatic. Then apply suction while removing catheter and airway at the same time. The client does not need to take a deep breath before deflating the cuff. A deep breath is not required before preparing the suction catheter. A deep breath is not required before untying the endotracheal tube ties.

QSEN Standard: III. A. 1. Demonstrate knowledge of basic scientific methods and processes; ANA Standard: 5. 5. Utilizes evidence-based interventions and treatments specific to the diagnosis or problem; Cognitive Level: Applying; Client Need: Physiological Integrity; Client Need Sub: Reduction of Risk Potential; Nursing/Integrated Concepts: Nursing Process: Implementation/Teaching/Learning

7. **4.** The tip of the catheter became contaminated when it touched the client's chin. The catheter is contaminated and cannot be used. The nurse needs to obtain another sterile catheter. Placing a contaminated tip into sterile lubricant will contaminate the lubricant. Hyperoxygenating the client is not part of the procedure when suctioning a client's nasopharyngeal airway. Placing a contaminated tip in sterile water will contaminate the sterile water.

QSEN Standard: III. A. 1. Demonstrate knowledge of basic scientific methods and processes; ANA Standard: 5. 5. Utilizes evidence-based interventions and treatments specific to the diagnosis or problem; Cognitive Level: Applying; Client Need: Physiological Integrity; Client Need Sub: Reduction of Risk Potential; Nursing/Integrated Concepts: Nursing Process: Implementation

8. **4.** The nurse should withdraw the catheter and permit the client to cough. After coughing has stopped, the nurse can resume suctioning to remove the secretions loosened by coughing. Hyperoxygenation should occur before suctioning and between each pass of the catheter to suction. Nothing should be instilled into the tube to loosen secretions. Continuing to suction could dramatically reduce the client's oxygen level.

QSEN Standard: V. B. 1. Demonstrate effective use of technology and standardized practices that support safety and quality; ANA Standard: 5. 5. Utilizes evidence-based interventions and treatments specific to the diagnosis or problem; Cognitive Level: Applying; Client Need: Physiological Integrity; Client Need Sub: Reduction of Risk Potential; Nursing/Integrated Concepts: Nursing Process: Implementation

9. **3.** Half-strength, not full-strength, hydrogen peroxide may be used to remove crusty secretions around the tracheostomy site. Hydrogen peroxide can be irritating to the skin and may inhibit healing if not thoroughly removed. The client should flex the neck before tying the ties to ensure that the ties are not too tight. Tap water may be used for rinsing the inner cannula. The hands should be washed before applying gloves and after removing gloves.

QSEN Standard: V. B. 1. Demonstrate effective use of technology and standardized practices that support safety and quality; ANA Standard: 5B. 3. Seeks opportunities for feedback and evaluation of the effectiveness of the strategies used; Cognitive Level: Analyzing; Client Need: Physiological Integrity; Client Need Sub: Reduction of Risk Potential; Nursing/Integrated Concepts: Nursing Process: Evaluation/Teaching/Learning

10. **4.** The absence of fluctuation of the fluid level in the water, or tidaling, may be due to outside pressure or kinks caused by the client lying on the tube. This check is what the nurse should do first. Milking the tube involves squeezing, kneading, or twisting the tube to create bursts of suction to move any clots. This should only be done with a healthcare provider's order since it could cause negative pressure in the intrapleural space. Stripping consists of compressing the tube between the fingers and thumb using a pulling motion down the rest of the tubing away from the chest. This should only be done with a healthcare provider's order since it could create negative pressure in the intrapleural space. Palpation would detect subcutaneous emphysema. There is no reason to suspect that the client is developing this complication.

QSEN Standard: V. B. 1. Demonstrate effective use of technology and standardized practices that support safety and quality; ANA Standard: 5. 5. Utilizes evidence-based interventions and treatments specific to the diagnosis or problem; Cognitive Level: Applying; Client Need: Physiological Integrity; Client Need Sub: Reduction of Risk Potential; Nursing/Integrated Concepts: Nursing Process: Implementation

11. **2.** Cloudy chest tube drainage is associated with infection or inflammation. A culture would be needed before starting antibiotics. Anticoagulants would be held if the drainage were blood-tinged. Airborne precautions would be appropriate if it is suspected that the client has tuberculosis. Nothing by mouth status would be appropriate if food particles were present in the drainage.

QSEN Standard: V. B. 1. Demonstrate effective use of technology and standardized practices that support safety and quality; ANA Standard: 4. 3. Includes strategies in the plan of care that address each of the identified diagnoses or issues; Cognitive Level: Applying; Client Need: Physiological Integrity; Client Need Sub: Reduction of Risk Potential; Nursing/Integrated Concepts: Nursing Process: Planning

12. **1.** Since the client is demonstrating signs of poor lung inflation after the removal of the chest tube, a chest

x-ray is needed to determine the best course of action. Incentive spirometry might be prescribed; however, it would occur after confirmation with a chest x-ray. A chest x-ray is needed before determining if the chest tube needs to be reinserted. Deep breathing and coughing would most likely be prescribed, but only after a chest x-ray is done to determine the best course of action for the client.

QSEN Standard: V. B. 1. Demonstrate effective use of technology and standardized practices that support safety and quality; ANA Standard: 4. 3. Includes strategies in the plan of care that address each of the identified diagnoses or issues; Cognitive Level: Applying; Client Need: Physiological Integrity; Client Need Sub: Reduction of Risk Potential; Nursing/Integrated Concepts: Nursing Process: Planning

Chapter 12

1. **2.** Vomiting is an indication of a transfusion reaction. The first thing to do is to stop the transfusion. After the transfusion is stopped and the intravenous tubing changed to infuse normal saline, the nurse should call for help. Although the client is uncomfortable and vomiting, an emesis basin in not a priority. The transfusion needs to be stopped and the client's hemodynamic status needs to be supported first. The saline infusion should continue, not be increased; however, new tubing is required.

QSEN Standard: V C. 3. Value own role in preventing errors; ANA Standard: 5. 5. Utilizes evidence-based interventions and treatments specific to the diagnosis or problem; Cognitive Level: Applying; Client Need: Physiological Integrity; Client Need Sub: Pharmacological and Parenteral Therapies; Nursing/Integrated Concepts: Nursing Process: Implementation

2. **2.** Since the UAP will be removing the devices for bathing, it is appropriate for the UAP to report the condition of the skin under the devices. The UAP is not responsible for assessing pulses in the feet of a client with sequential compression devices. This is the nurse's responsibility to assess. Although the devices should not be off for an extended period of time, it is not essential for the UAP to report the length of time the devices were turned off for bathing. Sensorimotor function assessment is a responsibility of the nurse. It is beyond the scope of practice for the UAP to assess for sensation and movement of the client's feet.

QSEN Standard: II. B. 4. Function competently within own scope of practice as a member of the health care team; ANA Standard: 11. 10. Demonstrates effective communication and information sharing across disciplines and throughout transitions in care; Cognitive Level: Applying; Client Need: Physiological Integrity; Client Need Sub: Reduction of Risk Potential; Nursing/Integrated Concepts: Nursing Process: Implementation/Communication and Documentation

3. **4.** The electrode pads should be located below the right clavicle and below the left nipple. After the AED delivers a shock, CPR should be resumed. The graduate should loudly state "clear" before discharging the AED. The AED will automatically prompt to reanalyze the client in 2–3 min. Chest compressions should be stopped during the analysis.

QSEN Standard: II. B. 4. Function competently within own scope of practice as a member of the health care team; ANA Standard: 1. 8. Uses appropriate evidence-based assessment techniques and instruments and tools; Cognitive Level: Analyzing; Client Need: Physiological Integrity; Client Need Sub: Reduction of Risk Potential; Nursing/Integrated Concepts: Nursing Process: Evaluation

4. **4.** V4, not V6, should be placed at the fifth intercostal space, left midclavicular line. It is correct to place the green lead on the client's left leg. It is correct to place the white lead on the client's right wrist. It is correct to place the V2 at the fourth intercostal space, left sternal border.

QSEN Standard: II. B. 4. Function competently within own scope of practice as a member of the health care team; ANA Standard: 1. 8. Uses appropriate evidence-based assessment techniques and instruments and tools; Cognitive Level: Applying; Client Need: Physiological Integrity; Client Need Sub: Reduction of Risk Potential; Nursing/Integrated Concepts: Nursing Process: Assessment

5. **2.** Atrial activity is best detected in Lead II. Atrial arrhythmic activity is poorly identified in Lead I. Left inferior wall function is best detected in Lead III. Lead aVL records activity between the center of the heart and left arm.

QSEN Standard: II. B. 4. Function competently within own scope of practice as a member of the health care team; ANA Standard: 1. 8. Uses appropriate evidence-based assessment techniques and instruments and tools; Cognitive Level: Applying; Client Need: Physiological Integrity; Client Need Sub: Reduction of Risk Potential; Nursing/Integrated Concepts: Nursing Process: Implementation

6. **1.** The client is demonstrating third degree heart block. One reason for this rhythm is digoxin toxicity. Thyroid hormone imbalance is not a reason for this rhythm. Arterial blood gases will not help determine the reason for this rhythm. An electrolyte imbalance is not a reason for this rhythm.

QSEN Standard: II. B. 4. Function competently within own scope of practice as a member of the health care team; ANA Standard: 1. 8. Uses appropriate evidence-based assessment techniques and instruments and tools; Cognitive Level: Applying; Client Need: Physiological Integrity; Client Need Sub: Reduction of Risk Potential; Nursing/Integrated Concepts: Nursing Process: Planning

7. **4.** The client should be informed of electromagnetic interference restrictions, which include not placing a cell phone over the generator. It is wise for the client to wear a medical alert band/bracelet at all times. Many clients use telephone transmission of the generator's

pulse rate to determine status of pacemaker function. Special equipment is used to transmit information concerning function of the pacemaker over the telephone to a receiving system in a pacemaker clinic. The client should carry a pacemaker information ID card in the wallet.

QSEN Standard: II. B. 4. Function competently within own scope of practice as a member of the health care team; ANA Standard: 5B. 3. Seeks opportunities for feedback and evaluation of the effectiveness of the strategies used; Cognitive Level: Analyzing; Client Need: Physiological Integrity; Client Need Sub: Reduction of Risk Potential; Nursing/Integrated Concepts: Nursing Process: Evaluation/Teaching/Learning

8. **4.** When leveling and calibrating the monitoring system, the first action is to adjust the head of the bed to be between flat to up to a 45-degree angle. Then the calibration process is completed. Readings will be inaccurately high or low if the stopcock above the transducer is not level with the client's phlebostatic axis, which is done when calibrating the monitor. However, calibration is done after the head of the bed is adjusted. The pressure bag setting has no impact on the monitor reading. The arterial site dressing has no impact on the monitor reading.

QSEN Standard: III. A. 1. Demonstrate knowledge of basic scientific methods and processes; ANA Standard: 1. 8. Uses appropriate evidence-based assessment techniques and instruments and tools; Cognitive Level: Applying; Client Need: Physiological Integrity; Client Need Sub: Reduction of Risk Potential; Nursing/Integrated Concepts: Nursing Process: Assessment

Chapter 13

1. **2.** Older adults are at greater risk for postoperative complications, such as pneumonia; breathing and coughing exercises should be reinforced. Although wound infection, postoperative hemorrhaging, and deep vein thrombus of the calf are postoperative complications, they are not identified as occurring at a higher rate in older clients.

QSEN Standard: III B. 3. Base individualized care plan on patient values, clinical expertise and evidence; ANA Standard: 5B. 1. Provides health teaching that addresses such topics as healthy lifestyles, risk-reducing behaviors, developmental needs, activities of daily living, and preventive self-care; Cognitive Level: Applying; Client Need: Physiological Integrity; Client Need Sub: Reduction of Risk Potential; Nursing/Integrated Concepts: Nursing Process: Planning/Teaching/Learning

2. **4.** After using circular movements to wash the palms and backs of the hands, the wrists, and the forearms, the nurse should next interlace the fingers and thumbs, and move the hands back and forth; this action should be continued for 20–25 seconds. Scrubbing each finger of both hands with a brush is a later step done after checking and cleaning the nails. Hands and arms are held under water after scrubbing with interlaced fingers and thumbs. The nurse should check the nails and

clean them with a file or an orange stick after the first wash and rinse.

QSEN Standard: III A. 1. Demonstrate knowledge of basic scientific methods and processes; ANA Standard: 5. 5. Utilizes evidence-based interventions and treatments specific to the diagnosis or problem; Cognitive Level: Applying; Client Need: Safe and Effective Care Environment; Client Need Sub: Safety and Infection Control; Nursing/Integrated Concepts: Nursing Process: Implementation

3. **3.** After removing the hair from the surgical area, antiseptic solution is applied; this solution is applied on 4 × 4 pads in widening circles, moving from the center to the most distant line of the area, and the scrub is to occur for 2–3 min. The area is rinsed with warm water after being cleansed with an antiseptic solution. A clean gown is applied last. Antimicrobial gel is not used when preparing a site for surgery.

QSEN Standard: III A. 1. Demonstrate knowledge of basic scientific methods and processes; ANA Standard: 5. 5. Utilizes evidence-based interventions and treatments specific to the diagnosis or problem; Cognitive Level: Applying; Client Need: Safe and Effective Care Environment; Client Need Sub: Safety and Infection Control; Nursing/Integrated Concepts: Nursing Process: Implementation

4. **2.** The flap closest to the nurse should be opened last. If it is opened first, then every hand movement is made reaching over the sterile field and would cause contamination. The two side flats should be grasped prior to opening them together. The flap farthest away should be opened first. The two side flaps should be extended together.

QSEN Standard: III A. 1. Demonstrate knowledge of basic scientific methods and processes; ANA Standard: 5. 5. Utilizes evidence-based interventions and treatments specific to the diagnosis or problem; Cognitive Level: Analyzing; Client Need: Safe and Effective Care Environment; Client Need Sub: Safety and Infection Control; Nursing/Integrated Concepts: Nursing Process: Evaluation

5. **3.** Moist or damp sterile fields are considered contaminated if the surface below them is not sterile. Since the field is being set up on the client's over-bed table, the field is considered contaminated and should be set up again. Air drying will not alter the level of contamination. Blotting the water with sterile gauze will not alter the level of contamination. Moving the container with the poured sterile water toward the edge of the field will increase the level of contamination, since the edges of a sterile field are considered contaminated. Sterile objects should be no closer than 2 cm (1 in.) from the edges of the sterile field.

QSEN Standard: III A. 1. Demonstrate knowledge of basic scientific methods and processes; ANA Standard: 5. 5. Utilizes evidence-based interventions and treatments specific to the diagnosis or problem; Cognitive Level: Applying; Client Need: Safe and Effective Care

Environment; Client Need Sub: Safety and Infection Control; Nursing/Integrated Concepts: Nursing Process: Implementation

6. **3.** The sleeves of a sterile gown should be considered sterile from above the cuff to 5 cm (2 in.) above the elbow. Moisture collection and friction areas such as the sleeve cuffs should be considered unsterile. Since the catheter tip touched the cuff, the catheter is contaminated and another one needs to be brought to the bedside. The gloves are not contaminated, so they do not need to be changed. The catheter is contaminated and should not be used for a sterile procedure. Placing the contaminated catheter onto the sterile field would contaminate the entire field. The sterile field would need to be re-established. The gown was not contaminated by the sterile catheter.

QSEN Standard: III A. 1. Demonstrate knowledge of basic scientific methods and processes; ANA Standard: 5. 5. Utilizes evidence-based interventions and treatments specific to the diagnosis or problem; Cognitive Level: Applying; Client Need: Safe and Effective Care Environment; Client Need Sub: Safety and Infection Control; Nursing/Integrated Concepts: Nursing Process: Implementation

7. **2.** A surgical case that involves a single organ, such as the lumbar spine, can be exempt from the marking procedure. Verification must include the client's name, agreement on the procedure to be done, and correct client position.

QSEN Standard: III A. 1. Demonstrate knowledge of basic scientific methods and processes; ANA Standard: 5. 5. Utilizes evidence-based interventions and treatments specific to the diagnosis or problem; Cognitive Level: Applying; Client Need: Safe and Effective Care Environment; Client Need Sub: Safety and Infection Control; Nursing/Integrated Concepts: Nursing Process: Implementation

8. **3.** Rings may be taped to the finger. They are taped to protect the skin from possible burns from electrical arcing generated by electrical cautery machines. Pinning the ring to the gown increases the risk of the ring being lost. The gown might need to be changed after the procedure and the ring could accidentally be left on the used gown. There are situations in which jewelry is worn in the operating room. However, the piece of jewelry must be covered with tape to secure the item to the body area. The surgeon does not need to discuss the client's refusal to remove a ring. The nurse can discuss this and secure the ring to the finger with tape.

QSEN Standard: III A. 1. Demonstrate knowledge of basic scientific methods and processes; ANA Standard: 5. 5. Utilizes evidence-based interventions and treatments specific to the diagnosis or problem; Cognitive Level: Applying; Client Need: Safe and Effective Care Environment; Client Need Sub: Safety and Infection Control; Nursing/Integrated Concepts: Nursing Process: Implementation

Chapter 14

1. **2.** Leopold maneuvers are used to determine fetal position. These maneuvers are conducted by palpating the abdomen. Once the nurse has located the fetal back, the next assessment step is to auscultate the fetal heartbeat. There is no reason to palpate the feet for edema after palpating the abdomen. The client's blood pressure was most likely measured earlier in the examination. Fundal height, not identification of the fetal back, is used to estimate the number of weeks gestation.

QSEN Standard: III A 1. Demonstrate knowledge of basic scientific methods and processes; ANA Standard: 1. 8. Uses appropriate evidence-based assessment techniques and instruments and tools; Cognitive Level: Applying; Client Need: Health Promotion and Maintenance; Nursing/Integrated Concepts: Nursing Process: Assessment

2. **3.** The nurse should assess deep tendon reflexes to test for the presence of hyperreflexia and clonus. These symptoms may indicate central nervous system irritability and pre-eclampsia or eclampsia in the pregnant woman. Fundal height will not help determine why the client is experiencing edema of the face and hands. Fetal heart rate will not help determine why the client is experiencing edema of the face and hands. Measuring the urine for protein, not measuring capillary blood glucose, would be appropriate to determine if the client is experiencing pre-eclampsia or eclampsia.

QSEN Standard: III A 1. Demonstrate knowledge of basic scientific methods and processes; ANA Standard: 1. 8. Uses appropriate evidence-based assessment techniques and instruments and tools; Cognitive Level: Applying; Client Need: Health Promotion and Maintenance; Nursing/Integrated Concepts: Nursing Process: Assessment

3. **1.** The client's Rh factor is required to determine whether Rh immune globulin is needed. Rh immune globulin is a blood product given as an intramuscular injection to a pregnant woman who is Rh negative to prevent an immune response when the baby is Rh positive. The client's blood type is not needed. Rh factor, not fundal height or number of weeks gestation, is needed prior to determining if the Rh immune globulin injection is required.

QSEN Standard: III A 1. Demonstrate knowledge of basic scientific methods and processes; ANA Standard: 1. 7. Prioritizes data collection activities based on the patient's immediate condition, or anticipated needs of the patient or situation; Cognitive Level: Applying; Client Need: Health Promotion and Maintenance; Nursing/Integrated Concepts: Nursing Process: Assessment

4. **2.** Ephedrine is used in the event of a hypotensive episode in this situation. This medication should be at the bedside and is administered according to unit protocol and MD/CNM orders. Naloxone is a medication used to reverse the effects of opioid medications. A bolus of

intravenous fluids should have been given before the epidural was started. Magnesium sulfate is used to treat eclampsia, not hypotension.

QSEN Standard: III A 1. Demonstrate knowledge of basic scientific methods and processes; ANA Standard: 4. 3. Includes strategies in the plan of care that address each of the identified diagnoses or issues; Cognitive Level: Applying; Client Need: Physiological Integrity; Client Need Sub: Pharmacological and Parenteral Therapies; Nursing/Integrated Concepts: Nursing Process: Planning

5. **2.** A fetal scalp electrode may be internally placed only after the amniotic sac has ruptured. The cervix must be dilated at least 2 cm before placing an internal fetal scalp electrode. The lithotomy position is used when placing this electrode. The monitoring cables are connected after the electrode is placed on the fetal skull.

QSEN Standard: V. B. 2. Demonstrate effective use of strategies to reduce risk of harm to self or others; ANA Standard: 4. 3. Includes strategies in the plan of care that address each of the identified diagnoses or issues; Cognitive Level: Applying; Client Need: Physiological Integrity; Client Need Sub: Reduction of Risk Potential; Nursing/Integrated Concepts: Nursing Process: Planning

6. **3.** Oxygen at 10 L/min via face mask should be applied to the client to support oxygenation of the fetus. The cord should not be handled since it could spasm and adversely affect fetal oxygenation. The client should be in bed; getting out of bed would put more pressure on the prolapsed cord and would compromise oxygenation further. Upon identification of the prolapsed cord, the client should be placed in the knee–chest position to use gravity to relieve umbilical cord pressure.

QSEN Standard: V. B. 2. Demonstrate effective use of strategies to reduce risk of harm to self or others; ANA Standard: 5. 5. Utilizes evidence-based interventions and treatments specific to the diagnosis or problem; Cognitive Level: Applying; Client Need: Physiological Integrity; Client Need Sub: Reduction of Risk Potential; Nursing/Integrated Concepts: Nursing Process: Implementation

7. **2.** Lochia that changes to clear does not need to be reported to the healthcare provider. The lochia should change from red to pink to clear. Clots and heavy bleeding should be reported to the healthcare provider. Heavy bleeding that saturates more than 4 to 8 perineal pads a day should be reported to the healthcare provider.

QSEN Standard: V. B. 4. Communicate observations or concerns related to hazards and errors to patients, families, and the health care team; ANA Standard: 5B. 3. Seeks opportunities for feedback and evaluation of the effectiveness of the strategies used; Cognitive Level: Analyzing; Client Need: Health Promotion and Maintenance; Nursing/Integrated Concepts: Nursing Process: Evaluation/Teaching/Learning

8. **4.** The REEDA scale is used to assess perineal tissue. Approximation of the episiotomy incision is a part of this assessment. The lochia is assessed prior to assessing the perineal tissue. Pain level is assessed prior to assessing the perineal tissue. Fundal height is assessed prior to assessing the perineal tissue.

QSEN Standard: III A 1. Demonstrate knowledge of basic scientific methods and processes; ANA Standard: 1. 7. Prioritizes data collection activities based on the patient's immediate condition, or anticipated needs of the patient or situation; Cognitive Level: Applying; Client Need: Health Promotion and Maintenance; Nursing/Integrated Concepts: Nursing Process: Assessment

9. **3.** If the fundus is not firm, massage the abdomen lightly until it becomes firm, and then check for bleeding. The nurse should have the client empty the bladder before palpating the uterine fundus. The perineal pad would be removed after the uterine fundus is massaged. Pushing on a uterus that is not firm is dangerous because it could cause the uterus to invert.

QSEN Standard: V. B. 2. Demonstrate effective use of strategies to reduce risk of harm to self or others; ANA Standard: 5. 5. Utilizes evidence-based interventions and treatments specific to the diagnosis or problem; Cognitive Level: Applying; Client Need: Health Promotion and Maintenance; Nursing/Integrated Concepts: Nursing Process: Implementation

10. **1.** Teach parents to apply petroleum gauze to the site. Parents should be instructed to use ointment such as A&D to prevent adherence of the diaper to the surgical site. Teach the parents that the glans is sensitive and to avoid placing the newborn on the stomach for the first day after the procedure. Dry gauze should not be used. This will adhere to the site and cause pain when removed.

QSEN Standard: V. B. 4. Communicate observations or concerns related to hazards and errors to patients, families, and the health care team; ANA Standard: 5B. 1. Provides health teaching that addresses such topics as healthy lifestyles, risk-reducing behaviors, developmental needs, activities of daily living, and preventive self-care; Cognitive Level: Applying; Client Need: Physiological Integrity; Client Need Sub: Reduction of Risk Potential; Nursing/Integrated Concepts: Nursing Process: Implementation/Teaching/Learning

11. **2.** If the newborn's temperature drops below 36.1°C (97°F), the nurse should remove all newborn's clothing except for the diaper first, then place the newborn under the radiant warmer. Removal of all clothing except the diaper happens before placing the newborn under the radiant warmer. The control probe is fastened onto the newborn's anterior abdominal wall once the newborn is under the radiant warmer. The newborn has a low temperature and needs to be placed under the radiant warmer. Double-wrapping outside the warmer is appropriate once the temperature has reached 37°C (98.6°F).

QSEN Standard: V. B. 2. Demonstrate effective use of strategies to reduce risk of harm to self or others; ANA Standard: 5. 6. Provides holistic care that addresses the needs of diverse populations across the lifespan; Cognitive Level: Applying; Client Need: Health Promotion and Maintenance; Nursing/Integrated Concepts: Nursing Process: Implementation

12. **1.** Turn the phototherapy lights off while the blood is drawn to ensure accurate serum bilirubin levels. The newborn should be weighed once per day, but this does not need to be done before the bilirubin level is drawn. The eye patches should be removed every 8 hours, but removal is not necessary before the test. Repositioning can occur after the blood has been drawn for the bilirubin level.

QSEN Standard: V. B. 2. Demonstrate effective use of strategies to reduce risk of harm to self or others; ANA Standard: 5. 6. Provides holistic care that addresses the needs of diverse populations across the lifespan; Cognitive Level: Applying; Client Need: Physiological Integrity; Client Need Sub: Reduction of Risk Potential; Nursing/Integrated Concepts: Nursing Process: Implementation

Chapter 15

1. **2.** The use of an assistive device to ambulate is an indication of increased risk for falling. Wearing eyeglasses does not increase a client's risk for falling. The specific diagnosis of diabetes does not increase a client's risk for falling. Hypertension is not identified as increasing a client's risk for falling. Orthostatic hypotension and syncope would increase the risk.

QSEN Standard: V.B. 4. Communicate observations or concerns related to hazards and errors to patients, families, and the health care team; ANA Standard: 2. 4. Identifies actual or potential risks to the patient's health and safety or barriers to health, which may include but are not limited to interpersonal, systematic, or environmental circumstances; Cognitive Level: Applying; Client Need: Safe and Effective Care Environment; Client Need Sub: Safety and Infection Control; Nursing/Integrated Concepts: Nursing Process: Planning

2. **4.** Nothing should be inserted into the client's mouth during a seizure. A padded tongue blade should not be at the bedside. Oxygen setup with flowmeter should be present because it may be needed to oxygenate the client after a seizure. Side rails should be padded to reduce the client's risk of injury if having a seizure while in bed. Suctioning may be needed to prevent aspiration of oral secretions.

QSEN Standard: V.B. 4. Communicate observations or concerns related to hazards and errors to patients, families, and the health care team; ANA Standard: 2. 4. Identifies actual or potential risks to the patient's health and safety or barriers to health, which may include but are not limited to interpersonal, systematic, or environmental circumstances; Cognitive Level: Applying; Client Need: Safe and Effective Care

Environment; Client Need Sub: Safety and Infection Control; Nursing/Integrated Concepts: Nursing Process: Implementation/Communication and Documentation

3. **1.** A throw rug could cause the client to trip and fall, particularly if using an assistive device to ambulate after major joint replacement surgery. Handrails should be present around the toilet and bathtub and mounted securely along stairways. A method to call for help, such as a telephone, should be present and functioning in the home.

QSEN Standard: V.B. 4. Communicate observations or concerns related to hazards and errors to patients, families, and the health care team; ANA Standard: 2. 4. Identifies actual or potential risks to the patient's health and safety or barriers to health, which may include but are not limited to interpersonal, systematic, or environmental circumstances; Cognitive Level: Applying; Client Need: Safe and Effective Care Environment; Client Need Sub: Safety and Infection Control; Nursing/Integrated Concepts: Nursing Process: Implementation/Communication and Documentation

4. **1.** Devices that require a high current should be plugged directly into a separate outlet, not attached through an extension cord. Because equipment with frayed cords has been tagged for removal, this situation does not still need to be addressed. Healthcare facilities do not allow the use of tobacco products or smoking in the facility. This is appropriately communicated throughout the facility through the use of No Smoking signs. Devices that require a high current should be plugged directly into a separate outlet, so no further action is needed.

QSEN Standard: V.B. 2. Demonstrate effective use of strategies to reduce risk of harm to self or others; ANA Standard: 2. 4. Identifies actual or potential risks to the patient's health and safety or barriers to health, which may include but are not limited to interpersonal, systematic, or environmental circumstances; Cognitive Level: Applying; Client Need: Safe and Effective Care Environment; Client Need Sub: Safety and Infection Control; Nursing/Integrated Concepts: Nursing Process: Evaluation

5. **1.** When using a safety monitoring device, the battery device and alarm sound should be tested every shift to ensure proper functioning. The top side rails should be raised. Raising all side rails is a form of physical restraint. The position and location of the leg band would be checked after the battery and alarm system are checked. Reminding the client to call for help to get out of bed should be the last thing that the nurse does before leaving the client's bedside.

QSEN Standard: V.B. 2. Demonstrate effective use of strategies to reduce risk of harm to self or others; ANA Standard: 5. 5. Utilizes evidence-based interventions and treatments specific to the diagnosis or problem; Cognitive Level: Applying; Client Need: Safe and Effective Care Environment; Client Need Sub: Safety and Infection Control; Nursing/Integrated Concepts: Nursing Process: Assessment

6. **4.** Range of motion should be provided to the restrained limb every 2 hr. A client in restraints should be assessed every 15 min, not every hour. Bony areas should be padded before applying a restraint. Food and fluids should be offered every 2, not 3, hours to the client in restraints.

QSEN Standard: V.B. 2. Demonstrate effective use of strategies to reduce risk of harm to self or others; ANA Standard: 5. 5. Utilizes evidence-based interventions and treatments specific to the diagnosis or problem; Cognitive Level: Applying; Client Need: Safe and Effective Care Environment; Client Need Sub: Safety and Infection Control; Nursing/Integrated Concepts: Nursing Process: Implementation

7. **1.** When using a vest restraint on a client in bed, the ties should be affixed to the bed frame. The ties of a vest restraint should not be affixed to the bed wheels, the upper side rails, or the lower side rails; these could move and tighten the restraint.

QSEN Standard: V.B. 2. Demonstrate effective use of strategies to reduce risk of harm to self or others; ANA Standard: 5. 5. Utilizes evidence-based interventions and treatments specific to the diagnosis or problem; Cognitive Level: Applying; Client Need: Safe and Effective Care Environment; Client Need Sub: Safety and Infection Control; Nursing/Integrated Concepts: Nursing Process: Implementation

8. **1.** If a change in status of a restrained extremity is assessed, the first thing to do is to remove the restraint. The extremity should be massaged after the restraint is removed. The extremity would be elevated after it is massaged. Requesting a different type of restraint is the last action for the nurse to take.

QSEN Standard: V.B. 2. Demonstrate effective use of strategies to reduce risk of harm to self or others; ANA Standard: 5. 5. Utilizes evidence-based interventions and treatments specific to the diagnosis or problem; Cognitive Level: Applying; Client Need: Safe and Effective Care Environment; Client Need Sub: Safety and Infection Control; Nursing/Integrated Concepts: Nursing Process: Implementation

Chapter 16

1. **1.** Pooled exudate is not cultured. These secretions contain a mixture of contaminants that are not the same as those causing the infection. The sample should be collected from the base of the wound. Microorganisms most likely to be responsible for a wound infection reside in viable tissue. The inner ampule containing the medium for organism growth is to be crushed to ensure that the swab with the specimen is surrounded by culture medium. The specimen tube should be opened and the cap placed upside down on a firm, dry surface so that the inside will not become contaminated.

QSEN Standard: V.B. 6. Participate appropriately in analyzing errors and designing system improvements; ANA Standard: 6. 7. Actively participates in assessing

and assuring the responsible and appropriate use of interventions in order to minimize unwarranted or unwanted treatment and patient suffering; Cognitive Level: Analyzing; Client Need: Safe and Effective Care Environment; Client Need Sub: Safety and Infection Control; Nursing/Integrated Concepts: Nursing Process: Evaluation

2. **3.** When securing the bulb, the bulb should be below the level of the wound to facilitate drainage. When caring for a Jackson-Pratt drain, the plug is inserted into the emptying port, the ends of the emptying port are cleansed, and the bulb is to be compressed with the port open.

QSEN Standard: V.B. 6. Participate appropriately in analyzing errors and designing system improvements; ANA Standard: 6. 7. Actively participates in assessing and assuring the responsible and appropriate use of interventions in order to minimize unwarranted or unwanted treatment and patient suffering; Cognitive Level: Analyzing; Client Need: Safe and Effective Care Environment; Client Need Sub: Safety and Infection Control; Nursing/Integrated Concepts: Nursing Process: Evaluation

3. **1.** The wound should be cleaned starting at the center and working toward the outside of the wound. A separate swab should be used for each stroke and should be discarded after use. Hydrogen peroxide is not used on acute wounds because it dries the wound bed. When cleaning a wound, sterile gloves are applied before picking up a pair of forceps.

QSEN Standard: V.B. 2. Demonstrate effective use of strategies to reduce risk of harm to self or others; ANA Standard: 5. 5. Utilizes evidence-based interventions and treatments specific to the diagnosis or problem; Cognitive Level: Applying; Client Need: Safe and Effective Care Environment; Client Need Sub: Safety and Infection Control; Nursing/Integrated Concepts: Nursing Process: Implementation

4. **1.** If the older dressing adheres to the suture line, wet it with sterile normal saline. The dressing should not be pulled off. Tape, not the dressing, is removed by pulling it toward the wound. Picking the dressing off could cause severe pain and may injure the suture line. Pulling away from the wound puts strain on the suture line.

QSEN Standard: V.B. 2. Demonstrate effective use of strategies to reduce risk of harm to self or others; ANA Standard: 5. 5. Utilizes evidence-based interventions and treatments specific to the diagnosis or problem; Cognitive Level: Applying; Client Need: Safe and Effective Care Environment; Client Need Sub: Safety and Infection Control; Nursing/Integrated Concepts: Nursing Process: Implementation

5. **2.** Moistened fluffed gauze should be pressed lightly into the depressions in the wound. Only the edges of the dressing should be taped. A moist sterile 4 × 8 pad should be applied over the wet fluffed gauze. Sterile normal saline solution is poured onto the gauze pads, not into the wound. The gauze is not applied first and then saturated.

QSEN Standard: V.B. 2. Demonstrate effective use of strategies to reduce risk of harm to self or others; ANA Standard: 5. 5. Utilizes evidence-based interventions and treatments specific to the diagnosis or problem; Cognitive Level: Applying; Client Need: Safe and Effective Care Environment; Client Need Sub: Safety and Infection Control; Nursing/Integrated Concepts: Nursing Process: Implementation

6. **3.** The bandage should be terminated above, not at, the joint, with two circular turns. The bandage should be anchored with two circular turns. The bandage should be carried above the joint, around it, and then below it, making a figure eight. The previous turns should be overlapped by two thirds of the width of the bandage.

QSEN Standard: V.B. 2. Demonstrate effective use of strategies to reduce risk of harm to self or others; ANA Standard: 5B. 3. Seeks opportunities for feedback and evaluation of the effectiveness of the strategies used; Cognitive Level: Analyzing; Client Need: Safe and Effective Care Environment; Client Need Sub: Safety and Infection Control; Nursing/Integrated Concepts: Nursing Process: Evaluation/Teaching/Learning

7. **2.** The dressing should be changed if a white blister appears under the dressing. A hydrocolloid dressing is changed every 3–4 days. Silk tape to window frame the dressing is appropriate and does not indicate that the dressing needs to be changed. The dressing should be placed one third above the wound and two thirds below the wound; this increases the absorption capacity of the dressing.

QSEN Standard: III.B. 3. Base individualized care plan on patient values, clinical expertise, and evidence; ANA Standard: 1. 8. Uses appropriate evidence-based assessment techniques and instruments and tools; Cognitive Level: Analyzing; Client Need: Safe and Effective Care Environment; Client Need Sub: Safety and Infection Control; Nursing/Integrated Concepts: Nursing Process: Assessment

8. **2.** The new dressing should be "walked on" starting at one edge of the area and gently laying the dressing down, keeping it free of wrinkles. Skin prep should be applied to the surrounding tissue and not directly on the wound since this agent contains alcohol. The dressing should have a 3.8-cm (1 ½-in.) margin beyond the wound edges to ensure coverage of the entire wound area. Hydrogen peroxide is too drying. The wound should be cleansed with sterile normal saline.

QSEN Standard: V.B. 2. Demonstrate effective use of strategies to reduce risk of harm to self or others; ANA Standard: 5. 5. Utilizes evidence-based interventions and treatments specific to the diagnosis or problem; Cognitive Level: Applying; Client Need: Safe and Effective Care Environment; Client Need Sub: Safety and Infection Control; Nursing/Integrated Concepts: Nursing Process: Implementation

9. **3.** Black foam has larger pores and is used to stimulate granulation tissue and wound contraction, so this is what the nurse would assess. White, not black, foam is used for wounds that are tunneled wounds, superficial wounds, or shallow chronic ulcers.

QSEN Standard: III.B. 3. Base individualized care plan on patient values, clinical expertise, and evidence; ANA Standard: 1. 8. Uses appropriate evidence-based assessment techniques and instruments and tools; Cognitive Level: Applying; Client Need: Safe and Effective Care Environment; Client Need Sub: Safety and Infection Control; Nursing/Integrated Concepts: Nursing Process: Assessment

10. **3.** To prevent further skin damage, the client should be positioned off the reddened area. Reddened skin areas are not massaged. Massaging can lead to deep tissue trauma. Hot water can further injure the skin. The head of the bed should be maintained at the lowest degree of elevation that is consistent with the client's medical problem. Below 30 degrees is the most desirable.

QSEN Standard: III.B. 3. Base individualized care plan on patient values, clinical expertise, and evidence; ANA Standard: 5. 5. Utilizes evidence-based interventions and treatments specific to the diagnosis or problem; Cognitive Level: Applying; Client Need: Safe and Effective Care Environment; Client Need Sub: Safety and Infection Control; Nursing/Integrated Concepts: Nursing Process: Implementation

11. **2.** Lying prone and contracting the gluteal muscles extends the stump to prevent the development of a hip contracture. Pressing the stump into a padded surface reduces pain and prepares the stump for a prosthesis; it does not help resolve a contracture. Placing the stump on a pillow encourages the development of a hip contracture. Squeezing a pillow placed between the thighs encourages hip adduction but does not help resolve a contracture.

QSEN Standard: V.B. 2. Demonstrate effective use of strategies to reduce risk of harm to self or others; ANA Standard: 5B. 1. Provides health teaching that addresses such topics as healthy lifestyles, risk-reducing behaviors, developmental needs, activities of daily living, and preventive self-care; Cognitive Level: Applying; Client Need: Health Promotion and Maintenance; Nursing/Integrated Concepts: Nursing Process: Implementation/Teaching/Learning

12. **1.** The tunneled areas need to be irrigated, so the nurse would flush the wound. The catheter is not removed until the irrigation solution becomes clear. Irrigation would not occur if the irrigating solution is simply poured over the wound. The catheter should not be forced since this could cause tissue damage.

QSEN Standard: III.B. 3. Base individualized care plan on patient values, clinical expertise, and evidence; ANA Standard: 5. 5. Utilizes evidence-based interventions and treatments specific to the diagnosis or problem; Cognitive Level: Applying; Client Need: Safe and Effective Care Environment; Client Need Sub: Safety and Infection Control; Nursing/Integrated Concepts: Nursing Process: Implementation

Appendix B
Guidelines for Laboratory and Diagnostic Assessment

Explain to the patient (or parent) the diagnostic test and type of specimen needed for the test. Follow specific procedures for specimen collection, or steps of the diagnostic test. Communicate these steps with the patient (or parent) and other interdisciplinary team members caring for the patient as appropriate.

Laboratory Test Guidelines

- Follow facility procedures.

- Observe strict aseptic technique when collecting specimen. Keep the outside of the specimen container clean.

- Collect the correct amount of specimen required for the test.

- Clearly label all specimen containers, including patient information, date, and time specimen collected, as well as any medications the patient is taking that may influence the test results.

- Note significant information about the patient relative to the lab test on the lab slip.

- If the patient needs to be NPO before the specimen is collected, instruct the patient not to eat or drink anything until after the specimen has been collected.

- For 24-hr specimens, follow specific procedures to maintain the specific cumulative specimen.

- For the specimen collected, send the specimen to the lab in an appropriate container and in a timely manner.

Diagnostic Test Guidelines

- Follow facility policies and procedures specific for the diagnostic test.

- Verify signed informed consent has been obtained from the patient and the form is located in the front of the medical record.

- If the patient needs to be NPO before the diagnostic test, instruct the patient not to eat or drink anything until after the diagnostic test is completed.

- Encourage the patient to void before the diagnostic test begins unless a full bladder is recommended.

- Ask the patient about any allergies to iodine, seafood, dye, or latex and verify this information in the medical record, if available. Communicate any allergies to the healthcare provider and others who will assist during the diagnostic test.

- Monitor vital signs before and after the diagnostic test, as prescribed.

- If the patient has been premedicated for the diagnostic test, maintain his or her safety.

Nursing Guidelines

- Explain all procedures to the patient (or parent) and answer any questions before the procedure begins. Discuss how the patient can participate.

- Explain why the test is being done and how the results will be used in planning further care or treatments.

- Assess the test results when available.
  - Compare the test results to reference values or expected values (these values may vary with equipment and calibration; may also vary by facility and lab/reference used).
  - If test results are critical (panic) values above or below the reference range of expected results or if they indicate an abnormality, notify the healthcare provider (or follow facility policy).

- Serial lab results should be assessed and monitored for value-trends.

Supplies Used to Collect and Contain Specimens for Laboratory Tests

- Cotton swabs (sterile) for wound or tissue swabs
- Glass slides and covers for smears
- Sterile glass containers for blood tests and sterile plastic containers for cultures
- Collection containers, including for urine, feces, sputum, and mucus
- Flat wooden sticks for collecting specimen
- Small plastic containers and strips (unsterile) to collect specimens for bedside testing

Types of Specimens Collected for Laboratory Tests

- Blood
- Urine
- Spinal fluid
- Feces
- Sputum
- Body fluids

Blood Specimens

Blood clots shortly after being obtained and leaves the blood serum separate. Most blood tests are done using the serum part of blood. If the specific test needs all components of blood to run the test, there must be an *anticoagulant* in the test collection tube to stop the blood from clotting. This is why blood collection tube stoppers are color coded, so the colors indicate whether the tube is to collect blood for the blood serum or whether the tube contains an anticoagulant to prevent clotting of the blood specimen. The list below provides examples of color-coded stopper collection tubes and types of tests that can be done with them.

Color Coded Stoppers of Blood Collection Tubes

Red top	Electrolytes, proteins, enzymes, lipids, hormones, drug levels, blood bank tests
Lavender top	CBC, chemistries
Gray top	Glucose tests
Blue top	Coagulation studies PT, PTT
Green top	ABGs, lupus erythematosus tests

Considerations for Blood Specimen Collection

Site	Venous blood is most often used for blood tests.
	Arms, hands, and fingersticks are frequently used to collect venous blood, and legs and feet are not used, if possible, to avoid circulation complications.
	Heel-stick tests of a newborn can be done for capillary blood samples.
	When blood is in the tube, use a gentle mixing motion, but *do not shake it*.
	Arterial blood is used for arterial blood gases tests.
	The radial artery is frequently the site of collection for arterial blood.
Time of collection	The best time for routine blood collection for tests is before breakfast.
	Fingerstick blood is used for accuchecks as prescribed, usually before meals and at bedtime.
Drug interference	Some medications can affect certain lab results.
	Include medication information on the specimen order slip.
Labeling	Each collection tube must be labeled, including patient's name, age, healthcare provider, room number, date, and time blood collected, and any other pertinent additional information.
Time	Blood collection tubes must get to the lab in a timely way in order to obtain accurate results.

References

Chapter 1

AHRQ. Agency for Healthcare Research and Quality. (2014). *Preventing Falls in Hospitals. Tool 3F: Orthostatic Vital Sign Measurement*. Retrieved from http://www.ahrq.gov/professionals/systems/hospital/fallpxtoolkit/fallpxtk-tool3f.html

American Academy of Ophthalmology. (2016). *Procedures for the Evaluation of the Visual System by Pediatricians: Clinical Report - 2016*. Retrieved from https://www.google.com/search?q=American+Academy+of+Ophthalmology.+(2016).+Procedures+for+the+Evaluation+of+the+Visual+System+by+Pediatricians%3A+Clinical+Report+-+2016&rlz=1C1QJDB_enUS610US620&oq=American+Academy+of+Ophthalmology.+(2016).+Procedures+for+the+Evaluation+of+the+Visual+System+by+Pediatricians%3A+Clinical+Report+-+2016&aqs=chrome..69i57.2659j0j8&sourceid=chrome&ie=UTF-8

American Cancer Society. (2015). *Do I Have Testicular Cancer?* Retrieved from http://www.cancer.org/cancer/testicularcancer/moreinformation/doihavetesticularcancer/do-i-have-testicular-cancer-self-exam.html

American Heart Association. (2017). *Monitoring Your Blood Pressure at Home*. Retrieved from http://www.heart.org/HEARTORG/Conditions/HighBloodPressure/KnowYourNumbers/Monitoring-Your-Blood-Pressure-at-Home_UCM_301874_Article.jsp#.WNFY2KJJlFY

Centers for Disease Control (CDC). (2014). *Non-Contact Temperature Measurement Devices: Considerations for Use in Port of Entry Screening Activities*. Retrieved from http://wwwnc.cdc.gov/travel/files/ebola-non-contact-temperature-measurement-guidance.pdf?action=NotFound&controller=Utility

Centers for Disease Control (CDC). (2015). *STEADI Stopping Elderly Accidents, Deaths & Injuries*. Retrieved from http://www.cdc.gov/steadi/patient.html

MedlinePlus. (2015). *U.S. National Library of Medicine, Breast Self-Exam*. Retrieved from https://www.nlm.nih.gov/medlineplus/ency/article/001993.htm

Medscape. (2015). *Normal Vital Signs*. Retrieved from http://emedicine.medscape.com/article/2172054-overview

NPR. (2014). *How a No-Touch Thermometer Detects a Fever*. Retrieved from http://www.npr.org/sections/health-shots/2014/10/15/356398102/how-a-no-touch-thermometer-detects-a-fever

U.S. Department of Health & Human Services. (2015). *Head Start. Tips for Keeping Children Safe: A Developmental Guide*. Retrieved from https://eclkc.ohs.acf.hhs.gov/hslc/tta-system/health/safety-injury-prevention/safe-healthy-environments/keep-children-safe.html#toddlers

World Health Organization (WHO). (2014). *WHO Interim Guidance for Ebola Virus Disease: Exit Screening at Airports, Ports, and Land Crossing*. Retrieved from http://apps.who.int/iris/bitstream/10665/139691/1/WHO_EVD_Guidance_PoE_14.2_eng.pdf

Chapter 2

American Academy of Dermatology (AAD). (2015). *Head lice: Overview, Symptoms, Causes, Treatment, Tips*. Retrieved from https://www.aad.org/public/diseases/contagious-skin-diseases/head-lice

American Dental Association (ADA). (2016). *Mouth Healthy. Flossing*. Retrieved from http://www.mouthhealthy.org/en/az-topics/f/flossing

American Diabetes Association. (2016). *Insulin & Other Injectables*. Retrieved from http://www.diabetes.org/living-with-diabetes/treatment-and-care/medication/insulin/?loc=lwd-slabnav

Centers for Disease Control and Prevention (CDC). (2015). *Epidemiology and Prevention of Vaccine-Preventable Diseases. The Pink Book. Vaccine Administration*. Retrieved from http://www.cdc.gov/vaccines/pubs/pinkbook/vac-admin.html

Centers for Disease Control and Prevention (CDC). (2015). *Parasites – Lice – Head Lice*. Retrieved from http://www.cdc.gov/parasites/lice/head/treatment.html

Community Hospitals of Indiana, Inc. (2016). *Medical Staff Policies & Procedures. Medication Orders*. Retrieved from https://www.ecommunity.com/sites/default/files/uploads/2016-09/chs_medication_orders.pdf

Grosch, S. (2015). *Improving Patient Safety and Cutting Costs with Healthcare Automation. Swisslog Healthcare Solutions*. Retrieved from http://docplayer.net/3496160-Improving-patient-safety-and-cutting-costs-with-healthcare-automation.html

Hettinger, D., & Jurkovich, P. (2013). *Featured EBP Project – June 2013. Evidence-based injection practice: To aspirate or not*. Retrieved from National Nursing Practice Network website: http://www.nnpnetwork.org/staff-nurses/latest-news/newsitem?nid=52

Institute for Safe Medication Practices. (2013). *Acute Care Medication Safety Alert, Independent Double Checks: Undervalued and Misused: Selective Use of This Strategy Can Play an Important Role in Medication Safety*. Retrieved from https://www.ismp.org/newsletters/acutecare/showarticle.aspx?id=51

Institute for Safe Medication Practices. (2014). *Reporting a medication or vaccine error or hazard to ISMP*. Retrieved from https://www.ismp.org/errorReporting/reportErrortoISMP.aspx

Institute for Safe Medication Practices. (2014). *List of High-Alert Medications in Acute Care Settings*. Retrieved from http://www.ismp.org/Tools/institutionalhighAlert.asp

Institute for Safe Medication Practices. (2015). *Oral Dosage Forms That Should Not Be Crushed 2015*. Retrieved from http://www.ismp.org/tools/donotcrush.pdf

Just Nebulizers. (2016). *Tips & Advice Center: Breathing Treatments & Kids*. Retrieved from http://justnebulizers.com/breathing-treatments-and-kids/

Occupational Safety and Health Administration (OSHA). (2015). *U.S. Department of Labor. Regulations (Standards – 29-CFR). Part Title: Occupational Safety and Health*

Standards. Title: Bloodborne Pathogens. Retrieved from https://www.osha.gov/pls/oshaweb/owadisp.show_document?p_table=FEDERAL_REGISTER&p_id=16265

Office on Women's Health, U.S. Department of Health and Human Services. (2015). *ePublications. Douching fact sheet.* Retrieved from http://womenshealth.gov/publications/our-publications/fact-sheet/douching.html

The Joint Commission. (2016). *The Joint Commission. Facts about the Official "Do Not Use" List of Abbreviations.* Retrieved from https://www.jointcommission.org/facts_about_do_not_use_list/

The Joint Commission. (2016). *The Joint Commission. Hospital National Patient Safety Goals Effective January 1, 2016. Hospital Accreditation Program.* Retrieved from http://www.jointcommission.org/assets/1/6/2016_NPSG_HAP_ER.pdf

National Eye Institute. (2015). *Facts about color blindness.* Retrieved from https://nei.nih.gov/health/color_blindness/facts_about

New Health Advisor. (2016). *10 Rights of Medication Administration.* Retrieved from http://www.newhealthadvisor.com/10-Rights-of-Medication-Administration.html

U.S. Food and Drug Administration (FDA). (2014). *U.S. Department of Health and Human Services. Medical Devices. A Guide to Bed Safety Bed Rails in Hospitals, Nursing Homes and Home Health Care: The Facts.* Retrieved from http://www.fda.gov/medicaldevices/productsandmedicalprocedures/generalhospitaldevicesandsupplies/hospitalbeds/ucm123676.htm

U.S. Food and Drug Administration. (2015). *U.S. Department of Health and Human Services. Medical Gloves.* Retrieved from http://www.fda.gov/MedicalDevices/ProductsandMedicalProcedures/GeneralHospitalDevicesandSupplies/PersonalProtectiveEquipment/ucm056077.htm

U.S. National Library of Medicine. (2014). *DailyMed. Nitrostat – nitroglycerin tablet.* Retrieved from https://dailymed.nlm.nih.gov/dailymed/drugInfo.cfm?setid=79ba021e-183c-4b4d-822e-4ff5ef54ca61

U.S. National Library of Medicine. (2014). *Medline Plus. Skin care and incontinence.* Retrieved from https://www.nlm.nih.gov/medlineplus/ency/article/003976.htm

U.S. National Library of Medicine. (2014). *Medline Plus. Wearing gloves in the hospital.* Retrieved from https://www.nlm.nih.gov/medlineplus/ency/patientinstructions/000452.htm

Chapter 3

Centers for Disease Control and Prevention (CDC). (2015). *National Health Statistics Report. Number 79. Trends in the Use of Complementary Health Approaches Among Adults: United States, 2002–2012.* Retrieved from http://www.cdc.gov/nchs/data/nhsr/nhsr079.pdf

Medscape News & Perspective. (2016). *New APS Guideline on Postoperative Pain. Medscape. Feb 26, 2016.* Retrieved from http://www.medscape.com/viewarticle/859492

Merkel, S. I., Voepel-Lewis, T., Shayevitz, J. R., & Malviya, S. (1997). The FLACC: A behavioral scale for scoring postoperative pain in young children. *Pediatric Nursing, 23*(3), 293–297.

Morrow, C. Reducing neonatal pain during routine heel lance procedures. *American Journal of Maternal Child Nursing, 35*(6), 346-354.

National Hospice and Palliative Care Organization (NHPCO). (2015). *NHPCO's Facts and Figures Hospice Care in America 2015 Edition.* Retrieved from https://webcache.googleusercontent.com/search?q=cache:t9KFylfsg3kJ;https://www.nhpco.org/sites/default/files/public/Statistics_Research/2015_Facts_Figures.pdf+&cd=1&hl=en&ct=clnk&gl=us

The Joint Commission (TJC). (2016). *Pain Management. Joint Commission Statement on Pain Management.* Retrieved from https://www.jointcommission.org/topics/pain_management.aspx

Chapter 4

American Association of Kidney Patients (AAKP). (2016). *The Facts of Peritoneal Dialysis.* Retrieved from https://aakp.org/dialysis/the-facts-of-peritoneal-dialysis/

Cafasso. J. (2015). *Urinary catheters: What are urinary catheters?* Retrieved from http://www.healthline.com/health/urinary-catheters#Overview1

Global Business Media. (2014). *Special Report: Managing constipation in the elderly.* Retrieved from https://issuu.com/globalbusinessmedia.org/docs/special_report_25_-_managing_consti

Health Communities.com. (2014). *Constipation in older adults.* Retrieved from http://www.healthcommunities.com/constipation/older-adults-elderly-constipation.shtml

Johns Hopkins Medicine. (2016). *Colostomy.* Retrieved from http://www.hopkinsmedicine.org/healthlibrary/test_procedures/gastroenterology/colostomy_92,p07727/

Kopac. M. (2014). Formula estimation of appropriate urinary catheter size in children. *Journal of Pediatric Intensive Care.* Retrieved from http://content.iospress.com/download/journal-of-pediatric-intensive-care/pic069?id=journal-of-pediatric-intensive-care%2Fpic069

MedlinePlus. U.S. National Library of Medicine. (2014). *Urostomy—stoma and skin care.* Retrieved from https://www.nlm.nih.gov/medlineplus/ency/patientinstructions/000477.htm

MedlinePlus. U.S. National Library of Medicine. (2015). *Suprapubic catheter care.* Retrieved from https://www.nlm.nih.gov/medlineplus/ency/patientinstructions/000145.htm

National Institute of Diabetes and Digestive and Kidney Diseases. U.S. Department of Health and Human Services. (2013). *Urinary diversion.* Retrieved from http://www.niddk.nih.gov/health-information/health-topics/urologic-disease/urinary-diversion/Pages/facts.aspx

National Kidney Foundation. (2016a). *African Americans and kidney disease.* Retrieved from https://www.kidney.org/news/newsroom/factsheets/African-Americans-and-CKD

National Kidney Foundation. (2016b). *Peritoneal dialysis: What you need to know.* Retrieved from https://www.kidney.org/atoz/content/peritoneal

Schuster, B., Kosar, L., & Kamrul, R. (2015). Constipation in older adults: Stepwise approach to keep things moving. *Canadian Family Physician.* Retrieved from http://www.cfp.ca/content/61/2/152.full

WebMD. (2014). *Care for an indwelling urinary catheter – Topic overview.* Retrieved from http://www.webmd.com/a-to-z-guides/care-for-an-indwelling-urinary-catheter-topic-overview

Chapter 5

Centers for Disease Control and Prevention (CDC). (2016). *National healthcare safety network (NHSN) overview.* Retrieved from http://www.cdc.gov/nhsn/pdfs/pscmanual/pcsmanual_current.pdf

EMedicineHealth. (2016). *Venous access devices*. Retrieved from http://www.emedicinehealth.com/venous_access_devices/article_em.htm

Ford, J. (2016). *Infusion therapy—requirements for flow control*. Retrieved from http://medidex.com/research/839-iv-pump-requirements.html

Goossens, G. A. (2015). Flushing and locking of venous catheters: Available evidence and evidence deficit. *Nursing Research and Practice*. Retrieved from http://www.hindawi.com/journals/nrp/2015/985686/

Infusion Nurse. (2015). Q&A: Dial-a-flow tubing. [Web blog comment]. Retrieved from https://infusionnurse.org/2015/09/08/qa-dial-a-flow-tubing/

Kienle, P. (2014). *Let's get clinical! Best practices for determining appropriate hang time for IV fluids*. Cardinal Health. Retrieved from http://www.cardinalhealth.com/en/thought-leadership/iv-fluid-hang-time.html

Kolecki, P. (2016). *Hypovolemic Shock Treatment & Management*. Retrieved from http://emedicine.medscape.com/article/760145-treatment

Med League. (2015). *Infusion therapy (IV) complications: Infiltration vs. extravasation*. Retrieved from http://www.medleague.com/infusion-therapy-iv-complications-infiltration-vs-extravasation/

MedlinePlus. (2014). *Heart failure—fluids and diuretics*. Retrieved from https://www.nlm.nih.gov/medlineplus/ency/patientinstructions/000112.htm

Medtronic. (2016). *Questions and answers – Drug pumps. Chronic pain*. Retrieved from http://www.medtronic.com/us-en/patients/treatments-therapies/drug-pump-cancer-pain/getting-the-device/questions-answers.html

Molin, D. (2016). Normal saline versus heparin solution to lock totally implanted venous access devices: Results from a multicenter randomized trial. *European Journal of Oncology Nursing 21*, 272–273.

The Joint Commission (TJC). (2013). *CVC maintenance bundles*. Retrieved from https://www.jointcommission.org/assets/1/6/CLABSI_Toolkit_Tool_3-22_CVC_Maintenance_Bundles.pdf

The Joint Commission (TJC). (2016). CLABSI Toolkit–Chapter 3. *CLABSI prevention strategies, techniques, and technologies*. Retrieved from https://www.jointcommission.org/topics/clabsi_toolkit__chapter_3.aspx

The Joint Commission (TJC). (2016). 2016 *Hospital national patient safety goals*. Retrieved from https://www.jointcommission.org/assets/1/6/2016_NPSG_HAP_ER.pdf

U.S. Food and Drug Administration (FDA). (2016). *General hospital devices and supplies. Infusion pumps*. Retrieved from http://www.fda.gov/MedicalDevices/ProductsandMedicalProcedures/GeneralHospitalDevicesandSupplies/InfusionPumps/

Wang, R., Zhang, M. G., Luo, O., He, L., Li, J. X., Tang, Y. J., … Chen, X. Z. (2015). *Heparin saline versus normal saline for flushing and locking peripheral venous catheters in decompensated liver cirrhosis patients: A randomized controlled trial*. Retrieved from https://www.ncbi.nlm.nih.gov/pubmed/26252305

Wayne, G. (2016). *Intravenous (IV) therapy technique. Nurseslabs*. Retrieved from http://nurseslabs.com/intravenous-iv-therapy-technique/

Chapter 6

Arrowsmith, V. A., & Taylor, R. (2014, August 4). *Removal of nail polish and finger rings to prevent surgical infection*. Abstract retrieved from http://www.ncbi.nlm.nih.gov/pubmed/25089848

Association for Professionals in Infection Control and Epidemiology. (2016). *Follow the rules for standard and isolation precautions*. Retrieved from http://professionals.site.apic.org/10-ways-to-protect-patients/follow-the-rules-for-isolation-precautions/

Centers for Disease Control and Prevention (CDC). (2013). *Handwashing: Clean hands save lives*. Retrieved from http://www.cdc.gov/handwashing

Centers for Disease Control and Prevention (CDC). (2014). *Ebola (Ebola Virus Disease). Procedures for Safe Handling and Management of Ebola-Associated Waste*. Retrieved from http://www.cdc.gov/vhf/ebola/healthcare-us/cleaning/handling-waste.html

Centers for Disease Control and Prevention (CDC). (2014). Healthcare Infection Control Practices Advisory Committee (HICPAC). *2007 Guideline for Isolation Precautions: Preventing Transmission of Infectious Agents in Healthcare Settings*. Retrieved from http://www.cdc.gov/hicpac/2007IP/2007ip_appendA.html

Centers for Disease Control and Prevention (CDC). (2015). NIOSH. The National Personal Protective Technology Laboratory (NPPTL). *Respirator Trusted-Source Information. Section 3: Ancillary Respirator Information*. Retrieved from http://www.cdc.gov/niosh/npptl/topics/respirators/disp_part/respsource3healthcare.html

Centers for Disease Control and Prevention (CDC). (2015). Table 20. *Leading causes of death and numbers of deaths, by age: U.S., 1980-2014*. Retrieved from http://www.cdc.gov/nchs/data/hus/2015/020.pdf

Centers for Disease Control and Prevention (CDC). (2016). *Hand Hygiene in Healthcare Settings. Clean Hands Count for Healthcare Providers*. Retrieved from http://www.cdc.gov/handhygiene/providers/index.html

MedlinePlus. (2015). *Isolation precautions*. Retrieved from https//medlineplus.gov/ency/patientinstructions/000446.htm

MedlinePlus. (2016). *Personal protective equipment*. Retrieved from https://www.nlm.nih.gov/medlineplus/ency/patientinstructions/000447.htm

Montana State Hospital. (2016). *Guidelines for isolation precautions*. Retrieved from http://dphhs.mt.gov/Portals/85/amdd/documents/MSH/volumei/infectioncontrol/GuidelinesForIsolationPrecautions.pdf

Nurse.com. (2014). *Strong suits: CDCs personal protective equipment guidelines get revamp*. Retrieved from https://www.nurse.com/blog/2014/10/31/strong-suits-cdc%C2%92s-personal-protective-equipment-guidelines-get-revamp/

Rutala, W. A. (2015). University of North Carolina at Chapel Hill, USA. *Bloodborne Pathogen Standard, OSHA's Final Rule*. Retrieved from http://spiceducation.unc.edu/wp-content/uploads/2015/01/05-LTC-BBP14.ppt

San Francisco Department of Public Health. (2016). Communicable Disease Control and Prevention. *How to put on and remove a face mask*. Retrieved from http://www.sfcdcp.org/facemask.html

University of Kentucky HealthCare. (2014). University of Kentucky/UK HealthCare Policy and Procedure. *Policy #NU10-19*. Retrieved from http://www.hosp.uky.edu/policies/viewpolicy.asp?PolicyManual=8&PolicyID=1920

University of Kentucky Hospital Department of Nursing. (2016).

Orientation handbook for nursing faculty. Retrieved from https://ukhealthcare.uky.edu/uploadedFiles/physicians-providers/Nursing/nurse-education/nursing-faculty-orientation-handbook.pdf

U.S. Department of Health & Human Services, Agency for Healthcare Research and Quality (2014). *Electronic hand hygiene monitoring system significantly reduces health care–associated infections.* Retrieved from https://innovations.ahrq.gov/profiles/electronic-hand-hygiene-monitoring-system-significantly-reduces-health-care-associated

U. S. Food and Drug Administration (FDA). (2015). Personal Protective Equipment for Infection Control. *Masks and N95 respirators.* Retrieved from http://www.fda.gov/MedicalDevices/ProductsandMedicalProcedures/GeneralHospitalDevicesandSupplies/PersonalProtectiveEquipment/ucm055977.htm

Washington State Hospital Association. (2015). *Contact enteric precautions (in addition to standard precautions).* Retrieved from http://www.wsha.org/wp-content/uploads/Standardization_Updated_ContactEntericPrecautions-March-2015.pdf

Western University of Health Sciences. (2015). *Biohazardous waste and sharps disposal.* Retrieved from http://www.westernu.edu/bin/students/biohazardous-waste-policy.pdf

Chapter 7

Das, J. M. (2016). *Slideshare. ICP waveforms & monitoring. Intracranial pressure-waveforms and monitoring.* Retrieved from http://www.slideshare.net/joemdas/intracranial-pressure-waveforms-and-monitoring

Gupta, G., & Nosko, M. G. (2015). Intracranial pressure monitoring. In J. Miller (Ed.), *Medscape.* Retrieved from http://emedicine.medscape.com/article/1829950-overview

Jalali, R., & Rezaei, M. (2014). A comparison of the Glasgow Coma Scale Score with Full Outline of Unresponsiveness scale to predict patients' traumatic brain injury outcomes in intensive care units, *Critical Care Research and Practice* (vol. 2014, Article ID 289803). doi:10.1155/2014/289803

MedlinePlus. (2015). *Intracranial pressure monitoring.* Retrieved from https://

www.nlm.nih.gov/medlineplus/ency/article/003411.htm

National Health Service (NHS). (2013). *Lumbar puncture—How it is performed.* Retrieved from http://www.nhs.uk/conditions/Lumbar-puncture/Pages/How-it-is-performed.aspx

Queens University. (2014). School of Medicine. *Lumbar puncture.* Retrieved from https://meds.queensu.ca/central/assets/modules/lumbar_puncture/introduction.html

Chapter 8

American Diabetes Association (ADA). (2015). *Visiting your health care team.* Retrieved from http://www.diabetes.org/living-with-diabetes/treatment-and-care/whos-on-your-health-care-team/visiting-your-health-care.html

American Heart Association. (2016). *Symptoms, diagnosis & monitoring of diabetes.* Retrieved from http://www.heart.org/HEARTORG/Conditions/Diabetes/SymptomsDiagnosisMonitoringofDiabetes/Symptoms-Diagnosis-Monitoring-of-Diabetes_UCM_002035_Article.jsp#.V2v6GPkrJD8

HealthCentral. (2015). *Hypoglycemia (diabetic) & hyperglycemia.* Retrieved from http://www.healthcentral.com/encyclopedia/hc/hypoglycemia---hyperglycemia-3168893

MedlinePlus. (2015). *Capillary sample.* Retrieved from https://www.nlm.nih.gov/medlineplus/ency/article/003427.htm

Modern Medicine Network. (2014). *Afrezza, fast-acting, inhaled insulin, is approved.* Retrieved from http://drugtopics.modernmedicine.com/drug-topics/content/tags/afrezza/afrezza-fast-acting-inhaled-insulin-approved?page=full

National Center for Complementary and Integrative Health (NCCIH). (2016). *Complementary, alternative, or integrative health: What's in a name?* Retrieved from https://nccih.nih.gov/health/integrative-health

National Institute of Health. (2013). *What are complementary health approaches?* Retrieved from http://nihseniorhealth.gov/complementaryhealthapproaches/whatarecomplementaryhealthapproaches/01.html

Pittas, A. G. (2015). *Inhaled insulin therapy in diabetes mellitus.* Retrieved from http://www.uptodate.com/contents/inhaled-insulin-therapy-in-diabetes-mellitus

Thompson, D. (2015). *Nasal spray may treat diabetics' low blood sugar.* Retrieved from WebMD website: http://www.webmd.com/diabetes/news/20151218/nasal-spray-may-give-diabetics-faster-treatment-for-low-blood-sugar

University of Connecticut. (2016). Korey Stringer Institute. Emergency Conditions. *Hypo/Hyperglycemia.* Retrieved from http://ksi.uconn.edu/emergency-conditions/hypohyperglycemia

Chapter 9

American Academy of Nursing. (2014). *Immobility ambulation.* Retrieved from http://www.aannet.org/initiatives/choosing-wisely/immobility-ambulation

Medical Center Healthsystem. (2015). *Proper body mechanics.* Retrieved from http://medicalcenterhealthsystem.com/wp…/2015/…/Proper-Body-Mechanics

MedlinePlus. (2015). *Pulling a patient up in bed.* Retrieved from https://medlineplus.gov/ency/patientinstructions/000429.htm

National Institute for Occupational Safety and Health (NIOSH). Centers for Disease Control and Prevention (CDC). (2016). *Safe patient handling and movement (SPHM).* Retrieved from https://www.cdc.gov/niosh/topics/safepatient/

Occupational Safety and Health Administration (OSHA). U.S. Department of Labor. (2013). *Caring for our caregivers. Facts about hospital worker safety.* Retrieved from https://www.osha.gov/dsg/hospitals/documents/1.2_Factbook_508.pdf

Occupational Safety and Health Administration (OSHA). U.S. Department of Labor. (2014). *Safety and Health Topics. Healthcare. Safe patient handling.* Retrieved from https://www.osha.gov/SLTC/healthcarefacilities/safepatienthandling.html

Sharecare Inc. (2016). *What is a cast?* Retrieved from https://www.sharecare.com/health/broken-bones/what-is-cast

Southwestern Pennsylvania Healthcare Quality Unit (APS HCQU). (2015). *Body mechanics and back pain.* Retrieved from https://hcqu.kepro.com/content/overview/PACKET%20-%20Body%20Mechanics%20and%20Back%20Pain%20-%208.15.pdf

Zwerdling, D. (2015). *Even 'proper' technique exposes nurses' spines to dangerous forces*. Retrieved from http://www.npr.org/2015/02/11/383564180/even-proper-technique-exposes-nurses-spines-to-dangerous-forces

Chapter 10

American Association of Critical-Care Nurses (AACN). (2016). *AACN Practice Alert. Initial and Ongoing Verification of Feeding Tube Placement in Adults.* Retrieved from https://www.aacn.org/clinical-resources/practice-alerts/initial-and-ongoing-verification-of-feeding-tube-placement-in-adults

Amirlak, B., Amirlak, I., Awad, Z. T., & Forse, R. (2014). *Pneumothorax following feeding tube placement: Precaution and treatment.* Retrieved from https://www.researchgate.net/publication/230573733_Pneumothorax_Following_Feeding_Tube_Placement_Precaution_and_Treatment

Fessler, T. (2015). *Blenderized foods for home tube feeding: Learn about the benefits, risks, and strategies for success.* Retrieved from http://www.todaysdietitian.com/newarchives/011315p30.shtml

Healthline. (2013). *Nasogastric intubation and feeding.* Retrieved from http://www.healthline.com/health/nasogastric-intubation-and-feeding#Overview1

Healthline. (2014). *Parenteral nutrition. What is parenteral nutrition?* Retrieved from http://www.healthline.com/health/parenteral-nutrition#Overview1

Ipatenco, S. (2015). *List of foods with no salt.* Retrieved from http://www.livestrong.com/article/351637-list-of-foods-with-no-salt/

Klek, S. (2016). Omega-3 fatty acids in modern parenteral nutrition: A review of the current evidence. *Journal of Clinical Medicine, 5,* 34.

Lehman, S. (2016). *What you can eat on a mechanical soft diet.* Retrieved from https://www.verywell.com/what-you-can-eat-on-a-mechanical-soft-diet-2507158

Loo, Y. (2015). *Pneumothorax from nasogastric feeding tube in a patient with tracheostomy tube.* Retrieved from http://jaccr.com/pneumothorax-from-nasogastric-feeding-tube-in-a-patient-with-tracheostomy-tube/

Lund M. (2013). Integrative medicine embraces nutrition. *Today's Dietitian 15,* 2:26.

National Heart, Lung, and Blood Institute (NHLBI). (1998). *Clinical guidelines on the identification, evaluation,* and treatment of overweight and obesity in adults: The evidence report. Bethesda, MD: Author.

Nestlé Nutrition Institute. (2016). *MNA mini nutritional assessment.* Retrieved from http://www.mna-elderly.com/default.html

Shapiro, J. (2016). *Bland diet foods to eat and avoid.* Retrieved from http://www.doctorshealthpress.com/food-and-nutrition-articles/bland-diet-foods

U.S. Department of Health and Human Services. (2016). *Low sodium foods: Shopping list. Office of Disease Prevention and Health Promotion.* Retrieved from https://healthfinder.gov/HealthTopics/Category/health-conditions-and-diseases/heart-health/low-sodium-foods-shopping-list

Chapter 11

American Speech-Language-Hearing Association. (2016). Clinical Topics and Disorders. *Frequently asked questions (FAQ) about tracheotomy and swallowing.* Retrieved from http://www.asha.org/SLP/clinical/Frequently-Asked-Questions-on-Tracheotomy-and-Swallowing/

Brauner, M . (2015). *Thoracentesis.* Retrieved from http://emedicine.medscape.com/article/80640-overview#a2

Byrd, R. (2016). *Mechanical ventilation. Indications for mechanical ventilation.* Retrieved from http://emedicine.medscape.com/article/304068-overview#a3

Celli, B. (2015).*Chest physiotherapy.* Retrieved from https://www.merckmanuals.com/professional/pulmonary-disorders/pulmonary-rehabilitation/chest-physiotherapy

Family Practice Notebook. (2016). Emergency Medicine Book. *Nasopharyngeal airway.* Retrieved from http://www.fpnotebook.com/er/procedure/NsphrynglArwy.htm

Family Practice Notebook. (2016). Emergency Medicine Book. *Oropharyngeal airway.* Retrieved from http://www.fpnotebook.com/er/procedure/OrphrynglArwy.htm

Garg, S. (2013). Noninvasive ventilation in premature infants: Based on evidence or habit? *Journal of Clinical Neonatology.* 2(4),155–159.

George, R., & Papagiannopoulos, K. (2016). Advances in chest drain management in thoracic disease. *Journal Thoracic Disease.* 8(Suppl 1), S55–S64.

Krucik. G. (2014). *What is oxygen therapy?* Retrieved from http://www.healthline.com/health/oxygen-therapy#Overview1

MedlinePlus. (2015). *Using an incentive spirometer.* Retrieved from https://www.nlm.nih.gov/medlineplus/ency/patientinstructions/000451.htm

Neuspiel, D. (2015). *Peak flow rate measurement.* Retrieved from http://emedicine.medscape.com/article/1413347-overview

Novant Health. Rowan Medical Center. (2016). *Instructions for proper sputum collection.* Retrieved from https://www.novanthealth.org/rowan-medical-center/services/laboratory/laboratory-test-catalog/instructions-and-testing-materials/instructions-for-proper-sputum-collection.aspx

Nursing Reviews. (2011). *Chest physiotherapy (CPT).* Retrieved from http://currentnursing.com/reviews/chest_physiotherapy.html

Safe Care Campaign. (2015). *Ventilator associated pneumonia.* Retrieved from http://www.safecarecampaign.org/vap.html

Salmon, N. (2013). AMN Healthcare Education Services. *Chest tube management.* Retrieved from https://lms.rn.com/getpdf.php/1933.pdf

Underwood, C., & Weatherspoon, D. (2015). *Endotracheal intubation. What is endotracheal intubation?* Retrieved from http://www.healthline.com/health/endotracheal-intubation#overview1

Chapter 12

American Heart Association. (2015). *What is an automated external defibrillator?* Retrieved from https://www.heart.org/idc/groups/heart-public/@wcm/@hcm/documents/downloadable/ucm_300340.pdf

American Heart Association. (2015). *What is a pacemaker?* Retrieved from https://www.heart.org/idc/groups/heart-public/@wcm/@hcm/documents/downloadable/ucm_300451.pdf

American Red Cross. (2016). *Blood types.* Retrieved from http://www.redcrossblood.org/learn-about-blood/blood-types

Armstrong, D., & Meyr, A. (2015). *Compression therapy for the treatment of chronic venous insufficiency*. Retrieved from http://www.uptodate.com/contents/compression-therapy-for-the-treatment-of-chronic-venous-insufficiency

Balentine, J. (2015). *Blood transfusion*. Retrieved from http://www.medicinenet.com/blood_transfusion/article.htm

Chia. P., & Foo, D. (2015). A practical approach to perioperative management of cardiac implantable electronic devices. *Singapore Medical Journal*, 56(10), 538–541.

Christakou, A. (2015). *Effectiveness of early mobilization in hospitalized patients with deep venous thrombosis*. Retrieved from http://www.hospitalchronicles.gr/index.php/hchr/article/view/553

Health Communities. (2015). *Pulmonary embolism/ DVT. Compression stockings & blood clots*. Retrieved from http://www.healthcommunities.com/pulmonary-embolism-dvt/compression-stockings.shtml

Health Sciences Authority. (2014). *Blood components and their uses*. Retrieved from http://www.hsa.gov.sg/content/hsa/en/Blood_Services/Blood_Donation/Why_Should_I_Donate/Blood_Components_and_Their_Uses.html

Johns Hopkins Medicine. (2015). *Pacemaker insertion*. Retrieved from http://www.hopkinsmedicine.org/healthlibrary/test_procedures/cardiovascular/pacemaker_insertion_92,p07980/

MedlinePlus. (2014). *Blood gases*. Retrieved from https://medlineplus.gov/ency/article/003855.htm

Ohio State University. (2015). *Deep venous thrombosis (DVT): Prevention*. Retrieved from https://evidencebasedpractice.osumc.edu/Documents/Guidelines/DVTPreventionGuideline.pdf

Remedy's Health Communities. (2015). *Compression stockings & blood clots*. Retrieved from http://www.healthcommunities.com/pulmonary-embolism-dvt/compression-stockings.shtml

Sovari, A. (2016). *Transvenous cardiac pacing*. Retrieved from http://emedicine.medscape.com/article/80659-overview#a3

Summit Medical Group. (2014). *Temporary cardiac pacing*. Retrieved from http://www.summitmedicalgroup.com/library/adult_health/car_temporary_cardiac_pacing/

Wellmark. Blue Cross and Blue Shield. (2015). *Pneumatic compression devices*. Retrieved from http://www.wellmark.com/Provider/MedPoliciesAndAuthorizations/MedicalPolicies/policies/Pneumatic_Compression_Devices.aspx

Chapter 13

Al Maqbali, M. (2016). Pre-operative hair removal: A literature review. *International Journal of Nursing & Clinical Practices* I163. Retrieved from http://dx.doi.org/10.15344/2394-4978/2016/163

Association of periOperative Registered Nurses (AORN). (2015). *Hand hygiene*. Retrieved from https://www.aorn.org/guidelines/clinical-resources/clinical-faqs/hand-antisepsis-hygiene

Association of periOperative Registered Nurses (AORN). (2015). *Patient skin antisepsis/prep*. Retrieved from https://www.aorn.org/guidelines/clinical-resources/clinical-faqs/patient-skin-antisepsis-prep

Brinkley, M. (2015). *Abdominal surgery postoperative complications*. Retrieved from http://www.livestrong.com/article/244440-abdominal-surgery-postoperative-complications/

Centers for Disease Control and Prevention (CDC). (2016). *Hand hygiene guideline*. Retrieved from http://www.cdc.gov/handhygiene/providers/guideline.html

Denu, Z. A., Yasin, M. O., Melekie, T. B., Berhe, A. (2015). Postoperative pulmonary complications and associated factors among surgical patients. *Journal of Anesthesia & Clinical Research (6)554*. doi:10.4172/2155-6148.1000554 Retrieved from http://www.omicsonline.org/open-access/postoperative-pulmonary-complications-and-associated-factors-among-surgical-patients-2155-6148-1000554.php?aid=59597

Ellrich, M. (2015). *The benefits of pre-surgery education*. Retrieved from http://www.gallup.com/businessjournal/183317/benefits-pre-surgery-education.aspx

Encyclopedia of Surgery. (2016). *Preoperative care*. Retrieved from http://www.surgeryencyclopedia.com/Pa-St/Preoperative-Care.html

Glick, D. (2016). *Overview of post-anesthetiv care for adult patients*. Retrieved from http://www.uptodate.com/contents/overview-of-complications-in-adults-admitted-to-the-post-anesthesia-care-unit

ICD10 Monitor. (2016). *Postoperative complications: It's complicated*. Retrieved from http://www.icd10monitor.com/enews/item/1599-postoperative-complications-it-s-complicated

NetCE. (2015). *#90761. Postoperative complications*. Retrieved from http://www.netce.com/coursecontent.php?courseid=1143

OrthoBuzz. (2016). *Preventing wrong-site surgery*. Retrieved from https://orthobuzz.jbjs.org/2016/01/28/jbjs-reviews-editors-choice-preventing-wrong-site-surgery/

Patient. (2013). *Common postoperative complications*. Retrieved from http://patient.info/doctor/common-postoperative-complications

Reference. (2016). *What is an Aldrete score?* Retrieved from https://www.reference.com/health/aldrete-score-25ef88e1192275a8

Tanner, J (2016). *Surgical hand antisepsis to reduce surgical site infection*. Retrieved from http://www.cochrane.org/CD004288/WOUNDS_surgical-hand-antisepsis-reduce-surgical-site-infection

The Joint Commission. (2016). *Universal protocol*. Retrieved from https://www.jointcommission.org/standards_information/up.aspx

Trichak, A. (2016). *Are you practicing proper pre-op skin preparation?* Retrieved from http://mkt.medline.com/advancing-blog/are-you-practicing-proper-pre-op-skin-preparation/

World Health Organization (WHO). (2016). *WHO surgical safety checklist*. Retrieved from http://www.who.int/patientsafety/safesurgery/checklist/en/

Chapter 14

American Congress of Obstetricians and Gynecologists (ACOG). (2013). *Study finds adverse effects of pitocin in newborns*. Retrieved from http://www.acog.org/About-ACOG/News-Room/News-Releases/2013/Study-Finds-Adverse-Effects-of-Pitocin-in-Newborns

American Congress of Obstetricians and Gynecologists (ACOG). (2017). *Delayed umbilical cord clamping after birth*.

Retrieved from http://www.acog.org/
Resources-And-Publications/
Committee-Opinions/Committee-on-
Obstetric-Practice/Delayed-Umbilical-
Cord-Clamping-After-Birth

American Pregnancy Association. (2015).
Inducing labor. Retrieved from http://
americanpregnancy.org/labor-and-
birth/inducing-labor

American Pregnancy Association. (2015).
Umbilical cord prolapse. Retrieved from
http://americanpregnancy.org/
pregnancy-complications/umbilical-
cord-prolapse

Children's Health. (2016).
Hyperbilirubinemia (Jaundice). Retrieved
from https://www.childrens.com/
specialties-services/specialty-centers-
and-programs/fetal-neonatal/
conditions-and-treatments/
hyperbilirubinemia#tab-3

Delisle, R. (2016). *Why you should delay
baby's first bath.* Retrieved from http://
www.todaysparent.com/baby/why-
you-should-delay-babys-first-bath

DovePress. (2014). *Role of effective
thermoregulation in premature neonates.*
Retrieved from https://www.dovepress.
com/role-of-effective-thermoregulation-
in-premature-neonates-peer-reviewed-
fulltext-article-RRN

EMedicineHealth. (2015). *Postpartum
perineal care.* Retrieved from http://www.
emedicinehealth.com/postpartum_
perineal_care/article_em.htm

Haelle, T. (2015). *Delayed umbilical cord
clamping may benefit children years later.*
Retrieved from http://www.npr.org/
sections/health-shots/2015/05/26/
409697568/delayed-umbilical-cord-
clamping-may-benefit-children-years-
later

Kim, K., Kwak, D. W., Ko, H. S., Park,
H. S., Seol, H. J., Hon, J. S.,... Kim, S. J.
(2014). *The clinical practice patterns of
fetal ultrasonography in the first-trimester:
A questionnaire survey of members of the
Korean Society of Ultrasound in Obstetrics
and Gynecology.* Retrieved from http://
www.ncbi.nlm.nih.gov/pmc/articles/
PMC4245337

Lewis, R. (2016). *Birth injuries. Pitocin for
induction and augmentation? Ask your
doctor to tell you the risks.* Retrieved
from http://www.lawrencefirm.com/
blog/2016/06/pitocin-for-induction-
and-augmentation-ask-your-doctor-to-
tell-you-the-risks.shtml

Lim, K. H. & Steinberg, G. (2016).
Preeclampsia. Retrieved from http://
emedicine.medscape.com/
article/1476919-overview

MedGadget. (2017). *Phototherapy
Equipment Market is expected to reach a
value of USD 788.7 million by 2025:
Radiant Insights.* Retrieved from,
https://www.medgadget.
com/2017/04/phototherapy-
equipment-market-is-expected-to-
reach-a-value-of-usd-788-7-million-by-
2025-radiant-insights.html

O'Connell, N. & Walker, B. (2014).
Amniotomy. Retrieved from http://
emedicine.medscape.com/
article/1997932-overview

O'Neill, E., & Thorp, J. (2013).
Antepartum evaluation of the fetus
and fetal well being. *Clinical Obstetrics
and Gynecology.* 55(3) 722–730.
Retrieved from http://www.ncbi.
nlm.nih.gov/pmc/articles/
PMC3684248

RxList. (2016). *RhoGAM.* Retrieved from
http://www.rxlist.com/rhogam-drug/
patient-images-side-effects.htm

Siddique, A. (2013). *Pitocin may have
adverse effects on newborn babies.*
Retrieved from http://www.
medicaldaily.com/pitocin-may-
have-adverse-effects-newborn-
babies-245641

Simpson, L., Deshmukl, S. P., Dudiak, K.
M., Harisinghani, M. G., Henrichsen, T.
L., Meyer, B. J., ... Khat, N. J. (2016).
Assessment of fetal well-being. Retrieved
from https://acsearch.acr.org/
docs/3094108/Narrative

Society for Maternal-Fetal Medicine
(SMFM). (2014). *SMFM consult – Delayed
umbilical cord clamping.* Retrieved from
http://contemporaryobgyn.
modernmedicine.com/contemporary-
obgyn/content/tags/maternal-fetal-
medicine/smfm-consult-delayed-
umbilical-cord-clamping?page=full

Stöppler, M. (2016). *Amniocentesis.*
Retrieved from http://www.
medicinenet.com/amniocentesis/
page3.htm

World Health Organization. (WHO).
(2014). *Delayed umbilical cord clamping,
for improved maternal and infant health
and nutrition outcomes.* Retrieved from
http://apps.who.int/iris/bitstream/
10665/148793/1/9789241508209_
eng.pdf?ua=1

World Health Organization. (WHO).
(2016). *Reproductive Health Library.
Oral misoprostol for induction of
labour.* Retrieved from https://
extranet.who.int/rhl/topics/
pregnancy-and-childbirth/induction-
labour/oral-misoprostol-induction-
labour

Chapter 15

Agency for Healthcare Research and
Quality (AHRQ). (2013). *Preventing falls
in hospitals. Which fall prevention
practices do you want to use?* Retrieved
from http://www.ahrq.gov/
professionals/systems/hospital/
fallpxtoolkit/fallpxtk3.html

American Foundation for Suicide
Prevention. (2016). *Suicide statistics.*
Retrieved from https://afsp.org/about-
suicide/suicide-statistics

AnteaGroup. (2015). *Healthcare in crisis:
Workplace safety at hospitals.* Retrieved
from http://us.anteagroup.com/
en-us/blog/healthcare-crisis-
workplace-safety-hospitals

Barr, D., Miller, H., Principe, A. J., Merandi,
J., & Catt, C. (2016). *Strategies for helping
employees stay healthy on the job.* Retrieved
from https://www.childrenshospitals.
org/newsroom/childrens-hospitals-
today/winter-2016/articles/strategies-
for-helping-employees-stay-healthy-on-
the-job

Calloway, S. (2017). Emergency Physicians
Insurance Exchange, EPIX. *Restraint and
seclusion.* Retrieved from http://www.
kyha.com/docs/Presentations/2017/
RestraintAndSeclusion.pdf

Centers for Disease Control and
Prevention (CDC). (2016a). *Prevent
child abuse & neglect* [Infographic].
Retrieved from http://www.cdc.gov/
violenceprevention/pub/technical-
packages/infographic/can.html

Centers for Disease Control and
Prevention (CDC). (2016b). *Ten leading
causes of death and injury.* Retrieved
from https://www.cdc.gov/injury/
wisqars/leadingcauses.html

Door County Memorial Hospital. (2013).
Restraints & safety staff education.
Retrieved from http://www.slideshare.
net/14021888/patient-restraints

EliteFire. (2015). *Common fire hazards
for the healthcare industry.* Retrieved
from http://www.elitefire.co.uk/
common-fire-hazards-healthcare-
industry

EMedicineHealth. (2016). *Seizures in
children.* Retrieved from http://www.
emedicinehealth.com/seizures_in_
children/page2_em.htm

Johns Hopkins Medicine. (2016). *Tonic-
clonic (grand mal) seizures.* Retrieved
from http://www.hopkinsmedicine.
org/neurology_neurosurgery/
centers_clinics/epilepsy/seizures/
types/tonic-clonic-grand-mal-seizures.
html

National Council on Aging (NCOA). (2017). *Falls Free® Initiative*. Retrieved from https://www.ncoa.org/healthy-aging/falls-prevention/falls-free-initiative

Oliver, R. (2015). *Five safety tips for health care workers*. Retrieved from https://ohsonline.com/blogs/the-ohs-wire/2015/05/five-safety-tips-for-health-care-workers.aspx

Schachter, S., Shafer, P., & Sirven, J. (2014). *What is a seizure?* Retrieved from http://www.epilepsy.com/learn/epilepsy-101/what-seizure

Stempniak, M. (2016). *Joint Commission shines spotlight on suicide in hospitals and other settings, with 8 steps to detect growing concern*. Retrieved from http://www.hhnmag.com/articles/6980-joint-commission-shines-spotlight-on-suicide-in-hospitals-and-other-settings-with-eight-steps-to-detect-growing-concern

Substance Abuse and Mental Health Services Administration (SAMHSA). (2015). *Suicide prevention*. Retrieved from http://www.samhsa.gov/suicide-prevention

Substance Abuse and Mental Health Services Administration (SAMHSA). (2015). *SAMHSA's suicide prevention mobile app to help health care providers save lives*. Retrieved from http://www.samhsa.gov/newsroom/press-announcements/201504020800

The Joint Commission. (2015). *Preventing falls and fall-related injuries in health care facilities*. Retrieved from http://www.jointcommission.org/assets/1/18/SEA_55.pdf

The Joint Commission. (2017). *Facts about patient safety*. Retrieved from http://www.jointcommission.org/facts_about_patient_safety

U.S. Department of Labor, Occupational Safety and Health Administration. (n.d.) *Healthcare*. Retrieved from https://www.osha.gov/SLTC/healthcarefacilities

U.S. National Library of Medicine. (2015). *Use of restraints*. Retrieved from MedlinePlus website: https://medlineplus.gov/ency/patientinstructions/000450.htm

White, J. (2015). *6 keys to reduce patient falls in hospitals*. Retrieved from http://www.healthcarebusinesstech.com/keys-reduce-falls

White, J. (2016). *What hospitals should do to prevent patient suicide*. Retrieved from http://www.healthcarebusinesstech.com/hospital-patient-suicide

Chapter 16

The American Apitherapy Society Inc. (2016). *About apitherapy*. Retrieved from http://www.apitherapy.org/about-apitherapy/what-is-apitherapy

British Columbia Provincial Nursing Skin and Wound Committee (BCPNSWC). (2014). *Guideline: Braden scale for predicting pressure ulcer risk in adults & children/infants*. Retrieved from https://www.clwk.ca/buddydrive/file/guideline-braden-risk-assessment

Dang. J. (2015). U.S. Food and Drug Administration (FDA). *Guidance for industry and FDA staff – Class II special controls guidance document: Non-powered suction apparatus device intended for negative pressure wound therapy (NPWT)*. Retrieved from https://www.fda.gov/RegulatoryInformation/Guidances/ucm233275.htm

Dhivya, S., Padma, V. V., & Santhini, E. (2015). National Center for Biotechnology Information. *Wound dressings – a review*. Retrieved from http://www.ncbi.nlm.nih.gov/pmc/articles/PMC4662938

Drugs.com. (2017). *Jackson-pratt drain care*. Retrieved from https://www.drugs.com/cg/jackson-pratt-drain-care.html

Encyclopedia of Surgery. (2017). *Stitches and staples*. Retrieved from http://www.surgeryencyclopedia.com/St-Wr/Stitches-and-Staples.html

Gabriel, A. (2015). *Wound irrigation*. Retrieved from http://emedicine.medscape.com/article/1895071-overview

Heale, M. (2014). *How "clean" is your clean dressing technique?* Retrieved from http://www.woundsource.com/blog/how-clean-your-clean-dressing-technique

Medical eStudy. (2016). *Collecting a specimen for wound culture*. Retrieved from http://www.medicalestudy.com/collecting-specimen-wound-culture

MedlinePlus. (2014). *Skin care and incontinence*. Retrieved from https://medlineplus.gov/ency/article/003976.htm

MedlinePlus. (2016). *Pressure sores*. Retrieved from https://medlineplus.gov/pressuresores.html

National Pressure Ulcer Advisory Panel. (2016). *National pressure ulcer advisory panel announces a change in terminology from pressure ulcer to pressure injury and updates the stages of pressure injury*. Retrieved from http://www.npuap.org/national-pressure-ulcer-advisory-panel-npuap-announces-a-change-in-terminology-from-pressure-ulcer-to-pressure-injury-and-updates-the-stages-of-pressure-injury

NHS Choices. (2016). *Venous leg ulcer*. Retrieved from http://www.nhs.uk/Conditions/Leg-ulcer-venous/Pages/Introduction.aspx

Ud-Din, S., & Bayat, A. (2014). *Electrical stimulation and cutaneous wound healing: A review of clinical evidence*. Retrieved from http://leonhardtventures.com/wp-content/uploads/2016/05/healthcare-02-00445-ES-and-Cutaneous-wound-healing-review-clnical-evidence.pdf

WebMD. (2015). *Find a vitamin or supplement. Bee venom*. Retrieved from http://www.webmd.com/vitamins-supplements/ingredientmono-972-bee%20venom.aspx?activeingredientid=972&

WebMD. (2015). *Pressure sores—Topic overview*. Retrieved from http://www.webmd.com/skin-problems-and-treatments/tc/pressure-sores-topic-overview

Wegner, L. (2015). *Physiopedia. Acute post-surgical management of the amputee*. Retrieved from http://www.physio-pedia.com/Acute_post-surgical_management_of_the_amputee

Woolston, C. (2016). *Bee venom therapy*. Retrieved from https://consumer.healthday.com/encyclopedia/holistic-medicine-25/mis-alternative-medicine-news-19/bee-venom-therapy-647499.html

Index